Pediatric Retina

Pediatric Retina

EDITOR-IN-CHIEF

Mary Elizabeth Hartnett, MD

Associate Professor of Ophthalmology
Department of Ophthalmology
University of North Carolina School of Medicine
Chapel Hill, North Carolina

SURGERY SECTION EDITORS

Michael Trese, MD

Associated Retinal Consultants
Clinical Professor of Biomedical Sciences
Eye Research Institute
  Oakland University
  Rochester, Michigan
Chief of Adult and Pediatric Vitreoretinal Surgery
  Department of Ophthalmology
  William Beaumont Hospital
  Royal Oak, Michigan

Antonio Capone, Jr., MD

Clinical Associate Professor
  Department of Biomedical Sciences
  Oakland University
  Auburn Hills, Michigan
Director, Fellowship in Vitreoretinal Diseases
  Department of Ophthalmology
  William Beaumont Hospital
  Royal Oak, Michigan

GENETICS SECTION EDITOR

Bronya J. B. Keats, PhD

Professor and Chair
  Department of Genetics
  Louisiana State University Health Sciences Center
  New Orleans, Louisiana

MEDICAL SECTION EDITOR

Scott M. Steidl, MD, DMA

Associate Professor
  Department of Ophthalmology
  University of Maryland School of Medicine
  Baltimore, Maryland
Director of Vitreoretinal Services
  Department of Ophthalmology
  University of Maryland Medical System
  Baltimore, Maryland

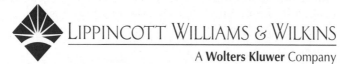

LIPPINCOTT WILLIAMS & WILKINS
A **Wolters Kluwer** Company

Philadelphia · Baltimore · New York · London
Buenos Aires · Hong Kong · Sydney · Tokyo

Acquisitions Editor: Jonathan Pine
Developmental Editor: Scott Scheidt
Marketing Manager: Kathy Neely
Production Editor: David Murphy
Compositor: Maryland Composition, Inc.
Printer: Quebecor-Kingsport

©2005 by LIPPINCOTT WILLIAMS & WILKINS
530 Walnut Street
Philadelphia, PA 19106-3780 USA
LWW.com

Printed in the USA

Library of Congress Cataloging-in-Publication Data

Pediatric retina:medical and surgical approaches / [edited by] Mary Elizabeth
   Hartnett—[et al.].
     p. ; cm.
   Includes bibliographical references.
   ISBN 0-7817-4782-1
   1. Pediatric ophthalmology. 2. Retina–Diseases. I. Hartnett, Mary Elizabeth.
   [DNLM: 1. Retinal Diseases–Child. 2. Retinal Diseases–Infant. 3. Ophthalmologic
Surgical Procedures–methods–Child. 4. Ophthalmologic Surgical Procedures–methods–
Infant. WW 270 P371 2005]
   RE48.2.C5P455 2005
   618.92'097735–dc22

10 9 8 7 6 5 4 3 2 1

CONTENTS

SECTION II: CLINICAL ASSESSMENT AND MANAGEMENT OF RETINAL DISEASES REQUIRING SURGERY IN INFANTS AND CHILDREN

CONTRIBUTORS

Thomas A. Aaberg, Sr, MD, MSPH Professor and Chair, Department of Ophthalmology, Emory University; Chief, Department of Ophthalmology, Emory University Hospital, Atlanta, Georgia

Thomas M. Aaberg, Jr, MD Assistant Clinical Professor, Department of Ophthalmology, Michigan State University, Grand Rapids, Michigan

Peep V. Algevere, MD, PhD Department of Ophthalmology, Örebro University Hospital, Örebro, Sweden

Y. Robert Barishak, MD Professor, Department of Ophthalmology, Tel Aviv University, Tel Aviv, Israel; Professor, Veterinary Faculty, Hebrew University of Jerusalem, University Veterinary Hospital, Jerusalem, Israel

J. Bronwyn Bateman, MD Professor and Chair of Ophthalmology, University of Colorado; Director, Department of Ophthalmology, Rocky Mountain Lions Eye Institute, Aurora, Colorado

Jean Bennett, MD, PhD Professor, Department of Ophthalmology, University of Pennsylvania, Philadelphia, Pennsylvania

Antonio Capone, Jr, MD Clinical Associate Professor, Department of Biomedical Sciences, Oakland University, Auburn Hills, Michigan; Director, Fellowship in Vitreoretinal Diseases, Department of Ophthalmology, William Beaumont Hospital, Royal Oak, Michigan

Cynthia de Almeida Carvalho Recchia, MD Department of Ophthalmology and Visual Sciences, Vanderbilt University Medical Center, Nashville, Tennessee

Marsha C. Cheung, MD Ophthalmology Resident, Department of Ophthalmology, University of California at San Francisco, San Francisco, California

Itay Chowers, MD Lecturer in Ophthalmology, Department of Ophthalmology, Hadassah School of Medicine, Hebrew University, Jerusalem, Israel

R. Max Conway, MD, PhD Senior Lecturer, Save Sight Institute, Department of Ophthalmology, University of Sydney; Consultant Ophthalmologist, Department of Ophthalmology, Sydney Eye Hospital, Sydney, NSW, Australia

Deborah Costakos, MD, MS Pediatric Ophthalmologist, Department of Ophthalmology, Columbia St. Mary's, Milwaukee, Wisconsin

Sven Crafoord, MD, PhD Associate Professor, Department of Ophthalmology, Örebro University Hospital; Senior Vitreo Retinal Surgeon, Department of Ophthalmology, Örebro University Hospital, Örebro, Sweden

Melanie H. Erb, MD Department of Ophthalmology, University of California at Irvine, Irvine, California; Department of Ophthalmology, UC Irvine Medical Center, Orange, California

C. Stephen Foster MD, FACS Professor of Ophthalmology, Harvard Medical School; Director, Ocular Immunology and Uveitis, Massachusetts Eye and Ear Infirmary, Boston, Massachusetts

Anne B. Fulton, MD Associate Professor, Ophthalmology, Harvard Medical School; Senior Associate in Ophthalmology, Ophthalmology, Children's Hospital, Boston, Massachusetts

Zein Ghassan, MD Senior Ophthalmic Specialist, Head of the Department of Ophthalmology, Ahmadi Hospital, Ahmadi, Kuwait

Clare Gilbert, MB, ChB, FRCOphth, MD, MSc Senior Lecturer, Clinical Research Unit, London School of Hygiene and Tropical Medicine, London, England

Ronald M. Hansen, PhD Instructor, Ophthalmology, Harvard Medical School; Research Associate, Ophthalmology, Children's Hospital, Boston, Massachusetts

Mary Elizabeth Hartnett, MD, FACS Associate Professor of Ophthalmology, Department of Ophthalmology, University of North Carolina School of Medicine, Chapel Hill, North Carolina

G. Baker Hubbard, III, MD Assistant Professor of Ophthalmology, The Emory Eye Center, Emory University School of Medicine, Atlanta, Georgia

Lea Hyvärinen, MD Apollonkatu 6 A 4, FIN-00100 HELSINKI, Finland

Bronya J.B. Keats, PhD Professor and Chair, Department of Genetics, Louisiana State University Health Sciences Center, New Orleans, Louisiana

John B. Kerrison, MD Assistant Professor, Department of Ophthalmology, Neurology, and Neurosurgery, Johns Hopkins University School of Medicine, Baltimore, Maryland

Ferenc Kuhn, MD, PhD Director of Clinical Research, Helen Keller Foundation for Research and Education, President, United States Eye Injury Registry, Associate Professor of Clinical Ophthalmology, University of Alabama at Birmingham, Birmingham, Alabama; Visiting Professor, Department of Ophthalmology, University of Pécs, Pécs, Hungary

Leila Kump, MD Clinical Fellow, Medical Retina and Uveitis Service, National Eye Institute, National Institutes of Health, Bethesda, Maryland

Baruch D. Kuppermann, MD, PhD Association Professor of Ophthalmology, Department of Ophthalmology, University of California, Irvine, Irvine, California

John I. Loewenstein, MD Assistant Professor, Department of Ophthalmology, Harvard Medical School; Surgeon, Department of Ophthalmology, Massachusetts Eye and Ear Infirmary, Boston, Massachusetts

Ian M. MacDonald, MD, CM Professor and Chairman, Department of Ophthalmology, University of Alberta; Chairman, Department of Ophthalmology, Royal Alexandra Hospital, Edmonton, Canada,

Albert M. Maguire, MD Associate Professor, Department of Ophthalmology, University of Pennsylvania; Director, Retina Service, Department of Ophthalmology, Scheie Eye Institute, University of Pennsylvania, Philadelphia, Pennsylvania

Michael Marble, MD Associate Professor of Clinical Pediatrics, Department of Pediatrics, Louisiana State University Health Sciences Center; Clinical and Biochemical Geneticist, Division of Clinical Genetics, Children's Hospital of New Orleans, New Orleans, Louisiana

Janet R. McColm, PhD Research Associate, Ophthalmology, University of North Carolina, Chapel Hill, North Carolina

Viktória Mester, MD Consultant Vitreoretinal Surgeon, Mafraq Hospital, Abu Dhabi, United Arab Emirates; Chairman, Hungarian Eye Injury Registry

P. Anthony Meza, MD Head Section of Pediatric Anesthesiology, Department of Anesthesiology, William Beaumont Hospital, Royal Oak, Michigan

Robert Morris, MD President, International Society of Ocular Trauma, Associate Professor of Ophthalmology, University of Alabama at Birmingham; President, Helen Keller Foundation for Research and Education, Birmingham, Alabama

Raghu C. Murthy, MD Clinical Instructor, Retina Service, Casey Eye Institute, Oregon Health Sciences University; Portland, Oregon

Natalie Nguyen, BA VMR Institute, Huntington Beach, California

Joan M. O'Brien, MD Associate Professor, Department of Ophthalmology, University of California, San Francisco; Associate Professor, Director of Ocular Oncology Ophthalmology, UCSF Medical Center, San Francisco, California

Kean T. Oh, MD Assistant Professor, Department of Ophthalmology, University of North Carolina, Chapel Hill, North Carolina; The Retina Eye Center, Augusta, Georgia

Anup Parikh BS Doris Duke Medical Resaearch Fellow, University of North Carolina (Medical Student), Chapel Hill, North Carolina

Franco M. Recchia, MD Assistant Professor, Vanderbilt Eye Institute, Vanderbilt University Medical Center, Nashville, Tennessee

Joseph F. Rizzo, MD Associate Professor of Ophthalmology, Harvard Medical School; Massachusetts Eye and Ear Infirmary, Boston, Massachusetts

Jerry Sebag, MD, FACS, FRCOphth Associate Clinical Professor of Ophthalmology, Department of Ophthalmology, Keck/USC School of Medicine, Los Angeles, California; Staff Surgeon, Department of Ophthalmology, Hoag Hospital, Newport Beach, California

Carol L. Shields, MD Professor, Department of Ophthalmology, Jefferson Medical College, Thomas Jefferson University; Associate Director/Attending Surgeon, Department of Oncology Service, Wills Eye Hospital, Philadelphia, Pennsylvania

Paul A. Sieving, MD, PhD Director, National Eye Institute, National Institutes of Health, Bethesda, Maryland; Professor of Ophthalmic Genetics, Department of Ophthalmology, University of Michigan, Ann Arbor, Michigan

Brian D. Sippy, MD, PhD Vitreo-Retinal Disease & Surgery, Rocky Mountain Eye Center, Affiliate Faculty, University of Montana, School of Pharmaceutical Sciences, Missoula, Montana

Abraham Spierer, MD Senior Lecturer, Department of Ophthalmology, Sackler School of Medicine, Tel Aviv University, Tel Aviv, Israel; Senior Lecturer, Department of Ophthalmology, Sheba Medical Center, Ramat Gan, Israel

Scott M, Steidl, MD, DMA Associate Professor, Department of Ophthalmology, University of Maryland School of Medicine; Director of Vitreoretinal Services, Department of Ophthalmology, University of Maryland Medical System, Baltimore, Maryland

J. Timothy Stout, MD, PhD Associate Professor, Department of Ophthalmology, Casey Eye Institute, Oregon Health Sciences University, Portland, Oregon

Michael T. Trese, MD Clinical Professor of Biomedical Sciences, Eye Research Institute, Oakland University, Rochester, Michigan; Chief of Adult and Pediatric Vitreoretinal Surgery, Department of Ophthalmology, William Beaumont Hospital, Royal Oak, Michigan

Albert T. Vitale, MD Associate Professor, Department of Ophthalmology and Visual Sciences, John A. Moran Eye Center, University of Utah; Chief, Uveitis Division, John A. Moran Eye Center, University of Utah, Salt Lake City, Utah

Scott M. Warden, MD Ophthalmology Resident, Massachusetts, Eye and Ear Infirmary, Boston, Massachusetts

FOREWORD

The last fifteen years have produced an explosion of information and technology that allow us to better understand and manage many pediatric conditions for which there had been no good answers. Clearly, much work lies ahead, but progress has been made. For example, the findings of the cryotherapy for retinopathy of prematurity study in the late 1980s and the refinements in laser therapy have allowed us to at last offer treatments for these tiny patients, many of whom would have become permanently blind.

The identification of gene mutations in hereditary conditions, including familial exudative retinopathy, choroideremia, and incontinentia pigmenti; provides knowledge that in the next few years may lead to more effective treatments over and above the exquisite surgical techniques that continue to evolve.

Thus, the timing could not be better for a book that comprehensively examines the management of pediatric vitreo-retinal disease. Clearly written by experts in the field—indeed, pioneers in pediatric retina, albeit young pioneers—this volume fills a void not recently addressed.

Thirty-three chapters run the gamut from embryology to visual rehabilitation in infants and children and contain a generous assortment of illustrations, 194 of which are in color. This book also includes a unique mini atlas reference at the end of the book that is comprised of nine appendices that categorize inheritance patterns associated with retinal disorders, macular abnormalities, white spot syndromes, and other conditions.

Pediatric Retina will be a valuable addition to the library of all ophthalmologists and an essential text for those who treat pediatric patients with vitreoretinal disease.

–William Tasman, M.D.

PREFACE

The pediatric patient requires a unique approach from the clinician in the diagnosis and management of retinal diseases that is often different from that used in adults, and often with genetic expertise. Because few, if any, texts address the combined knowledge and different perspectives needed for pediatric retinal care, we created *Pediatric Retina* as a comprehensive source for geneticists, scientists, physicians, and surgeons to address these needs. Experts within a wide range of subspecialties have compiled their knowledge and have followed a consistent outline for each disease to facilitate easy referencing by the reader.

The book is divided into three sections that address predominant management with cross-references where applicable: Section 1: Clinical Assessment and Management of Medical Retinal Diseases in Infants and Children, Section 2: Clinical Assessment and Management of Medical Retinal Diseases Requiring Surgery in Infants and Children, and Section 3: Visual Rehabilitation of Infants and Children with Low Vision. Featured in the appendices are a classification of pediatric retinal diseases based on inheritance pattern, gene mutation, and protein product; and a photographic atlas that categorizes diseases based on retinal appearance referring the reader to the appropriate text for specific diseases. Throughout the text, the genetics of pediatric diseases is addressed. Diagnosis and medical and surgical management are discussed for developmental abnormalities, retinal degenerations, infectious and inflammatory diseases, disorders in metabolism, tumors, and trauma. In addition, the text provides the current science using electrophysiologic and psychophysical evaluations to assess retinal development and disease, methods to measure visual function, methods to image the pediatric retina, experimental approaches to restore vision through ocular and cortical prostheses and retinal transplantation, and the current science of gene therapy techniques to address genetic disorders. Also covered are legal considerations in genetics and the leading causes of blindness throughout the world. A most comprehensive view of retinopathy of prematurity — the science, management including anesthetic considerations, and future directions of therapy — and the most current thinking and approaches to congenital retinoschisis, persistent fetal vasculature, and other surgical diseases are discussed.

The text is organized with special attention to health care providers working with infants and children with retinal disorders. Medical or surgical management is advised based on the specific disease stage and possible referrals suggested to address ancillary aspects of patient care. We also emphasize the quality of life as children grow to adults by addressing not only the diagnostics and acute management but also visual rehabilitation. Thanks to the multiple, talented contributors, this text will be a valuable source for the retina specialist, general and pediatric ophthalmologist, and geneticist in many areas throughout the world.

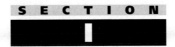

SECTION

I

CLINICAL ASSESSMENT AND MANAGEMENT OF MEDICAL RETINAL DISEASES IN INFANTS AND CHILDREN

1

EMBRYOLOGY OF THE POSTERIOR SEGMENT AND DEVELOPMENTAL DISORDERS

A. EMBRYOLOGY OF THE RETINA AND DEVELOPMENTAL DISORDERS

Y. ROBERT BARISHAK
ABRAHAM SPIERER

DEVELOPMENT OF THE RETINA

The development of the retina (Tables 1-1, 1-2, and 1-3) starts at the fourth week of gestation with the invagination of the optic vesicle and formation of the optic cup; the two layers of the optic cup constitute the anlage of the retina, the external layer of the retinal pigment epithelium (RPE), and the internal layer of the sensory retina (Fig. 1-1). The invagination involves the ventrocaudal wall of the optic vesicle and causes the formation of the embryonic fissure, which allows the hyaloid artery to enter into the developing optic cup cavity. By also involving the optic stalk and occluding progressively the optic vesicle cavity, which connects this cavity to the neural canal lumen, the invagination allows the axons of the first ganglion cells spreading in the retina to penetrate into the optic stalk and the narrowing optic vesicle cavity becomes the potential subretinal space. At the end of the fourth week, the vessels surrounding the neural tube spread over the optic cup and the cells of the external layer of the cup, the prospective RPE cells become pigmented. At this stage, the optic cup is surrounded by the secondary mesenchyme as migration of neural crest cells into the primary mesenchyme has already taken place.

At the fifth week, the RPE is made up of two or three layers of columnar, pseudostratified pigmented cells attached one to another with junctional complexes, the anlage of the membrane of Verhoeff. The inner layer of the optic cup, the prospective sensory retina is made of an external layer of nuclei (the proliferative or germinative zone) and an anuclear marginal zone. The outermost cells of the germinative zone have cilia projecting towards the potential subretinal space and are joined one with another by zonulae adherens, the anlage of the external limiting membrane of the retina. The anuclear, marginal zone is covered internally by a basal lamina, the anlage of the inner limiting membrane of the retina.

The sixth week is characterized by the closure of the embryonic fissure. The closure starts at the center of the fissure and proceeds anteriorly toward the anterior rim of the optic cup and posteriorly into the optic stalk. The RPE forms a one-cell-thick layer of cuboidal cells covered by a primitive Bruch's membrane made mostly by the basal membrane of the cells themselves. As to the sensory retina, it becomes thicker as a result of the proliferative activity of the germinal cells.

During the seventh week, the embryonic fissure closes completely and the anterior notch at the anterior rim of the optic cup and the posterior notch at the site of the prospective optic disc around the hyaloid artery disappear. The RPE cells extend posteriorly as the layer of the outer cells of the optic stalk, the precursors of the peripheral glial mantle of the optic nerve, which, later on, will constitute the barrier between the axons of the optic nerve and the surrounding mesenchyme (1). These cells also continue to differentiate and become almost mature: they develop apical villi, basal infoldings, smooth and rough endoplasmic reticulum, ribosomes, premelanosomes, and melanosomes (2). In the sensory retina, germinative cells proliferate and migrate inwards giving rise to the outer neuroblastic layer, the inner neuroblastic layer, and the layer of Chievitz in between (Fig. 1-2). The outermost cells of the outer neuroblastic layer develop short processes that point toward the potential subretinal space; they are the anlage of the photoreceptors. At the posterior pole, around the future optic disc, the innermost cells of the inner neuroblastic layer migrate inwards. The first cells to come out are the ganglion cells and the Müller cells follow them.

At the eighth week, the first ganglion cells develop axons, which extend toward the optic stalk (Fig. 1-3). These axons constitute the beginning of the nerve fiber layer. When the axons reach the optic stalk, they penetrate into it,

TABLE 1-1. STAGES OF RETINAL DEVELOPMENT

Fifth week	Invagination of optic vesicle, optic cup, and primary vitreous.
Sixth week	Retinal pigment epithelium (RPE), anlage of sensory retina, and primary vitreous.
Seventh week	Outer (ONB) and inner (INB) neuroblastic layers with layer of Chievitz in between. At INB layer, ganglion, and Müller cells migrate inward.
Eighth week	RPE cells mature. Ganglion cell axons penetrate into optic stalk. Bergmeister's papilla forms. Secondary vitreous develops.
Third mo	At INB layer first ganglion cells and then Müller cells migrate inward and form separate layers. Inner plexiform layer is formed. Müller cells attach to outer and inner limiting membranes of retina. At ONB layer, future bipolar and horizontal cells migrate inward obstructing the layer of Chievitz. The external plexiform layer is formed. Primary vitreous transforms into Cloquet's canal.
Fourth mo	Mitotic division of neurogenic cells ceases. Putative fovea appears at outer nuclear layer posteriorly. Mueller cells mature and produce hyaluronic acid. Outer cells of ONB layer, the future photoreceptors, start to differentiate and produce F-actin and alpha-tubulin but are in close contact with the RPE. Hyaloid vasculature starts to regress and retinal vascularization starts to develop. Bergmeister's papilla disintegrates and physiological cup appears.
Fifth mo	Photoreceptors further differentiate. The subretinal space forms and the interstitial retinol-binding protein appears. The photoreceptor plasma membrane develops infoldings and rhodopsin and S antigen appear. Horizontal cells form an irregular row. Apoptosis causes a marked decrease in ganglion cell number in the retina and their axons in the optic nerve. Retinal vascularization progresses rapidly.
Sixth mo	Photoreceptor differentiation involves mostly the cones. Outer and inner segments and primitive cone pedicles are recognizable. Rod differentiation lags behind. The macula appears to bulge. Ganglion cells mature and accumulate cytoplasm in conjunction with retinal vascular migration. Retinal vascularization progresses and perivascular capillary free zones appear. Myelin-associated glycoprotein is present. The ora serrata is established.
Seventh mo	Photoreceptor differentiation involves the rods and presents the same pattern as the cones. Photoreceptor terminals differentiate and develop synaptic vesicles and ribbons. Foveal development proceeds in the macula as a result of outward migration of ganglion cells and inward migration of photoreceptors. The fovea is avascular. Retinal vascularization progresses toward the periphery but does not extend to the ora serrata.
Eighth mo	Differentiation of the outer layers of the retina and the subretinal space extend to the ora serrata. Ganglion cells remain denser posteriorly as overall number decreases. The ora serrata appears as a circular retinal fold called the Lange fold.
Ninth mo	Retina is well differentiated. Its surface area increases considerably. Cells shift transversally and RPE cells accommodate themselves to increased area. Macula continues to differentiate, the foveolar depression forms, and a foveolar reflex appears. Retinal vessels extend to ora serrata.
After birth	Differentiation of the fovea continues until 45 months of postnatal age.

TABLE 1-2. TIME LINE OF RETINAL DEVELOPMENT: ORGANOGENESIS

	Fifth Week	Sixth Week	Seventh Week	Eight Week
Invagination	———	———	——	
Retinal pigment epithelium	———	———	———	———
Outer + inner neuroblastic layers			———	———
Ganglion cells migration			———	———
Müller cells radial fibers			———	———
Ganglion cell axons enter optic stalk				——
Bergmeister's papilla				——
Primary vitreous	———	———	———	———
Secondary vitreous			———	———
Prospective photoreceptors give outer short processes			———	———

TABLE 1-3. TIME LINE OF RETINAL DEVELOPMENT: DIFFERENTIATION

	Third Mo	Fourth Mo	Fifth Mo	Sixth Mo	Seventh Mo	Eighth Mo	Ninth Mo
Ganglion cells migrate	——						
Müller cells give radial fibers	——						
Inner plexiform layer	————————————————————————————————						
Bipolar + horizontal cells migrate	————————						
External plexiform layer	————————————————————————————————						
Hyaloid regresses		———————————————————————					
Retinal vessels develop		———————————————————————					
Physiological cup develops		———————————————————————					
Subretinal space appears		———————————————————————					
Interstitial retinol binding protein		———————————————————————					
Cones differentiate				———————————————			
Rods differentiate					———————————		
Macula					———————————		
Fovea					———————————		
Ora serrata		————————					
Decrease in number of ganglion cells			———————————————				

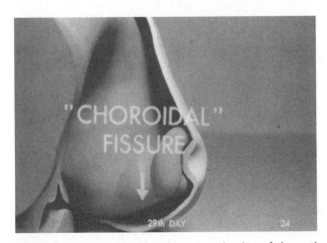

FIGURE 1-1. Four-week-old embryo. Invagination of the optic vesicle causes the formation of the optic cup and the embryonic fissure. (From *Embryology of the eye* [film] San Francisco: American Academy of Ophthalmology, 1950. Courtesy of Dr. Michael Hogan.)

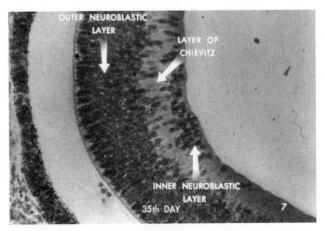

FIGURE 1-2. Seven-week-old embryo. Cells from the common neuroblastic layer of the retina arrange themselves into an outer and an inner neuroblastic layer causing the appearance of the layer of Chievitz in between. (From *Embryology of the eye* [film] San Francisco: American Academy of Ophthalmology, 1950. Courtesy of Dr. Michael Hogan.)

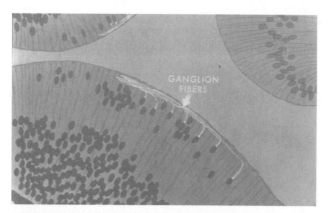

FIGURE 1-3. Seven-week-old embryo. Migration inwards of the ganglion cells and appearance of their axons. (From *Embryology of the eye* [film] San Francisco: American Academy of Ophthalmology, 1950. Courtesy of Dr. Michael Hogan.)

penetration made possible by the natural cell death (apoptosis) of the primitive neuroectodermal cells filling the optic stalk (3). As more ganglion cells differentiate and more axons penetrate into the optic stalk, Bergmeister's papilla forms as a conic mass of glial cells covering the future optic disc area. It is believed that proliferation of glial cells is the main factor in its appearance (4). The hyaloid artery becomes surrounded by the increasing number of axons and is isolated in the center of the optic nerve. At the same time, Müller cells develop their inner radial fibers that extend to the internal limiting membrane. Migrating retinal glioblasts, the future retinal astroglia, arrange themselves along the axons and onto the internal limiting membrane (5).

At the third month, the differentiation of the retina follows the same pattern as that of the neuroectoderm in the central nervous system. In the central nervous system, cellular proliferation starts at the inner layers and progresses externally while differentiation occurs in a reverse direction, starting externally from the outer layers and proceeding internally. In the retina, because of the invagination of the optic cup, the location of the layers is reversed: the proliferating cells are located externally and the acellular layer internally. That is why, in the retina, proliferation starts at the outer nuclear layer and progresses internally, while differentiation proceeds from the internal layers and proceeds externally. The internal ganglion cells are the first to differentiate and the external photoreceptors the last. The differentiation of the retina also starts at the posterior pole and progresses gradually toward the periphery; thus, the posterior retina differentiates at an early stage and the peripheral retina a short time before birth (6). The differentiation of the retina at the inner neuroblastic layer manifests with (i) the formation of a separate layer of ganglion cells, (ii) the development of external radial fibers at the Müller cells that extend to the site of the prospective external limiting membrane(iii) the appearance of glycogen granules in the cytoplasm of these Müller cells (7), (iv) the formation of dendrites by the ganglion cells, and (v) the migration of the first amacrine cells inwards. The differentiation of the outer neuroblastic layer, much less advanced, manifests itself by an inward migration of its most internal cells, the future bipolar cells, and of those external to them, the future horizontal cells. This migration causes the occlusion of the Chievitz layer and the formation of the external plexiform layer (the internal plexiform layer has been formed by the inward migration of the ganglion cells). The outermost cells of the outer neuroblastic layer, the future photoreceptors, do not migrate; they are connected to one another with adherens junctions, the prospective external limiting membrane of the retina.

At the fourth month, all the major constituents of the retina are present (Fig. 1-4). The ora serrata appears as a line of demarcation at the peripheral retina. At the posterior pole, the outer nuclear layer becomes the precursor of the rod free zone, the future fovea. The inner plexiform layer differentiates and acquires ribbon and conventional synapses. The maturation of neurons occurs together with the maturation of Müller cells, which acquire more

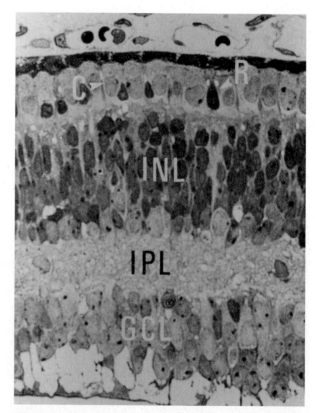

FIGURE 1-4. Four-month-old human fetus. All the major constituents of the retina are present. Cones (*c*), rods (*R*), external plexiform layer, internal nuclear layer (*INL*), internal plexiform layer (*IPL*), ganglion cell layer (*GCL*), nerve fiber layer, and internal limiting membrane can be clearly distinguished (×540). Reproduced from Hollenberg and Spira. (Reproduced from Hollenberg MJ, Spira AW. Early development of the human retina. *Can J Ophthalmol* 1972;7:472–491, with permission.)

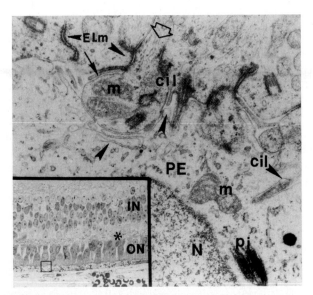

FIGURE 1-5. Five-month-old human fetus. The inset shows all the layers of the retina. Amacrine cells with large, light-colored nuclei; Müller cells with dark, angular nuclei; bipolar cells with small, oval nuclei of medium density; horizontal cells with large nuclei. ON, outer nuclear layer; IN = inner nuclear layer; asterisk, outer plexiform layer. The main figure shows the pigment epithelium–photoreceptor contact area. The blank arrow points to the beginning of an inner segment. The thin solid arrow indicates villi of a retinal pigment epithelial cell (*PE*). There are junctions between the retinal pigment epithelial cells and the photoreceptors. The Subretinal space is not yet present. cil, cilium; Elm, external limiting membrane; m, mitochondria; N = nucleus of pigment epithelial cell; pi, pigment granule; arrow heads, microvilli of pigment epithelial cell (×24,000). (Reproduced from Ozanics, Jakobiec. Prenatal development of the eye and its ednexae. In: *Ocular anatomy, embryology, and teratology.* Philadelphia: Harper & Row, 1982:11–96, with permission.)

glycogen, intermediate filaments, myelin-associated protein, and hyaluronic acid. The differentiation of the photoreceptors manifests with the production of F-actin and alpha-tubulin, components of the microtubules. There is not yet a subretinal space present. The most important event occurring at this stage is the appearance of retinal vascularization. Spindle shaped mesenchymal cells originating inside the optic disc from the walls of the two venous channels located on either side of the hyaloid artery and from the adventitia of the hyaloid artery proliferate and migrate into the inner retina. They differentiate into endothelial cells, make cords, and then canalize to form capillaries.

The fifth month is characterized by the conspicuous differentiation of the photoreceptors. Infolding of the photoreceptor membrane makes the tubular structures of the outer segments and rhodopsin and S antigen appear (8). The differentiation of the apical surfaces of the photoreceptors and of the apical villi of the RPE cells causes the breakdown of the junctions present between these two kinds of cells and the formation of the subretinal space (Fig. 1-5). This space contains the interphotoreceptor matrix, which includes, among others, the interstitial retinol

binding protein (IRBP), apparently secreted by the photoreceptors themselves. Following the development of the photoreceptors, horizontal cells become more conspicuous and are arranged in a row. At the internal layers of the retina, both amacrine and ganglion cells become located at their definitive locations. Apoptosis causes the appearance of cell debris between retinal cells and this debris become phagocytosed by the surrounding cells, not by macrophages, as retinal vasculature, the source of macrophages, has not yet completely developed. Apoptosis is also the cause of a marked decrease in the number of ganglion cells. This cell loss is not uniform; it is more pronounced at the periphery, creating in this way the centrifugal gradient of the distribution of the ganglion cells in the fetal retina. The beginning of the development of the pars plana renders the ora serrata more clearly distinguishable. Retinal vascularization progresses rapidly. Newly formed capillaries extend peripherally and form arteries and veins; the artery and veins present at the optic disc become the central retinal artery and veins. In the capillaries, the cells in contact with the blood flow become endothelial cells and the surrounding ones pericytes. Processes of astrocytes get attached to the collagenous matrix surrounding the capillaries.

At the sixth month, photoreceptor differentiation involves the cones. Cone nuclei are arranged in a row adjacent to the external limiting membrane and the rod nuclei are located more internally. Tubular structures increase in number, and mitochondria, ribosomes, and endoplasmic reticulum appear in the prospective inner segment while primitive cone pedicles without ribbon synapses but with conspicuous contact synapses form (9). For the first time, the macula appears as a bulging area with a thickened ganglion cell layer (Fig. 1-6). Most of the photoreceptors are cones. There is a

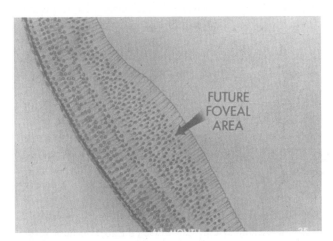

FIGURE 1-6. Six-month-old human fetus. The future fovea at the central bulging area of the retina. Ganglion cells present a multilayered arrangement. (From *Embryology of the eye* [film] San Francisco: American Academy of Ophthalmology, 1950. Courtesy of Dr. Michael Hogan.)

remnant of the layer of Chievitz. Ganglion cells mature and accumulate cytoplasm: this maturation starts at the posterior pole and progresses toward the periphery at the same rate as retinal vascularization. Ganglion cells posterior to the edge of advancing vessels are more mature than those anterior to them (10). Müller cells are well developed and strongly attached to the internal limiting membrane and myelin-associated protein is present throughout all the layers of the retina. Retinal vascularization continues its rapid progression. More capillaries appear. Arterial and venous channels develop while some of their side branches retract and atrophy, giving rise to the formation of capillary free perivascular zones; this is called remodeling of the retina. In all mammals with an intraretinal capillary system, one can see that the capillary-free zone around arteries is wider than that around veins. The width of the capillary-free zone depends on the oxygen concentration in the blood flow. Raising the oxygen concentration in the blood widens the periarterial capillary-free zone, while reducing it narrows the capillary-free zone (11). Weiter et al. (12) emphasize that the normal embryonal and fetal retina is avascular until the fourth month. Until then, choroidal circulation is sufficient for full-thickness oxygenation of the retina. With the development of the photoreceptors that require increased oxygen consumption, choroidal circulation becomes insufficient and retinal vascularization develops. Retinal maturation precedes vascular outgrowth. The inner retinal plexus forms initially and the deeper capillary plexus follows.

At the seventh month, the rods differentiate in the same way cones have previously differentiated (Fig. 1-7). In the cones, (i) tubular structures arrange as lamellar sacs, (ii) mitochondria aggregate at the ellipsoid, and (iii) cone and rod terminals develop synaptic vesicles and ribbons. The more the photoreceptors develop, the more the subretinal space enlarges. The ora serrata appears as a circular line covered by the Lange fold made up by the peripheral retina (13). The macula still bulges. No new cones are generated in this area. The fovea forms as a result of two kinds of migration. The first takes place in the inner retina and causes the formation of the foveal pit and foveal slope. It consists of the centrifugal displacement of the ganglion cells with their dendrites and their synapses, of the bipolar cells with their synapses, and of the axons of the associated photoreceptors, which elongate and form the fibers of Henle's layer. The second takes place in the external photoreceptor layer and consists of a centripetal migration of photoreceptors, cones and rods, and also of the adjacent RPE cells (14). There is no vascularization inside the foveal area. The macular area is encircled by capillaries, which do not proliferate over the center. Retinal vascularization advances toward the periphery but does not extend to the ora serrata and an avascular retinal zone persists at the periphery. The advancing edge of the retinal vasculature is made up of spindle-shaped mesenchymal cells, the vanguard of vasoformative tissue. There remains some controversy over the origin of the cells at the

advancing edge of the retinal vasculature. Early investigators believed these to be of neuroectodermal origin, but the current theory that the cells are of mesenchymal origin is more commonly accepted (15). Behind the vanguard, endothelial cells proliferate and form loops. The spindle-shaped cells are attached to one another with gap junctions. At a fully differentiated stage, these cells possess few gap junctions and capillaries continue to advance normally inside the nerve fiber layer. When the cells are active, the gap junctions increase in number and may constitute a barrier to further intraretinal capillary growth (16).

At the eighth month, the differentiation of the photoreceptors extends to the ora serrata. The photoreceptors be-

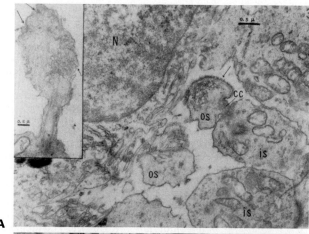

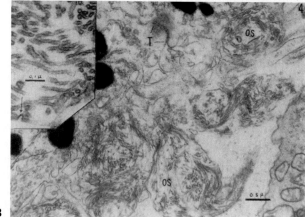

FIGURE 1-7. Seven-month-old human fetus. Development of the photoreceptor. **(A)** Two outer segments (*OS*) of which one is seen attached to an inner segment (*is*) by a connecting cilium (*cc*) and the other not; they contain tubular structures. N, nucleus of pigment epithelial cell. **Inset A**: Primitive outer segment shows an invaginated plasma membrane (*arrows*) at the lateral and apical surfaces. Some tubular structures show a swelling at their end. **(B)** The outer segments (*OS*) contain numerous tubular structures intermingled with each other; they are surrounded by the apical surface and processes of retinal pigment epithelial cells. I, terminal bar between two pigment epithelial cells. **Inset**: Tubular structures at higher magnification. (Reproduced from Yamada, Ishikawa. Submicroscopic morphogenesis of the human retina in the structure of the eye, symposium ii. Stuttgart: Verlag, 1965, with permission.)

come longer and the lamellar structures of their outer segments acquire their normal arrangement. The inner segments become mature. The subretinal space extends to the ora serrata. The ganglion cell density is the highest at the perifoveal region. In general, the ganglion cell population continues to decrease, but the density remains greater posteriorly whereas peripheral ganglion cells become rarer at the periphery. The macula continues to thin out and the retinal vessels extend to the ora serrata.

At the ninth month, the retina is well differentiated: both the RPE cells and the photoreceptors are mature. The retinal surface increases although mitotic activity has ceased and this is due to a transverse shifting of the retinal cells. The RPE accommodates itself to this increased retinal surface area by changing in regional densities. The differentiation of the macula continues and manifests itself with the following clinical signs: (i) first, some pigment appears in the macula; (ii) then, a perimacular reflex soon becomes annular; and, finally, (iii) the appearance of a concavity accompanies a foveolar light reflex. Macular pigmentation appears at the 34th gestational week, the perimacular annular reflex at the 36th (17). The foveolar reflex is due to the deepening of the foveal depression (18). During the formation of the foveolar depression, not only the ganglion cells, but also amacrine, bipolar, Müller, and horizontal cells move away from the fovea (19). Functional development accompanies the differentiation of the retina and expresses itself with the appearance of visual evoked response (20). The retinal vessels reach the temporal periphery. Deep in the retina, the retinal capillaries reach the internal nuclear layer and form the external capillary net, which itself does not reach the equator.

At birth, the development of the eye is complete except for the macula. The size of the immature fovea is 5 degrees (21). In the postnatal development of the fovea, two factors play a role: the inward migration of the cone cells toward the center and the elongation of the foveal cones. This elongation involves the outer segment and the basal axon and causes the narrowing of the foveal cones. The cone diameter decreases from 7.5 μm at birth to 2 μm at the age of 45 months. As a result, the foveal density increases from 18/100 μm. at birth to 42/100 μm in the adult eye. The foveola reaches its adult configuration at the age of 45 months (22). The development of the fovea coincides with the cortical neuronal dendritic growth and synapse formation. This central nervous system development continues during the 2 postnatal years at a slower rate (20,23).

DEVELOPMENTAL DEFECTS

Papillorenal Syndrome

Genetics

The *PAX* gene family plays an essential role in early mammalian development. *PAX2* is expressed during development in the optic and otic vesicles and in the kidney. The *Krd* (kidney and retinal defects) mouse carries a defect on chromosome 19, which includes the *PAX2* locus. The adult *Krd* mouse, which is heterozygous for this deletion, presents a variable semidominant phenotype characterized by structural anomalies in the kidney and retina similar to what appears in the papillorenal (renal coloboma) syndrome. Homozygosity causes embryonal death. The *Krd* mouse (*Krd/+*) constitutes a good model for the study of the embryonal basis of the ocular defects observed in the papillorenal syndrome in humans. In normal mouse embryos, *PAX2*-immunopositive cells (*PAX2+*) demarcate the embryonic fissure on the ventral side of the optic cup and optic stalk. With the closure of the fissure, these *PAX2+* cells disappear from the ventral retina but persist as a cuff of cells around the developing optic disc, at the site of exit of the axons of the developing ganglion cells. In the *Krd/+* mouse embryo, these *PAX2+* cells undergo abnormal morphogenetic movements and the embryonic fissure does not close normally giving rise to the retinal and optic disc defects that characterize the papillorenal (renal coloboma) syndrome (24).

The ocular manifestations described in the syndrome include optic nerve coloboma, abnormal vascular pattern of the optic disc (25), and optic disc dysplasia (26). Extraocular anomalies include renal hypoplasia, vesicoureteral reflux, and sensorineural hearing loss (27). Mutations in the *PAX2* gene were determined in some of the patients (28). Its mutations cause several different abnormalities. On the one hand, there is no correlation between the mutation and the phenotype; on the other, the same mutation can cause different ocular abnormalities. The *PAX2* gene is expressed in primitive cells of the kidney, ureter, eye, ear, and central nervous system. Therefore, *PAX* abnormalities include several syndromes involving both eyes and kidneys. Ocular manifestations described in this syndrome include morning glory anomaly (24), optic nerve coloboma, abnormal vascular pattern of the optic disc (25), and optic disc dysplasia (26). Extraocular abnormalities include renal hypoplasia, vesicoureteral reflux, and sensorineural hearing loss (27). A mutation of the *PAX2* gene was determined in some patients with these findings (28). Parsa et al. (29) hypothesized that a primary deficiency in the vascular development compromised the retinal and choroidal growth and accounted for the ocular anomalies found in this syndrome. In an analogous way, renal vascular anomalies could be the etiological factor responsible for the renal anomalies.

Optic Nerve and Choroidal Coloboma

During the seventh week the embryonic fissure closes completely. Failure of closure of the anterior (proximal) end of the embryonic fissure will result in coloboma of the iris, ciliary body and choroid at the inferonasal quadrant of the

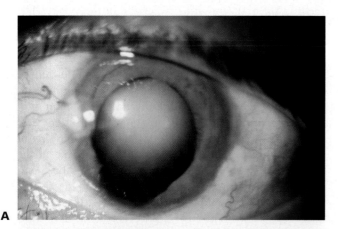

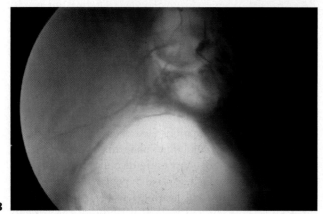

FIGURE 1-8. Coloboma of the iris **(A)** and the retina and choroid **(B)** in the same eye.

globe (Figs. 8 A and 8B). Failure of closure of the posterior end causes coloboma of the optic disc (15,30). These colobomas are defined as typical colobomas. In contrast, atypical colobomas can be located anywhere in the globe and, therefore, probably do not result from an embryonic fissure defect (31). Abnormally persistent vascularized strands of the tunica vasculosa lentis prevent the normal growth of the iris in a certain location and this results in atypical coloboma of the iris (32). Coloboma of the iris varies from a small notch at the pupillary margin to a large sector defect. The defect can take the shape of a pear with its broad base at the pupillary area or can have parallel margins extending peripherally. Eyes with isolated iris coloboma usually have normal visual acuities.

In optical nerve coloboma, there is a white bowl-shaped excavation of the optic disc, located usually inferonasally. The defect appears on funduscopy as a white area that may involve the retina and choroid adjacent to the optic disc, and even extend anteriorly to include the ciliary body and the iris (33). Microphthalmos is frequently present in cases of extensive coloboma and is called colobomatous microphthalmos. Optic nerve colobomas can be associated with systemic abnormalities (34,35). Ocular anomalies found in patients with chorioretinal coloboma include microcornea,

choroidal detachment, and retinal detachment (35). Several mechanisms for retinal detachment are speculated in these patients. One or more small breaks within the thin white membrane overlying the colobomatous defect can permit communication between liquefied vitreous and the subretinal space. Often vitreoretinal membranes can overlay these breaks making them difficult to appreciate preoperatively even with a contact lens evaluation. Another possible mechanism is similar to that reported of the association between optic nerve pit and serous detachment of the macula (30). Cerebrospinal fluid from the subarachnoidal space around the optic nerve passes through the defect and enters into the subretinal space (36). Finally, retinal detachments can result from vitreoretinal traction on one or more retinal breaks that occur in normal retina similar to what occurs in eyes without colobomas that develop rhegmatogenous retinal detachments. The prevalence of retinal or choroidal detachment was found to be 2.4% to 43% (37–40). The higher prevalence in some series likely results from the greater age range of the patients reported. Visual acuity may be mildly to severely affected, depending on the extent of damage to the optic disc and the retina. A coloboma that involves the macula often has markedly decreased visual acuity. Coloboma can be unilateral or bilateral and present sporadically or it may have an autosomal-dominant pattern (33).

MANAGEMENT

Treatment of shallow retinal detachment associated with breaks within the colobomatous defect can initially be attempted by placing laser spots along the area of normal retina that abuts the coloboma where the defect exists. If this fails, then laser can be placed all around the colobomatous area. If the defect is within the optic nerve coloboma, laser may initially be placed in certain quadrants in an attempt to avoid interference of nerve fibers from all quadrants. However, if this fails, laser can be placed around the entire optic nerve coloboma. If however, the retinal detachment is too highly elevated to permit absorption of the laser energy, attempts can be made to drain subretinal fluid before applying laser. However, if this fails, vitreoretinal surgery is often required to remove the membranes, drain subretinal fluid, and apply laser. Sometimes, silicone oil tamponade and occasionally cyanoacrylate placed onto the colobomatous defect to seal it from liquefied vitreous are needed. For eyes with breaks in normal peripheral retina, a scleral buckle may be adequate (41).

Lens Coloboma

Coloboma of the lens is characterized by a notching in the equator of the lens. As discussed previously, lack of absorption of part of the tunica vasculosa lentis lateralis causes a localized inhibition of the growth of the zonules and lens while the rest of the lens continues its normal development. The lens deprived of its normal pull in the defective region is thicker and more spherical. Lens coloboma can occur separately or in conjunction with colobomas of the ciliary body. Lens colobomas can be associated with complicated retinal detachments involving large peripheral retinal breaks, retinal attachments to the lens, and in some cases, are believed to be associated with nonattachment of the retina (42). Treatment usually requires complicated vitreoretinal surgery.

Morning Glory Anomaly

Morning glory anomaly is an enlarged excavated optic disc, orange in color with fibroglial tissue at its center. The disc is located at the center of a funnel shaped excavation of the posterior fundus. The blood vessels arise from the periphery of the disc. Peripapillary retinal pigmentation surrounds the disc. This is usually a unilateral defect, which presents sporadically. The embryonic defect of the morning glory anomaly is unknown, although an abnormal closure of the embryonic fissure (43) and a mesodermal defect were suggested (44). Kindler (45), who first described this anomaly, related it to an abnormal development of remnants of Bergmeister papilla. Visual acuity is usually decreased, ranging from 20/100 to hand motion. Amblyopia can develop and further reduce visual acuity (46). The morning glory disc anomaly has been described and part of trisomy 4q and found to be associated with transsphenoidal encephalocele (34). Retinal detachment developed in 26% to 38% of the patients (47,48). The pathogenesis of the retinal detachment has been attributed to subretinal exudation (45), traction from abnormal papilla (49), vitreoretinal traction (50), preretinal vitreous strands (51), or rhegmatogenous retinal detachment (52). Management often requires vitrectomy, sometimes with silicone oil tamponade.

Peripapillary Staphyloma

Peripapillary staphyloma is a posterior retinal excavation, at the bottom of which the optic disc is located. Atrophic pigmentary changes can be seen at the margin of the defect (53). Cases of contractile peripapillary staphyloma have been described; retinal pulsation may follow the respiratory rhythm (54) or occur at irregular intervals (53,55). This anomaly usually causes decreased visual acuity although some cases with normal vision have been also reported (56). Management often requires vitrectomy, sometimes with silicone oil tamponade.

Nonattachment of the Retina

During the formation of the optic vesicle, lack of contact between the surface ectoderm and the vesicle results in nondevelopment of the retina and the transformation of the cells of the optic vesicle into a layer similar to the RPE (57). Moreover, in cases of nonattachment of the retina, the presumptive retinal epithelium may form a sensory retina and the presumptive retina may form a RPE (58).

Patients and medical staff are often confronted with difficult ethical decisions involving the birth of a child whose vision might be severely afflicted. Questions arise: Is prenatal diagnosis always mandatory and what procedures are ethically justified? Should prenatal diagnosis be reserved for all couples who are at high risk of giving birth to children with serious genetic disease or only for children who have treatable conditions? The decisions must be based on the interests of the child, mother, and society. Prenatal medicine and the understanding of the genetics and pathogenesis of diseases have applied diagnostic methods as well as fetal therapy. Genetic screening, gene therapy, and other applications of genetic engineering may be used for the treatment, cure, or prevention of congenital diseases. Gene delivery *in utero* is an approach to gene therapy in children with genetic diseases. It is based on the concept that applying gene therapy vectors to the fetus in utero may prevent the development of a congenital disease.

A: REFERENCES

1. Hollenberg J, Spira AW. Human retinal development: ultrastructure of the outer retina. *Am J Anat* 1973;137:357–386.
2. Mund MI, Rodrigues MM. Embryology of the human retinal pigment epithelium. In: Zinn, Marmor, eds. *The retinal pigment epithelium.* Cambridge: Harvard University Press, 1979:45–52.
3. Ulshafer RJ, Clavert A. Cell death and optic fiber penetration into the optic stalk of the chick. *J Morphol* 1979;162:67–76.
4. Rhodes RH. Development of the optic nerve. In: Jakobiec, ed. *Ocular anatomy, embryology and teratology.* Philadelphia: Harper and Row, 1982:601–638.
5. Vrabec F. Early stages of development of the human retinal astroglia: a neurohistological study. *Folia Morphol (Praha)* 1988;36:250–255.
6. Siegelmann J, Ozanics V. Retina. In: Jakobiec, ed. *Ocular anatomy, embryology and teratology.* Philadelphia: Harper and Row, 1982:441–506.
7. Rhodes RH. Ultrastructure of Mueller cells in the developing human retina. *Arch Clin Exp Ophthalmol* 1984;221:171–178.
8. Donoso LA, Hammas H, Dietzschold B, et al. Rhodopsin and retinoblastoma: a monoclonal antibody histopathologic study. *Arch Ophthalmol* 1986;104:111–113.
9. Yamada F, Ishikawa T. Some observations on the submicroscopic morphogenesis of the human retina. In: Rohen, ed. *Eye structure II.* Schattauer: Stuttgart, 1965:5–16.
10. Provis JM, Bellson FA, Russell P. Ganglion cell topography in human fetal retina. *Invest Ophthalmol Vis Sci* 1983;24:1316–1320.
11. Ashton N. Retinal angiogenesis in the human embryo. *Br Med Bull* 1970;26:103–106.
12. Weiter JJ, Zuckerman R, Schepens CL. A model for the pathogenesis of retrolental fibroplasia based on the metabolic control of blood vessel development. *Ophthalmic Surg* 1982;13:1013–1017.
13. Barishak YR. The development of the angle of the anterior chamber in vertebrate eyes. *Doc Ophthalmol* 1978;45:329–360.

14. Hendrickson AE. Primate foveal development: a microcosm of current questions in neurobiology. *Invest Ophthalmol Vis Sci* 1994;35:3129–3133.

15. Barishak YR. *Embryology of the eye and its adnexae*, 2nd ed. Basel: Karger, 2001.

16. Kretzer FL, Hittner HM, Johnson AT, et al. Vitamin E and retrolental fibroplasias: ultrastructure support of clinical efficacy. *Ann N Y Acad Sci* 1982;393:145–166.

17. Isenberg SJ. Macular development in premature infant. *Am J Ophthal* 1986;101:74–80.

18. Hendrickson AE, Yuodelis C. The morphological development of the human fovea. *Ophthalmology* 1984;91:603–612.

19. Hendrickson AE, Kupfer C. The histogenesis of the fovea in the macaque monkey. *Invest Ophthalmol Vis Sci* 1976;15:746–756.

20. Mellor DH, Fielder AR. Dissociated visual development: electrodiagnostic studies in infants who are slow to see. *Dev Med Child Neurol* 1980;22:327–335.

21. Abramov I, Gordon J, Hendrickson AE, et al. The retina in new born infant. *Science* 1982;217:265–267.

22. Yuodelis c, Hendrickson AE. A qualitative and quantitative analysis of the human fovea during development. *Vision Res* 1986;26: 847–855.

23. Hoyt CS, Jastrzebski G, Marg E. Delayed visual maturation in infancy. *Br J Ophthalmol* 1983;67:127–130.

24. Otteson DC, Shelden E, Jones JM, et al. PAX2 expression and retinal morphogenesis in the normal and Krd mouse. *Dev Biol* 1998;192:209–224.

25. Weaver RG, Cashwell LF, Lorentz W, et al. Optic nerve coloboma associated with renal disease. *Am J Med Genet* 1988;29: 597–605.

26. Dureau P, Attie-Bitach T, Salomon R, et al. Renal coloboma syndrome. *Ophthalmology* 2001;108:1912–1916.

27. Schimenti LA, Cunliffe HE, McNoe LA, et al. Further delineation of renal coloboma syndrome in patients with extreme variability of phenotype and identical PAX 2 mutations. *Am J Hum Genet* 1997;60:869–878.

28. Sanyanusin P, McNoe LA, Sullican MJ, et al. Mutation of the PAX 2 in two siblings with renal coloboma syndrome. *Hum Mol Genet* 1995;4:2183–2184.

29. Parsa CF. Redefining papillorenal syndrome: an undiagnosed cause of ocular and renal morbidity. *Ophthalmology* 2001;108:738–749.

30. Savell J, Cook JR. Optic nerve colobomas of autosomal dominant heredity. *Arch Ophthalmol* 1979;94:395–400.

31. Duke-Elder ST. *System of ophthalmology, vol III, part 2. Congenital deformities.* London: Henry Kimpton:456–480.

32. Duke-Elder ST. *System of ophthalmology vol. III pt.2. Congenital anomalies.* London: Henry Kimpton:577–578.

33. Francois J. Colobomatous malformations of the ocular globe. *Int Ophthalmol Clin* 1968;8: 797–816

34. Brodsky MC. Congenital optic disk anomalies. *Surv Ophthalmol* 1994;39: 89–112.

35. Daufenbach DR, Ruttum MS, Pulido JS, et al. Chorioretinal coloboma in a pediatric population. *Ophthalmology* 1998;105: 1455–1458.

36. Gass JDM. Serous detachment of the macula secondary to congenital pit of the optic nervehead. *Am J Ophthalmol* 1969;67: 821–841.

37. Jesberg DO, Schepens CL. Retinal detachment associated with coloboma of the choroid. *Arch Ophthalmol* 1961;65: 163–173.

38. Patnaik B, Kalsi R. Retinal detachment with coloboma of the choroid. *Indian J Ophthalmol* 1981;29: 345–349.

39. Maumenee IH, Mitchell TN. Colobomatous malformations of the eye. *Trans Am Ophthalmol Soc* 1990;88:123–132.

40. Gopal L, Badrinath SS, Kumar KS, et al. Optic disk in fundus coloboma. *Ophthalmology* 1996;103:2120–2126.

41. Hartnett ME, Hirose T. Retinal detachment in the pediatric population. In: Schepens CL, Hartnett ME, Hirose T, eds. *Schepens' retinal detachment and allied diseases*, 2nd ed. Boston: Butterworth Heinemann, 2000.

42. Hovland KR, Schepens CL, Freeman HM. Developmental giant retinal tears associated with lens coloboma. *Arch Ophthalmol* 1968;80:325–331.

43. Mafee MF, Jampol LM, Langer BG, et al. Computed tomography of optic nerve colobomas, morning glory anomaly and colobomatous cyst. *Radiol Clin N Am* 1987;25:693–699.

44. Dempster AG, Lee WR, Forrester JV, et al. The morning glory syndrome. A mesodermal defect? *Ophthalmologica* 1983;187: 222–230.

45. Kindler P. Morning glory syndrome. Unusual optic disk anomaly. *Am J Ophthalmol* 1970;69:376–384.

46. Kushner BJ. Functional Amblyopia associated with abnormalities of the optic nerve. *Arch Ophthalmol* 1985;102:683–685.

47. Steinkuller PG. The morning glory disc anomaly. Case report and literature review. *J Pediatr Ophthalmol Strabismus* 1980;17: 81–87.

48. Haik BG, Greenstein SH, Smith ME, et al. Retinal detachment in the morning glory syndrome. *Ophthalmology* 1984;91:1638–1647.

49. Cogan DJ. *Neurology of the visual system.* Springfield: Thomas, 1966:153.

50. Jensen PE, Kalina RE. Congenital anomalies of the optic disk. *Am J Ophthalmol* 1976;82:27–31

51. Hamada S, Ellsworth RM. Congenital retinal detachment and the optic disk anomaly. *Am J Ophthalmol* 1971;71:460–464.

52. von Fricken MA, Dhungel R. Retinal detachment in the morning glory syndrome. *Retina* 1984;4:97–99

53. Wise JB, McLean AL, Gass JDM. Contractile peripapillary staphyloma. *Arch Ophthalmol* 1966;75:626–630.

54. Sugar HS, Beckman H. Peripapillary staphyloma with respiratory pulsations. *Am J Ophthalmol* 1969;68:895–897.

55. Kral K, Svarc D. Contractile peripapillary staphyloma. *Am J Ophthalmol* 1971;71:1090–1092.

56. Caldwell JBH, Sears ML, Gilman M. Bilateral peripapillary staphyloma with normal vision. *Am J Ophthalmol* 1971: 71:423–425.

57. Lopashov VG. *Development mechanisms of vertebrate eye rudiments.* New York: Pergamon Press/McMillan, 1963:142.

58. Coulombre AJ. *The eye in Dahaan Ursprung. Organogenesis.* New York: Holt, Rinehart and Winston, 1965:219–240.

B. VITREOUS EMBRYOLOGY AND VITREO-RETINAL DEVELOPMENTAL DISORDERS

JERRY SEBAG
NATALIE NGUYEN

INTRODUCTION

Invisible by design (Fig. 1-9), vitreous was long unseen as an important participant in the physiology and pathology of the eye. Yet recent studies have determined that vitreous plays a significant role in ocular health and disease. In particular, a number of important vitreoretinal disorders arise from abnormal embryogenesis. Vitreous embryology is presented in detail elsewhere in Part A of this chapter. Part B of this chapter will review vitreous biochemistry and structure, and will discuss the congenital disorders that arise from developmental biochemical abnormalities as well as the ways by which abnormalities in vitreous vascular embryogenesis result in significant vitreoretinal pathology.

VITREOUS BIOCHEMISTRY

That vitreous is now considered an important ocular structure with respect to normal physiology (1) and several important pathologic conditions (1,2) of the posterior segment is due in no small part to a better understanding of the biochemical organization of vitreous (3–5).

Collagens

Gloor (6) pointed out that the collagen content is highest where the vitreous is a gel. As shown in Fig. 1-10, individual vitreous collagen fibrils are organized as a triple helix of three alpha chains. The major collagen fibrils of the corpus vitreus are heterotypic, consisting of more than one collagen type. Recent studies of pepsinized forms of collagen confirm that the corpus vitreus contains collagen type II, a hybrid of types V/XI, and type IX (3,5).

Type II Collagen

Type II collagen, a homotrimer composed of three identical alpha chains designated as $[\alpha\ 1\ (II)]_3$, comprises 75% of the total collagen content in vitreous. When first synthesized as

a procollagen and secreted into the extracellular space, type II collagen is highly soluble. The activity of *N*-proteinase and *C*-proteinase enzymes reduces the solubility and enables type II collagen molecules to cross-link covalently in a quarter-staggered array. Within this array are likely to be *N*-propeptides, which probably extend outward from the surface of the forming fibril (4). This may influence the interaction of the collagen fibril with other components of the extracellular matrix. Recent studies (7) combined immunolocalization with Western blot analysis of macromolecules extracted from bovine vitreous collagen fibrils and found that the pN-type IIA procollagen is located on the surface of the vitreous collagen fibril. The finding (8) that type IIA procollagen propeptides specifically bind growth factors such as transforming growth factor-β1 (TGF-β1) and bone morphogenic protein (BMP-2) supports the concept that, in certain circumstances, such growth factors interact with vitreous fibrils to promote the cell migration and proliferation that could result in proliferative diabetic retinopathy and proliferative vitreoretinopathy.

Type IX Collagen

Type IX collagen is a heterotrimer that is disulfide-bonded with an $[\alpha\ 1\ (IX)\ \alpha\ 2\ (IX)\ \alpha\ 3\ (IX)]$ configuration. This heterotrimer is oriented regularly along the surfaces of the major collagen fibrils in a "D periodic" distribution, where it is cross-linked onto the fibril surface. Type IX is not a typical collagen, but is a member of the FACIT (fibrillar-associated collagens with interrupted triple helixes) group of collagens. It contains collagenous regions described as COL1, COL2, and COL3 interspersed between noncollagenous regions called NC1, NC2, NC3, and NC4 (9,10). In vitreous, as opposed to cartilage, the NC4 domain is small and, therefore, not highly charged and not likely to exhibit extensive interaction with other extracellular matrix components (11). In vitreous, type IX collagen always contains a chondroitin sulfate glycosaminoglycan chain (9,10), which is linked covalently to the α 2 (IX) chain at the NC3 domain;

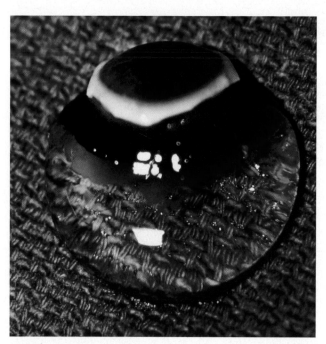

FIGURE 1-9. Vitreous from a 9-month-old child was dissected of the sclera, choroid, and retina. In spite of the specimen being on a surgical towel exposed to room air, the gel state is maintained. (Specimen is courtesy of the New England Eye Bank.)

this enables the molecule to assume a proteoglycan form. Electron microscopy of vitreous stained with cationic dyes enables visualization of the chondroitin sulfate chains of type IX collagen. In some of these studies, sulfated glycosaminoglycans are found distributed regularly along the surface of vitreous collagen fibrils (12), and often bridge between neighboring collagen fibrils. Duplexing of gly-

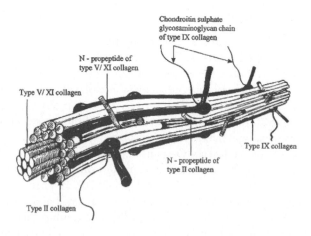

FIGURE 1-10. Schematic diagram of collagen fibril structure in the human vitreous. (From Bishop PN. Structural macromolecules and supramolecular organisation of the vitreous gel. *Prog Retin Eye Res* 2000;19:323–344, with permission.)

cosaminoglycans chains from adjacent collagen fibrils may result in a "ladderlike" configuration (13).

Type V/XI Collagen

Ten percent of vitreous collagen is a hybrid V/XI collagen that is believed to comprise the central core of the major collagen fibrils of vitreous (14). Type V/XI is a heterotrimer that contains α 1 (XI) and α 2 (V) in two chains, while the nature of the third chain is presently not known (15). Along with type II collagen, type V/XI is a fibril-forming collagen. While the interaction of the fibril with other extracellular matrix components is probably influenced by a retained *N*-propeptide that protrudes from the surface of the fibril in cartilage (14), it is not known whether this is the case in vitreous (5).

Type VI Collagen

Although there are only small amounts of type VI collagen in vitreous, the ability of this molecule to bind both type II collagen and hyaluronan suggests that it could be important in organizing and maintaining the supramolecular structure of vitreous gel.

Glycosaminoglycans

Glycosaminoglycans are polysaccharides of repeating disaccharide units, each consisting of hexosamine (usually N-acetyl glucosamine or N-acetyl galactosamine) glycosidically linked to either uronic (glucuronic or iduronic) acid or galactose. The nature of the predominant repeating unit is characteristic for each glycosaminoglycan and the relative amount, molecular size, and type of glycosaminoglycan are said to be tissue-specific (16). Glycosaminoglycans do not normally occur as free polymers *in vivo*, but are covalently linked to a protein core, the ensemble called a proteoglycan. A sulfated group is attached to oxygen or nitrogen in all glycosaminoglycans except hyaluronan (HA). Balazs (17) first documented the presence of sulfated galactosamine-containing glycosaminoglycans in bovine vitreous (less than 5% of total vitreous glycosaminoglycans), and others (18,19) identified these as chondroitin-4-sulfate and undersulfated heparan sulfate. Studies in the rabbit (20) found a total vitreous glycosaminoglycan content of 58 ng with 13% chondroitin sulfate and 0.5% heparan sulfate.

Hyaluronan

Although hyaluronan (HA) is present throughout the body, it was first isolated from bovine vitreous. In humans, HA first appeared after birth and then became the major vitreous glycosaminoglycan. Although it has been proposed that hyalocytes synthesize HA (2), other plausible candidates are the ciliary body and retinal Müller cells. Whereas the synthesis of hyaluronan seems to continue at a constant rate in the adult while no extracellular degradation occurs, hyaluronan levels are in a steady state because the molecule escapes via the anterior segment of the eye (17). Laurent and Fraser (21) showed that the passage of HA from the vitreous *to the* anterior segment is strongly molecular weight dependent, indicating a diffusion-controlled process. In contrast, disappearance of HA *from* the anterior chamber is independent of molecular weight, suggesting that this is controlled by bulk flow.

HA is a long, unbranched polymer of repeating glucuronic acid β-1,3-N,N-acetylglucosamine disaccharide moieties linked by β 1–4 bonds (22). It is a linear, left-handed, three-fold helix with a rise per disaccharide on the helix axis of 0.98 nm (23). Rotary shadowing electron microscopy of human and bovine vitreous detected lateral aggregates of HA that form an anastomosing three-dimensional network (24). This periodicity, however, can vary depending on whether the helix is in a "compressed" or "extended" configuration (25). Changes in the degree of "extension" of HA could be important in the role vitreous plays in retinal disease. Indeed, the volume of the unhydrated HA molecule is about 0.66 cm^3/g, whereas the hydrated specific volume is 2,000 to 3,000 cm^3/g (17). Thus, the degree of hydration has a significant influence on the size and configuration of the HA molecular network. Although there is no definitive evidence that adjacent hyaluronan chains bind to one another, Brewton and Mayne (26) first proposed such an arrangement. Recent rotary shadowing electron microscopy studies (27) of bovine and human vitreous found lateral aggregates of hyaluronan that formed three-dimensional latticelike networks. HA also interacts with the surrounding mobile ions and can undergo changes in its conformation that are induced by changes in the surrounding ionic milieu (28). A decrease in surrounding ionic strength can cause the anionic charges on the polysaccharide backbone to repel one another, resulting in an extended configuration of the macromolecule. An increase in surrounding ionic strength can cause contraction of the molecule and, in turn, the entire vitreous body. As a result of HA's entanglement and immobilization within the vitreous collagen fibril matrix, this mechanical force can be transmitted by collagen fibrils to the retina, optic disc, and other structures, such as neovascular complexes. In this way, changes in the ionic milieu of vitreous may be converted into mechanical energy via extension or contraction of the HA macromolecule. This can be important in certain pathologic conditions that feature fluctuations in ionic balance and hydration, such as diabetes mellitus (29).

The sodium salt of HA has a molecular weight of 3–4.5 $\times 10^6$ in normal human vitreous (17). Laurent and Granath (30) used gel chromatography and found the average molecular weight of rabbit vitreous to be 2 to 3 $\times 10^6$ and of bovine vitreous to be 0.5 to 0.8 $\times 10^6$. In these studies, there were age-related differences in the bovine vitreous, in which HA molecular weight varied from 3 $\times 10^6$ in the newborn calf to 0.5 $\times 10^6$ in old cattle. Furthermore, there may be several species of HA within vitreous that have polysaccharide chains of different lengths (31) with a variable distribution in different topographic regions within the corpus vitreus (32).

Chondroitin Sulfate

Vitreous contains two chondroitin sulfate proteoglycans. The minor type is actually type IX collagen, which was described earlier. The majority of vitreous chondroitin sulfate is in the form of versican. This large proteoglycan has a globular N-terminal that binds hyaluronan via a 45-kd link protein (27). Thus, in human, but not bovine, vitreous versican is believed to form complexes with hyaluronan as well as microfibrillar proteins, such as fibulin-1 and fibulin-2 (5). New research (33) has further determined the presence of small amounts of versicanlike proteoglycan in the human vitreous gel, with a concentration of 0.06 mg protein/ml of vitreous gel and is about 5% of the total protein content. It has a molecular mass of 380 kd and core protein substituted by chondroitin sulphate side chains. Like versican, these proteoglycan monomers bind hyaluronan and form large aggregates.

Heparan Sulfate

This sulfated proteoglycan is normally found in basement membranes and on cell surfaces throughout the body. It was first detected in bovine vitreous in 1977 (34), and in chick vitreous (as "agrin") in 1995 (35). However, it is not clear whether heparan sulfate is a true component of vitreous or a "contaminant" from adjacent basement membranes, such as the internal limiting lamina of the retina (36). As pointed out by Bishop (5) this may also be the case for nodogen-1, the aforementioned fibulins, and fibronectin.

Noncollagenous Structural Proteins

Fibrillins

Fibrillin-containing microfibrils are more abundant in vitreous than the type VI collagen microfibrils described earlier. They are found in vitreous gel as well as in the zonular fibers of the lens. This fact explains why in Marfan's syndrome the defects in the gene encoding fibrillin-1 (FBN1 on chromosome 15q21) result in both ectopia lentis and vitreous liquefaction (5). The latter probably plays a role in the frequent occurrence of rhegmatogenous retinal detachment in these patients.

Opticin

The major noncollagenous protein of vitreous is a leucine-rich repeat (LRR) protein which is bound to the surface of the heterotypic collagen fibrils, known as opticin (37). Formerly called vitrican, opticin is believed to be important in collagen fibril assembly and in preventing the aggregation of adjacent collagen fibrils into bundles. Thus, a breakdown in this property or activity may play a role in age-related vitreous degeneration (38). A recent study (39) attempted to determine the structure, location, and expression of the mouse opticin gene (*Optc*). The gene was found to be localized to mouse chromosome 1, consisting of seven exons. Additionally, in situ hybridization revealed that opticin mRNA is localized exclusively to the ciliary body during development and to the nonpigmented ciliary epithelium of the adult mouse eye. The researchers concluded that opticin may represent a marker for the differentiation of ciliary body. Besides regulating vitreous collagen fibrillogenesis, it may also have other functions as demonstrated by its continued expression in the adult mouse eye.

VIT1

Another novel vitreous protein is VIT1, a collagen-binding macromolecule (40). Because of its propensity to bind collagen, this highly basic protein may play an important role in maintaining vitreous gel structure.

Supramolecular Organization

As described by Mayne (41), vitreous is "organized" as a dilute meshwork of collagen fibrils interspersed with extensive arrays of long HA molecules. The collagen fibrils provide a scaffoldlike structure that is "inflated" by the hydrophilic HA. If collagen is removed, the remaining HA forms a viscous solution; if hyaluronan is removed, the gel shrinks (28) but is not destroyed. Early physiologic observations (42) suggested the existence of an interaction between HA and collagen that stabilizes collagen.

Bishop (5) has proposed that to understand how vitreous gel is organized and stabilized requires an understanding of what prevents collagen fibrils from aggregating and by what means the collagen fibrils are connected to maintain a stable gel structure. Studies (43) have shown that the chondroitin sulfate chains of type IX collagen bridge between adjacent collagen fibrils in a ladderlike configuration spacing them apart. This arrangement might account for vitreous transparency, in that keeping vitreous collagen fibrils separated by at least one wavelength of incident light would minimize light scattering and allow unhindered transmission of light to the retinal photoreceptors. However, depolymerizing with chondroitinases does not destroy the gel, suggesting that chondroitin sulphate side chains are not essential for vitreous collagen spacing. Complexed with HA, however, the chondroitin sulfate side chains might space apart the collagen fibrils (13,43), but Bishop believes that this form of collagen–HA interaction is "very weak." Instead, he proposes that the LRR protein opticin is the predominant structural protein in short-range spacing of collagen fibrils.

Concerning long-range spacing, Scott (13) and Mayne et al. (44) have claimed that HA plays a pivotal role in stabilizing the vitreous gel via this mechanism. However, studies (45) using hyaluronan lyase to digest vitreous HA demonstrated that the gel structure was not destroyed, suggesting that HA is not essential for the maintenance of vitreous gel stability and leading to the proposal that collagen alone is responsible for the gel state of vitreous (5).

VITREOUS STRUCTURE

Vitreous Body (Corpus Vitreus)

There is heterogeneity in the distribution of collagen throughout the vitreous body. Chemical (46,47) and light-scattering studies (48) have shown that the highest density of collagen fibrils is present in the vitreous base, followed by the posterior vitreous cortex anterior to the retina, and then by the anterior vitreous cortex behind the posterior chamber and lens. The lowest density is found in the central vitreous and adjacent to the anterior cortical gel. HA molecules have a different distribution from collagen. They are most abundant in the posterior cortical gel with a gradient of decreasing concentration as one moves centrally and anteriorly (49,50). Balazs (51) has hypothesized that this is due to the fact that vitreous HA is synthesized by hyalocytes in the posterior vitreous cortex and cannot traverse the internal limiting lamina of the retina, but leaves the vitreous to enter the posterior chamber by way of the annulus of the anterior vitreous cortex that is not adjacent to a basal lamina. Bound water (nonfreezable) has a distribution within the vitreous similar to that of HA (52), presumably due to HA binding.

Laboratory investigations of vitreous structure have long been hampered by the absence of easily recognized landmarks within the vitreous body. Consequently, removal of the vitreous from the eye results in a loss of orientation. The transparency of the vitreous renders observation in conventional diffuse light unrewarding. Attempts to study vitreous structure with opaque dyes (53) do visualize the areas filled by dye but obscure the appearance of adjacent structures. The use of histologic contrast-enhancing techniques usually involves tissue fixation, which often includes dehydration of the tissue. Since vitreous is 98% water, dehydration induces profound alteration of the internal morphology. Consequently, any investigation of vitreous structure must overcome these difficulties.

The sclera, choroid, and retina can be dissected and the "naked" vitreous body can be maintained intact and attached to the anterior segment of the eye. This enables study of internal vitreous morphology without a loss of intraocular orientation. However, depending on the person's age and consequently the degree of vitreous liquefaction (54), the dissected vitreous will remain solid and intact in young persons or will be flaccid and collapse in older indi-

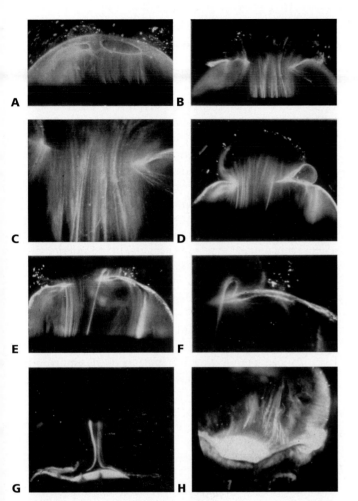

FIGURE 1-11. Dark-field slit microscopy of human vitreous in eyes dissected of the sclera, choroid, and retina. The anterior segment is below and the posterior pole is above in all specimens. (Courtesy of the New York Eye Bank for Sight Restoration.)

Recent studies have used these techniques to investigate human vitreous structure. Within the adult human vitreous there are fine, parallel fibers coursing in an anteroposterior direction (Figs. 1-11B, 1-11C) (2,58–60). The fibers arise from the vitreous base (Fig. 1-11H) where they insert anterior and posterior to the ora serrata. As the peripheral fibers course posteriorly they are circumferential with the vitreous cortex, while central fibers "undulate" in a configuration parallel with Cloquet's canal (61). The fibers are continuous and do not branch. Posteriorly, these fibers insert into the vitreous cortex (Figs. 1-11E and 1-11F).

Ultrastructural studies (62) have demonstrated that collagen fibrils are the only microscopic structures that could correspond to these fibers. These studies also detected the presence of bundles of packed, parallel collagen fibrils. It has been hypothesized that visible vitreous fibers form when HA molecules no longer separate microscopic collagen fibrils, resulting in the aggregation of collagen fibrils into bundles from which HA molecules are excluded. Eventually the aggregates of collagen fibrils attain sufficiently large proportions so as to be visualized *in vitro* (Fig. 1-11) and clinically.

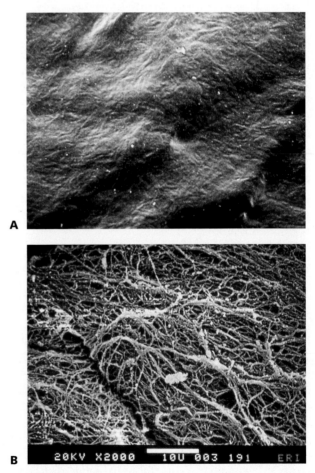

FIGURE 1-12. Scanning electron microscopy of the anterior surface of the internal limiting lamina of the retina (*top photo*) and the posterior aspect of posterior vitreous cortex in a human.

viduals. Consequently, vitreous turgescence must be maintained to avoid distortion of its inner structure. Immersion of a dissected vitreous specimen that is still attached to the anterior segment into a physiologic solution maintains vitreous turgescence and avoids structural distortion. The limitations induced by the transparency of the vitreous were overcome by Goedbloed (55), Friedenwald and Stiehler (56), and Eisner (57), who employed dark-field slit illumination of the vitreous body to achieve visualization of intravitreal morphology. Illumination with a slit-lamp beam directed into the vitreous body from the side and visualization of the illuminated portion from above produces an optical horizontal section of the vitreous body (58). The illumination/observation angle of 90 degrees that is achieved using this technique maximizes the Tyndall effect, and thus overcomes the limitations induced by vitreous transparency. Furthermore, the avoidance of any tissue fixation eliminates the introduction of many of the artifacts that flawed earlier investigations.

The areas adjacent to these large fibers have a low density of collagen fibrils separated by HA molecules and therefore do not scatter light as intensely as the larger bundles of aggregated collagen fibrils. These adjacent "channels" probably offer relatively less resistance to bulk flow through the vitreous body and are the areas visualized in studies (53,63) using India ink to fill the channels. There are changes occurring in these fibrous structures throughout life (38,58) that probably result from age-related biochemical alterations in the composition and organization of the molecular components that simultaneously result in vitreous liquefaction and fiber formation.

Both collagen and HA are synthesized during development into adulthood. The synthesis of collagen only keeps pace with increasing vitreous volume, thus the overall concentration of collagen within the corpus vitreus is unchanged during this period of life. Total collagen content in the vitreous gel decreases during the first few years of life and then remains at about 0.05 mg until the third decade (54). As collagen concentration does not appreciably increase during this time, and the size of the vitreous increases, the network density of collagen fibrils effectively decreases. This could potentially weaken the collagen network and destabilize the gel. However, since there is net synthesis of HA during this time, the dramatic increase in HA concentration "stabilizes" the thinning collagen network (17).

Recently, age-related liquefaction of the human vitreous body was evaluated using light and transmission electron microscopy (64). Based on these observations, the investigators claimed that the breakdown of collagen fibrils into smaller fragments is significant in the pathogenesis of vitreous liquefaction. However, the fragmentation-inducing mechanism of vitreous fibrils was not elucidated in these studies. The investigators tentatively proposed that an extracellular process is involved since cells and their fragments were absent in all specimens. It is conceivable that endogenous matrix metalloproteinases or other enzymes are involved in this process.

Vitreous Base

The vitreous base is a three-dimensional zone. It extends 1.5 to 2 mm anterior to the ora serrata, 1 to 3 mm posterior to the ora serrata (65), and several millimeters into the vitreous body itself (66). The posterior extent of the posterior border of the vitreous base varies with age (38,67). Vitreous fibers enter the vitreous base by splaying out to insert anterior and posterior to the ora serrata (Fig. 1-11H). The anterior-most fibers form the "anterior loop" of the vitreous base, a structure that is important in the pathophysiology of anterior proliferative vitreoretinopathy (2,68–70). In the posterior portion of the vitreous base, vitreous fibers are closer together than elsewhere. Gartner (71) has found that, in humans, the diameters of collagen fibrils in the vitreous base range from 10.8 to 12.4 nm, with a major period of cross-

striations of 50 to 54 nm. Hogan (65) demonstrated that just posterior to the ora serrata, heavy bundles of vitreous fibrils attach to the basal laminae of retinal glial cells. Studies by Gloor and Daicker (72) showed that cords of vitreous collagen insert into gaps between the neuroglia of the peripheral retina. They likened this structure to Velcro (a self-adhesive nylon material) and proposed that this would explain the strong vitreoretinal adhesion at this site. A recent investigation (73) confirmed that the anteroposterior dimension of the posterior vitreous base increases with age, but more so in men than in women. Ultrastructural studies revealed that bundles of collagen fibrils progressively invade the innermost peripheral retina, as "braids" splaying out beneath the internal limiting lamina (ILL) in the young and as a dense sublaminar "mat" in the elderly. In the anterior vitreous base, fibrils interdigitate with a reticular complex of fibrillar basement membrane material between the crevices of the nonpigmented ciliary epithelium (74). The vitreous base also contains intact cells that are fibroblastlike anterior to the ora serrata, and macrophagelike posteriorly. Damaged cells in different stages of involution and fragments of basal laminae, presumed to be remnants of the embryonic hyaloid vascular system, are also present in the vitreous base (74).

Vitreous Cortex

The vitreous cortex is the peripheral "shell" of the vitreous body that courses forward and inward from the anterior vitreous base to form the anterior vitreous cortex, and posteriorly from the posterior border of the vitreous base to form the posterior vitreous cortex. The anterior vitreous cortex, clinically referred to as the "anterior hyaloid face," begins about 1.5 mm anterior to the ora serrata. Fine and Tousimis (75) described that in this region the collagen fibrils are parallel to the surface of the cortex. Studies by Faulborn and Bowald (76) detected dense packing of collagen fibrils in the anterior cortex with looser collagen fibril packing in the subjacent vitreous, giving the impression of lamellae. Rhodes (77) studied mouse vitreous and found that the anterior vitreous cortex varied in thickness from 800 to 2,000 nm. He also found that there are connections between the loose fibrils in the anterior vitreous and the anterior vitreous cortex.

The posterior vitreous cortex is 100 to 110 μm thick (78) and consists of densely packed collagen fibrils (Fig. 1-12, bottom panel). It is this structure that is detected by dynamic light scattering as a source of very intense light scattering. There is no vitreous cortex over the optic disc (Fig. 1-11A), and the cortex is thin over the macula due to rarefaction of the collagen fibrils (78). The prepapillary hole in the vitreous cortex can sometimes be visualized clinically when the posterior vitreous is detached from the retina. If peripapillary glial tissue is torn away during posterior vitreous detachment and remains attached to the vitreous cortex around the prepapillary hole it is referred to as Vogt's or Weiss's ring.

Vitreous can extrude through the prepapillary hole in the vitreous cortex (Fig. 1-11A) but does so to a much lesser extent than through the premacular vitreous cortex.

Jaffe (79) has described how vitreous can extrude into the retrocortical space created following posterior vitreous detachment and has proposed that persistent attachment to the macula can produce traction and certain forms of maculopathy (80,81). Although there are no direct connections between the posterior vitreous and the retina, the posterior vitreous cortex is adherent to the internal limiting lamina of the retina, which is actually the basal lamina of retinal Müller cells. The exact nature of this adhesion between the posterior vitreous cortex and the internal limiting lamina is not known, but probably results from extracellular matrix molecules (58,82–83).

Hyalocytes

Reeser and Aaberg (66) consider the vitreous cortex to be the "metabolic center" of the vitreous because of the presence of hyalocytes. These mononuclear cells are embedded in the vitreous cortex (Fig. 1-13), widely spread apart in a single layer situated 20 to 50 μm from the internal limiting lamina of the retina posteriorly and the basal lamina of the ciliary epithelium at the pars plana and vitreous base. Quantitative studies of cell density in the bovine (84) and rabbit (85) vitreous found the highest density of hyalocytes in the region of the vitreous base, followed next by the posterior pole, with the lowest density at the equator. Hyalocytes are oval or spindle-shaped, 10 to 15 μm in diameter, and contain a lobulated nucleus, a well-developed Golgi complex, smooth and rough endoplasmic reticula, and many large periodic acid-Schiff–positive lysosomal granules and phagosomes (78,86). Hogan and colleagues (87) described that

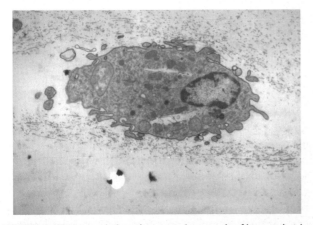

FIGURE 1-13. Transmission electron micrograph of human hyalocyte embedded in the posterior vitreous cortex characterized by the dense matrix of collagen fibrils (black "C"). N, lobulated nucleus; white "C", dense marginal chromatin; M, mitochondria; arrows, dense granules; V, vacuoles; Mi, microvilli. Original magnification ×11,670.

the posterior hyalocytes are flat and spindle-shaped, whereas anterior hyalocytes are larger, rounder, and at times star-shaped. Saga and co-workers (88) have described that different ultrastructural features can be present in different individual cells of the hyalocyte population in a single eye. Whether this relates to different origins for the different cells or different states of cell metabolism or activity is not clear. Balazs (89) pointed out that hyalocytes are located in the region of highest HA concentration and suggested that these cells are responsible for vitreous HA synthesis. There is experimental evidence in support of this hypothesis (90–94). Swann (22) claimed that there is no evidence that hyalocytes are responsible for the synthesis of vitreous HA. There is, however, evidence to suggest that hyalocytes maintain ongoing synthesis and metabolism of glycoproteins within the vitreous (95,96). Hyalocytes have also been shown to synthesize vitreous collagen (97) and enzymes (98). The phagocytic capacity of hyalocytes has been described in vivo (99) and demonstrated in vitro (100–101). This activity is consistent with the presence of pinocytic vesicles and phagosomes (86) and the presence of surface receptors that bind immunoglobulin G and complement (101). Balazs (51) has proposed that in their resting state, hyalocytes synthesize matrix glycosaminoglycans and glycoproteins and that the cells internalize and reutilize these macromolecules by means of pinocytosis. They become phagocytic cells in response to inducting stimuli and inflammation. HA may have a regulatory effect on hyalocyte phagocytic activity (102,103).

Vitreoretinal Interface

In the child, it is virtually impossible to mechanically detach the posterior cortical vitreous from the retina. This difficulty in releasing the cortical vitreous causes surgical complications in cases in which a retinal break occurs. Temporary silicone oil tamponade may be useful in some of these cases that detach, but that alone does not prevent proliferative vitreoretinopathy.

The interface between vitreous and the retina posteriorly, as well as the ciliary body and lens anteriorly, consists of a complex formed by the vitreous cortex and the basal laminae of adjacent cells. These basal laminae are firmly attached to their cells (87,104) and vitreous cortex collagen fibrils purportedly insert into the basal laminae (75). The only region not adjacent to a basal lamina is the annulus of the anterior vitreous cortex, which is directly exposed to the zonular fibers and the aqueous humor of the posterior chamber. Balazs (51) has pointed out the structural similarities between this zone and the surface of articular cartilage, which in joints is exposed to synovial fluid. The significance of such an arrangement in the vitreous is not known, although it probably enables aqueous to enter the vitreous and allows various substances (e.g., red blood cells, HA, growth factors) to exit the vitreous anteriorly.

The basal laminae surrounding the vitreous are composed of type IV collagen closely associated with glycoproteins (82,83,105). At the ciliary body, the basal lamina of the pars plicata is a meshwork of lamina densa that is 0.05 to 0.1 μm thick and is organized in a reticular, multilayered structure that is 2 to 6 μm thick and fills the spaces between the crevices of the ciliary epithelium. At the pars plana, the basal lamina has a true lamina densa with insertions of vitreous collagen fibrils. The basal lamina posterior to the ora serrata is actually the basement membrane of retinal Müller's cells, known as the ILL of the retina (Fig. 1-12). Immediately adjacent to the Müller cells is the lamina rara, which is 0.03 to 0.06 μm thick and demonstrates no species variations, nor changes with topography or age. The lamina densa is thinnest at the fovea (0.01 to 0.02 μm). It is thicker elsewhere in the posterior pole (0.5 to 3.2 μm) than at the equator or vitreous base. At the rim of the optic nerve head, the retinal ILL ceases, although the basement membrane continues as the inner limiting membrane of Elschnig (106). This membrane is 50 nm thick and is believed to be the basal laminae of the astroglia in the optic nerve head. At the central-most portion of the optic disc the membrane thins to 20 nm, follows the irregularities of the underlying cells of the optic nerve head, and is composed only of glycosaminoglycans and no collagen (107). This structure is known as the central meniscus of Kuhnt. Balazs (51) has stated that the Müller cell's basal lamina prevents the passage of cells as well as molecules larger than 15 to 20 nm. Consequently, the thinness and chemical composition of the central meniscus of Kuhnt and the membrane of Elschnig may account for, among other effects, the frequency with which abnormal cell proliferation arises from or near the optic nerve head (68,70). Zimmerman and Straatsma (108) claimed that there are fine, fibrillar attachments between the posterior vitreous cortex and the ILL and proposed that this was the source for the strong adhesion between vitreous and retina. The composition of these fibrillar structures is not known and their presence has never been confirmed. It is more likely that an extracellular matrix "glue" exists between the vitreous and retina in a fascial as opposed to focal apposition (82,83). These and other studies (109) have demonstrated the presence of fibronectin, laminin, and other extracellular matrix components. Certain extracellular matrix components that were found at the vitreoretinal interface were not present at the interface between the peripheral vitreous and the basal lamina of the ciliary epithelium at the pars plana. For example, N-acetylgalactosamine was present in the lamina rara externa of the retinal ILL, but not in the basal lamina of the ciliary epithelium, suggesting a specific role in mediating vitreoretinal adhesion. Of particular interest is the finding that there was intense reactivity of numerous antibodies directed against chondroitin sulfate glycosaminoglycan. The pattern of immunoreactivity was most intense at the vitreous base and optic disc margin, sites of strong vitreoretinal adhesion.

Western blots of separated proteins derived from dissected vitreoretinal tissues identified two chondroitin sulfate-containing proteoglycans of approximately 240-kd molecular weight that are believed to function as adhesive molecules at the vitreoretinal interface. These findings formed the rationale for experimental and clinical studies on pharmacologic vitreolysis (110) using ABC chondroitinase.

The vitreous is known to be firmly adherent to the vitreous base, optic disc/macula, and over retinal blood vessels. In the posterior pole vitreoretinal adhesion is not focal but extends as a sheet encompassing the disc, peripapillary region, and macula (58). So-called attachment plaques between the Müller cells and the ILL have been described in the basal and equatorial regions of the fundus but not in the posterior pole, except for the fovea. It has been hypothesized that these develop in response to vitreous traction upon the retina. It has also been proposed that the thick ILL in the posterior pole dampens the effects of vitreous traction except at the fovea where the ILL is thin. The thinness of the ILL and the purported presence of attachment plaques at the perifoveal central macula could explain the predisposition of this region to changes induced by traction.

There is an unusual vitreoretinal interface overlying retinal blood vessels. Kuwabara and Cogan (111) described "spider-like bodies" in the peripheral retina which coil around blood vessels and connect with the ILL. Pedler (112) found that the ILL was thin over blood vessels, while Wolter (113) noted the existence of pores in the ILL along blood vessels and found that vitreous strands inserted where the pores were located. Mutlu and Leopold (106) described that these strands extend through the ILL to branch and surround vessels in what they termed "vitreoretino-vascular bands." Physiologically, such structures may provide a shock-absorbing function, damping arterial pulsations. However, pathologically, this structural arrangement could also account for the hemorrhagic and proliferative events associated with vitreous traction upon retinal blood vessels during posterior vitreous detachment (2,114) and proliferative diabetic vitreoretinopathy (29).

ABNORMAL VITREOUS DEVELOPMENT

Biochemical Anomalies

At birth, vitreous is composed primarily of collagen. Thus, there is a dense appearance on dark-field slit microscopy (Fig. 1-14) because collagen scatters light quite significantly.

Following birth, there is considerable synthesis of HA as well as some ongoing synthesis of collagen. As a result of considerable hydrophilicity, HA generates a "swelling" pressure within the burgeoning vitreous that contributes to growth of the eye. The latter maintains pace with the enlarging eye. The primary role of hyaluronan is to spread apart the collagen fibrils by at least one wavelength of incident light so as to minimize scattering and induce trans-

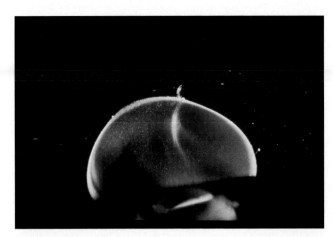

FIGURE 1-14. Dark-field slit microscopy of vitreous from a 33-week-gestational-age human. The anterior segment is below where the posterior aspect of the lens can be seen. Coursing through the central vitreous is the remnant of the hyaloid artery, destined to become Cloquet's canal. There is considerable light scattering by the gel vitreous.

parency (Fig. 1-9). This is evident when comparing the dark-field microscopy image of the human embryo (Fig. 1-14) with a similar image from a 4-year-old child (Fig. 1-15). In spite of intense illumination by the slit-lamp beam (note the high degree of light scattering from the lens) there is little scattering within the vitreous of the 4-year-old because HA has separated the collagen fibrils.

Vitreous Collagen Disorders

As vitreous is one of many connective tissues in the body, it is of interest to consider parallel phenomena occurring in the vitreous and connective tissues elsewhere, especially as related to collagen. Long ago, Gartner (115) pointed out the similarities between the intervertebral disk and the vitreous, in which age-related changes with herniation of the nucleus

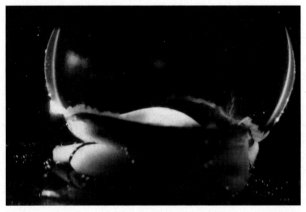

FIGURE 1-15. Dark-field slit microscopy of vitreous from a 4-year-old child. The posterior aspect of the lens is seen below. Other than the peripheral vitreous cortex that contains densely-packed collagen fibrils, there is little light scattering within the vitreous body.

pulposus was associated with presenile vitreous degeneration in 40% of cases. He proposed that a generalized connective tissue disorder resulted in disk herniation and presenile vitreous degeneration in these cases. Based on these findings, Gartner likened herniation of the nucleus pulposus in the disk to prolapse of vitreous into the retrohyaloid space by way of the posterior vitreous cortex following posterior vitreous detachment (Fig. 1-11D).

Maumenee (116) identified several different disorders with single-gene autosomal-dominant inheritance in which dysplastic connective tissue primarily involves joint cartilage. In these conditions, there is associated vitreous liquefaction, collagen condensation, and vitreous syneresis (collapse). Since type II collagen is common to cartilage and vitreous, Maumenee suggested that various arthroophthalmopathies might result from different mutations, perhaps of the same or neighboring genes, on the chromosome involved with type II collagen metabolism. In these disorders, probably including such conditions as Wagner's disease (117), the fundamental problem in the posterior segment of the eye is that the vitreous is liquefied and unstable, and becomes syneretic at an early age. However, there is no dehiscence at the vitreoretinal interface in concert with the changes inside the vitreous body, perhaps because the internal limiting lamina of the retina is composed of type IV collagen. Thus, in these cases, abnormal type II collagen metabolism causes destabilization of the vitreous and results in traction on the retina that can lead to large posterior tears and difficult retinal detachments.

Marfan's Syndrome

In Marfan's syndrome, an autosomal-dominant disorder featuring poor musculature, lax joints, aortic aneurysms, and arachnodactyly, there is lens subluxation, thin sclera, peripheral fundus pigmentary changes, and vitreous liquefaction at an early age. Myopia, vitreous syneresis, and abnormal vitreoretinal adhesions at the equator likely account for the frequency of rhegmatogenous retinal detachment caused by equatorial or posterior horseshoe tears (118).

Ehlers-Danlos Syndrome

Systemic Manifestations

Ehlers-Danlos syndrome has some similarities to Marfan's syndrome, most notably joint laxity, aortic aneurysms, and an autosomal-dominant pattern of inheritance. However, there are as many as six types of Ehlers-Danlos patients, and the genetics of this condition are probably more heterogeneous than in Marfan's syndrome. A further distinction from Marfan's patients is seen in hyperelastic skin and poor wound healing of all connective tissues, including cornea and sclera, in Ehlers-Danlos patients.

Ocular Manifestations

Ocular manifestations include lens subluxation, angioid streaks, thin sclera, and high myopia due to posterior staphyloma. Vitreous liquefaction and syneresis occur at a young age. Vitreous traction causes vitreous hemorrhage, perhaps also due to blood vessel wall fragility, and retinal tears with rolled edges, often causing bilateral retinal detachments (118).

Stickler Syndrome

Genetics

In 1965, Stickler and associates (119) described a condition in five generations of a family that was found to be autosomal dominant with complete penetrance and variable expressivity. Stickler syndrome arises from mutations in at least three collagen genes, the most common being COL2A1, a 54-exon–containing gene coding for type II collagen with 17 different mutations so far reported (118). In one instance (120,121) of a family with typical Stickler syndrome, posterior chorioretinal atrophy and vitreoretinal degeneration were found, even though they have been classically associated with Wagner disease. Vitreous findings from that study validated reports that mutations in the *COL2A1* gene result in an optically empty vitreous with retrolenticular membrane phenotype.

Systemic Manifestations

In general, the features of Stickler syndrome were a marfanoid skeletal habitus and orofacial and ocular abnormalities. Subsequent studies identified subgroups with short stature and a Weill-Marchesani habitus. The skeletal abnormalities now accepted as characteristic of Stickler's syndrome are radiographic evidence of flat epiphyses, broad metaphyses, and especially spondyloepiphyseal dysplasia (122).

Ocular Manifestations

Ocular abnormalities are high myopia, greater than–10 D in 72% of cases (123), and vitreoretinal changes characterized by vitreous liquefaction, fibrillar collagen condensation, and a perivascular laticelike degeneration in the peripheral retina believed to be the cause of a high incidence (greater than 50%) of retinal detachment (122).

More recent studies correlated specific gene defects with particular phenotypes, thereby enabling the classification of Stickler syndrome patients into four subgroups (124). Patients with abnormalities in the genes coding for type II procollagen and type V/XI procollagen are the ones who have severe vitreous abnormalities. Another study (125) analyzed the ultrastructural feature of a vitreous membrane with multiple fenestrations in a patient with a Stickler syndrome. A type 2 vitreous phenotype was found in the left eye whereas the other eye's vitreous abnormalities appeared to result from a conversion to a type 1 phenotype. In such a conversion, a fenestrated membrane may represent the posterior vitreous cortex in a complete posterior vitreous detachment. The fenestrated membrane is made of avascular fibrocellular tissue with cells arranged cohesively around the fenestration. Results from ultrastructural findings were characteristic of proliferating Müller cells, and collagen fibrils were shown to be similar to normal vitreous by ultrastructural examination. The authors concluded that collagen molecules are not functionally modified, but they are probably quantitatively insufficient during vitreous development.

Knobloch Syndrome

Knobloch (126) described a syndrome similar to Stickler's syndrome with hypotonia, relative muscular hypoplasia, and mild to moderate spondyloepiphyseal dysplasia causing hyperextensible joints. The vitreoretinopathy is characterized by vitreous liquefaction, veils of vitreous collagen condensation, and perivascular lattice-like changes in the peripheral retina. Retinal detachment in patients with Knobloch syndrome has been explained by loss-of-function mutations in collagen XVIII based on findings from one investigation (127) demonstrating that collagen XVIII is crucial for anchoring vitreous collagen fibrils to the inner limiting membrane.

Myopia

It is presently unknown whether myopia unrelated to the aforementioned arthroophthalmopathies should be considered a form of vitreous collagen disease as well. The extensive liquefaction of vitreous (*myopic vitreopathy*) and propensity for retinal detachment due to peripheral retinal traction and myopic peripheral retinal degeneration suggest that this postulate may deserve closer scrutiny.

Embryonic Vascular System

Many developmental vitreoretinal disorders result from abnormalities related to the embryonic vascular system of the vitreous (vasa hyaloidea propria) and lens (tunica vasculosa lentis). These attain maximum prominence during the ninth week of gestation or 40-mm stage (128). Atrophy of the vessels begins posteriorly with dropout of the vasa hyaloidea propria, followed by the tunica vasculosa lentis. Recent studies have detected the onset of apoptosis in the endothelial cells of the tunica vasculosa lentis as early as day 17.5 in the mouse embryo (129). At the 240-mm stage (seventh month) in the human, blood flow in the hyaloid artery ceases. Regression of the vessel itself begins with glycogen and lipid deposition in the endothelial cells and pericytes of the hyaloid vessels (130). Endothelial cell processes then fill the lumen, and macrophages form a plug that occludes the vessel. The cells in the vessel wall then undergo necrosis and are phagocytized by mononuclear phagocytes (131). Gloor (132) claimed that macrophages are not involved in vessel regression within the embryonic vitreous but that autolytic vacuoles form in the cells of the vessel walls, perhaps in response to hyperoxia. The sequence of cell disappearance from the primary vitreous begins with endothelial and smooth muscle cells of the vessel walls, followed by adventitial fibroblasts and lastly phagocytes (133), consistent with a gradient of decreasing oxygen tension. Recent studies have suggested that the vasa hyaloidea propria and the tunica vasculosa lentis regress via apoptosis (134). These studies concluded that macrophages are important in this process. Subsequent studies by a different group confirmed the importance of macrophages in promoting regression of the fetal vitreous vasculature and further characterized these macrophages as hyalocytes (135).

Regression of Fetal Vasculature

It is not known what stimulates regression of the hyaloid vascular system, but studies have identified a protein native to the vitreous that inhibits angiogenesis in various experimental models (136–138). Mitchell and colleagues (139) point out that the first event in hyaloidal vascular regression is endothelial cell apoptosis and propose that lens development separates the fetal vasculature from vascular endothelial growth factor–producing cells, decreasing the levels of this survival factor for vascular endothelium, inducing apoptosis. Following endothelial cell apoptosis, there is loss of capillary integrity, leakage of erythrocytes into the vitreous, and phagocytosis of apoptotic endothelium by hyalocytes. Meeson and colleagues (140) proposed that there are actually two forms of apoptosis that are important in regression of the fetal vitreous vasculature. The first ("initiating apoptosis") results from macrophage induction of apoptosis in a single endothelial cell of an otherwise healthy capillary segment with normal blood flow. The isolated dying endothelial cells project into the capillary lumen and interfere with blood flow. This stimulates synchronous apoptosis of downstream endothelial cells ("secondary apoptosis") and ultimately causes obliteration of the vasculature. Removal of the apoptotic vessels is achieved by hyalocytes.

Pathologies of the Primary Vitreous

Regression of the hyaloid artery usually occurs completely and without complications. Persistence of the hyaloid vascular system occurs in 3% of full-term infants but in 95% of premature infants (141) and can be associated with prepapillary hemorrhage (142). Anomalies involving incomplete regression of the embryonic hyaloid vascular system occur in more than 90% of infants born earlier than 36 weeks of gestation and in over 95% of infants weighing less than 5 lb at birth (143). There is a spectrum of disorders resulting from persistence of the fetal vasculature (144).

Mittendorf's dot is a remnant of the anterior fetal vascular system located at the former site of anastomosis of the hyaloid artery and tunica vasculosa lentis. It is usually inferonasal to the posterior pole of the lens and is not associated with any known dysfunction.

Bergmeister's papilla is the occluded remnant of the posterior portion of the hyaloid artery with associated glial tissue. It appears as a gray, linear structure anterior to the optic disc and adjacent retina and does not cause any known functional disorders. Exaggerated forms can present as prepapillary veils.

Vitreous cysts are generally benign lesions that are found in eyes with abnormal regression of the anterior (145) or posterior (146) hyaloid vascular system; otherwise normal eyes (147,148); and eyes with coexisting ocular disease, such as retinitis pigmentosa (149) and uveitis (150). Some vitreous cysts contain remnants of the hyaloid vascular system (151), supporting the concept that the cysts result from abnormal regression of these embryonic vessels (152). However, one histologic analysis of aspirated material from a vitreous cyst purportedly revealed cells from the retinal pigment epithelium (153). Vitreous cysts are generally not symptomatic and thus do not require surgical intervention. However, argon laser photocoagulation has been employed, and a report (154) described the use of neodymium:yttrium-aluminum-garnet (Nd:YAG) laser therapy to rupture a free-floating posterior vitreous cyst.

Persistent hyperplastic primary vitreous (PHPV) was first described by Reese (155) as a congenital malformation of the anterior portion of the primary vitreous. It has subsequently been renamed as persistent fetal vasculature (PFV) (144) and is known to include a broad spectrum of presentations. The initial description of PHPV/PFV was that of a plaque of retrolental fibrovascular connective tissue that was adherent to the posterior lens capsule. The membrane extended laterally to attach to the ciliary processes, which were elongated and displaced centrally. Although 90% of cases were unilateral, many of the fellow eyes had Mittendorf's dot or another anomaly of anterior vitreous development (156). A persistent hyaloid artery, often still perfused with blood, arose from the posterior aspect of the retrolental plaque in the affected eye. In severe forms, there can be microphthalmos with anterior displacement of the lens–iris diaphragm, shallowing of the anterior chamber, and secondary glaucoma. PHPV/PFV is believed to arise from abnormal regression and hyperplasia of the primary vitreous (155). Experimental data suggest that the abnormality begins at the 17-mm stage of embryonic development (157). The hyperplastic features result from generalized hyperplasia of retinal astrocytes and a separate component of glial hyperplasia arising from the optic nerve head (158). The fibrous component of the PHPV/PFV membrane is presum-

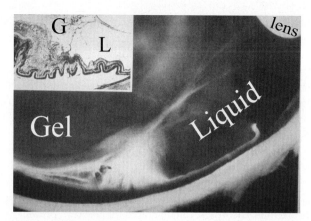

FIGURE 1-16. Photomicrograph of peripheral fundus in retinopathy of prematurity. The lens (*) is in the upper right hand corner. Below, a fibrovascular membrane is present at the interface between the posterior gel vitreous and the peripheral liquid vitreous. The inset shows the histopathology that clearly distinguishes between gel (G) and liquid (L) vitreous. (Courtesy of Maurice Landers, MD.)

ably synthesized by these astrocytes and glial cells (159). A recent case report with clinicopathologic correlation found that collagen fibrils in this fibrous tissue had diameters of 40 to 50 nm with a cross-striation periodicity of 65 nm. The investigators concluded that the collagen fibrils differed from those of the primary vitreous and suggested that they arose either from a different population of cells or were the result of abnormal metabolism by the same cells that synthesize vitreous collagen (160).

The retina is usually not involved in anterior PHPV. Indeed, previous studies have suggested that the anterior form is due to a primary defect in lens development and that vitreous changes are all secondary (161). This postulate has never been substantiated. There are rare instances of posterior PHPV/PFV in which opaque connective tissue arises from Bergmeister's papilla and persistent hyaloid vessels (159,162). These can cause congenital falciform folds of the retina and, if severe, can cause tentlike retinal folds, leading on rare occasions to tractional and/or rhegmatogenous retinal detachment. Font and investigators (163) demonstrated the presence of adipose tissue, smooth muscle, and cartilage within the retrolental plaque and suggested that PHPV/PFV arises from metaplasia of mesenchymal elements in the primary vitreous.

Familial Exudative Vitreoretinopathy (Dominant Exudative Vitreoretinopathy)

Familial exudative vitreoretinopathy (FEVR) was first described in 1969 by Criswick and Schepens (164) as a bilateral, slowly progressive abnormality of the vitreous and retina that resembles retinopathy of prematurity but without a history of prematurity or postnatal oxygen administration. Gow and Oliver (165) identified this disorder as an autosomal dominant condition with complete pene-

trance. They characterized the course of this disease in stages ranging from posterior vitreous detachment with snowflake opacities (stage I), to thickened vitreous membranes and elevated fibrovascular scars (stage II), and vitreous fibrosis with subretinal and intraretinal exudates, ultimately developing retinal detachment due to fibrovascular proliferation arising from neovascularization in the temporal periphery (stage III). Plager and coworkers (166) recently reported the same findings in four generations of three families, but found X-linked inheritance. Van Nouhuys (167–169) studied 101 affected members in 16 Dutch pedigrees and five patients with sporadic manifestations. He found that the incidence of retinal detachment was 21%, all but one case occurring prior to the age of 30. These were all tractional or combined traction-rhegmatogenous detachments, and there were no cases of exudative retinal detachment. Van Nouhuys (169) concluded that the etiology of FEVR lies in premature arrest of development in the retinal vasculature, since the earliest findings in these patients were nonperfusion of the peripheral temporal retina with stretched retinal blood vessels and shunting with vascular leakage. Thus, Van Nouhuys considers FEVR as a retinopathy with secondary vitreous involvement. However, Brockhurst and colleagues (170) reported that vitreous membrane formation began just posterior to the ora serrata and that it preceded retinal vessel abnormalities, suggesting a vitreous origin to this disorder. Others suggested that there may be a combined etiology involving anomalies of the hyaloid vascular system, primary vitreous, and retinovascular dysgenesis (171).

Retinopathy of Prematurity

Vitreous liquefaction, often unidentified (172) in stages 1 and 2 ROP, likely occurs as a result of reactive oxygen species (173) but also overlying the peripheral retina where immature Müller cells do not support typical gel synthesis and may account for the vitreous trough apparent during surgery for Stage 4 ROP (182). The disrupted composition may limit the inherent vitreous ability to inhibit cell invasion (136–138), thereby permitting neovascularization in stage 3 ROP to grow (174, 175) between posterior gel and peripheral liquid vitreous anteriorly (Fig. 1-16) (175). Instability at the interface between gel and liquid vitreous exerts traction on the underlying ridge. As ROP advances from stage 3 to 4, the neovascular tissue grows through the vitreous along the walls of the future Cloquet's canal or the tractus hyaloideus of Eisner toward Wiegert's ligament on the posterior lens capsule (176). Primary vitreous cells, responding to intraocular angiogenic stimuli, likely proliferate and migrate to help create the dense central vitreous stalk and retrolental membrane seen in the cicatricial stages. Further information on ROP pathophysiology and treatment is located in Chapters 26 and 27.

SUMMARY

Thus, numerous pathologic processes may involve the vitreous. Knowledge of the differences in the child's vitreous and that of the adult is important when determining the surgical management (Section 2). The vitreoretinal interface cannot be mechanically stripped from the retina; therefore, extra care is taken in the dissection of preretinal membranes from the surface of the child's or infant's retina to avoid creating retinal breaks. Future development of pharmacologic vitreolysis with enzymes to release the vitreous from the inner retina will be important in the management of complicated pediatric retinal detachments.

B: REFERENCES

1. Foulds WS. Is your vitreous really necessary? The role of the vitreous in the eye with particular reference to retinal attachment, detachment and the mode of action of vitreous substitutes. (The 2nd Duke-Elder Lecture). *Eye* 1987;1:641–664.
2. Sebag J. *The vitreous: structure, function and pathobiology.* New York: Springer-Verlag, 1989.
3. Sebag J. Macromolecular structure of vitreous. *Prog Polym Sci* 1998;23:415–446.
4. Sebag J. Vitreous—from biochemistry to clinical relevance. In: Tasman W, Jaeger EA, eds. *Duane's foundations of clinical ophthalmology*, vol 1. Philadelphia: Lippincott Williams & Wilkins, 1998;1–34.
5. Bishop PN. Structural macromolecules and supramolecular organisation of the vitreous gel. *Prog Retin Eye Res* 2000;19: 323–344.
6. Gloor BP. The vitreous. In: Moses RA, ed. *Adler's physiology of the eye.* St. Louis: Mosby, 1975:246–267.
7. Reardon A, Sandell L, Jones CJP, et al. Localization of pN-type IIA procollagen on adult bovine vitreous collagen fibrils. *Matrix Biol* 2000;19:169–173.
8. Zhu Y, Oganesian A, Keene DR, Sandell LJ. Type IIA procollagen containing the cysteine-rich amino propeptide is deposited in the extracellular matrix of prechondrogenic tissue and binds to TGFbeta-1 and BMP-2. J Cell Biol 1999;144:1069–1080.
9. Bishop PN, Crossman MV, McLeod D. Extraction and characterization of the tissue forms of collagens type II and IX from bovine vitreous. *Biochem J* 1994;299:497–505.
10. Bishop PN, Reardon AJ, McLeod D, et al. Identification of alternatively spliced variants of type II procollagen in vitreous. *Biochem Biophys Res Commun* 1994;203:289–295.
11. Brewton RG, Ouspenskaia MV, Van der Rest M, et al. Cloning of the chicken alpha 3 (IX) collagen chain completes the primary structure of type IX collagen. *Eur J Biochem* 1992;205:443–449.
12. Asakura A. Histochemistry of hyaluronic acid of the bovine vitreous body as studied by electron microscopy. *Acta Soc Ophthalmol Jpn* 1985;89:179–191.
13. Scott JE. The chemical morphology of the vitreous. *Eye* 1992;6:553–555.
14. Zhidkova NI, Justice S, Mayne R. Alternative in RNA processing occurs in the variable region of the pro-peptide. *J Biol Chem* 1995;270:9485–9493.
15. Swann DA, Caulfield JB, Broadhurst JB. The altered fibrous form of vitreous collagen following solubilization with pepsin. *Biochem Biophys Acta* 1976;427:365.

16. Toledo DMS, Dietrich CP. Tissue specific distribution of sulfated mucopolysaccharides in mammals. *Biochem Biophys Acta* 1977;498:114.
17. Balazs EA. The vitreous. In: Davson H, ed. *The eye,* vol la. London: Academic Press, 1984;533–589.
18. Breen M, Bizzell JW, Weinstein MG. A galactosamine-containing proteoglycan in human vitreous. *Exp Eye Res* 1977;24:409.
19. Allen WS, Otterbein EC, Wardi AH. Isolation and characterization of the sulfated glycosaminoglycans of the vitreous body. *Biochem Biophys Acta* 1977;498:167.
20. Kamei A, Totani A. Isolation and characterization of minor glycosaminoglycans in the rabbit vitreous body. *Biochem Biophys Res Comm* 1982;109:881.
21. Laurent UBG, Fraser JRE. Turnover of hyaluronate in aqueous humor and vitreous body of the rabbit. *Exp Eye Res* 1983; 36:493.
22. Swann DA. Chemistry and biology of vitreous body. *Int Rev Exp Pathol* 1980;22:1.
23. Sheehan JK, Atkins EDT, Nieduszynski IA. X-Ray diffraction studies on the connective tissue polysaccharides. Two dimensional packing scheme for threefold hyaluronic chains. *J Mol Biol* 1975;91:153–163.
24. Atkins EDT, Phelps CF, Sheehan JK. The conformation of the mucopolysaccharides—hyaluronates. *Biochem J* 1972;128:1255.
25. Chakrabarti B, Park JW. Glycosaminoglycans structure and interaction. *CRC Crit Rev Biochem* 1980;8:225–313.
26. Brewton RG, Mayne R. Mammalian vitreous humor contains networks of hyaluronan molecules. *Exp Eye Res* 1992;198: 237–249.
27. Reardon A, Heinegard D, McLeod D, et al. The large chondroitin sulphate proteoglycans versican in mammalian vitreous. *Matrix Biol* 1998;17:325–333.
28. Comper WD, Laurent TC. Physiological functions of connective tissue polysaccharides. *Physiol Rev* 1978;58:255.
29. Sebag J. Diabetic vitreopathy. *Ophthalmology* 1996;103: 205–206.
30. Laurent UBG, Granath KA. The molecular weight of hyaluronate in the aqueous humour and vitreous body of rabbit and cattle eyes. *Exp Eye Res* 1983;36:481.
31. Laurent TC, Ryan M, Pietruszkiewicz A. Fractionation of hyaluronic acid: The polydispersity of hyaluronic acid from the vitreous body. *Biochim Biophys Acta* 1960;42:476.
32. Berman ER. Studies on mucopolysaccharides in ocular tissues. 1. Distribution and localization of various molecular species of hyaluronic acid in the bovine vitreous body. *Exp Eye Res* 1963;2:1.
33. Theocharis AD, Papageorgakopoulou N, Feretis E, et al. Occurrence and structural characterization of versican-like proteoglycan in human vitreous. *Biochimie* 2002;84:1235–1241.
34. Allen WS, Ottenbein E, Wardi AH. Isolation and characterization of the sulphated glycosaminoglycans of the vitreous body. *Biochim Biophys Acta* 1977;498:167–175.
35. Tsen G, Halfter W, Kroger S, Cole GJ. Agrin is a heparan sulphate proteoglycans. *J Biol Chem* 1995;270:3392–3399.
36. Kroger S. Differential distribution of agrin isoforms in the developing and adult avian retina. *Mol Cell Neurosci* 1997;10: 149–161.
37. Reardon AJ, LeGoff M, Briggs MD, et al. Identification in vitreous and molecular cloning of opticin, a novel member of the family of leucine-rich repeat proteins of the extracellular matrix. *J Biol Chem* 2000;275:2123–2129.
38. Sebag J. Ageing of the vitreous. *Eye* 1987;1:254–262.
39. Takanosu M, Boyd TC, Le Goff M, et al. Structure, chromosomal location, and tissue-specific expression of the mouse opticin gene. *Invest Ophthalmol Vis Sci* 2001;42:2202–2210.

40. Mayne R, Ren Z-X, Liu J, Cook T, et al. VIT1—the second member of a new branch of the von Willebrand A domain superfamily. *Biochem Soc Trans* 1999;27:832–835.

41. Mayne R. The eye. In: Royce P, Steimann B, eds. *Connective tissue and its heritable disorders*. Wiley-Liss, 2001;131–141.

42. Jackson DS. Chondroitin sulphuric acid as a factor in the stability of tendon. *Biochem J* 1953;54:638–641.

43. Scott JE, Chen Y, Brass A. Secondary and tertiary structures involving chondroitin and chondroitin sulphate in solution, investigated by rotary shadowing electron microscopy and computer simulation. *Eur J Biochem* 1992;209:675–680.

44. Mayne R, Brewton RG, Ren Z-H. Vitreous body and zonular apparatus. In: Harding JJ, ed. *Biochemistry of the eye*. London: Chapman and Hall, 1997;135–143.

45. Bishop PN, McLeod D, Reardon A. The role of glycosaminoglycans in the structural organization of mammalian vitreous. *Invest Ophthalmol Vis Sci* 1999;40:2173–2178.

46. Balazs EA. The vitreous. *Int Ophthalmol Clin* 1973;15:53.

47. Balazs EA, Laurent TC, Laurent UBG, et al. Studies on the structure of the vitreous body. VIII. Comparative biochemistry. *Arch Biochem Biophys* 1959;81:464.

48. Bettelheim FA, Balazs EA. Light-scattering patterns of the vitreous humor. *Biochem Biophys Acta* 1968;158:309.

49. Osterlin SE, Balazs EA. Macromolecular composition and fine structure of the vitreous in the owl monkey. *Exp Eye Res* 1968; 7:534.

50. Berman ER, Michaelson IC. The chemical composition of the human vitreous body as related to age and myopia. *Exp Eye Res* 1964;3:9.

51. Balaz EA. Functional anatomy of the vitreous. In: Duane TD, Jaeger EA, eds. *Biomedical foundations of ophthalmology*, Vol 1. Philadelphia: Harper & Row, 1982;17:6–12.

52. Ali S, Bettelheim FA. Distribution of freezable and nonfreezable water in bovine vitreous. *Curr Eye Res* 1984;3:1233.

53. Worst JGF. Cisternal systems of the fully developed vitreous body in the young adult. *Trans Ophthalmol Soc UK* 1977;97:550–554.

54. Balaz EA, Denlinger JL. Aging changes in the vitreous. In: *Aging and Human Visual Function*. New York: Alan R Liss, 1982;45–47.

55. Goedbloed J. Studien am Glaskorper. I. Die Struktur des Glaskorpers. Albrecht von *Graefes Arch Klin Exp Ophthalmol* 1934;323.

56. Friedenwald IF, Stiehler RD. Structure of the vitreous. *Arch Ophthalmol* 1935;14:789.

57. Eisner G. *Biomicroscopy of the peripheral fundus*. New York: Springer-Verlag, 1973.

58. Sebag J. Age-related changes in human vitreous structure. *Graefes Arch Clin Exp Ophthalmol* 1987;225:89.

59. Sebag J, Balazs EA. Pathogenesis of CME: Anatomic consideration of vitreo-retinal adhesions. *Surv Ophthalmol* 1984; 28[Suppl]:493.

60. Sebag J, Balazs EA. Human vitreous fibres and vitreoretinal disease. *Trans Ophthalmol Soc UK* 1985;104:123.

61. Retzius R. Om membrana limitans retinae interna. *Norkdiskt Archiv III* 1871;2:1–34.

62. Sebag J, Balazs EA. Morphology and ultrastructure of human vitreous fibers. *Invest Ophthalmol Vis Sci* 1989;30:1867–1871.

63. Jongebloed WL, Worst JFG. The cisternal anatomy of the vitreous body. *Doc Ophthalmol* 1987;67:183.

64. Los LI, Van Der Worp RJ, Van Luyn MJ, et al. Age-related liquefaction of the human vitreous body: LM and TEM evaluation of the role of proteoglycans and collagen. *Invest Ophthalmol Vis Sci* 2003;44:2828–2833.

65. Hogan MJ. The vitreous: Its structure in relation to the ciliary body and retina. *Invest Ophthalmol* 1963;2:418.

66. Reeser FH, Aaberg T. Vitreous humor. In: Records PE, ed. *Physiology of the human eye and visual system*. Hagerstown, MD: Harper & Row, 1979;1–31.

67. Teng CC, Chi HH. Vitreous changes and the mechanism of retinal detachment. *Am J Ophthalmol* 1957;44:335.

68. Sebag J. Vitreous pathobiology. In: W Tasman, EA Jaeger, eds. *Duane's Clinical ophthalmology,* vol 5. Philadelphia: JB Lippincott Co, 1992;1–26.

69. Sebag J. Anatomy and pathology of the vitreo-retinal interface. *Eye* 1992;6:541–552.

70. Sebag J. Surgical anatomy of vitreous and the vitreo-retinal interface. In: Tasman W, Jaeger EA, eds. *Duane's Clinical ophthalmology,* vol 6. Philadelphia: JB Lippincott Co, 1994;1–36.

71. Gartner J. Electronmicroscopic study on the fibrillar network and fibrocyte-collagen interactions in the vitreous cortex at the ora serrata of human eyes with special regard to the role of disintegrating cells. *Exp Eye Res* 1986;42:21.

72. Gloor BP, Daicker BC. Pathology of the vitreo-retinal border structures. *Trans Ophthalmol Soc UK* 1975;95:387.

73. Wang J, McLeod D, Henson DB, et al. Age-dependent changes in the basal retinovitreous adhesion. *Invest Ophthalmol Vis Sci* 2003;44:1793–1800.

74. Gartner J. The fine structure of the vitreous base of the human eye and the pathogenesis of pars planitis. *Am J Ophthalmol* 1971;71:1317.

75. Fine BS, Tousimis A J. The structure of the vitreous body and the suspensory ligaments of the lens. *Arch Ophthalmol* 1961;65:95–110.

76. Faulborn J, Bowald S. Combined macroscopic, light microscopic, scanning and transmission electron microscopic investigation of the vitreous body. 1I: the anterior vitreous cortex. *Ophthalmic Res* 1982;14:117.

77. Rhodes RH. An ultrastructural study of complex carbohydrates in the posterior chamber and vitreous base of the mouse. *Histochem J* 1985;17:291.

78. Streeten BA. Disorders of the vitreous. In: Garner A. Klintworth GK, eds. *Pathobiology of ocular disease: a dynamic approach.* Part B. New York: Marcel Dekker, 1982;49:1381–1419.

79. Jaffe NS. Vitreous traction at the posterior pole of the fundus clue to alterations in the vitreous posterior. *Trans Am Acad Ophthalmol Otolaryngol* 1967;71:642.

80. Jaffe NS. Macular retinopathy after separation of vitreoretinal adherence. *Arch Ophthalmol* 1967;78:585.

81. Schachat AP, Sommer A. Macular hemorrhages associated with posterior vitreous detachment. *Am J Ophthalmol* 1986;102:647.

82. Sebag J, Hageman GS. Interfaces. *Eur J Ophthalmol* 2000;10:1–3.

83. Sebag J, Hageman GS. *Interfaces.* Rome: Fondazione G. B. Bietti, 2000:47–50.

84. Balazs EA, Toth LZ, Eckl EA, et al. Studies on the structure of the vitreous body. XII. Cytological and histochemical studies on the cortical tissue layer. *Exp Eye Res* 1964;3:57.

85. Gloor BP. Cellular proliferation on the vitreous surface after photocoagulation. *Graefes Arch Clin Exp Ophthalmol* 1969; 178:99.

86. Bloom GD, Balazs EA. An electron microscope study of hyalocytes. *Exp Eye Res* 1965;4:249.

87. Hogan MJ, Alvarado JA, Weddel JE. *Histology of the human eye: an atlas and textbook*. Philadelphia: WB Saunders, 1971:607.

88. Saga T, Tagawa Y, Takeuchi T et al. Electron microscopic study of cells in vitreous of guinea pig. *Jpn J Ophthalmol* 1984;28:239.

89. Balazs EA. Structure of vitreous gel. *Acta XVII Concil Ophthalmol* 1954;11:1019.

90. Balazs EA, Sundblad L, Toth LZJ. In vitro formation of hyaluronic acid by cells in the vitreous body and by comb tissue. *Abstr Red Proc* 1958;17:184.

91. Jacobson B, Osterlin S, Balazs EA. A soluble hyaluronic acid

synthesizing system from calf vitreous. *Proc Fed Am Soc Exp Biol* 1966;25:588.

92. Osterlin SE. The synthesis of hyaluronic acid in the vitreous. III. In vivo metabolism in the owl monkey. *Exp Eye Res* 1968;7:524.

93. Berman ER, Gombos GM. Studies on the incorporation of U-14 C-glucose into vitreous polymers in vitro and in vivo. *Invest Ophthalmol* 1969;18:521.

94. Bleckmann H. Glycosaminoglycan metabolism of cultured fibroblasts from bovine vitreous. *Graefes Arch Clin Exp Ophthalmol* 1984;222:90.

95. Rhodes RH, Mandelbaum SH, Minckler DS, et al. Tritiated glucose incorporation in the vitreous body, lens and zonules of the pigmented rabbit. *Exp Eye Res* 1982;34:921.

96. Jacobson B. Identification of sialyl and galactosyl transferase activities in calf vitreous hyalocytes. *Curr Eye Res* 1984;3:1033.

97. Newsome DA, Linsemayer TF. Trelstad RJ. Vitreous body collagen. Evidence for a dual origin from the neural retina and hyalocytes. *J Cell Biol* 1976;71:59.

98. Hoffmann K, Baurwieg H, Riese K. Uber gehalt und vertailang niederund hoch molekularer substanzen in glaskorper. II. Hock molekulare substanzen (LDH, MDH, GOT). *Graefes Arch Clin Exp Ophthalmol* 1974;191:231.

99. Teng CC. An electron microscopic study of cells in the vitreous of the rabbit eye. Part I. The macrophage. *Eye Ear Nose Throat Mon* 1969;48:91.

100. Szirmai JA, Balazs EA. Studies on the structure of the vitreous body. 111. Cells in the cortical layer. *Arch Ophthalmol* 1958; 59:34.

101. Grabner G, Baltz G, Forster O. Macrophage-like properties of human hyalocytes. *Invest Ophthalmol Vis Sci* 1980;19:333.

102. Forrester JV, Balazs EA. Inhibition of phagocytosis by high molecular weight hyaluronate. *Immunology* 1980;40:435.

103. Sebag J, Balazs EA, Eakins KE, et al. The effect of Na-hyaluronate on prostaglandin synthesis and phagocytosis by mononuclear phagocytes. *Invest Ophthalmol Vis Sci* 1981;20:33.

104. Cohen AI. Electron microscopic observations of the internal limiting membrane and optic fiber layer of the retina of the rhesus monkey. *Am J Anat* 1961;108:179.

105. Kefalides NA. The biology and chemistry of basement membranes. In: Kefalides NA, ed. *Proceedings of the first international symposium on the biology and chemistry of basement membranes.* New York: Academic Press, 1978:215–228.

106. Mutlu F, Leopold IH. Structure of the human retinal vascular system. *Arch Ophthalmol* 1964;71:93.

107. Heergaard S, Jensen OA. Prause JU. Structure of the vitread face of the monkey optic disc (*Macacca mulatta*): SEM on frozen resin-cracked optic nerve heads supplemented by TEM and immuno-histochemistry. *Graefes Arch Clin Exp Ophthalmol* 1988;226:377.

108. Zimmerman LE, Straatsma BR. Anatomic relationships of the retina to the vitreous body and to the pigment epithelium. In: Schepens CL, ed. *Importance of the vitreous body in retina surgery with special emphasis on reoperation.* St. Louis: CV Mosby, 1960;15–28.

109. Russell SR, Shepherd JD, Hageman GS. Distribution of glycoconjugates in the human internal limiting membrane. *Invest Ophthalmol Vis Sci* 1991;32:1986–1995.

110. Sebag J. Pharmacologic vitreolysis. *Retina* 1998;18:1–3.

111. Kuwabara T, Cogan DG. Studies of retinal vascular patterns. I. Normal architecture. *Arch Ophthalmol* 1960;64:904.

112. Pedler C. The inner limiting membrane of the retina. *Br J Ophthalmol* 1961;45:423.

113. Wolter JR. Pores in the internal limiting membrane of the human retina. *Acta Ophthalmol (Copenh)* 1964;42:971.

114. Sebag J. Guest editorial: Classifying posterior vitreous detachment: a new way to look at the invisible. *Brit J Ophthalmol* 1997;81:521–522.

115. Gartner J. Photoelastic and ultrasonic studies on the structure and senile changes of the intervertebral disc and of the vitreous body. *Mod Probl Ophthalmol* 1969;8:136.

116. Maumenee IH. Vitreoretinal degeneration as a sign of generalized connective tissue diseases. *Am J Ophthalmol* 1979;88:432.

117. Maumenee IH, Stoll HU, Meta MB. The Wagner syndrome versus hereditary arthroophthalmopathy. *Trans Am Ophthalmol Soc* 1982;81:349.

118. Schepens CL. *Retinal detachment and allied diseases.* Philadelphia: WB Saunders, 1983.

119. Stickler GB, Belau PG, Farrell FJ, et al. Hereditary progressive arthro-ophthalmopathy. *Mayo Clin Proc* 1965;40:443.

120. Donoso LA, Edwards AO, Frost AT, et al. Clinical variability of Stickler syndrome: role of exon 2 of the collagen COL2A1 gene. *Surv Ophthalmol* 2003;48:191–203.

121. Vu CD, Brown J Jr, Korkko J, Ritter R III, et al. Posterior chorioretinal atrophy and vitreous phenotype in a family with Stickler syndrome from a mutation in the COL2A1 gene. *Ophthalmology* 2003;110:70–77.

122. Spencer WH. Vitreous. In: Spencer WH, ed. *Ophthalmic Pathology: An Atlas and Text.* Vol 2. Philadelphia: WB Saunders, 1985;548–588.

123. Hermann J, France TO, Spranger JW, et al. The Stickler syndrome (hereditary arthro-ophthalmopathy). *Birth Defects* 1978;11:76.

124. Snead MP, Yates JRW. Clinical and molecular genetics of Stickler syndrome. *J Med Genet* 1999;36:353.

125. Betis F, Hofman P, Gastaud P. Vitreous changes in Stickler syndrome. *J Fr Ophthalmol* 2003;26:386–390.

126. Knobloch WH. Inherited hyaloideoretinopathy and skeletal dysplasia. *Trans Am Ophthalmol Soc* 1975;73:417.

127. Fukai N, Eklund L, Marneros AG, et al. Lack of collagen XVIII/endostatin results in eye abnormalities. *EMBO J* 2002;21:1535–1544.

128. Mann I. The vitreous and suspensory ligament of the lens. In: *The development of the human eye.* New York: Grune & Stratton, 1964:150.

129. Mitchell CA, Risau W, Drexler HC. Regression of vessels in the tunica vasculosa lentis is initiated by coordinated endothelial apoptosis: A role for vascular endothelial growth factor as a survival factor for endothelium. *Dev Dyn* 1998;213:322.

130. Jack RL. Regression of the hyaloid artery system: An ultrastructural analysis. *Am J Ophthalmol* 1972;74:261.

131. Balazs EA. Fine structure of the developing vitreous. *Int Ophthalmol Clin* 1973;15:53.

132. Gloor BP. Zur entwicklung des glaskorpers und der Zonula. III. Henkunft, Lebenszeit und ersatz der glaskorpezellen beim kaninchen. *Graefes Arch Clin Exp Ophthalmol* 1973;187:21.

133. Balazs EA, Toth LZ, Ozanics V. Cytological studies on the developing vitreous as related to the hyaloid vessel system. *Graefes Arch Clin Exp Ophthalmol* 1980;213:71.

134. Ito M, Yoshioka M. Regression of the hyaloid vessels and papillary membrane of the mouse. *Anat Embryol (Berl)* 1999;200:403.

135. McMenamin PG, Djano J, Wealthall R, et al. Characterization of the macrophages associated with the tunica vasculosa lentis of the rat eye. *Invest Ophthalmol Vis Sci* 2002; 43:2076.

136. Raymond L, Jacobson B. Isolation and identification of stimulatory and inhibiting growth factors in bovine vitreous. *Exp Eye Res* 1982;34:267.

137. Lutty GA, Mello RJ, Chandler C, et al. Regulation of cell growth by vitreous humour. *J Cell Sci* 1985;76:53.

138. Jacobson B, Dorfman T, Basu PK, et al. Inhibition of vascular endothelial cell growth and trypsin activity by vitreous. *Exp Eye Res* 1985;41:581.

139. Mitchell CA, Risau W, Drexler HC. Regression of vessels in the tunica vasculosa lentis is initiated by coordinated endothelial

apoptosis: a role for vascular endothelial growth factor as a survival factor for endothelium. *Dev Dyn* 1998;213:322.

140. Meeson A, Palmer M, Calfon M, et al. A relationship between apoptosis and flow during programmed capillary regression is revealed by vital analysis. *Development* 1996;122:3929.

141. Jones H. Hyaloid remnants in the eyes of premature babies. *Br J Ophthalmol* 1963;47:39.

142. Delaney WV. Prepapillary hemorrhage and persistent hyaloid artery. *Am J Ophthalmol* 1980;90:419.

143. Renz B, Vygantas C. Hyaloid vascular remnants in human neonates. *Ann Ophthalmol* 1977;9:179.

144. Goldberg M. Persistent fetal vasculature: An integrated interpretation of signs and symptoms associated with PHPV. *Am J Ophthalmol* 1997;124:587.

145. Lisch W, Rochels R. Zur pathogenese kongenitaler Glaskorperzysten. *Klin Monatsbl Augenheilkd* 1989;195:375.

146. Steinmetz RL, Straatsma BR, Rubin ML. Posterior vitreous cyst. *Am J Ophthalmol* 1990;109:295.

147. Bullock JD. Developmental vitreous cysts. *Arch Ophthalmol* 1974;91:83.

148. Fewan SM, Straatsma BR. Cyst of the posterior vitreous. *Arch Ophthalmol* 1974;91:328.

149. Perera P. Bilateral cyst of the vitreous: Report of a case. *Arch Ophthalmol* 1936;16:1015.

150. Brewerton EW. Cysts in the vitreous. *Trans Ophthalmol Soc UK* 1913;33:93.

151. Francois J. Pre-papillary cyst developed from remnant of the hyaloid artery. *Br J Ophthalmol* 1950;34:365.

152. Duke-Elder S. Anomalies in the vitreous body. In: Duke-Elder S (ed). *System of ophthalmology*, vol 3, part 2. London: Henry Klimpton, 1964:763–770.

153. Orellana J, O'Malley RE, McPherson AR, et al. Pigmented free floating vitreous cysts in two young adults: electron microscopic observations. *Ophthalmology* 1985;92:297.

154. Ruby AJ, Jampol LM. Nd:YAG treatment of a posterior vitreous cyst. *Am J Ophthalmol* 1990;110:428.

155. Reese AB. Persistent hyperplastic primary vitreous. *Am J Ophthalmol* 1955;40:317.

156. Awan KJ, Thumayam M. Changes in the contralateral eye in uncomplicated persistent hyperplastic primary vitreous. *Am J Ophthalmol* 1985;99:122.

157. Boeve MH, Stades FC. Glaucom big hond und Kat. Overzicht en retrospective evaluatie van 421 patienten. I. Pathobiologische achtergronden, indeling en raspredisposities. *Tijdschr Diergeneeskd* 1985;110:219.

158. Wolter JR, Flaherty NW. Persistent hyperplastic vitreous. *Am J Ophthalmol* 1959;47:491.

159. Manschot WA. Persistent hyperplastic primary vitreous. *Arch Ophthalmol* 1958;59:188.

160. Akiya S, Uemura Y, Tsuchiya S, et al. Electron microscopic study of the developing human vitreous collagen fibrils. *Ophthalmol Res* 1986;18:199.

161. Spitznas M, Koch F, Phols P. Ultrastructural pathology of anterior persistent hyperplastic primary vitreous. *Graefes Arch Clin Exp Ophthalmol* 1990;228:487.

162. Pruett RC, Schepens CL. Posterior hyperplastic primary vitreous. *Am J Ophthalmol* 1970;69:535.

163. Font RL, Yanoff M, Zimmerman LE. Intraocular adipose tissue and persistent hyperplastic primary vitreous. *Arch Ophthalmol* 1969;82:43.

164. Criswick VG, Schepens CL. Familial exudative vitreo-retinopathy. *Am J Ophthalmol* 1969;68:578.

165. Gow J, Oliver GL. Familial exudative vitreoretinopathy. *Arch Ophthalmol* 1971;86:150.

166. Plager DA, Orgel IK, Ellis FD, et al. X-linked recessive familial exudative vitreoretinopathy. *Am J Ophthalmol* 1992;114:145.

167. Von Nouhuys CE. Juvenile retinal detachment as a complication of familial exudative vitreoretinopathy. *Fortschr Ophthalmol* 1989;86:221.

168. Van Nouhuys CE. Dominant exudative vitreoretinopathy and other vascular developmental disorders of the peripheral retina. *Doc Ophthalmol* 1982;54:1.

169. Van Nouhuys CE. Signs, complications, and platelet aggregation in familial exudative vitreoretinopathy. *Am J Ophthalmol* 1991;111:34.

170. Brockhurst RJ, Albert DM, Zakov ZN. Pathologic findings in familial exudative vitreoretinopathy. *Arch Ophthalmol* 1981;99:2143.

171. Miyakubo H, Inohara N, Hashimoto K. Retinal involvement in familial exudative vitreoretinopathy. *Ophthalmologica* 1982;185:125.

172. Sebag J. Imaging vitreous. *Eye* 2002;16:429.

173. Ueno N, Sebag J, Hirokawa H, et al. Effects of visible-light irradiation on vitreous structure in the presence of a photosensitizer. *Exp Eye Res* 1987;44:863.

174. Machemer R. Description and pathogenesis of late stages of retinopathy of prematurity. *Ophthalmology* 1985;92:1000.

175. Foos RY. Chronic retinopathy of prematurity. *Ophthalmology* 1985;92:563.

176. Hirose T, Sang DA. Vitreous changes in retinopathy of prematurity. In: Schepens CL, Neetens A, eds. *The vitreous and vitreoretinal interface*. New York: Springer-Verlag, 1987;165–177.

2

VISUAL ASSESSMENT OF THE INFANT AND CHILD: ASSESSMENT OF VISION IN INFANTS AND CHILDREN WITH VISION LOSS

LEA HYVÄRINEN

Infants and children with retinal diseases can have normal vision in one or both eyes or be moderately to severely visually impaired or blind. It is difficult to predict the visual potential of the infant eye at the time of retinal diagnosis. Management may require appropriately timed surgical intervention, medical management, and well-organized pediatric low-vision services. These services involve comprehensive assessments preoperatively, immediately following surgery, and later on into postoperative follow-ups. Comprehensive evaluation is necessary to correctly evaluate the child's visual function and to maximize the child's visual outcome. Ultimately, it is the vision and function of a child that are important, not only the anatomic result.

Various aspects of visual function assessments have been discussed for early intervention and rehabilitation of children in a great number of papers (1–3).

At the outset of the visual function evaluation, it is important to define the goals of the visual assessment and what is to be assessed. Assessment of visual function of an infant or child can have two different purposes: (i) to record the effect of the intervention on the child's vision and what visual functions were affected, and (ii) to determine whether the infant or child has a visual impairment that requires early intervention, special education, and support for the family. This chapter presents the different tests and test conditions used for children with visual impairments. The classification of visual impairment and disability in children is covered in Chapter 33.

To have a common ground when discussing visual function assessment, vision will be defined as the use of visual information processed by the retina and interpreted within the brain combined with other functions like memory and attention. Visual information is composed of three components. *We see forms, colors, and motion.*

Detection or discrimination acuity is often clinically assessed using tests at high contrast. There are other aspects of visual function that are important and are not always measured

in standard assessments. For example, the functionally more important aspect of form perception measured at low contrast is not always assessed. The same is true of color vision. Motion perception is not measured at all because there are no clinical tests for pediatric use. Our clinical assessment of visual functioning is thus inadequate and requires well-planned observations in different vision-related tasks and activities.

FACTORS THAT MAY INFLUENCE ASSESSMENT OF VISION

When assessing vision of visually impaired children, especially vision of visually impaired children with other disabilities, numerous factors can affect children's responses (Fig. 2-1).

A child may be seriously ill, weak, or sleepy because of medications. It is wise to inquire when medications are given and choose a time when their effect on wakefulness is minimal. A better *time for assessment* is often during and after the midday meal or later in the afternoon.

Communication needs to be at the level of the child. During the first assessment, parents demonstrate how they communicate with the child. This information permits the pediatric ophthalmologist or vision specialist to choose the type of communication—visual, tactile, and auditory—with which the child is accustomed.

The child's *visual sphere* is observed, so that testing can be performed well within it. The visual sphere is the space in which the child uses vision and is dependent on the visual qualities of an object, its movement, and its emotional value. A milk bottle with dark stripes on it is recognized at a farther distance than is a square or round picture with similar stripes on it. A parent's face is one of the best objects to test the range of a child's visual sphere.

Visual attention might vary based on the area within the visual field. If clinical findings suggest that parts of the visual

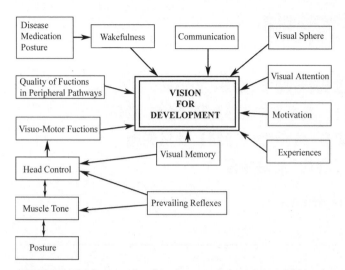

FIGURE 2-1. Diagram showing the most important variables affecting an assessment of vision for development.

field are missing or that visual acuity and contrast sensitivity are poor in certain parts of the visual field, then stronger stimuli can be presented in the best areas of the visual field.

Oculomotor functions are used as signs of visual responses. Therefore, it is important to know whether they are affected and to observe them for some time while the parents interact with the child. During presentation of test objects, it is essential not to adjust the speed and direction of movement of the test object to the movements of the child's eyes. The object is brought to a point in the child's visual field where it should be visible and then is moved in each of the cardinal directions to determine whether it elicits tracking movements.

Motor problems in arms and hands may make reaching impossible. However, an intention to move the hand in the correct direction provides valuable information. *Pathologic reflexes* may disturb head movements and may require a change of posture or support by the child's physiotherapist.

Motivation to participate in the test situation may be low if the child has unpleasant memories of unknown persons causing pain in previous treatments or examinations. Often the child's own therapist is the best person to start the test situation.

The first assessment is seldom very successful. We do not yet know the child and the child does not relate to us. It is important to inform the parents of this and to ask them to repeat the test situations together with the therapist later to determine how frequently the child's response is similar to that elicited during the assessment. Quite often parents or the therapist spontaneously will say, "This response is not his or her normal response."

VISUAL ACUITY MEASUREMENTS

Visual acuity can be measured with different tests that depict different qualities of vision. According to the Visual

Acuity Measurement Standard of the Consilium Ophthalmologicum Universale, Visual Function Committee (1984), *the basic visual acuity test is the line test* that has at least five optotypes (test symbols) on the test lines with spaces between the optotypes that are equal to the width of the optotypes of that line and where the distance between the test lines is equal to the height of the lower line (4). Even though the international recommendation was published more than ten years ago and was well known in the 1970s, few visual acuity tests have been designed that comply with its recommendations. Even with standardized tests, other important factors that are difficult to control may be overlooked and can affect the results. *Luminance level* is one important variable. If regular room illumination is used, luminance on the eye chart surfaces is lower than the recommended 85 or more candela/meter^2. In the 1970s, this problem was solved in large multicenter studies by using back illuminated tests in standardized lightboxes. The Early Treatment Diabetic Retinopathy Study (ETDRS)-lightbox has become a standard worldwide. However, it is big and heavy and thus difficult to move. Therefore, smaller lightboxes have been manufactured in several countries. The latest development is the use of visual acuity tests on computer screens. The tests can be presented as charts or single symbols and the luminance level varied by using filters in front of the test without changing the contrast of the optotypes.

Even when the tests, test situations, and luminance level are standardized, there is still one important variable that resists standardization, the tester. Every tester has his or her personal way of talking to the child, waiting for the response, and supporting the child. Therefore, visual acuity values measured by two people, well-trained and motivated to test in the same way, still vary. This needs to be accounted for when values from different test series are compared. The testers should follow the instructions exactly. Such "detail" as pointing or not pointing to the optotypes can cause surprising differences in measurements.

In pediatric services, visual acuity charts can be used to examine older children. For infants and young children and children with limited communication, other testing is needed.

Visual acuity measurements thus cover a broad area, including (i) detection acuity measured with small objects; (ii) grating acuity as detection acuity by preferential looking; (iii) grating acuity by resolving orientation of lines; (iv) recognition acuity using optotype tests: single optotype tests, line tests, and crowded tests; and (v) reading acuity.

Detection Acuity, Measured with Small Objects

To measure detection acuity, small and large objects are used at different distances to determine the smallest object the child sees at a certain distance. The objects can be small pieces of food with which the child is familiar. Families can provide suggestions for test materials. It is important to ask about food allergies so as to avoid these foods as test materials.

Dark colored cake decorations less than 2 mm in diameter on light colored surfaces are better than light colored sweets on dark surfaces. If the child has uncorrected hyperopia, light-colored small pieces on a dark surface can appear to be large blurred images like haloes. Thus, the size of the object does not give an accurate impression of detection acuity. The Sheridan rolling balls and balls on a wand are still used to assess detection acuity.

To perform the test, both hands are moved over the top of the light-colored surface in front of the child and one or a few pieces of sweets are dropped onto the surface without stopping the movement. Several observations are made: (i) how the child scans the surface to find the sweets, (ii) how regular and well planned the eye movements are, (iii) whether errors in localizing the small objects might be caused by defects in the central visual field, and (iv) whether there are differences in the visual behavior between the right and left visual field. This test situation is similar to the play situations used in occupational therapy where it can be repeated several times to determine possible variations in a child's responses.

Grating Acuity as Detection Acuity

In infants, children, and adults at an early developmental level, visual acuity may not be measured with optotype tests because of communication difficulties. An estimate of the function of some aspects of the visual pathways can be assessed using grating acuity measurements. When a striped pattern is presented in front of an infant simultaneously with a gray surface of the same size and luminance, the infant is likely to look at and prefer the striped pattern to the gray surface, a preferential looking test condition. Preferential looking has been used for twenty years as a routine clinical measurement. The Teller Grating Acuity Cards made the measurement popular because the responses could be elicited in very young infants and in infants and children with very little communication. When the card appears in front of the infant or child, the child usually turns the gaze to the striped pattern, if it is seen.

The child may or may not see the lines the way we see them. The lines can be seen quite badly distorted even though the child can detect them. If a child has motor functions adequate to follow a tactile line with his finger (i.e., has the concept of following a line), it is wise to ask the child to follow the lines of the grating test with his or her finger. If the child is able to follow tactile lines but not even the broadest lines of the grating test, then the response could be interpreted as a visual response without perception of line orientation.

Because a grating acuity value depicts the detection of large surfaces with stripes, it should not be converted into optotype acuity values. Grating acuity below 6 cpd (cycles per degree) may depict subcortical, and not cortical, function (5).

The Teller Acuity Cards function well in clinical situations but cannot be used in humid and dusty conditions, and are also heavy to carry to outreach operations. The Lea gratings (1,6) were designed to assess visual function for early intervention teams and for work in outreach clinics in Africa. The simple "paddles" can be presented like the Teller Acuity Cards, lifting them in front of the infant or sliding them apart with equal speed. In the latter case one can make observations about the infant's motion perception. If an infant does not track the moving grating but makes a quick saccade to the grating when it stops, it can be a sign of poor motion perception.

Gratings are defined by their spatial frequency (i.e., the number of pairs of black-and-white stripes or cycles) within 1 degree of visual angle. When grating is printed onto a surface, it can be defined also as the number of cycles per centimeter of surface. When a grating is held at 57 cm ($\sim$2 feet) from the infant's face, 1 cm equals 1 degree of visual angle. This is a convenient test distance because the number of cycles per centimeter corresponds to the grating acuity in cycles per degree.

Infants and children at an early developmental level may not respond to stimuli placed at 57-cm distance because their visual sphere might be limited to less than 30 cm ($\sim$1 foot). When the gratings are held at half the 57-cm distance, the number of cycles per degree is half that at 57 cm. If the infant's response can be elicited only at 15 cm ($\sim\frac{1}{2}$ foot), one-fourth of the 57-cm test distance, the frequency of the grating is one-fourth of the value printed on the test card. If the child responds to the stimuli at about 1 m (exactly 114 cm or $\sim$4 feet), the grating acuity values are twice the value printed on the test card.

Grating Acuity by Resolving Line Orientation

True grating acuity is measured when the subject needs to resolve the orientation of lines. This can be done by using computer-based grating tests or gratings printed on round cards that can be turned in different orientations. This test is used only in research laboratories. Even if this test situation is closer to discrimination acuity than grating stimuli used as detection tests, the values cannot be converted to optotype acuities. The grating can be seen badly distorted in its middle and yet its orientation can be perceived.

Recognition Acuity Using Optotype Tests

When testing adults, it is customary to test distance vision first, followed by near vision. When testing children, better results are obtained by starting with near-vision testing before proceeding to a distance-vision testing. This allows the child to learn the testing procedures and symbols. The examiner learns what to expect from the child under the most favorable conditions. Binocular vision is tested first, then each eye separately.

Before testing starts, a method of communication must be established, such as naming (signing) or matching. If the child does not spontaneously name the symbols, you may ask "What should we call this?" When the Lea symbol tests are used we can suggest, "Should we call it 'apple' or 'heart', 'house' or 'garage', 'window' or 'box' or 'TV', 'ball' or 'ring'?" (6). Any name that the child chooses to use is accepted: house may be garage, cottage, arrow, dog house, or bird house, and the apple gets the greatest variation of names. A child may also change the name of a symbol; the larger symbols may be apples and the smaller, berries. When the HOTV test is used, a young child needs to use a key card to match. Use of a key card makes testing slower and requires changes in accommodation when testing at a distance. There are numerous pediatric visual acuity tests with a variety of pictures. Because the tests have not been calibrated against the Landolt C, the reference optotype, and their layout does not follow the International Recommendation, visual acuity values measured with these tests are not comparable to those measured with calibrated tests. School-aged children are tested using letter or number charts.

If a child with multiple handicaps cannot point to a symbol or make a selection with his or her hand or foot, the single pictures of the keycard are arranged farther apart so the child can direct his or her eye gaze to indicate selection, as long as voluntary eye movements are accurate enough. The child can also indicate choice with head movements. If a child has only "yes" and "no" as responses, show one test card at a time asking "Is this . . . ?" and randomly show the optotype that you mention to get a "yes" answer and one that is not represented to get a "no".

Training of the test situation is often needed when testing young children and children with developmental delays. The child needs to develop the concept of *similar to or different from* when asked to match test symbols. This concept is learned first when comparing colors and then when comparing forms, so playing with colorful test optotypes can be used when training young children. The next concept to be learned is the concept of *pictures representing objects.* Here the tester can draw the test optotypes around the three-dimensional test symbols while the child watches. When this concept is developed, smaller and smaller pictures are drawn so the child learns that pictures with the same form have the same name even when they are of different sizes.

According to the Visual Acuity Measurement Standard, "A line of optotypes is generally considered to have been read correctly when more than 50% (e.g., 3 of 5, 4 of 6) of the optotypes presented have been read correctly." In follow-up testing and in amblyopia training, the −1, −2, and +1, +2 system should be used to give credit for minimal changes. For example, "20/32 (+1) or 0.63 (+1)" indicates

that the child met the 20/32 line criteria and also correctly named one symbol on the next smaller size, 20/25 (0.8). When pointing is used, it is recorded in the report.

During testing, the *test distance* should be kept as the standard distance of the test or carefully measured so that the visual acuity value can be calculated corresponding to the distance used. It is difficult to keep a child's head at exactly the same distance from the test during distance testing if there is not a bar that the child can lean his or her forehead against. This is rarely used except in research work. However, moving only 15 cm closer to the test decreases the distance by 5%. If a child bends forward the distance can be decreased 10%. During near testing, even small changes in head position can change the result notably. The parent can hold the end of a cord fixed on the near test at the level of the child's eye, without touching the child's face, to maintain the standard distance during near testing.

Because visual acuity tests are mainly used in amblyopia screening, it is important to remember that skipping symbols is a feature typical to amblyopic eyes. This finding can be found in amblyopia even if the visual acuity difference between the two eyes is less than two lines. If the child skips symbols when tested using one eye, but not the other, the tester should be alerted to the possibility that the child might have mild amblyopia developing.

Near-Vision Acuity

Near vision is functionally more important than distance vision in the life of a young child. The child is more accustomed to using vision at near than at greater distances. Therefore, introduction of the test situation at near familiarizes the child with the test before measurement of distance vision. In case of myopia, the parents are reassured that the child has useful vision at near and not alarmed when the child does not see as well during the distance visual acuity testing.

When examining normally sighted children, the card should be held at the standard distance of the test card. For visually impaired children, it is useful to allow the child to use their preferred distance and head posture during the first testing and later to measure their vision at the standard distance.

When teaching the team members of the low-vision team or when creating a protocol for a project, the test situation should be defined in detail:

- Establish a method of communication such as naming (signing) or pointing (matching). Decide with the child which names will be used to identify the symbols. When needed, train with the optotypes used.
- Start with binocular testing.
- Point to each of the symbols on the top line of the test or on the keycard; observe the baseline responses for comprehension, speed, and accuracy.

- Cover the line above the line to be read with a white card. Ask the child to identify only the first symbol on the line below the covering card.
- Repeat this procedure for each or every second line (moving quickly down the chart to avoid tiring the child) until the child hesitates or misidentifies a symbol.
- Move back up one line and ask the child to identify all the symbols on that line.
- If the child identifies all symbols correctly, go to the next line down and ask the child to identify all the symbols on that line.
- If the child skips a symbol, let the child read the line to the end and then ask the child to try again while briefly pointing to the skipped symbol.
- The visual acuity value is recorded as the last line on which at least three of the five symbols are read correctly. Always test until the threshold line.
- If the near-vision card is held at the standard distance, the visual acuity value is found in the margin adjacent to that line.
- After binocular testing, proceed with testing each eye separately.
- Use two pairs of plano glasses for occlusion of the child's eyes.
- For monocular testing, follow the same procedure as for binocular testing.

Older children can be tested using more crowded near-vision tests in which the same symbols are spaced closer together as in words or sentences. The testing procedure is the same as for binocular testing. The close spacing of the symbols makes it a sensitive test for detection of mild amblyopia in monocular testing and increased crowding due to brain damage in binocular testing.

Visual acuity measured with crowded symbols approximates the smallest text size that the child will be able to read, but is smaller than the size that is comfortably read. It is *not* equivalent to the print size used in learning because nobody likes to read at the level of a threshold. We usually read texts that are three to ten times larger than the threshold size.

Binocular visual acuity values are functionally important. Monocular near-vision values are important in the follow-up of vision disorders, especially during amblyopia treatment. Visual acuity values often improve at near first and at distance later. Before the age of 3 years it is usually easier to measure monocular near-vision values than distance visual acuity values. Worse visual acuity values at near than at distance need to be controlled using proper near correction to exclude insufficient accommodation as the cause of worse values at near.

A child with a visual impairment is allowed to choose any distance and is given a correction for that distance, if needed. If the chart is used at a distance other than the standard distance, the viewing distance and the symbol size read (the M value) or the visual acuity value printed adjacent to the threshold line are measured and recorded.

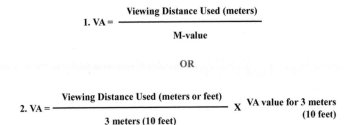

$$\text{1. VA} = \frac{\text{Viewing Distance Used (meters)}}{\text{M-value}}$$

OR

$$\text{2. VA} = \frac{\text{Viewing Distance Used (meters or feet)}}{\text{3 meters (10 feet)}} \times \begin{array}{c}\text{VA value for 3 meters}\\ \text{(10 feet)}\end{array}$$

FIGURE 2-2. Formulas for calculating visual acuity values measured at other than the standard distance. VA, Visual Acuity

The correct visual acuity value in distance visual acuity you can use formulas in Fig. 2.2 or choose the measurement distance to be 1/2, 1/3, or 1/4 of the standard distance. Then, the visual acuity is 1/2 to 1/4 of the value written next to the line that was the smallest line read correctly. The calculation is simple: multiply the denominator by 2, if the distance was 1/2 the standard, i.e., if the value on the threshold line was 20/32, then the visual acuity value is 20/63.

Similarly, when the near vision test is held at 8" (20 cm) instead of the standard 16" (40 cm) and the smallest line read correctly was the 20/25 (0.8) line, the visual acuity value is 20/25 (0.8) divided by 2, equal to 20/50 (0.4).

When the M-value is used, the calculation is simple: distance in meter, 0.2, divided by the M-value of the line read, 0.5M, is equal to 2 divided by 5, which is 2/5. This is easy to change to the American or the European notation 20/50 or 0.4. The calculation is based on metric measurements.

The visual acuity in the Snellen notation can be found on the visual acuity chart. If the exact corresponding Snellen value is not printed on the chart, it can be calculated as follows: 0.07 = 7/100 = [7 × 3/100 × 3] = 21/300 or approximately 20/300. You multiply both the numerator and the denominator by the number that makes the numerator closely equal to 20.

Distance Vision Acuity

When examining young children, introduce the distance chart to the child after near testing by saying, "Let's look at the same pictures a little farther away." Move the chart gradually back to 3 m (10 ft) while watching the child for signs of inattention. If the child loses interest, the chart is moved closer to the child to 2 m (80 in) or 1 m (40 in). *Testing always should be performed well within the visual sphere of the child.* Older children can be switched directly from a near vision test to a 3-m (10-ft) chart.

Distance testing follows exactly the same procedure as near-vision testing.

Even with standardized testing and visual acuity testers trained to perform precisely to the standard, there are still surprising variations in children's visual acuity values with repeated measures. We cannot standardize the most important variable in the test situations: the child. The mood and the concentration of the child can vary so much that the results can also vary two lines better or worse. Thus, a drop in a visual acuity value by two lines might be within normal variation and should be repeated the same day or within a few days before the child is referred for further evaluation.

In the measurement of optotype acuity, we should:

- Use age appropriate tests with correct layout and optotypes
- Use the correct luminance level
- Adjust communication to the level that is comfortable to the child
- Test first at near, then at distance
- Test with single, line, and crowded tests

Report visual acuity values as the exact threshold values (±1 or 2)

Even though much time is spent measuring visual acuity at high contrast, it depicts visual information that is rare in the life of a young child (i.e., small details at high contrast) until she or he becomes interested in letters and numbers. Therefore, visual acuity should always be measured at low contrast levels also, as discussed in Contrast Sensitivity.

Reading Acuity

Visual acuity measured with crowded symbols often depicts an approximate size of the text that a child might be able to read. When a child knows letters, reading acuity of visually impaired children should be measured using the size of the text that gives optimal reading speed. The test using random words, developed by Markku Leinonen, has a pediatric version at three different grade levels.

If a child can read but makes atypical *reading errors*, the cause might be a *small scotoma* on the right side of the fixation point. With eye movement, the scotoma could occasionally affect one or two letters, causing them to disappear. When the eye and therefore, the scotoma, moves to another location the child sees the missed letters and corrects the error. A small scotoma is an important differential diagnosis in each case of *atypical dyslexia* and should be sought. By increasing the size of the text to be read, the scotoma covers smaller and smaller parts of the word. At a certain text size, it no longer interferes with reading. *If errors disappear by increasing the size of the text, the child is likely to have a visual field problem, not dyslexia.*

Refraction must be corrected so that the best possible image is available to the child. Refractive errors should be tested for near vision in children. A child may use another preferred retinal locus (PRL) at near than at distance or may use one eye at distance, the other at near. When refraction cannot be measured using retinoscopy, subjective tests can be used to assess first graders and older children. The refractive power of that eye can be estimated by measuring at which distances the different meridians of the astigmatism wheel are clearest. First, suitable correction is used to bring the image within the arm's reach (i.e., the child is made approximately 2 D myopic in the least-myopic meridian). When the child looks at the astigmatism wheel while moving it closer and farther, the spokes either are all equally sharp at all distances or they are sharpest in one meridian at a certain distance and in another meridian at another distance. The difference in the dioptric values at each of these two distances where the spokes are clearest is the value of astigmatism in that eye. When the astigmatism is corrected with a cylinder lens, the astigmatism wheel can be used to observe whether the image is now clear in all meridians simultaneously. Irregularities in the optical media can cause some lines to appear double even after astigmatism is corrected.

CONTRAST SENSITIVITY

Contrast sensitivity measures the ability to see details at low contrast levels. Visual information at low contrast levels is particularly important (i) in communication, because faint shadows on our faces carry visual information related to facial expressions; ii) in orientation and mobility because curbs, faint shadows, and stairs can be of low contrast and provide valuable information; (iii) in everyday tasks at low contrast, like cutting an onion on a light-colored surface, pouring coffee into a dark mug, or checking for wrinkles on an ironed shirt; and (iv) in near-vision tasks that have low-contrast information, like reading a newspaper or writing with a pencil.

Measurement of contrast sensitivity resembles audiometry: a pure-tone audiogram determines the weakest pure tones that a person can hear at different frequencies. The contrast sensitivity curve or visuogram shows the faintest contrasts perceived by the person. If the stimulus is a sine wave grating, then the curve depicts a similar function, as does the pure-tone audiogram. If the stimuli are optotypes (i.e., letters, numbers, or pediatric symbols), the test resembles speech audiometry. As in audiometry, the result of the contrast sensitivity measurement is not one single value but rather a diagram (Fig. 2-3).

Contrast sensitivity measurements were first made using grating stimuli on oscilloscopes and later on computers. The detection of threshold using this testing paradigm requires several (five to eight) steps and can thus be difficult in children. Because we measure visual acuity at high contrast with optotypes, it is logical to measure low contrast visual acuity with the same optotypes.

Measurement Techniques for Contrast Sensitivity When Using Optotype Tests

There are several low-contrast tests in clinical use. The most common used to examine adult patients is the Pelli-Robson test. When used according to the instructions, the size of the Sloan optotypes corresponds to 0.04 (20/500). Therefore, it does not help to measure the upper end of the descending slope. The thresholds at very low contrast values at 0.04 depict vision in such situations as seeing faint shadows on white snow on a cloudy day.

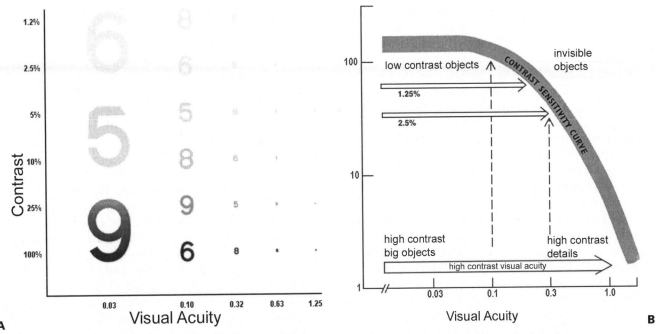

FIGURE 2-3. Contrast sensitivity curve. **(A)** Visual acuity is plotted along the horizontal axis and contrast along the vertical axis. The size of the symbols decreases along the horizontal axis and they become paler and paler in the vertical direction. **(B)** The boundary between symbols perceived and those that are too small or too pale and are thus not seen is depicted by a curve called the contrast sensitivity curve. Its declining right-hand slope is the most interesting part of the curve in clinical cases. To define the slope of the contrast sensitivity curve with a small number of thresholds we need two or three measurements. The first one defines the point at the x-axis, the visual acuity value determined in the usual way; the second is the definition of the upper end of the straight part of the slope usually located in the 1% to 5% contrast area. An additional measurement at low contrast is often of interest. This curve shows clearly why measurement at 10% contrast is insufficient in evaluation of low contrast vision. Changes in contrast sensitivity due to corneal haze, early cataractous changes, macular edema or degeneration, or lesions in the visual pathways are often measurable only at a 1% to 2% contrast level.

The threshold values can be measured with two different techniques when using optotype tests by using low-contrast visual acuity charts (moving horizontally in the diagram), or by using tests with one symbol size and several contrast levels, as in the Pelli-Robson test (vertically in the diagram).

The combination of high- and low-contrast visual acuity values defines the location of the slope of the contrast sensitivity curve. Diagnostically, the most important feature is a change over time.

Measurement of Contrast Sensitivity Using Low-Contrast Visual Acuity Charts

Testing of contrast sensitivity using low-contrast visual acuity charts is identical to the measurement of visual acuity at high contrast level (i.e., the smallest size of the optotypes that the person can recognize is measured). The threshold is defined as the line of optotypes on which at least three out of five optotypes are correctly recognized. The visual acuity chart at 2.5% contrast is the most practical test in clinical use. The resulting threshold point on the curve is far enough from the high contrast value so that the declination of the slope of the curve can be defined. In severe low vision, the tests must be performed quite close and this testing might require reading lenses. The number of optotypes read correctly is recorded; e.g., if on the 2.5% contrast chart one of the symbols was read incorrectly on line 20/63, the visual acuity value is recorded as 20/63 (−1) at 2.5%.

Measurement of Contrast Sensitivity Using Tests with One Symbol Size

In the pediatric LEA test, the 10 M size is convenient because at the most common testing distance of 1 m, it corresponds to visual acuity 0.1 (20/200), at 2 m to 0.2 (20/100), at 4 m to 0.4 (20/50), and at 0.3 m to 0.03 (20/600). These testing situations cover the low contrast visual acuity range of most children with vision problems. The contrast levels of the test lines on the four pages are 10%, 5%, 2.5%, and 1.2%.

Luminance variation can affect the threshold value. To provide a high enough luminance in a standardly lit room, the light source is directed toward the test. Then, the amount of light falling on the test is dependent on the distance of the test from the light source. For reliable follow-up measurements, the test should be at a fixed distance from the light source. In field surveys, the variation in the results caused by variation in illumination needs to be considered. Back-illuminated charts in lightboxes have standard luminance levels.

Among normally sighted people, both visual acuity and contrast sensitivity have a *wide range of variation*. In evaluating visual acuity, 20/25 (0.8) is a low normal value and 20/8 (2.5) is the highest normal value, three times higher. Similarly, the range of normal variation in contrast sensitivity values is great. Therefore, a value within the range of normal may not indicate that a particular child has normal contrast sensitivity if that child had a higher recorded contrast sensitivity previously. Contrast sensitivity can decrease to one-third its original value and still be in the "normal" range. Thus, careful longitudinal comparisons are important.

A change in contrast sensitivity is a diagnostically important feature that should be monitored in the future. Ideally, contrast sensitivity and visual acuity should be measured using optimal refractive correction when children leave their high school or secondary school or in young adulthood. These values should be recorded and saved as part of the patient's basic medical record. A change warrants an examination to find out the cause. Although the most common cause would be a small change in the refractive power of the eye—a benign finding—repeating the measurement of contrast sensitivity would be beneficial as a part of the routine health examination.

Measurement of contrast sensitivity helps explain the complaints of a child whose visual acuity at high contrast has not changed but whose vision at low contrast levels has decreased. It is important not to underestimate the importance of the child's complaint.

Hiding Heidi Low-Contrast Test for Vision in Communication

Contrast sensitivity needs to be assessed in children and adults who are unable to respond verbally or by pointing. If the child can follow a moving target, shift gaze, or perform a head turn to look at peripherally presented visual stimuli, preferential looking test situations can be used when testing with Hiding Heidi pictures.

Whenever contrast sensitivity has decreased, it is advisable to measure the visibility of facial features at different distances. Surprises are common. Because the area of the Heidi picture—and that of a face—is so much larger than the area of a symbol or even a grating stimulus, the low contrast pictures can be discerned at unexpectedly long distances. If the function of a healthy child is demonstrated at the same luminance level, the teachers and therapists will better understand the requirements of the visually impaired child's communication. If the child only shifts his or her gaze to the low-contrast picture, not much information is obtained about how the child interprets the picture. If the infant or child responds with a smile, we learn a great deal more. The child must have seen the picture well enough to perceive the smile and has developed a normal social smile.

Assessment of visual function at low contrast adds an important dimension to the evaluation of a child's capabilities. It should be a part of the visual evaluation in all low-vision services and diagnostic work. With the easy-to-use optotype tests, it is possible to assess the visibility of low contrast details quickly and reliably.

VISUAL FIELD

To assess visual field, the total area of the binocular visual field is determined using confrontation techniques. The quality of the central visual field is assessed with tests like the Damato campimeter, the Amsler grid to determine distortion, and text reading to detect whether letters in words disappear. The usual Amsler grid has such thin lines that a visually impaired child may not see them. In such a case, the public-domain extrafoveal fixation recorder (www.lea-test.fi/en/vistests/instruct/extrafov/extrafov.html) can be printed or a page of a regular college block can be used for visually impaired students.

Visual field is difficult to assess during the first few months of life because the infant's *attention* is directed to the center of the visual field. Peripheral stimuli need to be strong to cause a shift in attention. Small, illuminated toys in a dimly lit room can elicit a response better than the traditional white Sheridan balls used in assessing vision.

Peripheral Visual Field

Confrontation visual field can be measured using the tester's finger movements as the stimulus or a white Sheridan ball on a thin stick. The object or the fingers are moved forward from behind the child's head. As the stimulus appears in the peripheral visual field, a young child may turn their eyes to it. The approximate place where the stimulus is detected is recorded (e.g., 90 degrees to the right and left, 60 degrees up and down). When using Goldmann perimetry, young children respond better if asked to shift fixation from the central fixation target to the stimulus as soon as it becomes visible rather than to press a button.

Visual field defects include (i) hemianopias, half field defects in one or both eyes either on the same side (homonymous hemianopias) or on both temporal sides (bitemporal hemianopias); (ii) quadrantanopias, quarter of the visual field defects, again in one or both eyes; or (iii) a ring scotoma, loss of visual function in the "midperiphery" of the visual field.

The functional importance of the child's visual field defect should be carefully assessed. There are two aspects that are not always discussed in detail in medical reports. One is the affect of bitemporal visual field loss on a child's function. If both temporal halves are blind and the nasal halves of the visual fields functional, the child has approximately a 120-degree visual field when looking straight ahead in the distance. However, when the child looks at something at near, for example, at something on the desk, the objects in the midperiphery are lost when the eyes converge. An example of this is illustrated: when a child looks at something on the desk, he or she does not see a sector of the classroom in front of her or him. The same problem occurs in physical education and during games.

The second important feature often unreported and untested is the presence of motion perception in some "blind" areas. Flicker sensitivity may be present in the area of the scotoma and should be measured whenever possible (7).

Tunnel vision, in which the central visual field is only 10 to 20 degrees, can be tested using plain white paper at a distance of 57 cm and a dark pen. A cross is drawn in the middle of the paper and the child is asked to fixate on the cross. The pen is moved from the side of the paper toward the cross and the child is asked to indicate when the pen becomes visible at the edge of the tubular field. The extent of the field is measured from the right, left, up, down, and diagonally. A line is drawn through these points and the size of the visual field is depicted by the oval area. At 57 cm, each centimeter on the paper equals 1 degree of visual angle, so you can measure the size of the visual field simply by measuring the size of the area in centimeters. When the visual field is quite limited, a longer measuring distance, 114 cm or 228 cm, may be desired to obtain a more exact measurement. At 114 cm, 2 cm equals 1 degree of visual angle and at 228 cm, 4 cm equals 1 degree.

Children with tubular visual fields usually adapt poorly to low luminance levels so the effect of luminance level on the size of the field needs to be assessed. Most school children can tell where they see their hand movements at the luminance levels used in Goldmann perimetry (10 cd/m^2) and in daylight conditions.

If a child has nystagmus or difficulties maintaining fixation, visual field testing becomes inaccurate and an approximation must suffice.

Communication Field

The communication field of a child who uses visual sign language and who has a tubular visual field should be tested at the beginning of each school term. Each teacher and therapist should be able to measure it.

The measurement is performed as follows:

- Use the communication distance of 1.5 to 2 m.
- The child should fixate the tester's face ("nose") and say when he or she notices the tester's hand approaching from the side.
- The tester brings their outreached hand toward their head until the child notices it. The tester touches their shoulder to give a tactile reference for signing. Then the tester brings their hand from the other side, from above, and from below to measure the area in space within which the hands are visible at that particular distance. This space is

the child's communication field at that luminance level and distance. At a greater distance, the child's communication field will be larger and at shorter distances it will be smaller. The effect of the luminance level should be demonstrated to teachers so that they remember to check it in the school environment and during evening activities.

The communication field of children with central scotomas is best assessed by asking the child how much of the tester's face he or she sees without scanning. It is also wise to ask a child with a large central scotoma to describe in what manner the image of a face changes when fixation is moved from eccentric to central, i.e., when the child places the scotoma on the face of the tester. Many children give a vivid description of the *distortions and changes in color* of the face of the tester.

Central Visual Field

The quality of the central visual field is important to assess for sustained near vision tasks, like reading and using picture materials. In these tasks, small scotomas, areas of loss of sensitivity, and distortions of the image can disturb the perception of visual information.

In routine clinical work, scotomas are mapped using perimeters and tangent screens. Both are large and expensive. A campimeter developed by Dr. Bertil Damato is suitable for educational assessment. In it, the stimulus appears in the middle of the test screen while the subject looks at numbers placed at different locations on the screen. The untested eye is usually covered by the parent or another adult, because otherwise there are too many demanding functions disturbing the child's response to the visual stimulus.

Damato campimetry can be used starting at the age of about 5 years. Because few children at that age know numbers well enough to locate a particular number to fixate, a pointer with a ring at its end is placed on the number to help the child maintain fixation on it. It is wise to start the measurement with a few points in the middle and then measure the blind spot. If the blind spot can be mapped and determined, other small scotomas can also be detected. If a child has a central scotoma and fixation is shifted to a PRL, the blind spot is also shifted in the same direction and the child will have a visual response when the stimulus is shown in the area of the normal blind spot. This should not confuse the tester to believe that the child's responses are unreliable. The same is true for all visual field testing: if the child does not fixate with the fovea, the whole visual field map will be shifted in the direction opposite to the PRL, i.e. if the new fixation area is above the central lesion, the shadow of the lesion will be located above the area of fixation and the blind spot will be shifted up.

The extrafoveal fixation recorder was designed to measure shifts in fixation during reading by plotting the location of the blind spot. If there are several islands of useful vision, they are likely to be of different sizes and have different visual acuity and contrast sensitivity measurements. Thus, fixation might vary from one PRL to another depending on the type of visual task. The child might use a small island of vision during measurement of visual acuity and another one when reading long words. In that case, the reading text size would likely be larger than expected based on the visual acuity value. To demonstrate the use of PRLs, choose first as the fixation target a two- or three-letter word in the smallest size perceived by the child and map the location of the blind spot. Then use a six- to eight-letter word of the optimal size for reading as the fixation target and map the location of the blind spot. If its location is different from that in the first measurement, the child uses two different PRLs during visual acuity measurement and during reading. This test is advised whenever there is a *discrepancy between the measured visual acuity value and the magnification preferred for reading.*

Functions of the central visual field can also be disturbed by field defects extending to the midline. A field defect on the left side hinders one from finding the beginning of the next line. It is helpful to use a ruler or card under the line to be read in this situation. If the right-sided field loss is complete, with no macular sparing, reading toward the blind half field is difficult. In this situation there is a simple solution: turning the book upside down moves the blind half field behind the point of reading, which can be helped by the card or the ruler below the line while reading from right to left. If the child has learned to read before the accident the change in reading can occur during convalescence before the child returns to school. Children can also learn to fixate 1 or 2 degrees extrafoveally to gain reading field on the right.

Scanning is an important strategy to compensate for visual field defects. The child can be taught to use regular scanning of the surrounding world, the hemianopic child "throwing" their gaze to the blind side and then moving it smoothly back to midline. A child with a tunnel field defect can shift the gaze from side to side like a long cane.

COLOR VISION

Color vision testing is used for diagnostic purposes and to assess functional vision for early intervention and special education. Therapists and schools often use colors in their materials. Therefore, it is important for therapists and teachers to know if a child confuses certain colors so that the child's deviating responses are not misunderstood. In the early teens, color vision tests are needed for advice in career planning.

Inherited color vision defects are generally screened using pseudoisochromatic Ishihara-type tests and, in testing young children, the Waggoner test. Anomaloscopy is the criterion standard but rarely is the test available. Acquired color vision defects, dyschromatopsias, are caused by dis-

eases or trauma and can affect cone cells, inner retinal layers, optic nerve fibers, or the visual cortex. The structural and functional changes can be patchy or diffuse and can affect vision in one eye more than in the other. For diagnostic purposes, the eyes are tested separately. For functional purposes, binocular measurements are more informative.

Macular lesions often cause a defect in the blue-yellow, or tritan, axis because there are fewer S-cones (blue) than L- (red) and M-cones (green), and they are concentrated around the edge of the fovea. However, when the macular lesion is small or patchy, there can be no axis determined or it can vary from day to day.

Results in quantitative testing vary as a function of stimulus size. This is more pronounced in acquired color vision defects than in congenital color vision defects. Results using small stimuli depict function in the PRL used for fixation, whereas results using large stimuli give information on color perception in everyday life. In the peripheral retina, we all have "defective" color perception of small test stimuli. In everyday life, we are not aware of variations in color perception in different parts of our visual field, because of the complicated summation functions of the brain.

In diagnostic evaluations, the tester should be aware that reduced retinal illuminance due to unclear media from the cornea, lens, or vitreous distorts test results. In these cases, increased illumination can decrease the degree of the defect or make it disappear. *Illumination should be natural, overcast daylight* at a window facing the northern sky (in the northern hemisphere) or artificial light with a color temperature of approximately 6,774 K (standard illuminant C). The next best to natural overcast daylight is a daylight tube light fixture placed above the color-vision testing table. The testing table is covered with a black cloth. The grayish-blue light is often an unpleasant experience because it makes patients and the tester look sick. Therefore, other light fixtures in the room are usually chosen that have a warmer color temperature. However, these lights are turned off during the actual color vision evaluation.

Quantitative measurement of color vision is an important diagnostic test used to define the degree of hereditary color vision defects that are detected with pseudoisochromatic tests. These tests are used to evaluate deficient color vision from acquired disorders. Quantitative color vision tests in pediatric examinations are sorting tests like the Farnsworth Panel 15 and the Good-Lite Panel 16, and sometimes the Lanthony test with desaturated test colors. Panel 16 is unique from other quantitative color vision tests because it uses large cap sizes, and gives more information about color vision function both in normally sighted and low vision individuals. The color surface in Panel 16 has a protective coating, which decreases the risk of the stimulus area getting smudged.

The sorting tests consist of a set of a "pilot" and 15 test caps. The diameter of the stimulus area is 3.3 cm (1.3 in) in the Panel 16. The stimulus size can be reduced by using a dark-gray restriction ring with an opening of 1.2 cm (0.47 in) in diameter to give the same stimulus area as the Farnsworth Panel D-15. The large stimulus area corresponds to a visual angle of 3.8 degrees when testing at 50 cm (20 in) and to 6.3 degrees when testing at 30 cm (12 in). The small stimulus is seen as the recommended 1.5-degree stimulus at a distance of 46 cm (18 in). When testing young children or individuals with low vision, testing is often performed at a shorter distance than 30 cm. Thus, the size of the large stimulus becomes 9.5 degrees at 20 cm (8 in) and 19 degrees at 10 cm (4 in).

In adult testing, we ask the patient to choose a cap that is closest in color to the previously chosen cap. This is surprisingly easy for children. Generally, even 5-year-old children with normal color vision are able to arrange the whole test quickly. A child may train for the test situation with the Color Vision Game on the internet (in "Games" at www.lea-test.fi). During the games, the color confusion areas will be noticed. The degree of deficiency must be then investigated using a sorting test. Testing can be made easier by using the following technique:

Explain to the child, "I would arrange these colors in this order." Place the caps one after the other in the correct order. Then say, "This was my way of arranging. Now, let's sort the caps together."

Place the Pilot cap at the left edge of the test area and say," This is always the first cap." Then take it and move it above the other caps that are mixed on the table and ask, "Which one of these caps has nearly the same color?" When the child chooses one by pointing to it, place the Pilot on its place on the table and use the chosen cap the same way as the Pilot cap to find the next cap.

Continue until all caps are sorted. If one or two caps are left over, tell the child, "These we forgot to sort, where would you place them?"

When the child does not need to concentrate on the motor functions, sorting the colors becomes easier.

If the child cannot point, but can make a sound or tap with his hand or foot, place the caps in a row, move first the Pilot, then the other caps along the row and ask the child to indicate when you are at the cap that is closest in color to the one you are moving.

Fewer than four crossings across the color space are usually accepted as normal if there is no definitive axis. Color confusions that occur regularly in a certain direction across the color space, or *axis,* reveal the type of color vision defect. More than four crossings in an axis are recorded as deficient color perception in that axis. The border between mild and moderate color defects is not well defined. The border between moderate and severe color vision deficiencies is usually placed at ten crossings. Different employers and

P-1 ⊖ 15 ⊖ 2-3 ⊖ 14-13-12-11-10-9-8-7-6-5-4

P-1 ⊖ 15-14 ⊖ 2-3 ⊖ 13-12-11-10-9-8-7-6-5-4

FIGURE 2-4. Results of two measurements of color vision of a child. There are only two crossings across the color space with slight variation in the axis.

schools have different limits for color confusions tolerated for specific tasks and careers.

The three axes of color vision defects—*protan, deutan,* and *tritan*—are sometimes called red blindness, green blindness, and blue blindness, but these names are confusing. Persons with color vision deficiencies are not color blind—they just confuse some colors. For example, protanopes and deuteranopes, both confuse some blue and purple shades and certain brown, red, and green shades. Tritanopes match violet with green. It would be wise to discontinue the use of color blindness except in complete achromatopsia. Even then the name "complete achromatopsia" is far more positive than "color blindness."

Recording the Test Results

Lines are drawn to connect the numbers on the recording sheet in the order in which the child has arranged the caps. The results can also be recorded simply by writing down the numbers of the caps in the order that they are arranged. If the tester wants to mark the errors, the errors are circled. This is also the easiest way to record results in a case history. If the test is done twice, as it often is, the results can be written under each other to make it easier to see any variations. For example, please see Fig. 2-4. In this case, there is only a mild uncertainty in the arrangement of the colors, no stable axis, and fewer than four crossings.

ADAPTATION

Visual adaptation is not commonly used when assessing low vision. This is unfortunate because photophobia and delayed adaptation to lower luminance levels are among the most common visual problems in children with low vision. Photophobia can occur also in blind children.

Normally, we can see in bright daylight and in twilight. In daylight or *photopic* vision, we use cone cells while activity in the cone pathway inhibits the rod pathway. When the luminance level becomes lower, input from cone cells decreases and input from rod cells increases (*mesopic* vision). When the luminance level decreases further, the cone cells' contribution to vision stops, colors disappear, and the image is seen in different shades of gray because rod cells do not convey color differences (*scotopic* vision).

When we enter a darker place, it takes a few seconds before we start to see colors at the lower luminance level. This is called *cone adaptation time*. This rapid adaptation to a lower luminance level is possible because cone cells adapt quickly within the range of their adaptation capability. Rod cell adaptation to very dim light is much slower. In retinitis pigmentosa, rod cell adaptation to a threshold level after a sunny day may take more than 24 hours.

In retinal degenerations, cone cell adaptation time can become longer than normal quite early in the course of the degeneration. Therefore, the CONE Adaptation Test was designed to screen for retinitis pigmentosa and follow-up of retinal function in all retinal disorders. It is the only test that is available for testing young children.

The test consists of fifteen 5 × 5 cm (2 × 2 in) red, blue, and white plastic chips designed to help parents, teachers, and doctors become aware of a child's visual difficulties in twilight.

Instructions for the CONE Adaptation Test

1. If the child is able to sort colors, mix up the chips on a dark colored table or black cloth and direct him or her to put them into three separate groups: red, blue, and white. Explain that next time the chips should be sorted into these three groups as soon as possible after the lights have been dimmed.

2. Dim the lights so the child can still see the colors without difficulty and ask the child to sort the chips. Mix the chips again and turn up the lights to the usual room illumination. Tell the child that next time the lights will be very dim but the chips should be sorted as before.

3. Now dim the lights to a level where you can barely see the colors of the chips after an adaptation period of a few (four or five) seconds. The child will pick the white chips first because they are the easiest to see and then will try to separate the blue chips from the red chips. If the child makes a mistake, never say anything about it. Mix the chips while in the dark and then turn up the lights to normal room illumination to come back to photopic functioning and repeat the play situation. If the child has difficulties in the twilight level of illumination, increase the illumination until the colors can be recognized within a few seconds.

This test determines the minimum level of illumination that is adequate for comfortable visual communication and activities of daily life. A child with delayed cone adaptation needs to have a flashlight when sent to get something from a dark place. The way to school is assessed, environmental orientation marks improved, when possible, and the use of a flashlight and long cane techniques evaluated.

A practical test of cone adaptation in assessment of deaf children can be arranged after watching TV during a dark afternoon. When the program is over, the TV set is switched off and the room lights are not turned on. The children are assigned a short question or asked to do something immediately. The child who does not respond is examined for dark adaptation.

Photophobic children need absorptive lenses, regular dark spectacle lenses, or filter lenses, usually more than one pair, if nonphotochromatic lenses are used. Because of variations in the loss of sensory cells, there is no single lens type that can be recommended for all retinitis pigmentosa children. Several absorptive lenses should be tested, preferably by letting the child borrow them for a weekend or longer and deciding for himself or herself which is the best. If photochromatic lenses (Corning) are available, they may be a good choice.

Cosmetic factors are important, especially in teenaged children. It is possible to hide the socially unacceptable but otherwise good red filter lenses with a polarizing surface. Filter lenses with the polarized surface are a pleasant brown (Multilens, Sweden). They are plastic lenses and thus lighter and less breakable than glass lenses. Side shields and upper shields can be made inconspicuous.

Filter lenses should always be tested when there is a loss of cone function. Some of these filter lenses have transmission in blue, so blue cones adapt. If there is no transmission in blue, the sky and other blue surfaces appear dirty gray, which can be an unpleasant or even depressing experience for many people. Transmission of light within the range of rod absorption is minimal, so rods function at the mesopic level. Thus, the filter allows the child to use both cone and rod vision in daylight, which results in better quality of information than if regular absorption lenses were used. Specific absorption in the blue-green part of the spectrum leads to the surprising experience of higher subjective brightness although the filter reduces the amount of light entering the eye. The increase is due to the function of millions of rod cells at the same time as the cone cells are functioning. This can be explained to children as follows, "Rod cells believe that it is twilight and, therefore, function normally; cone cells know that it is daylight and function normally." Most children describe the effect of filter lenses as "the image becomes calm and easy to see." Some notice the decrease of diffraction of blue light and see details more sharply.

COGNITIVE VISION TESTS

In western countries and in some cities of the developing countries, the largest and increasing group of children with vision impairment is the group with cerebral vision impairment (CVI), also called cortical visual impairment or brain damage–related vision loss. The lesion can be only in the visual cortex but often involves both cortical and subcortical functions. The name cerebral visual impairment should be used in those cases. CVI is most common in children with cerebral palsy and intellectual disabilities but occurs also in children who have impaired vision caused by eye disorders like retinopathy of prematurity, or who may have "normal" vision.

CVI is often a hidden vision loss that can be understood first when all visual functions are carefully assessed. We have more than 30 specific cortical visual functions and each of them can be lost without changes in the other cortical visual functions. The *profile of the child's visual function is uneven*, some visual functions are normal, and other functions may be poor or totally lost.

Visual Functions Often Impacting Performance of Children with Cerebral Vision Impairment

When assessing a visually impaired child and in the clinical examination of all children with congenital strabismus or strabismus after encephalitis, asphyxia, or accident, symptoms of CVI should be sought. Among the many symptoms that children with CVI may have, the following ones are common and should be considered.

Oculomotor problems are assessed using regular clinical tests: *fixation, tracking, saccades, convergence, accommodation, and nystagmus.* These signs are described to therapists, teachers, and parents in clear language and preferably recorded on video. Each of these functions should be assessed again at the school or daycare or during therapies together with a vision teacher.

Strabismus is common but rarely a big problem because most children use the central vision of only one eye. A child with alternating use of the eyes can be disturbed by the shifts of fixation in demanding near work. This disturbance can often be avoided if one eye is fitted with a distance lens and the other with near correction. If accommodation is insufficient or spastic, a progressive near correction may lead to the best function.

Increased crowding is diagnosed with a near-vision test: there is better visual acuity with single symbols than with a line test and tightly crowded symbols. When this phenomenon is found in a child who is starting to read, text size for reading needs to be assessed using texts on a computer screen so that the child is allowed to choose the *size of the* that is easiest to see. After that the *spacing* between letters is increased stepwise until the child finds it good. Usually the text size can be decreased somewhat when the spacing is increased.

Contrast sensitivity or visual acuity at low contrast should always be measured because it may be much more affected than visual acuity at high contrast.

Color vision defects are assessed with quantitative tests because the changes are irregular and therefore are not defined by the screening tests. Testing children with different communication problems requires variation in the testing technique.

Photophobia is a common problem in children with optic atrophy. There are several good filter lenses and absorption lenses (sunglasses) that should be evaluated as a part of clinical examinations.

Visual field defects are the most difficult part of the assessment. We can measure the size of the visual field with confrontation perimetry. Often there is detection of movement in the "blind" field half and vision for planning hand movements, i.e., the parietal visual functions have not been lost (7). This is important to know for physical education. Changes within the visual field, small defects or *scotomas*, especially on the right side of the fixation point need to be evaluated if the child makes *unusual errors in reading*. If increasing the size of the text makes the errors to disappear, the child does not have dyslexia but changes in the central visual field. If the lesion is in the anterior visual pathway, the scotoma is in the visual field and may affect saccades, whereas if the lesion is in the posterior visual pathways, saccadic functions can be quite normal.

Motion perception or perceiving visual information that moves can be disturbed. Either the student would have difficulties seeing objects that stand still or difficulties seeing objects that move. If moving objects cannot be seen, traffic, and most games are nearly impossible to cope with. Orientation and mobility training of these children requires an instructor who is well trained in brain damage related functional problems.

Perception of length or orientation of lines can be lost. These visual functions can be assessed using easy test games (Lea Rectangles and Mailbox) and drawing lines of different lengths, parallel ones, and lines that form angles and crosses. A child may not see length or orientation of lines but could still be able to use this information for hand movements.

Recognition of facial features is a socially important function that can be lost. If the parents and the therapists are aware of this possibility, they can make the diagnosis often when the infant is 11 months old. An infant with loss of face recognition does not respond differently to known and unknown people when they approach without saying anything, but responds differently to voices of known and unknown people. It is important to recognize this early and work on training this ability and on compensating strategies to prevent frustrations in communication situations.

Recognition of facial expressions can be difficult either because the image quality is poor, contrast sensitivity is so low that the faint shadows that convey expressions are not seen, or that at the cortical level there is a loss of perception of expressions.

Perception of surface qualities is an often-missed problem, although it is easy to detect. Often, a child who does not perceive differences in surfaces will explore shadows with their feet before stepping onto them or onto irregular surfaces. Although this child may have "good" central vision measured by visual acuity and contrast sensitivity testing, he or she might find a benefit in using long cane techniques.

Picture perception and comprehension understanding vary and are important to assess, especially if pictures are used to support communication. A student may not be able to see complicated pictures although parts of the same picture can be perceived when shown in isolation. *Composing a whole picture of its parts* may be a lost ability in an otherwise well functioning student.

Perception of depth should not be confused with stereovision in that it can be achieved through a number of monocular skills. Stereovision is a small part of visual information that we use to experience three-dimensionality. Motion parallax or perception of relative movement of objects at different distances, shadowing, partial occlusion of objects behind other objects, and perspective, or relative size of known objects, convey information on depth and are important skills.

Spatial awareness and orientation in space are disturbed in parietal lobe lesions. These functions can also be poorly developed in children who cannot move but have always been moved passively. Orientation and mobility training of a student who has CVI and who uses a wheelchair is a special area that requires a well trained instructor willing to carefully observe what the child can perceive in the environment and how that information is interpreted. Careful testing of auditory spatial concepts and visual memory are an integral part of the assessment of vision.

Eye–hand coordination (vision–hand coordination) can also be affected in parietal lesions. These defects can be associated with a clumsiness that is caused by poor visual maps for hand movements. Some children with CVI turn their head away from the object they try to reach. This may be related to poor visual feedback during the movement. If the student is able to perform the task better with eyes closed than with eyes open, visual information disturbs motor performance instead of making it more precise.

Simultan agnosia occurs in CVI and means that the child can direct attention to only one detail or object at a time. This condition makes visual field measurement difficult because during the standard testing, the child must look straight ahead and observe when a light or fingers appears on the side.

Effect of posture on the use of vision needs to be assessed together with the child's therapist and teacher. When head control is poor, use of multimedia goggles (virtual reality glasses) can be considered.

Neuropsychological testing is important in each case of CVI although several difficulties can be observed and evaluated during therapies and in other teaching situations. Neuropsychological tests may need to be modified to meet the needs of the student in terms of contrast, size, and number of details to be seen at one time.

Step-by-step assessment by ophthalmologists, optometrists, psychologists, a child's special teachers, therapists, and, later, classroom teachers and teacher's aids guided by a vision teacher, is instrumental in completing the overall clinical visual assessment. The team at the school and in daycare needs only a few new tests to perform a comprehensive functional assessment when supported by a vision teacher and when working in collaboration with a pediatric ophthalmologist, retina specialist, and an intervention team.

If information about CVI is available at clinics, private offices, daycare centers, and schools for all those who are involved in the education and care of children with CVI, the services would improve without additional cost. In many cases, sound common sense is used to assess children's problems.

It is much easier to understand the often-puzzling behaviors of children with CVI if we know a few basic facts about the visual pathways (Fig. 2-5) and functions of the visual cortices (8). There are key features to know and to teach parents and those involved with the care and education of the child: (i) the parallel visual pathways make it possible for some parts of the brain to receive visual information when other parts are damaged, and (ii) the brain cortex has more than 30 specialized areas that handle specific parts of visual information. We do not need to know where exactly these specific small areas are located but we do need to know that each of these areas can be damaged by a localized lesion that does not interfere with the other visual areas.

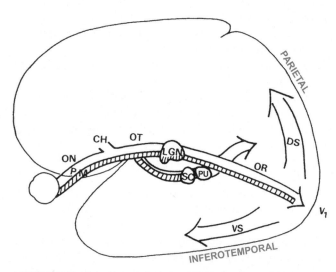

FIGURE 2-5. This picture is a simplified drawing of the visual pathways. We usually think of visual pathways as the retinocalcarine pathway, the pathway from the retina to the primary visual cortex, V$_1$, located at the calcarine sulcus in the back of the brain. Midway in this pathway is the lateral geniculate nucleus (LGN) where the first nerve cell passes the information to the second nerve cell. The other pathway, the tectal pathway, leaves the main pathway before the LGN and brings visual information to several nuclei. The most important among them is the superior colliculus (SC) the center for the rapid saccadic movements. Another important relay station is the pulvinar nucleus (PU) from where the information gets to the cortical areas in the parietal and occipital lobe, without having gone through the form analysis in V$_1$. Because of the presence of two parallel visual pathways, some areas of brain may get normal visual information via the tectal pathway when the main pathway is damaged in its posterior part. The two main directions of the flow of the visual information are called the dorsal stream (DS) toward the posterior parietal lobe where we have visual functions related to orientation in space and to eye–hand coordination, and the ventral stream (VS) toward the inferior temporal lobe where we have numerous recognition related functions.

REFERENCES

1. Hyvärinen L. Assessment of visually impaired infants. In: Colenbrander A, Fletcher DC, eds. *Low vision and vision rehabilitation. Ophthalmol Clin North Am* 1994:219–226.
2. Jacobson L. Visual dysfunction and ocular signs associated with periventricular leukomalacia in children born preterm [thesis]. Stockholm, 1998.
3. Jan JE, Groenveld M, Sykanda AM, et al. Behavioural characteristics of children with permanent cortical visual impairment. *Dev Med Child Neurol* 1987; 29:571–576.
4. Colenbrander A. Consilium Ophthalmologicum Universale Visual Functions Committee, visual acuity measurement standard. *Ital J Ophthalmol* 1988;2:5–19.
5. Humphrey NK. Vision in a monkey without striate cortex: a case study. *Perception* 1974;3:241–255.
6. Hyvärinen L. Paediatric visual acuity testing in low vision. In: Stuen C, Arditi A, Horowitz A, et al, eds. *Vision rehabilitation, assessment, intervention and outcomes.* Lissa: Swets & Zeitlinger, 2000.
7. Hyvärinen L, Raninen AN, Näsänen RE. Vision rehabilitation in homonymous hemianopia. *Neuroophthalmology* 2002;27:97–102.
8. Milner AD, Goodale MA. *The visual brain in action.* Oxford: Oxford University Press, 1995.

RECOMMENDED READING

1. Adelson E, Fraiberg S. Gross motor development in infants blind from birth. *Child Dev* 1974;45:114–126.
2. Ashmead DH, Hill EW, Talor CR. Obstacle perception by congenitally blind children. *Percept Psychophys* 1989;46:425–433.
3. Baird SM, Mayfield P, Baker P. Mothers' interpretations of the behavior of their infants with visual and other impairments during interactions. *J Vis Impair Blindness* 1997;91:467–483.
4. Barraga NC, Collins ME. Development of efficiency in visual functioning: rationale for a comprehensive program. *J Vis Impair Blindness* 1979;73:121–126.
5. Hof-van-Duin J, Heersema DJ, Groenendaal F, et al. Visual field and grating acuity development in low-risk preterm infants during the first 2.5 years after term. *Behav Brain Res* 1992;49:115–122.
6. McConachie HR, Moore V. Early expressive language of severely visually impaired children. *Dev Med Child Neurol* 1994;36:230–240.
7. Porro GL. Vision and visual behaviour in responsive and unresponsive neurologically impaired children. Utrecht: Brouwer Uithof, 1998.

EXAMINATION OF PEDIATRIC RETINAL FUNCTION

ANNE B. FULTON
RONALD M. HANSEN

This chapter describes the function of the immature retina in infants and children. Studies of function disclose information about activity of cells and even molecules in the living child's retina. On one hand, results of these studies may yield insights into the action of protein products of genes, and on the other hand, may explain visual behavior. The numeric data provide the basis for making comparisons over time in an individual patient, and for making comparisons between individuals or groups. Coupled with clinical examination, including careful ophthalmoscopy, studies of function lead to secure diagnoses, and support good management of infants and children with retinal diseases. Additionally, this combined approach has led to new knowledge about pediatric retinal disease and will continue to do so.

Ophthalmoscopy is primarily used to assess the retina in infants and children. Standardized systems have been developed to capture and categorize ophthalmoscopic observations (1–5). Analyses of these categorical data have led to tremendous advances in the understanding and management of diseases such as retinopathy of prematurity (ROP) (6–12). But it is the continuous, numeric data that result from tests of function that link the patient's condition to cellular and molecular events in the retina, and to visual behavior. Information about retinal function holds promise of further understanding of fundamental disease processes (13–26).

Retinal function depends on the physical properties of the eye and retina. The physical properties change with development. In this chapter we describe the physical development of the normal retina during the ages that are of direct clinical importance, from late gestation, when ROP has its onset, through infancy and early childhood. Investigations of function, constrained by physical immaturity, provide a body of information about the development of human retinal processes (27–39). Furthermore, these data define age-specific normal values of parameters of retinal function against which patients' data can be compared. In this chapter, we focus on those retinal functions that we use most frequently to assess our patients. We present some results from patients with ROP, retinal degenerative conditions, and the stationary conditions, achromatopsia and congenital stationary night blindness. These conditions cause visual impairment that brings infants to us as diagnostic dilemmas, the most basic dilemma being: Can this child's visual impairment be due to disease of the eye, the brain, or both?

NORMAL DEVELOPMENT

Development of Structure

Development of the retina (Table 3-1) continues after term as does growth of the eye (40–42). The retinal area in a preterm infant, aged 24 weeks, is less than a third of that of adults. By term, total retinal area is approximately 60% of the average retinal area in adults. And it follows that the volume of the globe increases enormously. The volume of the globe of a 6-year-old child is eight times that of the 24-week-old preterm infant.

Few mitoses are found in the retina at term, indicating nearly all retinal cells are present. Thus, with postterm growth of the globe, and in particular growth of the posterior segment, an expanding surface area is paved by the same number of retinal cells. The macular area remains constant through development, but the peripheral retinal area increases (43–45). A clinical consequence of this is observed. The indentation from encircling elements appears more posterior and surgical drainage sites placed quite posterior in early infancy appear more anterior at older ages.

The last cells to differentiate are the photoreceptors, and the photoreceptor outer segments are the last retinal structures to develop (46). Thus, the outer segments place a notable constraint on the development of retinal function. Hendrickson and colleagues have charted the development of simian photoreceptors (43–45,47,48), and found the major features are similar in human retina (44,49).

TABLE 3-1. EYE SIZE AND TOTAL RETINAL AREA 40–42

Age (weeks)	Corneal Diameter (mm)	Equatorial Diameter of Globe (mm)	Total Retinal Area (mm^2)	Volume of Globe (mm^3)
24	6.5	11.5	300	796
40 (term)	10	16.5	600	2,352
6 yr	11.5	23.0	900	6,371

The expansion of retinal area leads to a developmental redistribution of the photoreceptor cells. This creates a ring having a high density of rod cells (45). The rod ring is concentric with the fovea, and located 15 to 20 degrees eccentric to it at the location of the optic nerve head. At preterm ages, outer segments are first detectable at the posterior pole, then gradually appear in more peripheral retina. Developmental elongation of the outer segments becomes very rapid at preterm ages and continues postterm. The outer segments elongate by addition of newly manufactured discs to the base of the outer segments, that part nearest to the center of the cell. The elements of the discs are assembled in the inner segments. The discs at the tip of the outer segment are the oldest, and these are regularly discarded (50). In development, the net effect is the addition of new discs (51).

However, even in the immature outer segment, old discs are discarded from the tips as more are added at the base (52). The absorbance of light by the immature discs at the tip is less than at the base (53), possibly because the spacing between the most immature discs at the tip is large.

As each rod acquires more discs per outer segment, consequent axial density of rhodopsin and probability of photon capture increase (29,31,54–56). Photon capture activates rhodopsin and sets in motion the transduction cascade that activates the photoreceptor cell to signal the response to light (57–59). Contemporary electroretinogram (ERG) procedures assess the photoresponse (60,61).

Development of Function

Psychophysical and electrophysiological tests have been devised for assessment of retinal function in infants and children. The most important requirement of the tests is that the stimulus controls events in the retina, and thus controls the behavioral, or electrical, response of the patient's retina. Stimulus control depends on measurement of the stimulus in physical units, estimation of the effectiveness of the stimulus on the photoreceptors, and careful control of retinal adaptation. Developmental changes in eye size, media density, and visual pigment content must be taken into account (30–32,62,63).

Special expertise is required in the setup of an electrophysiology unit, procedures for performance of the tests, and analysis of the test results (64–66). The major components of a functioning unit are the equipment, the professional and physical requirements of the facility, housing the setup, and the knowledge and experience of the electrophysiologist gathering and interpreting the data. The designs of commercial systems are constantly being updated as technical advances are exploited for the good of the system and its application. The other ingredients (e.g., facility, electrophysiologist) can vary. All components must be considered in setting up the unit. In this chapter, the main concepts guiding tests of retinal function in pediatric patients are given.

Electroretinography

The molecular and cellular events in the photoreceptors and postreceptoral retina are registered in the components of the ERG. The responses of young infants and adults differ as the sample records in Figure 3-1 illustrate. The a- and b-waves are observed in the intact ERG response (Figs. 3-1 and 3-2), which is the sum of receptoral and postreceptoral retinal responses (67–70). The photoreceptors' response to light is now sufficiently understood that explicit mathematical models (Fig. 3-2) of the molecular events in the photoreceptors can be applied to the a-wave component of the ERG recorded from healthy subjects and those with retinal disease (23–25,59,71,72). Subtraction of the receptoral component, represented by the a-wave, from the intact ERG reveals postreceptoral retinal activity, and is designated P2 (23,24,69,70). The isolated P2 component may be a clearer representation of postreceptoral activity than the b-wave (23,24). The postreceptoral responses originate in bipolar and other second and third-order retinal cells (73–78). The on-bipolar cells have their own G-protein cascade (76,79).

Rod and cone photoreceptor activities and also postreceptoral activity undergo developmental changes that continue after term. For the rod and rod-mediated responses, it is known that developmental changes occur over the age range during which rhodopsin content increases (27,30). Developmental increases in rod cell sensitivity, rod-mediated postreceptoral sensitivity, and rod-mediated visual sensitivity are shown in Figure 3-3. Note the lag in development of parafoveal rod-mediated sensitivity (Fig. 3-3C) in accord with the lag in development of parafoveal rod outer segments (48).

Cone and cone-mediated ERG responses to full-field stimuli (Fig. 3-4A) mature earlier than rod- mediated responses (80,81). With the exception of those in the fovea, cones mature earlier than the rods (82,83). Foveal cones

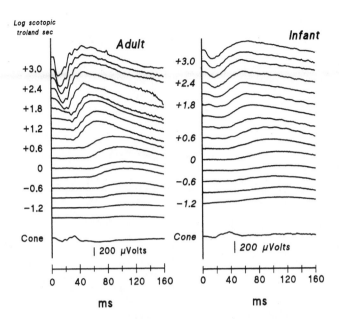

FIGURE 3-1. Normal ERG responses to a brief (<1 msec), blue (λ < 510 nm) flash. Sample records from an adult (left panel) and a 10-week-old infant (right panel) are shown. The numbers to the left of the traces indicate the stimulus in units of retinal illuminance, log scotopic troland seconds. For clarity, only every other trace is labeled. Specification of the stimulus took into account pupillary diameter, eye size, and transmissivity of the ocular media. The amplitude of the responses increases, and the time to the peak of deflections (implicit times) decreases with increasing flash intensity. Note that the amplitudes of the infant's responses are smaller, and are not evoked by such dim flashes as in the adult.

have a protracted course of development that extends into childhood (43,44,84). After early infancy, normal, developing acuity (Fig. 3-4B) is limited by the immaturity of the fovea (44,85–87).

Psychophysics

Psychophysical measures are actually specialized tests of vision. Psychophysical tests are designed to enable investigators to draw conclusions about processes in the visual system. For studies of pediatric retinal function, preferential looking methods are used (33). Psychophysical procedures sample function in selected, small retinal areas. This contrasts full-field electroretinography, which samples the function of the retina as a whole. Thus, the psychophysical thresholds are particularly suitable for assessment of regional variations in retinal sensitivity (Fig. 3-3C).

A number of laboratories find higher dark-adapted thresholds in young infants than in adults (33,88–92). Higher thresholds mean lower sensitivity. However, the evidence does not support higher infantile thresholds being caused by cone intrusion. For conditions in which the thresholds are rod mediated in adults, the spectral sensitivity function in infants is also described by the scotopic luminous efficiency function (35,63,90,91).

Psychophysical studies of adaptation to background light, temporal summation, spatial summation, and center-surround organization have demonstrated significant immaturities of rod and rod-mediated postreceptoral processes in young infants (28,36,37,89,92). The curious pattern of immature temporal summation is attributable to photoreceptor immaturity (28). Postreceptoral immaturities are demonstrated by the infantile patterns of spatial summation and center-surround organization (36,89,92,93). Larger receptive fields and larger excitatory centers appear to be the basis for the infantile results.

Psychophysical tests are noninvasive and readily applied to the study of pediatric patients with retinal disorders (3, 94–96). In cases with markedly attenuated ERG responses, reliable psychophysical responses can be obtained (3,94). ERG responses are exquisitely sensitive to photoreceptor dysfunction. Thus, the ERG responses may be nondetectable even when there is considerable visual function remaining. In patients with progressive disorders who are not able to participate in awake ERG testing, retinal function may be monitored by measuring the dark-adapted visual threshold, while ERG testing under anesthesia performed less frequently (97–99).

RETINAL FUNCTION IN RETINAL DISORDERS

Pediatric retinal disorders almost always have some impact on vision. Therefore, visual abnormalities are frequent presenting complaints, with the notable exception of ROP that is identified by ophthalmic examination in the nursery. With the exception of ROP, conspicuous visual inattention (apparent blindness), or nystagmus, may herald retinal disease. Ophthalmologists and neurologists are consulted about the visual inattention and nystagmus. The task is to determine if there is eye or brain disease, or some other disorder. Other less severely abnormal visual behaviors such as photosensitivity, night blindness, or holding things too close instigate referral. A coordinated approach that does not ignore the child's medical condition, and which includes evaluation of retinal function using electrophysiological and psychophysical tests, characterizes the child's vision and helps to secure a diagnosis. Application of this approach to pediatric retinal disorders is given in the following examples. Some of the disorders are acquired, such as ROP. Some are heritable and have stable vision while others have slowly progressive loss of vision. No matter what the final diagnosis, visually impaired infants and children must be given the benefit of educational and other support services.

Retinopathy of Prematurity

ROP has its onset at preterm ages during which outer segments grow long and rhodopsin content increases at a rapid pace (8,31,44) (Fig. 3-5A). Active ROP runs its course over

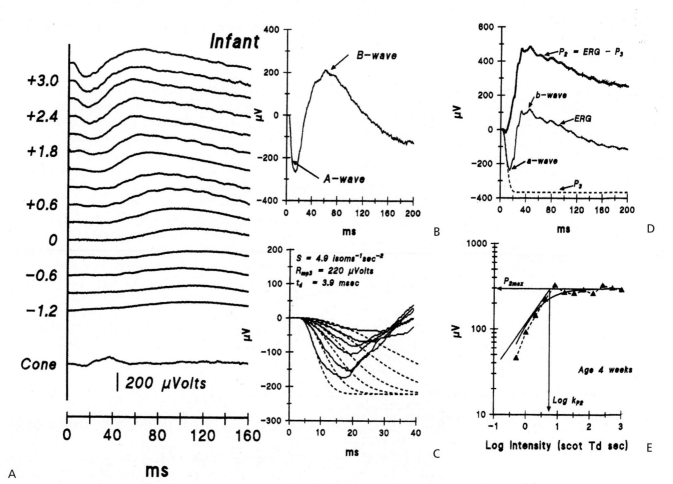

FIGURE 3-2. Sample ERG records. **(A)** Responses from a full-term 10-week-old infant to a series of flashes (replotted from Figure 1). **(B)** The intact ERG response. The corneal negative deflection, the a-wave, reflects the initial activity in the rod photoreceptor cells. The corneal positive b-wave represents the sum of the responses of the rod photoreceptor plus postreceptoral cells. **(C)** The a-wave is replotted with an expanded time scale. The dashed lines represent a model of the activation of phototransduction fit to these data (30,59,61,71). The a-wave results from a series of biochemical events that lead to the rod cell signaling a response to light. A photon isomerizes a molecule of rhodopsin, which is followed by sequential activation of the other proteins in the cascade with consequent closure of the cyclic nucleotide–gated (cG) channel in the outer segment membrane and a reduction in the current circulating the inner and outer segments. This produces the a-wave. A mathematical model of these events,

$$R(I,t) = R_{mp3} * (1 - \exp[-0.5\, S\, I\, (t - t_d)^2])$$

is fit to the a-wave (59,71,72). I is the flash intensity in isomerizations/rod/flash, and t_d a brief delay. S is a gain parameter that depends on the time constants of the reactions in the cascade, from photon capture by rhodopsin to closure of the cG-regulated channel in the outer segment membrane. R_{mp3} is the saturated amplitude of the rod response and reflects the number of channels in the outer segment membrane available for closure by light. **(D)** Postreceptoral responses. In an analysis reminiscent of that of Granit (67,68), the intact ERG waveform is considered to be the sum of the photoreceptor and post receptoral retinal responses (23–25,65,66,69,70). The rod photoreceptor response, derived from the a-wave, is digitally subtracted from the intact ERG waveform to obtain P_2, which represents postreceptoral activity. **(E)** The amplitude of the P_2 response is plotted as a function of stimulus intensity. The P_2 stimulus/response function is fit with

$$P_2/P_{2max} = I/(I + K_{p2})$$

where P_{2max} is the saturated amplitude and K_{p2} is the semisaturation constant.

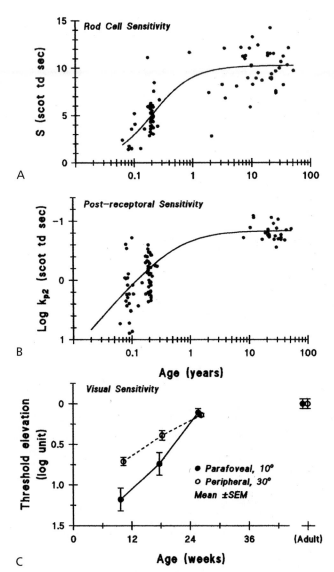

FIGURE 3-3. Development of rod and rod-mediated function. **(A)** Rod cell sensitivity, S, as a function of age; replotted from Fulton and Hansen (30). Data from 89 subjects are shown. S is obtained by analysis of the ERG a-wave responses to full field stimuli as described in Figure 2. The normal developmental increase in S, and also R_{mp3}, is indistinguishable from that for rhodopsin (30,31). **(B)** Postreceptoral sensitivity, represented by log kp2, is plotted as a function of age. Data from 92 subjects are shown. **(C)** Dark-adapted rod mediated visual thresholds as a function of age [replotted from Hansen and Fulton (38)]. Maturation at the parafoveal site lags that at the more peripheral site as does development of the rod outer segments (49,174). Thresholds at both sites approach adult levels by age 6 months. These thresholds are measured using a modification of the preferential looking procedures (33,35,66,68). Two 2° diameter retinal sites are tested, a parafoveal spot 10° eccentric, and a more peripheral spot, 30° eccentric. Test conditions were selected so that adults' thresholds at the two sites were equal.

the weeks during which development of the outer segments and rhodopsin content is most rapid. Involution of active ROP begins at about term and is complete a few weeks after that (7). Thus, it is not surprising that the photoreceptors are involved in the disease process.

Rod photoreceptor involvement in ROP has been demonstrated by ERG and psychophysical procedures (26,95,96, 100,101). For example, some children who had mild ROP showed elevated psychophysical thresholds years after the ROP resolved (96). In a study of background adaptation in adolescents with a history of mild ROP (95) parafoveal thresholds were shifted in such a fashion as to indicate involvement of the photoreceptors in the ROP disease process (95). Among infants and children with more severe ROP, threshold abnormalities appear more marked than in those with mild ROP (102). Furthermore, evidence of the retinal origins of threshold deficits lies in the ERG abnormalities documented in the same patients. (95,101,103,104).

In infants and children with a history of ROP (Fig. 3-5B), deficits in rod photoreceptor sensitivity, derived from ERG a-waves, varied significantly with severity of ROP (26). The basis for the photoreceptor dysfunction is demonstrated in experimental studies. In a rat model of ROP, the rod outer segments are disorganized (105). Additionally, experimental evidence suggests that the oxygen-greedy photoreceptors (106) are among the factors in the developing retina that instigate ROP (26,107).

Retinal Degenerations

Leber Congenital Amaurosis or Congenital Retinal Blindness

In Leber congenital amaurosis (LCA) or congenital retinal blindness, the patient has ERG responses that are markedly attenuated in infancy (94). The infant presents with roving eye movements, sluggish pupillary responses, and conspicuous visual inattention. Sluggish pupillary responses are the rule, but at times are difficult to judge. Nearly all are hyperopic (108) although not necessarily outside of the limits for normal infants (109). Ophthalmoscopic abnormalities may be minimal (94,110).

Nondetectable ERG responses are considered diagnostic of LCA (Fig. 3-6). Nevertheless, interpretation of the ERG responses from young infants must be done with caution because the young infants' ERG responses are normally small (80). Figure 3-1 reminds us of the importance of testing with a range of stimuli of sufficient intensity to evoke reliable responses. Signal averaging may also be helpful. Even repeating the ERG test a little later in infancy may be considered another strategy to obtain valid ERG records from infants (80,111). And, of course, the ERG equipment should include provision for a systems check that the equipment is functioning properly.

In our experience about a third of patients with LCA have no light perception and no measurable dark-adapted thresh-

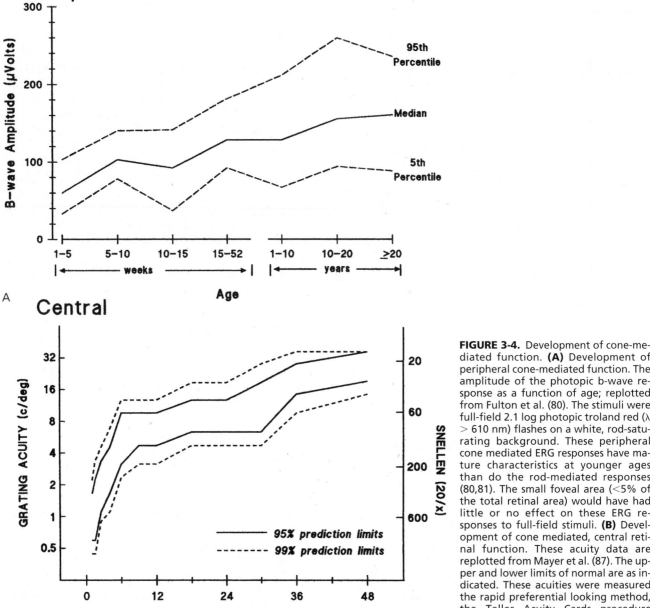

FIGURE 3-4. Development of cone-mediated function. **(A)** Development of peripheral cone-mediated function. The amplitude of the photopic b-wave response as a function of age; replotted from Fulton et al. (80). The stimuli were full-field 2.1 log photopic troland red (λ > 610 nm) flashes on a white, rod-saturating background. These peripheral cone mediated ERG responses have mature characteristics at younger ages than do the rod-mediated responses (80,81). The small foveal area (<5% of the total retinal area) would have had little or no effect on these ERG responses to full-field stimuli. **(B)** Development of cone mediated, central retinal function. These acuity data are replotted from Mayer et al. (87). The upper and lower limits of normal are as indicated. These acuities were measured the rapid preferential looking method, the Teller Acuity Cards procedure (87,175).

old (94). Among those with light perception and measurable thresholds, the dark-adapted thresholds are significantly elevated, but often remain stable for many years (94). In others, thresholds slowly worsen. Examples of longitudinal data in children with LCA are shown in Figure 3-6.

Several genes have been associated with uncomplicated LCA and more, surely, remain to be discovered (112–125). Uncomplicated LCA means disease limited to the eyes without metabolic or independent systemic abnormalities.

Metabolic disorders and neurological disease at times present with the ophthalmic and ERG constellation of congenital retinal blindness (23). Thus, MRI studies of the brain and consultation with a pediatric neurologist as well as with experts in metabolic disorders are indicated in some patients with congenital retinal blindness.

Bardet-Biedl Syndrome

In contrast to retinal degenerations due to diseases expressed only in the eyes, such as many forms of LCA or the common forms of retinitis pigmentosa, retinal degenerations can be associated with systemic disorders (e.g., the degeneration of the nervous system present in neuronal ceroid lipofuscinosis). Examples of syndromic retinal degenerations are

Alstrom, Cohen, and Bardet-Biedl syndromes. The visual difficulties or accompanying features lead to presentation in the pediatric age range. Altogether, these "retinal degenerations plus" disorders are seen more frequently in pediatric retinal practice than are the common forms of retinal degeneration without systemic involvement. Among children with syndromic retinal degenerations, behavioral or cognitive impairments can be present. Despite this, valid dark adapted thresholds can be obtained (3,126) and contemporary ERG recordings are feasible and valid even if best done under light anesthesia (127).

ERG and threshold (3) results in children with Bardet-Biedl syndrome (BBS) are illustrated in Figure 3-7. Signifi-

cant and often marked attenuation of ERG responses is found even in infancy and early childhood, and is often used to secure the diagnosis as the retinal degeneration is a nearly constant feature of BBS whereas polydactyly and genitourinary anomalies are less constant features (Fig. 3-7A) (see also Chapter 10). Thresholds from children with BBS are shown Figures 3-7B and 3-7C. The dark-adapted threshold provided a means of monitoring retinal function, even though from the time of the initial evaluation nearly all the patients had markedly attenuated ERG responses to full-field stimuli.

Minor but statistically significant ERG abnormalities are found in individuals heterozygous for BBS (24), and at times may pose a diagnostic issue as to whether a child has

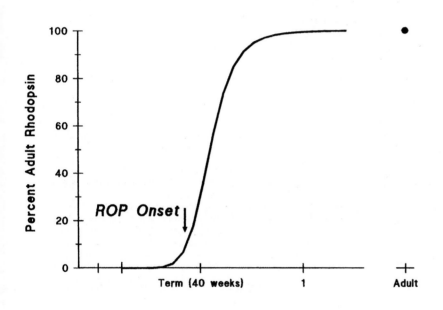

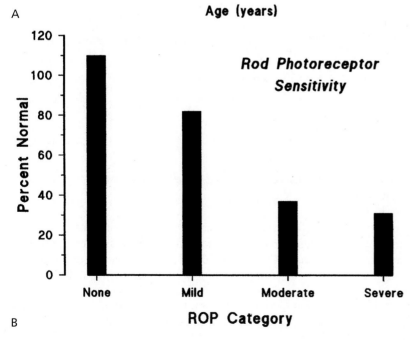

FIGURE 3-5. Retinopathy of prematurity (ROP). **(A)** A logistic growth curve represents the developmental increase in rhodopsin (31). The arrows indicate the age (32 weeks after conception) of onset of prethreshold ROP (8). Involution of ROP begins just before term and ends in the postterm weeks (7). **(B)** Mean rod cell sensitivity, S, for children with a history of ROP categorized as none, mild, moderate, or severe. Replotted from Fulton et al. (26).

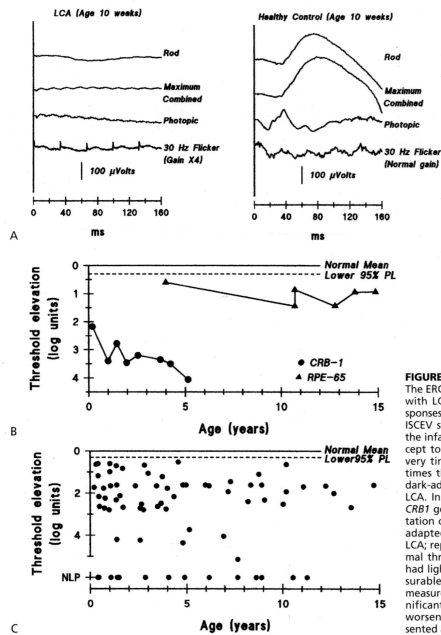

FIGURE 3-6. Leber congenital amaurosis (LCA). **(A)** The ERG responses of two infants, age 10 weeks, one with LCA and the other a healthy infant. The responses are to the selected stimuli designated by the ISCEV standards (176). Even with signal averaging, the infant with LCA had no detectable responses except to the 30-Hz flickering stimulus, and this was very tiny (barely visible when displayed with four times the gain). **(B)** Longitudinal measures of the dark-adapted visual threshold in two patients with LCA. In one, the disease is due to mutation of the *CRB1* gene (118). In the other, disease is due to mutation of the *RPE65* gene (121). **(C)** Results of dark-adapted visual threshold tests in 36 children with LCA; replotted from Fulton et al. (94). None had normal thresholds. About a third of the sample never had light perception (NLP). Among those with measurable thresholds, children had up to nine serial measurements of threshold. In most there was no significant worsening, but five did show significant worsening (94) as did the child with *CRB1* represented above.

early signs of the syndrome or is merely heterozygous for it. Studies of heterozygotes offer a strategy for studying molecular mechanisms in the living subject and disclosing the action of gene products, not only in BBS but also in other disorders in which the affected individual's retinal function is too compromised to be amenable to analysis of function.

Several genes have been associated with BBS syndrome (128–142). The variation in the genetic cause may account in part for the broad distribution of thresholds in BBS (Fig. 3-7C).

Anomalies of Retinal Function

Achromatopsia

In the infant with achromatopsia, rod-mediated scotopic ERG responses are essentially normal in infancy and remain normal. On the other hand, cone-mediated ERG responses assessed using red stimuli on a steady, white, rod-saturating background are significantly attenuated or nearly nondetectable (Fig. 3-8). Rod-mediated dark-adapted visual thresholds are normal and remain normal.

Infants with achromatopsia present with nystagmus and unusual visual behavior or inattention. The early infantile nystagmus in achromatopsia may not be the small amplitude, horizontal, high frequency "jelly-like" nystagmus that is quite typical in older patients with achromatopsia. The early nystagmus may look a bit chaotic and feature vertical components. Photophobia certainly becomes a main feature as the child begins to crawl or ambulate independently. The intensity of the photophobia may not be appreciated until the child is old enough to ambulate and is exposed to sunlight out-of-doors. Orientation and mobility instruction are important for such children.

Typically paradoxical pupillary constriction to darkness is present even after infancy. If the excursion of the paradoxical pupillary response is small, a simple infrared video system can be helpful in documenting it. Hyperopia is common. The fundi are considered normal although some may have diminished foveal reflexes. Ophthalmic and ERG fea-

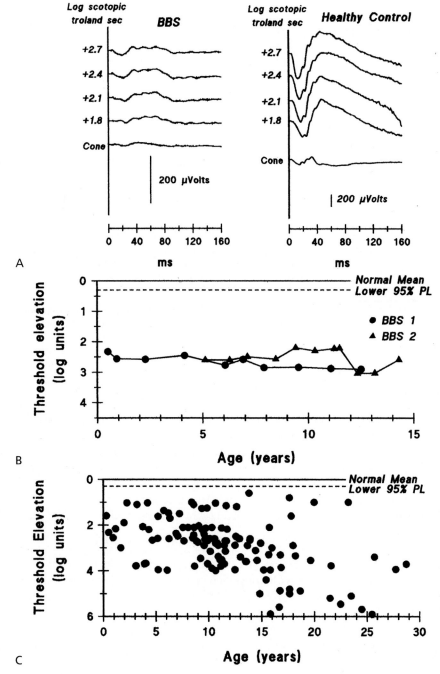

FIGURE 3-7. Retinal function in patients with Bardet-Biedl Syndrome (BBS). **(A)** Rod-mediated ERG responses of a child with BBS are compared to those of a healthy control subject. The responses to selected full-field stimuli illustrate the conspicuous difference in the responses of the two children. The stimuli are those designated in the ISCEV standards. Note the calibration bar for the BBS records is four times longer than the control. **(B)** The dark-adapted visual thresholds of two children with BBS1 (141). One has been followed since early infancy, one since age 5 years. There was significant impairment of night vision even at the initial measurements. However, for more than a decade, the thresholds have remained quite stable, within 1 log unit of the initial results. In both the ERG responses were markedly attenuated. The thresholds in these two children contrast those in some other children with BBS who show progressive worsening in the same age range. **(C)** Dark-adapted visual thresholds in 20 patients with BBS; replotted from Fulton et al. (3). Note that the horizontal axis spans twice as many years as in the middle panel. Over the long haul, a gradual decline in night vision with age is found.

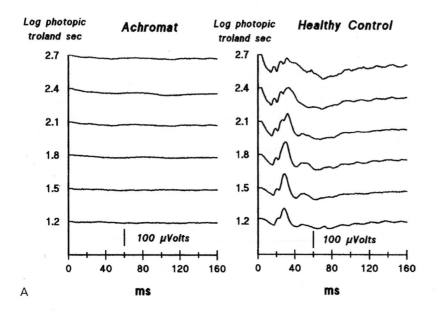

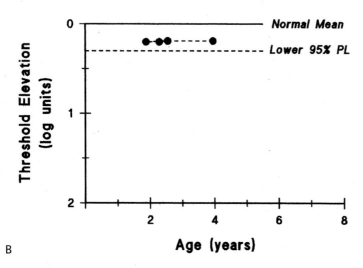

FIGURE 3-8. Cone-mediated ERG responses and dark-adapted thresholds in infants and children with achromatopsia. **(A)** The cone-mediated ERG response to red flashes was recorded while the patient was adapted to a steady white background that suppressed rod responses. The responses of the child with achromatopsia are markedly attenuated. **(B)** Longitudinal rod-mediated thresholds in a child with achromatopsia. The thresholds are normal and stable.

tures do not necessarily distinguish pediatric patients with achromatopsia from those with early cone–rod degenerations. Therefore, careful monitoring of the eyes and vision of children with achromatopsia is recommended.

In early infancy the acuity measured by preferential looking procedures may not be measurable, or may be near the lower limits of normal for age. A discrepancy between acuity measured in normal room light and that in dim room light is often observed with the better acuity being obtained in dim room light. Once the child reaches the age at which acuity can be measured with symbols or letters, moderate to marked reductions, at times to about 20/200 with correction are typically found. The ability to discriminate color is affected; the severity of the color vision deficit varies widely among those with the clinical diagnosis of achromatopsia, perhaps not surprising because detailed psychophysical studies of mature subjects with achromatopsia show a range of reductions in cone-mediated functions (143). Interestingly, functional

magnetic resonance imaging (MRI) studies demonstrate anomalous organization of the cortical maps in an adult with achromatopsia (144), suggesting that early, anomalous retinal inputs shape the organization of the cortex. Mutations in the genes for cone transducin (145,146) and the cone cyclic nucleotide gated cation channel (147–151) have been identified in individuals with achromatopsia.

Congenital Stationary Night Blindness

In common with the infants having achromatopsia, at times those with congenital stationary night blindness (CSNB) present with visual inattention and nystagmus. Whereas daytime vision is impaired in achromatopsia, night vision, that is vision in dim light, is impaired in those with CSNB. Infants with CSNB are reported to grope for their bottle in dim light, or to become content when the room lights are put on. Such a history, along with demonstration of a paradoxical pupillary constriction to darkness and myopia in infancy, is suggestive of CSNB. Among healthy, young children with normal eyes, any myopia is exceedingly rare (109).

Among infants with CSNB whom we have followed up, in early infancy only low myopia is found. Over the ensuing preschool years, the degree of myopia increases. In CSNB, the dark-adapted psychophysical threshold is elevated. The dark-adapted threshold is expected to remain stable, although some worsening of thresholds has been reported in adults with CSNB (152). Letter acuities are typically in the 20/40 to 20/60 range. Strabismus is common in CSNB. For patients with complete CSNB, the ERG response is characterized by a nearly normal a-wave, but a markedly attenuated b-wave whereas incomplete CSNB has more robust b-waves. The density and kinetics of rhodopsin bleaching and regeneration are normal (153,154).

The molecular bases for X-linked and autosomal forms of CSNB have been reported (155–160). Autosomally in-herited forms have been associated with mutations in three of the transduction cascade proteins including rhodopsin (161–164), transducin (165,166), and phosphodiesterase (167–169). The X-linked forms are separated into complete and incomplete CSNB based on retinal function of the affected males. However, overlap of phenotypes is recognized (170–173). The incomplete X-linked (*CSNB2*) is due to the calcium-channel gene *CACNA1F* on *Xp11.23*. B-waves are recordable, but have decreased amplitudes. Clinical variability even among individuals with the same mutation is documented; at least one of the major features (night blindness, myopia, nystagmus) was absent in 72% of the patients (170). Complete X-linked (*CSNB1*) is due to the gene *NYX*, "nyctalopin." The affected males have decreased scotopic b-wave amplitudes and mildly abnormal photopic ERG responses. There is absence of rod dark adaptation and elevated dark-adapted visual thresholds (Fig. 3-9).

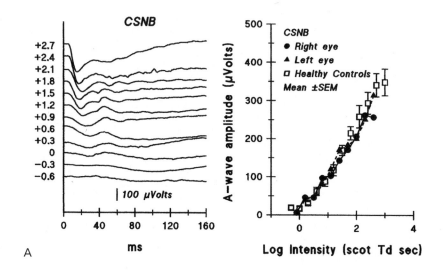

A

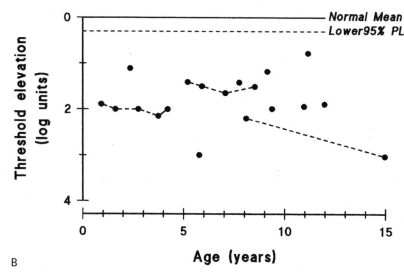

B

FIGURE 3-9. ERG responses and dark-adapted visual thresholds in children with congenital stationary night blindness (CSNB). **(A)** Rod and rod-mediated ERG responses in a child with CSNB. The responses have a waveform considered characteristic of complete CSNB with nearly normal a-waves and markedly attenuated b-waves (right panel). **(B)** Rod-mediated thresholds children with CSNB. Serial thresholds from an individual are connected by dashed lines.

SUMMARY

These results from patients with ROP, retinal degenerative conditions, and the stationary conditions (achromatopsia and CSNB), illustrate the use of ERG and dark-adapted visual thresholds to secure diagnoses and characterize retinal processes. In those who present with visual inattention, these characteristics document the role of the retina in the child's pathophysiology.

REFERENCES

1. Committee for the Classification of Retinopathy of Prematurity. An international classification of retinopathy of prematurity. *Arch Ophthalmol* 1984;102:1130–1134.
2. Committee for the classification of the late stages of retinopathy of prematurity. An international classification of retinopathy of prematurity: II. The classification of retinal detachment. *Arch Ophthalmol* 1987;105:906–912.
3. Fulton AB, Hansen RM, Glynn RJ. Natural course of visual functions in the Bardet-Biedl syndrome. *Arch Ophthalmol* 1993;111:1500–1506.
4. Summers CG. Vision and albinism. *Trans Am Ophthalmol Soc* 1996;94:1095–1155.
5. STOP ROP Study Group. Supplemental therapeutic oxygen for pre-threshold retinopathy of prematurity (STOP-ROP). A randomized, controlled trial: I. Primary outcomes. *Pediatrics* 2000;105:295–310.
6. McGregor ML, Bremer DL, Cole C, et al. Retinopathy of prematurity outcome in infants with prethreshold retinopathy of prematurity and oxygen saturation >94% in room air: the high oxygen percentage in retinopathy of prematurity study.[comment]. *Pediatrics* 2002;110:540–544.
7. Repka MX, Palmer EA, Tung B. Involution of retinopathy of prematurity. Cryotherapy for Retinopathy of Prematurity Cooperative Group. *Arch Ophthalmol* 2000;118:645–649.
8. Palmer EA, Flynn JT, Hardy RJ, et al. Incidence and early course of retinopathy of prematurity. *Ophthalmology* 1991;98:1628–1640.
9. Quinn GE, Dobson V, Repka MX, et al. Development of myopia in infants with birth weights less than 1251 grams. *Ophthalmology* 1992;99:329–340.
10. Dobson V, Quinn G, Tung B, et al. Comparison of recognition and grating acuities in very-low-birth-weight children with and without retinal residual of retinopathy of prematurity. *Invest Ophthalmol Vis Sci* 1995;1995:692–702.
11. Dobson V, Quinn GE, Saunders RA, et al. Grating acuity in eyes with retinal residua of retinopathy of prematurity. *Invest Ophthalmol Vis Sci* 1994;35(Suppl):1393.
12. Dobson V, Quinn G, Abramov I, et al. Color vision measured at five and a half years in eyes of children in the CRYO ROP study. *Invest Ophthalmol Vis Sci* 1996;37:2467–2474.
13. Cryotherapy for Retinopathy of Prematurity Cooperative G. Contrast sensitivity at age 10 years in children who had threshold retinopathy of prematurity.[comment]. *Arch Ophthalmol* 2001;119:1129–1133.
14. Repka MX, Summers CG, Palmer EA, et al. The incidence of ophthalmologic interventions in children with birth weights less than 1251 grams. Results through 5 1/2 years. Cryotherapy for Retinopathy of Prematurity Cooperative Group. *Ophthalmology* 1998;105:1621–1627.
15. Dobson V, Quinn GE, Abramov I, et al. Color vision measured with pseudoisochromatic plates at five-and-a-half years in eyes of children from the CRYO-ROP study. *Invest Ophthalmol Vis Sci* 1996;37:2467–2474.
16. Kivlin JD, Biglan AW, Gordon RA, et al. Early retinal vessel development and iris vessel dilatation as factors in retinopathy of prematurity. Cryotherapy for Retinopathy of Prematurity (CRYO-ROP) Cooperative Group [comment]. *Arch Ophthalmol* 1996;114:150–154.
17. Johnson L, Quinn GE, Abbasi S, et al. Severe retinopathy of prematurity in infants with birth weights less than 1250 grams: incidence and outcome of treatment with pharmacologic serum levels of vitamin E in addition to cryotherapy from 1985 to 1991 [comment]. *J Pediatr* 1995;127:632–639.
18. Dobson V, Quinn GE, Summers CG, et al. Effect of acute-phase retinopathy of prematurity on grating acuity development in the very low birth weight infant. The Cryotherapy for Retinopathy of Prematurity Cooperative Group. *Invest Ophthalmol Vis Sci* 1994;35:4236–4244.
19. Reynolds J, Dobson V, Quinn GE, et al. Prediction of visual function in eyes with mild to moderate posterior pole residua of retinopathy of prematurity. Cryotherapy for Retinopathy of Prematurity Cooperative Group. *Arch Ophthalmol* 1993;111:1050–1056.
20. Quinn GE, Dobson V, Barr CC, et al. Visual acuity in infants after vitrectomy for severe retinopathy of prematurity. [Published erratum appears in *Ophthalmology* 1991 Jul;98:1005]. *Ophthalmology* 1991;98:5–13.
21. Dobson V, Quinn GE, Biglan AW, et al. Acuity card assessment of visual function in the cryotherapy for retinopathy of prematurity trial. *Invest Ophthalmol Vis Sci* 1990;31:1702–1708.
22. Palmer EA. Results of U.S. randomized clinical trial of cryotherapy for ROP (CRYO-ROP). *Doc Ophthalmol* 1990;74:245–251.
23. Cooper LL, Hansen RM, Darras BT, et al. Rod photoreceptor function in children with mitochondrial disorders. *Arch Ophthalmol* 2002;120:1055–1062.
24. Cox G, Hansen R, Quinn N, et al. Retinal function in carriers of Bardet Biedl syndrome. *Arch Ophthalmol* 2003;121:804–811.
25. Elias ER, Hansen R, Irons M, et al. Rod Photoreceptor Responses in Children with Smith-Lemli-Opitz Syndrome. *Arch Ophthalmol* 2003 (in press).
26. Fulton AB, Hansen RM, Petersen RA, et al. The rod photoreceptors in retinopathy of prematurity: An electroretinographic study. *Arch Ophthalmol* 2001;119:499–505.
27. Fulton AB, Hansen RM. The rod sensitivity of dark adapted human infants. *Curr Eye Res* 1992;11:1193–1198.
28. Fulton AB, Hansen RM, Yeh Y-L, et al. Temporal summation in dark adapted 10-week-old infants. *Vision Res* 1991;31:1259–1269.
29. Fulton AB, Hansen RM. The relation of retinal sensitivity and rhodopsin in human infants. *Vision Res* 1987;27:697.
30. Fulton AB, Hansen RM. The development of scotopic sensitivity. *Invest Ophthalmol Vis Sci* 2000;41:1588–1596.
31. Fulton AB, Dodge J, Hansen RM, et al. The rhodopsin content of human eyes. *Invest Ophthalmol Vis Sci* 1999;40:1878–1883.
32. Hansen RM, Fulton AB. Psychophysical estimates of ocular media density of human infants. *Vision Res* 1989;29:687–690.
33. Hansen RM, Fulton AB, Harris SJ. Background adaptation in human infants. *Vision Res* 1986;26:771–779.
34. Hansen R, Fulton AB. Electroretinographic assessment of background adaptation in 10 week old human infants. *Vision Res* 1991;31:1501–1507.
35. Hansen RM, Fulton AB. Development of scotopic retinal sensitivity. In: Simons K, ed. *Early visual development, normal and abnormal.* New York: Oxford University Press; 1993:130–142.

36. Hansen RM, Hamer RD, Fulton AB. The effect of light adaptation on scotopic spatial summation in 10-week-old infants. *Vision Res* 1992;32:387–392.

37. Hansen RM, Fulton AB. Scotopic center surround organization in 10-week-old infants. *Vision Res* 1994;34:621–624.

38. Hansen RM, Fulton A. The course of maturation of rod mediated visual thresholds in infants. *Invest Ophthalmol Vis Sci* 1999;40:1883–1885.

39. Hansen RM, Fulton AB. Rod mediated increment threshold functions in infants. *Invest Ophthalmol Vis Sci* 2000;41:4347–4352.

40. Harayama K, Amemiya T, Nishimura H. Development of the eyeball during fetal life. *J Pediatr Ophthalmol Strabismus* 1981;18:37–40.

41. Harayama K, Amemiya T, Nishimura H. Development of the cornea during fetal life: comparison of corneal and bulbar diameter. *Anat Rec* 1980;198:531–535.

42. Robb RM. Increase in retinal surface area during infancy and childhood. *J Pediatr Ophthalmol Strabismus* 1982;19:16–20.

43. Hendrickson AE. Morphological development of the primate retina. In: Simons K, ed. *Early visual development, normal and abnormal.* New York: Oxford University Press, 1993:287–295.

44. Hendrickson AE. The morphologic development of human and monkey retina. In: Albert DM, Jakobiec FA, eds. *Principles and practice of ophthalmology: basic sciences.* Philadelphia: WB Saunders Co., 1994:561–577.

45. Packer O, Hendrickson AE, Curcio CA. Developmental redistribution of photoreceptors across the maccaca nemestrina (pigtail macaque) retina. *J Comp Neurol* 1990;298:472–493.

46. Grun G. The development of the vertebrate retina: a comparative survey. *Adv Anat Embryol Cell Biol* 1982;78:1–83.

47. Curcio C, Sloan KR, Packer O, et al. Distribution of cones in human and monkey retina: Individual variability and radial asymmetry. *Science* 1987;236:579–582.

48. Dorn EM, Hendrickson L, Hendrickson AE. The appearance of rod opsin during monkey retinal development. *Invest Ophthalmol Vis Sci* 1995;36:2634–2651.

49. Hendrickson AE, Drucker D. The development of parafoveal and midperipheral retina. *Behav Brain Res* 1992;19:21–32.

50. Rodieck R. *The first steps in seeing.* Sunderland, MA: Sinauer Associates, 1998.

51. LaVail M. Kinetics of rod outer segment renewal in the developing mouse retina. *J Cell Biol* 1973;58:650–661.

52. Tamai M, Chader GJ. The early appearance of disc shedding in the rat retina. *Invest Ophthalmol Vis Sci* 1979;18:913–7.

53. Dodge J, Fulton AB, Parker C, et al. Rhodopsin in immature rod outer segments. *Invest Ophthalmol Vis Sci* 1996;37:1951–1956.

54. Fulton AB, Baker BN. The relation of retinal sensitivity and rhodopsin in developing rat retina. *Invest Ophthalmol Vis Sci* 1984;25:647–651.

55. Fulton AB, Dodge J, Schremser J-L, et al. The quantity of rhodopsin in human eyes. *Curr Eye Res* 1990;9:1211–1216.

56. Fulton AB, Dodge J, Hansen RM, et al. The quantity of rhodopsin in young human eyes. *Curr Eye Res* 1991;10:977–982.

57. Ridge KD, Abdulaev NG, Sousa M, et al. Phototransduction: crystal clear. *Trends Biochem Sci* 2003;28:479–487.

58. Burns ME, Baylor DA. Activation, deactivation, and adaptation in vertebrate photoreceptor cells. *Ann Rev Neurosci* 2001;24:779–805.

59. Lamb TD, Pugh EN Jr. A quantitative account of the activation steps involved in phototransduction in amphibian photoreceptors. *J Physiol* 1992;449:719–758.

60. Breton ME, Schueller A, Lamb TD, et al. Analysis of ERG a-wave amplification and kinetics in terms of the G-protein cascade of phototransduction. *Invest Ophthalmol Vis Sci* 1994;35:295–309.

61. Hood DC, Birch DG. Rod phototransduction in retinitis pigmentosa: estimation and interpretation of parameters derived from the rod a-wave. *Invest Ophthalmol Vis Sci.* 1994;35:2948–2961.

62. Hansen R, Fulton A. Development of scotopic retinal sensitivity. In: Simons K, ed. *Early visual development, normal and abnormal.* New York: Oxford University Press, 1993:130–142.

63. Werner JS. Development of scotopic sensitivity and the absorption spectrum of the human ocular media. *J Opt Soc Am* 1982;72:247–258.

64. Fulton A, Hansen RM, Moskowitz A. Assessment of vision in infants and children. In: Celesia GC, ed. *Handbook of clinical neurophysiology.* New York: Elsevier, 2004.

65. Fulton A, Hansen RM. Stimulus response functions for the scotopic b-wave. In: Heckenlively J, Arden G, editors. Principles and practice of clinical electrophysiology of vision. Second Edition. Cambridge: MIT Press, 2003 *(in press).*

66. Fulton A, Hansen RM. Testing pediatric patients. In: Heckenlively J, Arden G, eds. *Principles and practice of clinical electrophysiology of vision.* 2nd ed. Cambridge: MIT Press, 2003 *(in press).*

67. Granit R. The components of the retinal action potential in mammals and their relation to the discharge in the optic nerve. *J Physiol* 1933;77:207–239.

68. Granit R. The components of the vertebrate electroretinogram. In: *Sensory mechanisms of the retina.* London: Hafner Publishing Company, 1963:38–68.

69. Hood DC, Birch DG. A computational model of the amplitude and implicit time of the b-wave of the human ERG. *Vis Neurosci* 1992;8:107–126.

70. Hood D, Birch D. Beta wave of the scotopic (rod) electroretinogram as a measure of the activity of human on-bipolar cells. *J Opt Soc Am A* 1996;13:623–33.

71. Pugh EN Jr, Lamb TD. Amplification and kinetics of the activation steps in phototransduction. *Biochem Biophys Acta* 1993;1141:111–149.

72. Pugh EN Jr, Lamb TD. Phototransduction in vertebrate rods and cones: Molecular mechanisms of amplification, recovery and light adaptation. In: Stavenga DG, de Grip WJ, Pugh EN Jr, eds. *Handbook of biological physics. Volume 3: molecular mechanisms of visual transduction.* New York: Elsevier Science, 2000:183–255.

73. Aleman T, LaVail MM, Montemayor R, et al. Augmented rod bipolar cell function in partial receptor loss: an ERG study in P23H rhodopsin transgenic and aging normal rats. *Vision Res* 2001;41:2779–2797.

74. Hanitzsch R, Lichtenberger T, Mattig W-U. The influence of MgCl2 and APB on the light induced potassium changes and the ERG b-wave of the isolated superfused retina. *Vision Res* 1996;36:499–507.

75. Robson J, Frishman L. Response linearity and kinetics of the cat retina: the bipolar cell component of the dark-adapted electroretinogram. *Vis Neurosci* 1995;12:837–850.

76. Robson JG, Frishman LJ. Photoreceptor and bipolar cell contributions to the cat electroretinogram: a kinetic model for the early part of the flash response. *J Opt Soc Am* 1996;13:613–622.

77. Robson JG, Frishman LJ. Dissecting the dark adapted electroretinogram. *Doc Ophthalmol* 1999;95:187–215.

78. Stockton R, Slaughter RM. B-wave of the electroretinogram: A reflection of ON-bipolar cell activity. *J Gen Physiol* 1989;93:101–121.

79. Robson JG, Frishman LJ. Response linearity and kinetics of the cat retina: The bipolar cell component of the dark-adapted electroretinogram. *Vis Neurosci* 1995;12:837–850.

80. Fulton AB, Hansen RM, Westall CA. The ISCEV rod, maximal and cone response in normal subjects. *Doc Ophthalmol* 2003 *(in press)*.

81. Hansen RM, Fulton AB. The development of cone mediated electroretinographic (ERG) responses in infants. *Invest Ophthalmol Vis Sci* 2000;41(Suppl):S499.

82. Young RW. The renewal of photoreceptor cell outer segments. *J Cell Biol* 1967;33:61–72.

83. Young RW. Visual cells and the concept of renewal. *Invest Ophthalmol Vis Sci* 1976;15:700–725.

84. Hendrickson AE. Primate foveal development: a microcosm of current questions in neurobiology. *Invest Ophthalmol Vis Sci* 1994;35:3129–3133.

85. Blakemore C. Maturation of mechanisms for efficient spatial vision. In: Blakemore C, ed. *Vision: coding and efficiency.* Cambridge: University Press, 1990:256–266.

86. Yuodelis C, Hendrickson AE. A qualitative and quantitative analysis of the human fovea during development. *Vision Res* 1986;26:847–855.

87. Mayer DL, Beiser AS, Warner AF, et al. Monocular acuity norms for the Teller acuity cards between ages 1 month and 4 years. *Invest Ophthalmol Vis Sci* 1995;36:671–685.

88. Hansen RM, Fulton AB. Behavioral measurement if background adaptation in infants. *Invest Ophthalmol Vis Sci* 1981; 21:625–629.

89. Hamer RD, Schneck ME. Spatial summation in dark-adapted human infants. *Vision Res* 1984;24:77–85.

90. Brown AM. Scotopic sensitivity of the two-month-old human infant. *Vision Res* 1986;26:707–711.

91. Powers MK, Schneck ME, Teller DY. Spectral sensitivity of human infants at absolute visual threshold. *Vision Res* 1981;21: 1005–1016.

92. Schneck ME, Hamer RD, Packer OS, et al. Area threshold relations at controlled retinal locations in 1-month-old human infants. *Vision Res* 1984;24:1753–1763.

93. Hansen RM, Fulton AB. Scotopic center surround organization on 10-week-old infants. *Vision Res* 1994;34:621–624.

94. Fulton AB, Hansen RM, Mayer DL. Vision in Leber congenital amaurosis. *Arch Ophthalmol* 1996;114:698–703.

95. Hansen RM, Fulton AB. Background adaptation in children with a history of mild retinopathy of prematurity. *Invest Ophthalmol Vis Sci* 2000;40:320–324.

96. Reisner DS, Hansen RM, Findl O, et al. Dark adapted thresholds in children with histories of mild retinopathy of prematurity. *Invest Ophthalmol Vis Sci* 1997;38:1175–1183.

97. Fulton AB, Hansen RM. Retinal adaptation in infants and children with retinal degenerations. *Ophthalmic Paediatr Genet.* 1983;2:69.

98. Fulton AB, Hansen RM. Electroretinography: application to clinical studies of infants. *J Pediatr Ophthalmol Strabismus* 1985; 22:251.

99. Fulton A, Hansen R, Mayer D, Rodier D. Clinical examination of infant visual status. In: K Simons, ed. *Early visual development, normal and abnormal.* New York: Oxford University Press, 1993: 309–317.

100. Fulton AB, Hansen RM. Photoreceptor function in infants and children with a history of mild retinopathy of prematurity. *J Opt Soc Am A* 1996;13:566–571.

101. Fulton AB, Hansen RM. ERG responses and refractive errors in patients with a history of ROP. *Doc Ophthalmol* 1996;91:87–100.

102. Jolesz M, Vanderveen DK, M HR, Fulton A. Development of rod mediated visual thresholds in infants with a history of mild retinopathy of prematurity. *Invest Ophthalmol Vis Sci* 2003: ARVO Abstract 2864.

103. Fulton A, Hansen R, Jolesz M. Retinal function and myopia in retinopathy of prematurity. *Invest Ophthalmol Vis Sci* 2003: ARVO Abstract 2863.

104. Fulton AB, Hanson RM. Photoreceptor function in infants and children with a history of mild retinopathy of prematurity. *J Opt Soc Am* 1996;13:566–571.

105. Fulton AB, Reynaud X, Hansen RM, et al. Rod photoreceptors in infant rats with a history of oxygen exposure. *Invest Ophthalmol Vis Sci* 1999;40:168–174.

106. Steinberg RH. Monitoring communications between photoreceptors and pigment epithelial cells: Effects of "mild" systemic hypoxia. *Invest Ophthalmol Vis Sci* 1987;28:2015–2025.

107. Reynaud X, Hansen RM, Fulton AB. Effect of prior oxygen exposure on the electroretinographic responses of infant rats. *Invest Ophthalmol Vis Sci* 1995;36:2071–2079.

108. Dagi LR, Leys MJ, Hansen RM, et al. Hyperopia in complicated Leber's congenital amaurosis. *Arch Ophthalmol* 1990;108: 709–712.

109. Mayer DL, Hansen RM, Moore BD, et al. Cycloplegic refractions in healthy children, aged 1 through 48 months. *Arch Ophthalmol* 2001;119:1625–1628.

110. Lambert SR, Taylor D, Kriss A. The infant with nystagmus, normal appearing fundi, but an abnormal ERG. *Surv Ophthalmol* 1989;34:173.

111. Fulton AB, Hansen RM. Stimulus/ response functions for the scotopic b-wave. In: Heckenlively J, Arden G, eds. *Handbook of clinical electrophysiology of vision.* Cambridge: MIT Press, 2004.

112. den Hollander AI, ten Brink JB, de Kok YJ, et al. Mutations in a human homologue of Drosophila crumbs cause retinitis pigmentosa (RP12). *Nat Genet* 1999;23:217–221.

113. Gregory-Evans K, Kelsell RE, Gregory-Evans CY, et al. Autosomal dominant cone-rod retinal dystrophy (CORD6) from heterozygous mutation of GUCY2D, which encodes retinal guanylate cyclase. *Ophthalmology* 2000;107:55–61.

114. Gu S, Thompson DA, Srikumari CR, et al. Mutations in RPE65 cause autosomal recessive childhood-onset severe retinal dystrophy. *Nat Genet* 1997;17:194–197.

115. Freund CL, Wang Q-L, Chen S, et al. De novo mutations in the CRX homeobox gene associated with Leber congenital amaurosis. *Nat Genet* 1998;18:311–312.

116. Jacobson SG, Cideciyan AV, Huang Y, et al. Retinal degenerations with truncation mutations in the cone-rod homeobox (CRX) gene. *Invest Ophthalmol Vis Sci* 1998;39:2417–2425.

117. Lewis CA, Batlle IR, Batlle KG, et al. Tubby-like protein 1 homozygous splice-site mutation causes early-onset severe retinal degeneration. *Invest Ophthalmol Vis Sci* 1999;40:2106–14.

118. Lotery AJ, Jacobson SG, Fishman GA, et al. Mutations in the CRB1 gene cause Leber congenital amaurosis [comment]. *Arch Ophthalmol* 2001;119:415–420.

119. Lorenz B, Gyurus P, Preising M, et al. Early-onset severe rod-cone dystrophy in young children with RPE65 mutations. *Invest Ophthalmol Vis Sci* 2000;41:2735–2742.

120. Marlhens F, Bareil C, Griffoin JM, et al. Mutations in RPE65 cause Leber's congenital amaurosis. *Nat Genet* 1997;17:139–141.

121. Morimura H, Fishman GA, Grover SA, et al. Mutations in the RPE65 gene in patients with autosomal recessive retinitis pigmentosa or Leber congenital amaurosis. *Proc Nat Acad Sci U S A* 1998;95:3088–3093.

122. Perrault I, Rozet JM, Gerber S, et al. A retGC-1 mutation in autosomal dominant cone-rod dystrophy. *Am J Hum Genet* 1998; 63:651–654.

123. Sohocki MM, Sullivan LS, Mintz-Hittner HA, et al. A range of clinical phenotypes associated with mutations in CRX, a photoreceptor transcription-factor gene. *Am J Hum Genet* 1998;63: 1307–1315.

124. Sohocki MM, Perrault I, Leroy BP, et al. Prevalence of AIPL1 mutations in inherited retinal degenerative disease. *Mol Genet Metab* 2000;70:142–150.

125. Sohocki MM, Bowne SJ, Sullivan LS, et al. Mutations in a new photoreceptor-pineal gene on 17p cause Leber congenital amaurosis. *Nat Genet* 2000;24:79–83.

126. Fulton AB, Hansen RM. Retinal sensitivity and adaptation in pediatric patients. *Behav Brain Res* 1983;10:59.

127. Wongpichedchai S, Hansen RM, Koka B, et al. Effects of halothane on children's electroretinograms. *Ophthalmology* 1992;99:1309–1312.

128. Kwitek-Black A, Carmi R, Duyk GM, et al. Linkage of Bardet-Biedl syndrome to chromosome 16q and evidence for non-allelic genetic heterogeneity. *Nat Genet* 1993;5:392–396.

129. Leppert M, Baird L, Anderson KL, et al. Bardet-Biedl syndrome is linked to DNA markers on chromosome 11q and is genetically heterogeneous. *Nat Genet* 1994;6:108–112.

130. Sheffield VC, Carmi R, Kwitek-Black A, et al. Identification of a Bardet-Biedl syndrome locus on chromosome 3 and evaluation of an efficient approach to homozygosity mapping. *Hum Mol Genet* 1994;3:1331–1335.

131. Carmi R, Elbedour K, Stone EM, et al. Phenotypic differences among patients with Bardet-Biedl syndrome linked to three different chromosome loci. *Am J Med Genet* 1995;59:199– 203.

132. Young TL, Penney L, Woods MO, et al. A fifth locus for Bardet-Biedl syndrome maps to chromosome 2q31. *Am J Hum Genet* 1998;64:900–904.

133. Beales PL, Elcioglu N, Woolf AS, et al. New criteria for improved diagnosis of Bardet-Biedl syndrome: results of a population survey. *J Med Genet* 1999;36:437–446.

134. Beales PL, Warner AM, Hitman GA, et al. Bardet-Biedl syndrome: a molecular and phenotypic study of 18 families. *J Med Genet* 1997;34:92–98.

135. Katsanis N, Beales PL, Woods MO, et al. Mutations in MKKS cause obesity, retinal dystrophy and renal malformations associated with Bardet-Biedl syndrome. *Nat Genet* 2000;26:67–70.

136. Katsanis N, Ansley J. Triallelic inheritance in Bardet-Biedl syndrome, a Mendelian recessive disorder. *Science* 2001;293(5538): 2256–2259.

137. Slavotinek AM, Stone EM, Mykytyn K, et al. Mutations in MKKS cause Bardet-Biedl syndrome. *Nat Genet* 2000;26: 15–16.

138. Slavotinek AM, Biesecker LG. Phenotypic overlap of McKusick-Kaufman syndrome with Bardet-Biedl syndrome: a literature review. *Am J Med Genet* 2000;95:208–215.

139. Slavotinek AM, Stone EM, Mykytyn K, et al. Mutations in MKKS cause Bardet-Biedl syndrome. *Nat Genet* 2000;26: 15–16.

140. Mykytyn K, Braun T, Carmi R, et al. Identification of the gene that, when mutated, causes the human obesity syndrome BBS4. *Nat Genet* 2001;28:188–191.

141. Mykytyn K, Nishimura DY, Searby CC, et al. Identification of the gene (BBS 1) most commonly involved in Bardet-Biedl syndrome, a complex human obesity syndrome. *Nat Genet* 2002; 31:435–438.

142. Nishimura DY, Searby CC, Carmi R, et al. Positional cloning of a novel gene on chromosome 16q causing Bardet Biedl syndrome (BBS). *Hum Mol Genet* 2001;10:865–874.

143. Hagerstrom-Portnoy G, Freidman N, Adams AJ, et al. Vision function of rod monochromats. I. Advanced clinical measures. Non-invasive assessment of the visual system. *Technical Digest Series, Opt Soc Am* 1988;3:13.

144. Baseler HA, Brewer AA, Sharpe LT, et al. Reorganization of human cortical maps caused by inherited photoreceptor abnormalities. *Nat Neurosci* 2002;5:364–370.

145. Aligianis IA, Forshew T, Johnson S, et al. Mapping of a novel locus for achromatopsia (ACHM4) to 1p and identification of a germline mutation in the alpha subunit of cone transducin (GNAT2). *J Med Genet* 2002;39:656–660.

146. Kohl S, Baumann B, Rosenberg T, et al. Mutations in the cone photoreceptor G-protein alpha-subunit gene GNAT2 in patients with achromatopsia. *Am J Hum Genet* 2002;71:422– 425.

147. Kohl S, Baumann B, Broghammer M, et al. Mutations in the CNGB3 gene encoding the beta-subunit of the cone photoreceptor cGMP-gated channel are responsible for achromatopsia (ACHM3) linked to chromosome 8q21. *Hum Mol Genet* 2000; 9:2107–2116.

148. Rojas CV, Maria LS, Santos JL, et al. A frameshift insertion in the cone cyclic nucleotide gated cation channel causes complete achromatopsia in a consanguineous family from a rural isolate. *Eur J Hum Genet* 2002;10:638–642.

149. Wissinger B, Gamer D, Jagle H, et al. CNGA3 mutations in hereditary cone photoreceptor disorders. *Am J Hum Genet* 2001;69:722–737.

150. Sundin OH, Yang JM, Li Y, et al. Genetic basis of total colourblindness among the Pingelapese islanders. *Nat Genet* 2000;25: 289–293.

151. Peng C, Rich ED, Varnum MD. Achromatopsia-associated mutation in the human cone photoreceptor cyclic nucleotide-gated channel CNGB3 subunit alters the ligand sensitivity and pore properties of heteromeric channels. *J Biol Chem* 2003;278: 4533–4540.

152. Nakamura M, Ito S, Piao C, et al. Atypical incomplete congenital stationary night blindness with retinal atrophy associated with CACNA1F mutation. Presented at the 40th symposium, International Society for the Clinical Electrophysiology of Vision, Leuvan, Belgium, 2002.

153. Carr RE, Ripps H, Siegel IM, et al. Rhodopsin and the electrical activity of the retina in congenital stationary night blindness. *Invest Ophthalmol* 1966;5:497–507.

154. Alpern M, Holland MG. Rhodopsin bleaching signals in essential night blindness. *J Physiol* 1972;225:457.

155. Dryja TP, Berson EL, Rao VR, et al. Heterozygous missense mutation in the rhodopsin gene as a cause of congenital stationary night blindness. *Nat Genet* 1993;4:280–283.

156. Dryja T. Molecular genetics of Oguchi disease, Fundus Albipunctatus, and other forms of stationary night blindness. *Am J Ophthalmol* 2000;130:547–563.

157. Gal A, Orth U, Baehr W, et al. Heterozygous missense mutation in the rod cGMP phosphodiesterase b-subunit gene in autosomal dominant stationary night blindness. *Nat Genet* 1994;7: 64–67.

158. Bech-Hansen NT, Naylor MJ, Maybaum TA, et al. Mutations in NYX, encoding the leucine-rich proteoglycan nyctalopin, cause X-linked complete congenital stationary night blindness. *Nat Genet* 2000;26:319–323.

159. Boycott KM, Maybaum TA, Naylor MJ, et al. A summary of 20 CACNA1F mutations identified in 36 families with incomplete X-linked congenital stationary night blindness, and characterization of splice variants. *Hum Genet* 2001;108:91–97.

160. McLaughlin ME, Sandberg MA, Berson EL, et al. Recessive mutations in the gene encoding the beta-subunit of rod phosphodiesterase in patients with retinitis pigmentosa. *Nat Genet* 1993;4:130–134.

161. al-Jandal N, Farrar GJ, Kiang AS, et al. A novel mutation within the rhodopsin gene (Thr-94-Ile) causing autosomal dominant congenital stationary night blindness. *Hum Mutat* 1999;13: 75–81.

162. Zvyaga TA, Fahmy K, Siebert F, et al. Characterization of the mutant visual pigment responsible for congenital night blindness: a biochemical and Fourier-transform infrared spectroscopy study. *Biochemistry* 1996;35:7536–7545.

163. Rao VR, Cohen GB, Oprian DD. Rhodopsin mutation G90D and a molecular mechanism for congenital night blindness. *Nature* 1994;367(6464):639–642.

164. Sieving PA, Richards JE, Naarendorp F, et al. Dark-light: model for nightblindness from the human rhodopsin Gly-90—>Asp mutation. *Proc Nat Acad Sci U S A* 1995;92:880–884.

165. Sandberg MA, Pawlyk BS, Dan J, et al. Rod and cone function in the Nougaret form of stationary night blindness. *Arch Ophthalmol* 1998;116:867–872.

166. Dryja TP, Hahn LB, Reboul T, et al. Missense mutation in the gene encoding the alpha subunit of rod transducin in the Nougaret form of congenital stationary night blindness. *Nat Genet* 1996;13:358–360.

167. Gal A, Xu S, Piczenik Y, Eiberg H, et al. Gene for autosomal dominant congenital stationary night blindness maps to the same region as the gene for the beta-subunit of the rod photoreceptor cGMP phosphodiesterase (PDEB) in chromosome 4p16.3. *Hum Mol Genet* 1994;3:323–325.

168. Gal A, Orth U, Baehr W, Schwinger E, et al. Heterozygous missense mutation in the rod cGMP phosphodiesterase beta-subunit gene in autosomal dominant stationary night blindness. [Published erratum appears in *Nat Genet* 1994;7:551]. *Nat Genet* 1994;7:64–68.

169. Dryja TP. Molecular genetics of Oguchi disease, fundus albipunctatus, and other forms of stationary night blindness: LVII

170. Boycott KM, Pearce WG, Bech-Hansen NT. Clinical variability among patients with incomplete X-linked congenital stationary night blindness and a founder mutation in CACNA1F. *Can J Ophthalmol* 2000;35:204–213.

171. Miyake Y, Yagasaki K, Horiguchi M, et al. Congenital stationary night blindness with negative electroretinogram: a new classification. *Arch Ophthalmol* 1986;104:1013.

172. Miyake Y, Horiguchi M, Suzuki S, et al. Complete and incomplete type congenital stationary night blindness as a model of 'off retina' and 'on retina'. In: LaVail MM, Hollyfield J, Anderson RE, eds. *Degenerative retinal diseases.* New York: Plenum Press, 1997:31–41.

173. Weleber RG. Infantile and childhood retinal blindness: a molecular perspective (The Franceschetti Lecture). *Ophthalmic Genet* 2002;23:71–97.

174. Drucker D, Henrickson AE. The morphological development of extrafoveal human retina. *Invest Ophthalmol Vis Sci* 1989;30 (Suppl):226.

175. McDonald MA, Dobson V, Sebris SL, et al. The acuity card procedure: a rapid test of infant acuity. *Invest Ophthalmol Vis Sci* 1985;26:1158–1162.

176. Marmor MF, Zrenner E. Standard for clinical electroretinography (1999 update). *Doc Ophthalmol* 1998;97:143–156.

Edward Jackson Memorial Lecture. *Am J Ophthalmol* 2000;130: 547–563.

GENETIC COUNSELING FOR RETINAL DISEASES

DEBORAH COSTAKOS
J. BRONWYN BATEMAN

With ever-increasing genetic information, it has become more complicated to provide accurate, timely, and compassionate counseling to patients or the families of a patient with a genetic retinal dystrophy. As our collective knowledge of the genetic bases for disease expands, application of this genetic information to clinical practice is increasingly important to allow patients to plan their lives and make decisions regarding reproduction. The availability of such scientific information forces the patient, physician, and society to consider aspects of medicine that have significant ramifications. Social, legal, and confidentiality issues abound, including insurance eligibility, family planning, prenatal diagnosis, and paternity/maternity. A team including geneticists, genetic counselors, scientists, and other physician members involved in the care of the patient, and family can most effectively address these issues. At times, social workers and psychiatrists may join the effort to help families cope with and address lifestyle and planning adjustments.

The Human Genome Project was begun in 1990 as a result of a coordinated effort between the US Department of Energy (DOE) and the National Institutes of Health (NIH); as executed, the project was international. The goals of the Human Genome Project included the following: (i) determining the human genome sequence; (ii) identifying all genes in human deoxyribonucleic acid (DNA) and managing the enormous database for use by geneticists, scientists, and those interpreting the information, including clinicians and genetic counselors; (iii) improving tools for data analyses and transferring related technologies to the private sector; and (iv) addressing the ethical, legal, and social issues that arise from the project. The annual budget devoted 3% to 5% of total funding to study ethical, legal, and social issues surrounding the increasing availability of genetic information.

The public has expressed substantial concerns regarding the potential use of this information by insurers to deny, limit, or cancel insurance policies and by employers to discriminate against existing workers or potential employees.

These concerns have yet to be addressed by federal legislation. Although several bills have been introduced, no law relating to genetic discrimination for individual insurance coverage or to genetic discrimination in the workplace has been passed. In 1999, former President Clinton signed an executive order prohibiting any federal agency from using genetic information in any hiring or promotion action. The American Medical Association, American College of Medical Genetics, National Society of Genetic Counselors, and the Genetic Alliance supported this order. Parts of the Americans with Disabilities Act of 1990, the Health Insurance Portability and Accountability Act (HIPAA) of 1996, and Title VII of the Civil Rights Act of 1964 may be interpreted to include some forms of genetic discrimination protection. A few states (IL, OR, KY, MI, NE, NY, WA, WI) have nondiscrimination laws that vary in terms of coverage, protection afforded, and enforcement schemes, but none is comprehensive. Despite the lack of protection against the discriminatory use of genetic information, more than 25 US jurisdictions recognize an action for wrongful birth (parents suing with the position they would not have given birth had they been properly informed of the genetic risks), and three recognize an action for wrongful life (the child suing with the position that no life would have been better than being born with the genetic defect). The claim in a wrongful birth/life action can arise when a physician fails to provide and document appropriate genetic counseling, fails to detect or inform the parents of a discoverable fetal defect, or fails to interpret test results properly. In 1986, a wrongful birth lawsuit was filed by parents alleging that their second blind child would not have been born had their first child's blindness been diagnosed as hereditary; the child also filed a claim for wrongful life alleging that, but for the physicians' negligent diagnosis, he would not have been born to suffer impairment (*Lininger v Eisenbaum,* 764 P2d 1202 [Colo 1988]). In this case, the first child was diagnosed with optic nerve hypoplasia. After the second child was born with visual impairment, Leber congenital amaurosis was diagnosed. On appeal, the Colorado Supreme Court held that the wrongful birth claim was a viable cause of action; the wrongful life claim was dismissed. This case established the precedent of wrongful birth in the state of Colorado.

In another case, *Weed v Meyers* (674 NYS2d 242 [NY App Div 1998]), an ophthalmologist treated Mr. Weed for retinoblastoma. Twenty-four years later, the patient went on to have two children affected with retinoblastoma. The patient alleged that the ophthalmologist failed to provide adequate genetic counseling at the time of the father's treatment. This case was dismissed, in part because the children (plaintiffs) could not maintain an action for a duty owed by the doctor to the father, and the father filed his lawsuit after the statute of limitations expired.

As such, in today's era of exponential growth of available genetic information, it is more important than ever for ophthalmologists to have a basic understanding of genetics, how it relates to medical practice, and their responsibility to ensure adequate genetic counseling. Additional resources can be obtained from geneticists and counselors by the American Board of Medical Genetics or the National Board of Genetic Counselors.

GENETIC TERMINOLOGY

Genetic conditions are classified with the understanding that as research progresses and insight into genetic mechanisms evolves, new terms are developed to explain previously unrecognized or unexplainable phenomena. Chromosomes (the structures in the cell nucleus) and mitochondria contain the DNA that transfers genetic information from cell to cell and from organism to organism. Inheriting an abnormal number of chromosomes results in well-defined systemic syndromes that involve multiple organ systems including the eye.

Single-gene or mendelian disorders are classified into autosomal dominant, autosomal recessive, X-linked recessive, or X-linked dominant conditions. An *autosomal dominant disorder* is one in which the heterozygote, a person having one copy of the abnormal gene, is symptomatic or has physical evidence (phenotype) of the abnormal copy. Both genders are equally "at risk," and the abnormal gene is transmitted from generation to generation. This mode of inheritance is complicated by penetrance and expressivity. *Penetrance* is the probability that a person with the abnormal gene has physical evidence of the presence of the gene; penetrance is commonly less than 100% in autosomal dominant disorders. *Expressivity,* on the other hand, describes the variation in phenotype among individuals carrying the abnormal gene and usually has a broader spectrum in autosomal dominant disorders compared to autosomal recessive and X-linked disorders.

Autosomal recessive disorders are fully expressed in homozygotes, those individuals carrying two copies of the mutant gene. *Carriers,* those who have only one copy of the mutant gene, usually are not symptomatic and have a normal phenotype. Parents are generally carriers, and each of their offspring has a 25% chance of having the disorder. Consanguinity of the parents is common unless the gene has a high frequency, such as in cystic fibrosis or sickle cell anemia. In general, autosomal recessive disorders show less clinical variability (expressivity) than autosomal dominant disorders; penetrance usually is complete.

An *X-linked recessive disorder* is one in which the mutant gene is on the X chromosome and is not expressed or is minimally expressed in the female. Because males have only one X chromosome, all males with the mutant gene are affected with the disorder, whereas females, because they have two X chromosomes, are carriers. Females have varying levels of expression as carriers because of the inactivation phenomenon describe by Mary Lyon (1) in 1962; one X chromosome is randomly inactivated in each cell. In the unusual event that a female has Turner syndrome (XO karyotype), she will be affected but also will be infertile. Male-to-male transmission is not seen in X-linked disorders. Sons of carrier females have a 50% risk of being affected, whereas daughters of carriers have a 50% chance of being carriers.

There are few *X-linked dominant disorders.* The gene usually is lethal in males, and generally only females are affected. Pedigrees may appear to represent autosomal dominant inheritance, except that there is no male-to-male transmission. Goltz syndrome (also known as Goltz-Gorlin syndrome or focal dermal hypoplasia) and microphthalmia with linear skin defects syndrome are examples of X-linked dominant conditions.

All genetic counseling should include the possibility that the gene may be identified soon (if not already known), treatment modalities may develop in the future, and preimplantation or prenatal diagnosis may be available.

Abnormalities of entire chromosomes, such as trisomy 13, occur and are generally associated with multiple congenital anomalies and developmental delay. The exceptions are sex chromosome abnormalities in which the Y chromosome contains little genetic information and the X chromosome where extra chromosomes may be inactivated (e.g., XYY or XXX). These karyotypes may be associated with anomalies, but they can be mild and developmental delay may or can not be present. Additionally, portions of chromosomes may be deleted or duplicated.

Sporadic refers to the case in which no other family members have the disorder. Sporadic conditions may be mendelian (caused by a single gene) or of unknown basis. Individuals with a sporadic form of a known genetic disorder are at risk of passing the disorder to their offspring if the mutation is present in the germinal or reproductive cells of the body. An example is a patient with isolated aniridia with normal biologic parents. Parents of a child with a sporadic new mutation are not at greater risk than the general population of having more children with the disorder. However, offspring of the affected individual may inherit the mutation and be affected with the disorder. Important exceptions include a parent without manifestation of the disorder who carries a mutation in his/her reproductive cells but not in the somatic (nonreproductive) cells. This parent would be considered a germline mosaic, and each child would be at increased risk of having the disorder. In addition, a somatic cell mosaic individual who carries the mutated gene in some somatic cells but not in others may have affected children if the germ line also is mosaic. Somatic cell mosaics may be affected or unaffected, presumably depending on the number of cells with the mutant gene.

Mitochondria contain DNA, and mutations may cause ocular disease such as Kearns-Sayre (associated with retinal degeneration) or Leber hereditary optic neuropathy (LHON). Mitochondria are exclusively inherited from the mother in the cytoplasm of the ovum. Both homoplasmy (uniform mitochondrial DNA within an individual cell) and heteroplasmy (more than one form of mitochondrial DNA within a cell) have been reported in LHON (2,3). The basis for male predominance in LHON is unknown. Expression of mitochondrial diseases is influenced by heteroplasmy, the proportion of mitochondria that contain the mutation; thus, mitochondrial diseases are quantitative. For instance, point mutations within the ATPase 6 gene result in neuropathy, ataxia, and retinal pigmentosa (NARP) or in Leigh syndrome, a progressive encephalopathy unassociated with retinal degeneration. Leigh syndrome occurs if the mutation is present in the majority (>90%) of mitochondria ("extreme heteroplasmy") (4,5).

Other exceptions to traditional mendelian inheritance have become evident as molecular biology methodology has advanced. Determining the parental origin of a gene or segment of DNA is feasible. *Uniparental disomy,* a phenomenon of an offspring inheriting both alleles of a gene or segment of DNA from one of the two parents, has been documented. As a result, an offspring may manifest an autosomal recessive disorder when, in fact, only one parent is a carrier.

Uniparental disomy has led to an understanding of the *imprinting* phenomenon (6). Imprinting defies mendelian patterns of inheritance. With imprinting, chromosomes are "marked" as to their parental origin. (7). Presumably, imprinting occurs prior to conception and is maintained throughout mitosis. With imprinted genes, the parent of origin is recognized by the cell transcription process, resulting in expression of only maternal or paternal alleles ("monoallelic expression"). Methylation of DNA may be a mechanism for imprinting because transcription patterns are blocked by methylation of DNA. Recruitment of a transcription repressor may be an alternative mechanism. Genes capable of imprinting are clustered throughout the genome, and studies suggest that 0.1% to 1.0% of mammalian genes undergo imprinting (8). For example, although both Prader-Willi and Angelman syndromes are associated with a deficiency in expression of genes within the 15q11q13 region, they are distinct phenotypes (9). This is because Prader-Willi syndrome is associated with a deficiency in paternal expression of genes within that region, whereas Angelman syndrome is caused by reduced maternal expression.

Some patients affected with a disorder that is generally caused by a deletion of a portion of DNA, but without identifiable chromosomal abnormalities, may have a mutation of a gene causing deleterious imprinting. Additionally, imprinting may affect gene expression in a tissue-specific manner. For example, in the mouse, ubiquitin-protein ligase (UBE3A) is exclusively maternally expressed in hippocampal neurons and Purkinje cells; thus, gender differences may have genetic/metabolic bases. In a mouse model of Angelman syndrome caused by paternal uniparental disomy (maternal deficiency), expression of UBE3A was undetectable in the hippocampus and cerebellum and caused ataxia, reduction in brain weight, and late-onset obesity. In other parts of the mouse brain, maternal and paternal expression of UBE3A was equivalent (10,11).

Anticipation, which is the process of a disorder becoming more severe in progressive generations, was believed in the nineteenth and early twentieth centuries to be a feature of genetic disease and was a justification for sterilization programs. In fact, most genetic disorders do not exhibit anticipation; however, there are exceptions. The phenomenon has been established in disorders including myotonic dystrophy and spinocerebellar atrophy 6 (SCA6) (12). The increase in severity of the disease in one generation to the next results from an unstable DNA triplet sequence which allows an increasing number of triplet repeats within the gene. In myotonic dystrophy, repeat sequences of the CTG triplet in the untranslated (not resulting in a protein product) region of the DNA accounts for the disorder. A CAG repeat within the CACNLIA4 gene is responsible for anticipation in SCA6 (13).

Heritable cancers, such as retinoblastoma, also defy a strict mendelian pattern of inheritance. Retinoblastoma appears to be inherited in an autosomal dominant fashion, but it is autosomal recessive at the cellular level. Because the retinoblastoma gene, located on 13q14, is a tumor suppressor gene, a defect in the second allele is required to allow tumors to develop. Therefore, a parent with retinoblastomas and a known genetic defect has only a 45% chance of having an affected offspring compared with 50% in a fully penetrant autosomal dominant disorder. This phenomenon was described originally by Knudson et al. (14,15) as a "two-hit hypothesis."

Anticipation, genetic heterogeneity, variable expressivity, penetrance, and phenotypic variability are all important concepts to understand when counseling patients about prognosis and risk to siblings and future children.

GENETIC COUNSELING

Family History

Taking a family history is an essential portion of the ophthalmologic examination and may allow insight into the diagnosis, inheritance, and variability of a disorder. Means of obtaining useful genetic information extend beyond the usual blood work or tissue biopsy of the "proband" (initial patient). Medical records, autopsy reports, family photo albums, laboratory tests on relatives, or clinical evaluation of family members may aid in establishing the diagnosis and the inheritance pattern. A *pedigree* is a graphic record of the family history. Patterns of familial transmission emerge as the pedigree is constructed (Fig. 4-1).

Testing

Decades of research endeavors have resulted in the sequencing of the three billion base-pair DNA sequence of the human genome completed in April 2003 *(www. doegenomes.org)*. Currently, more than 1,000 genetic tests are available from laboratories; information can be obtained from a Web site funded by the NIH and DOE *(www. genetests.org)*.

Prenatal Testing

Prenatal testing is now available for multiple genetic diseases. Molecular technologies (the manipulation of DNA) have allowed analyses by karyotyping, high-resolution chromosomal analysis, fluorescence *in situ* hybridization, polymerase chain reaction for copying small segments of DNA, quantitative fluorescence polymerase chain reaction for quantifying, linkage analysis, and cloning. Fetal samples can be obtained prior to implantation with *in vitro* fertilization or during gestation with amniocentesis, chorionic villus sampling, or periumbilical cord blood sampling. Ultrasound may aid in the diagnosis of associated anatomic fetal anomalies. In some cases, multiple family members must be stud-

ied to identify the genetic abnormality specific to a family ("private mutations" that are unique to the individual/ family) or to allow for accurate linkage studies. A geneticist or genetic counselor may be able to identify academic laboratories studying a particular disorder prior to commercial availability of genetic testing. The Web site *www.genetests.org* lists available genetic tests.

Hereditary Retinal Disorders

The prevalence of retinal degeneration/dystrophies is estimated to be 1 in 3,000. Vision is a complex phenomenon, and many genes are expressed in the visual pathway. Genetic disorders may alter the structure and function of the eye if the abnormal genes are expressed in ocular structures. Isolated retinal degenerations or dystrophies may be caused by mutations in single genes or by chromosomal deletions, duplications, or rearrangements that encompass genes encoding proteins that affect the visual cascade (photon conversion to neuronal signal). They include structural proteins, transcription factors, and catabolic enzymes, as well as mitochondrial proteins. Other unknown genes also may cause retinal degeneration/dystrophies. Retinal degenerations and dystrophies may be isolated ocular disorders or part of genetic disorders affecting multiple organs. These genes may cause abnormalities in photoreceptor cell transcription factors, in catabolic functions in the retina, and in mitochondria, thus, resulting in retinal dystrophies or degenerations. The same gene defect can cause significant phenotypic variation in retinal degeneration/dystrophy, even within the same family (16,17). To date, 149 loci and 99 cloned genes causing retinal diseases have been reported *(www.sph.uth. tmc.edu/RetNet/sum-dis.htm)*.

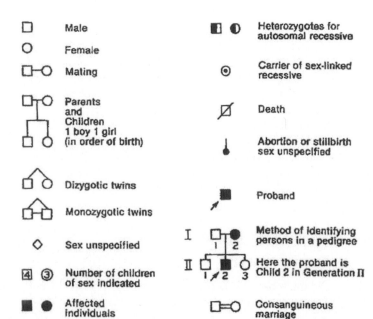

FIGURE 4-1. Common symbols used in pedigree construction.

Although chromosomal disorders are not usually associated with a retinal degeneration or dystrophy unless a gene expressed in the retina is disrupted, some may be associated with persistent hyperplastic primary vitreous or intrauterine retinal detachments (e.g., trisomy 13).

Management

Counseling of affected individuals and families requires a team approach. Genetic counseling may aid in assessing recurrence risk and establishing carrier status in other family members. For some disorders, DNA analysis may be available for identification of the specific mutation. Counselors can discuss reproductive options (sperm or egg donor); arrange for appropriate prenatal diagnosis, if available; explain more complicated concepts such as anticipation, variable expressivity, and penetrance; and assess recurrence risk in future offspring. They also can provide psychosocial and educational resources. These may include family counseling to support the acceptance of an individual with limited visual abilities with or without other handicaps. The affected individual may need information regarding low-vision aids, educational services, career counseling, and recreational opportunities. Medical intervention may be available.

REFERENCES

1. Lyon MF. Sex chromatin and gene action in the mammalian X chromosome. *Am J Hum Genet* 1962;14:135–148.
2. Black GC, Morton K, Laborde A, et al. Lebers hereditary optic neuropathy: heteroplasmy is likely to be significant in the expression on LHON in families with the 3460 ND1 mutation. *Br J Ophthalmol* 1996;80:915–917.
3. Cremers FPM, van den Hurk JAJM, den Hollander AI. Molecular genetics of Leber congenital amaurosis. *Hum Mol Genet* 2002;11:1169–1176.
4. Fryer A, Appleton R, Sweeney MG, et al. Mitochondrial DNA 8993 (NARP) mutation presenting with a heterogeneous phenotype including "cerebral palsy." *Arch Dis Child* 1994;71:419–422.
5. Santorelli FM, Mak SC, Vazquez-Memije E, et al. Clinical heterogeneity associated with the mitochondrial DNA T8993C point mutation. *Pediatr Res* 1996;39:914–917.
6. Ledbetter DH, Ballabio A. Molecular cytogenetics of contiguous gene syndromes: mechanisms and consequences of gene dosage imbalance. In: *The metabolic and molecular bases of inherited disease,* 7th ed. New York: McGraw-Hill, 1995:811—839.
7. Barlow DP. Genetic imprinting in mammals. *Science* 1995;270:1610–1613.
8. Pfeifer K. Mechanisms of genomic imprinting. *Am J Hum Genet* 2000;67:777–787.
9. Jiang Y, Tsai TF, Bressler J, et al. Imprinting in Angelman and Prader-Willi syndromes. *Curr Opin Genet Dev* 1998;8:334–342.
10. Albrecht U, Sutcliffe JS, Cattanach BM, et al. Imprinted expression of the murine Angelman syndrome gene, Ube3a, in hippocampal and Purkinje neurons. *Nat Genet* 1997;17:75–78.
11. Vu TH, Hoffman AR. Imprinting of the Angelman syndrome gene, UBE3A, is restricted to the brain. *Nat Genet* 1997;17:12–13.
12. Matsuyama Z, Kawakami H, Maruyama H, et al. Molecular features of the CAG repeats of SCA 6. *Hum Mol Genet* 1997;6:1283–1287.
13. Garcia-Planells J, Cuesta A, Vilchez JJ, et al. Genetics of the SCA6 gene in a large family segregating an autosomal dominant "pure" cerebellar ataxia. J Med Genet 36:148–51, 1999.
14. Knudson AG Jr. Mutation and cancer: statistical study of retinoblastoma. *Proc Natl Acad Sci USA* 1971;68:820–823.
15. Knudson AG Jr, Hethcote HW, Brown BW. Mutation and childhood cancer; a probabilistic model for the incidence of retinoblastoma. *Proc Natl Acad Sci USA* 1975;72:5116–5120.
16. Weleber RG, Carr RE, Murphey WH, et al. Phenotypic variation including retinitis pigmentosa, pattern dystrophy, and fundus flavimaculatus in a single family with a deletion of codon 153 or 154 of the peripherin/RDS gene. *Arch Ophthalmol* 1993;111:1531–1542.
17. Rivolta C, Sharon D, DeAngelis MM, et al. Retinitis pigmentosa and allied diseases; numerous diseases, genes, and inheritance patterns. *Hum Mol Genet* 2002;11:1219–1227.

5

POSTERIOR SEGMENT IMAGING IN INFANTS AND CHILDREN

CYNTHIA DE A. CARVALHO RECCHIA
CAROL L. SHIELDS
FRANCO M. RECCHIA
ANTONIO CAPONE, JR.

Ultrasonography, optical coherence tomography (OCT), and fundus photography are valuable adjuncts to ophthalmoscopy in infants and children with vitreoretinal pathologies. These imaging techniques are useful to diagnose conditions, to compare longitudinal examinations and measurements, to exchange clinical information, and to provide medicolegal documentation.

This chapter addresses the basic principles, clinical indications, advantages, and limitations of the most commonly used methods of posterior segment imaging in infants and children. Techniques not addressed herein including scanning laser ophthalmoscopy and radiologic imaging techniques (plain film, computerized tomography, magnetic resonance imaging) are specifically addressed in separate chapters on trauma (Chapter 33), tumors (Chapters 14, 15), and Coats disease (Chapter 29).

ECHOGRAPHY

Standardized ophthalmic ultrasound is a widely used, noninvasive, painless technique in which acoustic waves, reflected at different acoustic interfaces, provide dynamic images of ocular structures. Ophthalmic ultrasonography requires ultrasound frequencies ranging from 8 to 50 MHz. These frequencies provide the resolution necessary to image smaller ocular structures and are higher than those needed for larger organ systems. Several models of ophthalmic ultrasonographs that differ primarily in their probe frequencies are available. The standard ophthalmic ultrasound uses 8- to 10-MHz wavelengths that permit good resolution (typically 300–600 μm) and adequate penetration of acoustic waves for visualizing posterior ocular structures. Ultrasound biomicroscopy provides higher-resolution (20–60 μm) images of anterior segment structures but does not penetrate sufficiently to provide posterior segment images.

The processed echoes obtained by the ophthalmic ultrasound probes can be displayed as one-dimensional, graph-like images in which the different reflective structures (acoustic interfaces) are represented by vertical spikes of varying amplitudes (A-scan mode; Fig. 5-1, bottom), or as a two-dimensional gray-scale image depicting a cross-sectional representation of the intraocular and orbital structures (B-scan mode; Fig. 5-1). The amplitude of the ultrasound, and thus the appearance displayed as either an A or B scan, depends on the change in speed of the acoustic waves as they travel from one medium to another. The "boundary" representing different media and different acoustic velocities is referred to as an *acoustic interface*. This section addresses primarily the B-scan representation of major vitreoretinal conditions.

Opaque Media

In eyes with opaque media precluding adequate visualization of the posterior pole, ultrasonography is useful for detecting posterior segment pathology. For example, vitreous opacity from blood, uveitis, or tumor seeding can prevent visualization of an underlying retinal detachment, intraocular foreign body, or mass. B-scan ultrasonography performed in the office can provide important information leading to diagnosis and later management. In pediatric trauma patients with suspected ruptures or lacerations, ultrasonography often is avoided so as to reduce additional trauma to the eye.

In the office setting, pediatric ultrasonography can be challenging. Sedation or anesthesia might be considered in some cases; however, the loss of eye movement gained from dynamic scans precludes acquisition of valuable information, such as the identification of a mobile retinal detachment or characterization of vitreous or subretinal fluid. Therefore, when possible, gentle coaxing, warming of the methylcellulose gel, and wrapping of a young infant in a secure blanket can be calming and permit an awake examination.

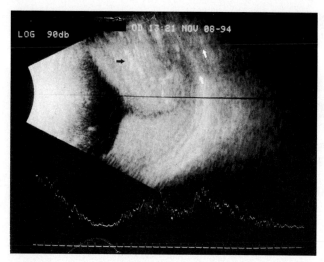

FIGURE 5-1. B-scan ultrasonographic image demonstrating a retinoblastoma with intralesional calcific deposits *(black arrow)* and Leukocoria associated acoustic shadowing *(white arrows)*.

Leukocoria

Leukocoria is a common indication for ultrasonography in pediatric ophthalmology. The differential diagnosis of leukocoria is extensive but most commonly includes congenital cataract, retinoblastoma, persistent fetal vasculature syndrome, retinopathy of prematurity (ROP), Coats disease, and toxocariasis (Table 5-1) (1). Other causes of leukocoria include corneal opacities, vitreous opacities (uveitis, blood, tumor seeding, endophthalmitis), choroidal coloboma, and other causes of retinal detachment.

Retinoblastoma can be unilateral or bilateral, and it can present with one or multiple tumors. On ultrasound, these tumors tend to have an irregular configuration and variable internal reflectivity. Noncalcified tumors are more likely to have low-to-medium internal reflectivity. The presence of calcium within a lesion results in spikes of very high reflectivity, which in some instances can cause shadowing of the

underlying structures (Fig. 5-1). The calcium deposits can be condensed and localized, or they can spread throughout the tumor. Extraocular extension of retinoblastoma can occur but is difficult to detect because of shadowing from intraocular calcifications.

Persistent fetal vasculature syndrome results from an abnormal involution of the tunica vasculosa lentis and primary vitreous. It usually is unilateral and associated with some degree of microphthalmia, most clearly apparent when both eyes are imaged simultaneously. On ultrasound, it is most common to find an extremely thin band, representing vascular or fibrous tissue in the region of the Cloquet canal that is difficult to detect throughout its entire extent. Occasionally, a total retinal detachment can be identified. The retinal detachment appears as a highly reflective retrolental membrane connected to the optic nerve by a vitreous band (Fig. 5-2A). Anatomically, the band represents persistent hyaloid vessels with the retina drawn up around them into a funnel-shaped detachment. The flow of the persistent hyaloid vessels occasionally can be demonstrated by color flow ultrasonography (Fig. 5-2B).

ROP typically is a bilateral disease of premature newborns arising as a consequence of arrested development of the retinal vasculature. The advanced stages are characterized by traction retinal detachment and are classified as partial (stage 4) or total (stage 5). The detachments can be associated with dense retrolental and transvitreous contractile membranes. Acoustic shadowing of the orbital fat and choroidal thickening are seen in about 30% of cases (1). Although indirect ophthalmoscopy and wide-angle fundus imaging are used for most ROP examinations, ultrasonography is helpful in the setting of dense fibrotic membranes behind the lens (seen in advanced stage 4 or stage 5 ROP) precluding posterior pole visualization. Ultrasonography reveals the configuration of the funnel detachment (anteriorly open–posteriorly open, anteriorly open–posteriorly closed, or closed both anteriorly and posteriorly) and whether dense

TABLE 5-1. DIFFERENTIAL DIAGNOSIS OF ECHOGRAPHIC FEATURES OF CONDITIONS CAUSING LEUKOCORIA

Condition	Laterality	Echographic Characteristic
Retinoblastoma	Unilateral or bilateral	One or multiple calcified tumors
Persistent fetal vasculature syndrome	Usually unilateral	Retrolental membrane
		Vitreous band from lens to optic nerve
		Microphthalmia
Retinopathy of prematurity	Usually bilateral	Total or partial retinal detachment
		Retrolental membrane
Coats disease	Usually unilateral	Low mobile retinal detachment
		Subretinal opacities (cholesterol)
Toxocariasis	Unilateral	Peripheral or posterior granulomas
		Vitreous band between granulomas and posterior pole
		Posterior traction retinal detachment or fold

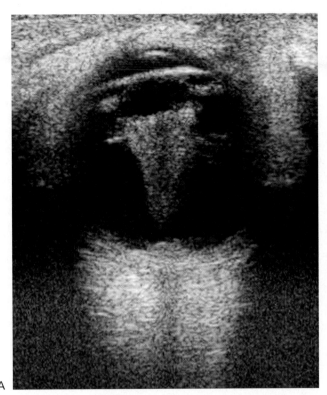
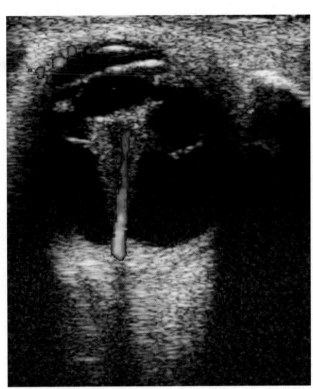

A B

FIGURE 5-2. Image of the left eye depicted in Fig. 5-2. **A:** Gray-scale, B-scan ultrasonographic image demonstrating funnel-shaped hyperreflective retrolental tissue extending to the optic nerve. **B:** Color flow image confirms the presence of blood flow in the funnel, which distinguishes this as persistent fetal vasculature versus a stage 5 retinopathy of prematurity-related retinal detachment.

subretinal blood or cholesterol crystals are present. The configuration of the funnel is associated with the likelihood of successful retinal reattachment after surgery, with closed funnels having the poorest prognoses (2–4). In addition, subretinal blood, fibrosis, and cholesterol are associated with a poor prognosis for visual outcome after surgery.

Coats disease is an idiopathic vascular condition that can cause exudative retinal detachment. It can present as leukocoria and is responsible for 16% of the cases that clinically simulate retinoblastoma (1). It can be difficult to distinguish by ultrasonography an exudative retinal detachment due to Coats disease from a noncalcified exophytic retinoblastoma. The exudative detachments of Coats disease are dome-shaped shallow retinal detachments (Fig. 5-3). By echography, highly reflective subretinal calcifications can be seen in cases of total funnel retinal detachment. More typically, moderately reflective opacities attributable to cholesterol deposits are seen in the subretinal spaces (5).

Ocular toxocariasis often presents with a posterior or peripheral granulomatous lesion that also can be associated with a chronic endophthalmitis. It is characterized ultrasonographically by a triad of findings: (i) mild to moderately elevated, solid, highly reflective peripheral lesions (usually from calcifications), (ii) vitreous band extending between the granulomatous lesion and the posterior pole, and (iii) traction retinal detachment or fold from the posterior pole to the mass (6).

OPTICAL COHERENCE TOMOGRAPHY

OCT is a relatively new diagnostic tool for cross-sectional retinal imaging. In principle it is analogous to ultrasound, although it uses an infrared (840-nm) light instead of acoustic waves to obtain the tomographic scans. The infrared

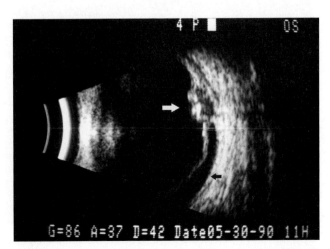

FIGURE 5-3. B-scan ultrasonographic image from a child with Coats disease demonstrating the vascular lesions *(white arrow)* and an underlying sloped exudative retinal detachment *(black arrow)*.

light avoids absorption by the ocular media and, through a technique called *low coherence interferometry,* results in high-resolution scans of approximately 10 to 15 μm. Retinal tissues can be seen *in vivo* in almost histologic detail. It is a noncontact, noninvasive procedure similar to slitlamp biomicroscopy. Although pharmacologic mydriasis is not required, pupil diameter of at least 3.2 mm is necessary to allow detailed examination of the macular anatomy.

Although OCT has been studied in posterior pole imaging, its value has yet to be fully realized in pediatric retinal diseases. Accurate OCT examination requires a cooperative child who is able to remain seated and maintain fixation. It is not a practical tool for imaging infants and some children. The dimensions and sensitivity of the machinery preclude examination of a child under anesthesia. Despite these limitations, OCT can provide valuable diagnostic information for selected pediatric conditions in children old enough to cooperate with the examination.

Foveal hypoplasia can be seen in isolation or in association with other ocular or systemic findings. Typical associated features include nystagmus, aniridia, cataract, skin hypopigmentation, and a poorly formed capillary-free zone. OCT examination demonstrates the absence of a normal foveal depression with preservation of multiple inner retinal layers where there should be only the cone photoreceptors (Fig. 5-4) (7,8). The examination in these patients can be compromised by nystagmus.

Goldman-Favre syndrome is an autosomal recessive vitreoretinal degeneration characterized by degenerative vitre-

ous changes, cystoid macular edema, retinoschisis, and atypical pigmentary dystrophy. OCT is capable of imaging the macular cystoid changes of the posterior retinal schisis (Fig. 5-5) (9).

X-linked congenital retinoschisis is a genetic disorder that has been localized to the short arm of the X chromosome (Xp22.1–p22.3). It presents clinically with typical phenotypic features (10,11), including a stellate-shaped maculopathy (Fig. 5-6A) and peripheral schisis cavities (12,13). The midperipheral retina is generally considered to be uninvolved in eyes with X-linked congenital retinoschisis. However, a unique OCT finding in the midperipheral retina is that of flat, lamellar schisislike abnormalities in areas of ophthalmoscopically normal retina (Fig. 5-6B) (14).

FUNDUS PHOTOGRAPHY

Imaging of the ocular fundus is important for documenting numerous retinal and choroidal conditions. Several fundus imaging systems are commercially available.

Conventional Fundus Photography

The most popular fundus camera systems are the nonportable, small-angle cameras (such as the Zeiss, Canon, and the Topcon) or the portable cameras (e.g., portable Nidek noncontact fundus camera, [Nidek Co., Gamagori, Aichi, Japan], Genesis portable camera for fundus photography and

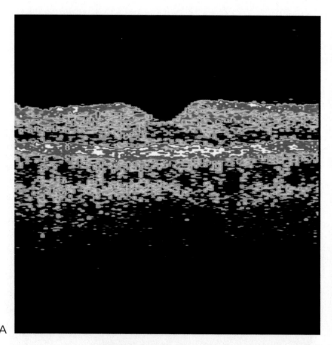
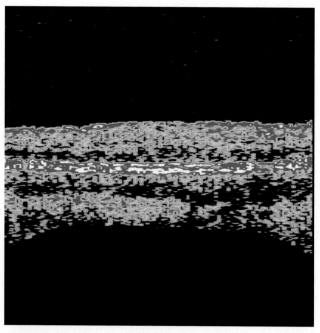

A   B

FIGURE 5-4. A: Optical coherence tomographic image of a normal macula. **B:** Image from a child with foveal hypoplasia (compare with panel **A**). Findings include absence of a normal foveal declivity and preservation of multiple inner retinal layers where there should be only the cone photo receptors.

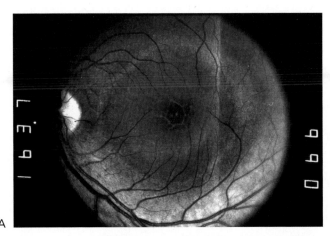

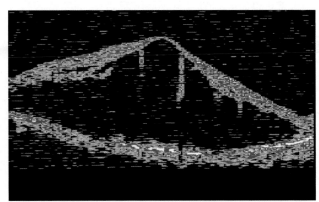

A   B

FIGURE 5-5. Red-free **(A)** and Optical coherence tomographic **(B)** images of the macula in a child with Goldmann-Favre syndrome. Optical coherence tomography confirmed the clinical impression of dramatic macrocystic macular edema and posterior retinal schisis, distinguishing it from macular hole with an associated annular neurosensory detachment.

fluorescein angiography [Kowa Company, Ltd, Nihonbashi-Honcho, Shuo-ku, Japan]). The portable systems are most useful for imaging infants, whereas the tabletop units can be used to image small children. Such small-angle systems typically have a light source mounted near the camera with light directed through the pupil into the posterior segment of the eye. These systems generally provide small-angle, high-resolution (approximately 1,500 pixels) fundus images with fields from approximately 20 to 80 degrees. The image size varies depending on whether film or a digital chip is used and, if the latter is used, on the size of the chip and the optics of the particular system. However, there is limited ability to image the retina anterior to the equator. Additionally, imaging of large fundus abnormalities is inadequate with small-angle systems because the abnormality is documented

in a piecemeal fashion without the desired broad perspective of the entire lesion.

During an examination with a child under anesthesia, the fundus can be imaged through a noncontact 60-diopter lens or through a small contact lens placed onto the cornea and photographed using a camera connected to the operating room microscope. The field of view is limited; however, imaging of the peripheral retina can be achieved by manipulating the position of the globe using a scleral depressor or lens loupe. In the case of the contact lens, focus is achieved by moving the microscope toward the cornea, whereas with a 60-diopter lens, focus is achieved by moving the microscope anteriorly away from the cornea. Fluorescein angiography also can be performed using a KOWA or standard office fluorescein angiography camera. With a tabletop

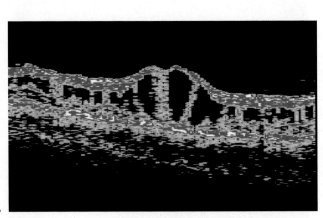

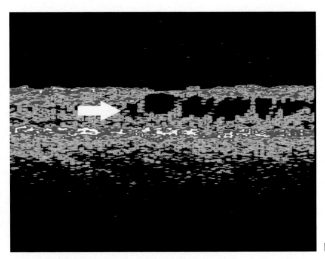

A   B

FIGURE 5-6. A: Typical foveal schisis in a child with congenital retinoschisis. **B:** Lamellar schisis **(arrow)** from an area of midperipheral retina—usually presumed to be normal clinically in light of the normal ophthalmoscopic appearance—in a child with congenital retinoschisis.

TABLE 5-2. WIDE-ANGLE FUNDUS IMAGING SYSTEMS

| | Camera System | | |
Parameter	Retcam 120	Panoramic200	Panoret-1000
Fundus illumination	Transpupillary	Transpupillary	Transscleral
Camera type	Contact	Noncontact	Contact
Degrees of fundus imaged	130	200	130
Image resolution	Good	High	High
Image distortion	No	Yes	No
Color match	Realistic	"Blue-free" aberration	Realistic
Camera portable	Somewhat	No	Somewhat
Fluorescein angiography	Yes	No	No[a]
Indocyanine green angiography	No	No	No[a]
Single operator	No	Yes	Yes

[a]Future plans for angiography.

fluorescein camera, the infant is placed onto his/her side. The infant's eye is moved close to the camera lens and kept open with a lid speculum. Balanced salt solution is dropped onto the cornea to maintain clarity of media. In children, the dose of sodium fluorescein is 35 mg per 10 pounds of body weight [*Physicians' Desk Reference for Ophthalmology (PDR 2000),* 28th ed. Montvale, NJ: Medical Economics, 1999:214].

Wide-Angle Fundus Imaging

Wide-angle systems have been devised to address the limitations of field of view of conventional fundus cameras. However, in gaining field of view, some wide-angle systems must sacrifice resolution. Their main uses are serial wide-angle documentation of fundus pathology (tumors, shaken baby syndrome) and fundus screening (15–17). Currently three systems are available: Retcam 120™, (Massie Laboratories, Inc., Pleasanton, CA, USA), Panoramic200™ (Optos Pic, Dunfermline, Fife, Scotland), and Panoret-1000™ (Medibell Medical Vision Technologies, Haifa, Israel) (Table 5-2).

Retcam 120

The Retcam 120 requires contact between the hand-held camera and the corneal surface (contact system) and uses transpupillary illumination to capture digital images of the fundus through a widely dilated pupil. The Retcam 120 provides high-resolution images using a 3-CCD (charged coupling device) digital camera coupled to a family of lens units, including a 130-degree unit designed for imaging ROP, a standard 120-degree unit, a high-magnification 30-degree unit, a high-contrast /adult 80-degree unit, and the flat-field portrait lens used for external photographs. The images are 640 × 480 pixels, approximately 900 kB in size, with a resolution of 72 pixels per inch and a realistic color match. Focus and illumination adjustments are manual and can be performed either on the base unit or with a foot pedal.

The Retcam 120 is most commonly used for infants and children because image quality degrades significantly with even mild degrees of nuclear sclerosis. Optimal image quality requires wide pupillary dilation, a clear crystalline lens, and light-to-medium fundus pigmentation. There are other factors that reduce image quality. Extreme prematurity with narrow palpebral fissures precludes good corneal contact with the lens nosepiece. Media opacity from corneal clouding, pseudophakia, or cataract or a stark white fundus lesions from excessive reflection of light can reduce image quality. Poor mydriasis results in a dark, round or ring-shaped artifact; and dark choroidal pigmentation can impair visualization of retinal vascular detail.

Although the Retcam 120 can be used on alert infants with topical anesthetic, in children younger than 5 years the best images are acquired when the children are under anesthesia. Anterior segment images of reasonable quality can be acquired with this system (Fig. 5-7). Retinal conditions well imaged with this system include retinoblastoma, ROP (Fig.

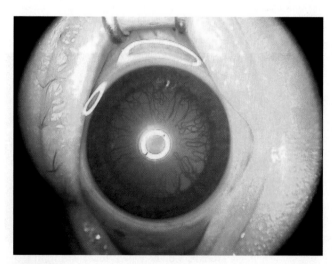

FIGURE 5-7. Retcam 120 anterior segment image demonstrating tunica vasculosa lentis in a premature infant.

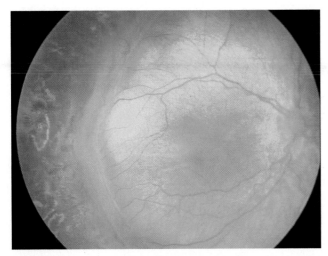

FIGURE 5-8. Retcam 120 fundus image demonstrating low-lying posterior macula-sparing (stage 4A) retinopathy of prematurity-related retinal detachment in a previously lasered eye.

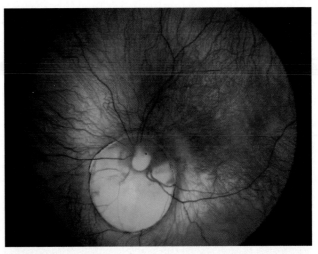

FIGURE 5-10. Retcam 120 fundus image demonstrating optic nerve and chorioretinal coloboma in an infant.

5-8), retinal hemorrhages (shaken baby syndrome, thrombocytopenic retinopathy), Coats disease (Fig. 5-9), and congenital ocular conditions (Fig. 5-10). Wide-angle fluorescein angiography (Fig. 5-11) can be performed with the Retcam 120, a feature not yet available on other wide-angle systems.

Panoramic200

The Panoramic200 is a noncontact, nonmydriatic scanning laser ophthalmoscopic system that uses transpupillary illumination to acquire 200-degree, high-resolution digital fundus images (Optomap^TM). Images are acquired using an ellipsoidal mirror to scan the retina with green laser (532 nm) for imaging the sensory retina to the retinal pigment epithelium and red laser (633 nm) for imaging the retinal pigment

epithelium and choroid. The result is a 2,000 × 2,000-pixel image, 12 MB in size, with resolution of up to 20 μm. The goal of nearly full-fundus imaging is to provide an effective tool for screening and routine posterior pole imaging.

Image acquisition is conceptually straightforward: the patient places his/her chin on a chin rest, focuses on a spot directly ahead, and presses a button. In practice, positioning the patient within the instrument is a bit awkward and correct fixation alignment can be tricky. Because of the level of cooperation required, pediatric imaging could be performed only in older children.

The image captured is indeed broad (Fig. 5-12). Both adult and pediatric eyes can be imaged. Although nonmydriatic, optimal imaging requires wide pupillary dilation. The image acquired is somewhat distorted due to elliptical aberration induced by the mirror within the system. No

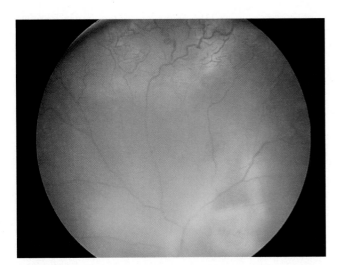

FIGURE 5-9. Retcam 120 fundus image demonstrating Coats disease with peripheral lesions superiorly accentuated by scleral indentation.

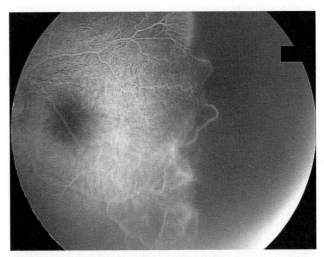

FIGURE 5-11. Retcam 120 fundus fluorescein angiographic image demonstrating incomplete peripheral retinal vascularization and retinal neovascularization (leaking superiorly) in an infant with incontinentia pigmenti.

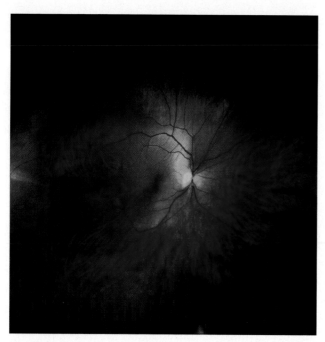

FIGURE 5-12. Panoramic200 fundus image. Note elliptical aberration and color variance compared to traditional fundus images.

TABLE 5-3. WIDE-ANGLE IMAGING IN SPECIAL CIRCUMSTANCES

	Camera System	
Clinical Situations	Retcam 120	Panoret-1000
Small pupil	Poor	Fair to good
Cataract	Poor	Fair to good
Media opacity	Poor	Fair to good
Dark uvea	Fair	Fair

from the "Equator Plus" camera popularized by Oleg Pomerantzeff, M.D., in the early 1970s (18–22). The Pomerantzeff film camera was the first to separate the illumination source from the camera and place it on the globe to illuminate the interior of the eye.

The Panoret-1000 captures approximately 130 degrees of the fundus using a CCD digital camera that acquires $1,024 \times 1,024$-pixel images with image resolution of 20 μm at a rate of 3 frames per second. This system allows imaging by a single operator because the focus and illumination levels are automatic, whereas in the Retcam 120, these parameters must be adjusted separately using a foot pedal. The light source is placed on the globe 180 degrees opposite the lesion to be imaged to illuminate the interior of the eye. Images are of high quality (Fig. 5-13).

As is true of the Retcam 120, the Panoret-1000 is somewhat portable. The Panoret-1000 has the additional capability of imaging both children and adults because the transscleral light provides adequate illumination in patients with small pupils, cataract, pseudophakia, and some corneal and media opacities. As with the Retcam 120, image quality is diminished in eyes with dark uveal pigmentation, and in children younger than 5 years the best images are acquired when the children are under anesthesia (Table 5-3).

blue laser is used in the system because all clinically relevant fundus detail is captured with green and red wavelengths. The result is a "blue-free" fundus image. One quickly becomes accustomed to the elliptical and color variances.

Panoret-1000

The Panoret-1000 differs from all other wide-angle imaging systems in that it uses transscleral rather transpupillary illumination. The idea for transscleral illumination derives

CONCLUSION

This chapter provides an overview of widely available technology for posterior segment imaging in infants and children. The technologies reviewed are complementary, each providing unique information useful in the diagnosis and management of pediatric posterior segment pathology.

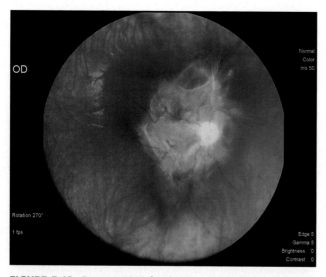

FIGURE 5-13. Panoret-1000 fundus image of combined hamartoma of the retina and retinal pigment epithelium in a 12-year-old boy.

REFERENCES

1. Shields JA, Shields CL, Parsons HM. Review: differential diagnosis of retinoblastoma. *Retina* 1991;11:232–243.
2. Shapiro DR, Stone RD. Ultrasonic characteristics of retinopathy of prematurity presenting with leukokoria. *Arch Ophthalmol* 1985;103:1690–1692.
3. Pulido JS, Byrne SF, Clarkson JG, et al. Evaluation of eyes with advanced stages of retinopathy of prematurity using standardized echography. *Ophthalmology* 1991;98:1099–1104.

4. Zilis JD, deJuan E, Machemer R. Advanced retinopathy of prematurity. The anatomic and visual results of vitreous surgery. *Ophthalmology* 1990;97:821–826.

5. Jabbour NM, Eller AE, Hirose T, et al. Stage 5 retinopathy of prematurity. Prognostic value of morphologic findings. *Ophthalmology* 1987;94:1640–1646.

6. Atta HR, Watson NJ. Echographic diagnosis of advanced Coats' disease. *Eye* 1992;6:80–85.

7. Wan WL, Cano MR, Pince KJ, et al. Echographic characteristics of ocular toxocariasis. *Ophthalmology* 1991;98:28–32.

8. Oliver MD, Dotan SA, Chemke J, et al. Isolated foveal hypoplasia. *Br J Ophthalmol* 1987;71:926–930.

9. Recchia FM, Carvalho Recchia CA, Trese MT. Optical coherence tomography in the diagnosis of foveal hypoplasia. *Arch Ophthalmol* 2002;120:1587–1588.

10. Theodossiadis PG, Koutsandrea CT, Kollia AC, et al. Optical coherence tomography in the study of the Goldman-Favre syndrome. *Am J Ophthalmol* 2000;129:542–544.

11. Alito T, Kruse TA, dela Chapelle A. Refined localization of the gene causing X-linked juvenile retinoschisis. *Genomics* 1991;9:505–510.

12. Sieving PA, Bingham EL, Roth MS, et al. Linkage relationship of X-linked juvenile retinoschisis with Xp22.1–p22.3 probes. *Am J Hum Genet* 1990;47:616–621.

13. Haas J. Ueber das Zusammenvorkommen von Veranderungen der Retina und Cohroidea. *Arch Augenheilkd* 1898;343–348.

14. Prenner JL, Capone A Jr, Ciaccia S, et al. Congenital retinoschisis: unique OCT findings and system of classification. 2004 (in press).

15. Shields CL, Materin M, Epstein J, et al. Wide-angle imaging of the ocular fundus. *Rev Ophthalmol* 2003;10:66–70.

16. Schwartz SD, Harrison SA, Ferrone PJ, et al. Telemedical evaluation and management of retinopathy of prematurity using a fiberoptic digital fundus camera. *Ophthalmology* 2000;107:25–28.

17. Roth DB, Morales D, Feuer WJ, et al. Screening for retinopathy of prematurity employing the Retcam 120: sensitivity and specificity. *Arch Ophthalmol* 2001;119:268–272.

18. Seiberth V, Woldt C. Wide angle fundus documentation in retinopathy of prematurity. *Ophthalmologe* 2001;98:960–963.

19. Pomerantzeff O. Equator-plus camera. *Invest Ophthalmol* 1975;4:401–406.

20. Ducrey N, Pomerantzeff O, Schepens CL, et al. Clinical trials with equator-plus camera. *Am J Ophthalmol* 1977;84:840–846.

21. Pomerantzeff O, Webb RH, Delori FC. Image formation in fundus cameras. *Invest Ophthalmol Vis Sci* 1979;18:630–637.

22. Pomerantzeff O. Wide-angle noncontact and small-angle contact cameras. *Invest Ophthalmol Vis Sci* 1980;19:973–979.

6

ALBINISM, LYSOSOMAL STORAGE DISEASES, AND OTHER METABOLIC CONDITIONS

MICHAEL MARBLE

ALBINISM

Albinism is a genetically and clinically heterogeneous group of disorders characterized by hypopigmentation of the skin, hair, and eyes. The hypopigmentation is due to deficiency of melanin production in specialized cells known as *melanocytes*. Oculocutaneous albinism (OCA) involves all three tissues, whereas ocular albinism (OA) is confined to the eyes. The ocular findings are important in the diagnosis of albinism. The major ocular features are decreased pigment of the retina and irides, foveal hypoplasia, and misrouting of optic nerve fibers. Patients typically have reduced visual acuity and have refractive errors, strabismus, and nystagmus (1–3).

Genetics and Classification

Advances in the molecular biology of albinism have helped to clarify the classification of these conditions (Table 6-1). Some disorders previously thought to be distinct entities now are considered to be part of the spectrum of defined etiologic groups. From a genetic and etiologic standpoint, albinism can be classified according to the following categories: tyrosinase deficiency (OCA1) (4); defects in the *P* gene (OCA2) (5,6); defects in the tyrosinase-related protein 1 (*TYRP1*) gene (OCA3) (7,8); defects in a membrane-associated transport protein (OCA4) (9); genes involved in vesicle formation [Hermansky-Pudlak syndrome (HPS)] (10–14), defects in a lysosomal trafficking regulator [Chediak-Higashi syndrome (CHS)] (15), and defects in the OA1 gene (ocular albinism) (16). Other than OA, which is X linked, these disorders are inherited in an autosomal recessive fashion. OCA1 to OCA4 and OA are disorders in which the metabolic problem is specific to melanocytes, either in the melanin biosynthesis pathway itself or in the melanosomal membrane. In contrast, the defects in HPS and CHS involve multiple cell types; therefore, OCA is only one component of these conditions. The corresponding mouse phenotype and locus have been - described for the albinism disorders discussed in this chapter.

Prevalence of Albinism

Albinism is a relatively common genetic condition. Its frequency varies considerably in the United States and around the world. The prevalence worldwide is about 1 in 10,000 to 1 in 20,000. In the United States, OCA2 is the most common in African-Americans and Caucasians, with a prevalence of about 1 in 10,000 (1). OCA2 has a high prevalence in some Native-American populations, such as the Hopi, Zuni (1), and Navajo. In the Navajo population, a unique deletion in the *P* gene is associated with an increased frequency of OCA2 (17). The prevalence of OCA1 is about 1 in 28,000 in African-Americans and Caucasians. OCA3 occurs in about 1 in 8,500 in South Africa (1). HPS is rare overall but is relatively common in Puerto Rico, occurring in about 1 in 1,800 (18). It also is relatively common in an isolated village in the Swiss Alps (19).

Pathophysiology: Biochemistry of Melanin Synthesis

To understand the different defects causing albinism, it is helpful to be familiar with the melanin biosynthetic pathway. This pathway takes place within lysosome-related organelles known as *melanosomes*. Tyrosinase catalyzes the initial and rate-limiting step in melanin synthesis. In this step, the amino acid tyrosine is converted to dihydroxyphenylalanine (DOPA) and then to DOPAquinone. DOPAquinone represents a branch point, which can go in the direction of either pheomelanin (yellow/red) synthesis or eumelanin (brown/ black) synthesis. The pheomelanin pathway can occur in the presence of sulfhydryls. In the eumelanin pathway, DOPAchrome is formed and is converted to either 5,6-dihydroxyindole (DHI) or 5,6-dihydroxyindole-2-carboxylic acid (DHICA). Further processing of DHI results in DHI melanin (black) formation, whereas further processing of DHICA results in DHICA melanin (brown) formation. Tyrosinase is involved in both the DHI melanin and DHICA melanin pathways; however, in the DHICA melanin pathway, another protein, TYRP1, is also

TABLE 6-1. GENES INVOLVED IN ALBINISM

Gene	Gene Product	Function	Disease	Mouse locus
TYR	Tyrosinase	Enzyme in melanin synthesis	OCA1	Albino (c)
Pgene	P protein	Melanosomal membrane protein involved in maintenance of acidity in melanosome	OCA2	Pink-eyed dilution (p)
TYRP1	Tyrosinase-related protein 1	Stabilizes melanosomal enzyme complex	OCA3	Brown (b)
MATP	Membrane-associated transporter protein	Transporter	OCA4	Underwhite (uw)
OA1	Melanosomal membrane glycoprotein	Melanosomal membrane	OA1	OA1 (moa)
HPS1	Transmembrane protein	Involved in development function of organelles (e.g., melanosome)	Hermansky-Pudlak syndrome	Pale ear (ep)
ADTB3A (HPS2)	β_3-adaptin subunit of the adaptor complex 3	Protein sorting in organelle biogenesis	Hermansky-Pudlak syndrome	Pearl (pe)
HPS3	HP3 protein	Involved in melanosome biogenesis and maturation	Hermansky-Pudlak syndrome	Cocoa (coa)
HPS4	HPS4 protein	Organelle biogenesis	Hermansky-Pudlak syndrome	Light ear (le)
HPS5	HPS5 protein	Biogenesis of lysosome-related organelles	Hermansky-Pudlak syndrome	Ruby-eye-2 (ru2)
HPS6	HPS6 protein	Biogenesis of lysosome-related organelles	Hermansky-Pudlak syndrome	Ruby-eye (ru)
CHSI	Membrane Protein	Lysosomal trafficking regulator	Chediak-Higashi syndrome	Beige (bg)

Adapted from King RA, Hearing VJ, Creel DJ, et al. Albinism. In: Scriver CR, Beaudet AL, Sly WS, et al., eds. *Metabolic and molecular bases of inherited disease,* 8th ed. New York: McGraw-Hill, 2001: 5587-5627.

believed to play a role as a stabilizer of the melanogenic enzyme complex. Another enzyme, DHICA polymerase, is believed to catalyze the final step in DHICA melanin production (1).

As discussed in the section on Phenotypic Patterns of Albinism, the different albinism phenotypes result from corresponding defects at different levels affecting the above pathway, including (i) enzymatic steps in the pathway, (ii) proteins important for the melanosomal organelle and transport, and (iii) proteins important for multiple organelles, including melanosomes.

Clinical Symptoms and Signs

Normally, melanin accumulates in the retinal pigment epithelium during the early embryonic stages. This is important for appropriate routing of optic nerve fibers and for eventual visual function. The ocular findings of albinism are characteristic. Decreased melanin causes iris translucency and retinal hypopigmentation (1–3).

Decreased visual acuity occurs in albinism and is due to foveal hypoplasia. Visual acuity may range from 20/40 to 20/400. Color vision is normal. A very characteristic finding in albinism is the misrouting of optic nerve fibers. Normally, fibers from the nasal retina cross at the optic chiasm and end up in the lateral geniculate nucleus on the contralateral side. Temporal fibers do not cross over. In albinism, the temporal fibers inappropriately cross at the chiasm. The result is that the proportion of crossed fibers is increased. Misrouting of the optic nerve fibers can sometimes be detected by visual evoked potential (1,2). Other ocular features of albinism include nystagmus, strabismus, and abnormal stereoscopic vision (1,2).

Phenotypic Patterns of Albinism

OCA1

Clinical Symptoms and Signs

Patients with OCA1 ("tyrosinase-related") are characteristically born with severe hypopigmentation of the skin and hair (1–3). In OCA1A, which is associated with complete absence of tyrosinase activity, the hypopigmentation does not significantly change over time. No freckles or other pigmented skin lesions develop. In contrast, OCA1B is associated with varying levels of residual tyrosinase activity. As in OCA1A, there is severe hypopigmentation of the skin and hair at birth; however, patients with OCA1B tend to develop some pigmentation over time. They may develop freckles and some tanning, and the hair may develop a brown or yellow coloration. The ocular features of OCA1B are generally milder than those in OCA1A. The varying levels of tyrosinase activity in OCA1B cause corresponding differences in phenotype. Some clinical entities, such as yellow albinism, temperature-sensitive albinism, and platinum or mixed or minimal pigment albinism, now are considered to be phenotypes within the OCA1B spectrum (1).

OCA2

Clinical Symptoms and Signs

As mentioned previously, OCA2 ("tyrosinase-positive") is the most common form of albinism in the United States and worldwide. In contrast to OCA1, some pigmentation usually is present at birth. Similar to OCA1B, patients may undergo some tanning and can develop freckles. OCA2 sometimes is referred to as *tyrosinase-positive OCA* because of the normal tyrosinase activity (1).

Genetics

The defect in these patients is in the *P* gene, which encodes for a protein thought to be involved in maintenance of acidic pH in the melanosomes (20). The *P*-gene product also may play a role in intracellular transport of tyrosinase and possibly a minor role in transport of TYRP1 (21). There is marked clinical variability within the spectrum of OCA2. In Africans and African-Americans, a classic phenotype has been described consisting of congenitally yellow hair and a creamy white skin color (Figs. 6-1 and 6-2). The irides are usually blue-gray, hazel, or tan (1). Some African-American and African patients have a phenotype called *brown OCA,* which also is due to mutations in the *P* gene (1,22,23).

The *P* gene maps to chromosome 15 within the Prader-Willi syndrome and Angelman syndrome region. Prader-Willi and Angelman syndrome are complex conditions with mental retardation (24,25). The majority of these patients have deletion of 15q11–q13, and a substantial proportion have hypopigmentation related to the

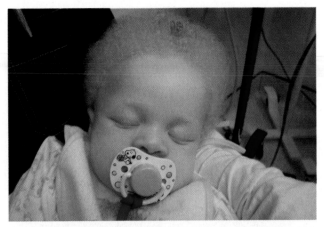

FIGURE 6-1. Three-month-old African-American boy with OCA2. Note the yellow hair color, which was present at birth.

P gene. The mouse locus for the *P* gene is "pink-eyed dilution" (*p*) (26).

OCA3

Clinical Symptoms and Signs

OCA3 has been described in a number of patients in South Africa. These individuals tend to have reddish hair color and hazel or brown eyes; the skin color is described as reddish-brown (Fig. 6-3). The ocular features are mild. Misrouting of optic fibers has not been described. The entity known as *rufous albinism* is now considered to be OCA3 (1,27).

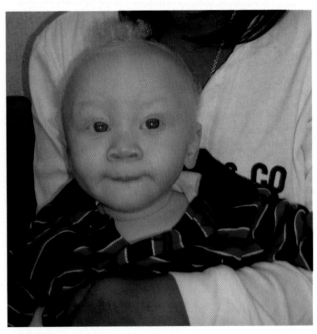

FIGURE 6-2. Six-month-old African-American boy with OCA2 phenotype.

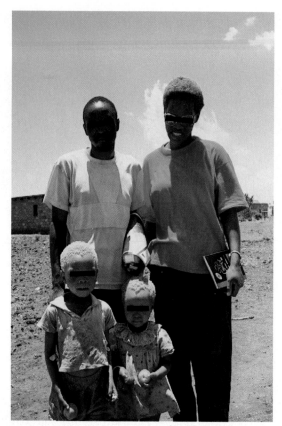

FIGURE 6-3. Two South-African siblings *(front)* with atypical oculocutaneous albinism (OCA). Mutation testing showed compound heterozygosity for mutations in the *TYRP1* gene but also a 2.7-kb deletion of the *P* gene. In addition, an unrelated woman *(back right)* reportedly has rufous OCA. Mutation testing showed compound heterozygosity for mutations in the *TYRP1* gene. (From Manga P, Kromberg JG, Box NF, et al. Rufous oculocutaneous albinism in southern African Blacks is caused by mutations in the *TYRP1* gene. *Am J Hum Genet* 1997;61:1095–1101, with permission.)

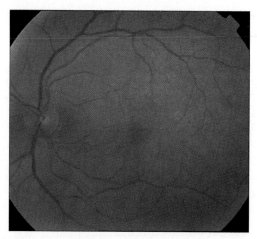

FIGURE 6-4. Left macula of OA1 carrier female. Note mottling and patchy hypopigmentation of the retinal pigment epithelium. (From Donsoff L, Yannuzzi D, Costa S, et al. X-linked ocular albinism: fundus of a heterozygous female retina. *J Retinal Vitreous Dis* 2003;23:410–411, with permission.)

Ocular Albinism (Nettleship-Falls Type)

Clinical Symptoms and Signs

The phenotype of OA1 is similar from an ocular standpoint to OCA. However, the skin and hair pigmentation are normal, although scattered hypopigmentation has been observed in some African-American patients. Giant melanosomes are found in the melanocytes of OA1 patients.

Genetics

OA is inherited in an X-linked recessive fashion; therefore, males are predominantly affected (1). However, carrier females may have a mosaic pattern of pigmentation of the fundus due to lyonization (Figs. 6-4 and 6-5) (31). The gene maps to Xp22 and is designated OA1 (32). OA1 encodes for

Genetics

The molecular basis of OCA3 is mutation in the *TYRP1* gene (28). The encoded protein TYRP1 is involved in the eumelanin pathway to form DHICA melanin (brown). TYRP1 is thought to stabilize the melanogenic enzyme complex. The corresponding mouse locus for TYRP1 is "brown" *(b)*. The precise function of TYRP1 is unclear. It may play a role in stabilizing tyrosinase, and it may affect the catalytic activity of tyrosinase. It also is thought to be involved in maintenance of melanosomal structure and proliferation (29).

OCA4

OCA4 is associated with a similar phenotype to that of OCA2 (9). The gene involved in OCA4 encodes for a membrane-associated transporter protein. The mouse homolog is underwhite *(uw)* (30).

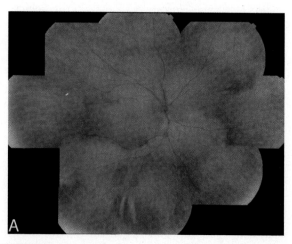

FIGURE 6-5. Composite photographs of the right eye of an OA1 carrier female. Note "mud-splattered" hyperpigmented streaks. (From Donsoff L, Yannuzzi D, Costa S, et al. X-linked ocular albinism: fundus of a heterozygous female retina. *J Retinal Vitreous Dis* 2003;23:410–411, with permission.)

an integral membrane protein. A number of mutations have been detected (16). The corresponding mouse locus for OA1 is "OA1" *(moa)* (32).

Hermansky-Pudlak Syndrome

Clinical Symptoms and Signs

HPS is a multisystem disorder, one component of which is OCA (1). The other major components of the phenotype are bleeding problems due to absent platelet dense bodies and ceroid storage in multiple tissues, an increased risk for granulomatous colitis, and pulmonary fibrosis. Patients tend to have a creamy-white skin color and may develop freckles. However, the degree of hypopigmentation of the skin and hair is quite variable (Fig. 6-6). Visual acuity is decreased, and the other typical ocular features of albinism are present. Platelets in HPS do not undergo appropriate secondary aggregation. This leads to bleeding problems, which usually are mild (1,33,34).

Genetics

HPS is genetically heterogeneous and involves genes that encode for proteins important for the formation of vesicles such as melanosomes, lysosomes, and platelet dense bodies (1,33,34).

Chediak-Higashi Syndrome

Clinical Symptoms and Signs

CHS patients have hypopigmentation of the skin, hair, and eyes. The hair tends to have a metallic silver-gray sheen (Fig. 6-7). The skin may have a white-creamy appearance. There

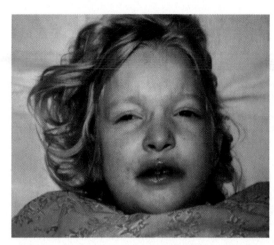

FIGURE 6-7. Patient with Chediak-Higashi syndrome. (From Weinberg S, Prose N, Kristal L. *Color atlas of pediatric dermatology*, 3rd ed. McGraw-Hill, New York. 1998:237, with permission.)

is variable pigmentation in the iris and variable presence of nystagmus and photophobia. Immunologic problems are characteristic and include defects in natural killer cell activity and defective chemotaxis. Recurrent pyogenic bacterial infections are common. Platelet dense bodies are abnormal, and there is a tendency to bleeding. Multiple neurologic problems develop over time (35,36).

Genetics

The product of the Chediak-Higashi gene is thought to be involved in regulation of lysosomal trafficking and the corresponding mouse locus is "beige" *(bg)*. CHS is considered to be a disorder of lysosomes and lysosome-related organelles (35,36).

Diagnosis of Albinism

Diagnosis of albinism usually is based on the clinical features, which include oculocutaneous or ocular hypopigmentation along with the characteristic ocular abnormalities in albinism. If necessary, visual evoked potential studies should be done to detect misrouting. Other aspects of evaluation include general ophthalmologic assessment for decreased visual acuity, nystagmus, strabismus, foveal hypoplasia, and abnormalities in depth perception (1).

An important clinical distinction between OCA1 and OCA2 is the presence of visible pigmentation at birth in OCA2, whereas in both types of OCA1 the newborn appears to have white skin and hair. DNA diagnostic testing is now clinically available for OCA1A, OCA2, and OA1. For OA1, electron microscopic evaluation of skin or hair bulb melanocytes can be performed to detect macromelanosomes to help in the diagnosis of this condition (1).

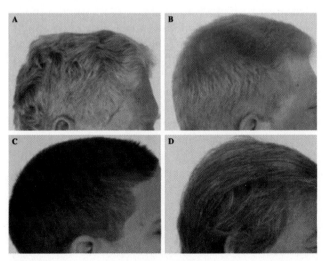

FIGURE 6-6. Hypopigmentation of the skin and hair in different types of Hermansky-Pudlak syndrome: **A:** HPS-1; **B:** HPS-2; **C:** HPS-3; **D:** HPS-4. (From Huizing M, Boissy R, Gahl W. Hermansky-Pudlak syndrome: vesicle formation from yeast to man. *Pigment Cell Res* 2002;15:405–419, with permission.)

The diagnosis of HPS is based on the presence of OCA in combination with the other characteristic features of HPS. The absence of platelet dense bodies on electron microscopy is diagnostic of HPS. DNA diagnostic testing is clinically available for HPS1 and HPS3. The diagnosis of CHS is based mainly on the clinical features (1). Huge lysosomes and cytoplasmic granules are important diagnostic findings for CHS (35).

Differential Diagnosis: Disorders with Hypopigmentation Not Classified as Albinism

Besides albinism, there are a number of other genetic conditions associated with skin hypopigmentation. Hypopigmentation of Ito consists of whirls of hypopigmentation along Blaschko lines, as well as mental retardation and other clinical features. This condition is associated with chromosomal mosaicism (37,38). Some inborn errors of metabolism are associated with hypopigmentation. These include Menkes disease, which is due to abnormal copper metabolism, and phenylketonuria before treatment was available (39,40). Waardenburg syndrome is an autosomal dominant condition with hearing loss, specific facial characteristics, and localized hypopigmentation including white forelock of the hair (41). Other disorders such as Griscelli syndrome (42), Tietz syndrome (43), and Cross syndrome (44) are associated with generalized skin hypopigmentation but do not have the characteristic eye findings typically seen in albinism. The term *albinoidism* has been used in reference to some of the conditions with hypopigmentation that do not fit the overall ocular phenotype of albinism, such as nystagmus, decreased visual acuity, and visual pathway abnormalities (45).

Management

Ongoing care with the ophthalmologist and dermatologist is important. Ocular management is through low-vision rehabilitation and filters (see Chapter 33). However, future treatments may be developed to correct the genetic defect, such as through gene therapy (see Chapter 13). Dermatology is important mainly to advise the patient on measures to take for protection against the sun.

Although a diagnosis of albinism is evident in most cases, it is useful to refer the patient to a clinical geneticist to help determine the type of albinism and to provide appropriate genetic counseling, pedigree analysis, and deoxyribonucleic acid (DNA) testing if warranted. Genetic evaluation can be helpful in ruling out or diagnosing complex syndromes with albinism, such as HPS or CHS. If either is diagnosed, other consultations are needed, depending on complications and monitoring. The care for these patients may be coordinated by the clinical geneticist or other physicians experienced in the management of rare diseases.

LYSOSOMAL DISEASES

The lysosomes are cytoplasmic organelles that serve as the cellular compartments where macromolecules are degraded into their individual constituents. To perform this function, lysosomes contain hydrolytic enzymes to carry out the digestion of these macromolecules. Numerous diseases due to deficiency of various lysosomal enzymes have been described. The result of individual defects is the accumulation of the macromolecule substrate for which the enzyme was responsible for degrading. The clinical phenotype is determined by the specific substrate and the effect of its accumulation on various tissues. From a clinical standpoint, a consistent characteristic of most lysosomal storage diseases is developmental regression. This is caused by the ongoing damage due to accumulation of the undegraded substrate.

The major groups of macromolecules degraded in the lysosomes include glycoproteins, glycolipids, and glycosaminoglycans (mucopolysaccharides).

Glycoproteins are compounds with varying proportions of carbohydrate molecules, such as fucose, mannose, sialic acid, and galactose attached to proteins. Disorders of glycoprotein breakdown include fucosidosis, mannosidosis, aspartylglucosaminuria, sialidosis, and galactosialidosis (46).

A variety of complex lipid-containing compounds are degraded in the lysosomes. Sphingomyelin is a phospholipid and contains ceramide attached to phosphocholine and a long chain fatty acid. The term "glycolipid" refers to compounds with a glucosy or galactosyl group attached to ceramide. Defects in the degradation of the above compounds include Niemann-Pick disease, Tay-Sachs disease, Sandhoff disease, G_{M1} gangliosidosis, Krabbe-disease, Gaucher disease and others. Farber disease is due to a defect in the degradation of ceramide which is a core component of phospholipids and glycolipids (46).

Glycosaminoglycans (mucopolysaccharides) consist of polymers of hexuronic acid attached to amino sugars. The glycosaminoglycans are important components of connective tissue ground substance. Disorders in this category are called *mucopolysaccharidoses* and include Hurler syndrome, Hunter syndrome, Sanfilippo syndrome, Scheie syndrome, Morquio syndrome, Maroteaux-Lamy syndrome, and Sly syndrome (46).

Retinal abnormalities are common in lysosomal storage disease. For example, cherry-red spot in the macula is a consistent feature of several of the disorders of glycolipid and glycoprotein degradation (Table 6-2). Retinal abnormalities along with other ocular problems such as corneal clouding and glaucoma are common in the mucopolysaccharidoses.

TABLE 6-2. LYSOSOMAL DISORDERS CONSISTENTLY ASSOCIATED WITH CHERRY-RED SPOT MACULA

Disorder	Deficient Enzyme	Inheritance
Niemann-Pick, type A	Acid sphingomyelinase	Autosomal recessive
Niemann-Pick, type B	Acid sphingomyelinase	Autosomal recessive
GM1 gangliosidosis	β-galactosidase	Autosomal recessive
Tay-Sachs disease	Hexosaminidase A α-subunit	Autosomal recessive
Sandhoff disease	Hexosaminidase B β-chain	Autosomal recessive
Galactosialidosis	Protective protein/cathepsin A	Autosomal recessive
Farber lipogranulomatosis	Ceramidase	Autosomal recessive
Sialidosis	α-Neuraminidase	Autosomal recessive

Defects in Glycoprotein Metabolism

Sialidosis

Symptoms and Signs

Sialidosis is an autosomal recessive disorder of glycoprotein degradation. Clinically, this disorder can be classified into a less severe form, type 1, and a more severe phenotype, type 2. Type 2 is itself divided into congenital, infantile, and juvenile subtypes. A cherry-red spot macula occurs commonly in sialidosis, especially in type I subtypes (47).

Type 1 sialidosis has been referred to as *cherry-red spot myoclonus syndrome.* Patients with this disorder may have normal development for the first 2 to 3 decades of life and then manifest visual and neurologic problems. Night blindness and problems with color vision are relatively common. Funduscopic evaluation demonstrates a cherry-red spot in the macula (48). Other ocular features may include nystagmus or opacities of the lenses or corneas. Neurologic problems occur including seizures, ataxia, and dysarthria (47,49).

Type 2 sialidosis has an earlier onset and includes a congenital form, which can present with hydrops. In contrast to type 1, somatic features are characteristic. These may include enlarged liver and spleen, ascites, abnormal facies, and a radiographic pattern known as *dysostosis multiplex.* A cherry-red spot is seen in the majority, but not all, of type 2 patients (47).

Diagnosis

The defect in sialidosis is neuraminidase deficiency. The diagnosis is based on a characteristic oligosaccharide pattern in the urine and assay of the neuraminidase enzyme (47).

Defects in Metabolism of Sphingomyelin, Gangliosides, and Other Complex Lipids

Niemann-Pick Disease Types A and B

Symptoms and Signs

Type A Niemann-Pick disease is an autosomal recessive disorder caused by deficiency of acid sphingomyelinase.

Normally, this enzyme is involved in the lysosomal degradation of sphingomyelin. Patients present in early infancy with hepatosplenomegaly, hypotonia, and weakness. Developmental delay is evident by about 6 months of age. Development regresses, and patients become rigid and spastic and lose contact with their environment. During the first 12 to 24 months of life, many patients are found to have cherry-red spots in their macula and abnormal electroretinograms (ERGs). Some patients develop a gray granular appearance to the macula referred to as the *macular halo syndrome* (50,51).

Type B Niemann-Pick disease also is due to acid sphingomyelinase deficiency; however, the clinical spectrum is much milder. Clinical presentation is later and, in some patients, splenomegaly is not apparent until adulthood. Respiratory problems due to alveolar infiltration may occur at 15 to 20 years of age. The central nervous system is usually spared. A few type B patients have cherry-red spots in the macula.

Diagnosis

The diagnosis of Niemann-Pick type A and B is suspected based on the clinical features and bone marrow findings (Nieman-Pick disease [NPD] "foam" cells). Confirmatory enzyme studies for acid sphingomyelinase, such as from peripheral leukocytes, cultured fibroblasts, and lymphoblasts, are necessary for diagnosis (50).

Genetics

Molecular diagnosis for detection of mutations in the gene for acid sphingomyelinase is possible (50).

Disorders of Ganglioside Degradation: G_{M1} Gangliosidosis

Symptoms and Signs

G_{M1} gangliosidosis is an autosomal recessive neurodegenerative disease due to deficiency of β-galactosidase. The clinical presentation is variable and includes infantile, late infantile/juvenile, and adult/chronic forms. Most patients present in early infancy, usually with arrested development several months after birth. This is followed by developmental regression. Exaggerated startle response and seizure are common. Rigidity, spasticity, and seizures are frequent. Dysmorphic features, skeletal dysplasia, and hepatomegaly are characteristic, and patients eventually regress to a vegetative state. Ophthalmologic evaluation reveals optic atrophy, corneal clouding, retinal edema, and macular cherry-red spot. In the late infantile/juvenile form, the onset is later, but developmental regression leads to early death. There are dysmorphic facial features and the skeletal pattern of dysostosis multiplex. Cherry-red spots in the macula occur in the late infantile form but not as consistently as in the early infantile presentation (52,53).

Diagnosis
Enzyme assay for β-galactosidase is performed for diagnostic confirmation (52,53).

Disorders of Ganglioside Degradation: G_{M2} Gangliosidosis (Tay-Sachs Disease)

Tay-Sachs disease is an autosomal recessive condition due to a deficiency of β-hexosaminidase A (Hex A), which normally participates in the hydrolysis of ganglioside G_{M2}. Hex A deficiency results in the accumulation of ganglioside G_{M2} in the lysosomes of the nervous system causing progressive tissue damage. There is marked variability in the clinical patterns, ranging from the classic infantile disease to later onset and even an adult form of the condition.

Symptoms and Signs
In the acute infantile presentations, patients develop some degree of motor weakness by age 3 to 5 months. Exaggerated startle responses, seizures, and rapid developmental regression occur. A cherry-red spot is seen on funduscopic examination. ERG is normal; however, visual evoked responses are abnormal early on. The disease progresses rapidly after about 8 to 10 months of age as the infant becomes less responsive to the environment. Ultimately, Tay-Sachs patients become vegetative and usually do not survive beyond age 3 to 5 years (54).

Diagnosis
The diagnosis is confirmed by assay of β-hexosaminidase A in serum, leukocytes, or other tissues.

G_{M2} Gangliosidosis (Sandhoff Disease)

Sandhoff disease is due to deficiency of both Hex A and Hex B. The clinical course is very similar to that of Tay-Sachs disease. As in Tay-Sachs disease, a cherry-red spot macula is characteristic (54,55).

Galactosialidosis

Galactosialidosis is an autosomal recessive lysosomal disease due to deficiency of protective protein/cathepsin A (PPCA), which leads to deficiency of two lysosomal enzymes, β-galactosidase and neuraminidase. The disorder is subdivided into early infantile, late infantile, and juvenile/adult presentations.

Symptoms and Signs
The early infantile form can present as hydrops fetalis or, in the neonatal period, with edema, proteinuria, telangiectasia, inguinal hernia, and coarse facial features. Skeletal changes, hepatosplenomegaly, and developmental delay are present. Death due to heart failure usually occurs by age 20 months. Ophthalmologic findings can include corneal clouding and a cherry-red spot in the macula. In the late infantile form, similar features are noted but with a later onset (usually in early infancy). A more chronic course is noted, with a mean age of death at about 15 years. Cherry-red spots are seen in the juvenile/adult form of galactosialidosis, which is mainly seen in individuals of Japanese background. The mean age of onset is 16 years but can be much later. In some cases, intelligence is normal. Age of death usually is between 13 and 45 years.

Diagnosis
Diagnosis is based on an enzyme assay, which shows combined deficiency of β-galactosidase and neuraminidase (56,57).

Farber Disease

Farber disease is an autosomal recessive condition due to deficiency of acid ceramidase. This is a lysosomal enzyme that normally is responsible for the degradation of ceramide, a component of glycolipids. In this condition, ceramide accumulates in lysosomes and leads to an array of clinical problems (58).

Symptoms and Signs
Classic Farber disease usually presents in early infancy with painful swollen joints, subcutaneous nodules, and progressive hoarseness. Enlarged liver and spleen may develop. There is significant variability of the phenotype (59,60). Because of respiratory involvement, pulmonary infiltrates are frequently seen. A cherry-red spot is seen in the macula. One may see granulomatous lesions of the conjunctiva. A "neurologic progressive" form of Farber disease has been described. This condition, like the classic form, has a cherry-red spot in the macula as a feature.

Diagnosis
Farber disease is diagnosed by clinical presentation and is confirmed by assay of ceramidase activity in leukocytes, plasma, skin fibroblasts, or other tissues (58).

Genetics

The gene encoding ceramidase has been identified and mutations have been detected (58).

Fabry Disease

Fabry disease is a rare X-linked disease due to deficiency of α-galactosidase A. Because of its inheritance pattern, mainly males are affected. The enzyme defect results in an accumulation of glycosphingolipids.

Symptoms and Signs

The typical clinical features include pain of the extremities, angiokeratomas, and hypohidrosis. Renal failure eventually develops and is a common cause of death. There are a number of eye findings in Fabry disease, including subepithelial corneal whorls, corneal verticillata, lens opacities, conjunctival vascular lesions, and retinal tortuosity. The phenotype is variable; some patients have later onset and overall milder features (61,62).

Diagnosis

Diagnostic confirmation is based on enzyme assay showing deficiency of α-galactosidase A in leukocytes, plasma, serum, fibroblasts, and other tissues.

Mucopolysaccharide Diseases

Mucopolysaccharide diseases are listed in Table 6-3.

Hurler Syndrome

Symptoms and Signs

Hurler syndrome (MPS IH) is characterized by severe multiorgan involvement due to accumulation of mucopolysaccharides. In early to middle infancy, multiple problems become evident, which may include hepatosplenomegaly, macroglossia, coarse face, and skeletal features (dysostosis multiplex) (Figs. 6-8 to 6-11). Developmental delay is evident by age 1 year, and after a period of developing some milestones, developmental regression occurs. Neurosensory and conductive hearing loss is frequent. Hydrocephalus may occur (63,64). Death due to respiratory and cardiac problems usually occurs in childhood.

Ocular features include corneal clouding, glaucoma, and retinal degeneration. Night blindness and decreased peripheral vision have been described.

Pathophysiology

Hurler syndrome is caused by α-L-iduronidase deficiency. Normally, this enzyme participates in the degradation of heparan and dermatan sulfate (63,64).

Genetics

Hurler syndrome is an autosomal recessive condition.

Scheie Syndrome

Scheie syndrome (MPS IS) is also due to deficiency of α-L-iduronidase. However, this is a much milder condition than Hurler syndrome.

Symptoms and Signs

Onset of symptoms typically is seen after age 5 years, and the disease may not be diagnosed until much later. The findings may include joint stiffness, carpal tunnel syndrome, cardiac valvular disease, and coarse facial features. Obstructive sleep apnea and cervical cord compression have been described.

As in Hurler syndrome, ocular problems such as glaucoma, retinal degeneration, and corneal clouding can occur (63,64).

Genetics

The inheritance of Scheie syndrome is autosomal recessive.

Hurler-Scheie

Hurler-Scheie syndrome (MPS I H/S) is an intermediate type due to deficiency of α-L-iduronidase deficiency (63,64) and is autosomal recessive.

Hunter Syndrome

Symptoms and Signs

Hunter syndrome (MPS II) has a severe form and a mild presentation. The severe presentation is similar to that of Hurler syndrome with respect to the somatic and developmental characteristics.

As in Hurler syndrome, there is retinal degeneration and problems with night vision and peripheral vision. However, in contrast to Hurler syndrome, there is no corneal clouding (63,64).

Pathophysiology

Hunter syndrome is due to deficiency of iduronate sulfatase deficiency. This enzyme is involved in heparan and dermatan sulfate metabolism.

Genetics

The inheritance of Hunter syndrome is X linked. This is in contrast to the other known mucopolysaccharide disorders, which are autosomal recessive (63,64).

Sanfilippo Syndrome

Sanfilippo syndrome (MPS III) consists of four conditions (type A through D) that are all due to defects in heparan sulfate metabolism.

TABLE 6-3. MUCOPOLYSACCHARIDOSES

Disorder	Clinical	Inheritance	Enzyme	Mucopolyssacharide(s) Accumulated
Hurler (MPS IH)	Severe presentation: hepatosplenomegaly, coarse facies, dysostosis multiples, developmental regression; corneal clouding, glaucoma, retinal degeneration	Autosomal recessive	α-L-Iduronidase	Heparan, dermatan sulfate
Scheie (MPS IS)	Mild, later presentation; joint stiffness, valvular disease, coarse face; corneal clouding, glaucoma, retinal degeneration	Autosomal recessive	α-L-iduronidase	Heparan, dermatan sulfate
Hurler/Sheie (MPS I H/S)	Intermediate	Autosomal recessive	α-L-iduronidase	Heparan, dermatan sulfate
Hunter (MPS II)	Severe form similar to Hurler, but no corneal clouding; mild form also exists	X linked	Iduronate sulfatase	Heparan, dermatan sulfate
Sanfilippo (MPS III)	Hyperactivity, behavior problems, development delay, neurologic regression, retinal degeneration	Autosomal recessive	Heparan N-sulfatase (sulfaminidase) (Sanfilippo A), α-N-acetyl-glucosaminidase (Sanfilippo B), acetyl-CoA:α-glucosaminide acetyltransferase (Sanfilippo C), N-acetylglucosamine 6-sulfatase (Sanfilippo D)	Heparan sulfate
Morquio (MPS IVA)	Multiple skeletal anomalies: short trunk and neck, kyphosis, genu valgum, odontoid hypoplasia; mild corneal clouding, glaucoma	Autosomal recessive	N-acetylgalactosamine-6 sulfatase	Keratan sulfate, chondroitin-6-sulfate
Morquio (MPS IVB)	Similar to Morquio A but milder	Autosomal recessive	β-galactosidase	Keratan sulfate
Maroteaux-Lamy (MPS VI)	Dysostosis multiplex; corneal clouding; normal intelligence	Autosomal recessive	Arylsulfatase B	Dermatan sulfate
Sly (MPS VII)	May present with hydrops or later with Hurler-like features including dysostosis multiplex	Autosomal recessive	β-Glucuronidase	Chondroitin-4,6-sulfates, dermatan sulfate, heparan sulfate

Adapted from Neufeld EF, Muenzer J. The mucopolysaccharidoses. In Scriver CR, Beaudet AL, Sly WS, et al., eds. The metabolic and molecular bases of inherited disease, 8th ed. New York: McGraw-Hill, 2001: 3421–3452.

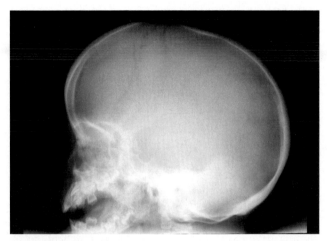

FIGURE 6-8. Skull film of a patient with Hurler syndrome showing J-shaped sella turcica.

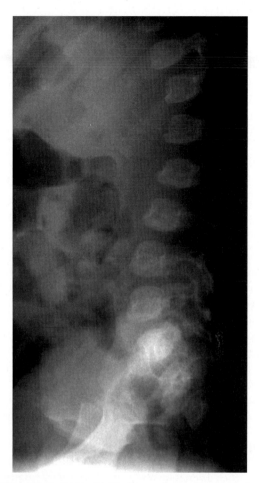

FIGURE 6-10. Patient with Hurler syndrome. Note anterior inferior beaking and kyphosis of thoracolumbar junction.

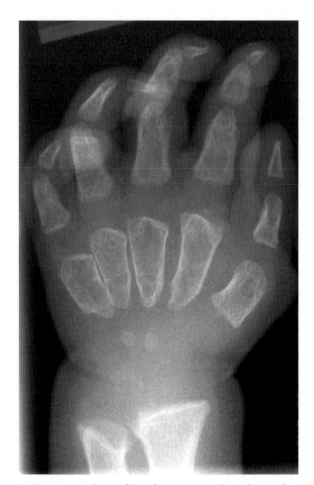

FIGURE 6-9. Hand x-ray film of a patient with Hurler syndrome. Note bullet-shaped metacarpals.

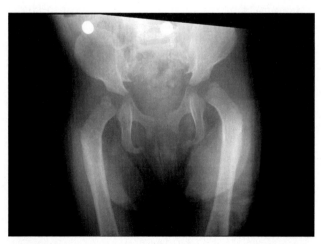

FIGURE 6-11. Patient with Hurler syndrome. Note pelvic dysplasia consisting of flared iliac wings, hypoplastic basilar portion of iliac wings, and slightly shallow acetabula.

Symptoms and Signs

These disorders are characterized by mild somatic features and severe neurologic decline by age 6 to 10 years. Patients may present with developmental delay, hyperactivity, and aggressive behavior. Somatic features are relatively mild and include mild hepatosplenomegaly, hirsutism, and coarse hair.

Ocular features include retinal degeneration, decreased night vision, and decreased peripheral vision (63,64).

Genetics

Sanfilippo syndrome is inherited in an autosomal recessive fashion.

Morquio Syndrome

Symptoms and Signs

Morquio syndrome (MPS IV) is characterized by multiple skeletal anomalies. Patients have a short trunk, short neck, kyphosis, genu valgum, and a waddling gait. Odontoid hypoplasia is an important feature, which increases the risk of atlantoaxial subluxation and neurologic complications. Morquio patients may have mild hepatosplenomegaly, hearing loss, upper airway obstruction, and cardiac valvular problems.

Ocular features of Morquio syndrome include mild corneal clouding and an increased risk for glaucoma (63,64).

Pathophysiology

Two different enzyme deficiencies can cause Morquio syndrome. The enzymes involved are *N*-acetylgalactosamine-6-sulfatase (IV-A) and β-galactosidase (IV-B).

Maroteaux-Lamy

Symptoms and Signs

Maroteaux-Lamy syndrome (MPS VI) is similar to Hurler syndrome with respect to somatic features. However, intelligence is normal.

Visual impairment due to corneal opacities are common.

Pathophysiology

The enzyme deficiency for MPS VI is *N*-acetyl-galactosamine 4-sulfatase (arylsulfatase B), which is involved in dermatan sulfate degradation (63,64).

Genetics

The gene for arylsulfatase B has been, identified and a feline model of MPS VI has been created (see Chapter 13).

Sly Syndrome

Symptoms and Signs

Sly syndrome (MPS VII) is a clinically variable mucopolysaccharide disorder, which may present with hydrops fetalis or later with Hurler-like features.

Corneal opacities are associated with this condition.

Pathophysiology

The enzyme β-glucuronidase is deficient in Sly syndrome (63,64).

Genetics

The gene for β-glucuronidase has been identified, and murine, feline, and canine models of MPS VII have been created (Chapter 13).

Diagnosis of Mucopolysaccharide Disorders

Diagnostic confirmation of mucopolysaccharide disease is accomplished by assay of the deficient enzyme of the respective disorders. A variety of tissues can be used, including leukocytes, serum, and fibroblasts, depending on the specific enzyme and the laboratory performing the test.

ERG testing has demonstrated variable retinal involvement in mucopolysaccharide diseases I, II, and III. The involvement is reported to be in a pattern characteristic of rod-cone degeneration, especially with regard to rod-mediated responses (65). Mild changes in retinal pigment epithelium can be found on funduscopic examination. As noted earlier, glaucoma and corneal clouding are common findings in several mucopolysaccharide disorders (66–69). In a retrospective study of patients with mucopolysaccharide disease treated by bone marrow transplantation, 81% of patients had improvements in ERG in the first year. However, this was followed by decline of ERG over the long term. Corneal clouding was shown to improve in some patients after bone marrow transplantation (70).

Management of Lysosomal Storage Diseases

Until fairly recently, the treatment of lysosomal storage diseases was mainly supportive and dealt with the various complications. However, major advances have occurred over the past decade or so. Enzyme replacement therapy is now available for some lysosomal storage diseases, such as Fabry disease, Hurler syndrome, and Gaucher disease (71). Enzyme replacement therapy also is being evaluated for Maroteaux-Lamy syndrome, Hunter syndrome, and other lysosomal storage diseases (72). Bone marrow transplantation is a treatment modality for some conditions (73). In addition, there is ongoing research into the possibilities of gene therapy (74). As effective treatments have become more feasible for lysosomal storage diseases, early diagnosis and referral to metabolic treatment centers are imperative.

All patients with or suspected to have lysosomal storage disease should be referred to a metabolic geneticist for diagnostic confirmation and clinical management. Ideally, the patient should go to a metabolic center. Prompt referral is especially important because of the advances in treatment of some of these conditions, such as enzyme replacement therapy and bone marrow transplantation. Genetic counseling should also be offered. This typically is done by the genetic counselor associated with the geneticist managing the patient. Depending on the specific disease, there may be ongoing clinical trials, and the patient/family should be made aware of options for possible participation. Monitoring and treatment of complications of lysosomal diseases require referrals to appropriate specialists and can be arranged by the geneticist, primary care physician, or other health care providers involved in the patient's care.

AMINO ACID DISORDERS

Gyrate Atrophy of the Choroid and Retina

Gyrate atrophy of the choroid and retina is a rare autosomal recessive disorder characterized by a slow visual decline resulting in blindness by the fifth decade of life (75,76).

Prevalence
This condition has been reported in a number of ethnic groups and countries. Finland has the highest incidence, at about 1 in 50,000 (76). Gyrate atrophy is very rare in the United States.

Pathophysiology
The etiology is deficiency of ornithine aminotransferase (OAT). The normal function of OAT is to catalyze the conversion of the amino acid ornithine to pyrroline-5 carboxylate (P5C), which is an intermediate in the biosynthesis of glutamate and proline. Ornithine accumulates, which can be detected on plasma amino acid analysis. Ornithine is an intermediate in several pathways, including the urea cycle, and the synthesis of polyamines, proline, and glutamate (76). The pathophysiology of gyrate atrophy most likely is due to high levels of ornithine. However, it is possible that deficiency of P5C or other metabolites play a role. A mouse model for OAT deficiency has been developed and has provided evidence for direct toxicity of ornithine (77).

Ocular Signs and Symptoms
Patients with OAT deficiency usually have decreased night vision and myopia beginning in childhood. At this point, punched-out areas of degeneration can be noted in the mid periphery of the fundus. The findings progress until in the older adult patient there is complete chorioretinal degeneration. The intervening period is characterized by progressive decline in peripheral visual fields and visual acuity and the development of subcapsular cataracts (76,78). Ophthalmologic testing shows progressively abnormal

ERGs, electrooculogram, and dark adaptometry testing. In addition to the eye findings, some patients have proximal muscle weakness.

Diagnosis
Diagnosis is based on the characteristic findings in the fundus (which can be pathognomonic in the early stages) and supported by plasma amino acid analysis, which shows a marked increase in ornithine, but also low levels of lysine, glutamate, and glutamine. Plasma levels of creatine and guanidinoacetate are low. Enzyme assay confirms OAT deficiency (76).

Management
Various treatments of OAT deficiency have been investigated, including reduced arginine diet, administration of pharmacologic doses of vitamin B_6, creatine supplementation, and proline supplementation (76). Studies in the mouse model have demonstrated that correction of ornithine levels in the mouse, via a low-arginine diet, can completely prevent retinal degeneration (77). These results and experience with a low-arginine diet in humans suggest that this therapy helps to slow the retinal deterioration and even may prevent further decline.

Patients diagnosed with OAT deficiency should be promptly referred to a metabolic center experienced in the dietary and metabolic management and confirmatory testing for this condition.

Cystinosis

Cystinosis is an autosomal recessive disorder caused by a defect in carrier-mediated transport of the amino acid cystine. Cystinosis can be considered an amino acid disorder. However, it also is a lysosomal storage disorder and is more commonly thought of in this category. Due to the transport defect, cystine accumulates in the lysosomes, and its storage causes damage to multiple tissues, including the eye (Table 6-4).

Prevalence
The incidence of cystinosis varies considerably around the world. The infantile form occurs in about 1 of 100,000 to 1 of 200,000 live births in North America (79).

TABLE 6-4. CLINICAL ASPECTS OF CYSTINOSIS

Ocular	Corneal crystals, pigmentary retinopathy
Kidney	Renal Fanconi syndrome, glomerular damage
Growth	Proportionate growth deficiency
Endocrine	Risk of hypothyroidism and other endocrine disturbances
Gastrointestinal	Gastrointestinal complications

Genetics

There is significant clinical variability in cystinosis. Several clinical phenotypes have been described, including "classic" nephropathic cystinosis, later-onset variants, and a type that clinically affects only the eye. Cystinosis is caused by mutation in the *CTNS* gene, which encodes the protein cystinosin.

Symptoms and Signs

Kidney damage is a major part of the morbidity in cystinosis. The renal tubules are damaged by continued lysosomal storage of cystine. Therefore, the patient can present in infancy with the renal Fanconi syndrome and have bouts of acidosis, dehydration, and electrolyte disturbances. Glomerular damage also occurs and leads to end-stage kidney disease. The onset of renal failure occurs during childhood if the condition is left untreated. Growth deficiency is characteristic and includes proportionate decreases in height and weight but normal head circumference. There is an increased risk of primary hypothyroidism, insulin-dependent diabetes mellitus, and delayed puberty. Patients usually have normal neurologic examinations but may have some degree of cerebral atrophy. Myopathy and gastrointestinal and hepatic complications may occur (79–81).

Ocular Symptoms and Signs

There is major ocular involvement in cystinosis. Cystine crystals accumulate in the cornea and usually are present by about 12 months of age. Eventually the corneas have a hazy appearance. Pain and photophobia are common. The conjunctiva, uvea, and sclera are other sites of crystal deposition. Patients develop a characteristic pigmentary retinopathy. The retinopathy is generally described as bilateral, symmetrical, and mainly affecting the periphery. On funduscopic examination, there may be a mottled appearance to the periphery of the retina. Patchy areas of depigmentation and pigment clumps may be noted. In young patients, the ERG, electrooculogram, and visual fields typically are normal; however, visual impairment becomes evident with increasing age (79,82,83).

Diagnosis

Diagnosis of cystinosis is confirmed by leukocyte cystine measurement, which is done by a cystine binding protein assay (84).

Genetics

Mutation analysis for the *CTNS* mutation can also be performed for diagnostic purposes (85,86).

Management

Treatment of cystinosis involves management of the individual organ problems and reducing cystine levels to decrease and prevent damage. Regarding the former, close monitoring for potential complications of cystinosis is imperative. Regarding the latter, oral cysteamine (β-mercaptoethylamine) has been shown to be beneficial. Cysteamine therapy removes cystine from cells and has been shown to markedly improve the outcome with respect to renal function and other clinical parameters of the disease (87–89). However, this therapy does not prevent the accumulation of corneal crystals. Cysteamine eyedrops have been developed for this purpose. Studies have demonstrated that the drops (cysteamine hydrochloride) dissolve corneal crystals and can relieve photophobia (90,91).

Patients with cystinosis are referred to a geneticist and metabolic center for diagnostic confirmation and specific therapy. Other physicians, such as nephrologists, may be consulted if complications arise.

GENETIC COUNSELING AND OTHER RESOURCES FOR METABOLIC CONDITIONS

Genetic counseling is an important component of the overall services for patients with metabolic conditions. The issues vary considerably in their complexity and importance, depending on the specific disease. Patients and/or their families should be offered genetic counseling services to help in the process of becoming more informed about the disease in question and to assist in making medical and personal decisions. The genetic counselor can play a key role in discussions with the family regarding expected clinical course, recurrence risk, carrier testing, benefits and limitations of DNA testing, options for prenatal testing, reproductive options, and other issues.

RESOURCES

A helpful Web site to find out about available genetics laboratory testing and clinics is GeneTest at *www.geneclinics.org*.

The Web site for the National Society for Genetic Counselors is *www.nsgc.org*.

A number of support groups and other resources are available for the disorders discussed in this chapter. Some of these resources are listed here:

The National Organization of Albinism and Hypopigmentation (NOAH)
P.O. Box 959
East Hampstead, NH 03826-0959
www.albinism.org

The National MPS Society, Inc.
45 Packard Drive
Bangor, ME 04401
www.mpssociety.org

National Tay-Sachs and Allied Diseases Association, Inc.
2001 Beacon Street, Suite 204
Brighton, MA 02135
www.ntsad.org

Fabry Support and Information Group
108 NE 2nd Street, Suite C
P.O. Box 51
Concordia, MO 64020
www.fabry.org

The Cystinosis Foundation
604 Vernon Street
Oakland, CA 94610
www.cystinosisfoundation.org

The Cystinosis Research Network, Inc.
8 Sylvester Road
Burlington, Ma 01803
www.cystinosis.org

REFERENCES

1. King RA, Hearing VJ, Creel DJ, et al. Albinism. In: Scriver CR, Beaudet AL, Sly WS, et al., eds. *Metabolic and molecular bases of inherited disease,* 8th ed. New York: McGraw-Hill, 2001: 5587–5627.

2. Russell-Eggit I. Albinism. In: Stamper RL, Lambert S, eds. *Ophthalmology clinics of North America,* vol. 14, no. 3. WB Saunders, 2001:533–546.

3. Kinnear PE, Jay B, Witkop CJ Jr. Albinism. *Surv Ophthalmol* 1985;30:75–101.

4. Oetting WS, King RA. Molecular basis of type I (tyrosinase-related) oculocutaneous albinism: mutations and polymorphisms of the human tyrosinase gene. *Hum Mutat* 1993; 2:1–6.

5. Lee ST, Nicholls RD, Bundey S, et al. Mutations of the P gene in oculocutaneous albinism, ocular albinism, and Prader-Willi syndrome plus albinism. *N Engl J Med* 1994;330:529–534.

6. Rinchik EM, Bultman SJ, Horsthemke B, et al. A gene for the mouse pink-eyed dilution locus and for human type II oculocutaneous albinism. *Nature* 1993;361:72–76.

7. Boissy RE, Zhao H, Oetting WS, et al. Mutation in and lack of expression of tyrosinase-related protein-1 (TRP-1) in melanocytes from an individual with brown oculocutaneous albinism: a new subtype of albinism classified as "OCA3." *Am J Hum Genet* 1996;58:1145–1156.

8. Manga P, Kromberg JG, Box NF, et al. Rufous oculocutaneous albinism in southern African Blacks is caused by mutations in the TYRP1 gene. *Am J Hum Genet 1997;*61:1095–1101.

9. Newton JM, Cohen-Barak O, Hasiwaran N, et al. Mutations in the human orthologue of the mouse underwhite gene (uw) underlie a new form of oculocutaneous albinism, OCA4. *Am J Hum Genet* 2001;69:981–988.

10. Oh J, Bailin T, Fukai K, et al. Positional cloning of a gene for Hermansky-Pudlak syndrome, a disorder of cytoplasmic organelles. *Nat Genet* 1966;14:300–306.

11. Dell'Angelica EC, Shotelersuk V, Aguilar RC, et al. Altered trafficking of lysosomal proteins in Hermansky-Pudlak syndrome due to mutations in the beta-3A subunit of the AP-3 adaptor. *Mol Cell* 1999;3:11–21.

12. Anikster Y, Huizing M, White J, et al. Mutation of a new gene causes a unique form of Hermansky-Pudlak syndrome in a genetic isolate of central Puerto Rico. *Nat Genet* 2001;28:376–380.

13. Suzuki T, Li W, Zhang Q, et al. Hermansky-Pudlak syndrome is caused by mutations in HPS4, the human homolog of the mouse light-ear gene. *Nat Genet 2002;*30:321–324.

14. Zhang Q, Zhao B, Li W, et al. Ru2 and Ru encode mouse orthologs of the genes mutated in human Hermansky-Pudlak syndrome types 5 and 6. *Nature Genet* 2003;33:145–154.

15. Nagle DL, Karim MA, Woolf EA, et al. Identification and mutation analysis of the complete gene for Chediak-Higashi syndrome. *Nat Genet* 1996;14:307–311.

16. Oetting WS. New insights into ocular albinism type I (OAI): mutation and polymorphisms of the OAI gene. *Hum Mutat* 2002;19:85–92.

17. Yi Z, Garrison N, Cohen-Barak O, et al. A 122.5-kilobase deletion of the P gene underlies the high prevalence of oculocutaneous albinism type 2 in the Navajo population. *Am J Hum Genet* 2002;72:62–72.

18. Wildenberg SC, Oetting WS, Aldmodovar C, et al. A gene causing Hermansky-Pudlak syndrome in a Puerto Rican population maps to chromosome 10q2. *Am J Hum Genet* 1995;57: 755–765.

19. Schrallreuter KU, Frenk E, Wolfe LS, et al. Hermansky-Pudlak syndrome in a Swiss population. *Dermatology* 1993;187: 248–256.

20. Brilliant MH. The mouse p (pink-eyed dilution) and human P genes, oculocutaneous albinism type 2 (OCA2), and melanosomal pH. *Pigment Cell Res* 2001;14:86–93.

21. Toyofuku K, Valencia JC, Kushimoto T, et al. The etiology of oculocutaneous albinism (OCA) type II: the pink protein modulates the processing and transport of tyrosinase. *Pigment Cell Res* 2002;15:217–224.

22. Lee ST, Nicholls RD, Schnur RE, et al. Diverse mutations of the P gene among African-Americans with type II (tyrosinase-positive) oculocutaneous albinism (OCA2). *Hum Mol Genet* 1994;3:2047–2051.

23. Manga P, Kromberg J, Turner A, et al. In Southern Africa, brown oculocutaneous albinism (BOCA) maps to the OCA2 locus on chromosome 15q: P-gene mutations identified. *Am J Hum Genet* 2001;68:782–787.

24. Cassidy SB. Prader-Willi syndrome. *J Med Genet* 1997;34: 917–923.

25. Saitoh S, Harda N, Jinno Y et al. Molecular and clinical study of 61 Angelman syndrome patients. *Am J Med Genet* 1994;52: 158–163.

26. Rosemblat S, Durham-Pierre D, Gardner JM, et al. Identification of a melanosomal membrane protein encoded by the pink-eyed dilution (type II oculocutaneous albinism) gene. *Proc Natl Acad Sci USA* 1994;91:12071–12075.

27. Manga P, Kromberg JGR, Box NF, et al. Rufous oculocutaneous albinism in Southern African Blacks is caused by mutations in the TYRP1 gene. *Am J Hum Genet* 1997;61:1095–1101.

28. Boissy RE, Zhao H, Oetting WS, et al. Mutation in and lack of expression of tyrosinase-related protein-1 (TRP-1) in melanocytes from an individual with brown oculocutaneous albinism: a new subtype of albinism classified as "OCA3." *Am J Hum Genet* 1996;58:1145–1156.

29. Sarangarajan R, Boissy RE. Tyrp1 and oculocutaneous albinism type 3. *Pigment Cell Res* 2001;14:437–444.

30. Costin GE, Valencia JC, Viera WD, et al. Tyrosinase processing and intracellular trafficking is disrupted in mouse primary melanocytes carrying the underwhite (uw) mutation. A model for oculocutaneous albinism (OCA) type 4. *J Cell Sci* 2003;116[Pt 15]: 3203–3212.

31. Costa DLL, Huang SJ, Donsoff IM, et al. X-Linked ocular albinism: fundus of a heterozygous female. *Retina* 2003;23:410–411.

32. Newton JM, Orlon SJ, Barsh GS. Isolation and characterization of a mouse homolog of the X-linked ocular albinism (OA1) gene. *Genomics* 1996;37:219–225.

33. Huizing M, Anikster Y, Gahl WA. Hermansky-Pudlak syndrome and related disorders of organelle formation. *Traffic* 2000;1:823–835.

34. Huizing M, Boissy RE, Gahl W. Hermansky-Pudlak syndrome: vesicle formation from yeast to man. *Pigment Cell Res* 2002.; 15:405–419.

35. Shiflett SL, Kaplan J, Ward DM. Chediak-Higashi syndrome: a rare disorder of lysosomes and lysosome related organelles. *Pigment Cell Res* 2002;15:251–257.

36. Introne W, Boissy RE, Gahl WA. Clinical, molecular, and cell biological aspects of Chediak-Higashi syndrome. *Mol Genet Metab* 1999;68:283–303.

37. Ruiz-Maldonado R, Toussaint S, Tamayo L, et al. Hypomelanosis of Ito: diagnostic criteria and report of 41 cases. *Pediatr Dermatol* 1992;9:1–10.

38. Donnai D, Read AP, McKeown C, et al. Hypomelanosis of Ito: a manifestation of mosaicism on chimerism. *J Med Genet* 1988; 25:809–818.

39. Hart DB. Menkes syndrome: an updated review. *J Am Acad Dermatol* 1983;9:145–152.

40. Farishian P, Shittaker J. Phenylalanine lowers melanin synthesis in mammalian melanocytes by reducing tyrosine uptake: implications for pigment reduction in phenylketonuria. *J. Invest Dermatol* 1980;74:85–89.

41. Winship L, Beighton P. Phenotypic discriminants in the Waardenburg syndrome. *Clin Genet* 1992;41:181–188.

42. Griscelli C, Durandy A, Guy-Grand D, et al. A syndrome associating partial albinism and immunodeficiency. *Am J Med* 1978; 65:619–702.

43. Tietz W. A syndrome of deaf-mutism associated with albinism showing autosomal dominant inheritance. *Am J Hum Genet* 1963;15:259.

44. Fryns JP, Dereymaeker AM, Heremans G, et al. Oculocerebral syndrome with hypopigmentation (Cross syndrome). Report of two siblings born to consanguineous parents. *Clin Genet* 1988;34:81–84.

45. Abadi R, Pascal E. The recognition and management of albinism. *Ophthalmic Physiol Opt* 1989;9:3–15.

46. Pennock CA. Lysosomal storage disorders. In: Holton JB, ed. *The inherited metabolic disorders,* 1st ed. New York: Churchill Livingstone, 1987:59–95.

47. Thomas GH. Disorders of glycoprotein degradation: alpha-mannosidosis, beta-mannosidosis, fucosidosis and sialidosis. In: Scriver CR, Beaudet AL, Sly WS, et al., eds. *Metabolic and molecular bases of inherited disease,* 8th ed. New York: McGraw-Hill, 2001:3507–3533.

48. Thomas GH, Tipton RE, Ch'ien LT, et al. Sialidase (alpha-N-acetyl neuraminidase) deficiency: the enzyme defect in an adult with macular cherry-red spots and myoclonus without dementia. *Clin Genet* 1978;13:369.

49. Federicko A, Battistini S, Ciacci G, et al. Cherry-red spot myoclonus syndrome (type I sialidosis). *Dev Neurosci* 1991;13:320–326.

50. Schuchman EH, Desnick RJ. Niemann-Pick Disease types A and B: acid sphingomyelinase deficiencies. In: Scriver CR, Beaudet AL, Sly WS, et al., eds. *The metabolic and molecular bases of inherited disease,* 8th ed. New York: McGraw-Hill, 2001:3589–3610.

51. Cogan DG, Chu FC, Barranger JA, et al. Macula halo syndrome. Variant of Niemann-Pick disease. *Arch Ophthalmol* 1983;101:1698–1700.

52. Suzuki Y, Oshima Akihiro, Nanba E: Beta-galactosidase deficiency (beta galactosidosis): G_{m1} gangliosidosis and Morquio disease. In: Scriver CR, Beaudet AL, Sly WS, et al., eds. *The metabolic and molecular bases of inherited disease,* 8th ed. New York: McGraw-Hill, 2001:3775.

53. Fricker H, O'Brien JS, Vassella F, et al. Generalized gangliosidosis: Acid β-galactosidase deficiency with early onset, rapid mental deterioration and minimal bone dysplasia. *J Neurol* 1976;-213:273–281.

54. Gravel RA, Kaback MM, Proia RL, et al. The G_{m2} gangliosidoses. In: Scriver CR, Beaudet AL, Sly WS, et al., eds. *The metabolic and molecular bases of inherited disease,* 8th ed. New York: McGraw-Hill, 2001:3827–3876.

55. Okada S, Veath ML, Leroy J, et al. Ganglioside GM2 storage diseases: hexosaminidase deficiencies in cultured fibroblasts. *Am J Hum Genet* 1971;23:55–61.

56. Strisciuglio P, Sly WS, Dodson WE, et al. Combined deficiency of β-galactosidase and neuraminidase: natural history of the disease in the first 18 years of an American patient with late infantile onset form. *Am J Med Genet* 1990;37:573–577.

57. Zhou X-Y, van der Spoel A, Rottier R, et al. Molecular and biochemical analysis of protective protein/cathepsin A mutations: correlation with clinical severity in galactosialidosis. *Hum Mol Genet* 1996;5:1977–1987.

58. Moser HW, Linke T, Fensom AH, et al. Acid ceramidase deficiency: Farber lipogranulomatosis. In: Scriver CR, Beaudet AL, Sly WS, et al., eds. The metabolic and molecular basis of inherited disease, 8th ed. New York: McGraw-Hill, 2001: 3573–3588.

59. Antonorakis SE, Valle D, Moser HW, et al. Phenotypic variability in siblings with Farber disease. *J Pediatr* 1984;104:406.

60. Qualman SJ, Moser HW, Valle D, et al. Farber disease: pathologic diagnosis in sibs with phenotypic variability. *Am J Med Genet Suppl* 1987;3:233–241.

61. Sher NA, Letson RD, Desnick RJ. The ocular manifestations in Fabry's disease. *Arch Ophthalmol* 1979;97:671–676.

62. Spaeth GL, Frost P. Fabry's disease. Its ocular manifestations. *Arch Ophthalmol* 1965;74:760.

63. Neufeld EF, Muenzer J. The mucopolysaccharidoses. In: Scriver CR, Beaudet AL, Sly WS, et al., eds. *The metabolic and molecular bases of inherited disease,* 8th ed. New York: McGraw-Hill, 2001:3421–3452.

64. Spranger J. Mucopolysaccharidoses. In: Rimoin DL, Connor JM, Pyeritz RE, eds. *Emery and Rimoin's principles and practice of medical genetics,* 3rd ed. New York: Churchill-Livingstone, 1996:2071–2079.

65. Caruso RC, Kaiser-Kupfer MI, Muenzer J, et al. Electroretinographic findings in the mucopolysaccharidoses. *Ophthalmology* 1986;93:1612–1616.

66. Sugar J. Corneal manifestations of the systemic mucopolysaccharidoses. *Ann Ophthalmology* 1979;11:531–535.

67. Nowaczyk MJ, Clarke JTR, Morin JD. Glaucoma as an early complication of Hurler's disease. *Arch Dis Child* 1988;63:1091–1093.

68. Cantor LB, Disseler JA, Wilson FM. Glaucoma in the Maroteaux-Lamy syndrome. *Am J Ophthalmol* 1989;108:426–430.

69. Cahane M, Treister G, Abraham FA, et al. Glaucoma in siblings with Morquio syndrome. *Br J Ophthalmol* 1990;74:382–383.

70. Gullingsrud EO, Krivit W, Summers CG. Ocular abnormalities in the mucopolysaccharidoses after bone marrow transplantation: longer follow-up. *Ophthalmology* 1998;105:1099–1105.

71. Mehta AB, Lewis S, Laverey C. Treatment of lysosomal storage disorders. *BMJ* 2003;327:462–463.

72. Muenzer J, Lamsa JC, Garcia A, et al. Enzyme replacement therapy in mucopolysaccharidosis type II (Hunter syndrome): a preliminary report. *Acta Paediatr Suppl* 2002;91:98–99.

73. Wraith JE. Advances in the treatment of lysosomal storage diseases. *Dev Med Child Neurol* 2001;43:639–646.

74. Cheng SH, Smith AE. Gene therapy progress and prospects: gene therapy of lysosomal storage disorders. *Gene Ther* 2003;10:1275–1281.

75. Takki K, Milton RC. The natural history of gyrate atrophy of the choroid and retina. *Ophthalmology* 1981;88:292–301.

76. Valle D, Simell O. The hyperornithinemias. In: Scriver CR, Beaudet AL, Valle D, et al., eds. *The metabolic and molecular bases of inherited disease,* 8th ed. New York: McGraw-Hill, 2001:1857–1895.

77. Wang T, Steel G, Milam AH, et al. Correction of ornithine accumulation prevents retinal degeneration in a mouse model of gyrate atrophy of the choroid and retina. *Proc Natl Acad Sci* 2000;97:1224–1229.

78. Kaiser-Kupfer MI, Kuwahara T, Uga S, et al. Cataracts in gyrate atrophy: clinical and morphologic studies. *Invest Ophthalmol Vis Sci* 1983;24:432.

79. Gahl WA, Thoene J, Schneider JA. Cystinosis: a disorder of lysosomal membrane transport. In: Scriver CR, Beaudet AL, Sly WS, et al., eds. *The metabolic and molecular bases of inherited disease,* 8th ed. New York: McGraw-Hill, 2001:5085–5108.

80. McDowell GA, Town MM, van't Hoff W, et al. Clinical and molecular aspect of nephropathic cystinosis. *J Mol Med* 1998;76:295.

81. Gahl WA. Cystinosis coming of age. *Adv Pediatr* 1986;33:95–126.

82. Kaiser-Kupfer MI, Caruso RC, Minkler DS, et al. Long-term ocular manifestations in nephropathic cystinosis. *Arch Ophthalmol* 1986;104:706–711.

83. Francois J, Hanssens M, Coppleters R, et al. Cystinosis: a clinical and histopathologic study. *Am J Ophthalmol* 1972;73:643–650.

84. Smith ML, Furlong CE, Greene AA, et al. Cystine: binding protein assay. *Methods Enzymol* 1987;143:144.

85. Anikster Y, Lucero C, Touchman JW, et al. Identification and detection of the common 65-kb deletion breakpoint in the nephropathic cystinosis gene (CTNS). *Mol Genet Metab* 1999;66:111–116.

86. Forestier L, Jean G, Attard M, et al. Molecular characterization of CTNS deletions in nephropathic cystinosis: development of a PCR-based detection assay. *Am J Hum Genet* 1999;65:353–359.

87. Gahl WA, Charnas L, Markello TC, et al. Parenchymal organ cystine depletion with long-term cysteamine therapy. *Biochem Med Metab Biol* 1992;48:275–285.

88. Kimonis VE, Troendle J, Rose SR, et al. Effects of early cysteamine therapy on thyroid function and growth in nephropathic cystinosis. *J Clin Endocrinol Metab* 1995;80:3257–3261.

89. Markello TC, Bernardini IM, Gahl WA. Improved renal function in children with cystinosis treated with cysteamine. *N Engl J Med 1993;*328:1157–1162.

90. Kaiser-Kupfer MI, Fujikawa L, Kuwabara T, et al. Removal of corneal crystals by topical cysteamine in nephropathic cystinosis. *N Engl J Med* 1987;316:775–779.

91. Gahl WA, Kuehl EM, Iwata F, et al. Corneal crystals in nephropathic cystinosis: natural history and treatment with cysteamine eyedrops. *Mol Genet Metab* 2000;71:100–120.

GENERALIZED RETINAL AND CHOROIDAL DYSTROPHIES

KEAN T. OH
ANUP PARIKH

In 1990, evidence that rhodopsin mutations caused retinitis pigmentosa (RP) heralded a new perception of the pathophysiology and an evolving approach to retinal dystrophies. Since then, an ever-increasing number of genes have been identified as causative in retinal and choroidal dystrophies. Molecular diagnoses dispel doubt in many conditions that have a wide range of phenotypic expressions. Furthermore, with the identification of disease-causing genes, ophthalmologists have elucidated the pathophysiology of ocular diseases and have suggested therapies for previously untreatable diseases. For example, a mutation in *RPE65* causes Leber congenital amaurosis (LCA) and rod-cone dystrophy in adults. Gene therapy using viral vectors to introduce working copies of the gene has induced long-term visual function in Briard dogs that have canine retinal degeneration and blindness (1).

The advent of treatments for genetic diseases will likely be specific for certain gene products. Therefore, clinical diagnoses will be important to identify patients with phenotypes who would benefit from specific therapies. Furthermore, understanding and characterizing the natural history of disease will be necessary to accurately interpret future clinical trials.

The goal of this chapter is to provide the clinical descriptions, genetics, differential diagnoses, and pathophysiologies of inherited retinal and choroidal disorders that may present in infancy and early childhood. Ancillary studies, such as electroretinography and perimetry, and molecular pathophysiology are reviewed for specific diseases. Diagnostic studies (see Chapter 3), visual rehabilitation (see Chapter 33), worldwide impact of disease (see Chapter 18), ethical issues and the roles of other professionals (see Chapter 4), and future therapies (see Chapters 12, 13) are covered in greater depth elsewhere in the text as indicated.

GENERALIZED RETINAL AND CHOROIDAL DYSTROPHIES

Retinitis Pigmentosa

RP describes a heterogeneous set of conditions that share progressive rod loss initially, followed by cone loss in most cases. The loss of photoreceptors results in characteristic symptoms and fundus findings. The term *retinitis pigmentosa* was first used by Donders in 1855 to describe patients with night blindness, although the first fundus description of RP preceded this, shortly after the invention of the ophthalmoscope in 1851.

Clinical Presentation and Disease Course

Pediatric patients most commonly present with symptoms of nyctalopia. In children, this symptom may manifest as extreme fear of the dark. Parents also may perceive that their child has a difficulty navigating in low-light conditions. Children with autosomal recessive RP are more likely to present at an earlier age (median age 10.7 years) than are patients with autosomal dominant RP (median age 23.4 years) (2). Awareness of RP within a family might lead to earlier identification of an affected child than would occur for cases that become apparent only after symptoms arise. Peripheral vision loss is another hallmark of RP, with the classic ring scotoma 30 to 50 degrees from fixation. However, changes in children may be subtle, with mild constriction of central isopters or early subtle superior field loss (3). Some parents may note that a child appears clumsy, e.g., tripping on objects frequently, or they may report that a child has difficulty seeing objects within plain view. Patients also may have decreased central vision and dyschromatopsia, although these tend to be later findings in RP. Color vision abnormalities appear to be associated with visual acuity and are unusual while central vision remains 20/40 or better (3).

The classic clinical signs of RP are the triad of bone spicule pigmentation, arteriolar attenuation, and waxy pallor of the optic nerve. However, clinical signs in children may be more subtle, with the classic signs of RP becoming apparent only with increasing age (Fig. 7-1). Previously described *retinitis pigmentosa sine pigmento* now is believed to be an early stage of RP, with minimal fundus changes that may last for decades prior to the development of the more classic signs (3). Another clinically described phenotype in children is *retinitis punctata albescens,* in which white dots at

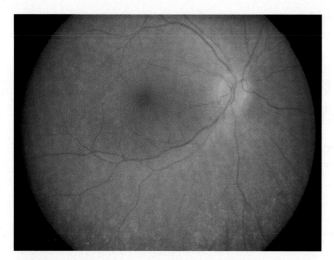

FIGURE 7-1. Early retinitis pigmentosa. Right fundus image of a 9-year-old boy from a family with autosomal dominant retinitis pigmentosa. He reported nyctalopia for as long as he could remember. Note arteriolar narrowing and pigmentary abnormalities but the absence of bone spicules and waxy optic nerve pallor.

the level of the retinal pigment epithelium (RPE) are present throughout the fundus. Although many forms of RP demonstrate subtle white dots as a stage of disease, such as rhodopsin-related RP (4), the finding of subtle white dots has become most closely associated with Bothnia dystrophy. Bothnia dystrophy is characterized by an early onset of nyctalopia, widespread white dots, development of macular changes by young adulthood, and late chorioretinal atrophy throughout the fundus (5,6). Other posterior segment findings, in general, include cystoid macular edema, epiretinal membranes, optic disc drusen, and vitreous cells. Anterior segment findings associated with RP include cataracts, but this finding is age dependent and more likely to present in early adulthood than childhood (7,8).

Even with subtle fundus findings, electroretinography will demonstrate reduced b-wave amplitudes and, frequently, delays in implicit time in patients with RP. Ultimately, with disease progression the electroretinogram (ERG) will become nonrecordable, but depending on the type of RP, this may not happen until late in the course of the disease.

Differential Diagnosis

The differential diagnosis of early-onset RP includes other conditions described here and elsewhere in this text. LCA (see also Chapters 3, 13) is a congenital form of blindness characterized by a markedly reduced or nonrecordable full-field ERG. Congenital stationary night blindness (CSNB) may also present with nyctalopia but is marked by normal visual fields and characteristic fundus or electroretinographic abnormalities (see also Chapter 3). Enhanced S-cone syndrome (ESCS) (p. 108), achromatopsia (p. 107), and cone-rod dystrophies (p. 95) are also most easily distin-

guished from one another based on electroretinographic abnormalities. Noninherited conditions such as inflammatory disease (see Chapter 17), trauma (Chapter 32), and infectious processes (see Chapter 16) may also mimic symptoms and fundus changes associated with RP. Rubella retinopathy (see Chapter 16) presents with a pigmentary retinopathy from birth that often is associated with congenital deafness. Electroretinography demonstrates only minimal changes. Syphilitic retinopathy (see Chapter 16) also will cause significant pigmentary changes, vitreous cells, and reduced electroretinographic recordings. Finally, drug toxicity can mimic RP and typically is the result of extended consumption of antipsychotic medications, such as thioridazine, or antimalarial medications, such as chloroquine or quinine. Hence, the presentation of drug toxicity in the pediatric age group would be unusual.

Molecular Genetics of Retinitis Pigmentosa

Simplex cases, i.e., those without a family history, make up the largest proportion of patients with RP. Up to 63% of cases worldwide are simplex. Studies performed in the United States and England reported incidences of 35% and 42%, respectively (3). When definite autosomal recessive cases are combined with simplex cases, this number accounts for approximately 70% of patients with RP. Autosomal dominant cases represent 15% to 20% of all RP, and X-linked RP represent 10% to 15% of all cases of RP.

Multiple genes have been implicated in RP, the first being rhodopsin, which was identified in 1990 (RetNet: *http://www.sph.uth.tmc.edu/Retnet/*) (Tables 7-1 and 7-2). It should be noted that just as different gene mutations can cause phenotypic RP, the same gene mutation can be associated with different phenotypic expressions (Table 7-2).

Mutations in the rhodopsin gene (*RHO*; RP4) represent a large proportion of all genotypically identified RP and are estimated to cause approximately 30% of all autosomal dominant RP cases in the United States (9,10). Other genes associated with autosomal dominant RP include *RP1, IMPDH1* (RP10), *RGR, NRL, FSCN2,* and peripherin/*RDS* (RP7), which can cause RP alone or a digenic form of RP in association with changes in the *ROM1* gene (11,12). Most recently, mutations in posttranscriptional processing-related genes *PRPF31, HPRP3,* and *PRPF8* have been identified as the cause of autosomal dominant RP types RP11, RP18, and RP13, respectively (13–19). An estimated 50% of all cases of autosomal dominant RP has been reported as having an identified genetic cause (20).

There are three X-linked forms of RP (RP2, RP3, RP6), and the genes have been identified for two of them (Table 7-1). Mutations in the *RPGR* gene are associated with RP3, whereas mutations in a novel gene that encodes a plasma membrane-associated protein are associated with RP2. Together they account for 70% (*RPGR*) and 10% (RP2)

TABLE 7–1. IDENTIFIED GENES ASSOCIATED WITH NONSYNDROMIC PIGMENTOSA

Disease Designation	Chromosome	Gene Name (Gene Product)
Autosomal Dominant		
RP1	8	*RP1*
RP4	3	*RHO* (rhodopsin)
RP7	6	*RDS* (peripherin)
RP10	7	*IMPDH* (inosine monophosphate dehydrogenase)
RP9	7	*PIM1-K* (PIM1-kinase)
RP11	19	*PRPF31* (pre-mRNA splicing factor 31)
RP13	17	*PRPF8* (pre-mRNA splicing factor C8)
RP18	1	*HPRP3* (pre-mRNA splicing factor 3)
RP27	14	*NRL* (transcription factor of the leucine zipper family)
RGR	10	*RGR* (RPE-retinal G-protein–coupled receptor)
CRX	19	*CRX* (transcription factor)
X-Linked Recessive		
RP2	X	*RP2* (plasma membrane protein homologous to cofactor C)
RP3 (RP15)	X	*RPGR* (retinitis pigmentosa GTPase regulator)
Autosomal Recessive		
RP12	1	*CRB1*[a] (RP with paraarteriolar preservation of RPE)
RP14	6	*TULP1* (tubby-like protein 1)[a]
RP19	1	*ABCA4* (ATP-binding cassette transporter)[a]
RP20	1	*RPE65*[a]
USH2A	1	*USH2A* (Usherin)[a]
MERTK	2	*MERTK* (c-mer protooncogene, receptor tyrosine kinase)
SAG	2	*SAG* (Arrestin)[a]
RHO	3	*RHO* (rhodopsin)
PDE6A	5	*PDE6A* (phosphodiesterase α-subunit)
PDE6B	4	*PDE6B* (phosphodiesterase β-subunit)
CNGA1	4	*CNGA1* (rod cGMP-gated channel α-subunit)
CNGB1	16	*CNGB1* (rod cGMP-gated channel β-subunit)
LRAT	4	*LRAT* (lecithin retinol acyltransferase)
RGR	10	*RGR* (RPE-retinal G-protein–coupled receptor)
NR2E3	15	*NR2E3* (nuclear receptor subfamily 2 group E3)[a]
RLBP1	15	*RLBP1* (cellular retinaldehyde binding protein)[a]

[a] Other specific disease associations such as Leber congenital amaurosis (*RPE65, CRB1, TULP1*), Stargardt disease (*ABCA4*), Oguchi disease (*SAG*), Enhanced S-cone syndrome/Goldmann-Favre syndrome (*NR2E3*), and Bothnia dystrophy (*RLBP1*).

of all X-linked RP (21). As *RPGR* accounts for such a significant fraction of X-linked RP, it also is a primary cause of all RP. Nevertheless, the ORF15 region of *RPGR* has presented technical difficulties in screening because of its repetitive nature and the high rate of variability within the normal population (22). RP6 has been linked to Xp21.3-21.2, but no causative gene has yet been identified.

Multiple genes have been associated with autosomal recessive RP (Table 7-1) (10). Specifically, Bothnia dystrophy and Newfoundland rod-cone dystrophies, both of which demonstrate a very clear retinitis punctata albescens phenotype, are caused by changes in the *RLBP1* gene that codes for cellular retinaldehyde binding protein (CRALBP) (5,6,23). A rare cause of RP in the United States, this gene accounts for a large proportion of retinal degenerations (5,6,24) in

certain geographic regions, such as northern Sweden and Newfoundland.

Cone-Rod Dystrophy

The definition of the group of cone-rod dystrophies is based on electrophysiologic characteristics and has come to include a number of phenotypic expressions once believed to represent entirely separate diseases. Cone-rod dystrophies are generalized photoreceptor disorders characterized on electroretinography by a greater loss of cone function than rod function and consequently have common symptomatic presentations (25). Like RP, cone-rod dystrophies are heterogeneous, with a wide range of presentations, disease courses, and severity.

TABLE 7–2. OTHER DISEASE ASSOCIATIONS LINKED TO GENES KNOWN TO CAUSE NONSYNDROMIC RETINITIS PIGMENTOSA

Gene Name (Gene Product)	Disease Associations (Phenotypes)
Autosomal Dominant Retinitis Pigmentosa Genes	
RHO	Autosomal recessive retinitis pigmentosa
	Autosomal dominant congenital stationary night blindness
RDS/peripherin	Autosomal dominant pattern dystrophy
	Autosomal dominant cone-rod distrophy
	Digenic retinitis pigmentosa
CRX	Autosomal dominant cone-rod dystrophy
	Leber congenital amaurosis
RGR	Autosomal recessive retinitis pigmentosa
X-Linked Retinitis Pigmentosa Genes	
RPGR	X-linked cone-rod dystrophy
	X-lined macular degeneration
	X-linked congenital stationary night blindness
Autosomal Recessive Retinitis Pigmentosa Genes	
CRB1	Leber congenital amaurosis
TULP1	Leber congenital amaurosis
RPE	Leber congenital amaurosis
ABCA4	Stargardt disease
	Fundus flavimaculatus
	Autosomal recessive cone-rod dystrophy
SAG	Oguchi disease
NR2E3	Enhanced S-cone syndrome
	Goldmann-Favre syndrome
RLBP1	Bothnia dystrophy
	Newfoundland rod-cone dystrophy

Clinical Presentation and Disease Course

Most cone-rod dystrophies (Table 7-3) present late in the second decade of life to early adulthood, e.g., *RPGR*-ORF15-associated X-linked cone-rod dystrophy typically presents by the age of 45 years (26,27). However, some cone-rod dystrophies present earlier in life. Autosomal dominant cone-rod dystrophy caused by mutations in the *CRX* gene may present in the first decade of life with symptoms of decreased central vision and dyschromatopsia. However, the *CRX* gene also has been associated with both LCA and a late onset of RP in which patients remain asymptomatic until the sixth decade of life (28). Autosomal recessive cone-rod dystrophy can be caused by the adenosine triphosphate (ATP)-binding cassette transporter *(ABCA4)* gene and present in conjunction with, or in the absence of, classic findings associated with Stargardt disease/fundus flavimaculatus in childhood (29–32).

Presenting symptoms of cone-rod dystrophy include decreased central vision, dyschromatopsia, and light sensitivity (25). Patients typically report that they are most comfortable in low ambient light settings such as dawn or twilight.

Early in the course, patients may not have nyctalopia, but with progression of disease, they will develop nyctalopia and peripheral vision loss. Typically, fundus changes are similar to RP with bone spicules and RPE atrophy. However, fundus changes tend to occur in the macula and posterior pole before the retinal periphery. Macular changes include geographic atrophy, a beaten bronze appearance (Fig. 7-2), a bull's-eye maculopathy, and a tapetal sheen.

The characteristic ERG demonstrates greater involvement of the cone system than the rod system with full-field testing. Further attempts have been made to characterize cone-rod dystrophies based on their dark-adapted perimetry characteristics (33). Finally, the multifocal ERG is diffusely abnormal and may be nonrecordable in patients with cone-rod dystrophies. Patients with focal macular changes, such as seen in Stargardt disease, will have greater central loss (Fig. 7-3).

Clinical diseases once believed to be separate from cone-rod dystrophies are now included within the broad group because of shared electrophysiologic characteristics. Foremost among these is Stargardt disease. The presence of cone dysfunction has been noted °to be mild to severe and may

TABLE 7–3. IDENTIFIED GENES ASSOCIATED WITH CONE-ROD DYSTROPHIES

Disease Designation	Chromosome	Gene Name (Gene Product)
Autosomal Dominant		
CRX	19	*CRX* (transcription factor)
(GUGY2D) (CORD5-6, RETGC)	17	Retinal guanylate cyclase gene
GUCA1A (COD3, GCAP1)	6	Guanylate cyclase activator 1A gene
Peripherin/RDS	6	*RDS* (peripherin)
CORD7 (RIM1, RIMS1)	6	Rab3A-interacting molecule
HGR4 (UNC119)	17	Human analog of caenorhabditis elegans UNC119
Autosomal Recessive		
RP19	1	*ABCA4* (ATP-binding cassette transporter)[a]
RDH5	12	*RDH5* (11-*cis* retinol dehydrogenase)
ACHM4	1	*GNAT2* (G-protein cone-specific transducin α-subunit)
X-Linked Recessive		
COD1	X	*RPGR*-ORF15 (retinitis pigmentosa GTPase regulator)

[a]: Other specific disease associations: Stargardt disease, autosomal recessive RP, fundus flavimaculatus.

present at any point in the course of a classic clinical appearance of Stargardt disease/fundus flavimaculatus. Although derangements in electroretinographic function are more common in late stages of this disease, patients have presented with minimal fundus changes and severe cone dysfunction early in the course of the disease. Lois et al. (29) suggested that the presence of advanced electroretinographic derangements may be an indicator of a poor long-term outcome. Itabashi et al. (34) reported that patients with a clinical phenotype of fundus flavimaculatus, i.e., pisciform changes involving the midperipheral and posterior

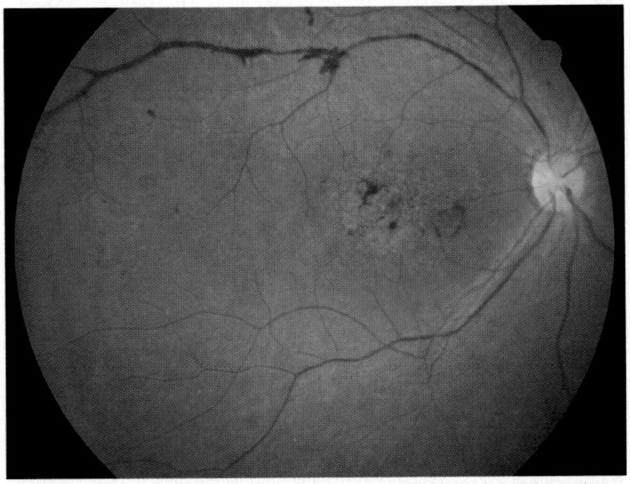

FIGURE 7-2. Cone-rod dystrophy. The patient is a 20-year-old woman with 20/400 OU and a markedly reduced electroretinogram for both cone and rod function. Note the beaten bronze appearance of the macula and bone spicule changes along the arterioles.

retina rather than disease limited to the macula, tended to present with worse electroretinographic dysfunction. Thus, a substantial fraction of patients with fundus flavimaculatus/Stargardt disease demonstrates some degree of cone dysfunction, although the largest proportion still has normal full-field ERGs. Another condition with severe cone dysfunction at presentation is fundus albipunctatus. Although fundus albipunctatus is classically considered to be nonprogressive, some patients will develop cone dysfunction accompanied by macular changes in midadulthood (35).

Systemic disease associations with cone-rod dystrophies are rare. Spinocerebellar ataxia has been associated with cone-rod dystrophies (36). There are two reported cases of thiamine-responsive megaloblastic anemia and cone-rod dystrophy (37,38) and a reported case of achondroplasia with cone-rod dystrophy (39). Alstrom syndrome also demonstrates a cone-rod dystrophy phenotype with cardiomyopathy and type 2 diabetes mellitus (40). Finally, Bardet-Biedl syndrome causes a pigmentary retinopathy and photoreceptor degeneration that may have a cone-rod electroretinographic phenotype because of associated central macular atrophy.

Molecular Genetics of Cone-Rod Dystrophies

Like RP, cone-rod dystrophies can be inherited in an autosomal dominant, autosomal recessive, or X-linked recessive manner (Tables 7-2 and 7-3). There are reports of potential associations with mitochondrial disease and cone dystrophies as well (41). Eight genes have been identified to cause cone-rod dystrophies and 11 loci mapped.

Genes associated with autosomal dominant cone-rod dystrophy are *CRX* (28), retinal guanylate cyclase gene

FIGURE 7-3. Stargardt disease. **A:** Note the classic appearance of pisciform flecks in the macula and beaten bronze appearance centrally. **B:** Multifocal electroretinography. The **top image** represents trace arrays for the central 40 degrees of the patient's field of vision. Note the loss of amplitude centrally. This is depicted in a graphic format in the **bottom image** as a response density plot. The central depression represents the loss of function due to Stargardt disease. The peripheral, shallower depression represents the blind spot.

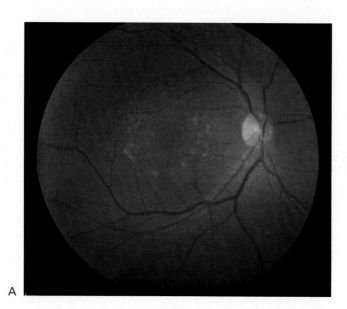

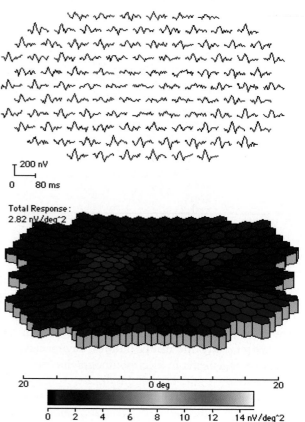

A   B

(*GUCY2D*), peripherin/*RDS* (42), Rab3A-interacting molecule *(RIM1)* gene in CORD7 (43), and guanylate cyclase activator 1A gene (*GUCA1A*) (26). Mutations in *GUCY2D* have been associated with both CORD5 and CORD6, now recognized as representing the same disease (44).

Genes associated with autosomal recessive cone-rod dystrophies are *ABCA4* (45), *GNAT2* (46,47), and *RDH5*. Some groups suggest that in up to 35% of patients with autosomal recessive cone-rod dystrophy, the cause may be mutations in the *ABCA4* gene (48,49). It is entirely possible that these groups are identifying patients who would otherwise be characterized as having Stargardt disease or fundus flavimaculatus at different stages in the evolution of their clinical disease and not as having *ABCA4*-related cone-rod dystrophy. The distinction between these diseases given their clinical features and molecular genetics remains to be clarified.

The gene thus far identified to cause X-linked cone-rod dystrophy (COD1) is the RP GTPase regulator *(RPGR)*, with the mutations occurring specifically in its ORF15 exon (27,50). This exon seems to be a mutation hotspot, probably because the sequence is highly repetitive rendering it difficult to screen. In addition, in-frame deletions and duplica-

tions, i.e., those that add or remove amino acids but do not change the remaining amino acid sequence of the protein product, are estimated to occur in up to 34% of the normal population. Thus, these changes do not seem to affect the function of the protein (22,27). One other locus for cone-rod dystrophy has been linked to the X chromosome but has not yet been identified (COD2).

Several genes associated with cone-rod dystrophies cause other retinal or macular dystrophies. Included among these are pattern dystrophies of the macula (peripherin/*RDS*), LCA (*CRX*, *GUCY2D*), RP (*CRX*, peripherin/*RDS*, *ABCA4*, *RPGR*), macular degeneration without full-field electroretinographic abnormalities (*RPGR*) (51), CSNB (*RDH5*), complete achromatopsia (*GNAT2*), and Stargardt disease (*ABCA4*). Cone-rod dystrophies, like RP, demonstrate that mutations in the same gene can cause different clinical appearances, which were previously considered to be entirely separate disease entities.

Choroideremia

Choroideremia is an X-linked disorder resulting in choroidal degeneration with subsequent loss of retinal function. It was first described in 1871 by Mauthner. The gene

(CHM) was identified in 1992. Late-stage choroideremia has an unmistakable appearance of widespread loss of RPE, choriocapillaris, and larger choroidal vessels, with occasional patches of pigment and sparing of a small patch of RPE and retina in the macula. When choroideremia presents in childhood and adolescence, its symptoms and clinical appearance can be very similar to those of RP.

Clinical Presentation and Disease Course

Because of its X-linked inheritance, choroideremia typically presents in males in the second to third decade of life with the primary symptom of nyctalopia (52). On occasion, patients report symptoms as early as the first decade of life. Early in the course of the disease, nummular patches of RPE atrophy appear in the midperipheral retina. These areas become confluent with progressive loss of choriocapillaris initially and larger choroidal vessels subsequently (Fig. 7-4). The end stage results in bare sclera extending from the posterior pole to the periphery. In one study, Roberts et al. (53) found that 84% of patients younger than 60 years had 20/40 or better central vision, whereas 33% of patients older than 60 years had 20/200 or worse vision. Thus, patients often maintain central vision until late in the course of disease but lose peripheral fields steadily from the time of diagnosis onward. As expected, the ERG shows progressive loss of retinal function throughout the disease course, eventually becoming nonrecordable in the late stages.

Female carriers of choroideremia demonstrate a spectrum of clinical manifestations ranging from essentially no findings to symptomatic loss of retinal function and apparent retinal degeneration (52). This spectrum likely is dependent on the degree of mosaicism and X inactivation. In general, carriers of the *CHM* gene demonstrate a moth-eaten appearance of RPE, with RPE clumping and atrophy. Many carriers also will demonstrate drusenoid deposition and peripapillary atrophy. However, some individuals will have a completely normal fundus. The degree of dysfunction on ancillary tests corresponds with the apparent clinical involvement.

Differential Diagnosis

Choroideremia can closely mimic the presentation of X-linked RP in its early stages. Both conditions have nearly identical clinical manifestations and symptoms, and present at approximately the same age (i.e., second decade of life). Examination of the carriers (preferably, the mother of the patient) is helpful because the carrier state of X-linked RP can manifest with a tapetal macular sheen or with patches of retina characteristic of RP. Gyrate atrophy can also resemble choroideremia in its early stages; however, gyrate atrophy has an autosomal recessive inheritance pattern, hyperornithinemia, and a milder course than choroideremia.

Molecular Findings

The *CHM* gene was identified in 1993 by Sankila and further characterized by Seabra and van Bokhoven (54–58). The *CHM* gene codes for a Rab escort protein (REP-1) for the enzyme geranylgeranyl transferase, which is involved in adding a geranylgeranyl moiety to the end of Rab proteins (54–56,59,60). Nearly all disease-causing changes in the *CHM* gene were found to prevent translation or result in significant truncation of the protein product. There was one reported case of a missense mutation resulting in disease (61), although in a recent review of 57 families with choroideremia, missense mutations did not account for a significant fraction of disease-causing changes. Transitions and transversions in the *CHM* gene accounted for more than 40% of identified changes, small deletions [<5 base pairs (bp)] an additional 28% of the mutations, partial deletions 9%, and complete deletions 4% (62). At this time, the severity of the mutation does not appear to correlate with either disease severity or carrier state manifestations. Finally, the pathophysiology of disease from mutations in the *CHM* gene has yet to be elucidated. Syed examined the retina of an 88-year-old symptomatic carrier of the *CHM* gene and found changes suggesting that rod photoreceptors were the primary site of disease. In addition, REP-1 was localized to rods but not cones, further supporting rods as the primary site in disease pathophysiology. The choriocapillaris was atrophic in areas where the retina was severely degenerated but normal elsewhere (63). Thus, the prior clinical assumption that choroideremia was

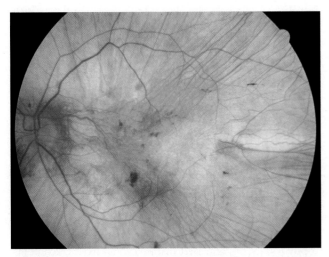

FIGURE 7-4. Choroideremia. Left fundus image of a 28-year-old man with choroideremia. He has severely constricted visual fields, and his central vision is 20/80 OD and finger-counting vision OS. Note the absence of retinal pigment epithelium and choriocapillaris throughout the fundus. Large-caliber choroidal vessels are easily visible.

primarily a choroidal dystrophy may be called into question in the future.

MACULAR DYSTROPHIES

Best Disease

Best disease was first described by Adams in 1883. However, it was named for Frederick Best, who described eight members of one family with the classic macular changes in 1905. The mode of inheritance is autosomal dominant with incomplete penetrance, as some patients have the abnormal allele and a normal-appearing fundus. Consequently, the true prevalence of this condition is unknown. Still, it is not a common disease; it has a reported prevalence of less than 1 in 10,000 in Iowa (64).

Clinical Findings

The clinical appearance of Best disease is highly variable and includes a normal-appearing fundus (5%–32%), macular RPE atrophy, or a gliotic scar from choroidal neovascularization (65,66). The classic ophthalmoscopic appearance of Best disease is symmetrical, bilateral, yellow-orange vitelliform lesions (Fig. 7-5) (65). The vitelliform lesion represents lipofuscin pigment and has been reported as early as shortly after birth and as late as age 64 years (67). The vitelliform appearance appears to be the least stable of the range of fundus manifestations seen in Best disease. Vitelliform lesions evolve into one of several appearances depending on the resorption of lipofuscin and include (i) a well-circumscribed gliotic scar, (ii) a pseudohypopyon, (iii) a "vitelliruptive" scrambled, scattered distribution of lipofuscin, and (iv) simple macular atrophy. Attempts had been made to classify the various findings into stages (66). Staging, however, implies a chronologic progression from one

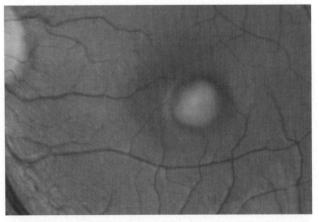

FIGURE 7-5. Best disease. Left macula of a 19-year-old man with Best disease. Note the vitelliform lesion in the macula. The other eye demonstrates a smaller vitelliform lesion than the left eye. Visual acuity is 20/30 OD and 20/40 OS.

appearance to another that is not necessarily true in Best disease. Eccentric vitelliform lesions (ectopic vitelliform lesions) and midperipheral flecklike deposits also can be seen in these patients (64). Multifocal Best disease may occur as a variant or represent a completely different condition (65). Gliotic nodules were previously thought to be preceded by choroidal neovascularization because classic choroidal neovascularization has been documented in Best disease (68,69). However, choroidal neovascularization does not necessarily precede gliotic lesions and is not ever even required to be present when hemorrhage is noted clinically. Incidental trauma has been documented to cause subretinal hemorrhage in the absence of choroidal neovascularization in patients with vitelliform lesions. Many of these patients will spontaneously recover vision, depending on the amount of hemorrhage and degree of vision loss. However, demonstration of a definite choroidal neovascular complex or severe vision loss associated with hemorrhage may be an indication for intervention to surgically evacuate the hemorrhage and extract the choroidal neovascular complex. (Fig. 7-6) (69).

The visual prognosis for patients with Best disease is good; 75% of patients maintain 20/40 or better vision in one eye through age 50 years (70). From a series in Iowa, the average visual acuity was 20/25 for patients younger than 30 years, 20/30 for patients aged 30 to 60 years, and 20/40 for patients older than 60 years (71). Even in the presence of a large vitelliform lesion, patients typically retained relatively good visual acuity.

Lipofuscin blocks fluorescence on fluorescein angiography. Thus, vitelliform lesions will block background fluorescence through most of the angiogram. With evolution of the lesion, hyperfluorescence can be seen as a window defect from RPE atrophy or as leakage from a choroidal neovascular membrane (65). The ERG is normal in patients with Best disease, whereas the electrooculogram (EOG), which measures the standing electrical potential across the RPE, is markedly abnormal. The EOG is reported as a ratio between the highest amplitude measured in a light adapted state and the lowest amplitude measured in the dark adapted state. The EOG normally is greater than 1.7, but in patients with Best disease it is below 1.5 and often 1.0 (65).

Differential Diagnosis

The differential diagnosis relates to the variable clinical appearances of Best disease. Pattern dystrophy can present with a small vitelliform lesion or atrophy. However, pattern dystrophy rarely presents with visual symptoms or clinical signs in childhood. Stargardt disease, North Carolina macular dystrophy (NCMD), and Best disease can all have macular atrophy. Family history and examination of family members can help to differentiate these conditions. Multifocal Best disease has also been described as an autosomal dominant disease with classic vitelliform lesions and a normal EOG.

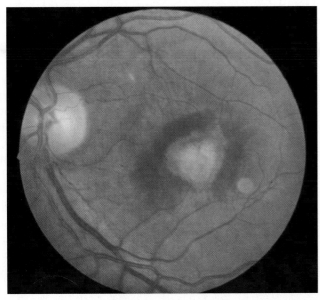
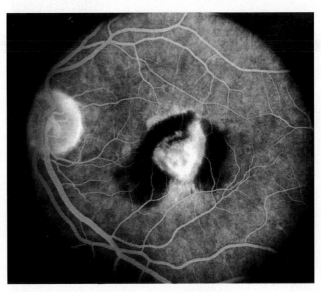

FIGURE 7-6. Best disease with choroidal neovascularization. **A:** Right eye demonstrates retinal pigment epithelium elevation and subretinal hemorrhage. **B:** Fundus fluorescein angiography in the late phases shows leakage consistent with choroidal neovascularization. Early phases clearly demonstrated lacy choroidal neovascularization. (From Chung M, et al. *Retina* 2001;21:575–580, with permission).

Molecular Genetics

Best disease was linked to chromosome 11q13 in 1992 (72), and the gene was identified by Marquardt and colleagues in 1998. The gene product was called bestrophin (73). Marmorstein and colleagues (74) were able to localize bestrophin to the basolateral plasma membrane of the RPE, supporting it in the pathogenesis of the reduced EOG. Sun et al. (75) and Gomez et al. (76) hypothesized that bestrophin functions as a chloride channel or a putative ion exchanger and provided further insight. Others have suggested that bestrophin might function as an intracellular messenger rather than an ion channel (77). The presence of a family history of macular disease in a patient suspected of having Best disease was a strong predictor of identifying a disease-causing sequence variation in the gene (78). Without a family history, only 28% of samples from patients clinically diagnosed with Best disease demonstrated a change in the bestrophin gene (E.M. Stone, *personal communication,* 2000).

North Carolina Macular Dystrophy

First described in 1971 by Lefler et al. (79) and later in 1984 by Hermsen and Judisch (80) as central areolar pigment epithelial dystrophy, NCMD was renamed by Gass in 1987. Each of the families described in these initial publications was related to the same family in the mountains of North Carolina. The family was traced back to 1715 and now consists of more than 5,000 individuals throughout the United States. NCMD was the first macular dystrophy demonstrating an inherited pattern, but, thus far, no causative gene has been identified (81).

Clinical Findings

NCMD is an autosomal dominant congenital macular disorder believed to be completely penetrant with variable expressivity. Patients typically have much better vision than would be predicted by their clinical appearances, with visual acuities ranging from 20/20 to 20/400 and a median visual acuity of 20/60 (82). The fundus appearance can vary from a few scattered macular drusen (Fig. 7-7) to a large excavated macular staphyloma. The staphyloma frequently has associated gliotic tissue involved in or at its rim (83–87) and has been documented in a patient as young as age 3 months. In general, NCMD is considered nonprogressive or, at worst, minimally progressive. Choroidal neovascularization has been documented and appears to be most common in patients who present with extensive drusen in the central macular area. The presence of choroidal neovascularization may result in severe vision loss (83–86).

Differential Diagnosis

For patients without the large bilateral macular staphylomata, the differential diagnosis can include other macular dystrophies, such as Stargardt disease or Best disease. Cone dystrophies may also present with macular changes but will have characteristic symptoms and a diagnostic ERG.

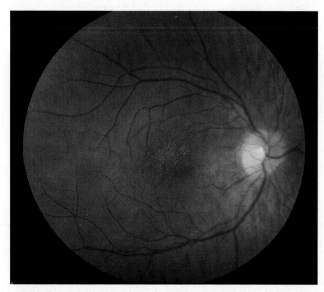

FIGURE 7-7. North Carolina macular dystrophy. Right eye of a man from a family with North Carolina macular dystrophy. He demonstrates relatively mild findings with drusen in the maculae of both eyes. Visual acuity is 20/20 OU.

Molecular Genetics

NCMD was first linked to chromosome 6 in 1991, with subsequent refinement of its locus to 6q16–21 (MCDR1) (83,85,86). Since its first description, families in France and Belize have been described with very close linkage to the MCDR1 locus and a clinical appearance consistent with that of the originally described family.

Other Macular Dystrophies

Other macular dystrophies covered elsewhere in the textbook include the following:

- Stargardt disease (see Chapter 8)
- X-linked or congenital retinoschisis (see Chapter 25)

CONGENITAL STATIONARY DISEASES

Congenital Stationary Night Blindness

CSNB includes a broad number of conditions marked by early-onset night blindness and a relatively stable clinical course (Table 7-4). The first description of CSNB was reported in 1838 by Cunier in a seven-generation French family (88). CSNB is subdivided into two categories based on the presence or absence of characteristic fundus changes. The forms of CSNB with characteristic findings display either white spots (fundus albipunctatus) or a greenish metallic sheen (Oguchi disease), whereas other forms of CSNB have minimal fundus changes. Most forms of CSNB have characteristic findings on dark adaptation and electroretinography and have a relatively good visual prognosis.

Normal Fundus Congenital Stationary Night Blindness

X-Linked Congenital Stationary Night Blindness: Complete and Incomplete

Both complete and incomplete X-linked CSNB are generally characterized by significant refractive changes, nystagmus, and nyctalopia, although reports indicate that many patients with X-linked CSNB may not present with nyctalopia (89). Best corrected visual acuity usually is in the range from 20/40 to 20/50 (90); however, vision can be worse.

Complete CSNB is characterized by severe progressive axial myopia and severe nyctalopia. Visual acuity may be relatively good, even 20/20 early in life (91). However, visual acuity subsequently is limited by myopia and astigmatic changes. Fundus findings are those consistent with high myopia, such as posterior staphyloma, scleral crescents, and tilted optic discs.

Incomplete CSNB demonstrates similar findings, although not all of these features need be present in each case. A study of 15 families with incomplete CSNB reported that 72% of patients lacked at least one major feature, up to 40% did perceive nyctalopia, and 60% lacked nystagmus. Visual acuity ranged from 20/25 to 20/400 (91–94), with poorer visual acuities present in patients with nystagmus. Finally, some patients were hyperopic rather than myopic.

Both forms of CSNB demonstrate selective loss of the b wave with an essentially normal a wave, classically know as a Schubert-Bornschein response (95). This response differs from that in other conditions, such as X-linked retinoschisis or severe intraretinal ischemia, with a reduced b/a ratio in which the a wave can be abnormal. Electroretinographic findings distinguish complete from incomplete CSNB (Fig. 7-8) (96). Incomplete CSNB demonstrates relatively well-preserved rod function and abnormalities in the cone response, such as loss of the cone b-wave amplitude and a double-peaked 30-Hz flicker response. Complete CSNB demonstrates severely abnormal rod-isolated responses with normal or mildly subnormal cone responses (96).

The differential diagnosis for a patient with CSNB overlaps and includes RP, LCA, and achromatopsia. Electroretinographic findings coupled with relatively normal –visual fields distinguish CSNB from these other conditions (97,98). Although almost pathognomonic for CSNB, the characteristic Schubert-Bornschein response can be seen in Duchenne muscular dystrophy and has been reported in a family with autosomal dominant inherited negative ERG (99).

Two different genes on the X chromosome cause complete and incomplete CSNB. The gene for incomplete CSNB was identified first in 1998 (100). It is known as the *CACNA1F* gene and codes for the α subunit of the calcium channel, which affects both the on pathway and, to a greater degree, the off pathway of the bipolar cells (101). Recently, the gene for complete CSNB was identified as nyctalopin

TABLE 7–4. GENES ASSOCIATED WITH CONGENITAL STATIONARY NIGHT BLINDNESS AND ACHROMATOPSIA

Disease Designation	Chromosome	Gene Name (Gene Product)
Autosomal Dominant Congenital Stationary Night Blindness		
RHO	3	*RHO* (rhodopsin)
GNAT1 (Nougaret)	3	*GNAT1* (rod transducin α-subunit)
PDE6B (Rambusch)	4	*PDE6B* (phosphodiesterase β-subunit)
Autosomal Recessive Congenital Stationary Night Blindness		
RDH5 (fundus albipunctatus)	12	*RDH5* (11-*cis* retinol dehydrogenase)
SAG (Oguchi disease)	2	*SAG* (Arrestin)[a]
RHOK (Oguchi disease)	13	*RHOK* (rhodopsin kinase)
X-linked Congenital Stationary Night Blindness		
CACNA1F (incomplete)	X	L-Type voltage-gated calcium channel α_1-subunit
NYX (complete)	X	Nyctalopin
RPGR (incomplete)	X	Retinitis pigmentosa GTPase regulator
Rod Monochromacy (Complete Achromatopsia)		
ACHM2	2	*CNGA3* (cone cGMO-gated cation channel α_3-subunit)
ACHM3	8	*CNGB3* (cone cGMP-gated cation channel β_3-subunit)
ACHM4	1	*GNAT2* (G-protein cone-specific transducin α-subunit)
Blue Cone Monochromacy		
OPN1MW	X	Green cone opsin
OPN1LW	X	Red cone opsin

[a]: Other specific disease associations such as autosomal recessive RP.

(NYX) (102). Mutations in nyctalopin are believed to disrupt the development of the on pathways of the bipolar cells (91–94,102).

Autosomal Dominant Congenital Stationary Night Blindness

Autosomal dominant CSNB is characterized by a stable course, normal visual acuity, and normal visual fields. The fundus appearance also appears normal, although some patients with rhodopsin-related CSNB may develop bone spicules in the midperiphery after middle age (35). Electroretinographic findings in the autosomal dominant form differ from X-linked CSNB in that a reduced response is present only under scotopic testing. Regardless of the molecular cause, the rod-isolated responses in autosomal dominant CSNB are absent, whereas cone-isolated responses are normal. However, late in the course of disease, some patients with rhodopsin-related autosomal dominant CSNB can demonstrate mild cone dysfunction (35). In contrast to forms of CSNB associated with an abnormal fundus, the reduction in electroretinographic response does not

reverse with continued dark adaptation. The final dark-adapted threshold for rods is markedly elevated. The primary distinguishing features of autosomal dominant CSNB from milder forms of autosomal dominant RP are the stability of visual acuity, visual fields, and cone function.

Mutations in three genes have been associated with autosomal dominant CSNB. Mutations in codon 90, 94, or 292 of rhodopsin *(RHO)* are associated with a nonprogressive condition with normal vision and visual fields under mesopic or photopic situations and a reduced rod-isolated response as the major characteristic of nyctalopia (35,103,104). Evidence suggests that the associated changes in rhodopsin disrupt a critical salt bridge, thus changing the tertiary structure of the protein, and result in an opsin that is constitutively active. Consequently, the retina is desensitized and night blindness results (105). Finally, one change, Gly90Asp, has been associated with late onset of bone spicules (35). Changes in the genes for both the α subunit of transducin *(GNAT1)* and the β subunit of the rod cGMP phosphodiesterase enzyme *(PDE6B)* have also been associated with autosomal dominant CSNB (88,106). *GNAT1* has been implicated in the Nougaret

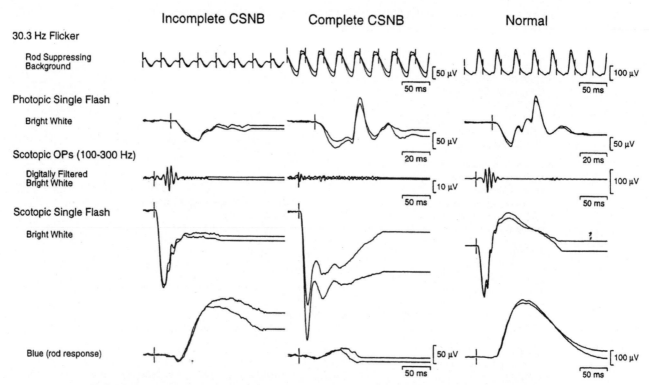

FIGURE 7-8. Full-field electroretinography comparing complete and incomplete congenital stationary night blindness. Electroretinograms of a 16-year-old boy with incomplete congenital stationary night blindness (CSNB; from $R_{50}X$ mutation of CACNAIF), a 6-year-old boy with complete CSNB (from common in-phase 24-nt deletion of NYX), and an 18-year-old normal for comparison. (From Weleber RG. Infantile and childhood retinal blindness: a molecular perspective [The Franceschetti Lecture]. *Ophthalmic Genet* 2002;23:71–97, with permission.)

pedigree from France first described by Cunier. *PDE6B* was found associated with the large Rambusch pedigree from Denmark (35,106,107).

Abnormal Fundus Congenital Stationary Night Blindness

Fundus Albipunctatus

Fundus albipunctatus was first described as a variant of retinitis punctata albescens by Lauber (108) in 1910. This condition is characterized by fine small white-yellow dots throughout the retina in association with a stationary, nonprogressive form of night blindness. In 1999, Yamamoto identified mutations in the gene encoding 11-*cis*-retinol dehydrogenase *(RDH5)* in patients with fundus albipunctatus (113). Although multiple mutations in the *RDH5* gene have been associated with fundus albipunctatus, some families with a classic clinical appearance have not exhibited mutations in *RDH5*.

Clinical Features

The most characteristic feature of this condition is the presence of widespread white-yellow dots that are present in a radial pattern extending from the macula. These dots can

fade as a patient reaches the fourth to fifth decade of life (35). This condition is characterized by subnormal rod-isolated responses with standard dark adaptation. Patients will frequently demonstrate an electronegative response with selective loss of the b wave for the maximum combined response with standard dark adaptation. However, with extended dark adaptation, electroretinographic responses improve and become essentially normal (Fig. 7-9) (35). Although this condition is classically considered to be a form of CSNB, evidence exists that, later in life, often the fourth to fifth decade (109), macular atrophy and an electroretinographic phenotype consistent with cone-rod dystrophy can develop and persist even after prolonged dark adaptation (35,110). Many of these patients also demonstrate other macular changes, such as a bull's-eye appearance. Typically, these changes occur in the fourth to fifth decades of life. Nakamura and Miyake identified a 9-year-old boy with atrophic foveal lesions, widespread white dots, and a compound heterozygous mutation in the *RDH5* gene (111). This patient also demonstrated normalization of his ERG with no apparent residual cone dysfunction after 3 hours of dark adaptation (111,112). Thus, macular disease is not necessarily associated with cone dysfunction and may be present earlier in life, although these findings are more common in late adulthood.

The differential diagnosis for fundus albipunctatus includes other forms of flecked retinas (Appendix 2) such as Stargardt disease, pattern dystrophies, and retinitis punctata albescens. In many of these cases, the flecks are distinctly different. Nevertheless, there is some degree of phenotypic overlap among these conditions. Dark adaptation, fluorescein angiography, and electroretinographic characteristics can help to distinguish these conditions. However, at one isolated visit in time, it may be difficult to separate these conditions even with clinical testing; therefore, repeated visits and the use of molecular genetic testing are useful.

Molecular Genetics

Fundus albipunctatus is caused by changes in the gene that codes for 11-*cis*-retinol dehydrogenase *(RDH5)* (113). This enzyme regenerates 11-*cis*-retinal in retinoid metabolism and is believed to play a particularly critical role. However, to date, no other conditions besides fundus albipunctatus have been associated with mutations in this gene. Furthermore, Driessen et al. (114) described two normal families with frameshift mutations in the *RDH5* gene that predicted essentially no function of the *RDH5* gene. From their work, they concluded that *RDH5* gene mutations would not be associated with more widespread retinal dystrophies other than fundus albipunctatus. Cideciyan et al. (115) also evaluated the consequences of a null mutation in *RDH5* on the visual cycle. Both of these groups ultimately concluded that other biochemical pathways besides 11-*cis*-retinol dehydrogenase exist for the production of 11-*cis*-retinal, the product of 11-*cis*-retinol dehydrogenase. The presence of these alternative pathways would explain, in part, the normalization of the ERG following prolonged

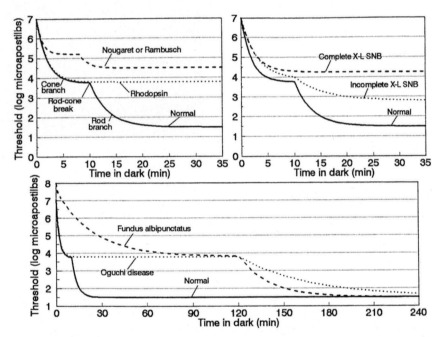

FIGURE 7-9. Dark adaptation curves for patients with congenital stationary night blindness (CSNB). Schematic dark-adaptation curves in normal individuals and in patients with stationary night blindness. In all three graphs, the y axis is the minimal intensity of a perceptible spot of light (logarithmic scale, units are microapostilbs) at the time (in minutes) designated on the x axis after exposure to light that bleaches 25% or more of the rhodopsin in each rod photoreceptor. The *solid curve* in each panel represents the normal dark-adaptation curve. The **top left graph** has the normal curve labeled with its components: the initial cone branch that ends at the rod-cone break and is followed by the cone branch. **Top left:** Dark-adaptation curves found in patients with the Nougaret or Rambusch forms of dominant stationary night blindness (similar forms of CSNB, represented by a *single dashed line*) and in a patient with the dominant rhodopsin mutation Ala292Glu causing stationary night blindness *(dotted line,* based on unpublished observations of E.L. Berson and M. Sandberg). **Top right:** Dark-adaptation curves from patients with complete *(dashed line)* or incomplete *(dotted line)* X-linked stationary night blindness. **Bottom:** Dark-adaptation curves characteristic of fundus albipunctatus *(dashed line)* and Oguchi disease *(dotted line)*. The rod-cone break in both fundus albipunctatus and Oguchi disease has been arbitrarily placed at the 2-hour time point; the actual time point depends on the degree of light exposure preceding the evaluation of dark adaptation. (From Dryja TP. Molecular genetics of Oguchi disease, fundus albipunctatus and other forms of stationary night blindness: LVII Edward Jackson Memorial Lecture. *Am J Ophthalmol* 2000;130:547–563, with permission.)

dark adaptation. Cideciyan et al. also demonstrated that recovery of the cone response after a bleaching stimulus was unexpectedly slower than the recovery of the rod response. In fact, following a weak bleaching stimulus, the rate of recovery of rod sensitivity was independent of *RDH5*. Finally, some families with fundus albipunctatus have no abnormalities in the *RDH5* gene, suggesting that there is some degree of genetic heterogeneity for fundus albipunctatus (116).

Oguchi Disease

This condition was first described by Oguchi (117) in 1907 as a cause of night vision loss. The majority of reported cases still originate in Japan. In 1995, this condition was found associated with mutations in the Arrestin gene and, shortly thereafter, with mutations in the rhodopsin kinase gene. It is commonly classified as a cause of CSNB with an abnormal fundus.

Clinical Features

Oguchi disease is characterized by the presence of a greenish metallic sheen in the fundus of a light-adapted patient. This sheen slowly fades with dark adaptation. After prolonged dark adaptation, the metallic sheen disappears completely but reappears following a few minutes of light adaptation; this is known as the Mizuo-Nakamura phenomenon. It has been hypothesized that excessive extracellular potassium in the retina due to overstimulation of rod photoreceptors plays a role in this clinical phenomenon (Fig. 7-10) (118). One group demonstrated by scanning laser ophthalmoscopy the formation and disappearance of fine dots in association with the Mizuo-Nakamura phenomenon and proposed these dots are related to the clinically observed metallic sheen and electroretinographic findings (119). The ERG shows the presence of abnormal rod-isolated responses and an electronegative waveform on electroretinographic testing. With prolonged dark adaptation of more than 4 hours, the electroretinographic responses normalize and dark adaptation resumes normal rod thresholds. However, following a single flash stimulus, prolonged dark adaptation is once again required for a normal electroretinographic response (Fig. 7-9) (35) and for patients to see in a dark environment (35). Visual function under mesopic conditions is essentially normal with vision ranging from 20/25 to 20/50 (120,121). Beyond the Mizuo-Nakamura phenomenon, the fundus appearance in Oguchi disease is otherwise unremarkable, with no evidence of bone spicules, macular changes, or chorioretinal atrophy. However, some patients with Arrestin mutations have family members with the symptoms and clinical signs of RP. Patients with Arrestin-related RP also exhibit the Mizuo-Nakamura phenomenon early in their disease (121).

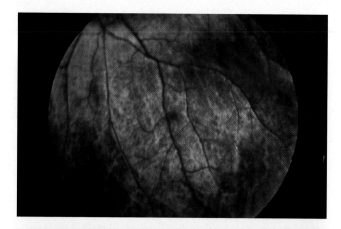

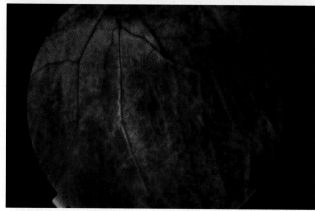

FIGURE 7-10. Mizuo phenomenon in Oguchi' disease. **Top:** Superior nasal view of the right eye in the state of light adaptation. **Bottom:** Same area of eye after 2 hours of dark adaptation. The choroidal vessels are more prominent and the retina has a more normal color. (From Bergsma DR Jr, Chen CJ. The Mizuo phenomenon in Oguchi disease. *Arch Ophthalmol* 1997;115:560–561, with permission.)

Molecular Genetics and Pathophysiology

Oguchi disease has been associated with mutations of the rhodopsin kinase gene or the Arrestin gene (35,122,123). No other retinal dystrophies have been associated with changes in the rhodopsin kinase gene. However, a mutation in Arrestin, specifically 1147delA, has also been associated with RP that manifests with decreased central vision, peripheral visual field constriction, midperipheral bone spicule pigmentation, and macular atrophy (124,125). The electrophysiologic and dark adaptation phenomena observed in Oguchi disease are directly related to the underlying molecular pathology of the disease. Rhodopsin activation occurs in the dark. Persistently activated rhodopsin (bleached rhodopsin) maintains rods in a desensitized state until all of the 11-*trans*-retinal, from previous light stimulation, is replaced with 11-*cis*-retinal. The inability to interrupt the phototransduction cascade due to defects in Arrestin or rhodopsin kinase permits a minimal amount of active rhodopsin to maintain rods desensitized. It takes approximately 2 or more hours to completely regenerate bleached rhodopsin molecules (126); thus, the patient experiences a prolonged dark adaptation.

Achromatopsia

Achromatopsia is a congenital inability to discriminate color. It is a rare condition estimated to have a prevalence of 3 in 100,000. However, the prevalence of achromatopsia on the island of Pingelap in Micronesia is 4% to 10% due to a sharp reduction in the population after a typhoon that struck in the late 1700s. All affected individuals trace their lineage back to 1 of about 20 survivors who was a carrier of the gene (127). Huddart first described in 1777 a patient with achromatopsia from a family with two affected brothers and three unaffected siblings (128). However, Daubeney is credited with the first overall description of achromatopsia in 1684 (128).

Achromatopsia is divided into two groups: complete achromatopsia (rod monochromacy) and incomplete achromatopsia (blue cone monochromacy). Complete achromatopsia is autosomal recessive and results in loss of all cone function, whereas incomplete achromatopsia is X-linked recessive and results in loss of red and green opsins only.

Clinical Characteristics

Both complete and incomplete achromatopsia are marked by poor color discrimination from birth, photosensitivity or photoaversion, decreased vision, and relative clinical stability. Nystagmus occurs in both forms of achromatopsia. However, by the time a patient presents for evaluation in late childhood or early adulthood, nystagmus may be barely noticeable. Patients with either form of achromatopsia tend to be myopic, sometimes with oblique astigmatism (3).

The two forms of achromatopsia are distinguished by the apparent inheritance pattern, although patients with incomplete achromatopsia can have better visual acuity [as good as 20/50 (3,91)], some color discrimination on certain clinical tests (129), such as the Sloan achromatopsia test (3), and macular changes with progression late in the course of the disease. In contrast, patients with complete achromatopsia tend to have visual acuity of 20/200 or worse.

Fundus findings in achromatopsia are relatively normal, with a reduced foveal light reflex in some cases. Some report macular atrophy in both forms of achromatopsia late in the course of the disease (91). Nathans et al. (130) have documented progression of disease in incomplete achromatopsia with macular atrophy. Nevertheless, both conditions have remarkably normal-appearing retinas and vessels. Electrophysiologic testing demonstrates loss of cone responses in the presence of essentially normal rod responses. In incomplete achromatopsia, minimal residual cone function can be detected with specialized testing, but under standard electroretinographic testing, cone function typically is nonrecordable (Fig. 7-11).

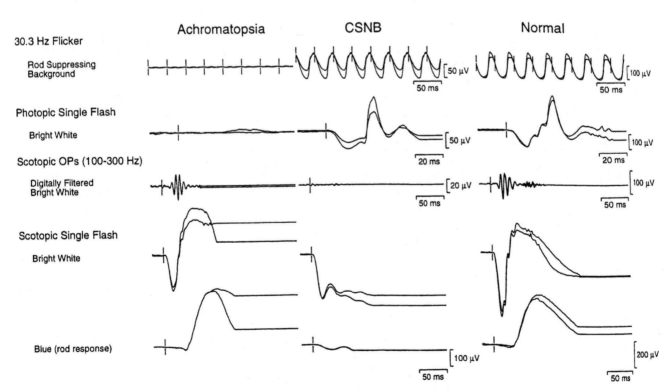

FIGURE 7-11. Full-field electroretinogram (ERG) of achromatopsia and enhanced S-cone syndrome. ERGs of a 12-year-old girl with congenital achromatopsia, a 4-year-old patient with autosomal recessive complete congenital stationary night blindness, and a normal for comparison. (From Weleber RG. Infantile and childhood retinal blindness: a molecular perspective [The Franceschetti Lecture]. *Ophthalmic Genet* 2002;23:71–97, with permission.)

The differential diagnosis for a child with decreased vision and nystagmus includes LCA, achromatopsia, CSNB, choroidal coloboma, peroxisomal disorders, optic nerve hypoplasia, and central nervous system causes. Electroretinographic characteristics and a patient's presenting symptoms are useful in differentiating among conditions. A study by Lambert and others documented the misdiagnosis of LCA in 40% of patients (98). The most common misdiagnoses were CSNB, Joubert syndrome (retinal dystrophy with hypoplasia of the cerebellar vermis), RP, and achromatopsia. Other conditions that have been misdiagnosed as LCA include infantile Refsum disease, Zellweger syndrome, Senior-Loken syndrome (nephrophthisis and retinal dystrophy), cone-rod dystrophy, and Alstrom syndrome (97,98).

Molecular Genetics of Achromatopsia

Complete achromatopsia (rod monochromacy) is an autosomal recessive condition caused by defects in the cone photoreceptor cGMP-gated cation channel. The channel complex is composed of two α subunits and two β subunits. Mutations in the genes that code for each subunit have been implicated in the pathogenesis of rod monochromacy. The gene for the α subunit *(CNGA3)* was the first gene identified and is located on chromosome 2q11 (131,132). Complete achromatopsia caused by changes in the *CNGA3* gene is called complete achromatopsia type 2 and accounts for up to 25% of all patients with complete achromatopsia. The β subunit is coded for by the gene *CNGB3* and is believed to cause 40% to 50% of complete achromatopsia (131). *CNGB3* is found on chromosome 8q21 and is called achromatopsia type 3. The inhabitants of the island of Pingelap carry a serine to phenylalanine missense change (Ser322Phe) that results in their disease (127). The final gene implicated in complete achromatopsia is *GNAT2* located on chromosome 1p13. *GNAT2* codes for the transducin α subunit in cone photoreceptors. *(GNAT1* codes for the α subunit of transducin in rods.) Kohl identified five families with complete achromatopsia caused by homozygous changes in *GNAT2* (91,133).

Incomplete achromatopsia (blue cone monochromacy) is caused by loss of the medium- (green) and long- (red) wavelength cone opsins encoded by genes that are found together on the X chromosome. Three mechanisms have been identified as causing incomplete achromatopsia. First, a locus control region (LCR) was identified 4.02 kb upstream from the start of the red opsin gene and more than 42 kb upstream from the start of the green opsin gene. The LCR region is responsible for unwinding the DNA prior to transcription regulated by the separate promoters of each respective opsin gene. A 579-bp deletion in the LCR has been identified in 18.2% of patients with incomplete achromatopsia studied; this mutation prevents transcription of either the red or green opsin (130). The second mechanism is related to unequal recombination of a red opsin gene with a mutant green opsin gene resulting in nonfunctional proteins. The final mechanism resulted from deletion of the green opsin gene with a missense mutation in the remaining red opsin gene (134). In incomplete achromatopsia, a region up to 4,000 bp upstream from the 5′ initiation site of the red opsin gene could have a potential effect on the transcription and subsequent translation of a gene.

Enhanced S-Cone Syndrome/Goldmann-Favre Disease

The enhanced S-cone syndrome (ESCS) was first described by Marmor et al. (135) based on specific electrophysiologic findings. Patients with ESCS presented with nyctalopia at an early age, cystoid changes in the macula, and an annular pigmentary retinopathy involving the region around and just outside the temporal vascular arcades. Visual acuity could be as good as 20/20, but with the onset of cystoid changes of the macula it could be as severe as 20/200. Color vision generally is unaffected, and the ERG shows a characteristic appearance. Rod-isolated responses are nonrecordable. However, the maximum combined response and photopic responses closely mirror each other in amplitude and waveform morphology. Spectral testing of the cones under photopic conditions demonstrate decreased function of long- (L; red) and medium- (M; green) wavelength sensitive cones and enhancement of short- (S; blue) wavelength sensitive cones (Fig. 7–11) (135). Several patients with Goldmann-Favre syndrome also had these electroretinographic characteristics. The gene for ESCS was identified as the *NR2E3* gene in 2000 (136). This gene codes for a retinal orphan nuclear receptor, a transcription factor that plays a role in determining cone photoreceptor phenotype in embryogenesis. Without this receptor, cones remain as S cones without differentiating into L/M cones. However, some cones are still able to differentiate despite the loss of *NR2E3* gene product, which accounts for the normal color vision and relatively good visual acuity that can be exhibited by these patients. *NR2E3* also is associated with a retinal degeneration described in Crypto-Jews from Portugal (137). These individuals demonstrate nyctalopia and constricted visual fields with a phenotype resembling ESCS and Goldman-Favre syndrome. Unfortunately, these patients were not studied with spectral ERGs to determine whether they also had ESCS (91).

Leber Congenital Amaurosis

LCA was first described by Theodore Leber in 1869 as an autosomal recessive condition that presented before age 1 year with severely affected vision, nystagmus, and poor pupillary reactions. Franceshetti subsequently showed that a markedly reduced or nonrecordable ERG was associated with these patients. The scope of this condition included any cause of infantile blindness with a reduced ERG and encompassed several recognized syndromic causes of retinal degeneration. In 1985 Foxman proposed subdividing patients into four groups based on their onset and associated systemic findings. Group 1 was considered uncomplicated LCA with ophthalmic findings but no systemic disease. Group 2 included patients with retinal disease and systemic findings such as Senior-Loken syndrome or cerebrohepatorenal syndrome of Zellweger. Groups 3 and 4 consisted of children with initially normal vision but with very early onset of symptoms consistent with RP (138). Later, studies focused on Group 1, using criteria for the diagnosis of LCA that included a markedly abnormal ERG, severe visual deficit since infancy, and, most importantly, the absence of another specific retinal or multisystem disorder (98). In this chapter, LCA will be considered synonymous with "uncomplicated LCA" and refers only to patients without other retinal or systemic disease.

Today, LCA is recognized as a heterogeneous group of disorders that together are estimated to account for approximately 5% of all retinal dystrophies and approximately 10% to 18% of all cases of congenital blindness (146).

To date, seven genes have been implicated in the pathophysiology of LCA and together account for almost 40% of patients presenting with this condition (Table 7-5). Identification of these genes may potentially lead to therapeutic interventions for this cause of childhood blindness in the near future.

Clinical Presentation and Disease Course

Patients present in the first year of life with visual inattention and sensory nystagmus. One study noted that parents observed visual inattention by 3 to 6 months of age. When examined, the infants frequently did not fixate to bright light (138). Clinical findings can be highly variable, from a normal-appearing fundus to macular changes such as colobomas or chorioretinal atrophy. Bull's-eye macular changes have also been reported in *TULP1*-related LCA (139). Peripheral findings vary from bone spicule pigmentation recognized as early as 9 months of age to diffuse fine

white dots at the level of the RPE (98). Some patients demonstrate paradoxical pupillary responses to light (Flynn pupils) and may exhibit an oculodigital response or vigorous eye rubbing in visually impaired children (140). Other associated clinical findings include keratoconus, high hyperopia and myopia, and cataracts (138).

Children with LCA may present with a wide range of visual acuity measurements once they are old enough to have accurate measurements made. Visual acuity may range from 20/200 to NLP. Fulton et al. (141) evaluated visual function in patients with LCA and was able to document stability of vision in the majority of patients (71%), with smaller fractions both improving and worsening over follow-up. Median visual acuity for the group was noted to be equivalent to 20/500 and one third of patients were designated no light perception (NLP). Children with LCA caused by mutations in the *RPE65* gene have demonstrated relatively better visual function and even minimal visual recovery with age (142). In one series of patients, a child with LCA due to *RPE65* had vision documented as good as 20/50 (143). Patients with *GUCY2D-* and *CRX*-related LCA, however, tend to have more severe visual impairment (142–145).

Because of the overlap with other conditions that can cause decreased vision early in life and the associated nystagmus, clinical testing with electrophysiology is indicated and demonstrates a markedly reduced or nonrecordable ERG for all test settings.

Differential Diagnosis

When considering a visually inattentive infant with sensory nystagmus, the differential diagnosis includes conditions causing both nystagmus and visual dysfunction. It is most important not to overlook conditions for which further systemic care by other services may be necessary. Furthermore, some conditions that may mimic LCA may carry significant mortality for the infant, and the correct diagnosis would allow parents to receive appropriate genetic counseling prior to having more children. One study documented misdiagnosis of LCA in 40% of patients (98). The most common

TABLE 7–5. ASSOCIATED GENES IDENTIFIED IN LEBER CONGENITAL AMAUROSIS

LCA Type	Gene	Chromosome	Protein
LCA 1	*RetGC1* (*GUCY2D*)	17 (17p13)	Photoreceptor-specific guanylate cyclase
LCA2	*RPE65*	1(1p31)	RPE65
CRX	*CRX*	19 (19q13.3)	Transcription factor
LCA 4	*AIPL1*	17 (17p13.1)	Arylhydrocarbon-interacting protein-like 1
LCA 6	*RPGRIP1*	14q11	Retinitis pigmentosa GTPase regular interacting protein
RP12	*CRB1*	1q31–q32.1	CRB1
RP14	*TULP1*	6p21.3	Tubby-like protein 1

misdiagnoses were CSNB, Joubert syndrome (retinal dystrophy with hypoplasia of the cerebellar vermis), RP, and achromatopsia. Other conditions that have been misdiagnosed as LCA include infantile Refsum disease, Zellweger syndrome, Senior-Loken syndrome (nephrophthisis and retinal dystrophy), cone-rod degeneration, and Alstrom syndrome (98). Late infantile and infantile neuronal ceroid lipofuscinosis may also present with visual inattention and nystagmus (101). In many of these situations, associated systemic findings, such as seizures, failure to thrive, and other neurologic or systemic signs, will lead the diagnosis away from LCA, but the potential exists for the ophthalmologist to be the primary point of contact. Imaging studies, metabolic/ biochemical studies, and a pediatric evaluation are indicated in these cases (97). Finally, distinguishing between LCA and early-onset RP may be more of a semantic issue at this time. However, very-early-onset RP will frequently lack searching nystagmus, a slightly older age of onset, and better central vision (138,146). The ERG in LCA patients shows an essentially nonrecordable study for all stimuli, whereas there may be relative sparing of the photopic component early in RP. Fazzi et al. suggest that the visual impairment in LCA is more stable compared to RP, which manifests as a more progressive pathology. However, some of the genes implicated in LCA (e.g., *RPE65, CRX, TULP1*) may also be a cause of RP. Finally, the inheritance pattern in LCA is almost exclusively autosomal recessive, whereas RP has varied forms of transmission (161).

Molecular Genetics of Leber Congenital Amaurosis

Although there is a wide range of clinical appearances and severity, it is easy to recognize the consequent genetic heterogeneity shown by this condition (Table 7-5). The first gene identified to be associated with LCA was the retinal-specific guanylate cyclase gene *(GUCY2D)* in 1996 (147). This was subsequently followed by *RPE65,* a gene expressed in the RPE and involved in retinoid metabolism (148). Other genes later identified include *CRX* (149), *TULP1* in one Dominican family (150), *AIPL1* (151), and *CRB1* (152). Together, these six genes were believed to account for 25% to 35% of all cases of LCA. Most recently, the *RPGRIP* gene was identified in families with LCA and believed by two separate groups to account for another 5% to 6% of families with LCA (153).

These genes represent a wide range of function, and many are associated with later-onset retinal dystrophies. *TULP1* is considered by some to represent early-onset RP rather than LCA (139,146,154). *CRX* (8,22) and *GUCY2D* (155) are both associated with autosomal dominant cone-rod dystrophies, whereas *CRB1* is the cause for RP12 with the particular phenotype of preservation of periarteriolar RPE (152,156). *RPE65* also is associated with later-onset retinal dystrophies (157). Recent studies conducted in

RPE65-null mice (a model of LCA) showed that activation of sensory transduction by unliganded opsin, and not the accumulation of retinyl esters, causes light-independent retinal degeneration in LCA. This study clearly identified opsin activity as a mechanism of retinal degeneration in human LCA resulting from mutations in *RPE65* (162).

Although LCA is classically believed to be autosomal recessive, many patients appear to be heterozygous for changes in their specific genes. Lotery described four possible explanations for the presence of these heterozygous changes (143). These changes may represent a dominant disease-causing allele; it may be the only detectable member of a pair of recessive disease causing alleles; it may be part of a pair of genes involved in causing digenic disease; and the change may not be associated with disease at all and represent only a nondisease-causing polymorphism (143). Among these explanations, *CRX* has been shown to be associated with a high degree of sporadic sequence mutations, and some authors suggest that these changes may cause disease in the heterozygous state (158,159). The *de novo* nature of these mutations results in the clinical appearance of autosomal recessive inheritance but may have further implications regarding potential inheritance of disease caused by *CRX* (159). However, one family demonstrated a null mutation for *CRX,* where the gene is completely not expressed, that was present in a normal-sighted father and an affected daughter. The absence of disease in the father argues strongly against the ability of this gene to cause disease in the heterozygous state (160).

REFERENCES

1. Acland GM, et al. Gene therapy restores vision in a canine model of childhood blindness. *Nat Genet* 2001;28:92–95.
2. Tanino T, Ohba N. Studies on pigmentary retinal dystrophy. I. Age of onset of subjective symptoms and mode of inheritance. *Jpn J Ophthalmol* 1976;20:474–481.
3. Carr RE. Abnormalities of cone and rod function. In: Ogden TE, Hinton DR, eds. *Retina.* St. Louis: Mosby, 2001:471–481.
4. Souied E, et al. Retinitis punctata albescens associated with the Arg135Try mutation in the rhodopsin gene. *Am J Ophthalmol* 1996;121:19–25.
5. Burstedt MS, et al. Bothnia dystrophy caused by mutations in the cellular retinaldehyde-binding protein gene (RLBP1) on chromosome 15q26. *Invest Ophthalmol Vis Sci* 1999;40:995–1000.
6. Burstedt MS, et al. Ocular phenotype of bothnia dystrophy, an autosomal recessive retinitis pigmentosa associated with an R234W mutation in the RLBP1 gene. *Arch Ophthalmol* 2001;119:260–267.
7. Heckenlively JR. The frequency of posterior subcapsular cataract in hereditary retinal degenerations. *Am J Ophthalmol* 1982;93:733–798.
8. Berson EL, Rosner B, Simonoff E. Risk factors for genetic typing and detection in retinitis pigmentosa. *Am J Ophthalmol* 1980. 89:763–775.
9. Sohocki MM, et al. Prevalence of mutations causing retinitis pigmentosa and other inherited retinopathies. *Hum Mutat* 2001;17:42–51.

10. Wang Q, et al. Update on the molecular genetics of retinitis pigmentosa. *Ophthalmic Genet* 2001;22:133–54.

11. Bessant DA, et al. A mutation in NRL is associated with autosomal dominant retinitis pigmentosa. *Nat Genet* 1999;21:355–356.

12. Wada Y, et al. Mutation of human retinal fascin gene (FSCN2) causes autosomal dominant retinitis pigmentosa. *Invest Ophthalmol Vis Sci* 2001;42:2395–2400.

13. Vithana EN, et al. A human homolog of yeast pre-mRNA splicing gene, PRP31, underlies autosomal dominant retinitis pigmentosa on chromosome 19q13.4 (RP11). *Mol Cell* 2001;8:375–381.

14. Martinez-Gimeno M, et al. Mutations in the pre-mRNA splicing-factor genes PRPF3, PRPF8, and PRPF31 in Spanish families with autosomal dominant retinitis pigmentosa. *Invest Ophthalmol Vis Sci* 2003;44:2171–2177.

15. Deery EC, et al. Disease mechanism for retinitis pigmentosa (RP11) caused by mutations in the splicing factor gene PRPF31. *Hum Mol Genet* 2002;11:3209–3219.

16. McKie AB, et al. Mutations in the pre-mRNA splicing factor gene PRPC8 in autosomal dominant retinitis pigmentosa (RP13). *Hum Mol Genet* 2001;10:1555–1562.

17. Kondo H, et al. Diagnosis of autosomal dominant retinitis pigmentosa by linkage-based exclusion screening with multiple locus-specific microsatellite markers. *Invest Ophthalmol Vis Sci* 2003;44:1275–1281.

18. van Lith-Verhoeven JJ, et al. Clinical characterization, linkage analysis, and PRPC8 mutation analysis of a family with autosomal dominant retinitis pigmentosa type 13 (RP13). *Ophthalmic Genet* 2002;23:1–12.

19. Chakarova CF, et al. Mutations in HPRP3, a third member of pre-mRNA splicing factor genes, implicated in autosomal dominant retinitis pigmentosa. *Hum Mol Genet* 2002;11:87–92.

20. Wada Y, et al. Frequency and spectrum of IMPDH1 mutations associated with autosomal dominant retinitis pigmentosa. *Invest Ophthalmol Vis Sci Abstract CD ROM Supplement* 2003:2307.

21. Miano MG, et al. Identification of novel RP2 mutations in a subset of X-linked retinitis pigmentosa families and prediction of new domains. *Hum Mutat* 2001;18:109–119.

22. Bader I, et al. X-linked retinitis pigmentosa: RPGR mutations in most families with definite X linkage and clustering of mutations in a short sequence stretch of exon ORF15. *Invest Ophthalmol Vis Sci* 2003;44:1458–1463.

23. Maw MA, et al. Mutation of the gene encoding cellular retinaldehyde-binding protein in autosomal recessive retinitis pigmentosa. *Nat Genet* 1997;17:198–200.

24. Morimura H, Berson EL, Dryja TP. Recessive mutations in the RLBP1 gene encoding cellular retinaldehyde-binding protein in a form of retinitis punctata albescens. *Invest Ophthalmol Vis Sci* 1999;40:1000–1004.

25. Simunovic MP, Moore AT. The cone dystrophies. *Eye* 1998; 12[Pt 3b]:553–565.

26. Downes SM, et al. Autosomal dominant cone and cone-rod dystrophy with mutations in the guanylate cyclase activator 1A gene-encoding guanylate cyclase activating protein-1. *Arch Ophthalmol* 2001;119:96–105.

27. Yang Z, et al. Mutations in the RPGR gene cause X-linked cone dystrophy. *Hum Mol Genet* 2002;11:605–611.

28. Sohocki MM, et al. A range of clinical phenotypes associated with mutations in CRX, a photoreceptor transcription-factor gene. *Am J Hum Genet* 1998;63:1307–1315.

29. Lois N, et al. Phenotypic subtypes of Stargardt macular dystrophy-fundus flavimaculatus. *Arch Ophthalmol* 2001;119: 359–369.

30. Paloma E, et al. Analysis of ABCA4 in mixed Spanish families segregating different retinal dystrophies. *Hum Mutat* 2002; 20:476.

31. Birch DG, et al. Visual function in patients with cone-rod dystrophy (CRD) associated with mutations in the ABCA4 (ABCR) gene. *Exp Eye Res* 2001;73:877–886.

32. Briggs CE, et al. Mutations in ABCR (ABCA4) in patients with Stargardt macular degeneration or cone-rod degeneration. *Invest Ophthalmol Vis Sci* 2001;42:2229–2236.

33. Yagasaki K, Jacobson SG. Cone-rod dystrophy. Phenotypic diversity by retinal function testing. *Arch Ophthalmol* 1989;107: 701–708.

34. Itabashi R, et al. Stargardt's disease/fundus flavimaculatus: psychophysical and electrophysiologic results. *Graefes Arch Clin Exp Ophthalmol* 1993;231:555–562.

35. Dryja TP. Molecular genetics of Oguchi disease, fundus albipunctatus and other forms of stationary night blindness: LVII Edward Jackson Memorial Lecture. *Am J Ophthalmol* 2000;130: 547–563.

36. Jbour AK, et al. Hypogonadotrophic hypogonadism, short stature, cerebellar ataxia, rod-cone retinal dystrophy, and hypersegmented neutrophils: a novel disorder or a new variant of Boucher-Neuhauser syndrome? *J Med Genet* 2003;40:e2.

37. Kipioti A, et al. Cone-rod dystrophy in thiamine-responsive megaloblastic anemia. *J Pediatr Ophthalmol Strabismus* 2003; 40:105–107.

38. Meire FM, et al. Thiamine-responsive megaloblastic anemia syndrome (TRMA) with cone-rod dystrophy. *Ophthalmic Genet* 2000;21:243–250.

39. Guirgis MF, et al. Cone-rod retinal dystrophy and Duane retraction syndrome in a patient with achondroplasia. *J AAPOS* 2002;6:400–401.

40. Hearn T, et al. Mutation of ALMS1, a large gene with a tandem repeat encoding 47 amino acids, causes Alstrom syndrome. *Nat Genet* 2002;31:79–83.

41. Porto FB, et al. Isolated late-onset cone-rod dystrophy revealing a familial neurogenic muscle weakness, ataxia, and retinitis pigmentosa syndrome with the T8993G mitochondrial mutation. *Am J Ophthalmol* 2001;132:935–937.

42. Fishman GA, et al. Serine-27-phenylalanine mutation within the peripherin/RDS gene in a family with cone dystrophy. *Ophthalmology* 1997;104:299–306.

43. Johnson S, et al. Genomic organisation and alternative splicing of human RIM1, a gene implicated in autosomal dominant cone-rod dystrophy (CORD7). *Genomics* 2003;81: 304–314.

44. Udar N, et al. Identification of GUCY2D gene mutations in CORD5 families and evidence of incomplete penetrance. *Hum Mutat* 2003;21:170–171.

45. Maugeri A, et al. Mutations in the ABCA4 (ABCR) gene are the major cause of autosomal recessive cone-rod dystrophy. *Am J Hum Genet* 2000;67:960–966.

46. Aligianis IA, et al. Mapping of a novel locus for achromatopsia (ACHM4) to 1p and identification of a germline mutation in the alpha subunit of cone transducin (GNAT2). *J Med Genet* 2002;39:656–660.

47. Wissinger B, et al. CNGA3 mutations in hereditary cone photoreceptor disorders. *Am J Hum Genet* 2001;69:722–737.

48. Klevering BJ, et al. Phenotypic spectrum of autosomal recessive cone-rod dystrophies caused by mutations in the ABCA4 (ABCR) gene. *Invest Ophthalmol Vis Sci* 2002;43:1980–1985.

49. Klevering BJ, et al. Phenotypic variations in a family with retinal dystrophy as result of different mutations in the ABCR gene. *Br J Ophthalmol* 1999;83:914–918.

50. Demirci FY, et al. X-linked cone-rod dystrophy (locus COD1): identification of mutations in RPGR exon ORF15. *Am J Hum Genet* 2002;70:1049–1053.

51. Ayyagari R, et al. X-linked recessive atrophic macular degeneration from RPGR mutation. *Genomics* 2002;80:166–171.

52. Karna J, Choroideremia. A clinical and genetic study of 84 Finnish patients and 126 female carriers. *Acta Ophthalmol Suppl* 1986;176:1–68.

53. Roberts MF, et al. Retrospective, longitudinal, and cross sectional study of visual acuity impairment in choroideraemia. *Br J Ophthalmol* 2002;86:658–662.

54. Schwartz H, et al. Identification of mutations in Danish choroideremia families. *Hum Mutat* 1993;2:43–47.

55. Seabra MC, et al. Purification of component A of Rab geranylgeranyl transferase: possible identity with the choroideremia gene product. *Cell* 1992;70:1049–1057.

56. Seabra MC, Brown MS, Goldstein JL. Retinal degeneration in choroideremia: deficiency of Rab geranylgeranyl transferase. *Science* 1993;259:377–381.

57. van Bokhoven H, et al. Mutation spectrum in the CHM gene of Danish and Swedish choroideremia patients. *Hum Mol Genet* 1994;3:1047–1051.

58. van Bokhoven H, et al. Mapping of the choroideremia-like (CHML) gene at 1q42-qter and mutation analysis in patients with Usher syndrome type II. *Genomics* 1994;19:385–387.

59. Sankila E-M, et al. Aberrant splicing of the CHM gene is a significant cause of choroideremia. *Nat Genet* 1992;1:109–113.

60. Seabra MC. New insights into the pathogenesis of choroideremia: a tale of two REPs. *Ophthalmic Genet* 1996;17:43–46.

61. Donnelly P, et al. Missense mutation in the choroideremia gene. *Hum Mol Genet* 1994;3:1017.

62. McTaggart KE, et al. Mutational analysis of patients with the diagnosis of choroideremia. *Hum Mutat* 2002;20:189–196.

63. Syed N, et al. Evaluation of retinal photoreceptors and pigment epithelium in a female carrier of choroideremia. *Ophthalmology* 2001;108:711–720.

64. Park DW, et al. Best's disease: molecular and clinical findings. In: Guyer DR, et al., eds. *Retina-vitreous-macula.* Philadelphia: WB Saunders, 1999;989–1005.

65. Blodi CF, Stone EM. Best's vitelliform dystrophy. *Ophthalmic Paediatr Genet* 1990;11:49–59.

66. Mohler CW, Fine SL. Long-term evaluation of patients with Best's vitelliform dystrophy. *Ophthalmology* 1981;101: 1409–1421.

67. Sorr EM, Goldberg RE. Vitelliform dystrophy in a 64 year old man. *Am J Ophthalmol* 1976;82:256–258.

68. Miller SA, Bresnick GH, Chandra SR. Choroidal neovascular membrane in Best's vitelliform macular dystrophy. *Am J Ophthalmol* 1976;82:252–255.

69. Chung M, et al. Visual outcome following subretinal hemorrhage in Best's disease. *Retina* 2001;21:575–580.

70. Fishman GA, et al. Visual acuity in patients with Best vitelliform macular dystrophy. *Ophthalmology* 1993;100: 1665–1670.

71. Nichols BE, et al. Refining the locus for Best vitelliform macular dystrophy and mutation analysis of the candidate gene ROM1. *Am J Hum Genet* 1994;54:95–103.

72. Stone EM, et al. Genetic linkage of vitelliform macular degeneration (Best's disease) to chromosome 11q13. *Nat Genet* 1992;1:246–250.

73. Marquardt A, et al. Mutations in a novel gene, VMD2, encoding a protein of unknown properties cause juvenile-onset vitelliform macular dystrophy (Best's disease). *Hum Mol Genet* 1998;7:1517–25.

74. Marmostein AD, et al. Bestrophin, the product of the Best vitelliform macular dystrophy gene (VMD2) localizes to the basolateral plasma membrane of the retinal pigment epithelium. *Proc Natl Acad Sci USA* 2000;97:12758–12563.

75. Sun H, et al. The vitelliform macular dystrophy protein defines a new family of chloride channels. *Proc Natl Acad Sci USA* 2002;99:4008–4013.

76. Gomez A, et al. The gene causing the Best's macular dystrophy (BMD) encodes a putative ion exchanger. *DNA Seq* 2001;12: 431–435.

77. Marmorstein LY, et al. Bestrophin interacts physically and functionally with protein phosphatase 2A. *J Biol Chem* 2002;277: 30591–30597.

78. Lotery AJ, et al. Allelic variation in the VMD2 gene in best disease and age-related macular degeneration. *Invest Ophthalmol Vis Sci* 2000;41:1291–1296.

79. Lefler WH, Wadsworth JAC, Sidbury JB. Hereditary macular degeneration and aminoaciduria. *Am J Ophthalmol* 1971;71: 224–230.

80. Hermsen VM, Judisch GF. Central areolar pigment epithelial dystrophy. *Ophthalmologica* 1984;189:69–72.

81. Small KW. North Carolina macular dystrophy. In: Traboulsi E, ed. *Genetic diseases of the eye.* New York: Oxford University Press, 1998:367–371.

82. Rohrschneider K, et al. Macular function testing in a German pedigree with North Carolina macular dystrophy. *Retina* 1998;18:453–459.

83. Small KW, et al. North Carolina macular dystrophy is assigned to chromosome 6. *Genomics* 1992;13:681–685.

84. Small KW, et al. North Carolina macular dystrophy and central areolar pigment epithelial dystrophy. *Arch Ophthalmol* 1992; 110:515–518.

85. Small KW, et al. Genetic analysis of additional families with North Carolina macular dystrophy (MCDR1). *Am J Hum Genet* 1993;53:1079.

86. Small KW, et al. North Carolina macular dystrophy (MCDR1). A review and refined mapping to 6q14–q16.2. *Ophthalmic Paediatr Genet* 1993;14:143–150.

87. Small KW, et al. North Carolina macular dystrophy (MCDR1) in Texas. *Retina* 1998;18:448–452.

88. Dryja TP, et al. Missense mutation in the gene encoding the alpha subunit of rod transducin in the Nougaret form of congenital stationary night blindness. *Nat Genet* 1996;13:358–365.

89. Price MJ, Judisch GF, Thompson HS. X-linked congenital stationary nightblindness with myopia and nystagmus without clinical complaints of nyctalopia. *J Pediatr Ophthalmol Strabismus* 1988;25:33–36.

90. Heckenlively JR. Congenital stationary night blindness. In: Traboulsi EI, ed. *Genetic diseases of the eye.* New York : Oxford University Press, 1998:389–396.

91. Weleber RG. Infantile and childhood retinal blindness: a molecular perspective (The Franceschetti Lecture). *Ophthalmic Genet* 2002;23:71–97.

92. Bech-Hansen NT, Moore BJ, Pearce WG. Mapping of locus for X-linked congenital stationary night blindness (CSNB1) proximal to DXS7. *Genomics* 1992;12:409–411.

93. Bech-Hansen NT, Pearce WG. Manifestations of X-linked congenital stationary night blindness in three daughters of an affected male: demonstration of homozygosity. *Am J Hum Genet* 1993;52:71–77.

94. Bech-Hansen NT, et al. Loss-of-function mutations in a calcium-channel alpha1-subunit gene in Xp11.23 cause incomplete X-linked congenital stationary night blindness. *Nat Genet* 1998;19:264–267.

95. Auerbach E, Godel V, Rowe H. An electrophysiologic and psychophysical study of two forms of congenital stationary night blindness. *Invest Ophthalmol Vis Sci* 1969;8:332–345.

96. Miyake Y, et al. Congenital stationary night blindness with negative electroretinogram. A new classification. Arch Ophthalmol 1986;104:1013–1020.

97. Lambert SR, Taylor D, Kriss A. The infant with nystagmus, normal appearing fundi, but an abnormal ERG. *Surv Ophthalmol* 1989;34:173–186.

98. Lambert SR, et al. Follow-up and diagnostic reappraisal of 75 patients with Leber's congenital amaurosis. *Am J Ophthalmol* 1989;107:624–631.

99. Cibis GW, Fitzgerald KM. The negative ERG is not synonymous with nightblindness. *Trans Am Ophthalmol Soc* 2001;99: 171–175, discussion 175–176.

100. Bech-Hansen NT, et al. Loss of function mutations in a calcium channel alpha 1 subunit gene in Xp11.23 cause incomplete X-linked congenital stationary night blindness. *Nat Genet* 1998; 19:264–267.

101. Weleber RG. Neuronal ceroid lipofuscinosis. *Eye* 1998;12: 580–590.

102. Bech-Hansen NT, et al. Mutations in NYX, encoding the leucine-rich proteoglycan nyctalopin, cause X-linked complete congenital stationary night blindness. *Nat Genet* 2000;26: 319–323.

103. Dryja TP, et al. Heterozygous missense mutation in the rhodopsin gene as a cause of congenital stationary night blindness. *Nat Genet* 1993;4:280–283.

104. Sieving PA, et al. Dominant congenital complete nyctalopia and Gly90Asp rhodopsin mutation. *Invest Ophthalmol Vis Sci* 1992;33[Suppl]:1397.

105. Gross AK, Rao VR, Oprian DD. Characterization of rhodopsin congenital night blindness mutant T94I. *Biochemistry* 2003;42: 2009–2015.

106. Gal A, et al. Heterozygous missense mutation in the rod cGMP phosphodiesterase subunit gene in autosomal dominant congenital stationary night blindness. *Nat Genet* 1994;7:64–68.

107. Rosenberg T, et al. Autosomal dominant stationary night-blindness: a large family rediscovered. *Acta Ophthalmol Scand* 1991;69:694–702.

108. Lauber H. Die sogenannte Retinitis punctata albescens. *Klin Monatsbl Augenheilkd* 1910;48:133–148.

109. Miyake Y, et al. Fundus albipunctatus associated with cone dystrophy. *Br J Ophthalmol* 1992;76:375–379.

110. Hirose E, et al. Mutations in the 11-cis retinol dehydrogenase gene in Japanese patients with fundus albipunctatus. *Invest Ophthalmol Vis Sci* 2000;41:3933–3935.

111. Nakamura M, Miyake Y. Macular dystrophy in a 9-year-old boy with fundus albipunctatus. *Am J Ophthalmol* 2002;133:278–280.

112. Nakamura M, et al. A high association with cone dystrophy in Fundus albipunctatus caused by mutations of the RDH5 gene. *Invest Ophthalmol Vis Sci* 2000;41:3925–3932.

113. Yamamoto H, et al. Mutations in the gene encoding 11-cis-retinol dehydrogenase cause delayed dark adaptation and fundus albipunctatus. *Nat Genet* 1999;22:188–191.

114. Driessen CA, et al. Disruption of the 11-cis-retinol dehydrogenase gene leads to accumulation of cis-retinols and cis-retinyl esters. *Mol Cell Biol* 2000;20:4275–4287.

115. Cideciyan AV, et al. Rod and cone visual cycle consequences of a null mutation in the 11-cis-retinol dehydrogenase gene in man. *Vis Neurosci* 2000;17:667–678.

116. Hirose E, et al. Mutations in the 11-cis retinol dehydrogenase gene in Japanese patients with Fundus albipunctatus. *Invest Ophthalmol Vis Sci* 2000;41:3933–3935.

117. Oguchi C. Uber eine Abart von Hemeralopie. *Acta Soc Ophthalmol Jpn* 1907;11:123–134.

118. de Jong PTVM, et al. Mizuo phenomenon in X-linked retinoschisis. *Arch Ophthalmol* 1991;109:1104–1108.

119. Usui T, et al. Mizuo phenomenon observed by scanning laser ophthalmoscopy in a patient with Oguchi disease. *Am J Ophthalmol* 2000;130:359–361.

120. Krill AE. Congenital stationary night blindness. In: Krill AE, ed. *Krill's hereditary retinal and choroidal diseases.* Hagerstown, MD: Harper & Row Publishers, 1977:391–420.

121. Yoshii M, et al. Visual function and gene analysis in a family with Oguchi's disease. *Ophthalmic Res* 1998;30:394–401.

122. Fuchs S, et al. A homozygous 1 base pair deletion in the arrestin gene is a frequent cause of Oguchi disease in Japanese. *Nat Genet* 1995;10:360–362.

123. Yamamoto S, et al. Defects in the rhodopsin kinase gene in the Oguchi form of stationary night blindness. *Nat Genet* 1997;15:175–178.

124. Nakazawa M, Wada Y, Tamai M, Arrestin gene mutations in autosomal recessive retinitis pigmentosa. *Arch Ophthalmol* 1998;116:498–501.

125. Nakazawa M, et al. Oguchi disease: phenotypic characteristics of patients with frequent 1147delA mutation in the arrestin gene. *Retina* 1997;17:17–22.

126. Cideciyan AV, et al. Null mutation in the rhodopsin kinase gene slows recovery kinetics of rod and cone phototransduction in man. *Proc Natl Acad Sci USA* 1998;95:328–333.

127. Sundin OH, et al. Genetic basis of total colour blindness among the Pingelapese islanders. *Nat Genet* 2000;25:289–293.

128. Traboulsi E. Cone dystrophies. In: Traboulsi E, ed. *Genetic diseases of the eye.* New York: Oxford University Press, 1998: 357–365.

129. Berson EL, et al. Color plates to help identify patients with blue cone monochromatism. *Am J Ophthalmol* 1983;95:741–747.

130. Nathans J, et al. Molecular genetics of human blue cone monochromacy. *Science* 1989;245:831–838.

131. Wissinger B, et al. Human rod monochromacy: linkage analysis and mapping of a cone photoreceptor expressed candidate gene on chromosome 2q11. *Genomics* 1998;51:325–31.

132. Kohl S, et al. Total colour blindness is caused by mutations in the gene encoding the alpha-subunit of the cone photoreceptor cGMP-gated cation channel. *Nat Genet* 1998;19:257–259.

133. Kohl S, et al. Mutations in the cone photoreceptor G-protein alpha-subunit gene GNAT2 in patients with achromatopsia. *Am J Hum Genet* 2002;57:422–425.

134. Nathans J, et al. Genetic heterogeneity among blue-cone monochromats. *Am J Hum Genet* 1993;53:987–1000.

135. Marmor MF, et al. Diagnostic clinical findings of a new syndrome with night blindness, maculopathy and enhanced S cone sensitivity. *Am J Ophthalmol* 1990;110:124–134.

136. Haider NB, et al. Mutation of a nuclear receptor gene, NR2E3, causes enhanced S cone syndrome, a disorder of retinal cell fate. *Nat Genet* 2000;24:127–131.

137. Gerber S, et al. The photoreceptor cell-specific nuclear receptor gene (PNR) accounts for retinitis pigmentosa in the Crypto-Jews from Portugal (Marranos), survivors from the Spanish Inquisition. *Hum Genet* 2000;107:276–284.

138. Foxman SG, et al. Classification of congenital and early onset retinitis pigmentosa. *Arch Ophthalmol* 1985;103:1502–1506.

139. Lewis CA, et al. Tubby-like protein 1 homozygous splice-site mutation causes early-onset severe retinal degeneration. *Invest Ophthalmol Vis Sci* 1999;40:2106–2114.

140. Franceschetti A. Rubeola pendant la grossesse et cataracte congenitale chez l'enfant accompagnee du phenomene digito-oculaire. *Ophthalmologica* 1947;83:27–31.

141. Fulton AB, Hansen RM, Mayer DL. Vision in Leber congenital amaurosis. *Arch Ophthalmol* 1996;114:698–703.

142. Lorenz B, et al. Early-onset severe rod-cone dystrophy in young children with RPE65 mutations. *Invest Ophthalmol Vis Sci* 2000;41:2735–2742.

143. Lotery AJ, et al. Mutation analysis of 3 genes in patients with Leber congenital amaurosis. *Arch Ophthalmol* 2000;118: 538–543.

144. Perrault I, et al. Different functional outcome of RetGC1 and RPE65 gene mutations in Leber congenital amaurosis. *Am J Hum Genet* 1999;64:1225–1228.

145. Koenekoop RK, et al. Visual improvement in Leber congenital amaurosis and the CRX genotype. *Ophthalmic Genet* 2002;23: 49–59.

146. Cremers FP, Van Den Hurk JA, Den Hollander AI. Molecular genetics of Leber congenital amaurosis. *Hum Mol Genet* 2002;11:1169–1176.

147. Perrault I, et al. Retinal-specific guanylate cyclase gene mutations in Leber's congenital amaurosis. *Nat Genet* 1996;14:461–4.

148. Marlhens F, et al. Mutations in RPE65 cause Leber's congenital amaurosis. *Nat Genet* 1997;17:139–141.

149. Freund CL, et al. De novo mutations in the CRX homeobox gene associated with Leber congenital amaurosis. *Nat Genet* 1998;18:311–312.

150. Banerjee P, et al. TULP1 mutation in two extended Dominican kindreds with autosomal recessive retinitis pigmentosa. *Nat Genet* 1998;18: 177–179.

151. Sohocki MM, et al. Mutations in a new photoreceptor-pineal gene on 17p cause Leber congenital amaurosis. *Nat Genet* 2000;24:79–83.

152. Lotery AJ, et al. Mutations in the CRB1 gene cause Leber congenital amaurosis. *Arch Ophthalmol* 2001;119:415–420.

153. Gerber S, et al. Complete exon-intron structure of the RPGR-interacting protein (RPGRIP1) gene allows the identification of mutations underlying Leber congenital amaurosis. *Eur J Hum Genet* 2001;9:561–571.

154. Hagstrom SA, et al. Recessive mutations in the gene encoding the tubby-like protein TULP1 in patients with retinitis pigmentosa. *Nat Genet* 1998;18:174–176.

155. Kelsell RE, et al. Mutations in the retinal guanylate cyclase (RETGC-1) gene in dominant cone-rod dystrophy. *Hum Mol Genet* 1998;7:1179–1184.

156. den Hollander AI, et al. Mutations in a human homologue of Drosophila crumbs cause retinitis pigmentosa (RP12). *Nat Genet* 1999;23:217–221.

157. Hamel CP, et al. Retinal dystrophies caused by mutations in RPE65: assessment of visual functions. *Br J Ophthalmol* 2001; 85:424–427.

158. Rivolta C, et al. Novel frameshift mutations in CRX associated with Leber congenital amaurosis. *Hum Mutat* 2001;18: 550–551.

159. Nakamura M, Ito S, Miyake Y. Novel de novo mutation in CRX gene in a Japanese patient with Leber congenital amaurosis. *Am J Ophthalmol* 2002;134:465–467.

160. Silva E, et al. A CRX null mutation is associated with both Leber congenital amaurosis and a normal ocular phenotype. *Invest Ophthalmol Vis Sci* 2000;41:2076–2079.

161. Fazzi E, Signorini SG, Scelsa B, et al. Lebers congenital amaurosis: An update. *Eur J Paediatr Neurol* 2003;7:13–22.

162. Rohrer B, Goletz P, Znoiko S, et al. Correlation of regenerable opsin with rod ERG signal in RPE 65-/- mice during development and aging. *Invest Ophthalmol Vis Sci* 2003;44:310–315.

8

STARGARDT DISEASE/FUNDUS FLAVIMACULATUS

BRIAN D. SIPPY
THOMAS A. AABERG, SR.

Karl Bruno Stargardt, in 1909, described seven patients from two families with a familial, progressive, bilateral, and symmetrical affliction of the foveal region leading to partial or complete loss of central vision. The pedigrees suggested an autosomal recessive inheritance pattern. Stargardt documented the progression from an early stage with reduced visual acuity in spite of an ophthalmoscopically normal fovea to the appearance of a characteristic horizontal oval area of atrophy of the retinal pigment epithelium (RPE) in the foveal region. This now "classic" Stargardt's lesion displayed a beaten-bronze appearance. In most cases, small yellow-white flecks surrounded the atrophic area and were separated from the central lesion by a zone of apparently unaffected pigment epithelium (1). Stargardt and others continued to observe and modify the characteristics of this entity, which has been referred to as Stargardt disease, Stargardt juvenile macular degeneration, juvenile macular degeneration, or simply Stargardt maculopathy.

During the first half of the twentieth century, interest in Stargardt disease primarily focused on the foveal/macular lesion, even though the two colored drawings in the original 1909 report showed perimacular white flecks. Little to no attention was given to the fleck component of the disorder until Franceschetti began discussing them in 1963 (2,3). He used the term "fundus flavimaculatus" to describe the appearance of irregularly shaped yellow-white flecks within the RPE. Emphasis on the flecked component of the disorder continued to increase in part due of the development of improved diagnostic techniques, such as fluorescein angiography (4).

For years to follow, Stargardt disease and fundus flavimaculatus were described as two related, but distinct, entities. Eventually, after careful clinical observation, the concept that Stargardt disease and fundus flavimaculatus were perhaps the same condition was renewed (5–8). Deutman (5,9) may have been the first author to use the term "Stargardt's flavimaculatus." In the mid 1980s, Aaberg (10) reported that Stargardt disease and fundus flavimaculatus

coexist within families as different phenotypic expressions of the same genotype. A study of 39 family pedigrees, containing 56 affected individuals, showed (i) that family members may demonstrate either maculopathy or diffuse flecks; (ii) that the flecks are of the same morphologic appearance in the two conditions; and (iii) that there is a tendency toward progressive retinal degeneration in some but certainly not all affected individuals.

Although the debate about whether Stargardt disease and fundus flavimaculatus are separate entities or whether they are part of a spectrum of the same disease will undoubtedly persist, genetic studies have now demonstrated a relationship between the two diseases (11). Indeed, previous clinical studies, together with more recent molecular studies evaluating genotype–phenotype correlation, suggest that Stargardt disease and fundus flavimaculatus are variable expressions of the same disorder (10–13). This does not, however, mean that these diseases are necessarily one entity. Other disorders including retinitis pigmentosa, cone–rod dystrophy, and age-related macular degeneration have been associated with similar genetic mutations. Deutman (14) recently coauthored a chapter on macular dystrophies in *Retina* in which Stargardt disease was presented in a photoreceptor and RPE dystrophy subcategory and in which fundus flavimaculatus was described under a related but separate subcategory of RPE dystrophies.

These two entities are historically divided in the following manner: (i) fundus flavimaculatus with no or only late macular involvement and presenting in adult life, and (ii) Stargardt disease with atrophic macular changes together with subtle or obvious fundus flavimaculatus flecks and presenting in children or young adults. However, the evidence overwhelmingly supports grouping these conditions into the same disease. In modern genetic databases, recessive Stargardt disease has been given the designation of STGD1. Therefore, throughout this chapter, Stargardt disease and fundus flavimaculatus will be addressed as one entity: STGD1/FF.

PREVALENCE

Although STGD1/FF has been referred to as the most common recessively inherited macular degeneration, it is still a rare disease having an estimated prevalence of 1:10,000 (15). In recessive disease, an affected parent can transmit only a single disease allele to his or her offspring, making the likelihood of having an affected child usually less than 1%.

Modern molecular genetic "chip" analysis of 100 healthy control subjects suggested a high carrier frequency (up to 10%) in the general population (16). Importantly, it should be noted that not all of the identified genetic variants necessarily cause disease in a particular family or individual. They may simply represent naturally occurring allelic polymorphisms (17).

ENVIRONMENTAL FACTORS

The relative role of genetic and environmental influences on STGD1/FF is still unknown. The disorder is clearly inherited in an autosomal recessive pattern, but with variable expression. Environmental influences could undoubtedly influence the disease phenotype. Because the accumulation of abnormal catabolic debris in the RPE is believed to lead to oxidative damage at the cellular level, studies addressing the influence of anti-oxidants will continue to further our understanding. Oxidative damage from light exposure and smoking can influence other macular diseases, such as age-related macular regeneration, and therefore, it seems reasonable to recommend that one quit smoking and reduce sunlight exposure (18). Because STGD1/FF is a relatively rare disorder, there have been no controlled cohort studies that implicate any particular environmental influence. Conversely, it has been suggested that having a particular mutation may make patients more susceptible to iatrogenic complications associated with medical therapy (19). Indeed, if allelic mutations do make an individual susceptible to environmental influences, behavior modification at an early age could slow disease progression and therefore help preserve visual function.

GENETICS

This section addresses recent advances and the current understanding of the genetics that influence a STGD1/FF phenotype. STGD1/FF is inherited in an autosomal recessive fashion because it is caused by recessive mutations in the ATP-binding cassette transporter, the *ABCA4(ABCR)* gene on the short arm of chromosome 1 (20). The same team later reported that the locus for fundus flavimaculatus mapped precisely to the same region (21). These stud-

ies provided further evidence that STGD and FF are likely the same genetic disease with allelic variation impacting phenotype.

Allikmets et al.'s (22) initial mutational analysis of the *ABCA4(ABCR)* gene in STGD1/FF families revealed a total of 19 different mutations. A recent survey of 493 individuals showed 1,321 instances of 147 distinct changes in the consensus sequence of the coding region and adjacent intronic regions of the *ABCA4(ABCR)* gene (23). In interpreting such findings, it is often prudent to assume that all sequence variants are non-disease causing polymorphisms until convincingly proven otherwise, ideally by multiple, complementary techniques. For instance, there have been repeatable, strong associations of STGD1/FF with certain *ABCA4(ABCR)* mutations. Specifically, the Gly1961Glu variation appears to be the most common mutation in Euro-American descendents, and the second most common might be Ala1038Val (12,23).

ABCA4(ABCR) mutational variants can be seen in other macular dystrophies. A phenomenon known as "gene sharing" occurs when different or the same mutations in a gene causes clinically related, but different, inherited diseases. For instance, the *ABCA4(ABCR)* gene may be shared with cone–rod degeneration and retinitis pigmentosa (RP) (24–26). Although the most obvious way that a single gene could be associated with multiple clinical phenotypes is through the existence of a number of different mutations, another important mechanism could also exist: the interaction of the mutated, "disease" gene with the approximately 100,000 other genes that make up the genetic framework of the individual.

Carriers of *ABCA4(ABCR)* mutations may account for some cases of age-related macular degeneration (ARMD) (27,28). Souied et al. (29) have described three unrelated families with STGD1/FF and grandparents with ARMD. Compound heterozygous missense mutations were found in the STGD patients, and complementary heterozygous missense mutations were observed in the grandparents with ARMD. Lewis et al. (30) evaluated 150 families and reported that compound heterozygous *ABCR* mutations may be responsible for STGD1/FF and that some heterozygous *ABCR* mutations might enhance susceptibility to ARMD. Indeed, heterozygous mutations in only one allele could lead to ARMD or no disease symptoms, independent of whether the mutations are mild, moderate, or severe (31). The idea that a heterozygous carrier of a mutation may be predisposed to a clinically similar, but phenotypically unique, disease than that of a patient with either a homozygous or a compound heterozygous state is not unique to STGD1/FF.

Van Driel et al. (32) have proposed a phenotype–genotype correlation model with (i) severe mutations which completely disrupt ABCA4(ABCR) protein activities and (ii) moderate and mild mutations with remaining partial ABCA4(ABCR) activities. One severe and one moderate mutation could cause cone–rod dystrophy, whereas one severe and one mild or two moderate mutations may provoke the STGD1/FF phenotype. Two severe mutations affecting both alleles could result in RP.

More recently, Yatsenko and others (33,34) have attempted to account for other molecular mechanisms of *ABCA4(ABCR)* gene alteration. They reported various missense mutations and one genomic deletion. A rare genetic event called uniparental isodisomy (UPID) could account for homozygosity of polymorphisms in and near the *ABCA4(ABCR)* gene on chromosome 1. A STGD1/FF patient was recently reported to be homozygous for all chromosome 1 markers. Specifically, all alleles on chromosome 1 of the proband were compatible with the paternal haplotype (35).

Transgenic mice can be created by "deleting" the mouse homologue of the human gene of interest from the mouse genome, giving rise to so-called knockout mice. To investigate the molecular etiology of STGD1/FF and potentially to develop new treatments, Travis et al. (35a) generated mice with a knockout mutation in *abcr*: the mouse homologue to *ABCA4(ABCR)*. The biochemical, morphological, and physiological phenotype in $abcr^{-/-}$ mice is strikingly similar to that in STGD1/FF patients, including accumulation of an oxidative cellular degradation product called A2E (N-retinylidene-N-retinylethanolamine). This toxic accumulation is thought to play a critical role in the photoreceptor degeneration of STGD1/FF.

If these mice are sheltered from bright light, the retinal degeneration may be attenuated (36). Studies like these support the concept that lifestyle modifications may delay the progression of disease and perhaps preserve useful vision for the life of the patient. Unfortunately, photoreceptor degeneration is very slow in $abcr^{-/-}$ mice, making it a cumbersome model for monitoring potential treatment effects (37). Newer mouse models or variations on the established $abcr^{-/-}$ mouse could lead to better understanding of the pathogenesis of STGD1/FF and to potential behavioral or medical interventions.

WORLDWIDE IMPACT

STGD1/FF affects males and females equally and spans all ethnic populations. Certain ethnic populations may eventually be found to harbor similar allelic variations that predispose to disease. In any isolated populations of people, the chance of consanguineous reproduction increases the likely expression of a recessively inherited disease, including STGD1/FF. Genetic studies may guide the development of population-specific screening protocols and perhaps customized therapeutic intervention. Certainly, the nutritional, environmental and genetic makeup of a given population could influence phenotypic expression of STGD1/FF.

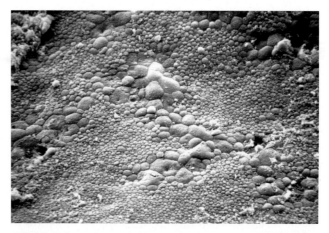

FIGURE 8-1. Scanning electron micrograph of a retinal pigment epithelial (RPE) monolayer from a patient with STGD1/FF. Note the marked heterogeneity of the RPE cells engorged with lipofuscin. Aggregates of engorged cells may correspond to flecks identified on clinical examination. (Courtesy of Ralph C. Eagle, Jr., MD, Department of Pathology, Wills Eye Hospital, Philadelphia, PA.)

PATHOPHYSIOLOGY

The primary pathologic defect in STGD1/FF is believed to be an abnormal accumulation of toxic lipofuscin pigments, such as A2E, in the RPE cells. Eagle et al. (38) suggested that the massive amounts of lipopigment seen the RPE of these young patients point toward a disorder in lipopigment metabolism. Lipofuscin-laden RPE cells from a patient with STGD1/FF demonstrate tremendous distension and loss of hexagonal architecture (Fig. 8-1). These hypertrophied RPE cells show abundant periodic acid-Schiff—positive material in the apical compartment (Fig. 8-2). This accumulation

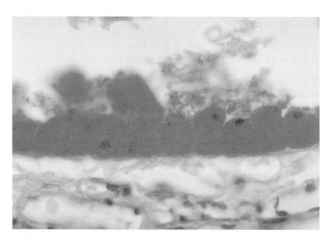

FIGURE 8-2. Histophotomicrograph of an intact monolayer of retinal pigment epithelium from a patient with STGD1/FF. The enlarged RPE cells demonstrate abundant periodic acid-Schiff—positive material in the apical compartment, consistent with lipofuscin-like material. (Periodic acid-Schiff stain, original magnification ×250, Courtesy of Ralph C. Eagle, Jr., MD, Department of Pathology, Wills Eye Hospital, Philadelphia, PA.)

appears to be responsible for RPE dysfunction with eventual photoreceptor death and severe vision loss in STGD1/FF patients (39).

An extensive review of RPE cellular structure and function is presented in *The Retinal Pigment Epithelium: Function and Disease* (40). Briefly, the apical surface of the RPE cell extends microvilli to encompass the rod and cone outer segments. The apex of the RPE cell is responsible for the phagocytosis of shed photoreceptor outer segment discs forming phagosomes in the apical RPE cell cytoplasm. The eventual fate of the phagosome is to be incorporated into the lysosomal system for degradation and partial recycling. Cathepsin D is an important protease involved in digestion of the rhodopsin-rich disk membranes. Perturbation of cathepsin D, or other catabolic enzyme systems such as ubiquitination, can lead the buildup of intracellular and extracellular debris (41,42).

Lipofuscin normally accumulates in the RPE in an apparent biphasic pattern with one peak occurring between 10 and 20 years of age and the second peak occurring around 50 years of age (43,44). Lipofuscin buildup is greatest in the posterior pole, especially in the macula, but sparing the fovea (45). Macular pigments composed of lutein and zeaxanthin may influence the accumulation of lipofuscin in the fovea (46). Moreover, specialized cones that reside in the fovea may have cellular membrane properties or different visual pigments that preclude the formation of lipofuscin in this region.

Lipofuscin is contained within granules of relatively uniform size. It is a lipid–protein aggregate that autofluoresces when excited by short wavelength light. The composition of RPE lipofuscin is controversial, but most believe that partially degraded outer segment disks and autophagy processes contribute to the bulk of lipofuscin (47–49). There is a growing body of evidence that lipofuscin may actually induce oxidative damage by acting as a photosensensitizing agent generating reactive oxygen species (50–52). As a design of function, the macula is exposed to a lifetime of light irradiation, including blue light wavelengths that have been shown to induce reactive oxygen intermediates (53,54). In addition, biochemical properties of lipofuscin may actually interfere with the enzymatic pathways of degradation by influencing lysosomal pH (55,56). Thus, as lipofuscin accumulates, the cellular catabolic machinery may be damaged or inhibited leading to more accumulation. This cycle would theoretically continue throughout life until the RPE cell is overwhelmed and cellular death and atrophy occur.

The *ABCA4(ABCR)* gene encodes a protein that is member of a well-characterized superfamily of proteins known as the ATP-binding cassette (ABC) transporters. *ABCA4(ABCR)* is believed to encode a protein that is involved in the transport of all-*trans* retinal from the photoreceptors to the RPE. Using knockout mice ($abcr^{-/-}$), studies have suggested that ABCA4(ABCR) functions as an export flippase for retinyl derivatives (57). This transport reaction is part of a larger cycle that replenishes the supply of the critical light-sensing form of vitamin A, 11-*cis* retinal, in the photoreceptor outer segments. The process of light absorption in the photoreceptors converts 11-*cis* retinal to a derivative called all-*trans* retinal, which is released into the disk membrane and then chemically modified and transported to an RPE cell. Defects in the ABCA4(ABCR) protein, however, slow the chemical modification of all-trans retinal, resulting in a buildup of this compound. Unfortunately, all-*trans* retinal spontaneously reacts at a low rate with membrane lipids to form a substance known as A2E. Sparrow et al. (58,59) have continued to provide evidence that A2E impairs RPE viability by sensitizing the cells to light damage.

Earlier work suggested that *ABCA4(ABCR)* produced a retina-specific transporter protein exclusively confined to the disk membrane of rod outer segments (60,61). Yet clinically STGD1/FF can severely impact central macular function, and some patients experience symptoms associated with cone function. In the foveal region, photoreceptor density approximates 200,000 cells/mm². These densely packed neuronal cells are primarily cones but have specialized architecture that resembles rods (62). Molday et al. (63) have recently suggested that ABCA4(ABCR) protein is present in both rod and cone photoreceptors. They conclude that the loss in central vision experienced by many STGD1/FF patients arises directly from ABCA4(ABCR)-mediated foveal cone degeneration. Elegant work by Scholl et al. (64,65) has shown altered electrophysiology in both the rod and cone systems in patients with confirmed genotyping for STGD1/FF.

CLINICAL SYMPTOMS AND SIGNS

The spectrum of disease that can occur even in the same family is broad. Sometimes obligate carriers of a mutant allele appear to be completely unaffected by the disease traits. This is referred to as *incomplete penetrance*. Sensitive modern equipment, however, can sometimes detect subclinical alterations in function that are suggestive of some degree of penetrance. The term *variable expressivity* is used when there is variable severity of phenotype between individuals with identical mutations. As mentioned earlier, the "classic" STGD1/FF patient has a bull's-eye maculopathy with a beaten-bronze appearance. In most cases, small yellow-white flecks with a pisciform shape surround the atrophic area and can be separated from the central lesion by a zone of apparently unaffected RPE (Figs. 8-3 and 8-4).

In patients with STGD1/FF, the age of disease onset and the age of presentation can vary slightly because patients often present only after central visual deterioration has impacted their lifestyle or ability to function. A hallmark of presentation is, however, that the visual function was at one time entirely normal. Children with STGD1/FF have reported visual complaints very early in life, as early as 3 years

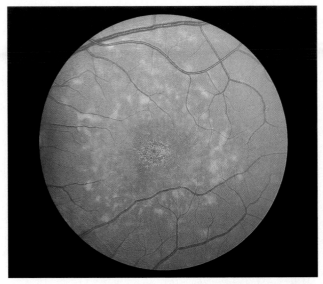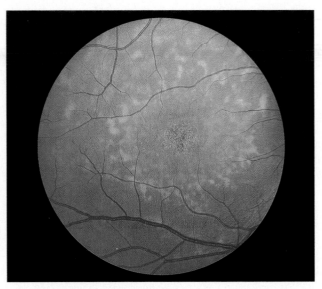

FIGURE 8-3. Left and right: Color fundus photographs of a typical STGD1/FF patient with pisciform yellow-white flecks and a central beaten-bronze bull's-eye maculopathy. There usually is symmetry in clinical appearance when comparing eyes within an individual. (Courtesy of James Gilman, CRA, Ophthalmic Photography, Department of Ophthalmology, Emory Eye Center, Atlanta, GA.)

of age. The mean age of symptomatic visual impairment in patients with central macular involvement appears to be in the early to mid teens. With specific questioning, many of these young patients will report visual symptoms that began several years prior to presentation. This hindsight reporting suggests that children may have delayed diagnosis that could impact future interventions. Patients without obvious atrophic macular involvement and only peripheral flecks usually present in early or mid adult life (14).

At presentation, there is a general symmetry of the fellow eyes in regard to function and clinical findings; however, there are always exceptions. In the initial stage, there may be no clinical findings associated with visual disturbance. Of the 56 patients followed by Aaberg Sr., all but 1 patient demonstrated symmetric ophthalmologic appearance, and 15 patients (26%) had a difference in visual acuity between fellow eyes of two or more lines on the Snellen distance chart. The asymmetry of visual acuity was present not only in those pa-

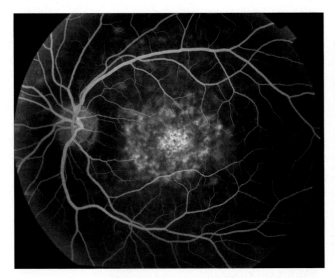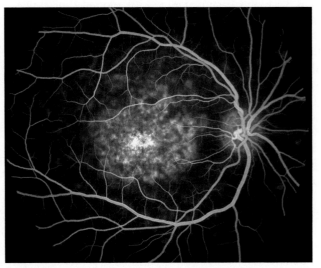

FIGURE 8-4. Left and **Right**: Fluorescein angiography of the same patient as shown in Figure 8-3 shows central areas of hyperfluorescence consistent with window defects, indicating pigment epithelial atrophy. Note the lack of hyperfluorescence corresponding to the flecks. Very late in an angiogram, these flecks may stain. (Courtesy of James Gilman, CRA, Ophthalmic Photography, Department of Ophthalmology, Emory Eye Center, Atlanta, GA.)

tients presenting with central lesions, but also in those with paracentral and diffuse flecks without a typical central lesion. As the patients were followed over 3 or more years, visual acuities between fellow eyes became more symmetrical. Typically, visual acuity gradually decreases, and once 20/200 is reached, further change rarely occurs (10,66). Almost 50 years after Stargardt's 1909 report, two of the original patients were reexamined and reported to be essentially unchanged except for an increased area of macular degeneration. Apparently, neither had significant loss of peripheral field nor complaints of night blindness (67). Of course, there are rare patients that do progress to more advanced stages of the disease. Patients that present with the fundus flavimaculatus phenotype are more likely to suffer from severe visual field loss and reduced visual acuity to counting fingers. These patients can eventually have clinical findings that resemble those seen in RP; and they can experience profound functional decline. As further studies are done on genetically identified cohorts, there will be a better understanding of the natural history of this disease.

Important to family members of a STGD1/FF patient, extensive psychophysical testing does not appear to have predictive value as to which family members will develop progressive retinal degeneration. Yet, for an affected individual, patients presenting with paracentral and diffuse flecks with or without a typical central lesion (characteristics of FF) have a greater tendency to progress to more advanced stages (10). Armstrong et al. (66) have also supported the concept that characteristics of presentation may be predictive of disease. They concluded that morphologic changes and deterioration of retinal function are more severe in patients with FF than in patients with STGD and that the duration of the disease has a greater effect on patients with FF than on patients with STGD progression.

It has been shown that a wide variation in clinical phenotype can occur in patients with sequence changes in the *ABCR* gene (12). More recently, 16 patients from 13 families with signs of STGD1/FF and known mutations on both alleles of the *ABCA4* gene (15 compound heterozygous, 1 homozygous) were characterized. In the majority of patients, the type and combination of *ABCA4* mutations in compound heterozygotes were compatible with the severity of the phenotype as to age of onset and the functional consequences. Unexplained phenotypic differences indicate the influence of other factors (13). The identification of correlations between specific mutations in the *ABCR* gene and clinical phenotypes will facilitate the counseling of patients regarding their visual prognoses. This information will also influence future therapeutic trials for STGD1/FF patients.

DIAGNOSTIC STUDIES

Fluorescein Angiography

Fluorescein angiography (FA), in the very early stages of STGD1/FF with a beaten-bronze macula, shows a central

ovoid area of hypofluorescence surrounded by a zone of blotchy hyperfluorescence. With increasing age, the central lesion may lose the metallic sheen and develop areas of atrophy and hyperfluorescence. The surrounding ring of paramacular white flecks often shows hypofluorescence initially but later hyperfluorescence, indicating staining by the fluorescein dye. The paramacular flecks later disappear leaving hyperfluorescent spots of RPE atrophy. Leakage on fluorescein does not occur unless it is associated with a secondary process, such as choroidal neovascularization.

The peripheral flecks are transient, usually becoming manifest in the second decade but then appearing and disappearing in various locations over several decades. The flecks may hypofluoresce or exhibit a pattern of hyperfluorescence in a zone surrounding the actual flecks. The variation in FA characteristics probably is related to the age of the fleck, the amount of pigment within the fleck, and degree of RPE involvement (Fig. 8-4).

The lack of choroidal fluorescence (dark choroid) in STGD1/FF has been suggested to be related to the presence of short-wavelength–absorbing chromophores in the RPE layer (68). The phenomenon of dark choroid is evident in approximately half of patients with STGD1/FF (Fig. 8-5). The hypofluorescent choroid appears dark throughout most of the angiogram and may highlight the overlying retinal circulation. The dark choroid effect has been thought to be caused by blockage of the choroidal fluorescence by lipofuscin-laden RPE; however, recent indirect measurements of lipofuscin by autofluorescence have little or no correlation with the presence or lack of a dark choroid on FA (see the section on the scanning laser ophthalmoscope later in this chapter) (69,70).

Aaberg and Han (71) have reported that the presence or absence of choroidal hypofluorescence does not correlate with the phenotypic expression of STGD1/FF. Although there may be considerable variability in phenotypic expression of the disease within a pedigree, there was a more uniform intrafamilial consistency of the dark choroid phenomenon. Moreover, as an individual with STGD1/FF ages, there may be consistent variation in the dark choroid, likely secondary to progressive RPE atrophy.

Other dye-based imaging techniques, such as indocyanine green angiography, may further our understanding of STGD1/FF by revealing different tissue characteristics specifically related to terminal choroidal arterioles and choriocapillaris perfusion defects in the diseased macula (72).

Electrophysiologic Evaluation

Electroretinogram

Abnormalities in the electroretinogram (ERG) parallel the degree of morphologic effect (stage of the disease). The most frequently described ERG abnormality is a decrease in the b-wave amplitude, usually with a normal implicit time.

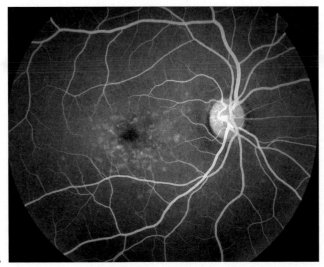
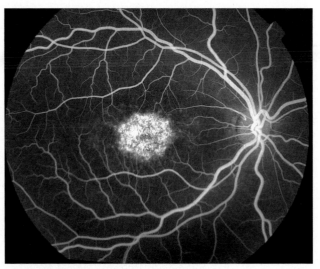

A　　　　　　　　　　　　　　　　　　　　　　　　　　　　　　　　　　　　　　　B

FIGURE 8-5. Fluorescein angiography of two different STGD1/FF patients demonstrating the variable phenomenon of the "dark choroid." **A:** shows a uniform choroidal blush that is typical of a "normal" angiogram, whereas (**B**) shows a relative hypofluorescence of the choroid (dark choroid) that can often highlight the overlying fine retinal capillary structure. Both angiograms are in the late arteriovenous phase. (Courtesy of James Gilman, CRA, Ophthalmic Photography, Department of Ophthalmology, Emory Eye Center, Atlanta, GA.)

However, in most patients with primarily central macular involvement, the ERG is normal. With increasing amounts of peripheral flecks and central atrophy, the ERG can be moderately reduced. This has been shown to be especially the case in patients with diffuse flecks and vision loss beginning in childhood (73). Comprehensive studies have shown that ERG abnormalities are more prevalent when flecks are clinically evident (74).

Electrooculogram

The electrooculogram (EOG) is typically normal, but can be reduced when extensive RPE changes are present. The more extensive the disease process, the lower the light peak/dark trough (L/D) ratio (14). Fast oscillations and slow oscillations of the standing potential of the eye are generated by light stimulus induced hyperpolarization or depolarization of the RPE basal membrane, respectively. Recent studies have shown that abnormalities in both fast and slow oscillations of the EOG can be present in patients with STGD1/FF. The disease affects the amplitude more than the time course of these oscillations. These results may reflect abnormalities in photoreceptor/RPE function (75).

Dark-Adaptation Amplitudes

Dark adaptation can be normal or slightly delayed in STGD1/FF patients, possibly as a result of altered RPE metabolism. Rod amplitudes might need increased time to reach total adaptational amplitudes (76). No frank abnor-malities in dark adaptation should be seen in younger, less severely affected patients.

Pattern Visual Evoked Potential

As described earlier in this chapter, rod adaptation kinetics have been reported to be abnormal in patients with STGD1/FF, but cone kinetics have been more recently studied by utilizing pattern visual evoked potential (VEP) recovery testing after macular bleaching. Altered recovery of pattern VEPs after macular bleaching in patients with STGD1/FF was detected in patients with relatively mild clinical impairment (77).

Visual Fields

Visual fields are generally normal, but progressive macular atrophy can give a relative and eventual absolute central scotoma. Annular (ring) scotomata and generalized peripheral field constriction can be seen in patients with more advanced disease and diffuse RPE atrophy.

Color Testing

In a majority of cases, there can be abnormal general color discrimination. Aaberg (10) found an acquired dyschromatopsia of the blue-yellow axis predominant, but noted that all forms of color discrimination dysfunction can be present. Gerth et al. (13) recently evaluated genotypically confirmed STGD1/FF patients and found various color discrimination anomalies in all patients tested. Therefore, color vision dysfunction should not be used as a diagnostic criterion for STGD1/FF, but its presence can help in understanding a patients' overall visual function. If severely affected color vision is found early in the clinical presentation, the diagnosis of cone dystrophy should be considered.

Optical Coherent Tomography

Optical coherent tomography (OCT) generates high-resolution cross-sectional tomograms of ocular tissue, and it has been particularly useful in evaluating and understanding diseases affecting the macula. Recent data suggest that OCT can be helpful in better understanding the structural changes associated with macular dystrophies. Extensive foveolar thinning and macular volume loss can be observed in STGD1/FF (78). Ultrahigh-resolution OCT scans of patients with STGD1/FF showed a diffuse retinal atrophy with a reduction in the thickness of all retinal layers, sub-RPE deposits corresponding with the flecks, and a focal loss of photoreceptor inner and outer segments (79).

Scanning Laser Ophthalmoscope

The lipofuscin or lipofuscinlike material that accumulates in RPE cells has intrinsic autofluorescence properties. Spectral characteristics of *in vivo* fundus autofluorescence (excitation at 510 to 550 nm with emission between 630 and 750 nm) are consistent with those of lipofuscin (80,81). Confocal scanning laser ophthalmoscopes (SLOs) have been used to detail autofluorescence as an index of lipofuscin in the living eye (82). The normal fundus shows a consistent pattern in patients older than 6 years, with diffuse autofluorescence that is most intense between 5 and 15 degrees from the fovea center (83,84).

Heritable macular dystrophies, such as STGD1/FF, have been shown to have more autofluorescence consistent with accelerated lipofuscin accumulation (70). The entire fundus of patients with STGD1/FF shows abnormally intense autofluorescence, suggesting a generalized biochemical abnormality of the RPE despite the discrete flecks seen on clinical examination. Interestingly, when correlating FA with SLO findings, high levels of autofluorescence may be present with or without the classic finding of a dark choroid on FA (70). Studies utilizing single-wavelength ultraviolet-absorbance high-performance liquid chromatography have examined the autofluorescence properties of A2E in a rat model (85) Calibration of an SLO to this wavelength might allow for *in vivo* detection of damaging A2E accumulation to assess disease progression.

Interestingly, foveal macular pigment has been related to foveal cone acuity in STGD1/FF, and these pigments may serve as reliable markers for the presence of foveal cones. Infrared light may serve as a sensitive screening tool for detection of early STGD1/FF (86).

Microchip Gene Array

Allikmets et al. (22) have designed a genotyping microarray (gene chip) for the *ABCA4(ABCR)* gene to enable comprehensive screening of populations with ABCA4(ABCR)-associated retinal pathology, including STGD1/FF. The chip includes greater than 400 sequence variants described thus far in this gene, allowing the detection of all known variants in one reaction. The ABCR400 array was constructed by the allele-specific primer extension technology (described at: http://www.asperbio.com). In tested STGD1/FF patient cohorts, the array detected between 54% and 78% of all possible disease-associated alleles (16).

Differential Diagnosis

In more advanced stages of STGD1/FF that usually present in adult life, the differential diagnosis is extensive. For a comprehensive review of macular dystrophies, readers can refer to Dr. Gass' *Stereoscopic Atlas of Macular Disease* (87). In the future, genetic characterization, like the gene chip microarray, may aid in routine diagnosis of STGD1/FF. But until these techniques are readily available and shown be reproducible and reliable, clinical findings remain the mainstay for making the diagnosis. For the purposes of this pediatric retina reference, the clinical differential can be limited to other macular diseases that typically present in childhood, including but not limited to, dominant Stargardt-like macular dystrophy [*STGD2 13q34* (88), *STGD3 6q11-q15* (89), Kniazeva (90), *STGD4 4p* (91)], cone–rod dystrophy, pericentral retinitis pigmentosa, pattern dystrophy, vitelliform dystrophy (Best disease), X-linked juvenile retinoschisis, dominant cystoid macular dystrophy, solar retinopathy, acute macular neuroretinopathy, central areolar choroidal dystrophy, and fundus albipunctatus.

MANAGEMENT
Trauma

RPE cells engorged with lipofuscin may predispose patients with STGD1/FF to subretinal fibrosis and outer retinal damage in the setting of minor contusion trauma (92–95). Sports activities should minimize contact-related activities when possible. The incidence of minor blunt trauma may be reduced with polycarbonate safety glasses.

Motor vehicles present their own problems. Szlyk et al. (96) have shown that the proportion of individuals with juvenile macular dystrophies, including STGD1/FF, involved in accidents was comparable to matched controls. However, for 13 of the 20 subjects with central vision loss who did not restrict their driving to daylight hours, there was a greater likelihood of involvement in nighttime accidents than in the control group. Motor vehicle accidents can be complicated by secondary trauma associated with airbag safety devices (97). Airbags combined with seat belts are an effective means of reducing injury and death during motor vehicle accidents. It is hoped that safety-industry researchers will be able to develop modifications that can continue to save lives and minimize ocular risk.

Medical/Surgical

In addition to limitations of central vision inherent to the natural course of STGD1/FF, patients may also suffer from secondary processes that further limit visual potential. Choroidal neovascularization has been reported in patients with STGD1/FF (98–100). More recently, photodynamic therapy has been employed to retard progression of subfoveal CNVM in a patient with STGD1/FF (101). Potter et al. (102) have recently reported surgical intervention for a patient with STGD1/FF who suffered further visual impairment from a prominent epiretinal membrane. The authors caution that surgical intervention in eyes with preexisting degenerative changes may lead to atypical complications or outcomes.

VISION REHABILITATION
School-Age Issues

In children and teens with STGD1/FF, it is very important to employ adequate low vision care and modify behavioral and environmental factors to maximize visual performance. For example, these students may have light and glare control problems in their classrooms. Adaptations such as sitting away from the window or shutting the curtains may be necessary. Moreover, these students should have permission from school administrators to wear special sun filters (sunglasses) in classrooms and on campus when needed to decrease glare and light sensitivity.

Because the vision loss may progress over time, each student should have a Teacher of the Visually Impaired (VI). A VI teacher can assess the classroom and educational plan for the child. With the low vision specialist's recommendations, the VI teacher makes adaptations including low vision devices, large-print materials, and other special services the child will need each year in school. Some students may require extended time on reading assignments and tests. Computer software is also available to convert standard programs into more user-friendly formats for people with low vision

As mentioned earlier, there are also safety issues to address in young active students. Eyewear with polycarbonate lenses should be worn for protection of the eyes from unexpected injury. Counseling includes safety issues in physical education. Low impact and minimal contact sports such as swimming and track are good options. Sports with fast-moving projectiles may put young patients at undo risk.

Protective face shields are essential if patients are to participate in such sports.

Preventive steps should be exercised when this condition manifests during early life. However, it should be noted that STGD1/FF rarely causes legal blindness during childhood years.

Low-Vision Care

Young patients with STGD1/FF respond well to magnification, and simple bifocals may be used in the early stages. In later stages, closed-circuit television systems are helpful. Mobility is usually minimally affected. Some young adults with STGD1/FF can drive with the assistance of bioptic devices, but it may be for a limited time. In deciding on low-vision devices for children and especially adolescents, it is important to maintain good cosmetic appearance.

ROLES OF OTHER PHYSICIANS AND HEALTH CARE PROVIDERS

Since the Americans with Disabilities Act passed in 1990, attempts have been made to determine the functional limitations imposed by various types of visual impairment. Szlyk et al. (103) have better defined real and perceived functional limitations of patients with juvenile macular degeneration. Their work has provided insight into the difficulties of performing everyday tasks in these patients. From a clinical perspective, it is important to be aware of the varying profiles of functional impairment produced by different visual disorders in order to be more sensitive to the individual needs of patients with vision loss. It is also important for the clinician to be prepared to direct patients and parents to information and support resources at the time of diagnosis to minimize uncertainty and emotional distress (Table 8-1).

There are no special or unique ethical considerations associated with STGD1/FF except that testing and treatment of dependent minors requires appropriate parental or guardian consent. It should be mentioned, however, that children complaining of visual symptoms are often thought to be malingering if the results of an eye examination are reported to be "within normal limits." Ophthalmologists need to be aware that early in the disease process the fundus examination may not reveal a typical macular sheen and flecks may be discrete or absent.

TABLE 8-1. INFORMATION AND SUPPORT SITES FOR STGD1/FF PATIENTS ON THE WORLD WIDE WEB

http://www.nei.nih.gov/health/organizations.htm
http://www.blindness.org
http://www.maculardegeneration.org

FUTURE TREATMENTS

Basic research into the biochemical and cellular defects responsible for STGD1/FF will lay the groundwork for developing therapies or cures for this heredodegeneration. Specifically, studies into the biochemical properties of the ABCA4(ABCR) protein may help in developing pharmacologic therapies for STGD1/FF. Sun and Nathans (60,61, 104,105) have given extensive effort in characterizing the biochemical properties of the ABCA4(ABCR) protein. Some of these *in vitro* studies have looked into ways to stimulate the biochemical activity of the wild-type ABCA4 (ABCR) protein, and several compounds have been identified. Interestingly, the ATPase activity of the ABCA4 (ABCR) protein can be enhanced by a commonly used antiarrhythmic drug, amiodarone (106). Others have suggested that known compounds may have a deleterious effect on the natural history of patients with STGD1/FF. For example, it has been reported that some individuals who have ABCA4 (ABCR) mutations may be predisposed to develop retinal toxicity when exposed to chloroquine/ hydroxychloroquine (19). Studies like these on compounds that positively or negatively impact the disease course will further our understanding of STGD1/FF pathophysiology. As drugs are characterized that interact with the *ABCA4(ABCR)* gene or its protein, it is hoped that therapies may be designed to slow or arrest the course of the disease.

Isotretinoin (Accutane) has been shown to slow the synthesis of 11-*cis*-retinaldehyde and regeneration of rhodopsin by inhibiting 11-*cis*-retinol dehydrogenase in the visual cycle. Recently, the effects of isotretinoin on lipofuscin accumulation in $abcr^{-/-}$ knockout mice were studied. Isotretinoin appeared to block the formation of A2E and the accumulation of lipofuscin pigments, and ERG parameters remained stable. Isotretinoin also blocked the slower, age-dependent accumulation of lipofuscin in wild-type mice. These results suggest that treatment with isotretinoin may inhibit lipofuscin accumulation and thus delay the onset of visual loss in STGD1/FF patients (39).

The retina contains high concentrations of several antioxidant chemicals that efficiently neutralize free radicals. Two of the antioxidants, zeaxanthin and lutein, are highly concentrated in the macula. Vitamin E is present at high concentrations in photoreceptor outer segments and also in the RPE. Other defenses employed by the body's cells include the zinc-containing enzyme superoxide dismutase and a second enzyme, catalase, both of which inactivate various free radicals. Observational and experimental data suggest that antioxidant and/or zinc supplements may delay progression of ARMD and vision loss (107). Biochemical studies on the mechanism of oxidative damage to the RPE cell may lead to other therapeutic interventions (108). It is not unreasonable to suppose that scientists will find a naturally occurring or synthetic compound that improves the function or extends the viability of RPE cells. Such a compound could protect the RPE from photooxidative damage, for example, or improve its efficiency in degrading abnormal photoreceptor outer segments.

To date, most, if not all, of the genetic analysis and genetic association studies on *ABCA4(ABCR)* and STGD1/FF have focused on coding regions or exon/intron boundaries within the gene. Further work defining the regulatory regions of the *ABCA4(ABCR)* gene will include sequencing promoter, terminator, and introns. These types of studies may help define potential targets for therapeutic intervention. For example, drugs might be developed that influence the expression of the *ABCA4(ABCR)* gene by targeting regulatory regions. These drugs could minimize the accumulative deleterious effect of the mutant gene over the lifetime of the individual. Transgenic animals will undoubtedly play a role in the development of such novel therapies.

REFERENCES

1. Stargardt K. Ueber familiare, progressive degeneration in der makulagegend des auges. *Graefes Arch Klin Exp Ophthalmol* 1909;71:534–550.
2. Franceschetti A. Ueber tapeto-retinale degeneration im kindesalter (kongenitale form [Leber]), Amaurotische idiotie, rezessive-geschlecht sgebundene tapeto-retinale degenerationen, fundus flavimaculatus. In: Enke F, editor. *Entwicklung und Fortschritt in der Augenheilkunde.* Stuttgart, 1963:107–120.
3. Franceschetti A. A special form of tapetoretinal degeneration: fundus flavimaculatus. *Trans Am Acad Ophthalmol Otolaryngol* 1965;69:1048–1053.
4. Ernest JT, Krill AE. Fluorescein studies in fundus flavimaculatus and drusen. *Am J Ophthalmol* 1966;62:1–6.
5. Krill AE, Deutman AF. The various categories of juvenile macular degeneration. *Trans Am Ophthalmol Soc* 1972;70:220–245.
6. Irvin AR, Wergeland FL Jr. Stargardt's hereditary progressive macular degeneration. *Br J Ophthalmol* 1972;56:817–826.
7. Hadden OB, Gass JDM. Fundus flavimaculatus and Stargardt's disease. *Am J Ophthalmol* 1976;82:527–539.
8. Noble KG, Carr RE. Stargardt's disease and fundus flavimaculatus. *Arch Ophthalmol* 1979;97:1281–1285.
9. Deutman AF. Stargardt's Disease. In: Deutman AF, editor. *The Hereditary Dystrophies of the Posterior Pole of the Eye*, Assen (The Netherlands): Van Gorcum, 1971:100–171.
10. Aaberg TM. Stargardt's disease and fundus flavimaculatus: evaluation of morphologic progression and intrafamilial co-existence. *Trans Am Ophthalmol Soc* 1986;84:453–487.
11. Souied EH, Ducroq D, Rozet JM, et al. A novel ABCR nonsense mutation responsible for late-onset fundus flavimaculatus. *Invest Ophthalmol Vis Sci* 1999;40:2740–2744.
12. Fishman GA, Stone EM, Grover S, et al. Variation of clinical expression in patients with Stargardt dystrophy and sequence variations in the ABCR gene. *Arch Ophthalmol* 1999;117:504–510.
13. Gerth C, Andrassi-Darida M, Bock M, et al. Phenotypes of 16 Stargardt macular dystrophy/fundus flavimaculatus patients with known ABCA4 mutations and evaluation of genotype-phenotype correlation. *Graefes Arch Clin Exp Ophthalmol* 2002;240:628–638.
14. Deutman AF, Hoyng CB. Macular dystrophies. In: Ryan SJ, Schachat AP, editors. *Retina*, 3rd ed. St. Louis: Mosby, 2001: 1210–1257.
15. Blacharski PA. Fundus Flavimaculatus. In: Newsome DA, ed.

Retinal dystrophies and degenerations. New York: Raven Press, 1988:135–159.

16. Zernant J, Jaakson K, Lewis RA, et al. Molecular diagnostics of Stargardt disease by genotyping patients on the ABCR (ABCA4) microarray. ARVO Abstract 2003; Program No. 5107.

17. Maugeri A, van Driel MA, van de Pol DJ, et al. The 2588G—>C mutation in the ABCR gene is a mild frequent founder mutation in the Western European population and allows the classification of ABCR mutations in patients with Stargardt disease. *Am J Hum Genet* 1999;64:1024–1035.

18. Cai J, Nelson KC, Wu M, et al. Oxidative damage and protection of the RPE. *Prog Retin Eye Res* 2000;19:205–221.

19. Shroyer NF, Lewis RA, Lupski JR. Analysis of the ABCR (ABCA4) gene in 4-aminoquinoline retinopathy: is retinal toxicity by chloroquine and hydroxychloroquine related to Stargardt disease? *Am J Ophthalmol* 2001;131:761–766.

20. Kaplan J, Gerber S, Larget-Piet D, et al. A gene for Stargardt's disease (fundus flavimaculatus) maps to the short arm of chromosome 1. *Nat Genet* 1993;5:308–311.

21. Gerber S, Rozet J-M, Bonneau D, et al. A gene for late-onset fundus flavimaculatus with macular dystrophy maps to chromosme 1q13. *Am J Hum Genet* 1995;56:396–399.

22. Allikmets R, Singh N, Sun H, et al. A photoreceptor cell-specific ATP-binding transporter gene (ABCR) is mutated in recessive Stargardt macular dystrophy. *Nat Genet* 1997;15:236–246.

23. Stone EM, Webster AR, Vandenburgh K, Streb LM, et al. Allelic variation in ABCR associated with Stargardt disease but not age-related macular degeneration. *Nat Genet* 1998;20:328–329.

24. Cremers FP, van de Pol DJ, van Driel M, et al. Autosomal recessive retinitis pigmentosa and cone-rod dystrophy caused by splice site mutations in the Stargardt's disease gene ABCR. *Hum Mol Genet* 1998;7:355–362.

25. Martinez-Mir A, Paloma E, Allikmets R, et al. Retinitis pigmentosa caused by a homozygous mutation in the Stargardt disease gene ABCR. *Nat Genet* 1998;18:11–12.

26. Shroyer NF, Lewis RA, Yatsenko AN, et al. Null missense ABCR (ABCA4) mutations in a family with Stargardt disease and retinitis pigmentosa. *Invest Ophthalmol Vis Sci* 2001;42:2757–2761.

27. Allikmets R. Further evidence for an association of ABCR alleles with age-related macular degeneration. The International ABCR Screening Consortium. *Am J Hum Genet* 2000;67:487–491.

28. Allikmets R. Simple and complex ABCR: genetic predisposition to retinal disease. *Am J Hum Genet* 2000;67:793–799.

29. Souied EH, Ducroq D, Gerber S, et al. Age-related macular degeneration in grandparents of patients with Stargardt disease: genetic study. *Am J Ophthalmol* 1999;128:173–178.

30. Lewis RA, Shroyer NF, Singh N, et al. Genotype/Phenotype analysis of a photoreceptor-specific ATP-binding cassette transporter gene, ABCR, in Stargardt disease. *Am J Hum Genet* 1999;64:422–434.

31. Efferth T. The human ATP-binding cassette transporter genes: from the bench to the bedside. *Curr Mol Med* 2001;1:45–65.

32. van Driel MA, Maugeri A, Klevering BJ, et al. ABCR unites what ophthalmologists divide(s). *Ophthalmic Genet* 1998;19:117–122.

33. Yatsenko AN, Shroyer NF, Lewis RA, et al. Late-onset Stargardt disease is associated with missense mutations that map outside known functional regions of ABCR (ABCA4). *Hum Genet* 2001;108:346–355.

34. Yatsenko AN, Shroyer NF, Lewis RA, et al. An ABCA4 genomic deletion in patients with Stargardt disease. *Hum Mutat* 2003;21:636–644.

35. Eliason DA, Affitagato LM, Haines HL, et al. A case of Stargardt macular dystrophy caused by uniparental isodisomy (UPID) and subsequent analysis of 830 Stargardt macular dystrophy cases for UPID. ARVO Abstract 2003; Program No. 5109.

35a.Weng J, Mata NL, Azarian SM, et al. Insights into the function of Rim protein in photoreceptors and etiology of Stargardt's disease from the phenotype in abcr knockout mice. *Cell* 1999;98:13–23.

36. Mata NL, Tzevor RT, Liu X, et al. Delayed dark adaptation and lipofuscin accumulation in abcr +/- mice:implications for involvement of ABCR in age-related macular degeneration. *Invest Ophthalmol Vis Sci* 2001;42:1685–1690.

37. Radu RA, Mata NL, Bagla A, et al. A2E accumulation and photoreceptor degeneration in pigmented and albino abcr−/−mice. ARVO Abstract 2003; Program No. 3519.

38. Eagle RC Jr, Lucier AC, Bernardino VB Jr, et al. Retinal pigment epithelial abnormalities in fundus flavimaculatus: a light and electron microscopic study. *Ophthalmology* 1980;87:1189–1200.

39. Radu RA, Mata NL, Nusinowitz S, et al. From the cover: treatment with isotretinoin inhibits lipofuscin accumulation in a mouse model of recessive Stargardt's macular degeneration. *Proc Natl Acad Sci U S A* 2003;100:4742–4747.

40. Marmor MF. Structure, function, and disease of the retinal pigment epithelium. In: Marmor MF, Wolfensberger TJ, eds. *The retinal pigment epithelium: function and disease*, 2nd ed. Oxford: Oxford University Press, 1998:3–12.

41. Verdugo ME, Ray J. Age-related increase in activity of specific lysosomal enzymes in the human retinal pigment epithelium. *Exp Eye Res* 1997;65:231–240.

42. Loeffler KU, Mangini NJ. Immunolocalization of ubiquitin and related enzymes in human retina and retinal pigment epithelium. *Graefes Arch Clin Exp Ophthalmol* 1997;235:248–254.

43. Wing GL, Blanchard GC, Weiter JJ. The topography and age relationship of lipofuscin concentration in the retinal pigment epithelium. *Invest Ophthalmol Vis Sci* 1978;17:601–607.

44. Feeney-Burns L, Hildebrande ES, et al. Aging human RPE: morphometric analysis of macular, equatorial and peripheral cells. *Invest Ophthalmol Vis Sci* 1984;25:195–200.

45. Weiter JJ, Delori FC, Wing GL, et al. Retinal pigment epithelial lipofuscin and melanin and choriodal melanin in human eyes. *Invest Ophthalmol Vis Sci* 1986;27:145–152.

46. Hammond BR Jr, Wooten BR, Snodderly DM. Individual variations in the spatial profile of human macular pigment. *J Opt Soc Am A* 1997;14:1187–1196.

47. Dorey CK, Wu G, Ebenstein D, et al. Cell loss in the aging retina. *Invest Ophthalmol Vis Sci* 1989;30:1691–1699.

48. Burke JM, Skumatz CMB. Autofluorescent inclusions in long-term postconfluent cultures of retinal pigment epithelium. *Invest Ophthalmol Vis Sci* 1998;39:1478–1486.

49. Wassell J, Ellis S, Burke J, et al. Fluorescence properties of autofluorescent granules generated by cultured human RPE cells. *Invest Ophthalmol Vis Sci* 1998;39:1487–1492.

50. Beatty S, Koh H, Phil M, et al. The role of oxidative stress in the pathogenesis of age-related macular degeneration. *Surv Ophthalmol* 2000;45:115–134.

51. Winkler BS, Boulton ME, Gottsch JD, et al. Oxidative damage and age-related macular degeneration. *Mol Vis* 1999;5:32.

52. Frank RN. "Oxidative protector" enzymes in the macular retinal pigment epithelium of aging eyes and eyes with age-related macular degeration. *Trans Am Acad Ophthalmol Otolaryngol* 1998;96:634–689.

53. Rozanowska M, Jarvis-Evans J, Korytowski W, et al. Blue light-induced reactivity of retinal age pigment: in vitro generation of oxygen-reactive species. *J Biol Chem* 1995;270:18825–18830.

54. Sparrow JR, Nakanishi K, Parish CA. The lipofuscin fluorophore A2E mediates blue light-induced damage to retinal pigmented epithelial cells. *Invest Ophthalmol Vis Sci* 2000;41:1981–1989.

55. Holz FG, Schutt F, Kopitz J, et al. Inhibition of lysosomal degradative functions in RPE cells by a retinoid component of lipofuscin. *Invest Ophthalmol Vis Sci* 1999;40:737–743.

56. Sparrow JR, Parish CA, Hashimoto M, et al. A2E, a lipofuscin fluorophore, in human retinal pigmented epithelial cells in culture. *Invest Ophthalmol Vis Sci* 1999;40:2988–2995.

57. Weng J, Mata NL, Azarian SM, et al. Insights into the function of Rim protein in photoreceptors and etiology of Stargardt's disease from the phenotype in abcr knockout mice. *Cell* 1999;98:12–23.

58. Sparrow JR, Zhou J, Ben-Shabat S, et al. Involvement of oxidative mechanisms in blue-light-induced damage to A2E-laden RPE. *Invest Ophthalmol Vis Sci* 2002;43:1222–1227.

59. Sparrow JR, Zhou J, Cai B. DNA is a target of the photodynamic effects elicited in A2E-laden RPE by blue-light illumination. *Invest Ophthalmol Vis Sci* 2003;44:2245–2251.

60. Sun H, Nathans J. Stargardt's ABCR is localized to the disc membrane of retinal rod outer segments. *Nat Genet* 1997;17:15–16.

61. Sun H, Nathans J. ABCR: rod photoreceptor-specific ABC transporter responsible for Stargardt disease. *Methods Enzymol* 2000;315:879–897.

62. Green RW. Retina. In: Spencer WH, ed. *Ophthalmic pathology: an atlas and textbook*, 4th ed. Philadelphia: WB Saunders, 1996:674–676.

63. Molday LL, Rabin AR, Molday RS. ABCR expression in foveal cone photoreceptors and its role in Stargardt macular dystrophy. *Nat Genet* 2000;25:257–258.

64. Scholl HP, Kremers J, Vonthein R, et al. L- and M-cone-driven electroretinograms in Stargardt's macular dystrophy-fundus flavimaculatus. *Invest Ophthalmol Vis Sci* 2001;42:1380–1389.

65. Scholl HP, Besch D, Vonthein R, et al. Alterations of slow and fast rod ERG signals in patients with molecularly confirmed Stargardt disease type 1. *Invest Ophthalmol Vis Sci* 2002;43:1248–1256.

66. Armstrong JD, Meyer D, Xu S, Elfervig JL. Long-term follow-up of Stargardt's disease and fundus flavimaculatus. *Ophthalmology* 1998;105:448–458.

67. Rosehr K. Ueber den weiteren Verlauf der von Stargardt und Behr beschriebenen familiaren degeneration der macula. *Klin Monatsbl Augenheilkd* 1954;124:171–175.

68. Fish G, Grey R, Sehmi KS, et al. The dark choroid in posterior retinal dystrophies. *Br J Ophthalmol* 1981;65:359–363.

69. Delori FC, Staurenghi G, Arend O, et al. In vivo measurement of lipofuscin in Stargardt's disease-fundus flavimaculatus. *Invest Ophthalmol Vis Sci* 1995;36:2327–2331.

70. von Rückmann A, Fitzke FW, Bird AC. In vivo fundus autofluorescence in macular dystrophies. *Arch Ophthalmol* 1997;115:609–615.

71. Aaberg TM, Han DP. Evaluation of phenotypic similarities between Stargardt flavimaculatus and retinal pigment epithelial pattern dystrophies. *Trans Am Ophthalmol Soc* 1987;85:101–119.

72. Schwoerer J, Secretan M, Zografos L, et al. Indocyanine green angiography in fundus flavimaculatus. *Ophthalmologica* 2000;214:240–245.

73. Itabashi R, Katsumi O, Mehta MC, et al. Stargardt's disease/fundus flavimaculatus: psychophysical and electrophysiological results. *Graefes Arch Clin Exp Ophthalmol* 1993;231:555–562.

74. Stavrou P, Good PA, Misson GP, et al. Electrophysiological findings in Stargardt's–fundus flavimaculatus disease. *Eye* 1998;12:953–958.

75. Caruso RC, Lopez P, Ayres LM, et al. Fast and slow oscillations of the electro-oculogram in Stargardt's disease. ARVO Abstract 2003; Program No. 5110.

76. Fishman GA, Farbman JS, Alexander KR. Delayed rod dark adaptation in patients with Stargardt's disease. *Ophthalmology* 1991;98:957–962.

77. Parisi V, Canu D, Iarossi G, et al. Altered recovery of macular function after bleaching in Stargardt's disease-fundus flavimaculatus: pattern VEP evidence. *Invest Ophthalmol Vis Sci* 2002;43:2741–2748.

78. Hargitai J, Somfai G, R.Vámos R, et al. Foveal thickness and macular volume changes in Stargardt macular dystrophy. ARVO Abstract 2003. Program No. 554.

79. Ergun E, Wirtitsch M, Hermann B, et al. Ultrahigh resolution optical coherence tomography in Stargardt's disease. ARVO Abstract 2003; Program No. 5108.

80. Eldred GE, Katz ML. Fluorophores of the human retinal pigment epithelium: separation and spectral characterization. *Exp Eye Res* 1988;47:71–86.

81. Delori FC, Dorey CK, Staurenghi G, et al. In vivo fluorescence of the ocular fundus exhibits retinal pigment epithelium lipofuscin characteristics. *Invest Ophthalmol Vis Sci* 1995;36:718–729.

82. von Rückmann A, Fitzke FW, Bird AC. Autofluorescence imaging of the human fundus. In: Marmor MF, Wolfensberger TJ, eds. *The retinal pigment epithelium: function and disease*, 2nd ed. Oxford: Oxford University Press, 1998:224–234.

83. von Rückmann A, Fitzke FW, Bird AC. Distribution of fundus autofluorescence with a scanning laser ophthalmoscope. *Br J Ophthalmol* 1995;79:407–412.

84. Delori FC, Goger DG, Dorey CK. Age-related accumulation and spatial distribution of lipofuscin in RPE of normal subjects. *Invest Ophthalmol Vis Sci* 2001;42:1855–1866.

85. Reinboth JJ, Gautschi K, Munz K, et al. Lipofuscin in the retina: quantitative assay for an unprecedented autofluorescent compound (pyridinium bis-retinoid, A2-E) of ocular age pigment. *Exp Eye Res* 1997;65:639–643.

86. Zhang X, Hargitai J, Tammur J, et al. Macular pigment and visual acuity in Stargardt macular dystrophy. *Graefes Arch Clin Exp Ophthalmol* 2002;240:802–809.

87. Gass JDM. *Stereoscopic atlas of macular diseases: diagnosis and treatment*, 4th ed. St. Louis: Mosby, 1997.

88. Zhang K, Bither PP, Park R, et al. A dominant Stargardt's macular dystrophy locus maps to chromosome 13q34. *Arch Ophthalmol* 1994;112:759–764.

89. Stone EM, Nichols BE, Kimura AE, et al. Clinical features of a Stargardt-like dominant progressive macular dystrophy with genetic linkage to chromosome 6q. *Arch Ophthalmol* 1994;112:765–772.

90. Kniazeva MF, Chiang MF, Cutting GR, et al. Clinical and genetic studies of an autosomal dominant cone-rod dystrophy with features of Stargardt disease. *Ophthalmic Genet* 1999;20:71–81.

91. Kniazeva M, Chiang MF, Morgan B, et al. A new locus for autosomal dominant Stargardt-like disease maps to chromosome 4. *Am J Hum Genet* 1999;64:1394–1399.

92. Del Buey MA, Huerva V, Minguez E, et al. Posttraumatic reaction in a case of fundus flavimaculatus with atrophic macular degeneration. *Ann Ophthalmol* 1993;25:219–221.

93. De Laey JJ, Verougstraete C. Hyperlipofuscinosis and subretinal fibrosis in Stargardt's disease. *Retina* 1995;15:399–406.

94. Ober RR, Limstrom SA, Simon RM. Traumatic retinopathy in Stargardt's disease. *Retina* 1997;17:251–254.

95. Gass JD, Hummer J. Focal retinal pigment epithelial dysplasia associated with fundus flavimaculatus. *Retina* 1999;19:297–301.

96. Szlyk JP, Fishman GA, Severing K, et al. Evaluation of driving performance in patients with juvenile macular dystrophies. *Arch Ophthalmol* 1993;111:207–212.

97. Pearlman JA, Au Eong KG, Kuhn F, et al. Airbags and eye injuries: epidemiology, spectrum of injury, and analysis of risk factors. *Surv Ophthalmol* 2001;46:234–242.

98. Klein R, Lewis R, Meyer S, et al. Subretinal neovascularization associated with fundus flavimaculatus. *Arch Ophthalmol* 1978; 96:2054.

99. Leveille A, Morse P, Burch J. Fundus flavimaculatus and subretinal neovascularization. *Ann Ophthalmol* 1982;14: 331–334.

100. Bottoni F, Fatigati G, Carlevaro D, et al. Fundus flavimaculatus and sudretinal neovascularization. *Graefes Arch Clin Exp Ophthalmol* 1992;230:498–500.

101. Valmaggia C, Niederberger H, Helbig H. Photodynamic therapy for choroidal neovascularization in fundus flavimaculatus. *Retina* 2002;22:111–113.

102. Potter MJ, Lee AS, Moshaver A. Improvement in macular function after epiretinal membrane removal in a patient with Stargardt disease. *Retina* 2000;20:560–561.

103. Szlyk JP, Fishman GA, Grover S, et al. Difficulty in performing everyday activities in patients with juvenile macular dystrophies: comparison with patients with retinitis pigmentosa. *Br J Ophthalmol* 1998;82:1372–1376.

104. Sun H, Nathans J. Mechanistic studies of ABCR, the ABC transporter in photoreceptor outer segments responsible for autosomal recessive Stargardt disease. *J Bioenerg Biomembr* 2001;33:523–530.

105. Sun H., Nathans J. ABCR, the ATP-binding cassette transporter responsible for Stargardt macular dystrophy, is an efficient target of all-trans-retinal-mediated photooxidative damage in vitro: implications for retinal disease. *J Biol Chem* 2001;276:11766–11774.

106. Sun H, Molday RS, Nathans J. Retinal stimulates ATP hydrolysis by purified and reconstituted ABCR, the photoreceptor-specific ATP-binding cassette transporter responsible for Stargardt disease. *J Biol Chem* 1999;274:8269–8281.

107. Jampol LM. Antioxidants, zinc, and age-related macular degeneration: results and recommendations. *Arch Ophthalmol* 2001;119:1533–1534.

108. Sparrow JR, Vollmer-Snarr HR, Zhou J, et al. A2E-epoxides damage DNA in retinal pigment epithelial cells. Vitamin E and other antioxidants inhibit A2E-epoxide formation. *J Biol Chem* 2003;278:18207–18213.

MITOCHONDRIAL AND PEROXISOMAL DISORDERS

ITAY CHOWERS
JOHN B. KERRISON

THE MITOCHONDRIA

Mitochondria are cytoplasmic organelles that synthesize adenosine triphosphate (ATP), the energy currency of the cell, through the process of oxidative phosphorylation. In oxidative phosphorylation, an electrochemical gradient is established across the inner mitochondrial membrane by passing electrons to successively lower energy states while transferring hydrogen into the intermembrane space. ATP is produced as hydrogen passes down this electrochemical gradient, back into the mitochondrial matrix, in a reaction coupled to the phosphorylation of adenosine diphosphate.

The mitochondria are thought to originate from bacteria that developed a symbiotic relationship with larger cells. Human cells contain many mitochondria, and each mitochondrion contains several circular DNA molecules of approximately 16,000 base pairs (16 kilobases or 16 kb). The mitochondrial genome encodes 13 proteins involved in ATP synthesis, two ribosomal RNAs, and 22 transfer RNAs involved in mitochondrial protein synthesis. However, the vast majority of mitochondrial proteins are encoded by nuclear DNA, synthesized in the cytoplasm, and transported to the mitochondria.

Mitochondria and mitochondrial DNA (mtDNA) are transmitted to a fertilized oocyte exclusively from the mother. Thus, the pattern of inheritance does not conform to classic rules of Mendelian inheritance, the law of segregation, and the law of independent assortment. All offspring of female carriers of an mtDNA mutation are at risk for the disease while offspring of male carriers are not at risk. In transmitting a population of mitochondria to the cytoplasm of each oocyte, maternal germ cells may contribute both normal and mutated mtDNA to a single offspring, a characteristic termed heteroplasmy (as opposed to homoplasmy, which means that all are normal or all have the mutation). In some cases, the proportion of mutated mtDNA may influence susceptibility to disease or penetrance.

Mitochondrial Disorders

Both optic neuropathy and retinopathy can be caused by mtDNA mutations. While Leber hereditary optic neuropathy (LHON) is caused by mtDNA point mutations, the importance of the mitochondria in optic nerve function is further underscored by the discovery that autosomal dominant optic atrophy is caused by mutations in a nuclear gene encoding a mitochondrial protein. Degenerative retinopathies can also be associated with mtDNA mutations (1–11). Pigmentary retinopathy is observed in Kearns-Sayre syndrome (KSS) (7,9,10), chronic progressive external ophthalmoplegia (CPEO), mitochondrial myopathies without external ophthalmoplegia (12,13), mitochondrial encephalomyopathy overlap syndrome (5), and neuropathy ataxia retinitis pigmentosa (NARP) syndrome (6,14,15). Salt-and-pepper retinopathy is the predominant fundus phenotype in these diseases, but a typical retinitis pigmentosa (RP)-like retinopathy, other types of retinal pigment epithelium (RPE) changes, and choriocapillaris atrophy may occur (5,12,13,16). Macular abnormalities are frequently associated with the pigmentary retinopathy, usually as hyperpigmentation and/or hypopigmentation (8).

LEBER'S HEREDITARY OPTIC NEUROPATHY
Prevalence

The prevalence of LHON was estimated to be in the range of 1:25,000 to 1:40,000 in two studies preformed in northern Europe. LHON is considered as the most common mitochondrial disease in caucasians (16a,16b).

Leber's hereditary optic neuropathy, named after the German ophthalmologist Theodor Leber (1840–1917), was recognized as a familial neuroophthalmologic disease in the late 1800s. Like other mitochondrial diseases, LHON is maternally inherited. It is characterized by bilateral, simultaneous or sequential, acute vision loss, typically occurring in young adult males.

Genetics and Pathophysiology

LHON is associated with 18 different mtDNA missense mutations, occurring in genes encoding Complex I, III, or IV subunit proteins of the mitochondrial respiratory chain (17). Of the 18 alleles associated with LHON, those at nucleotide positions 3460 (18), 11778 (19–21), and 14484 (22,23) are found in more than 90% of the patients (24) and may be present alone or in combination with additional mutations in LHON patients. These three mutations (3460, 11778, and 14484) are considered the primary mutations associated with LHON, with the 11778 mutation being the most common.

Many patients harboring mtDNA mutations do not have a family history of LHON. The percentage of patients with affected family members is 43%, 78%, and 65% for mutations in nucleotides 11778, 3460, and 14484, respectively (20,23).

Some functional studies performed on tissues from LHON patients harboring the 11778 or 3460 mutations have revealed reduced respiration in muscle, lymphoblast lines, and platelets, demonstrating the functional significance of these mutations. However, other studies failed to show any functional significance for these mutations (17,25), and thus the pathophysiology of LHON is still not well understood.

Environmental Factors and Additional Modifying Factors

An intriguing phenomenon in LHON is the higher risk of developing vision loss in male carriers in comparison with female carriers of the pathogenic mtDNA mutations (24,26). This characteristic is also associated with specific mutations, observed to be 80% for the 11778 mutation, 33% to 67% for the 3460 mutation, and 68% for the 14484 mutation (20,23,27). Of note, although more than 90% of the LHON patients in Asia harbor the 11778 mutation, only 58% of the patients are males (28).

Although a genetic modifier on the X chromosome is an attractive hypothesis, linkage analysis has failed to identify influential genes on the X chromosome that may explain the male predominance (29–32). Hormonal factors may contribute to gender bias in LHON, although this hypothesis has not been proven. Smoking, alcohol consumption, and diet have also been proposed (18,33) as additional risk factors for vision loss in LHON patients, but there is no evidence to support these as risk factors, particularly in children (26,34,35).

Ocular Manifestations

Visual loss typically occurs in the third or fourth decade but has been observed as early as age 1 year to as late in life as the eighth decade. Vision loss often begins painlessly in one eye but may be bilateral and simultaneous. Some individuals subjectively describe vision loss as sudden and complete, others describe progression over the course of a few weeks,

and yet others experience gradually deteriorating visual acuity over years (20). In almost all patients vision loss develops in the fellow eye, usually within 6 months of the vision loss in the first eye. Typically, no other symptoms occur at the time of vision loss.

The final visual acuity may range from 20/50 to no light perception but is commonly worse than 20/200 in each eye and associated with bilateral central scotomata (18,20,23,24). Both the final visual acuity and the recovery rate are associated with specific mutations. For example, patients affected by the more common 11778 mutation are more likely to have final visual acuity of no light perception and have only 4% chance for visual recovery, while patients with the 14484 mutation, which is associated with a more favorable outcome, are more likely to have a final visual acuity in the range of counting fingers and have up to a 36% chance of visual recovery (20,23,36). Prognosis for visual recovery is also higher in patients with onset of vision loss in the first or second decade of life (24).

On ophthalmoscopy, the optic nerve may appear normal or have a characteristic appearance described as a triad of circumpapillary telangiectasia, swelling of the nerve fiber layer around the disc, and absence of leakage on fluorescein angiography (1) (Fig. 9-1). The optic neuropathy progresses to optic atrophy with nonglaucomatous cupping, pallor, and arteriolar attenuation (37). Interestingly, some of the nonaffected carriers of mutations associated with LHON may show some of the ophthalmoscopic abnormalities characterizing their affected relatives

Systemic Manifestations

Neurologic abnormalities such as pathologic reflexes, mild cerebellar ataxia, tremor, movement disorders, muscle wasting, and distal sensory neuropathy might be associated with LHON. In some pedigrees, more severe neurologic deficits

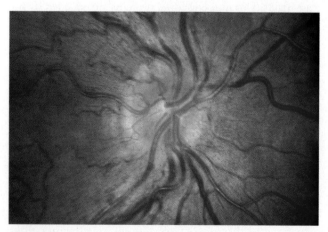

FIGURE 9-1. Leber's optic neuropathy disc in a patient harboring the 11778 mtDNA mutation demonstrating circumpapillary telangiectasia and swelling of the nerve fiber layer around the disc. (Photo courtesy of N. R. Miller.)

can be present including dystonia, spasticity, and encephalopathic episodes (38,39). In addition to neurologic abnormalities, some patients and their maternal relatives can have cardiac conduction defects including preexcitation syndromes (Wolff-Parkinson-White, Lown-Ganong-Levine) (40) or QT interval prolongation (37). Thus, LHON patients should undergo electrocardiography.

Differential Diagnosis

The differential diagnosis includes optic neuritis, ischemic optic neuropathy, compressive optic neuropathy, infiltrative optic neuropathy, and neoplasm. Definitive diagnosis is made by genetic testing.

Management

No treatments are available at the present time to prevent vision loss, arrest the progression of vision loss, or restore vision. However, a clinical trial is underway to assess the efficacy of brimonidine tartrate ophthalmic solution 0.15% (Alphagan P) in the prevention of vision loss in patients who have experienced unilateral vision loss from LHON and are at high risk for vision loss in the fellow eye.

Another potential future treatment technique for LHON is gene therapy. A gene-replacement technique in cell culture has been described in which a defect in complex I function in cells harboring the 11778 mutation was restored (41). The *in vivo* feasibility, efficacy, and safety of such a technique are unclear.

NEUROPATHY ATAXIA RETINITIS PIGMENTOSA AND LEIGH SYNDROMES

The NARP and Leigh syndromes are rare diseases with a few dozen of cases reported in the literature. Both diseases are associated with the same mtDNA mutation at nucleotide position 8993, although Leigh syndrome is also associated with mutations in several nuclear genes.

Genetics and Systemic Manifestations

The T to G point mutation at nucleotide 8993 of mtDNA causes a substitution of a highly conserved leucine by an arginine residue in the ATPase 6 protein (15). This is a heteroplasmic mutation, meaning that both normal and mutant mtDNA are found in the same subject, but the proportion of the mutant mtDNA is different among patients. Usually, a high proportion of mutant mtDNA is associated with severe clinical manifestations (2,42,43). Two clinical syndromes were described in association with the 8993 mtDNA mutation. The first, subacute necrotizing encephalomyopathy or Leigh syndrome, is a severe disease, with patients showing developmental delay, ataxia, psy-

chomotor regression, seizures, peripheral neuropathy, and optic atrophy. Onset is usually during infancy with progression to death within months to years. The 8993 mutation was found to be a common cause of Leigh syndrome, and most of the patients had more than 90% of mutant mtDNA (3,42). The second entity, NARP syndrome, first reported by Holt et al. in 1990 (15), is usually milder than Leigh syndrome. Patients show a variety of clinical manifestations such as migraine, sensory neuropathy, proximal muscle weakness, ataxia, seizures, dementia, and pigmentary retinopathy (2,8,15,16,44). Patients with the NARP syndrome usually carry around 80% of mutant mtDNA. At levels below 75% carriers may show pigmentary retinopathy, suffer from migraines, or be totally asymptomatic (2,43).

In some patients with Leigh syndrome, mutations have also been found in nuclear genes, including *Surf1* and other cytochrome oxidase assembly genes (45,46). However, mutations have not been found in many Leigh syndrome patients even after extensive molecular testing.

Ocular Manifestations

The ocular abnormalities in NARP syndrome were reported in most cases as typical RP or as pigmentary retinopathy (2,15,43,44) (Fig. 9-2). Puddu et al. (47) described three patients with NARP syndrome, two of whom had ocular manifestations. The fundus examination showed bone spicule pigmentation in the midperiphery and despite being described as RP, the electroretinogram (ERG) findings were normal except for subnormal photopic responses. In another report, Ortiz et al. (16) described eight patients from two families with the 8993 mutation in whom the ocular manifestations ranged from a mild salt-and-pepper retinopathy to severe RP-like changes with maculopathy. Four of these patients underwent ERG examination. One showed normal results and three revealed rod–cone-type dysfunction. In five patients who had perimetry, four had normal visual fields and one had a paracentral scotoma.

Chowers et al. (6) described three members from a family harboring the 8993 mtDNA mutation in whom great variability in the clinical manifestations of the disease was observed. Two of the three patients had ocular abnormalities that were different from classic RP. The clinical findings, visual fields, and ERG were typical of cone–rod dystrophy in one of the patients and progressive cone dystrophy in another patient. Other retinal findings in NARP include a bull's eye maculopathy and rod–cone type of retinal dystrophy (16).

As discussed, there is great variability in the ocular and systemic manifestations among patients carrying the mtDNA 8993 mutation. Several factors could account for the spectrum of abnormalities observed. First, the burden of mutant mtDNA in a particular tissue may vary thus influencing phenotype with a higher proportion of mutant

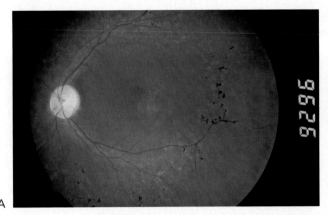
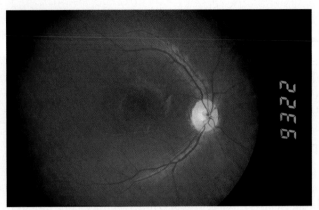

A   B

FIGURE 9-2. Color fundus photographs of two NARP patients demonstrating the variable ocular manifestation of the disease. **(A)** A 16-year-old male NARP patient with blots of pigment along with multiple small retinal scars, narrowing of the blood vessels, and pigmentary changes in the fovea. The optic disc appears normal. This patient had reduced visual acuity, nyctalopia, and showed bull's eye maculopathy on fluorescein angiogram. The visual field of this eye had central and paracentral scotomas, and ERG showed decreased cone- and rod-derived amplitudes. **(B)** The sister of the patient presented in panel A was 12 years old at that time. She manifested a bull's eye maculopathy with temporal optic disk pallor. No pigmentary changes were apparent. This patient had mild reduction of visual acuity and decreased cone-derived (but not rod-derived) ERG responses. This patient also had episodic ataxia and mild mental retardation.

mtDNA in blood lymphocytes being a marker for more severe clinical manifestations. However, Chowers et al. (6) observed that patients with a lower percentage of mutant mtDNA in the blood lymphocytes can have a more severe ocular disease compared with patients with higher proportion of mutant mtDNA. This can be partially explained if the proportion of mutant mtDNA in the retinas differ from that in the blood or other tissues, especially the central nervous system (CNS), but such differences have not yet been demonstrated (43). Differences among patients may also depend on age. Ortiz et al. (16) described two patients, aged 12 and 14 years, who suffered from NARP syndrome and had a rod–cone type of ERG dysfunction. The retinopathy of these patients was much less advanced than that of patients reported by Chowers et al. who were of a similar age but with a predominantly cone dysfunction. Thus, patients with the NARP syndrome may manifest either rod- or cone-dominant retinal dystrophy at a similar age. It is likely that other factors, not yet understood, modulate the phenotypic expression of the 8993 mtDNA mutation. In support of this, two of the three reported NARP pedigrees undergoing ERG had predominantly cone dysfunction, while the third pedigree had predominantly rod dysfunction. This finding cannot be explained by the differences in age, stages of the disease, or percentage of mutant mtDNA among families.

Diagnosis

Diagnosis is based on identification of the typical combination of ocular and systemic manifestations along with the mitochondrial inheritance pattern. Ancillary tests may in-

clude ERG, color vision, and fluorescein angiography. Definitive diagnosis is made by identification of the 8993 mtDNA mutation.

Management

No treatment has been shown to be of benefit in arresting the progression of retinal dystrophy in patients carrying the mtDNA 8993 mutation. Although controversial, one may consider extending from the findings of a potential beneficial effect for vitamin A palmitate in slowing the progression of retinal degeneration in patients with retinitis pigmentosa, but no evidence supports this. In addition, patients should be referred to a clinical geneticist for evaluation of medical and family history because although the 8993 mutation is transmitted from mother to each of her offspring, the proportion of mutant mtDNA in each offspring can differ considerably from that of the mother and with it the clinical manifestations.

KEARNS-SAYRE SYNDROME

Genetics and Pathogenesis

A mitochondrial defect was suspected to underlie the KSS based on the inheritance pattern observed in several affected families (48). Indeed, it was later found that these disorders are associated with mitochondrial DNA deletions (10,49). The deletions typically are 1.3 to 7.6 kb in length, but there is an increased prevalence of the 4.9-kb deletion. Interestingly, identical mtDNA deletions can lead to CPEO or KSS (with its additional systemic manifestations), and this may at least in part depend on the distribution of mtDNA deletions in different tissues.

It is noteworthy that PEO associated with mitochondrial DNA deletions can be transmitted in autosomal-dominant or autosomal-recessive modes of inheritance. Three genes are associated with autosomal-dominant PEO: adenine nucleotide translocator-1 (*ANT1*), which is located on chromosome 4 and encodes a muscle-specific adenine nucleotide translocator; Twinkle, which is located on chromosome 10 and encodes a helicase; and polymerase gamma (*POLG*), which is located on chromosome 15 and encodes the alpha subunit of polymerase gamma. Mutations in *POLG* are also associated with the autosomal-recessive form of PEO. All three genes are involved in mtDNA replication; thus, alterations in their function might lead to mtDNA deletions (49a). Genetic analysis in these patients usually finds multiple concurrent mitochondrial mutations, suggesting that the nuclear DNA mutation induces instability of mitochondrial DNA replication (50–52).

Ocular Manifestations

KSS is characterized by triad of external ophthalmoplegia (CPEO), pigmentary retinopathy, and heart block (9,53). Onset is in the first or second decade of life. CPEO is characterized by a bilateral symmetric ptosis associated with ophthalmoplegia and orbicularis oculi weakness. In addition, KSS patients manifest an atypical pigmentary retinopathy in which the macula is often the first part of the retina to be affected followed by the retina periphery. In some patients, all parts of the retina are affected simultaneously. Histology of a retina from KSS patient showed atrophy of the retinal pigment epithelium and outer retina that was most marked posteriorly (7). In addition to the different retinal involvement pattern, KSS also differs from classic RP in that there is usually no blood vessel attenuation and no waxy optic nerve appearance accompanying the pigmentary retinopathy. Furthermore, visual acuity, visual fields, and ERG are usually only mildly affected.

Systemic Manifestations

Neurologic manifestations in KSS may include cerebellar ataxia, hearing loss, dementia, and weakness of facial, pharyngeal, trunk and extremity muscles. Heart block is a characteristic finding (9,53,54).

Diagnosis

Diagnosis is based on the typical ocular, neurologic, and cardiac manifestations. Lumbar puncture can demonstrate an increased cerebrospinal fluid protein level (the underlying cause of which is still unknown). Electrocardiography is useful in identifying heart block, and genetic testing can establish the diagnosis in cases of doubt.

Management

While there is no cure, careful correction of ptosis or strabismus may be beneficial in selected cases. The cardiac conduction defect may be life threatening and is treated with a pacemaker.

MITOCHONDRIAL ENCEPHALOMYOPATHY, LACTIC ACIDOSIS, AND STROKELIKE EPISODES SYNDROME

While vision loss in mitochondrial genetic disorders more commonly occurs from retinal degeneration or optic nerve disease, vision loss can occur from damage to the retrochiasmal visual pathways as in mitochondrial encephalomyopathy, lactic acidosis, and strokelike episodes (MELAS) (55,56), a condition that is caused by a mutation at nucleotide position 3243 affecting the mitochondrial encoded gene for leucine tRNA. Other features included diabetes mellitus and deafness. Of note, the *A3243G* mutation may also be associated with a pigmentary retinopathy or optic neuropathy as well as CPEO (57).

Ocular Manifestations

Patients can have ptosis, external ophthalmoplegia, iris atrophy, cataract, pigmentary retinopathy with maculopathy, RPE and choroidal atrophy, and optic atrophy (58). Rummelt and colleagues have demonstrated histologic findings corroborating the clinical manifestations in two eyes of a patient with the MELAS syndrome and the mtDNA 3243 mutation, including posterior subcapsular cataract, photoreceptor degeneration, and RPE atrophy and hyperpigmentation. In addition, multiple cell types showed enlarged and abnormal mitochondria.

THE PEROXISOMES

Peroxisomes are cytoplasmic organelles that encompass several biochemical pathways, some related to energy production. Unlike mitochondria, peroxisomes do not contain DNA although they do replicate by division. Both catabolic and anabolic processes take place within the peroxisomes. Major functions of the peroxisomes are oxidation of very long fatty acids and amino acids. These reactions lead to the production of hydrogen peroxide, which is used for oxidation of additional molecules or converted to water and oxygen by the enzyme catalase.

Proteins required for peroxisome assembly are targeted to the peroxisome by either carboxy (peroxisome targeting signal 1 or PTS1) or amino (PTS2) terminus targeting signals. Specific translocation complexes then mediate their transport into the peroxisome.

Peroxisomal Disorders

Peroxisomal diseases are rare disorders affecting multiple tissues including the eye. These diseases have overlapping clinical manifestations and are classified into two categories. In peroxisome biogenesis disorders (PBD), peroxisomal assembly is defective due to abnormal localization of proteins normally targeted to the peroxisomes. This results in severe diseases, three of which commonly affect the retina: Zellweger syndrome (ZS), neonatal adrenoleukodystrophy (NALD), and infantile Refsum disease (IRD). While these three diseases were described as separate entities before the underlying peroxisomal defect was realized, recent advances in identifying the underlying molecular defects as well as better understanding of the resulting biochemical defects, suggest that all three are part of one spectrum in which ZS represents the more severe form, NALD an intermediate form, and IRD the least severe form (59).

A second group of peroxisomal disorders results from a defect in a single gene that results in abnormal function of the peroxisome but does not affect its assembly. This group includes entities such as X-linked adrenoleukodystrophy, primary hyperoxaluria type 1, and classical Refsum disease. X-linked adrenoleukodystrophy is associated with mutation in the *ABCD1* gene, which results in a defect in peroxisomal beta oxidation. This leads to the accumulation of saturated very-long-chain fatty acids in all tissues of the body with clinical manifestations which are primarily related to the adrenal cortex, CNS myelin (including visual disturbance), and Leydig cell dysfunction.

Prevalence

Peroxisomal disorders are rare. Moser recorded (60) the relative prevalence of the different peroxisomal disorders in 1345 patients with peroxisomal diseases. In his series, X-linked adrenoleukodystrophy was the most common disorder (1184 cases), followed by ZS (105 cases) and NALD (54 cases). Refsum disease and several other rare peroxisomal disorders were diagnosed in the remaining patients.

The following paragraphs will consider the three PBDs affecting the retina combined, followed by description of other peroxisomal disorders affecting the retina.

PEROXISOMAL BIOGENESIS DISORDERS AFFECTING THE RETINA

Genetics and Pathogenesis

PBDs are autosomal recessive diseases associated with defects in several different peroxins (PEX), which are proteins required for peroxisome biogenesis. More than 20 genes related to peroxisome biogenesis have been identified. PBDs have been associated with mutations in several of these genes, including peroxin-1 (*PEX1*) on chromosome 7, per-

oxin-2 (*PEX2*) on chromosome 8, peroxin-3 (*PEX3*) on chromosome 6, peroxin-5 (*PEX5*) on chromosome 12, peroxin-6 (*PEX6*) on chromosome 6, and peroxin-12 (*PEX12*) on chromosome 17. It is also suspected that additional loci for PBD exist, although the causative genes have not been identified so far.

In many instances, mutations in the same peroxin can lead to any of the PBD phenotypes, although defects in some peroxins are only associated with the more severe ZS phenotype (59). Failure of peroxisome biogenesis is thought to lead to the severe clinical manifestations resulting from absence of basic metabolic functions normally carried by peroxisomes.

The generation of mouse models for PBD has provided interesting insights into the pathogenesis of these diseases. Disruption of *Pex2, Pex5,* and *Pex11b* in mouse models can result in findings similar to PBD in humans including neuronal migration defects, hypotonia, developmental delay, and neonatal lethality (61). However, in mice with *Pex11b* disruption, there is no detectable defect in peroxisomal protein import, and only mild defects in peroxisomal fatty acid beta-oxidation and peroxisomal ether lipid biosynthesis are present (61). These findings are intriguing in that the PBD phenotype can manifest in association with PEX mutations with apparently intact peroxisomal biogenesis.

Ocular Manifestations

Patients with ZS show a variety of ocular manifestations including corneal clouding, posterior embryotoxon, glaucoma, cataract, RPE clumping, attenuation of retinal blood vessels, and optic disc pallor or hypoplasia (62). In IRD, the predominant findings are in the posterior segment where arteriolar attenuation and pigment clumping are present.

The histopathology in ZS, NALD, and IRD shows loss of photoreceptors and other retinal cells and infiltration of macrophages laden with cytoplasmic inclusion bodies. Similar finding were detected in other areas of the CNS.

Systemic Manifestation

ZS (cerebro–hepato–renal) and NALD present at infancy while IRD can manifest during the first decade of life. All PBD are associated with variety of severe systemic and ocular abnormalities. Death in ZS occurs within a few months of birth, while NALD patients live 4 years on average.

ZS patients present with skeletal and dysmorphic features including talipes equinovarus, limb contractures, high forehead, epicanthal folds, hypoplastic supraorbital ridge, micrognathia, high arched palate, and hypertelorism. While some of these findings can be present in IRD, they are absent in NALD. Neurologic manifestations include seizures, psychomotor retardation, hypotonia, and reduced hearing. Additional abnormalities include hepatomegaly, jaundice, and congenital heart defects. NALD is characterized by milder manifestations compared with ZS. Patients have adrenal and cortical atrophy but do not develop adrenal insufficiency. IRD patients share similar systemic findings but are less severe (59).

Differential Diagnosis/Diagnosis

The differential diagnosis includes a long list of other inborn errors of metabolism sharing the systemic manifestations. NALD may be confused with other causes of decreased vision in infancy including Leber's congenital amaurosis and neuronal ceroid lipofuscinosis.

Diagnosis is based on identifying the combination of typical systemic and ocular manifestations mentioned previously. Ancillary tests may include an ERG, which is severely reduced or extinguished in all three diseases. Measurements of plasma very-long-chain fatty acids, pipecolic acid, bile acid, and phytanic acid are typically increased while the plasmalogen level in red blood cells is reduced. Genetic testing and identification of the characteristic mutations can establish the diagnosis but are not available as a clinical diagnostic service in most cases.

Management

There is no treatment for PBD. Management is mainly supportive.

REFSUM DISEASE

Genetics and Pathogenesis

Refsum disease is an autosomal-recessive disorder associated with mutations in either phytanoyl–coenzyme A hydroxylase (*PAHX*) or the peroxin-7 (*PEX7*) genes (63–66). The resulting biochemical defects leads to accumulation of the branched chain fatty acid–phytanic acid (3,7,11,15-tetramethyl-hexadecanic acid) by perturbation of its normal degradation pathway.

Ocular Manifestations

Ocular manifestations are characterized by RP-like changes including nyctalopia, progressively constricted visual fields, granular type of pigmentary retinopathy, and attenuated blood vessels (62,67–70). Retinal histology shows atrophy of the retinal RPE and lipid-laden RPE cells in areas were RPE has not yet atrophied. The outer nuclear and plexiform layers are also atrophic, the inner nuclear layer thinned, and the ganglion cell number is decreased (71–73).

Systemic Manifestations

Refsum disease usually manifests between the first and third decades. Multiple systems are involved. Neurologic manifestations include peripheral polyneuropathy and cerebellar signs such as ataxia, anosmia, and decreased hearing. Additional manifestations are cardiac arrhythmia (that can be life threatening), skeletal malformations (mostly epiphyseal dysplasia), and ichthyosislike skin changes (68–70,73–75).

Diagnosis

Diagnosis is based on typical clinical findings. Ancillary tests may include kinetic perimetry, which is useful in documenting visual field loss and in following its progression, and ERG, which shows decreased photopic and scotopic responses. Blood levels of phytanic acid are typically elevated (76,77). Mutation detection is possible, but is still performed mainly as a research tool.

Management

Refsum disease is a rare case of an RP-like disease that is amenable to treatment. As phytanic acid cannot be synthesized in humans, its accumulation in Refsum disease patients depends on exogenous intake. Accordingly, a diet free of foods containing phytol, phytanic acid, or their precursors leads to reduced phytanic acid levels in the blood and to clinical improvement. Plasmapheresis to remove phytanic acid can be an alternative effective approach to diet in preventing the clinical manifestations of Refsum disease (78–81). It is thus imperative that Refsum disease diagnosis be made as early as possible.

PRIMARY HYPEROXALURIA TYPE 1

Primary hyperoxaluria type 1 (PHT1) is a rare peroxisomal autosomal-recessive disease in which a defect in the gene encoding the enzyme alanine-glyoxylate aminotransferase (*AGXT*), which is normally present only in liver peroxisomes, results in accumulation of oxalate (82).

Urologic manifestations first predominate with high urinary oxalate excretion and nephrolithiasis, which are followed by nephrocalcinosis and renal failure. Oxalate also deposits in additional organs including the eye. Untreated, the disease leads to death from renal failure in childhood or early adulthood.

The characteristic ocular findings are retinal pigmentary changes. These were found in 8 of 24 PHT1 patients in one large series, and were not associated with significantly decreased visual acuity (83). The findings range from multiple small parafoveal subretinal black rings with a white center in mild cases, to a large black geographic shape lesion underling the macula area with a whitish subretinal area in more severe cases (83). These black areas represent hyperplastic and hypertrophic RPE reaction to oxalate deposition, while the white center may represent choroidal neovascularization (84–86). Optic disc pallor was also reported in patients with PHT1 and may be associated with papilledema or vascular decompensation secondary to oxalate deposition. In cases in which the optic nerve is involved, visual acuity was markedly reduced (83). Histologic findings in the eye demonstrated oxalate crystal deposition in multiple tissues among them the RPE, retina, choroid, and conjunctiva. While as predicted by the clinical findings, histology showed that oxalate is primarily found in the RPE, but in some eyes, oxalate deposition may be primarily in the outer retina layers (85–87).

Management

Decreasing oxalate load in the body is one approach, although kidney transplantation is associated with a high recurrence rate, liver transplantation, when successful, is a definitive treatment for this disease (88).

SUMMARY

Mitochondrial and peroxisomal disorders have been the subject of intense research in recent years. Multiple genes associated with these disorders have been identified, and significant insight into the pathogenesis has been gained, leading to new classifications and to development of diagnostic genetic tests to many of these disorders. On the other hand, the pathogenesis of the disease described in this chapter is still unclear in many instances despite the discovery of the causative gene. The variable disease course in carriers of the same mutations suggests that additional yet unrecognized modifying factors play an important role in these disorders.

Furthermore, the complex and unique inheritance mode of mitochondrial disorders, heteroplasmy in particular, hampered the potential for prenatal diagnosis in many instances. For example, although all offspring of a mother carrying the NARP-causing mtDNA 8993 point mutation will also carry the same defect, the phenotype may vary considerably between offspring, so that while some may be asymptomatic, others may be severely affected. In this instance, determining the fraction of mitochondria carrying the mutation by prenatal diagnostic testing will not necessarily reliably reflect the fraction in target tissue for this disorder such as the retina and brain. Thus, basing pregnancy termination on such diagnostic testes raises complex ethical and moral issues.

REFERENCES

1. Nikoskelainen EK, Huoponen K, Juvonen V, et al. Ophthalmologic findings in Leber hereditary optic neuropathy, with special reference to mtDNA mutations. *Ophthalmology* 1996;103: 504–514.
2. Tatuch Y, Pagon RA, Vlcek B, et al. The 8993 mtDNA mutation: heteroplasmy and clinical presentation in three families. *Eur J Hum Genet* 1994;2:35–43.
3. Santorelli FM, Shanske S, Macaya A, et al. The mutation at nt 8993 of mitochondrial DNA is a common cause of Leigh's syndrome. *Ann Neurol* 1993;34:827–834.
4. Santorelli FM, Mak SC, Vazquez-Acevedo M, et al. A novel mitochondrial DNA point mutation associated with mitochondrial encephalocardiomyopathy. *Biochem Biophys Res Commun* 1995; 216:835–840.
5. Chang TS, Johns DR, Walker D, de la Cruz Z, et al. Ocular clinicopathologic study of the mitochondrial encephalomyopathy overlap syndromes. *Arch Ophthalmol* 1993;111:1254–1262.
6. Chowers I, Lerman-Sagie T, Elpeleg ON, et al. Cone and rod dysfunction in the NARP syndrome. *Br J Ophthalmol* 1999; 83:190–193.
7. Eagle RC, Jr., Hedges TR, Yanoff M. The atypical pigmentary retinopathy of Kearns-Sayre syndrome. A light and electron microscopic study. *Ophthalmology* 1982;89:1433–1440.
8. Heher KL, Johns DR. A maculopathy associated with the 15257 mitochondrial DNA mutation. *Arch Ophthalmol* 1993;111: 1495–1499.
9. Kearns T, Sayre G. Retinitis pigmentosa, external ophthalmoplegia and complete heart block; unusual syndrome with histologic study in one of two cases. *Arch Ophthalmol* 1958;60:280–289.
10. Moraes CT, DiMauro S, Zeviani M, et al. Mitochondrial DNA deletions in progressive external ophthalmoplegia and Kearns-Sayre syndrome. *N Engl J Med* 1989;320:1293–1299.
11. Santorelli FM, Tanji K, Kulikova R, et al. Identification of a novel mutation in the mtDNA ND5 gene associated with MELAS. *Biochem Biophys Res Commun* 1997;238:326–328.
12. Mullie MA, Harding AE, Petty RK, et al. The retinal manifestations of mitochondrial myopathy. A study of 22 cases. *Arch Ophthalmol* 1985;103:1825–1830.
13. Bosche J, Hammerstein W, Neuen-Jacob E, Schober R. Variation in retinal changes and muscle pathology in mitochondriopathies. *Graefes Arch Clin Exp Ophthalmol* 1989;227:578–583.
14. Kerrison JB, Biousse V, Newman NJ. Retinopathy of NARP syndrome. *Arch Ophthalmol* 2000;118:298–299.
15. Holt IJ, Harding AE, Petty RK, et al. A new mitochondrial disease associated with mitochondrial DNA heteroplasmy. *Am J Hum Genet* 1990;46:428–433.
16. Ortiz RG, Newman NJ, Shoffner JM, et al. Variable retinal and neurologic manifestations in patients harboring the mitochondrial DNA 8993 mutation. *Arch Ophthalmol* 1993;111: 1525–1530.
16a. Huoponen K. Leber hereditary optic neuropathy: clinical and molecular genetic findings. *Neurogenetics* 2001;3:119–125.
16b. Man PY, Griffiths PG, Brown DT, et al. The epidemiology of Leber hereditary optic neuropathy in the North East of England. *Am J Hum Genet* 2003;72:333–339.
17. Larsson NG, Andersen O, Holme E, et al. Leber's hereditary optic neuropathy and complex I deficiency in muscle. *Ann Neurol* 1991;30:701–708.
18. Johns DR, Smith KH, Miller NR. Leber's hereditary optic neuropathy. Clinical manifestations of the 3460 mutation. *Arch Ophthalmol* 1992;110:1577–1581.
19. Wallace DC, Singh G, Lott MT, et al. Mitochondrial DNA mutation associated with Leber's hereditary optic neuropathy. *Science* 1988;242:1427–1430.
20. Newman NJ, Lott MT, Wallace DC. The clinical characteristics of pedigrees of Leber's hereditary optic neuropathy with the 11778 mutation. *Am J Ophthalmol* 1991;111:750–762.
21. Singh G, Lott MT, Wallace DC. A mitochondrial DNA mutation as a cause of Leber's hereditary optic neuropathy. *N Engl J Med* 1989;320:1300–1305.
22. Johns DR, Neufeld MJ, Park RD. An ND-6 mitochondrial DNA mutation associated with Leber hereditary optic neuropathy. *Biochem Biophys Res Commun* 1992;187:1551–1557.
23. Johns DR, Heher KL, Miller NR, et al. Leber's hereditary optic neuropathy. Clinical manifestations of the 14484 mutation. *Arch Ophthalmol* 1993;111:495–498.

24. Riordan-Eva P, Sanders MD, Govan GG, et al. The clinical features of Leber's hereditary optic neuropathy defined by the presence of a pathogenic mitochondrial DNA mutation. *Brain* 1995;118(Pt 2):319–337.

25. Majander A, Huoponen K, Savontaus ML, et al. Electron transfer properties of NADH:ubiquinone reductase in the ND1/3460 and the ND4/11778 mutations of the Leber hereditary optic neuroretinopathy (LHON). *FEBS Lett* 1991;292: 289–292.

26. Kerrison JB, Miller NR, Hsu F, et al. A case-control study of tobacco and alcohol consumption in Leber hereditary optic neuropathy. *Am J Ophthalmol* 2000;130:803–812.

27. Johns DR, Smith KH, Savino PJ, et al. Leber's hereditary optic neuropathy. Clinical manifestations of the 15257 mutation. *Ophthalmology* 1993;100:981–986.

28. Mashima Y, Hiida Y, Oguchi Y, et al. High frequency of mutations at position 11778 in mitochondrial ND4 gene in Japanese families with Leber's hereditary optic neuropathy. *Hum Genet* 1993;92:101–102.

29. Chalmers RM, Davis MB, Sweeney MG, et al. Evidence against an X-linked visual loss susceptibility locus in Leber hereditary optic neuropathy. *Am J Hum Genet* 1996;59:103–108.

30. Jacobi FK, Leo-Kottler B, Mittelviefhaus K, et al. Segregation patterns and heteroplasmy prevalence in Leber's hereditary optic neuropathy. *Invest Ophthalmol Vis Sci* 2001;42:1208–1214.

31. Oostra RJ, Kemp S, Bolhuis PA, et al. No evidence for 'skewed' inactivation of the X-chromosome as cause of Leber's hereditary optic neuropathy in female carriers. *Hum Genet* 1996;97: 500–505.

32. Sweeney MG, Davis MB, Lashwood A, et al. Evidence against an X-linked locus close to DXS7 determining visual loss susceptibility in British and Italian families with Leber hereditary optic neuropathy. *Am J Hum Genet* 1992;51:741–748.

33. Cullom ME, Heher KL, Miller NR, et al. Leber's hereditary optic neuropathy masquerading as tobacco-alcohol amblyopia. *Arch Ophthalmol* 1993;111:1482–1485.

34. Charlmers RM, Harding AE. A case-control study of Leber's hereditary optic neuropathy. *Brain* 1996;119(Pt 5):1481–1486.

35. Newman NJ, Torroni A, Brown MD, et al. Epidemic neuropathy in Cuba not associated with mitochondrial DNA mutations found in Leber's hereditary optic neuropathy patients. Cuba Neuropathy Field Investigation Team. *Am J Ophthalmol* 1994;118:158–168.

36. Newman NJ. Leber's hereditary optic neuropathy. New genetic considerations. *Arch Neurol* 1993;50:540–548.

37. Ortiz RG, Newman NJ, Manoukian SV, et al. Optic disk cupping and electrocardiographic abnormalities in an American pedigree with Leber's hereditary optic neuropathy. *Am J Ophthalmol* 1992;113:561–566.

38. Shoffner JM, Brown MD, Stugard C, et al. Leber's hereditary optic neuropathy plus dystonia is caused by a mitochondrial DNA point mutation. *Ann Neurol* 1995;38:163–169.

39. Jun AS, Brown MD, Wallace DC. A mitochondrial DNA mutation at nucleotide pair 14459 of the NADH dehydrogenase subunit 6 gene associated with maternally inherited Leber hereditary optic neuropathy and dystonia. *Proc Natl Acad Sci U S A* 1994; 91:6206–6210.

40. Nikoskelainen E, Wanne O, Dahl M. Pre-excitation syndrome and Leber's hereditary optic neuroretinopathy. *Lancet* 1985;1 (8430):696.

41. Guy J, Qi X, Pallotti F, Schon EA, et al. Rescue of a mitochondrial deficiency causing Leber hereditary optic neuropathy. *Ann Neurol* 2002;52:534–542.

42. Tatuch Y, Christodoulou J, Feigenbaum A, et al. Heteroplasmic mtDNA mutation (T—G) at 8993 can cause Leigh disease when the percentage of abnormal mtDNA is high. *Am J Hum Genet* 1992;50:852–858.

43. Makela-Bengs P, Suomalainen A, Majander A, et al. Correlation between the clinical symptoms and the proportion of mitochondrial DNA carrying the 8993 point mutation in the NARP syndrome. *Pediatr Res* 1995;37:634–639.

44. Fryer A, Appleton R, Sweeney MG, et al. Mitochondrial DNA 8993 (NARP) mutation presenting with a heterogeneous phenotype including 'cerebral palsy'. *Arch Dis Child* 1994;71:419–422.

45. Shoubridge EA. Cytochrome c oxidase deficiency. *Am J Med Genet* 2001;106:46–52.

46. Sacconi S, Salviati L, Sue CM, et al. Mutation screening in patients with isolated cytochrome c oxidase deficiency. *Pediatr Res* 2003;53:224–230.

47. Puddu P, Barboni P, Mantovani V, et al. Retinitis pigmentosa, ataxia, and mental retardation associated with mitochondrial DNA mutation in an Italian family. *Br J Ophthalmol* 1993;77: 84–88.

48. Egger J, Wilson J. Mitochondrial inheritance in a mitochondrially mediated disease. *N Engl J Med* 1983;309:142–146.

49. Zeviani M, Moraes CT, DiMauro S, et al. Deletions of mitochondrial DNA in Kearns-Sayre syndrome. *Neurology* 1988; 38:1339–1346.

49a. Filosto M, Mancuso M, Nishigaki Y, et al. Clinical and genetic heterogeneity in progressive external ophthalmoplegia due to mutations in polymerase gamma. *Arch Neurol* 2003, 60: 1279–1284.

50. Spelbrink JN, Li FY, Tiranti V, et al. Human mitochondrial DNA deletions associated with mutations in the gene encoding Twinkle, a phage T7 gene 4-like protein localized in mitochondria. *Nat Genet* 2001;28:223–231.

51. Suomalainen A, Kaukonen J. Diseases caused by nuclear genes affecting mtDNA stability. *Am J Med Genet* 2001;106:53–61.

52. Kaukonen JA, Amati P, Suomalainen A, et al. An autosomal locus predisposing to multiple deletions of mtDNA on chromosome 3p. *Am J Hum Genet* 1996;58:763–769.

53. Kearns T. External ophthalmoplegia, pigmentary degeneration of the retina, and cardiomyopathy: a newly recognized syndrome. *Trans Ophthalmol Soc U K* 1965;63:559–625.

54. Ross A, Lipschutz D, Austin J, et al. External ophthalmoplegia and complete heart block. *N Engl J Med* 1969;280:313–315.

55. Pavlakis SG, Phillips PC, DiMauro S, et al. Mitochondrial myopathy, encephalopathy, lactic acidosis, and strokelike episodes: a distinctive clinical syndrome. *Ann Neurol* 1984;16:481–488.

56. Kuchle M, Brenner PM, Engelhardt A, et al. Ocular changes in MELAS syndrome. *Klin Monatsbl Augenheilkd* 1990;197: 258–264.

57. Hwang JM, Park HW, Kim SJ. Optic neuropathy associated with mitochondrial tRNA(Leu(UUR)) A3243G mutation. *Ophthalmic Genet* 1997;18:101–105.

58. Rummelt V, Folberg R, Ionasescu V, et al. Ocular pathology of MELAS syndrome with mitochondrial DNA nucleotide 3243 point mutation. *Ophthalmology* 1993;100:1757–1766.

59. Moser HW. Genotype-phenotype correlations in disorders of peroxisome biogenesis. *Mol Genet Metab* 1999;68:316–327.

60. Moser H. Peroxisomal diseases. *Adv Pediatr* 1989;36:1–38.

61. Li X, Baumgart E, Morrell JC, et al. PEX11 beta deficiency is lethal and impairs neuronal migration but does not abrogate peroxisome function. *Mol Cell Biol* 2002;22:4358–4365.

62. Folz SJ, Trobe JD. The peroxisome and the eye. *Surv Ophthalmol* 1991;35:353–368.

63. Jansen GA, Ofman R, Ferdinandusse S, et al. Refsum disease is caused by mutations in the phytanoyl-CoA hydroxylase gene. *Nat Genet* 1997;17:190–193.

64. Jansen GA, Wanders RJ, Watkins PA, et al. Phytanoyl-coenzyme A hydroxylase deficiency—the enzyme defect in Refsum's disease. *N Engl J Med* 1997;337:133–134.

65. Wierzbicki AS, Mitchell J, Lambert-Hammill M, et al. Identification of genetic heterogeneity in Refsum's disease. *Eur J Hum Genet* 2000;8:649–651.

66. van den Brink DM, Brites P, Haasjes J, et al. Identification of PEX7 as the second gene involved in Refsum disease. *Am J Hum Genet* 2003;72:471–477.

67. Rinaldi E, Cotticelli L, Di Meo A, et al. Ocular findings in Refsum's disease. *Metab Pediatr Ophthalmol* 1981;5:149–154.

68. Refsum S. Heredopathia atactica polyneuritiformis phytanic-acid storage disease, Refsum's disease:" a biochemically well-defined disease with a specific dietary treatment. *Arch Neurol* 1981;38:605–606.

69. Rake M, Saunders M. Refsum's disease: a disorder of lipid metabolism. *J Neurol Neurosurg Psychiatry* 1966;29:417–422.

70. Gordon N, Hudson R. Refsum's syndrome heredopathia atactica polyneuritiformis: a report of three cases, including a study of the cardiac pathology. *Brain* 1959;82:41–55.

71. Toussaint D, Danis P. An ocular pathologic study of Refsum's syndrome. *Am J Ophthalmol* 1971;72:342–347.

72. Flament-Durand J, Noel P, Rutsaert J, et al. A case of Refsum's disease: clinical, pathological, ultrastructural and biochemical study. *Pathol Eur* 1971;6:172–191.

73. Refsum S. Heredopathia atactica polyneuritiformis. A familial syndrome not hitherto described. *Acta Psychiatr Scand Suppl* 1946;38:1–303.

74. Leys D, Petit H, Bonte-Adnet C, et al. Refsum's disease revealed by cardiac disorders. *Lancet* 1989;1 (8638):621.

75. Plant GR, Hansell DM, Gibberd FB, et al. Skeletal abnormalities in Refsum's disease (heredopathia atactica polyneuritiformis). *Br J Radiol* 1990;63:537–541.

76. Herndon JH Jr, Steinberg D, Uhlendorf BW, et al. Refsum's disease: characterization of the enzyme defect in cell culture. *J Clin Invest* 1969;48:1017–1032.

77. Steinberg D, Avigan J, Mize CE, et al. The nature of the metabolic defect in Refsum's disease. *Pathol Eur* 1968;3:450–458.

78. Steinberg D, Mize CE, Herndon JH Jr, et al. Phytanic acid in patients with Refsum's syndrome and response to dietary treatment. *Arch Intern Med* 1970;125:75–87.

79. Eldjarn L, Try K, Stokke O, et al. Dietary effects on serum-phytanic-acid levels and on clinical manifestations in heredopathia atactica polyneuritiformis. *Lancet* 1966;1(7439):691–693.

80. Gibberd FB, Billimoria JD, Page NG, et al. Heredopathia atactica polyneuritiformis (Refsum's disease) treated by diet and plasma-exchange. *Lancet* 1979;1(8116):575–578.

81. Gibberd FB. Plasma exchange for Refsum's disease. *Transfus Sci* 1993;14 :23–26.

82. Danpure CJ. Primary hyperoxaluria type 1 and peroxisome-to-mitochondrion mistargeting of alanine:glyoxylate aminotransferase. *Biochimie* 1993;75:309–315.

83. Small KW, Letson R, Scheinman J. Ocular findings in primary hyperoxaluria. *Arch Ophthalmol* 1990;108:89–93.

84. Theodossiadis PG, Friberg TR, Panagiotidis DN, et al. Choroidal neovascularization in primary hyperoxaluria. *Am J Ophthalmol* 2002;134:134–137.

85. Meredith TA, Wright JD, Gammon JA, et al. Ocular involvement in primary hyperoxaluria. *Arch Ophthalmol* 1984;102:584–587.

86. Small KW, Scheinman J, Klintworth GK. A clinicopathological study of ocular involvement in primary hyperoxaluria type I. *Br J Ophthalmol* 1992;76:54–57.

87. Sakamoto T, Maeda K, Sueishi K, et al. Ocular histopathologic findings in a 46-year-old man with primary hyperoxaluria. *Arch Ophthalmol* 1991;109:384–387.

88. Latta K, Brodehl J. Primary hyperoxaluria type I. *Eur J Pediatr* 1990;149:518–522.

HEREDITARY RETINITIS PIGMENTOSA

RAGHU C. MURTHY
J. TIMOTHY STOUT

Retinitis pigmentosa (RP) is a heterogeneous group of diseases that present as symmetric, bilateral, inherited, progressive photoreceptor and retinal pigment epithelium (RPE) dystrophies. Often, rods are affected early in the disease process. This group of dystrophies was initially named retinitis pigmentosa by Donders (1) in 1855 when he described pigmentary changes in the midperipheral fundus that mimicked inflammation around vessels in a patient with night blindness. Retinal dystrophies were classified according to morphology before the molecular biology era provided criteria for division into peripheral and central degenerations. The former was classified as RP with initial and predominant changes in the postequatorial fundus. The latter were named macular dystrophies. The classic triad of RP was coined bone spicules in the midperiphery, arteriolar attenuation, and waxy pallor of the disc. Loss of the scotopic response early and the photopic response later in the disease as determined by electroretinogram (ERG) was discovered in the 1940s by Karpe (2), and these criteria were added to the diagnosis. Morphologic exceptions were made for patients presenting with nyctalopia, loss of peripheral visual field (VF), and loss of ERG without bone spicules in the midperiphery. RP without bone spicules was termed RP *sine pigmento* or retinitis punctata albescens, if whitish flecks or dots were seen in the midperiphery. These morphologic classifications were useful to group dystrophies. The analysis of pedigrees further subdivided them into autosomal dominant (AD), autosomal recessive (AR), and X-linked (XL) modes of inheritance. This subdivision helped with genetic counseling, and some level of visual prognostication. We now know that forms of RP can also be inherited mitochondrially, digenically (involving two genes), via a process that requires multiple alleles of different genes for the disease phenotype, or in syndromic forms. Often, the family history reveals no affected family members; this is commonly termed *simplex* disease.

Dystrophies can be stationary or progressive. Stationary dystrophies like congenital stationary night blindness (CSNB) were classified separately from RP. Some forms of CSNB are caused by mutations in the rhodopsin gene, which has been implicated in over 100 forms of RP. Although there is variability in the phenotypes of a disease within a pedigree and a genotype, it is clear that different genotypes can produce similar fundus findings. Careful phenotypic descriptions of patients with these diseases will be needed to establish meaningful phenotype-genotype relationships.

In typical RP, probands will often present with RPE mottling and atrophy with intraretinal migration of pigment. Bone spicule–like pigmentary accumulations are present in the midperiphery (Fig. 10-1). Rod degeneration in this area will often lead to a "ring scotoma" on initial VF testing. Epiretinal membranes may form on the internal limiting membrane, making a sheen visible on biomicroscopy of the fundus. The arterioles may become attenuated with time and the optic nerve may appear to have a "waxy" pallor (Fig. 10-2). As the disease progresses, cone function deteriorates with a concomitant loss of central vision.

Retinitis pigmentosa may occur in isolation or as part of a multiorgan syndrome. This provides a convenient method of division; we will divide the discussion of the pigmentosas into nonsyndromic RP and syndromic RP. Although syndromic RP is noted in the presence of systemic neurologic or metabolic diseases, in nonsyndromic disease, the eyes are affected in isolation. Syndromic RP should be excluded by a thorough history, physical examination, and appropriate laboratory studies because some patients require nonocular clinical intervention. Certain inflammatory and infectious conditions affecting the retina and choroid can mimic the RP fundus findings. Drug toxicity can produce an RP-like fundus picture, along with old ophthalmic artery occlusion. These pseudo-RP conditions should be excluded by history and appropriate workup. To explore each of these entities, this review will first examine the nonsyndromic forms of RP and will correlate these diseases with recent genetic information. We will also explore pseudo-RP conditions and their clinical and laboratory features. We will then review the syndromic RP conditions presenting with neurologic and metabolic diseases. We will discuss presentation, workup and diagnosis, genetics, natural history, and management of these diseases.

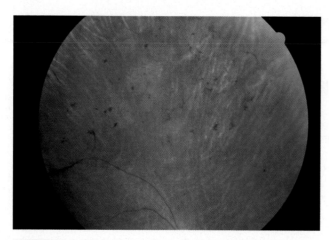

FIGURE 10-1. Pigmentary retinopathy vessel attenuation.

NONSYNDROMIC RETINITIS PIGMENTOSA

Retinitis pigmentosa most often occurs as an isolated ocular condition. RP conditions are caused by genetic defects in the visual phototransduction cascade, RPE and vitamin A metabolism, transcription factors, and structural defects in photoreceptors. Because of the genetic heterogeneity of these defects, there is great phenotypic variability. Furthermore, there are many mutations within each of these individual genes, and digenic inheritance is possible. This creates variability in age of presentation, inheritance, and phenotype. In this chapter, we will discuss typical RP, retinitis punctata albescens, and mimickers of RP.

Clinical Symptoms and Signs

Isolated RP represents a majority of patients with inherited retinal disease. Patients present with difficulty or clumsiness in dim light. Questions eliciting information about activity in low light or nighttime can reveal nyctalopia. The classic findings of RP includes nyctalopia, bone

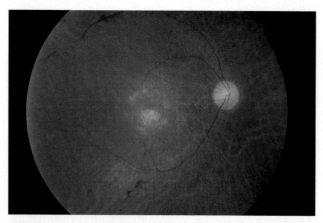

FIGURE 10-2. "Waxy pallor" of optic nerve in autosomal-dominant retinitis pigmentosa. Note narrowed arterioles.

spicules in the midperiphery, attenuated arterioles, waxy pallor of the optic disc, VF constriction, and a depressed scotopic and later photopic ERG patterns. Early clinical examination might only reveal subtle changes. These include RPE mottling, a fine layer intraretinal pigment, clumping of pigment in the retinal layers, focal RPE atrophy, and mild attenuation of vessels (Fig. 10-2). Even at this early stage, there can be significant ERG abnormalities. A diminished scotopic response, diminished combined photoreceptor response, and a delayed implicit time are typical.

Isolated RP can be subdivided into three common inheritance patterns: XL, AR, and AD. Cases, which do not have a known inheritance pattern, are referred to as *simplex*. Most *simplex* cases of RP reflect AR inheritance or incomplete penetrance. Along with these inheritance patterns, digenic transmission (via two AR genes) has also been documented. As of 2003, five XL RP genes have been mapped, and two of these have been cloned. Fifteen recessive loci have been mapped, and 10 of these have been cloned. There have been 12 AD RP loci mapped, and 11 of these have been cloned. There have also been two forms of digenic and one form of mitochondrial transmission reported, but these were in syndromic RP.

Prevalence/Incidence

The overall incidence of RP in the United States has been calculated to be approximately 1:3,700 (3). This makes RP the most prevalent of all retinal dystrophies. The reported proportions of each pattern of inheritance vary, with a US study estimating 10% AD, 84% AR (including *simplex* cases), and 6% XL (3), whereas a UK study found approximately 20% AD, 70% AR, and 10% XL (4). The highest recorded prevalence of RP is 1:1,800 in the Navajo of the southwestern United States (5). *Simplex* cases can account for 50% of all cases. AR inheritance is presumed to account for most of these cases. Incompletely penetrant AD RP, new AD RP mutations, digenic, and XL RP are purported to account for a small percentage of these cases.

Autosomal-Dominant Retinitis Pigmentosa

Autosomal-dominant RP typically presents in the second to the fourth decades and is often the mildest form of the disease. It may be unrecognized because of its slow progression, subtle clinical findings, and late onset. Reduced penetrance may give the illusion of "generation skipping." These patients are often asymptomatic into their second and third decades of life. Dominant RP is thought to account for 10% to 25% of all RP cases. Proteins responsible for AD RP include rhodopsin, peripherin/retinal degeneration slow (RDS), neural retina leucine zipper (NRL), cone–rod homeobox (CRX), retinal fascin (FSCN2), precursor RNA-processing complex C (PRPC8), and precursor RNA-processing factor 31 (PRPF31) (Table 10-1).

Autosomal-Recessive Retinitis Pigmentosa

Autosomal-recessive RP presents in the first two decades of life and generally has a more fulminant course and poorer prognosis than AD RP. Vision will typically deteriorate below 20/200, with significant loss of VF. Field loss can be a more significant contributor to visual dysfunction than acuity and often is first noted 30 to 50 degrees from fixation.

These scotomas enlarge, deepen, and coalesce forming a ring of peripheral VF loss, sparing small islands of temporal field. These islands of vision might contribute to some visual function initially, but they soon become smaller or not contiguous enough to be useful. Carrier state can be detected by clinical exam and ERG studies. There can be subtle changes in the fundus showing pigment disturbance, migration, and clumping. A golden-metallic tapetal reflex can be seen in some patients in the temporal periphery. ERG will reveal subnormal scotopic and photopic responses. Consanguinity suggests AR RP, if no other form of transmission is suggested by the pedigree.

TABLE 10-1. PROTEINS, GENES, AND LOCI IDENTIFIED IN NON-SYNDROMIC RETINITIS PIGMENTOSA

Protein	Gene	Locus	Inheritance
RP19	ABCA4, ABCRS, TG D1, FFM, RP19	1p21–p13	AR
RP18	HPRP3, RP18	1q21.2	AD
RP20	RPE65, RP20	1p31	AR
Crums homolog	CRB1	1q31–q32.1	AR
RP28	RP28	2p15–p11	AR
c-mer receptor tyrosine kinase	MERTK	2q14.1	AR
RP26		2q31–q33	AR
Rhodopsin	RHO	3q21–q24	AD
Prominin	PROM1	4p	AR
cGMP-gated channel	CNGCa	4p14–q13	AR
cGMP PDE-β	PDE-β	4p16.3	AR
Photoreceptor cGMP-gated channel-α	CNGA1, CNCG1	4p21-cen	AR
RP29		4q32–q34	AR
cGMP PDE-α	PDEα	5q31.2-qter	AR
Peripherin/RDS	RDS, RP7, PRPH2, PRPH	6p21.1	AD, digenic
Tubby-like protein	TULP1, RP14	6p21.3	AR
RP25	RP25	6q14–q21	AR
RP9	RP9	7p14.2	AD
RP10	RP10	7q31–q35	AD
Inosine-5-prime-monophosphate dehydrogenase	IMPD1	7q31.3–q32	AD
RP1	RP1	8p11–q13	AD
RPE-retinal G protein coupled receptor	RGR	10q23	AD
Rod outer mem protein-1	ROM-1	11q13	Digenic
Neutral retina leucine zipper	NRL	14q11.1–q11.2	AD
Photoreceptor-specific nuclear receptor	NR2E3, PNR, ESCS	15q23	AR
Retinaldehyde-binding protein	RLBP1	15q26	AR
RP22	RP22	16p12.3–p12.1	AR
Photoreceptor c-GMP gated channel β and γ subunit	CNGB1, CNCG3L, CNCG2	16q13	AR
Arylhydrocarbon interacting receptor protein-like 1	AIPL1, LCA4	17p13.1	
RP13	PRPF8, PRPC8, RP13	17p13.3	AD
RP17		17q22	AD
RP30	FSCN2, RFSN	17q25	AD
Cone–rod homeobox-containing gene	CRX, CORD2, CRD	19q13.3	AD
RP11	PRPF31, PRP31	19q13.4	AD
RP23		Xp22	XL
RP6	RP6	Xp21.3–p21.2	XL
RP GTPase regulator	RPGR, RP3, CRD, RP15, COD1	Xp21.1	XL
RP2	RP2	Xp11.3	XL
RP24	RP24	Xq26–q27	XL
Not cloned	RPY	Chromosome Y	YL

AR, autosomal recessive; AD, autosomal dominant; XL, X-linked; YL, Y-linked.

Many of the genes associated with AR RP are involved with photoreceptor development, the phototransduction cascade, and vitamin A metabolism. Mutations in the catalytic domain of the beta subunit of rod cyclic guanosine monophosphate (cGMP) phosphodiesterase (PDEβ) result in a loss of function cGMP phosphodiesterase (PDE) and lead to accumulation of cGMP levels, which may be toxic to rods (6). Mutations within this protein are the most common of the identified changes in patients with AR RP and account for 4% to 5% of cases. Mutations in the alpha subunit of cGMP PDE have also been identified as causing AR RP (7). The cGMP-gated cation channel proteins are heterotetramers of two homologous alpha and beta subunits. Mutations in the alpha (CNCG1) and the beta (CNGB1) subunit have also been found in ARRP (8,9).

Recessive RP may be caused by mutations of RPE65, a microsomal protein found exclusively in the RPE, where it accounts for 10% of total membrane proteins (10). Mutations in RPE65 have been reported in Leber's congenital amaurosis, recessive cone-rod dystrophy and AR RP (11,12). Murine studies have shown that although opsin apoprotein is present in the rod outer segment (ROS), no rhodopsin is present. Administration of oral 9-*cis*-retinal to RPE65-knockout mice resulted in rhodopsin formation with an improvement in ERGs, providing hope for pharmacologic intervention for individuals with this gene defect (13).

X-Linked Retinitis Pigmentosa

X-linked RP usually presents within the first decade of life, and is typically the most severe form of RP. These children can present in the first few years of life and can progressively lose VF and acuity over the next decade, and show profound impairment of vision (14). X-linked RP was the first type of RP to be linked to a specific locus by Bhattacharya in 1984 (15). There are now five distinct X-linked RP loci and two responsible genes have been cloned. The RP GTPase regulator gene has been identified in 20% to 30% of X-linked RP cases (16). This gene is expressed in many tissues, and is thought to play a role in membrane transport, possibly involving the shedding and regeneration of ROS, by regulating retinal GTPase activity. Clinically, affected males show early onset and severe retinal degeneration. Heterozygote female carriers can show mild to no effect to severe expression of the disease, depending on the lyonization of their cells. Rods and cones appear equally affected by ERG in this type of RP (17).

Phenotypic Variation

There is considerable variability in the RP phenotype. This variation is the result of four factors: (i) locus heterogeneity, which means that mutations in different genes are associated with the phenotype; (ii) allelic heterogeneity, which means that different mutations in the same gene are associated with the phenotype; (iii) modifier genes that affect phenotypic expression; and (iv) environmental factors that affect phenotypic expression. The RP phenotype can also vary in disease stages, penetrance, and expressivity.

Proteins

Proteins important in the pathogenesis of RP may be divided into four categories: (i) photoreceptor structural proteins; (ii) phototransduction cascade proteins; (iii) proteins that regulate photoreceptor and RPE metabolism (including vitamin A metabolism); and (iv) transcription factors.

Pathophysiology

The Visual Cycle

To understand the mutations in RP, one has to be familiar with photoreceptor anatomy, phototransduction pathway, and vitamin A metabolism (Fig. 10-3). Photoreceptors are the light-sensitive cells comprising the outer most layer of the neurosensory retina. They are highly specialized ciliated neuroepithelial cells that convert light into chemical signals. Their distal parts are specialized to capture light, and their proximal parts are specialized to transmit nerve signals. There are two types: rod and cone cells. They are so named because of the cylindrical (rod) or cone shape (cone) of their photon capturing apical membranes. There are approximately 92 million rods responsible for vision in low light conditions, and 5 million cones responsible for day vision and color vision. Rods are present throughout the fundus. Cones are concentrated especially in the center of the macula, although they are also found in the rest of the fundus. Rods also reach a peak density 20 degrees from the foveola (18). These specialized neuroepithelial cells have a cell body, an inner segment, connecting stalk, and an outer segment. The stalk has the structure of a cilium with nine tubules arising from a basal body in the inner segment and reaching varying heights in the outer segment. All rods contain rhodopsin, the light-sensitive chromophore. Cones contain three opsins sensitive to three different regions of the visual spectrum: blue, green, and red. The ROS is a modified cilium made up of approximately 600 to 1,000 flat disks piled on top of each other. The plasma membrane is extended and flattened into many disks and provides an extensive surface area for capturing incoming photons. At the end of the rims of the disks are lobules. Filaments connect disks to each other and lobules within the same disk (19). After light strikes the apical tips of the outer segments of rods, the outer disks are shed the following morning and phagocytosed by the RPE, which surround the apical portion of the outer segments. New disks are added at the base of the ROS daily.

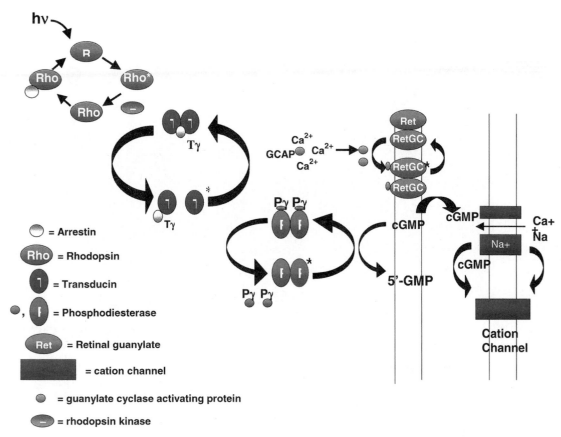

FIGURE 10-3. Phototransduction cascade. (Courtesy of Thomas E. Stout)

Rhodopsin (RHO) contains seven transmembrane domains and is found on the lamellar side of rod disks (Fig. 10-4). It is the most abundant protein found in rods, constituting up to 85% of the total amount of protein present, is the ROS. Rhodopsin is composed of a rod-specific opsin bound to the chromophore 11-*cis*-retinal. It is important for the initiation of the visual transduction cascade and might be important in ROS structure. Mice lacking a copy of the *rho* gene have ROSs that are short and disorganized and develop a slow retinal degeneration much like the peripherin/RDS mice (20). In the rim of the ROS, peripherin/RDS and retinal outer segment membrane protein 1 (ROM1) are found as transmembrane proteins. These two proteins are very homologous in structure and function, but are expressed in different cells. Peripherin/RDS is expressed in rods and cones, whereas ROM1 is only found in rods. These two proteins form dimers, which interact to form tetramers.

The phototransduction cascade begins when a photon strikes a ROS and is absorbed by 11-*cis*-retinal transforming it into all-*trans* retinal (Fig. 10-3). This event induces a conformational change in rhodopsin, which catalyzes the activation of the G-protein transducin. Many molecules of transducin are activated by a single rhodopsin, starting this signal amplification cascade. Transducin activates

cGMP phosphodiesterase to hydrolyze cGMP. The resulting decrease in cGMP concentration closes the cGMP-gated cation channels in the cell membrane, which results in the hyperpolarization of the cell, slowing the neurotransmitter release at the synaptic terminal (21). Deactivation of RHO starts with phosphorylation by rhodopsin kinase and capture by arrestin. The binding of arrestin to RHO prevents further activation of transducin and releases 11-*trans*-retinal from rhodopsin (22). The regeneration of the 11-*cis*-retinal from the all-*trans*-retinal is mediated by the interphotoreceptor retinoid-binding protein (IRBP), which transports it from the ROS to the RPE cell. Here it is transferred to the cellular retinoid-binding protein (CRBP) and is converted to 11-*cis*-retinol by RPE-specific isomerase. Lastly, 11-*cis*-retinol binds cellular retinaldehyde-binding protein (CRALBP) and is oxidized to 11-*cis*-retinal, which is released from the RPE cells. It is then transported to the ROS by IRBP, where 11-*cis*-retinal binds rhodopsin all over again. The RPE specific protein and RPE65 protein, which are involved in this regeneration process, constitute up to 10% of the total amount of protein in the RPE cells (23).

The daily shedding of photoreceptor outer segments and renewal of the 11-*cis*-retinal places a burden on the multi-

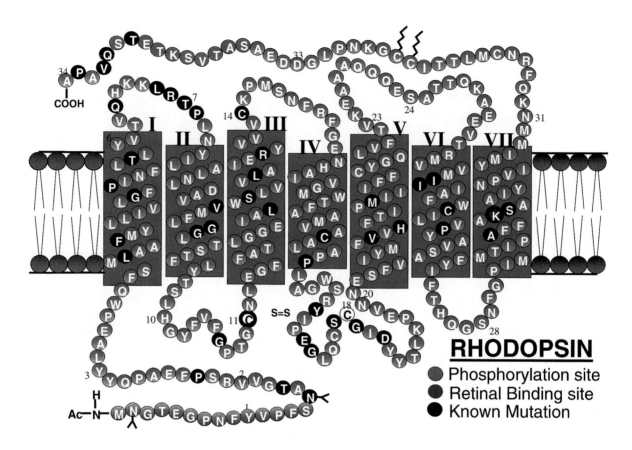

FIGURE 10-4. The complete amino acid sequence of human rhodopsin (RHO) is shown. The protein contains seven transmembrane domains and is found embedded in the billpid membranes that make up the intracellular photoreceptor discs. (Adapted from Hargrave PA [2001], Bird AC [1995], and Kolb H et al, with permission, www.webvision.med.utah.edu)

functional RPE cells. Any malfunction in this cycle can lead to an accumulation of shed outer segments, all-*trans*-retinal, and deposits between the RPE and photoreceptor layers.

Genetics

Rhodopsin

This light activated protein, part of the G-protein coupled receptor superfamily, consists of the apoprotein opsin with 348 amino acid residues and the chromophore 11-*cis*-retinal covalently bound to Lys-296 in the seventh transmembrane helix via a protonated Schiff base (PSB) linkage. The rhodopsin gene, located on chromosome 3q, was the first in which mutations associated with RP were identified. Over 100 different mutations in the opsin gene have been described since the initial Pro23His mutation in the intradiscal domain of the protein was reported in 1990. Almost all of these mutations result in the synthesis of an abnormal protein due to a single amino acid substitution (24). Mutations in the rhodopsin gene account for 25% of all AD RP in the United Kingdom, Europe, and the United States (25–27). The Pro23His mutation is the only one to have a

sizable number of cases. It has been detected in 12% of the RP population in the United States, although it has not yet been found in any of the European cases (28). A new mutation (Pro23Ala) has been recently reported. It is much less frequent than the Pro23His mutation, and causes a more benign form of AD RP, with greater preservation of ERG amplitudes at presentation and a milder course (29). Most mutations have been found only in a small number of patients and are associated with AD RP. Misfolding of the rhodopsin protein has been proposed as one of the main biochemical consequences resulting from mutations in the rhodopsin gene (30). Molecular chaperones have also been implicated as a source of dysfunction (31). The partial or complete misfolding of rhodopsin can result in the inability of the mutant protein to bind 11-*cis*-retinal. Other rhodopsin mutations include Thr58Arg and Gly106Asp. These two mutations produce a sectoral AD RP, characterized by loss of the superior VF with a corresponding inferior retinal degeneration (32). Rare cases of AR RP have been reported, including a proband from a consanguineous marriage who was homozygous for the Glu249Ter mutation. This mutation causes premature termination and would be expected to result in complete absence of functional protein. The heterozygous parents and siblings did not have RP, but abnormalities in rod photoreceptor function were noted (33,34).

Three rhodopsin mutations that cause both AD CStNBl and AR RP have been reported. Gly90Asp, Thr94Ile, and Ala292Glu are located in the region of the protein that is involved with the PSB linkage to 11-*cis*-retinal (35,36). The resulting phenotype is a stationary retinal dystrophy. These mutations do not seem to cause the gross structural misfolding that is predicted for other rhodopsin mutations (37), which may explain the more benign phenotype.

Functional and expression studies of mutations in rhodopsin *in vitro* have defined three classes of mutants based on the synthesis of rhodopsin, regeneration of 11-*cis*-retinal, and the glycosylation pattern (38,39). Class I mutants (15%) cluster in the first transmembrane region toward the C-terminus end of the molecule. These molecules resembled the wild type in terms of yield, regeneration with 11-*cis*-retinal, and subcellular location. Class II mutants (85%) were unstable or folded improperly, accumulating in the rough endoplasmic reticulum. Although cell-culture studies showed two classes of mutants, no direct correlation was observed between classes and the phenotype of the patients with either class of mutation. This study showed a different mechanism than had been hypothesized in earlier studies that speculated a constitutive activation of the phototransduction cascade. Animal studies have shown that continuous exposure to light leads to retinal degeneration (40). Examination of a constitutively activated codon 296 mutation at the binding site of 11-*cis*-retinal in humans, which might turn on the cascade continuously, actually revealed in a mouse model that it was the continuous shutoff of the visual cascade that triggered the degeneration of the photoreceptors (41).

As mentioned earlier, rhodopsin is a major constituent of ROS, accounting for 85% of the protein content. As such, it has an important structural role in the ROS. Generation of mice with a targeted disruption of the rhodopsin gene showed that homozygous knockouts did not have ROS and they lost their photoreceptors within 3 months. Heterozygotes, on the other hand, retained most of their photoreceptors, but they developed short, stubby ROS and underwent inexorable retinal degeneration as they got older, much like that seen in peripherin-deficient/RDS mice (42).

The abundance of rhodopsin, its importance for structure of the ROS, and the findings from animal studies suggest that the accumulation of most forms of mutant rhodopsin in subcellular structures may cause disruption of cellular processes necessary for the proper renewal and shedding of ROS and thus result in photoreceptor cell death.

Peripherin/RDS and ROM1

Peripherin is a transmembrane protein abundant in the outer disk rims in both rods and cones, while ROM1 is a transmembrane protein abundant only in rods. They are structural

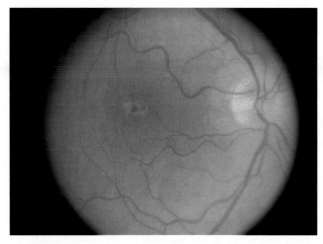

FIGURE 10-5. Autosomal-recessive pattern dystrophy.

proteins of the outer segment, and are estimated to be abnormal in 5% of all AD RP cases (43). The genes that encode peripherin/RDS and ROM1 are located on chromosome 6 and chromosome 11, respectively. These proteins play an important role in maintaining disk curvature and possibly anchoring these disks to the plasma membrane (44). More than 40 different mutations in the human peripherin/*RDS* gene have been identified. These are usually inherited in an AD fashion. Studies of *rds* mice have demonstrated that heterozygous mice with a 50% reduction of peripherin/RDS develop short and stubby photoreceptors that slowly degenerate (45). Homozygous mice do not develop any outer segments. Mutations in this gene in humans often result in a slow retinal degeneration, with a delayed onset. There is a slow dysfunction of both the rod and cone photoreceptors with the appearance of yellow deposits in the RPE. A variety of phenotypes have been observed within the same family, including RP, pattern dystrophy (Fig. 10-5), fundus flavimaculatus (Fig. 10-6), and retinitis punctata albescens (46–48). Transgenic mice with specific mutations in both copies of the peripherin/RDS gene

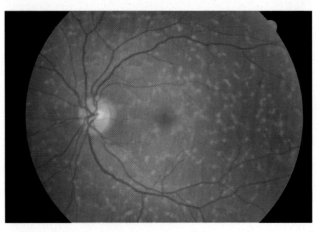

FIGURE 10-6. Fundus flavimaculatus. (Photograph courtesy of Richard Weleber, MD.)

have outer segment dysplasia and accelerated photoreceptor cell death compared with heterozygous mice (49).

The relationship between peripherin/ RDS and ROM1 was elucidated by families in which members with RP were heterozygous for the Leu185Pro mutation in the peripherin/*RDS* gene and a mutation in the *ROM1* gene, suggesting a digenic pattern of inheritance. Those who were heterozygous for only one of these two genes did not have the phenotype (50).

Differential Diagnosis

The diagnosis of RP is made by the clinical presentation of nyctalopia, fundus findings, loss of peripheral VF, family history and examination, and ERG testing. RP does not present in the first year of life. If an infant presents with wandering eyes from birth and no visual behavior, oculodigital reflex, or paradoxical pupillary response to light, other diagnoses should be considered including Leber's congenital amaurosis. Genetic testing for molecular diagnosis of RP is not yet routinely done, but it is available in difficult cases. Syndromic causes should be excluded by careful history and physical examination. An increased incidence of optic nerve head drusen (Fig. 10-7), pigmented vitreous cells (as a result of RPE migration), cystoid macular edema (CME), posterior subcapsular cataract, and epiretinal membranes may also provide clues to the diagnosis.

Diagnostic Studies

Electroretinogram (ERG) testing is useful, even in the first year of life. If testing is done before 6 months of age, this should be repeated after 6 months because visual maturation might not have been completed at the time of initial

testing. Standard ERG testing is performed according to the guidelines established by the International Society for Clinical Electrophysiology of Vision. Tested responses include: (i) a bright white flash, which elicits a mass response of combined cone and rod function; (ii) a scotopic response of rods after 45 minutes of dark adaptation; and (iii) a photopic response and a 30-Hz flicker, which measures the cone function. RP may cause a reduction in any of these responses. The implicit time may also be delayed, which measures the onset of the photopic b wave after a flash of white light. Pattern ERG testing may help evaluate macular function.

The electrooculogram, which measures the standing potential of the RPE, may also be abnormal, showing an absence of the light rise. Dark adaptometry, which measures quantitatively the kinetics of cone and rod recovery following a bright flash, can be useful to confirm RP in difficult cases. The rod–cone break will be abnormal. The confocal scanning laser ophthalmoscope (cSLO) can image the autofluorescence of the fundus, which results mostly from the RPE. Increased autofluorescence can indicate increased RPE dysfunction, as a result of overloading of these RPE cells in areas of excessive shedding of photoreceptor outer segments (51).

Fluorescein angiography, often not necessary for diagnosis, can reveal diffuse hyperfluorescence from the RPE window defects and hypofluorescence in areas of pigment clumping and leakage from cystoid macular edema, which may be responsible for potentially reversible loss of vision in RP patients.

Management

Although no clearly effective therapy is currently available for patients with RP, patients should be periodically monitored for disease progression and the possible development of reversible causes of vision loss. All patients suspected to have RP should be periodically assessed by kinetic perimetry. In addition to providing useful information about disease progression, serial perimetry has practical influences on driving ability, blind registration, and eligibility for disability funding. Serial ERGs can be followed if the diagnosis is suspected in the first few years of life. RP will result in a diminution of the scotopic and combined responses. Consultation with a low-vision specialist for optical devices that optimize contrast, increase magnification, or provide a dark background for reading text may be helpful. Patients with decreased central vision should be evaluated for CME that may be responsive to systemic carbonic anhydrase inhibitors. Because cataracts may reduce vision, cataract extraction with intraocular lens placement may improve central visual acuity in select cases. Vision loss may also accompany a Coats-like exudative process with retinal detachment that may respond to laser or cryo ablative therapy (Fig. 10-8). Limiting light exposure might be beneficial to some patients. Use of sun-

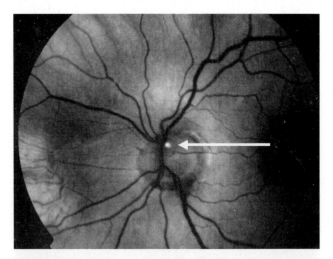

FIGURE 10-7. Red-free photograph of optic disc drusen (arrow) in autosomal-recessive retinitis pigmentosa demonstrating autofluorescence.

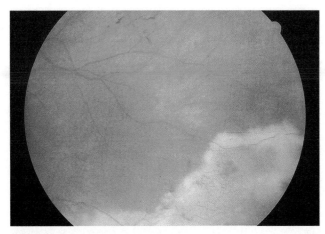

FIGURE 10-8. Retinitis pigmentosa with Coats-like exudative peripheral retinal detachment.

glasses may decrease light sensitivity. Although controversial, many physicians treat RP patients with 15,000 IU of oral vitamin A per day (51A). Somatic gene transfer may play a therapeutic role in the future as many genes responsible for RP are cloned and methods for gene transfer into terminally differentiated retinal and RPE cells improve. *In vitro* fertilization with zygote screening may be an option for parents who plan to have additional children.

Genetic counseling plays an important role in patient and family management. Disease risk and progression should be clearly explained and molecular analysis, when possible and appropriate, may be of use.

RETINAL PUNCTATA ALBESCENS

Clinical Symptoms and Signs

Mooren (52) first described this condition in 1882. It was characterized by finding discrete white or yellowish dots in the fundus, which lie under the retinal blood vessels and do not involve the macula. These dots fan out from the posterior pole often in a radial pattern, with a high concentration of spots in the equatorial region (53). This description was elaborated upon by Lauber (54), who noted in 1910 that there were two forms of the disease, stationary and progressive, in his case series of 25 patients with this disorder. He noted that in the progressive form there were disc and vessel changes, as well as development of abnormal pigmentation in addition to the white dots. Visual fields showed that the stationary form had constricted but fixed fields, while the progressive form has changing and progressive field changes. Nettleship (55) also described two cases with this entity that he followed over 26 years. In one case, he described a stationary form with no field changes over this time period. In the other case, the peripheral white dots began to disappear, and bone-spicule clumping began to appear in the retina. He also showed that this condition could be transmitted to offspring. Histologically, these lesions are lipid deposits. Reports exist of cases in which these punctate lesions have increased, decreased, or completely disappeared with time (56).

In the past, there has been a distinction made between the diagnosis of fundus albipunctatus and retinitis punctata albescens. Although both have been noted to have similar white lesions in the fundus, retinitis punctata albescens has been noted to either have or develop subsequent RPE changes, as well as changes in the vessels and optic disc. Retinitis punctata albescens is thought to be a progressive dystrophy, whereas fundus albipunctatus has been thought of as a stationary and more benign dystrophy, much in the way RP and CSNB have been classified, respectively. Retinitis punctata albescens has also been associated with a syndromic RP disorder, Bardet-Biedl syndrome, in an isolated community in Northern Territories in Canada (57).

Patients present with the same symptoms seen in classic RP. Night blindness is the most common symptom. Early in the disease they may have punctate white lesions in the equatorial region, sparing the macular area. Electroretinography may document a decreased scotopic response and combined response. Ophthalmoscopically, diffuse RPE disturbances and retinal pigment migration may be evident. Peripheral VF loss is common.

Inheritance/Prevalence

Autosomal-dominant and AR pattern of inheritance have been reported. Case series have been too few to give accurate percentages of inheritance patterns or the prevalence of this disorder.

Genetics

Retinitis punctata albescens has been associated with the Arg135Trp mutation in the rhodopsin gene in a large consanguineous French family. There is clinical heterogeneity in this family with some members presenting with retinitis punctata albescens and one member presenting with typical features of RP. There was an AD pattern of inheritance. Also, the apolipoprotein E e4 allele cosegregated with the Arg135Trp mutation in the individuals with the retinitis punctata albescens phenotype in this family (58).

A null mutation in the peripherin/*RDS* gene has been associated with retinitis punctata albescens in a family showing an AD pattern of inheritance. Peripherin/RDS is a structural protein found in the outer segments of both rods and cones. The mutation is a 2-bp deletion (frameshift) that leads to a premature stop codon, which substantially reduces the number of amino acid residues and is predicted to result in a nonfunctional protein (59).

Mutations in *RLBP1*, the gene encoding cellular retinaldehyde-binding protein, which is involved in vitamin A metabolism, have also been associated with retinitis punctata albescens. Several mutations have been reported, including a missense mutation, Arg234Trp, in patients belonging to a large pedigree from Northern Sweden on the Gulf of Bothnia; this form of retinitis punctata albescens is termed Bothnia dystrophy (60).

RETINITIS PIGMENTOSA MASQUERADE CONDITIONS

Other causes of pigmentary retinopathy should be considered (Table 10-2) prior to the diagnosis of RP. RP is a progressive, bilateral, inherited retinal dystrophy. It is important to get a detailed family history, examining in detail all forms of vision loss. Additionally, systemic inherited diseases should also be evaluated. Unilateral cases should be evaluated for monocular conditions, or unilateral presentations of systemic inflammatory, vascular, or infectious disease. Bilateral cases should be evaluated especially for any systemic neurologic, traumatic, or metabolic associations by history and physical exam. Maternal and perinatal history is important to evaluate for infectious causes, especially rubella (Fig. 10-9) and syphilis, both of which are pleiomorphic diseases that can closely mimic RP. Lung carcinoma and skin melanoma may result in a similar pigmentary retinopathy. Exposure to psychiatric medications like phenothiazines and antirheumatologic medicines like chloroquine might present as pseudo-RP. History of avitaminosis A might also provide a nutritional cause for this pigmentary retinopathy. Because the RPE has a limited repertoire of reactions to insult, inflammatory conditions

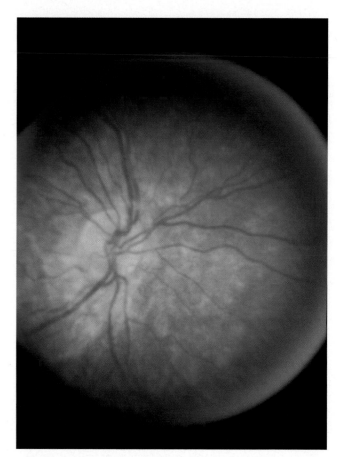

FIGURE 10-9. Rubella retinopathy in a 1 month old.

such as Vogt-Koyanagi-Harada syndrome and other causes of recurrent exudative retinal detachment can manifest as RP and should be considered in the differential diagnosis. Electroretinographic studies may be useful in distinguishing masqueraders from true dystrophic disease. Serial ERG studies can be useful in suspicious cases. With greater knowledge of the molecular mechanisms in RP, appropriate genetic analysis will become available for accurate diagnosis.

SYNDROMIC RETINITIS PIGMENTOSA

Retinitis pigmentosa can present with systemic symptoms in childhood; these are generally referred to as the syndromic RPs and often involve neurologic and metabolic disease. The fundus changes in syndromic RP are protean and may present with hyperpigmentary or hypopigmentary alterations. Often the fundus changes reveal pigmentary disturbances with RPE atrophy with vessel attenuation. The patients will typically manifest ERG changes. Although rare, these conditions should be carefully evaluated because of their high morbidity and mortality. Some of these conditions are amenable to treatment, and all have important implications for genetic counseling (Table 10-3).

TABLE 10-2. DIFFERENTIAL DIAGNOSIS OF RETINITIS PIGMENTOSA

Unilateral
Syphilis
DUSN
Vascular occlusion
Siderosis
Trauma
Reattachment of
   exudative retinal
   detachment

Bilateral

Infectious	Congenital rubella/syphilis/CMV/herpes
Inflammatory	Vogt-Koyanagi-Harada syndrome
	Exudative retinal detachment
Neoplastic	Cancer-associated retinopathy
	Melanoma-associated Retinopathy
Toxic	Phenothiazine
	Chloroquine
Nutritional	Avitaminosis A

DUSN, diffuse unilateral subacute neuroretinitis; CMV, cytomegalovirus.

TABLE 10-3. SYNDROMIC RETINITIS PIGMENTOSA

	Disease/Pathobiology	Primary Manifestations	Inheritance/Gene	Protein	Diagnosis	Treatment
Neurologic diseases	Usher/hair cell in organ of Corti (Type 1: some noted problem with decreased sperm motility and mucus clearance)	Type 1: profound sensorineural deafness and vestibular dysfunction Type 2: Mild sensineural deafness Type 3: progressive sensineural deafness ± vestibular dysfunction	AR Type 1: MYO7A, USH1C, CDH23, PCDH15, SANS Type 2: USH2A Type 3: ?	Type 1: myosin VIIA, harmonin, cadherin 23, protocadherin 15, Sans Type 2: Usherin Type 3:?	Audiometry Imbalance Infertility Bronchiectasis	Hearing aid
	Bardet-Biedl	Polydactyly in former only, mental retardation Hypogonadism Obesity, renal anomalies	AR BBS1-7 BBS 1 (most common)	BBS 6: homology to chaperonins	4/5 Primary manifestations ERG, IVP, BUN, Cr, BP	Renal dialysis Secondary HTN Speech therapy
	Kearns-Sayre/ Ragged red fibers	Ataxia CPEO, ptosis Sensineural deafness Cardiomyopathy Heart block White matter dz in brain	Mitochondrial		ECG Biopsy of muscle for electron microscopy	Pacemaker
	Friedreich's ataxia/ like vitamin E deficiency	Ataxia, Sensory loss Cerebellar dysfunction	AR	α-Tocopherol transfer protein	Neurologic examination Imbalance Abnormal cerebellar examination	Vitamin E supplementation
Lipid metabolism diseases	Abetalipoproteinemia (Bassen-Kornzweig)/ no betaliproproteins, lipid transport, low fat-soluble vitamins	Acanthocytosis Ataxia Fat intolerance Sensory neuropathy	AR 4q22–24	Microsomal triglyceride transfer protein	Neurologic examination Imbalance Serum lipoproteins Serum vitamin E, A, K levels	Vitamin E, A, K supplementation Fat-free diet Monitor serum level of vitamins
	Refsum's disease/ (phytanic acid α-hydroxylase deficiency)	Polyneuropathy Ataxia, ichthyosis Cardiomyopathy	AR	Phytanic acid α-hydroxylase	Serum phytanic acid level	Avoid phytanic acid in diet
	Neuronal ceroid lipofuscinosis (Batten)/ deposits of lipoproteins in neural tissues	Seizures Ataxia Mental retardation Hypotonia Cardiomyopathy Dry skin	AR AD: sporadic (Perry type) CLN1-8		ERG, EEG, VEP, SEP, MRI brain, conjunctival/ muscle/skin biopsy	Supportive care Genetic counseling

ERG, electroretinogram; ECG, electrocardiogram; IVP, intravenous pyleogram; BUN, blood urea nitrogen, BP, blood pressure; Cr, creatinine; HTN, hypertension.

As an ophthalmologist, one might be asked to evaluate the fundus for RP-like bone spicule changes, granular "salt-and-pepper" changes, or patchy degeneration of the RPE and choroid. Examples of the pigmentary retinopathy with neurologic dysfunction include Usher disease, which is associated with hearing loss and possible vestibular dysfunction; Bardet-Biedl syndrome (Fig. 10-10), which is associated with obesity, polydactyly, mental retardation, and hypogonadism; Laurence-Moon Syndrome, which is associated with spastic paraplegia, mental retardation, and hypogenitalism; Friedreich ataxia, which is associated with progressive cerebellar degeneration, ataxia, dysarthria, abolished deep-tendon reflexes, and cardiomyopathy; olivopontocerebellar degeneration, which is associated with ataxia and cerebellar degeneration; and Kearns-Sayre Syndrome, which is associated with chronic progressive external ophthalmoplegia, ptosis, heart block, and white matter disease in the brain. Usher syndrome is by far the most common syndrome associated with RP; it accounts for 50% of those persons that are both deaf and blind (61), and perhaps 18% of RP patients (62).

Examples of syndromic RP related to metabolic diseases are often disorders of lipid metabolism; they include abetalipoproteinemia (Bassen-Kornzweig disease, Fig. 10-11), which is associated with fat intolerance, acanthocytosis in which peripheral red blood cells take on membranous changes, ataxia, and sensory neuropathy; neuronal ceroid lipofuscinosis (Batten's disease, Fig. 10-12), which is associated with hypotonia, mental retardation, and ataxia; and Refsum's disease (phytanic acid hydroxylase deficiency), which is associated with cardiomyopathy, cerebellar ataxia, and ichthyosis (Chapter 19).

BARDET-BIEDL SYNDROME

Clinical Symptoms and Signs

Bardet described a patient in 1920 that had features of congenital obesity, polydactyly, and RP (63) (Fig. 10-10). Two

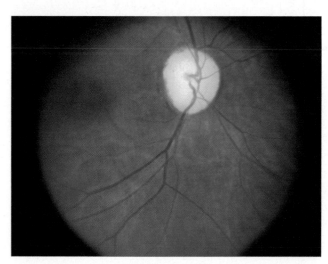

FIGURE 10-11. Late infantile neuronal ceroid lipofuscinosis (Batten's disease) with optic pallor in a 2 year old.

years later, Biedl saw two patients who had these features and exhibited mental retardation, hypogenitalism, anal atresia, and skull deformities (64). Additional reports have shown possible renal dysfunction secondarily from ureteral reflux (65). On the basis of a review of the literature, Schachat and Maumenee proposed the following criteria for the diagnosis of Bardet-Biedl syndrome (BBS): presentation of at least four of the following five cardinal symptoms: tapetoretinal degeneration, mental retardation, obesity, polydactyly, and hypogenitalism (66). Unlike typical RP, early changes may include cone–rod retinal dystrophy and central visual loss from macular involvement (Fig. 10-13).

Recently, Beales et al. (67) examined 109 patients with BBS and proposed a set of diagnostic criteria based on primary and secondary features; the presence of four primary features or three primary plus two secondary features are required for the diagnosis of BBS. Primary features include

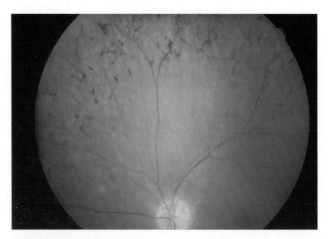

FIGURE 10-10. Peripheral pigmentary retinopathy in patient with Bardet-Biedl syndrome.

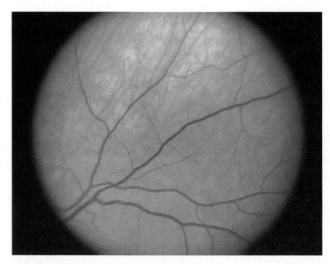

FIGURE 10-12. Peripheral pigmentary changes in abetalipoproteinemia (Bassen-Kornzweig syndrome).

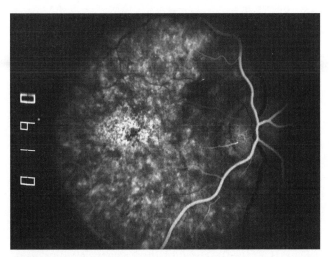

FIGURE 10-13. Fluorescein angiogram of a patient with Bardet-Biedl demonstrating speckled macular hyperfluorescence.

postaxial polydactyly, obesity, learning disabilities, hypogonadism in males, renal anomalies, and "rod–cone dystrophy." Secondary features include developmental delay, nephrogenic diabetes insipidus, diabetes mellitus, hepatic fibrosis, congenital heart disease, and "strabismus/cataract/astigmatism." In this large study, they found the average age of diagnosis of BBS to be 9 years. Postaxial polydactyly was present in 69% of the patients at birth. Obesity began to develop between 2 and 3 years of age in most of these patients. The mean age of diagnosis of the retinal degeneration was 8.5 years. In a study by Klein and Ammann (68), obesity and pigmentary retinopathy were detected in 96% and 92% of the cases. Hypogenitalism, mental retardation, and polydactyly were detected in 83%, 79%, and 69% of the cases. The patients can also present with short stature and renal anomalies. The macula can be involved early in the course of the disease and often will reflect a granular change in the RPE. The tapetoretinal degeneration can progress as an atrophic pigmentary retinopathy associated with a diffuse RPE atrophy, gliosis of the optic nerve, and attenuation and sheathing of the vessels. Mental retardation can be quite mild and is often inappropriately unrecognized. The hypogenitalism in female patients can be difficult to distinguish from normal female genitalia, though the microphallus in males is usually more obvious.

Inheritance

Bardet-Biedl syndrome is an AR condition. Carriers can have changes on ERG. In one study, all of 26 parents whose children had BBS showed decreased P2 sensitivity (see also Chapter 3). 60% of these parents also showed decreased b-wave sensitivity (69). Carriers are also at increased risk for diabetes, hypertension, obesity, and renal disease (70,71).

Triallelic inheritance has been reported in BBS, the first such pattern of inheritance in humans (72).

Prevalence/Incidence

This is a rare disease with a prevalence range of 1 in 140,000 to 160,000 in North America and Europe (73,74). There is a higher incidence in selected populations in Kuwait, the Bedouin in Saudi Arabia (75), and Newfoundland (76). There is a male preponderance of more than two to one in a large survey of reported cases (77).

Genetics

Seven different loci for BBS have been localized (*BBS1–7*). *BBS1* has been mapped to *11q13* (78). *BBS2* has been mapped to *16q21* (79). *BBS3* has been mapped to *3p13-12* (80). *BBS4* has been mapped to *15q22.3–23* (81). *BBS5* has been mapped to *2q31* (82). *BBS6* has been mapped to *20p12* (83). *BBS7* has been mapped to *4q27* (84). Four of the BBS genes have been identified (*BBS1, BBS2, BBS4, BBS6*). The predicted protein products of *BBS1, BBS2,* and *BBS4* show no obvious homology to known proteins. The protein encoded by *BBS6* shares homology with a group of proteins called chaperonins, which are involved in the transport and folding of membrane proteins (85). Mutations in *BBS1* are the most common cause of BBS; in one series of affected white families, 45% had *BBS1* mutations (74). *BBS4* mutations are the next most common cause of BBS (86).

Diagnosis

Diagnosis of BBS is made by the presence of four out of five cardinal characteristics of BBS per Schachat and Maumenee. The cardinal characteristics are tapetoretinal degeneration, mental retardation, obesity, polydactyly, and hypogenitalism. Initial investigation of patient suspected of having BBS should include a detailed history and physical exam that may involve ERG, visually evoked responses, renal ultrasound, intravenous pyelogram, electrocardiogram, and exclusion of Prader-Willi syndrome by molecular testing. Other studies that can be considered include brain and renal magnetic resonance imaging (MRI) or computed tomography scans and cognitive functioning and speech assessment.

Differential Diagnosis

In patients without pigmentary retinopathy, a diagnosis of Prader-Willi syndrome (Froelich's adiposogenital dystrophy) should be considered. Laurence Moon syndrome, a separate disorder often confused with BBS, includes spastic paraplegia without polydactyly and obesity. The retinopathy of Laurence-Moon syndrome has more associated choroidal atrophy than BBS (77, 87). McKusick-Kaufman syndrome, initially described in an Amish population, presents with postaxial polydactyly, congenital heart disease, and hydrometrocolpos (accumulation of loculated fluid in the uterus and vagina); it is associated with the *BBS6* gene, but it has no retinal changes (88). Alstrom's syndrome, which presents with retinal degeneration, obesity, deafness, hyperlipidemia and diabetes mellitus, is distinguished from BBS by the presence of infantile cardiomyopathy (89,90). Biemond's syndrome presents with mental retardation, obesity, hypogenitalism, postaxial polydactyly, and iris coloboma (91,92).

Management

Patients with BBS may have secondary hypertension from renal artery stenosis. They can also develop secondary renal failure requiring dialysis or renal transplantation. Therefore, BBS patients should have a urinalysis done every 6 months; blood pressure and renal function should be monitored annually. Speech therapy and special education may be quite beneficial.

NEURONAL CEROID-LIPOFUSCINOSES (BATTEN'S DISEASE)

Clinical Symptoms and Signs

Batten's disease is one of the most common neurogenetic diseases of childhood. It is characterized by accumulation of ceroid lipopigment in lysosomes in various tissues of the body, especially neuronal tissue. The first description of this disease was by Stengel (93) in 1826, who described four siblings developing progressive blindness, epilepsy, cognitive and motor dysfunction. In 1903, Batten demonstrated an intraneuronal storage disease in juvenile patients presenting with the symptoms that Stengel (94) described. Zeman and Dyken (95) in 1969 coined the term neuronal ceroid-lipofuscinosis to distinguish Batten's disease from other gangliosidoses. Four subtypes of Batten's disease were recognized by age of onset: infantile (first year of life), late infantile (2 to 4 years), juvenile (6 to 8 years), and adult (96). These were named infantile neuronal ceroid-lipofuscinoses (INCL), late infantile neuronal ceroid-lipofuscinoses (LINCL), juvenile neuronal ceroid-lipofuscinoses (JNCL) and adult neuronal ceroid-lipofuscinoses (ANCL).

Inheritance

Batten's disease is AR. There are a few reports of autosomal dominance or "Parry type," named after a family from southern New Jersey exhibiting this form of inheritance (97).

Prevalence/Incidence

The incidence of Batten's disease is 1 in 12,500 births, making it the most common of all the lysosomal storage diseases

(98). Mutations in the *CLN1* gene are the most common genetic defects in Batten's disease. They account for about 20% of all Batten's disease cases in the United States; half of these cases present within the first year of life (99). There is an incidence of 1 in 20,000 of CLN1-associated Batten's disease in the Finnish population with a carrier frequency of 1 in 70. The classical infantile form (INCL) is by far the most common. The incidence of LINCL is 0.46 per 100,000 live births in Germany (100); the prevalence is 0.6 to 0.7 per million in Scandinavia. The incidence of JNCL is 7 per 100,000 in Scandinavia (101).

Genetics

Mutations in eight genes have been associated with Batten's disease (*CLN1–8*). Three of these genes encode lysosomal/endosomal membrane proteins. Two others, *CLN1* and *CLN2*, encode enzymes: palmitoyl protein thioesterase 1 and tripeptidyl peptidase 1, respectively. *CLN1* mutations have been detected worldwide and are found in all four age-of-onset subtypes of Batten's disease, but most commonly in INCL, which occurs in the first year of life. Although the children seem to develop normally in the first year, the rate of head growth decreases after 5 months of age, resulting in microcephaly. They also have muscular hypotonia and fail to develop normal motor control. The neurological development of patients with INCL begins to slow during the second year, when hyperkinesis of the hands, myoclonic jerks of the limbs, and seizures appear. There is a deterioration of motor abilities, truncal ataxia, and progressive loss of vision. There may be a brownish appearance to the macula, attenuation of the retinal vessels, and optic nerve pallor. By age 3 years, INCL patients typically will have lost their motor function and vision. They usually die between the ages of 8 and 13 years (99,102).

Mutations in the *CLN2* gene are reported to cause most cases of classic LINCL. It seems to have a worldwide distribution, but more commonly in the northern European population. The onset of LINCL is heralded by seizures that occur between the ages of 2 and 4 years. Seizures may be either partial, generalized tonic–clonic, or secondarily generalized. These seizures can be followed by ataxia, myoclonus, and developmental regression. These children lose their ability to walk, sit without support, and speak. They are often completely blind by age 5 or 6 years and are noted to have severe, progressive optic atrophy (Fig. 10-12). They die within a few years after the onset of blindness (103,104).

A defect in the *CLN3* gene causes JNCL. More than 30 *CLN3* mutations have been reported. JNCL patients first develop visual failure between the ages of 4 and 7 years. Profound vision loss can occur by age 10 years. There is also progressive deterioration of short-term memory and cognitive functions by age 8 years. Dysarthria, seizures, and parkinsonism may occur. Death may ensue by age 30 to 40 years (103,105,106).

Diagnosis

The diagnosis of NCL is dependent on a thorough history and physical examination, emphasizing the neurologic examination. Hypotonia, poor motor control, presence of seizures, developmental delay, and progressive visual loss are all characteristics of NCL. Electroencephalograms (EEGs), ERGs, and MRI are important in the initial workup.

In INCL, the EEG may reveal seizure activity as well as hypoactivity in certain parts of the brain. After age 3 years, the EEG may become severely, permanently depressed. Electroretinography often demonstrates early decreases in the scotopic and photopic responses and may become completely extinguished by age 3 years. Brain MRI usually reveals hypointense thalamic structures in T2-weighted images even in the first 7 to 10 months of life in INCL, before the presentation of clinical symptoms. After age 3 years, MRI can show extensive cerebral and cerebellar atrophy, with high intensity signal in the white matter (99).

In LINCL, brain imaging is relatively nonspecific, but the clinical neurophysiologic findings are characteristic of LINCL. The EEG shows an occipital photosensitive response using flash rates of 1 or 2 Hz. The visually evoked potentials (VEPs) and the somatosensory evoked potentials (SEPs) can be grossly enhanced in LINCL patients. The ERG can be diminished early and extinguished later in the disease process.

In JNCL, the EEG shows nonspecific abnormalities. ERG, however, shows severe changes with the b-wave being affected early. VEPs are reduced or extinguished. SEPs are enhanced. MRI shows progressive atrophy mostly in the cerebrum by age 12 (103,105).

Historically, NCL was diagnosed by frontal lobe biopsy, which revealed autofluorescent collections of ceroid and lipofuscin. Rectal biopsies have been similarly informative. More recently, less invasive methods such as conjunctival biopsy, skin biopsy, muscle biopsy, and isolation of circulating leukocytes have been used for pathologic diagnosis (107–110). Inclusion bodies have been found in these tissues. Ceroid and lipofuscinlike materials were often found within lysosomes; they are found to be Sudan and Periodic acid-Schiff stain positive. They have actually been found to be a complex mixture of lipoprotein and hydrophobic peptides. These storage deposits take on characteristic patterns on light and electron microscopy, and are useful for classification and diagnosis. In INCL, ANCL, and some atypical forms of JNCL, granular inclusions are seen on light microscopy. Curvilinear inclusions are predominantly seen in LINCL, with rare fingerprint inclusions. Fingerprint inclusions are predominantly seen in JNCL, with rare curvilinear inclusions (107,111).

Management

There is no effective treatment for NCL at present. Supportive care and genetic counseling are the mainstays of present management of this disease. NCL is an AR disease, so *in vitro* fertilization with zygote prescreening and/or amniocentesis may be of value.

ABETALIPOPROTEINEMIA (BASSEN-KORNZWEIG DISEASE)

Clinical Symptoms and Signs

Bassen and Kornzweig described a syndrome in 1950, which consisted of retinal degeneration associated with malabsorption syndrome, ataxia, neuromuscular degeneration, and acanthocytosis. At that time some people characterized this syndrome as comprising of Freidreich's ataxia, RP, and red blood cells of bizarre shapes (112). Further investigation led to the characterization of the defect in the secretion of apolipoproteins B-100 and B-48 (113). Due to the lack of these apolipoproteins, there is marked inability to absorb fat-soluble vitamins, triglycerides and cholesterol from the small intestine, resulting in low plasma level of cholesterol and triglycerides. There is a more than 50% reduction in all major plasma lipids, and a total absence of very-light-density lipoproteins and chylomicrons. There are also very low serum vitamin A and vitamin E levels, which are fat-soluble vitamins. Patients can present with mild fat malabsorption with steatorrhea, progressive ataxia with spinocerebellar symptoms, acanthocytosis with abnormally shaped red blood cells, marked serum lipid abnormalities, atypical pigmentary retinopathy, and death if untreated by the fourth decade (114,115). The fundus changes usually appear in the teen years, between the ages of 13 and 19 years (116). The retinoscopic changes can be variable and may be similar to the appearance of typical RP with bone spicules (Fig. 10-10), retinitis punctata albescens, or even patchy hypopigmentation without spicules (117,118). The neuropathologic changes in abetalipoproteinemia resemble those seen in vitamin E deficiency; the affected structures include the posterior columns, the spinocerebellar tracts, the medulla, and the cerebellum (119).

Inheritance

This disease is AR.

Prevalence/Incidence

This is a rare disease with an undefined prevalence.

Genetics

Mutations in the gene (*MPT*) encoding the large subunit of microsomal triglyceride transfer protein are associated with this disease. The *MPT* gene is located on *4q22–24* (120). The protein catalyzes the transport of triglycerides, cholesteryl ester and phospholipids from membrane surfaces. Wetterau et al. (121) showed that it was not present in four abetalipoproteinemic patients in contrast to control subjects. They suggested that these findings proved that *MTP* is the site of the defect in abetalipoproteinemia and that microsomal triglyceride transfer protein is required for lipoprotein assembly.

Diagnosis

History and physical examination are important in the detection of the neurologic changes; these include onset during middle childhood of ataxia, loss of fine motor control, peripheral neuropathy, progressive loss of visual acuity, failure to thrive, and steatorrhea. The serum triglyceride and cholesterol levels will be below 1.5 mmol/L. Furthermore, circulating beta-lipoproteins, chylomicrons, very-low-density lipoproteins, and low-density lipoproteins are virtually absent in the plasma (115). Peripheral blood smears will show acanthocytosis (from the Greek word "thorny") in which peripheral blood erythrocytes are transformed into "burr" cells; the cell membrane becomes spiculated in appearance, likely secondary to vitamin E deficiency. It is important to differentiate true acanthocytosis from artifactual causes attributable to anionic drugs, high pH, and contact with glass (122).

Management

This disease mimics vitamin E deficiency. It has been shown in a mammalian model that vitamin E deficiency causes atrophy of the posterior columns, the spinocerebellar tracts, the medulla, and the cerebellum, and that early treatment with supplemental vitamin E can prevent neurologic sequelae (123). Patients treated with vitamin A were reported to have reversal of ERG abnormalities (117,118). Vitamin A therapy alone may not halt the progression in the long term. Treatment with both vitamin E and vitamin A has been shown to be more effective, as long as treatment is initiated early in the disease process. The muscular sequelae are more difficult to reverse with vitamin supplementation. Current recommendations for treatment include 300 IU/kg of water-soluble vitamin A and 100 IU/kg of vitamin E daily (124). Individuals with coagulopathies from vitamin K deficiency may benefit from 0.5mg/kg of vitamin K daily (125). It is important to monitor the serum level of these vitamins once therapy has been instituted. Dietary restriction of fat will lessen steatorrhea.

REFERENCES

1. Donders FC. Beitrage zur pathologischen anatomie des auges. *Graefes Arch Klin Exp Ophthalmol* 1855;1:139.
2. Karpe G. The basis of clinical electroretinography. *Acta Ophthalmol* 1945;24[Suppl]:84.
3. Boughman JA, Conneally PM, Nance WE. Population genetic studies of retinitis pigmentosa. *Am J Hum Genet* 1980;32:223.
4. Jay M. On the heredity of retinitis pigmentosa. *Br J Ophthalmol* 1982;66:405.
5. Heckenlively JR,, et al. Retinitis Pigmentosa in the Navajo. *Metab Pediatr Ophthalmol* 1980;4:155.
6. McLaughlin ME, et al. Recessive mutations in the gene encoding the beta-subunit of rod phosphodiesterase in patients with retinitis Pigmentosa. *Nat Genet* 1993;4:130.
7. Huang SH, et al. Autosomal recessive retinitis Pigmentosa caused by mutations in the alpha subunit of rodcGMP phosphodiesteraswe. *Nat Genet* 1995;11:468.
8. Bareil C, et al. Segregation of a mutationin CNGB1 encoding the beta-subunit of the rod cGMP-gated channel in a family with autosomal recessive retinitis pigmentosa. *Hum Genet* 2001;108:328
9. Dryja TP, et al. Mutations in the gene encoding the alpha subunit of the rod cGMP-gated channel in autosomal recessive retinitis pigmentosa. *Proc Natl Acad Sci U S A* 1995;92:10177.
10. Hamel CP, et al. Molecular cloning and expression of RPE65, a novel retinal pigment epithelial-specific microsomal protein that is post-transcriptionally regulated in vitro. *J Biol Chem* 1993;268:15751.
11. GU S-M, et al. Mutations in RPE65 cause autosomal recessive severe onset retinal dystrophy. *Nat Genet* 1997;17:194.
12. Marlhens F, et al. Mutations in RPE65 cause Leber's congenital Amaurosis. *Nat Genet* 1997;17:139.
13. Battacharya SS, et al. Close genetic linkage between X-linked retinitis pigmentosa and a restriction fragment length polymorphism identified by recombinant DNA probe L1.28. *Nature* 1984;309:253.
14. Bird AC. X-linked Retinitis Pigmentosa. *Br J Ophthalmol* 1975;59:177.
15. Battacharya SS, et al. Close genetic linkage between X-linked retinitis pigmentosa and a restriction fragment length polymorphism identified by recombinant DNA probe L1.28. *Nature* 1984;309:253.
16. Fujita R, Buraczynaka M, Gieser L, et al. Analysis of the RPGR gene in 11 pedigrees with the retinitis pigmentosa type 3 genotype: paucity of mutations in the coding region but splice defects in two families. *Am J Hum Genet* 1997;61:571–580.
17. Andreasson S, Ponjavic V, Abrahamson M, et al. Phenotypes in three Swedish families with X-linked retinitis pigmentosa caused by different mutations of the RPGR gene. *Am J Ophthalmol* 1997;124:95–102.
18. Kaufman PL, Alm A, eds. *Adler's physiology of the eye*, 10th ed. St. Louis: Mosby, 2003:327.
19. Kajimura N, Harada Y, Usukura J. High-resolution freeze etching replica images of the disk and the plasma membrane surfaces in purified bovine rod outer segments. *J Electron Microsc (Tokyo)* 2000;49:691.
20. Humphries MM, Rancourt D, Farrar GJ, et al. Retinopathy induced in mice by targeted disruption of the rhodopsin gene. *Nat Genet* 1997;15:216–219.
21. Stryer L. Visual excitation and recovery. *J Biol Chem* 1991; 266:10711–10714.
22. Sagoo MS, Lagnado L. G-Protein deactivation is a rate-limiting for the shut-off of the phototransduction cascade. *Nature* 1997;389:392–395.
23. Simon A, Hellman U, Wenstedt C, et al. The retinal pigment epithelial-specific 11-cis-retinal dehydrogenase belongs to a family of short chain alcohol dehydrogenases. *J Biol Chem* 1995;270:1107–1112.
24. Gal A, et al. Rhodopsin mutations in inherited retinal dystrophies and dysfunctions. *Prog Retin Eye Res* 1997;16:51.
25. Inglehearn CF, et al. A complete screen for mutations of the rhodopsin gene in a panel of patients with autosomal dominant retinitis Pigmentosa. *Hum Mol Genet* 1992;1:41.

26. Bunge S, et al. Molecular analysis and genetic mapping of the rhodopsin gene in families with autosomal dominant retinitis Pigmentosa. *Genomics* 1993;17:230.

27. Inglehearn CF, Tarttelin EE, Plant C, et al. A linkage survey of 20 dominant retinitis Pigmentosa families: frequencies of nine known loci and evidence for further heterogeneity. *J Med Genet* 1998;35:1–5.

28. Dryja TP, McGee T, Reichel E, et al. A point mutation in the rhodopsin gene in one form of retinitis Pigmentosa. *Nature* 1990;343:364–366.

29. Oh KT, Weleber RG, Lottery A, et al. Description of a new mutation in rhodopsin, pro23 to ala, and comparison with electroretinographic and clinical characteristics of the pro23-to-his mutation. *Arch Ophthalmol* 2000;118:1269–1276.

30. Garriga P, Liu X, Khorana HG. Structure and function in rhodopsin: correct folding and misfolding in point mutants at and in proximity to the site of the retinitis pigmentosa mutation Leu-125—>Arg in the transmembrane helix C. *Proc Natl Acad Sci U S A* 1996;93:4560–4564.

31. Chapple JP, Grayson C, Hardcastle AJ, et al. Unfolding retinal dystrophies: a role for molecular chaperones? *rends Mol Med* 2001;7:414–421.

32. Berson EL, Howard J. Temporal aspects of the electoretinogram in sector retinitis pigmentosa. *Arch Ophthalmol* 1971; 86:653.

33. Rosenfeld JR, Cowley GS, McGee TL, et al. A null mutation in the rhodopsin gene causes rod photoreceptor dysfunction and autosomal recessive retinitis Pigmentosa. *Nat Genet* 1992; 1:209–213.

34. Rosenfeld PJ, Hahn LB, Sandberg MA, et al. Low incidence of retinitis pigmentosa among heterozygous carriers of a specific rhodopsin splice mutation. *Invest Ophthalmol Vis Sci* 1995;36: 2186–2192.

35. Rao VR, Cohen GB Oprian DD. Rhodopsin mutation G90D and a molecular mechanism for congenital night blindness. *Nature* 1994; 367:639–642.

36. Al-Jandal N, Farrar GJ, Kiang AS, et al. *Hum Mutat* 1999; 13:75–81.

37. Garriga P, Manyosa J. The eye photoreceptor protein rhodopsin: structural implications for retinal disease. *FEBS Lett* 2002;528:17–22.

38. Kaushal S, Khorana HG. Structure and function in rhodopsin: point mutations associated with autosomal dominant retinitis pigmentosa. *Biochemistry* 1994;33:6121.

39. Sung C-H, Davenport C, Nathans J. Rhodopsin mutations responsible for autosomal dominant retinitis Pigmentosa. *J Biol Chem* 1993;268:26645.

40. Fain GL, Lisman JE. Photoreceptor degeneration in vitamin A deprivation and retinitis Pigmentosa: the equivalent light hypothesis. *Exp Eye Res* 1993;57:335–340.

41. Tiansen L, Franson WK, Gorden, et al. Constitutive activation of the phototransduction by K296E opsin is not a cause photoreceptor degeneration. *Proc Natl Acad Sci U S A* 1995;92: 3551–3555.

42. Humphries M, et al. Retinopathy induced in mice by targeted disruption of the rhodopsin gene. *Nat Genet* 1997;15:216.

43. Kajiwara K, et al. Mutations in the human retinal degeneration slow gene in autosomal dominant retinitis Pigmentosa. *Nature* 1991;354:450.

44. Travis GH, Sutcliffe G, Bok D. The re5tinal degeneration slow gene product is a photoreceptor disc membrane associated glycoprotein. *Neuron* 1991;6:61.

45. Hawkins RK, Jansen HG, Sanyal S. Development and degeneration of retina in rds mutant mice: photoreceptor abnormalities in heterozygotes. *Exp Eye Res* 1985;41:701–720.

46. Weleber RG, Carr RE, Murphey WH, et al. Phenotypic variation including Retinitis Pigmentosa, Pattern Dystrophy, and Fundus Flavimaculatus in a single family with the deleation of codon 153 or 154 of the peripherin/ RDS gene. *Arch Ophthalmol* 1993;111:1531–1542.

47. Apfelstedt-Sylla E, Theischen M, Ruther K, et al. Extensive intrafamilial and interfamilial phenotypic variation among patients with autosomal dominant retinal dystrophy and mutations with the human RDS/ peripherin gene. *Br J Ophthalmol* 1995;79:28–34.

48. Kajiwara K, Sandberg MA, Berson EL, et al. A null mutation in the human peripherin/ RDS gene in a family with autosomal dominant retinitis punctata albescens. *Nat Genet* 1993; 3:208–212.

49. Kedzierski W, Lloyd M, Birch DG, et al. Generation and analysis of transgenic mice expressing P216L-substituted Rds/ peripherin in rod photoreceptors. *Invest Ophthalmol Vis Sci* 1997;38:498–509.

50. Kajiwara K, Berson EL, Dryja TR. Digenic retinitis Pigmentosa due to mutations at the unlinked peripherin/ RDS and ROM1 loci. *Science* 1994;264:1604.

51. von Ruckmann A, Fitzke FW, Bird AC. Distribution of fundus autofluorescence with a scanning laser ophthalmoscope. *Br J Ophthalmol* 1995;79:407.

51A. Berson EL, Rosner B, Sandberg MA, et al. A randomized trial of vitamin A and vitamin E supplementation for retinitis pigmentosa. *Arch Ophthalmol* 1993;111:761–772.

52. Mooren A. *Funf lustren ophthalmologischer wirksamkeit.* Wiesbaden: Bergmann, 1882:216–229.

53. Duke-Elder S. *Textbook of ophthalmology: diseases of the inner eye.* St. Louis: Mosby, 1941:2784.

54. Lauber H. Die sogenaunte retinitis Puntata Albescens. *Klin Monatsbl Augenhenkd* 1910;48:133.

55. Nettleship E. A history of congenital stationary night blindness in nine consecutive generations. *Trans Ophthalmol Soc U K* 1907;27:269.

56. Francois J. The differential diagnosis of tapetoretinal degenerations. *Arch Ophthalmol* 1958;59:86–120.

57. Pearce WG, Gillan JG, Brosseau L. Bardet-Biedl syndrome and retinitis Puntata Albescens in an isolated northern Canadian community. *Can J Ophthalmol* 1984;19:115–118.

58. Souied E, Soubrane G, Benlian P, et al. Retinitis Puntata Albescens associated with the Arg135Trp mutation in the rhodopsin gene. *Am J Ophthalmol* 1996;121:19–25.

59. Kajiwara K, Sandbergh MA, Berson EL, et al. A null mutation in the human peripherin/RDS gene in a family with autosomal dominant retinitis punctata Albescens. *Nat Genet* 1993;3: 208–212.

60. Burnstedt MSI, Sandgren O, Holmgren G, et al. Bothnia dystrophy caused by mutations in the cellular retinaldehyde-binding protein gene (RLBP1) on chromosome 15q26. *Invest Ophthalmol Vis Sci* 1999;40;5:995–1000.

61. Vernon M. Usher's syndrome: deafness and progressive blindness. Clinical cases, prevention, theory and literature survey. *J Chronic Dis* 1969;22:133–151.

62. Boughman JA, Vernon M, Shaver KA. Usher syndrome: definition and estimate of prevalence from two high-risk populations. *J Chronic Dis* 1983;36:595–603.

63. Bardet G. Sur un syndrome d'obesity congenital avec polydactlie et retinite pigmentaire. Contribution a l'etude des formes cliniques de l'obesity hypophasaire [thesis]. Paris. Theses de Paris (Le Grand), 1920.

64. Biedl A. Ein geschwisterpaar mit adipose genitals dystrophie. *Dtsch Med Wochenchr* 1922;48:1630.

65. Campo RV, Aaberg TM. Ocular and systemic manifestations of the Bardet-Biedl syndrome. *Am J Ophthalmol* 1982;94: 750–756.

66. Schachat AP, Maumenee IH. Bardet-Biedl syndrome and related disorders. *Arch Ophthalmol* 1982;100:285–288.

67. Beales PL, Elcioglu N, Woolf AS, et al. New criteria for improved diagnosis of Bardet-Biedl syndrome: results of a population survey. *J Med Genet* 1999; 36:437–446.

68. Klein D, Ammann F. The syndrome of Laurence-Moon-Bardet-Biedl and allied diseases in Switzerland. Clinical, genetic, and epidemiological studies. *J Neurol Sci* 1969;9:479.

69. Cox GF, Hansen RM, Quinn N, et al. Retinal function in carriers of Bardet-Biedl Syndrome. *Arch Ophthalmol* 2003;121: 804–810.

70. Croft JB, Swift, M. Obesity, hypertention and renal disease ion relatives of Bardet-Biedl syndrome sibs. *Am J Med Genet* 1990;55:12–15.

71. Baskin E, Balkanci F, Cekirge S, et al. Renal vascular abnormalities in Bardet-Biedl syndrome. *Pediatr Nephrol* 1999;13: 787–789.

72. Katsanis N, Ansley SJ, Badano JL, et al. Triallelic inheritance in Bardet-Biedl syndrome, a Mendelian recessive disorder. *Science* 2001;293:2256–2259.

73. Beales PL, Warner AM, Hitman GA, et al. Bardet-Biedl syndrome: a molecular and phenotypic study of 18 families. *J Med Genet* 1997;34:92–98.

74. Croft JB, Morrell D, Chase CL, et al. obesity in heterozygous carriers of the Bardet-Biedl syndrome. *Am J Med Genetet* 1995;55:12–15.

75. Farag TI, Teebi AS. High incidence of Bardet-Biedl sndrome among the Bedouin. *Clin Genet* 1989;36:4463–4464.

76. Green JS, Parfrey PS, Harnett JD, et al. the cardinal namifestations of Bardet-Biedl syndrome, a form of Lawrence-Moon_Bardet-Biedl syndrome. *N Engl J Med* 1989;321: 1002–1009.

77. Stiggelbout W. The Bardet-Biedl syndrome, including Hutchinson-Laurence-Moon syndrome. In: Vinkin PJ, Bruyn GW, eds. *Handbook of clinical neurology.* New York: Elsevier North Holland, 1977:380–412.

78. Leppert M, Baird L, Anderson KL, et al. Bardt-Biedl syndrome is linked to DNA markers on chromosome 11q and is genetically heterogeneous. *Nat Genet* 1994; 6:108–112.

79. Kwitek-Black A, Carmi R, Kuk GM, et al. Linkage of Bardet-Biedl syndrome to chromosome 16q and evidence for non-allelic genetic heterogeneity. *Nat Genet* 1993; 5:392–396.

80. Sheffield VC, Carmi R, Kwitek-Black A, et al. Identification of a Bardet-Biedl syndrome locus on chromosome 3 and evaluation of an efficient approach to homozygosit mapping. *Hum Mol Genet* 1994;3:1331–1335.

81. Carmi R, Rokhlina T, Kwitek-Black AE, et al. Use of a DNA pooling strategy to identify a human obesity syndrome locus (Bardet-Biedl) on chromosome 15. *Hum Mol Genet* 1995;4:9–13.

82. Young TL, Penney L, Woods MO, et al. A fifth locus for Bardet-Biedl syndrome maps to chromosome 2q31. *Am J Hum Genet* 1998;64:900–904.

83. Slavotinek AM, Stone EM, Mykytyn K, et al. Mutations in MKKS cause Bardet-Biedl syndrome. *Nat Genet* 2000;26: 15–16.

84. Badano JL, Ansley SJ, Leitch CC, et al. Identification of a novel Bardet-Biedl syndrome protein, BBS7, that shares structural features with BBS1 and BBS2. *Am J Hum Genet* 2003;72: 650–658.

85. Katsanis N, Beales PL, Woods MO, et al. Mutations in MKKS cause obesity, retinal dystrophy and renal malformations associated with Bardet-Biedl syndrome. *Nat Genet* 200;26:67–70.

86. Bruford EA, Riise R, Teague PW, et al. Linkage mapping in 29 Bardet-Biedl syndrome families confirms loci in chromosomal regions 11q13, 15q22.3–q23, and 16q21. *Genomics* 1997; 41:93–99.

87. Laurence J Moon R. Four cases of "retinitis pigmentosa," occurring in the same family and accompanied by general imperfections of development. *Ophthalmol Rev* 1866;2:32.

88. Slavotninek AM, Searby C, Al-Gazali, et al. Mutation analysis of the MKKS gene in McKusick-Kaufman syndrome and selected Bardet-Biedl syndrome patients. *Hum Genet* 2002; 110:561–567.

89. Alstrom C, Hallgren G, Wilson L, et al. Retinal degeneration combined with obesity, diabetes mellitus and neurogenic deafness. A specific syndrome (not hitherto described) distinct from the Laurence-Moon-Bardet-Biedl syndrome. A clinic endocrinological and genetic examination based on a large pedigree. *Acta Psychiatr Neurol Scand* 1959;129[Suppl]:1.

90. Rusell-Eggitt IM, Clayton PT, Coffey RK, et al. Alstrom syndrome: report of 22 cases and literature review. *Ophthalmology* 1998; 105:1274–1280.

91. Biemond A. Het syndrome van Laurence-Biedl en een niew aanverwant syndroom. *Ned Tijdschr Geneeskd* 1934;78:1801.

92. Verloes A, Temple IK, Bonnet S, et al. Coloboma, mental retardation, hypogonadism, and obesity: critical review of the so-called Biemond syndrome type 2, updated nosology, and delineation of three 'new' syndrome. *Am J Med Genetet* 1997; 69:370–379.

93. Stengel C. Beretning om et maerkeligt sygdomstilfaelde hos fire Soedskende I Naerheden af Roeraas. *Eyr Med Tidskrift* 1826;1:347–352.

94. Batten FE. Cerebral degeneration with symmetrical changes in the maculae in two members of a family. *Trans Ophthalmol Soc U K* 1903;23:386–390.

95. Zeman W, Dyken P, neuronal ceroid-lipofuscinosis (Batten's disease) relationship to amaurotic family idiocy. *Pediatrics* 1969;44:570–583.

96. Goebel HH. The neuronal ceroid-lipofuscinoses. *J Child Neurol* 1995;10:424–437.

97. Boehme DH, Cottrrrell JC, Leonberg SC, et al. A dominant form of neuronal ceroid-lipofuscinosis. *Brain* 1971;94: 745–760.

98. Rider JA, Rider DL, Batten disease: past, present, and future. *Am J Med Genet* 1988;[Suppl]5:21–26.

99. Santavuori P, Gottlov I, Haltia M, et al. CLN1. Infantile and other types of NCL with GROD. In: Goebel HH, Mole SE, Lake BD, eds. *The neuronal ceroid lipofuscinoses (Batten disease).* Amsterdam: IOS Press, 1999:16–36.

100. Claussen M, Heim P, Knisper J, et al. incidence of neuronal ceroid-lipofuscinoses in West Germany: Variation of a method for studying autosomal recessive disorders. *Am J Med Genet* 1992;42:536–538.

101. Uvebrant P, Hagberg B. Neuronal ceroid-lipofuscinoses in Scandinavia: Epidemiology and clinical pictures. *Neuropediatrics* 1997;28:6–8.

102. Santavuori P, Haltia M, Rapola J, et al. infantile type of so called neuronal ceroid-lipofuscinosis. 1. A clinical study of 15 patients. *J Neurol Sci* 1973;18:257–267.

103. Wisniewski KE, Kida E, Golabek AA, et al. Neuronal ceroid-lipofuscinoses: classification and diagnosis. In: Wisniewski KE, Zhong N, eds. *Batten disease: ciagnosis, treatment and research.* San Diego: Academic Press, 2001:1–34.

104. Williams RE, Gottlob I, Lake BD, et al. Classic late infantile NCL. In: Goebel HH, Mole SE, Lake BD, eds. *The neuronal ceroid lipofuscinoses (Batten disease).* Amsterdam: IOS Press, 1999:37–54.

105. Hofmann I, Kohlschuetter P, Santavuori P, et al. CLN3. Juvenile lipofuscinoses (Batten disease). Amsterdam: IOS Press, 1999:55–76.

106. Wisniewski KE, Zhong N, Kaczmarski W, et al. Compound heterozygous genotype is associated with protracted juvenile neuronal ceroid lipofuscinosis. *Ann Neurol* 1998; 43: 106–110.

107. Libert J. Diagnosis of lysosomal storage disease by the ultrastructural study of conjunctival biopsies. *Pathol Annu* 1980; 15:37–66.

108. Rapola J, Santavuori P, Savilahti B. Suction biopsy of rectal mucosa in the diagnosis of infantile and juvenile types of neuronal ceroid0lipofuscinosis. *Hum Pathol* 1984;15:352–360.

109. Markesbery WR, Shield LK, Egel RT, et al. Late-infantile neuronal ceroid-lipofuscinosis: an ultrastructural study of lymphocyte inclusions. *Arch Neurol* 1976; 33:630–635.

110. Dom R, Brucheer JM, Ceuterick C, et al. Adult ceroid-lipofuscinosis (Kufs' disease) in two brothers: retinal and visceral storage in one, diagnostic muscle biopsy in the other. *Acta Neuropathol* 1979;45:67–72.

111. Arsenio-Nunes ML, Goutieres F, Aicardi J. An ultramicroscopic study of skin and conjunctival biopsies in chronic neurological disorders of childhood. *Ann Neurol* 1981;9:163–173.

112. Bassem FA. Lprmzweog AL. Malformation of erythrocytes in a case of atypical retinitis pigmentosa. *Blood* 1950;5:381–387.

113. Salt HB, Wolff OH, Lloyd JK, et al. On having no betalipoprotein. A syndrome comprising A-beta-lipoproteinemia, acanthocytosis and steatorrhea. *Lancet* 1960; 2: 325.

114. Kornzweig AL, Bassen FA. Retinitis pigmentosa, acanthocytosis, and heredodegenerative neuromuscular disease. *Arch Ophthalmol* 1957;58:183.

115. Kane JP, Havel RJ. Disorders of the biogenesis and secretion of lipoproteins containing the B apolipoproteins. In: Scriver CR, Beaudet AL, Sly WS, et al., eds. *The metabolic bases of inherited disease*, 7th ed. New York: McGraw-Hill, 1995:1853–1885.

116. Francois J. Metabolic tapetoretinal degenerations. *Surv Ophthalmol* 1982;26:293.

117. Gouras P, Carr RE, Gunkel RD. Retinitis pigmentosa in abetalipoproteinemia: effects of vitamin A. *Invest Ophthalmol* 1971;10:784.

118. Wolff OH, Lloyd JK, Tonks EL. A-B-lipoproteinemia with special reference to the visual defect. *Exp Eye Res* 1964;3:439.

119. Harding AE. Vitamin E and the nervous system. *Crit Rev Neurobiol* 1987;3:89–103.

120. Narcisi TM, Shoulders CC, Chester SA, et al. Mutations of the microsomal triglyceride-transfer-protein gene in abetalipoproteinaemia. *Am J Hum Genet* 1995;57:1298–1310.

121. Wetterau JR, Aggerbeck LP, Bouma ME, et al. Absence of microsomal triglyceride transfer protein in individuals with abetalipoproteinemia. 1992;258:999–1001.

122. Stevenson VL, Hardie RJ. Acanthocytosis and neurological disorders. *J Neurol* 2001;248:87–94.

123. Muller DP, Lloyd JK, Wolff OH. The role of vitamin E in the treatment of neurological features of abetalipoproteinemia and other disorders of fat absorption. *J Inherit Metab Dis* 1985;8[Suppl 1]:88–92.

124. Grant CA, Berson EL. Treatable forms of retinitis pigmentosa associated with systemic neurological disorders. *Int Ophthalmol Clin* 103–110.

125. Schaefer EJ. Diagnosis and management of ocular abnormalities in abetalipoproteinemia: possible role of vitamin E. *Arch Dis Child* 1977;52:509.

11

USHER DISEASE

BRONYA J. B. KEATS

Usher disease (or syndrome) is a group of genetic disorders with an autosomal recessive pattern of inheritance. The initial clinical finding is bilateral sensorineural hearing loss followed by retinitis pigmentosa, which usually manifests in late childhood or adolescence and may lead to total blindness. Siblings with congenital hearing loss and progressive pigmentary dystrophy were first reported in 1858 by von Graefe (1,2). However, the disorder was named after the British ophthalmologist, Charles Usher, who documented the frequency of hearing loss among patients with retinitis pigmentosa and recognized that there were at least two clinical types of Usher disease, the differences being in the degree of hearing loss and the age of onset of the visual loss (3). Since then, the clinical heterogeneity has been described in numerous publications (4,5) and the Usher Consortium (6) delineated comprehensive diagnostic criteria. Usher disease is genetically heterogeneous, and over the past 10 years remarkable progress has been made in the identification and functional characterization of the Usher disease genes, of which there are at least 11. For reviews of these advances, see references 7–9.

It is important to realize that a child with Usher disease is likely to be given the misdiagnosis of nonsyndromic congenital hearing loss with the correct diagnosis not entertained until the onset of visual loss. Thus, use of effective ophthalmologic and genetic diagnostic tools is critical for every child with sensorineural hearing loss who may be at risk for Usher disease. An early diagnosis provides time for careful preparation for the physical and emotional impact of the approaching visual loss (10), following satisfactory management of the hearing loss (11).

PREVALENCE

More than 50% of the deaf–blind population and about 18% of individuals with retinitis pigmentosa have Usher disease (12). The prevalence has been estimated in numerous northern European countries as well as the United Kingdom, the United States, and Colombia, and the range is 2 to 6.2 per 100,000 (7). Of great significance is the per-

centage of children born with severe to profound hearing loss who have Usher disease. In a 1969 study, Vernon (13) estimated between 3% and 6%, and a more recent ophthalmologic study found that 10.4% of children with severe to profound hearing loss had Usher disease (11). The percentage in some ethnic groups such as the Ashkenazi Jews (14) may be considerably higher.

WORLDWIDE IMPACT ON PUBLIC HEALTH

As the major cause of deafness and blindness, Usher disease is an important public health problem, particularly from the standpoint of early identification of hearing impaired children with Usher disease. It is an autosomal recessive disorder, meaning that affected children have two abnormal copies of the gene, one inherited from each parent. The parents are carriers but show no signs of the disease. The frequency of carriers may be as high as 1 in 50 in some populations. If both parents are carriers, then each child has a 25% chance of having Usher disease, and the probability that an unaffected child is a carrier is two-thirds (Fig. 11-1). Note that a positive family history is not expected with an autosomal recessive disorder such as Usher disease because the abnormal allele may be passed on from one (unaffected) carrier to the next for many generations before a couple, who by chance both carry an abnormal allele for the same genetic form of Usher disease, has an affected child.

The significance of developing effective approaches to management and therapy, and providing relief for the tremendous personal burden imposed by loss of both vision and hearing cannot be underestimated.

CLINICAL FINDINGS

Three clinical types of Usher disease have been defined (Table 11-1) with detailed diagnostic criteria (6). In Usher type I, the hearing loss is severe to profound across all frequencies and the onset of retinitis pigmentosa is during childhood. Vestibular function is generally absent although

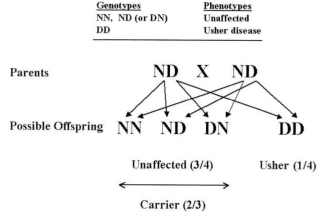

Autosomal Recessive Inheritance

Genotypes	Phenotypes
NN, ND (or DN)	Unaffected
DD	Usher disease

Parents   **ND X ND**

Possible Offspring   **NN   ND   DN   DD**

Unaffected (3/4)   Usher (1/4)

Carrier (2/3)

FIGURE 11.1. Autosomal-recessive inheritance. Both parents are carriers and the probabilities of each of the possible offspring genotypes are 1/4NN, 1/2ND, and 1/4DD. Shown in parentheses are the probabilities of the two phenotypes (unaffected and Usher) and the probability that an unaffected offspring is a carrier.

some Usher type I patients with normal response to bithermal vestibular testing have been reported (15). Hearing aids are usually not helpful, but cochlear implantation is proving to be beneficial for an increasing number of individuals with Usher type I (16). The degree of hearing loss in patients diagnosed with Usher type II increases from moderate in the low frequencies to severe in the high frequencies and tends to remain stable; carefully-fitted hearing aids usually work well for them. They have normal vestibular function and the age of onset of retinitis pigmentosa is usually during the teenage years. Usher type III is distinguished from the other two types by the progressive nature of the hearing loss. The age of onset of retinitis pigmentosa and the degree of vestibular dysfunction are variable.

The development of pigmentary retinopathy distinguishes Usher disease from nonsyndromic hearing loss, with night blindness often being the first indication of retinal degeneration. Vision loss gradually increases as a result of progressive degeneration of rod photoreceptor cells, and may progress to total blindness by the third or fourth decade. An

TABLE 11-1. CLINICAL TYPES OF USHER SYNDROME

	Type I	Type II	Type III
Bilateral sensorineural hearing loss	Severe to profound (stable)	Moderate to severe (stable)	Progressive
Vestibular function	Absent	Normal	Variable
Onset of visual loss	First decade	Second decade	Variable

early diagnosis can be made with an electroretinogram (ERG) and is recommended for all children with sensorineural hearing loss who may be at risk for Usher disease (16,17). Some minor clinical differences in ocular manifestations between Usher type I and type II have been reported (18,19), but none of them was found to distinguish between the two types besides age of onset of night blindness (20). However, Seeliger et al (21) recently demonstrated significant ERG implicit time differences between Usher type I and type II, which may reflect underlying structural differences.

Aberrant findings that have been reported in studies of the retinal photoreceptor cells include a high proportion of abnormal axonemes (22) and abnormal connecting cilia of photoreceptors in the macula (23). Studies of temporal bone histopathology have shown extensive degeneration of the hair cells of the organ of Corti and spiral ganglion cells with atrophy of the stria vascularis (24–26). Other clinical anomalies that have been reported in Usher patients are reviewed by Keats and Corey (7). They include olfactory loss (27), structural abnormalities of nasal cilia (28), and decreased sperm motility (22).

GENETICS

Eleven different Usher disease loci have been mapped and seven genes have been identified (Table 11-2). However, for at least three of these genes, some mutations cause Usher syndrome and others result in nonsyndromic hearing loss. As with many other phenotypes, mouse models have facilitated identification of Usher disease genes. Mutations in the murine homologs of four of these genes are responsible for the mouse mutants, *shaker 1, waltzer, Ames-waltzer,* and *Jackson shaker.*

Seven different Usher type I loci have been mapped to chromosomal regions and five (*USH1B, USH1C, USH1D, USH1F, USH1G*) have been identified. The other two loci, *USH1A* and *USH1E,* have been mapped to chromosome 14q32 (29) and chromosome 21q21 (30), respectively. Three Usher type II loci have been localized, but only the *USH2A* gene has been isolated. *USH2B* has been mapped to chromosome 3p23–24.2 (31) and *USH2C* is located on chromosome 5q14.3–21.3 (32). The only Usher type III locus reported so far (*USH3*) is on chromosome 3q and it was recently identified.

USH1B

Approximately 75% of Usher type I patients have USH1B. It is caused by mutations in the *MYO7A* gene on chromosome 11q, which encodes the unconventional myosin VIIa protein (33), a member of the large superfamily of myosin motor proteins that move along cytoplasmic actin filaments in an ATP-dependent manner. Mutations in the

TABLE 11-2. USHER GENES, PROTEINS, AND MOUSE MODELS

Locus	Gene	Protein	Phenotype	Mouse Model
USH1A (14q32)	—	—	Usher type I	—
USH1B (11q13)	*MYO7A*	Myosin VIIa	Usher type I, DFNA12, DFNB2	*shaker-1*
USH1C (11p15)	*USH1C*	Harmonin	Usher type I, DFNB18	—
USH1D (10q)	*CDH23*	Cadherin 23	Usher type I, DFNB12	*waltzer*
USH1E (21q21)	—	—	Usher type I	—
USH1F (10)	*PCDH15*	Protocadherin 15	Usher type I	*Ames waltzer*
USH1G (17q)	*SANS*	Sans	Usher type I	*Jackson shaker*
USH2A (1q41)	*USH2A*	Usherin	Usher type II type III, RP	—
USH2B (3p23–24)	—	—	Usher type II	—
USH2C (5q14–21)	—	—	Usher type II	—
USH3A (3q21–25)	*USH3A*	Clarin	Usher type III	—

DFNA* and DFNB* designate forms of autosomal dominant and recessive nonsyndromic hearing loss, respectively, that are due to mutations in an Usher gene. RP designates nonsyndromic retinitis pigmentosa.

orthologous mouse gene cause the deafness mutant *shaker-1*, and the gene was identified through studies of this mutant (34). *MYO7A* has 48 coding exons extending over 100 kb and it is expressed in several alternative splice forms. More than 80 different mutations have been reported in *MYO7A*. Although most of these mutations are in Usher type IB patients, some are associated with autosomal recessive (*DFNB2*) and autosomal dominant (*DFNA12*) nonsyndromic deafness. These mutations occur throughout the gene, although they do tend to cluster in the exons encoding important conserved domains of the protein (35).

Scanning electron micrographs of the cochlea of *shaker-1* mice show disorganization of the sensory hair bundles, which are normally highly organized structures with precisely arranged rows of stereocilia on the apical surface of the hair cells (36). *Shaker-1* mice do not show retinal degeneration, but there are subtle defects in their retinas. For example, their retinal pigmented epithelial cells do not transport pigment granules in the microvilli (37) and the opsin protein is observed in the connecting cilium, suggesting a failure of transport to the outer segment (38).

Myosin VIIa is a 254-kd protein consisting of 2,215 amino acids. As is typical of myosins, it has a motor head domain containing ATP- and actin-binding motifs and a long tail with two large repeats (FERM) of about 460 amino acids (7,8). It is expressed in the cochlear hair cells and both the RPE-cells and the photoreceptor cells of the retina, and has also been detected in testis, lung, kidney, intestine, and olfactory epithelium. In all of these epithelial tissues, highest expression is associated with the cilia and microvilli of the apical surfaces (39).

Myosin VIIa has been studied extensively; the findings point to a role in transport of membrane-associated proteins at apical surfaces of cells and, in the inner ear, it may be essential for adhesion between stereocilia. Boeda et al. (40) and Siemens et al. (41) suggest that several of the Usher type I proteins, including myosin VIIa, interact to form a functional unit needed for transport and adhesion (Fig. 11-2).

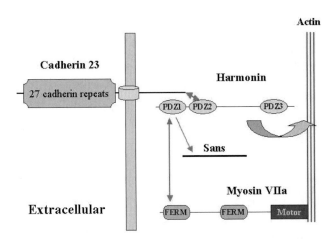

FIGURE 11.2. Schematic diagram depicting a proposed way in which harmonin, myosin VIIa, cadherin 23 and sans may interact with one another and actin via the PDZ domains in harmonin. A mutation in a gene encoding any one of these proteins may disrupt this functional unit and result in Usher syndrome type I. (Adapted from Weil D, El-Amraoui A, Masmoudi S, et al. Usher syndrome type IG (USH1G) is caused by mutations in the gene encoding SANS, a protein that associates with the USH1C protein, harmonin. *Hum Mol Genet* 2003;12:463–471, with permission.)

USH1C

Usher type IC was first described in the Acadian population of Louisiana, and the *USH1C* gene on chromosome 11p was recently shown to encode a PDZ-domain protein called harmonin (42,43). The *USH1C* gene contains 28 coding exons spanning 51 kb, and three subclasses of harmonin isoforms are found as a result of alternative splicing of eight exons. In patients of Acadian ancestry a mutation that introduces a cryptic splice site in exon 3 (216G>A) was detected, as well as a nine-repeat VNTR with an unusual structure in intron 5. These two events are in complete linkage disequilibrium in the Acadian population and neither was found in 340 unrelated controls from five different ethnic groups (44). Whether both of these events are necessary for abnormal gene expression remains to be determined. Several other mutations have been reported in patients of non-Acadian ancestry (42–45), and one of 44 Acadian patients was found to be a compound heterozygote, demonstrating admixture in this population (44). A second patient with an Acadian father and a non-Acadian mother was also a compound heterozygote. For this child, family history suggested a possible diagnosis of Usher disease (Fig. 11-3). If this had not been the case, the child would probably have been misdiagnosed as nonsyndromic bilateral profound hearing loss. When the diagnosis of Usher disease was made by genetic testing, the parents were proactive in obtaining a cochlear implant for their 18-month-old son. This child is now 3 years old and has excellent oral language. Mutations in *USH1C* have also been associated with nonsyndromic hearing loss (DFNB18).

The major protein isoform of harmonin contains 552 amino acids and three PDZ domains. These domains are involved in the organization of protein complexes (46), and may be essential components in the proposed functional unit composed of Usher type I proteins depicted in Fig. 11.2 (40,41).

USH1D

Usher type ID was recently shown to be associated with mutations in a novel cadherinlike gene (*CDH23*) on chromosome 10q (47). It is probably the second most common form of Usher type I. Mutations in this gene were also found in the mouse mutant *waltzer* (48), in which the hair bundles are disorganized just as in *shaker-1* mice. *CDH23* has 69 coding exons and spans more than 300 kb. Numerous mutations have been reported and there is a loose correlation between phenotype and type of mutation (48). As with *MYO7A* and *USH1C*, mutations in *CDH23* are also found in patients with nonsyndromic hearing loss (DFNB12).

The protein encoded by the *CDH23* gene has 3354 amino acids and 27 extracellular cadherin repeats. Cadherins are a large protein family, which contain extracellular calcium binding domains and are involved in intercellular adhesion. Boeda et al. (40) and Siemens et al. (41) have shown that cadherin 23, as well as myosin VIIa, binds to harmonin by means of PDZ-domain interactions, suggesting that myosin VIIa may convey harmonin along the actin core of developing stereocilia where harmonin may anchor cadherin 23 to the actin filaments (Fig. 11-2).

USH1F

Mutations in another cadherinlike gene, *PCDH15*, on chromosome 10 were found in patients with Usher type IF. The murine homolog of this protocadherin gene was shown to be defective in the *Ames waltzer* mouse, in which the disorganized hair bundles are very similar to those in *shaker-1* and *waltzer*. Subsequent analyses revealed the presence of splice site and nonsense mutations in the *PCDH15* gene in two families from Pakistan (49,50). More recently, a novel mutation (R245X) that appears to account for a large proportion of cases of Usher type I in the Ashkenazi Jewish population was reported (14).

Protocadherin 15 is a large transmembrane protein (216 kd) with 1955 amino acids and 11 cadherin repeats. It may be a mediator of protein–protein interactions through the proline-rich regions in its cytoplasmic domain, and a similar functional role to that of cadherin 23 seems plausible.

USH1G

The USH1G locus was mapped to chromosome 17q in a consanguineous Jordanian family (51) and the causative

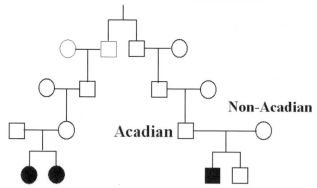

USH1C Compound Heterozygote
[238-239insC / 216G>A, 9VNTR(t,t)]

Non-Acadian

Acadian

FIGURE 11.3. Pedigree of Usher type IC male with Acadian ancestry on the paternal side but not the maternal side. The parents are carriers of two different mutations, D_1 [216G>A/9VNTR(t,t)] and D_2 (238–239insC) and the child is a compound heterozygote with the genotype D_1D_2. His unaffected sibling is a carrier of D_2 and the affected female relatives both have the genotype D_1D_1.

gene was quickly identified as *SANS*, which is mutated in the *Jackson shaker* mouse (52,53). As might be anticipated, these mice have disorganized hair bundles. *SANS* contains three exons, two of which are coding, and spans 7.2 kb. It encodes a novel 460-amino acid scaffoldlike protein that was shown to associate with harmonin in cotransfection experiments (53).

USH2A

Usher type IIA accounts for about 70% of all Usher syndrome patients. The *USH2A* gene is on chromosome 1q and encodes a novel 171-kd protein named usherin with 1,551 amino acids (54). Usherin shows homology with extracellular matrix and cell–cell adhesion proteins, and has ten laminin epidermal growth factor motifs arranged in tandem as well as four tandem repeats of a fibronectin type III motif in the carboxy terminal region. The *USH2A* transcript is expressed primarily in the cochlea and the cells of the outer nuclear layer of the retina (55).

At least 20 different mutations are found in *USH2A*, which consists of 21 exons (the first of which is noncoding), spanning at least 105 kb. The most frequent mutation, 2299delG, may be present in more than 20% of Usher type IIA patients in Europe and the United States, as well as some Usher type III patients (56). In addition, the 2299delG mutation has been observed in patients whose primary disorder is retinitis pigmentosa and who report minimal hearing loss, and another *USH2A* mutation, Cys759Phe, was found in about 4.5% of nonsyndromic autosomal recessive retinitis pigmentosa (57).

USH3

Most cases of Usher type III have been described in the Finnish population, and mutations in a novel gene (*USH3A*) on chromosome 3 were recently shown to be associated with Usher type III (58). This gene encodes a 232 amino acid protein called clarin, which contains four transmembrane domains and may be required for normal synaptic transmission by sensory cells.

PATHOPHYSIOLOGY

Degeneration of the hair cells underlies the hearing loss observed in Usher disease. The inner ears of each of the mouse models for Usher type I (*shaker-1*, *waltzer*, *Ames-waltzer*, and *Jackson shaker*) show disorganization of the hair bundles, which progressively increases after birth. The stereocilia of the *mariner* zebrafish mutant, also a model for Usher type IB, has similar disarray of stereocilia (59). Therefore, it seems likely that disorganization of the hair bundles

plays a major role in Usher type I as far as hearing loss is concerned.

The retinitis pigmentosa that affects Usher patients results from progressive degeneration of the rod photoreceptor cells. Myosin VIIa is found in the vicinity of the connecting cilium that joins the inner and outer segments of photoreceptor cells. Although *shaker-1* mice show no signs of retinal degeneration, electroretinographic anomalies (a reduction of the a-and b-wave amplitudes) have been reported (60), and opsin flow at the connecting cilium is significantly reduced (38).

DIAGNOSTIC TOOLS

A child diagnosed with moderate to profound hearing impairment may in fact have Usher disease. Among profoundly hearing impaired infants, approximately 3% to 6% are likely to have Usher type I, and the percentage is likely to be higher in some populations such as the Ashkenazi Jews (14) and the Acadians (44). An early diagnosis can be made with an ERG. This should be done, at a minimum, for all profoundly hearing impaired children who do not begin walking until after the age of 18 months or who have a family history of Usher disease (16,17). In the near future, genetic testing is likely to provide a definitive diagnosis at an earlier age than an ERG. Such testing is already feasible for profoundly hearing impaired infants of Ashkenazi Jewish and Acadian ancestry because specific mutations in the *PCDH15* and *USH1C* genes, respectively, are associated with the Usher I phenotype. In other populations, testing for a carefully selected set of mutations in *MYO7A*, *CDH23*, and *PCDH15* may provide an accurate diagnosis for more than 50% of the hearing impaired children who have Usher syndrome. Early diagnosis of Usher syndrome would substantially increase the length of preparation time for the gradual visual loss. In particular, the development of communication skills through interventions that provide effective management of profound hearing loss without reliance on vision could be initiated at an early age.

MANAGEMENT AND REHABILITATION

Effective management and rehabilitation for patients with Usher syndrome requires a team approach. Hearing loss in an infant may be suspected by the parents or the pediatrician, or it may be detected through newborn hearing screening, which is mandated in some states. In each suspected case, an audiologist should be the health care professional who confirms the diagnosis and develops a management plan. As with all forms of hearing loss, a clinical geneticist and a genetic counselor need to be part of the team (61), together with an ophthalmologist if testing indicates that the child has Usher disease. Pretest and post-test genetic counseling sessions are essential for preparing parents for the possibility of a diagnosis of Usher disease. Psychosocial counseling with a social worker who has experience in working with Usher patients (10) is important for the parents and critical for the child as vision begins to diminish. All professionals working with Usher patients and their family members need to be sensitive to their cultural orientation and emotional needs. Early consultation with an otolaryngologist will identify those infants with Usher type 1 who are most likely to benefit from cochlear implants. A child who has received a cochlear implant at an early age is likely to be able to maintain oral communication skills that do not rely on ability to see. However, a child whose mode of communication is visual sign language will need to adapt to a tactile form of sign language with loss of vision.

ETHICAL CONSIDERATIONS

Genetic testing is providing the ability to establish etiologic diagnosis in infants. Interpretation of the test results is not always straightforward, especially as mutations in the same gene may result in different phenotypes. The ability of the parents to accept an unfavorable result may vary dramatically depending on their emotional state (62). In addition, finding a mutation in a child has medical implications for all family members who share genes with the child. The ethical issue of genetic privacy for relatives is immediately obvious (63). Additionally, the issue of genetic discrimination is raised with loss of health insurance being a common concern.

Another ethical question is that of presymptomatic testing. Although this is of greater concern for later age of onset dominant genetic diseases such as Huntington disease and spinocerebellar ataxia, it is also of some relevance to Usher disease, where vision loss is predicted well in advance of deterioration in sight. The fact that an effective management and rehabilitation plan for an infant diagnosed with Usher disease is likely to be different from that for a child with nonsyndromic hearing loss is an argument in favor of genetic testing for Usher disease. Discussion of these issues is recommended for all patients so that an informed decision can be made as to whether or not to proceed with genetic testing.

FUTURE TREATMENTS BASED ON RESEARCH

Increasing knowledge of the abnormal genes associated with Usher disease means that accurate diagnoses, more effective management, and possibly, early intervention can be provided for affected children. New technologies that allow high-throughput and accurate genetic testing are evolving and will lead to routine molecular diagnostic screening.

Identification of genes for Usher disease provides an important step toward understanding the molecular mechanisms of hearing and vision. Research is providing insight into the function of the proteins encoded by these genes, and as a consequence, understanding of the auditory and visual systems is advanced. Animal models, in particular mouse mutants, which may be spontaneous, transgenic, or induced by N-ethyl-N-nitrosourea (ENU) mutagenesis, are essential for many developmental and functional studies of the abnormal gene and protein.

In addition, research is demonstrating the vast amount of variation at both the phenotypic and genotypic levels. The goal, which is to characterize all of the genetic and non-genetic factors that play a role in Usher disease, and to determine the interactions among them, is within reach. Effective molecular intervention therapies for some forms of Usher disease may be achievable in the near future.

Acknowledgment: Support for this work was provided by The Foundation Fighting Blindness.

REFERENCES

1. von Graefe A. Vereinzelte Beobachtungen und Bemerkungen. Exceptionelle Verhalten des Gesichtsfeldes bei Pigmentenartung des Netzhaut. *Graefes Arch Klin Ophthalmol* 1858;4:250–253.
2. Gorlin RJ, Toriello HV, Cohen MM. *Hereditary hearing loss and its syndromes.* Oxford: Oxford University Press, 1995.
3. Usher CH. On the inheritance of retinitis pigmentosa, with notes of cases. *R Lond Ophthalmol Hosp Rep* 1914;19:130–236.
4. Hallgren B. Retinitis pigmentosa combined with congenital deafness with vestobulo-cerebellar ataxia and mental abnormality in a proportion of cases. A clinical and genetico-statistical study. *Acta Psychiatr Scand Suppl* 1959;138:5–101.
5. Davenport SLH, Omenn GS. *The heterogeneity of Usher syndrome.* Publication 426. Amsterdam: Excerpta Medica Foundation, International Congress Series, 1977. Abstract 215:87–88.
6. Smith RJH, Berlin CI, Hejtmancik JF, et al. Clinical diagnosis of the Usher syndromes. *Am J Med Genet* 1994;50:32–38.
7. Keats BJB, Corey DP. The Usher syndromes. *Am J Med Genet* 1999;89:158–166.
8. Petit C. Usher Syndrome: From Genetics to Pathogenesis. *Ann Rev Genomics Hum Genet* 2001;2:271–297.
9. Call LM, Morton CC. Continuing to break the sound barrier: genes in hearing. *Curr Opin Genet Dev* 2002;12:343–348.
10. Miner ID. Psychosocial implications of Usher syndrome, Type I, throughout life cycle. *J Visual Impair Blindness* 1995;89:287–296.
11. Mets MB, Young NM, Pass A, et al. Early diagnosis of Usher syndrome in children. *Trans Am Ophthalmol Soc* 2000;98:237–242.
12. Boughman JA, Vernon M, Shaver KA. Usher syndrome: definition and estimate of prevalence from two high-risk populations. *J Chronic Dis* 1983;36:595–603.
13. Vernon M. Usher's syndrome–deafness and progressive blindness. Clinical cases, prevention, theory and literature survey. *J Chronic Dis* 1969;22:131–151.
14. Ben-Yosef T, Ness SL, Madeo AC, et al. A mutation of PCDH15 among Ashkenazi Jews with the type 1 Usher syndrome. *New Engl J Med* 2003;348:1664–1670.

15. Otterstedde CR, Spandau U, Blankenagel A, et al. A new clinical classification for Usher's syndrome based on a new subtype of Usher's syndrome type I. *Laryngoscope* 2001;111:84–86.
16. Loundon N, Marlin S, Busquet D, et al. Usher syndrome and cochlear implantation. *Otol Neurotol* 2003;24:216–221.
17. Young NM, Mets MB, Hain TC. Early diagnosis of Usher syndrome in infants and children. *Am J Otol* 1996;17:30–34.
18. Fishman GA, Kumar A, Joseph ME, Torok N, Anderson R. Usher's syndrome: Ophthalmic and neuro-otologic findings suggesting genetic heterogeneity. *Arch Ophthalmol* 1983;101: 1367–1374.
19. Seeliger M, Pfister M, Gendo K, et al. Comparative study of visual, auditory, and olfactory function in Usher syndrome. *Graefes Arch Clin Exp Ophthalmol* 1999;237:301–307.
20. Tsilou ET, Rubin BI, Caruso RC, et al. Usher syndrome clinical types I and II: could ocular symptoms and signs differentiate between the two types? *Acta Ophthalmol Scand* 2002;80:196–201.
21. Seeliger M, Zrenner E, Apfelstedt-Sylla E, et al. Identification of Usher syndrome subtypes by ERG implicit time. *Invest Ophthalmol Vis Sci* 2001;42:3066–3071.
22. Hunter DG, Fishman GA, Mehta RS, et al. Abnormal sperm and photoreceptor axonemes in Usher's syndrome. *Arch Ophthalmol* 1986;104:385–389.
23. Berson EL, Adamian M. Ultrastructural findings in an autopsy eye from a patient with Usher's syndrome type II. *Am J Ophthalmol* 1992;114:748–757.
24. Cremers CW, Delleman WJ. Usher's syndrome, temporal bone pathology. *Int J Pediatr Otorhinolaryngol* 1988;16:23–30.
25. Nadol JB. Application of electron microscopy to human otopathology. Ultrastructural findings in neural presbycusis, Meniere's disease and Usher's syndrome. *Acta Otolaryngol* 1988; 105:411–419.
26. van Aarem A, Cremers WR, Benraad-van Rens MJ. Usher syndrome. A temporal bone report. *Arch Otolaryngol Head Neck Surg* 1995;121:916–921.
27. Zrada SE, Braat K, Doty RL, et al. Olfactory loss in Usher syndrome: another sensory deficit? *Am J Med Genet* 1996;64: 602–603.
28. Arden GB, Fox B. Increased incidence of abnormal nasal cilia in patients with retinitis pigmentosa. *Nature* 1979;279:534–536.
29. Kaplan J, Gerber S, Bonneau D, et al. A gene for Usher syndrome type I (USH1) maps to chromosome 14q. *Genomics* 1992;14: 979–988.
30. Chaib H, Kaplan J, Gerber S, et al. A newly identified locus for Usher syndrome, USH1E, maps to chromosome 21q21. *Hum Mol Genet* 1997;6:27–31.
31. Hmani M, Ghorbel A, Boulila-Elgaied A, et al. A novel locus for Usher syndrome type II, USH2B, maps to chromosome 3 at p23–24.2. *Eur J Hum Genet* 1999;7:363–367.
32. Pieke-Dahl S, Moller CG, Kelley PM, et al. Genetic heterogeneity of Usher syndrome type II: localisation to chromosome 5q. *J Med Genet* 2000;37:256–262.
33. Weil D, Blanchard S, Kaplan J, et al. Defective myosin VIIA gene responsible for the Usher syndrome type 1B. *Nature* 1995;374: 60–61.
34. Gibson, F, Walsh, J, Mburu, P, et al. A type VII myosin encoded by the mouse deafness gene Shaker-1. *Nature* 1995;374:62–64.
35. Liu XZ, Hope CI, Walsh J, et al. Mutations in the myosin VIIA gene cause a wide phenotypic spectrum, including atypical Usher Syndrome. *Am J Hum Genet* 1998;63:909–912.
36. Self T, Mahony M, Fleming J, et al. Shaker-1 mutations reveal roles for myosin VIIA in both development and function of cochlear hair cells. *Development* 1998;125:557–566.
37. Liu X, Ondek B, Williams DS. Mutant myosin VIIa causes defective melanosome distribution in the RPE of shaker-1 mice. *Nat Genet* 1998;19:117–118.

38. Liu X, Udovichenko, IP, Brown SDM, et al. Myosin VIIa is required for normal opsin transport in photoreceptor cells. *J Neurosci* 1999;19:6267–6274.
39. Wolfrum U, Liu X, Schmitt A, et al. Myosin VIIa as a common component of cilia and microvilli. *Cell Motil Cytoskeleton* 1998;40:261–271.
40. Boeda B, El-Amraoui A, Bahloul A, et al. Myosin VIIa, harmonin and cadherin 23, three Usher I gene products that cooperate to shape the sensory hair cell bundle. *EMBO J* 2002; 21:6689–6699.
41. Siemens J, Kazmierczak P, Reynolds A, et al. The Usher syndrome proteins cadherin 23 and harmonin form a complex by means of PDZ-domain interactions. *Proc Natl Acad Sci U S A* 2002;99:14946–14951.
42. Bitner-Glindzicz M, Lindley KJ, Rutland P, et al. A recessive contiguous gene deletion syndrome causing infantile hyperinsulinism, enteropathy and deafness identifies the Usher type 1C gene. *Nat Genet* 2000;26:56–60.
43. Verpy E, Leibovici M, Zwaenepoel I, et al. A defect in harmonin, a PDZ domain-containing protein expressed in the inner ear sensory hair cells, underlies Usher syndrome type 1C. *Nat Genet* 2000;26:51–55.
44. Savas S, Frischhertz B, Pelias MZ, et al. The USH1C 216G>A mutation and the 9-repeat VNTR(t,t) allele are in complete linkage disequilibrium in the Acadian population. *Hum Genet* 2002;110:95–97.
45. Zwaenepoel I, Verpy E, Blanchard S, et al. Identification of three novel mutations in the USH1C gene and detection of thirty-one polymorphisms used for haplotype analysis. *Hum Mutat* 2001;17:34–41.
46. Sheng M, Sala C. PDZ domains and the organization of supramolecular complexes. *Annu Rev Neurosci* 2001;24:1–29.
47. Bork JM, Peters LM, Riazuddin S, et al. Usher syndrome 1D and nonsyndromic autosomal recessive deafness DFNB12 are caused by allelic mutations of the novel cadherin-like gene CDH23. *Am J Hum Genet* 2001;68:26–37.
48. Bolz H, von Brederlow B, Ramirez A, et al. Mutation of CDH23, encoding a new member of the cadherin gene family, causes Usher syndrome type 1D. *Nat Genet* 2001;27:108–112.
49. Ahmed ZM, Riazuddin S, Bernstein SL, et al. Mutations of the Protocadherin Gene PCDH15 cause Usher syndrome type 1F. *Am J Hum Genet* 2001;69:25–34.
50. Alagramam KN, Murcia CL, Kwon HY, et al. The mouse Ames waltzer hearing-loss mutant is caused by mutation of Pcdh15, a novel protocadherin gene. *Nat Genet* 2001;27:99–102.
51. Mustapha M, Chouery E, Torchard-Pagnez D, et al. A novel locus for Usher syndrome type I, USH1G, maps to chromosome 17q24–25. *Hum Genet* 2002;110:348–350.
52. Kikkawa Y, Shitara H, Wakana S, et al. Mutations in a new scaffold protein Sans cause deafness in Jackson shaker mice. *Hum Mol Genet* 2003;12:453–461.
53. Weil D, El-Amraoui A, Masmoudi S, et al. Usher syndrome type IG (USH1G) is caused by mutations in the gene encoding SANS, a protein that associates with the USH1C protein, harmonin. *Hum Mol Genet* 2003;12:463–471.
54. Eudy JD, Weston MD, Yao S, et al. Mutation of a gene encoding a protein with extracellular matrix motifs in Usher syndrome type IIa. *Science* 1998;280:1753–1757.
55. Huang D, Eudy JD, Uzvolgyi E, et al. Identification of the mouse and rat orthologs of the gene mutated in Usher syndrome type IIA and the cellular source of USH2A mRNA in retina, a target tissue of the disease. *Genomics* 2002;80:195–203.
56. Liu XZ, Hope C, Liang CY, et al. A mutation (2314delG) in the Usher syndrome type IIA gene: high prevalence and phenotypic variation. *Am J Hum Genet* 1999;64:1221–1225.

57. Rivolta C, Sweklo EA, Berson EL, Dryja TP. Missense mutation in the USH2A gene: association with recessive retinitis pigmentosa without hearing loss. *Am J Hum Genet* 2000;66: 1975–1978.

58. Joensuu T, Hamalainen R, Yuan B, et al. Mutations in a novel gene with transmembrane domains underlie Usher syndrome type 3. *Am J Hum Genet* 2001;69:673–684.

59. Ernest S, Rauch GJ, Haffter P, et al. Mariner is defective in myosin VIIA: a zebrafish model for human hereditary deafness. *Hum Mol Genet* 2000;9:2189–2196.

60. Libby RT, Steel KP. Electroretinographic anomalies in mice with mutations in Myo7a, the gene involved in human Usher syndrome type IB. *Invest Ophthalmol Vis Sci* 2001;42:770–778.

61. Genetic Evaluation of Congenital Hearing Loss Expert Panel. Genetics evaluation guidelines for the etiologic diagnosis of congenital hearing loss. *Genet Med* 2002;4:162–171.

62. Suter SM. Whose genes are these anyway? Familial conflicts over access to genetic information. *Mich Law Rev* 1993;91:1854–1908.

63. Miller H. DNA blueprints, personhood, and genetic privacy. *Health Matrix* 1998;8:179–221.

METHODS TO RESTORE VISION
A. VISUAL PROSTHESES

JOHN I. LOEWENSTEIN
SCOTT M. WARDEN
JOSEPH F. RIZZO

In blinding retinal diseases, at least some portion of the neural architecture that supports visual perception usually remains. In retinitis pigmentosa (RP), for example, inner retinal cells such as bipolar and ganglion cells seem to survive longer than photoreceptors (1–3). Even in diseases where all retinal neural cells are destroyed, cortical elements remain. It has also been known for many years that electrical stimulation of neural tissue in the visual pathways, from the retina to the cortex, can produce phosphenes or luminous impressions. The hope of researchers in the field of visual prostheses is that appropriate electrical (or other) stimulation of remaining neural elements can produce artificial vision (4,5).

TYPES OF VISUAL PROSTHESES
Retinal Prostheses

Two major types of retinal prostheses have been suggested. One uses electrodes that contact the epiretinal (vitreous) side of the retina, and the other has electrodes in the subretinal space. Epiretinal prostheses were initially conceived to stimulate retinal ganglion cells, although recent work suggests that properly designed stimuli may stimulate deeper cells (6–8). Subretinal prostheses were conceived to stimulate bipolar and horizontal cells that may remain in degenerated retinas. Some authors have suggested that chemical, rather than electrical, stimulation by prostheses may be possible (9,10).

The simplest retinal prostheses is a one piece, subretinal device consisting of multiple small photodiodes (Fig. 12-1). When light is absorbed by a photodiode, it is converted to electricity. Each photodiode acts like an artificial photoreceptor, receiving ambient light and converting it to a graded electrical response, which may then stimulate adjacent nerve cells (11,12). Since the incident light arrives in a topographically appropriate distribution and also could supply power, this type of device is very simple in design. There is concern, though, that these device designs might not produce enough electricity from ambient illumination to be useful (13,14). Some research groups are, therefore, developing subretinal prosthesis designs that utilize additional power sources (15,16).

Epiretinal device designs typically are more complex, as they rely on external imaging devices and power sources. In one example of an epiretinal device, an external television camera converts ambient light to an electrical signal. This signal is transmitted, along with additional electrical power, by an induction coil on the temple. A second coil on the scleral surface receives the power and signal, and transmits these via a small cable to a microchip. The chip generates electrical pulses that are distributed to an electrode array on the retina (Fig. 12-2). Designs vary according to how much of the required electronic circuitry is contained in an intraocular device versus extraocular elements. Power and signal transmission may be accomplished by penetrating wires, induction coils, or lasers. Wyatt and Rizzo (17) suggested placing the intraocular electronic components inside a modified intraocular lens, away from the retinal surface, and running a ribbon of electrodes from this device to the retinal surface.

Optic Nerve Prosthesis

A visual prosthesis could also stimulate the optic nerve, which contains the myelinated axons of all surviving retinal ganglion cells. Stimulating a 2-mm-diameter circular area of the retina or visual cortex would only correspond to a fraction of a patient's visual field. The same area, however, would encompass the entire visual field of one eye if targeting its optic nerve. This unique advantage of optic nerve stimulation can also be interpreted as a significant limitation. The ability to elicit specific phosphenes in a localized area of visual space may be difficult due to the high density of axons within the optic nerve. Verrart et al. (18–22) have implanted one subject with an optic nerve prosthesis. They have carried out computer controlled stimulation of the electrodes, and recently have connected the prosthesis to an

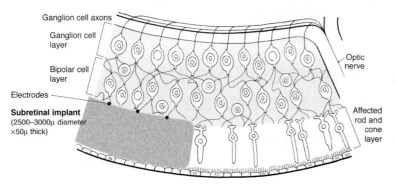

FIGURE 12-1. Schematic drawing of a subretinal implant placed under a retina with photoreceptor degeneration. The small electrodes on the implant are designed to stimulate inner retinal cells. (Reproduced with permission from *Archives of Ophthalmology*.)

imaging device. Despite the limitations suggested previously, and the fact that their electrodes are positioned outside the dura mater, they have created reproducible phosphenes within each quadrant of the visual field.

Cortical Prostheses

Electrically stimulating the visual cortex directly is yet another approach to a visual prosthesis. This technique has the greatest therapeutic potential of any visual prosthesis since it bypasses lesions in the retina, optic nerve, or optic tract. Visual cortex stimulation, therefore, could help the vast majority of blind patients. It has the disadvantage, however, of not utilizing any of the intricate neural processing that normally occurs in the retina and to a lesser extent in the lateral geniculate body.

Devices may have dural or intracortical electrodes. The earliest devices utilized surface electrodes, but subsequent devices with indwelling electrodes produced substantially

lower thresholds (23,24). Wires connected to these electrodes are typically brought through the skull to a connector. They may then be connected to the output of an imaging device such as a television camera (Fig. 12-3).

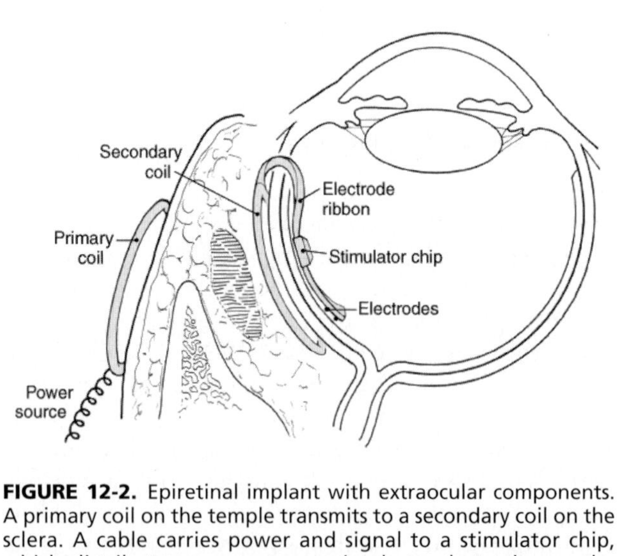

PROBLEM AREAS

Neural Cell Viability

A retinal or optic nerve prosthesis requires the presence of some viable retinal ganglion cells. The minimum number, type, and location of ganglion cells that would be required

FIGURE 12-2. Epiretinal implant with extraocular components. A primary coil on the temple transmits to a secondary coil on the sclera. A cable carries power and signal to a stimulator chip, which distributes energy appropriately to electrodes on the epiretinal surface. (Reproduced with permission from *Archives of Ophthalmology*.)

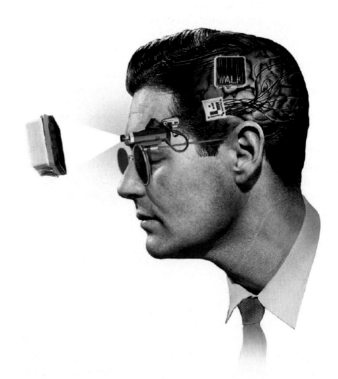

FIGURE 12-3. Artist's conception of a cortical prosthesis. A miniature television camera mounted on a spectacle frame sends images to a processor. Signals are then distributed by the processor to electrodes imbedded in the visual cortex. (Courtesy of Philip Troyk, PhD.)

for a useful prosthesis are currently unknown. Although histologic studies show that numerous retinal ganglion cells remain even in advanced RP (Fig. 12-4), the viability of these cells is unknown (1–3). There is currently no noninvasive method to test ganglion cell viability in the absence of functioning photoreceptors.

Similarly, the number and viability of cortical neurons in patients blind from a variety of disorders are unknown, and there is no method to assess the viability of the visual cortex noninvasively in blind patients.

Biocompatibility

A device that will remain in the body for any length of time must be biocompatible. Chemical, biophysical, and immunologic reactions to the implant materials and the effects of surgery may all conspire to limit biocompatibility. The device should be made of materials that are not toxic to neural tissue, and that do not elicit a significant inflammatory response. The natural reaction of the body to any foreign material is encapsulation with fibrous tissue, and such reactions from the retinal pigment epithelium (RPE) do occur around subretinal implants. Such tissue could disrupt the close contact of implant electrodes with the target tissue. This could result in an unacceptable increase in stimulation threshold or misalignment of the electrodes. For electrically active devices, the tissue reaction to electrical stimulation must be evaluated. Safe stimulation parameters for chronic stimulation of the retina have not yet been definitively determined. Finally, heating of the tissue must be considered. The transfer of electrical energy from electrodes to tissue, across a resistance, will dissipate heat. This could result in unacceptable heating of neurons.

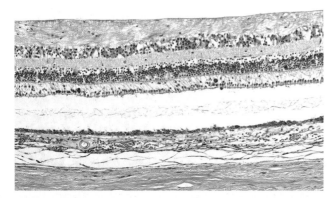

FIGURE 12-4. Cross section of paramacular retina of a patient with retinitis pigmentosa. Note the reduced number of photoreceptors with loss or degeneration of outer segments. In contrast, there are numerous cells in the inner nuclear and bipolar cell layers. (Slide courtesy of Thaddeus Dryja MD, and Jessica Fernandez-Suntay MD, Cogan Eye Pathology Laboratory, Massachusetts Eye and Ear Infirmary. Reproduced with permission from *Archives of Ophthalmology*.)

Power Requirements

For retinal prostheses, there are concerns that it may be difficult to achieve adequate power levels to stimulate a sufficient number of electrodes to yield detailed perceptions (13, 14). These concerns regarding simple subretinal devices were addressed earlier. For more complex devices, there are limits on coil size, proximity, and alignment for wireless power transmission. Using lasers for power transmission is fraught with problems of alignment and possible tissue injury.

Device Encapsulation

Any device placed in the eye must be able to survive the saline environment without corrosion or degradation (25). This necessitates encapsulation of the device. There will be areas of the device, such as electrodes, that cannot be completely encapsulated. The areas where such elements pass through the encapsulant are vulnerable to leakage. In addition, substances that make good encapsulants are usually hydrophobic, preventing entry of water molecules (26). Biocompatibility, on the other hand, generally requires hydrophilic materials, as proteins will denature on contact with hydrophobic materials.

Signal Encoding

Coding electrical (or other) stimuli and targeting them to the appropriate neurons is a major challenge for any type of visual prosthesis. Our knowledge of the physiology of the retina and visual cortex is meager, which compounds the problem. The section on visual results of prosthesis experiments addresses this question.

Testing of Implant Subjects

The early subjects for visual prosthesis implantation have had very poor or no vision. Early generation implants are capable of only limited resolution. Testing of vision in such circumstances is difficult, because the examiner can not just use a Snellen chart as in most clinical trials. We also know from experience in clinical trials that subjective measurements of visual function produce variable results. Subjects in trials therefore routinely have baseline and periodic post-intervention visual function measurements determined in a standardized manner by a masked examiner. While the specific methods used in most ophthalmic clinical trials are not appropriate for implant subjects, the general principles should be followed. This important experience from previous trials has not yet been applied to testing of implant subjects. Thus, new methods for assessing the visual results of implants for severely impaired subjects will have to be developed. The following section examines reports of visual results of prosthesis experiments to date.

VISUAL RESULTS OF PROSTHESIS EXPERIMENTS

Visual Cortex

Bartholow (27) is credited with being the first to electrically stimulate the human brain in 1874. In the late 1920s, the German neurosurgeon Foerster found that electrically stimulating points on exposed occipital cortex would result in the perception of a spot of light fixed in the visual field (28). In addition, he discovered there was a topographical nature to the visual cortex, as stimulation of different areas caused sensations in specific points in visual space. By studying a patient who had unilateral hemianopia for over 8 years after severe damage to the left optic radiation, Krause in 1931 showed that phosphenes could still be elicited by direct stimulation of the left visual cortex (29). He demonstrated that cortical tissue retains some functionality after many years of limited visual input. These early findings provided the framework for future research in the field.

Brindley and Lewin (30) significantly advanced the field in 1968 by implanting the first cortical visual prosthesis in a blind patient. An electronic device with 80 square electrodes each measuring 0.8 mm was placed over the medial surface of the right occipital pole. Wires connected each electrode to extracranial radio receivers that could be stimulated with the appropriate radiofrequency from an oscillator. The patient was able to see phosphenes in the left half of the visual field and could distinguish two phosphenes when the stimulation sites were as close as 2.4 mm. The sensations were always that of light, would not fade with continued stimulation, and would usually quickly cease after the stimulus stopped. In addition, the location of the perceptions in the visual field roughly corresponded to a retinotopic map that had been developed earlier from studies of visual field deficits in patients with war wounds. Brindley's efforts were continued by his contemporary, Dobelle, who demonstrated the ability to achieve pattern vision by implanted 64-electrode hexagonal grids onto the visual cortex of blind patients (31–33). By interpreting patterned stimulation, one patient could read aloud "cortical Braille," such as the phrase "he had a cat and ball," in just under a minute with few mistakes. Using an updated computer controller linked to an image-processing camera many years later, Dobelle (34) reported that a patient could recognize 2-inch-high letters at a distance of 5 feet (an acuity of 20/400).

These extracortical experiments were noted to have many associated difficulties and limitations. The need for relatively high currents caused headaches, believed to be secondary to stimulation of meningeal pain fibers (35). The large amount of electrical power required to feed extracortical systems raised important safety issues. There were also many inconsistencies while evoking phosphenes from the cortical surface. Dobelle (32) found that at times, stimulation of a single electrode could produce multiple phosphenes. Conversely, another group found difficulty in producing more than one phosphene when multiple electrodes were stimulated (36). It became evident that surface stimulation was too distant from the target neurons.

Since over 67% of the striate cortex is buried below the surface (37), researchers began studying whether direct intracortical stimulation would result in more precise control of neuronal function. Advances in technology and micromanufacturing allowed for the production of smaller electrodes that could be used for intracortical studies. Researchers at the National Institutes of Health used microstimulation electrodes with diameters of only 2 μm to study normally sighted patients undergoing occipital craniotomies for excision of epileptic foci (23). Examinations lasted approximately 1 hour, during which time phosphenes were elicited with intracortical stimulation using currents 10 to 100 times lower than that of surface stimulation. In addition, the quality of the phosphenes was improved. Extracortical stimulation often resulted in flickering phosphenes. On the other hand, intracortically evoked phosphenes were consistent and corresponded more closely to the onset and offset of the stimulus.

These preliminary data from short-term experiments were followed by the evaluation of a chronic intracortical implant in a blind patient in 1996 (24). Thirty-eight microelectrodes were implanted in the right visual cortex of a 42-year-old woman who had no light perception for 22 years. During the 4 months that the electrodes were left in place, many important phosphene characteristics were described. Thirty-four of the microelectrodes produced phosphenes with a threshold range of 1.9 to 80 μA, with the majority of the thresholds being under 25 μA. These thresholds were approximately two to three orders of magnitude less than that obtained by Dobelle using surface stimulation. The sizes of the phosphenes ranged from "pinpoint" to a "nickel" held at arm's length, and usually decreased as current increased and length of stimulus shortened. Phosphenes tended to be colorful when the current approached threshold, and at higher thresholds became whiter. Phosphene brightness could be modified by adjusting the stimulus amplitude, frequency, and duration. Three or more simultaneous stimuli would generate phosphenes that appeared to be coplanar, and move in synchrony in the direction of eye movements. Separate phosphenes were elicited when intracortical electrodes were spaced as close as 500 μm, a resolution five times that obtained by surface electrodes. Increased resolution, reduced power requirements secondary to lower phosphene thresholds, and improved quality of phosphenes indicated that intracortical stimulation had more potential to become an effective visual prosthesis than its surface counterpart.

Current work has focused on the ability to develop pattern recognition with intracortical stimulation. One limitation of the previous study is that the 38 electrodes did not appear to involve enough visual cortex to form pattern vision. One solution might be the use of high electrode count microelectrode arrays, which cover larger cortical areas with greater electrode density (38). There are, however, multiple problems that first must be overcome. Safe methods of inserting microelectrode arrays deeper into cortical structures need to be developed. Normann et al. (39) have shown that pneumatically inserting electrodes into cortical tissue at high speeds appears to avoid tissue injury and significant inflammation. Intracortical devices implanted for longer periods of time must also prove to be biocompatible, an issue that was noted by Brindley and Lewin (30) during their initial experiments. Finally, more recent studies with cats are indicating that the mapping of visual space onto electrode grids is difficult when interelectrode distances become very small (40). Though the global visuotopic map is generally conformal, the topographical correlation between cortical space and visual space is limited with 0.4-mm interelectrode spacing. As a result, there likely will be a need for better image processing software that can transform a visual image into a coherent group of electrode stimulations.

Troyk et al. (41) are beginning to study the perceptual results of *in vivo* intracortical stimulation in a chronic primate model. They have trained monkeys to generate saccadic eye movements in the direction of a small light flash, after the flash is extinguished. Once the monkeys have learned the task, the researchers stimulate intracortical-implanted electrodes. After a period of time, the animals are able to generate saccadic movements in response to the electrical stimuli. They hope to further develop this model to improve cortical stimulation paradigms.

Optic Nerve

One of the first documented cases of optic nerve stimulation in humans involved a 38-year-old man who underwent right-eye enucleation secondary to maxillary cancer in 1962 (42). When the optic nerve was stimulated directly with a platinum electrode 1 day after surgery, the patient reported colorful phosphenes in various locations in the visual field. Though there was little consistency, changing the location of the 0.5-mm-diameter electrode and its associated current levels resulted in different perceptions that at times would form colorful patterns.

Nearly all progress in the field of optic nerve stimulation for the development of a visual prosthesis has been described by the Veraart group in Brussels, Belgium (18–22). They proposed the use of a spiral cuff electrode to encircle the optic nerve. Spiral cuff electrode technology was developed to carefully regulate peripheral nerve stimulation and has the capability of activating regions within a nerve (43,44). The Veraart group selected a 59-year-old volunteer who was totally blind from RP. A spiral cuff electrode, containing four contacts located 90° apart around the right optic nerve, was intracranially implanted in 1998. Studies over the first 4 months of electrical stimulation documented over 1,400 phosphenes perceived over a large portion of the visual field

(18). Phosphenes were described as clusters of dots often arranged in rows or arrays. Typically a few dots were described. Various color combinations were elicited. Individual stimulation of each contact resulted in phosphenes generally localized to the corresponding quadrant of the visual field. This retinotopy corresponded very closely to previous studies of fiber organization within the optic nerve (45). Contrary to cortical stimulation described earlier, more recent work has demonstrated that adjusting phosphene brightness is difficult with optic nerve stimulation (20).

The major strength of research from Veraart and colleagues involved the implications of long-term follow-up. Thirty months after the initial operation, the transcutaneous leads were replaced with an antenna and telemetry system equipped with an image processing camera. The patient was subsequently able to recognize simple patterns (19). Performance improved incrementally with practice, demonstrated by quicker recognition and more accurate readings. Recent studies have evaluated object recognition, localization, and grasping in an attempt to simulate real-life activities (21,22). Images from a camera mounted on the patient's glasses were reduced to 32 by 64 pixels with 1° resolution. Six objects were used, including a large and small bottle, a cup, a CD box, a knife, and a toothpaste box. After several months of training, the patient was able to discriminate among several of the objects and then subsequently grasp the selected item. These experiments demonstrated that camera images could be transformed into useful visual information through an optic nerve prosthesis, even with a small number of electrodes. The process of learning associated with chronic implantation allows the patient to adapt to new visual stimuli. This may prove helpful to all prosthetic approaches.

Epiretinal

Several groups are investigating whether epiretinal implants can successfully bypass lesions in the outer retina (46–54). Researchers have elicited visual perceptions through external electrical stimulation in patients who have outer retinal degeneration (55–57). Potts and Inoue (55,56) were among the first to demonstrate this by passing electrical current through the eye using electrodes placed on the surface of the cornea. Scalp electrodes were used to detect cortical activity after an electrical stimulus (electrically evoked response or EER) or a light stimulus (visual evoked response or VER). The investigators noted that the EER was detected earlier than the VER after each respective stimulus, indicating that electrical stimulation bypassed a part of the visual pathway in the retina. Since a few RP patients were noted to have EERs disproportionately larger than VERs, the layer of cells circumvented was likely the degenerated photoreceptors. The patients described the electrically induced phosphenes as large areas of light that enveloped their entire visual fields.

Although these earlier studies demonstrated the ability to elicit phosphenes and EERs in blind subjects through electrical stimulation of the retina, there was no evidence to suggest that useful pattern vision could be obtained. Humayun et al. (48) addressed this issue by providing "pixelized visual input" to blind RP and age-related macular degeneration (ARMD) patients through focal stimulation of the retina. Using a three-port pars plana surgical procedure, stimulating electrodes were handheld at approximately 0.5 mm over the retinal surface. Phosphenes were elicited in all five patients tested and correlated with the timing of the electrical stimulation. Phosphene size and brightness increased with higher amplitude and longer pulse duration. Four of the subjects were always successful at localizing phosphenes to the retinotopically correct quadrants, and two could successfully describe the direction of probe movement. Based on the ability to detect separate phosphenes when electrodes were placed as close as 435 μm, one subject's visual acuity was estimated to be 4.5/200 (a visual angle of 1.5°). The Humayun group followed this study with another experiment to further test pattern vision utilizing multielectrode arrays (47). Electrode arrays (3 × 3 or 5 × 5) were hand-held on the retinal surface of two blind patients with RP. One patient could successfully distinguish between a horizontal line and a vertical line of stimulated electrodes. When the perimeter electrodes of the 3 × 3 electrode array were activated, the second patient described the percept as an outline of a matchbox with an empty center. These results suggested that it was possible to elicit form perceptions by selectively stimulating patterns of epiretinal electrodes.

Findings from more recent experiments by others have not been consistent with these initial studies (51,52,58). Electrode arrays in contact with the retina were stimulated in five blind RP patients and one normally sighted subject who was scheduled for enucleation due to orbital cancer. Stimulating a single electrode within the array often resulted in multiple phosphenes in the blind subjects. Using

geometric patterns of electrode stimulation, the investigators tested whether subjects could achieve simple pattern vision. Definite form perception that matched the stimulation pattern was not obtained by any of the five RP patients or the normally sighted subject. Descriptions of the phosphenes were then judged as accurate if they reasonably correlated with the pattern of the stimulus (Fig. 12-5). During trials with multiple electrodes, three of the five RP patients accurately described phosphenes 32% (average) of the time, compared with 43% of the time with the normally sighted individual. This relatively poor outcome was largely due to the limited two point discrimination among the subjects, which may be the result of interference created by interelectrode electrical fields. The investigators reported tentative two point discrimination with electrode spacing at 600 μm and 1,960 μm for two blind patients (a visual angle of 2.25–4.5°). In addition, there was less of a correlation between increased phosphene size and higher stimulus charge as compared with earlier studies. It was encouraging, however, that perceptions were reproducible, even if they did not conform to the stimulus pattern. This finding suggests that some unknown methodical adjustment could potentially lead to consistently accurate phosphenes.

The significant disparities among the research groups are difficult to explain based on different patient populations, since many of the subjects studied were severely blind. Different methods utilized could explain some of the variation. Electrodes held above the retinal surface (48) seemingly elicited more consistent phosphenes than electrode arrays directly in contact with the retina (58). Electrical stimulation on the surface of the retina might have the disadvantage of activating passing axons from distant ganglion cells, although the more elongated and diffuse percepts that could be expected from axonal stimulation were not found (50). This could explain the difficulties in obtaining pattern vision, since numerous phosphenes would be elicited from one electrode. Other studies with electrode arrays in contact

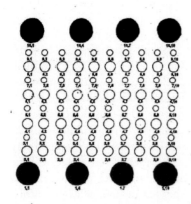 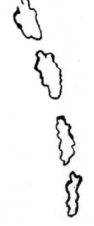

FIGURE 12-5. Results of a single trial of electrical stimulation with a microelectrode array on the retina in an acute experiment. Pattern of electrical stimulation delivered through the electrode array (*left*) and patient's drawing of the induced perception (*right*). The array was in the peripheral retina and was tilted such that only four electrodes along one edge of the array contacted the retina. Stimulation was a 196-μA, 8-msec pulse at 6 Hz. Only the darkened electrodes received current. (Reproduced with permission from *Investigative Ophthalmology and Visual Science*.)

with the retina, however, were reported to achieve simple pattern vision (47). Rizzo et al. (51,52,58) also studied a normally sighted individual. Though the subject performed on average better than blind patients, she could only describe phosphenes accurately less than half of the time. This control emphasizes that stimulation methods, and not merely retinal pathology, are likely responsible for the relatively poor outcomes.

Eckmiller et al. (46) have suggested that more accurate perceptions could be derived from a "learning" epiretinal implant that can be adjusted over time. Using a neural network model that simulates receptive field properties of retinal neurons, stimulus parameters can be adjusted to achieve pattern vision. The learning model has been tested with the use of a computer simulation that generates both stimulation input and phosphene output (59). Normally sighted volunteers adjust one or more of the 256 tunable elements to produce a percept that matches the input image. Future work will focus on applying this concept to long-term epiretinal devices in blind subjects.

Some data have been gathered from chronically implanted epiretinal constructs in two blind RP patients (49,53,54). The prosthesis consists of a 4 × 4 electrode array secured to the retina with a single retinal tack and linked by a multiwire cable to an extraocular microelectronic device. A custom computer interface or a head-worn video camera acts as the source for the stimulus. Devices were implanted without complication, and have been in place for 4 and 10 months in two patients. Both patients reported phosphenes from all 16 electrodes and could detect whether room lights were on or off. Using the camera as the stimulus source, one patient could determine the correct orientation of a tumbling "L" 75% of the time. The patients could also count and localize up to two white objects using images from the head-worn camera. Although sizes of the objects and other specifics were not described, it appeared that the implanted epiretinal prosthesis had some functionality.

Many important issues have to be addressed as researchers work towards developing a useful epiretinal implant in the future. One limitation involves the location of epiretinal prostheses. The goal of any retinal implant should be to activate viable cells that are most proximal in the afferent visual pathway. This would ensure the greatest use of innate neural processing. Compared with subretinal prostheses, epiretinal microelectrodes are farther from the outer retinal cell layers where the visual impulse is initiated. Investigators have recently offered a possible solution to this issue by showing that longer pulse durations selectively stimulate outer retinal cells (6,7). Epiretinal implants must also be effectively secured in order to withstand counter forces from ocular rotational speeds that can reach 700° visual angle/sec (50). Retinal tacks have been used in several subjects with early generation epiretinal implants, and have been successful for at least 10 months.

Subretinal

Surgically placed between the RPE and the photoreceptors, subretinal devices have the advantage of being located near outer retinal cell layers. A greater amount of downstream neural processing is utilized, thereby allowing for a clearer topographical relationship between stimulus patterns and perceived images. Designs for this type of intraocular implant are simpler than epiretinal prostheses. Subretinal devices consist solely of multiple photodiodes that convert absorbed light into electric impulses that activate overlying cells. Most designs do not require extraocular imaging or power sources.

Chow et al. (60,61) is the only group thus far to perform human clinical studies with subretinal devices. They surgically placed artificial silicon retina (ASR) microchips into the subretinal space of ten patients with RP. Each ASR chip is 25 μm thick, measures 2 mm in diameter, and consists of approximately 3,500 microphotodiodes. The implant procedures were surgically successful, and patients denied discomfort after surgical recovery. ASR microchips implanted for up to 2.5 years have continued to function electrically and appear to be safely tolerated without evidence of migration, degradation, or inflammation. Subjective and objective improvements in visual function have been described, but specific data have not been documented. Interestingly, the investigators reported that areas of improved visual function do not correspond to the location of the subretinal implant. As a result, they believe that chronic electrical stimulation (or the mere placement of a subretinal device) might have a neurotrophic or neuroprotective effect (62). This is one theory that could explain retinal cell rescue distant from the implant. Overall, the research by Chow and colleagues has demonstrated that chronic subretinal devices can be implanted in humans and appear to retain some functionality over time.

CONCLUSIONS

The scientific basis for developing a visual prosthesis is that the vast majority of blind patients still retain some functional neurons along the visual pathway. Investigators are developing ways to stimulate the visual cortex, optic nerve, and retina in order to utilize these cells and restore useful vision to blind patients. Each area of targeting has its own advantages and limitations. They all, however, share the need to emulate the normal sensory input at their respective levels. Although many obstacles still remain, a great deal of progress has been made since Brindley and Lewin's first visual prosthesis in 1968.

A few generalizations on the perception of phosphenes can be made after reviewing the human studies using different visual prostheses. Stimulating one electrode tends to elicit a distinct phosphene in visual space, and often will elicit multiple phosphenes. Modulating signal parameters, such as amplitude, often changes phosphene characteristics. Transferring electricity through several electrodes leads to the perception of multiple percepts. Although results are still preliminary, some subjects can detect two phosphenes using approximately similar separations between two intra-cortical or two epiretinal electrodes (500–1,000 μm). More easily appreciated with retinal implants, a topographical relationship exists between the location of stimuli and the position of phosphenes. This leads to a simple concept, that activating specific electrodes within an array, much like illuminating particular lights within a scoreboard, could elicit similarly shaped phosphenes. Difficulties arise, however, when arranging multiple electrodes in order to obtain pattern vision. Results have been largely inconsistent. Evidence does suggest, however, that simple patterns can be perceived through other recognizable and reproducible features. Future research efforts will focus on eliciting phosphenes that more accurately represent visual images. Over many years of work in this area, technological progress has been substantial. The quality of the perceptions in implant subjects, however, has not kept pace.

Human vision requires several years to fully develop with the need for recurrent visual stimuli. Achieving useful vision with a prosthesis will likely require long-term adaptation to novel electronic input. Advancements in microelectronics and improved methods of communicating with the visual pathway will hopefully allow for more successful attempts in the future.

PART A REFERENCES

1. Humayun MS, Prince M, de Juan E Jr, et al. Morphometric analysis of the extramacular retina from postmortem eyes with retinitis pigmentosa. *Invest Ophthalmol Vis Sci* 1999;40:143–148.
2. Santos A, Humayun MS, de Juan E Jr, et al. Preservation of the inner retina in retinitis pigmentosa. A morphometric analysis. *Arch Ophthalmol* 1997;115:511–515.
3. Stone JL, Barlow WE, Humayun MS, et al. Morphometric analysis of macular photoreceptors and ganglion cells in retinas with retinitis pigmentosa. *Arch Ophthalmol* 1992;110:1634–1639.
4. Margalit E, Maia M, Weiland J, et al. Retinal prosthesis for the blind. *Surv Ophthalmol* 2002;47:335–356.
5. Loewenstein J, Montezuma S, Rizzo JF. Outer retinal degeneration: an electronic retinal prosthesis as a treatment strategy. *Arch Ophthalmol* 2003 *(in press)*.
6. Jensen RJ, Ziv OR, Rizzo JF. Thresholds for direct and indirect activation of ganglion cells with an epiretinal electrode: effect of stimulus duration and electrode size. Fort Lauderdale: ARVO, 2003.
7. Greenberg RJ. Analysis of electrical stimulation of the vertebrate retina- work towards a retinal prosthesis. Wilmer Ophthalmological Institute. Baltimore: Johns Hopkins University, 1998.
8. Ziv OR, Jensen RJ, Rizzo JF III. In vitro activation of ganglion cells in rabbit retina: effects of glutamate receptor agents. *Invest Ophthalmol* 2002;43:178.
9. Iezzi R, Safadi M, Miller J, et al. Feasibility of retinal and cortical prosthesis based upon spatiotemporally controlled release of L-glutamate. *Invest Ophthalmol* 2001;42(S):941.

10. Fishman HA, Peterman MC, Leng T, et al. The artificial synapse chip: A novel interface for a retinal prosthesis based on neurotransmitter stimulation and nerve regeneration. *Invest Ophthalmol* 2002;43(S):114.
11. Zrenner E, Miliczek KD, Gabel VP, et al. The development of subretinal microphotodiodes for replacement of degenerated photoreceptors. *Ophthalmic Res* 1997;29:269–280.
12. Chow AY, Chow VY. Subretinal electrical stimulation of the rabbit retina. *Neurosci Lett* 1997;225:13–16.
13. Zrenner E, Stett A, Weiss S, et al. Can subretinal microphotodiodes successfully replace degenerated photoreceptors? *Vision Res* 1999;39:2555–2567.
14. Chow AY, Pardue MT, Chow VY, et al. Implantation of silicon chip microphotodiode arrays into the cat subretinal space. *IEEE Trans Neural Syst Rehabil Eng* 2001;9:86–95.
15. Schubert MB, Hierzenberger A, Lehner H, et al. Optimizing photodiode arrays for the use as retinal implants. *Sens Actuators* 1999;74:193–197.
16. Zrenner E. Will retinal implants restore vision? *Science* 2002;296(5557):1022–1025.
17. Rizzo JF III, Wyatt J. Retinal prosthesis. In: *Age-related macular degeneration.* St. Louis: Mosby, 1998.
18. Veerart C, Raftopoulos C, Mortimer JT, et al. Visual sensations produced by optic nerve stimulation using an implanted self-sizing spiral cuff electrode. *Brain Res* 1998;813:181–186.
19. Veerart CG, Wanet-Defalque MC, Delbeke J, et al. Assessment of the MIVIP optic nerve visual prosthesis. *Invest Ophthalmol Vis Sci* 2001;42:S942.
20. Delbeke J, Oozeer M, Veerart C. Position, size and luminosity of phosphenes generated by direct optic nerve stimulation. *Vision Res* 2003;43:1091–1102.
21. Delbeke J, Gerard B, Lambert V, et al. A first attempt to translate images in optic nerve stimuli for a visual prosthesis. Fort Lauderdale: ARVO, 2003.
22. Lambert V, Laloyaux C, Schmitt C, et al. Localization, discrimination, and grasping of daily life objects with an implanted optic nerve prosthesis. Fort Lauderdale: ARVO, 2003.
23. Bak M, Girvin JP, Hambrecht FT, et al. Visual sensations produced by intracortical microstimulation of the human occipital cortex. *Med Biol Eng Comput* 1990;28:257–259.
24. Schmidt EM, Bak M, Hambrecht FT, et al. Feasibility of a visual prosthesis for the blind based on intracortical microstimulation of the visual cortex. *Brain* 1996;119:507–522.
25. Donaldson PE. The encapsulation of microelectronic devices for long-term surgical implantation. *IEEE Trans Biomed Eng* 1976; 23:281–285.
26. Donaldson ND. Low-technology sealing method for implantable hermetic packages. *Med Biol Eng Comput* 1988;26:111–116.
27. Bartholow R. Experimental investigation into the functions of the human brain. *Am J Med Sci* 1874;67:305–313.
28. Foerster O. *J Psychol Neurol* 1929;39:463.
29. Krause F, Schum H. Neue deutsche chirurgie 1931;49a:482–486.
30. Brindley GS, Lewin WS. The sensations produced by electrical stimulation of the visual cortex. *J Physiol* 1968;194:54–55.
31. Dobelle WH, Mladejovsky MG, Girvin JP. Artificial vision for the blind: electrical stimulation of visual cortex offers hope for a functional prosthesis. *Science* 1974;183:440–444.
32. Dobelle WH, Mladejovsky MG. Phosphenes produced by electrical stimulation of human occipital cortex; and their application to the development of a prosthesis for the blind. *J Physiol* 1974;243:553–576.
33. Dobelle WH, Mladejovsky MG, Evans JR. Braille reading by a blind volunteer by visual cortex stimulation. *Nature* 1976;259: 111–112.
34. Dobelle WH. Artificial vision for the blind by connecting a television camera to the visual cortex. *ASAIO J* 2000;46:3–9.

35. Brindley GS. Effects of electrical stimulation of the visual cortex. *Hum Neurobiol* 1982;1:281–283.

36. Talalla A, Bullara L, Pudenz R. Electrical stimulation of the human visual cortex. *Can J Neurol Sci* 1974;1:236–238.

37. Stensaas SS, Eddington DK, Dobelle WH. The topography and variability of the primary visual cortex in man. *J Neurosurg* 1974;40:747–755.

38. Normann RA, Maynard EM, Rousche PJ, et al. A neural interface for a cortical vision prosthesis. *Vision Res* 1999;39:2577–2587.

39. Rousche PJ, Normann RA. A method for pneumatically inserting an array of penetrating electrodes into cortical tissue. *Ann Biomed Eng* 1992;20:413–422.

40. Warren DJ, Fernandez E, Normann RA. High-resolution two-dimensional spatial mapping of cat striate cortex using a 100-microelectrode array. *Neuroscience* 2001;105:19–31.

41. Troyk PR, Bradley D, Towle V, et al. Experimental results of intracortical electrode stimulation in Macaque V1. Fort Lauderdale: ARVO, 2003.

42. Nakagawa J. Experimental study on visual sensation by electric stimulation of the optic nerve in man. *Br J Ophthalmol* 1962;46:592–596.

43. Naples GG, Mortimer JT, Scheiner A, et al. A spiral cuff electrode for peripheral nerve stimulation. *IEEE Trans Biomed Eng* 1988;35:905–916.

44. Walter JS, Griffith P, Sweeney J, et al. Multielectrode nerve cuff stimulation of the median nerve produces selective movements in a raccoon animal model. *J Spinal Cord Med* 1997;20:233–243.

45. Miller N. *Walsh and Hoyt's clinical neuroophthalmology,* 4th ed. Baltimore, 1988.

46. Eckmiller R. Learning retina implants with epiretinal contacts. *Ophthalmic Res* 1997;29:281–289.

47. Humayun MS, de Juan E, Weiland JD, et al. Pattern electrical stimulation of the human retina. *Vision Res* 1999;39:2569–2576.

48. Humayun MS, de Juan E, Dagnelie G, et al. Visual perception elicited by electrical stimulation of retina in blind humans. *Arch Ophthalmol* 1996;114(1):40–6.

49. Humayun MS, Greenberg RJ, Mech BV, et al. Chronically implanted intraocular retinal prosthesis in two blind subjects. Fort Lauderdale: ARVO, 2003.

50. Rizzo JF, Wyatt J. Prospects for a visual prosthesis. *Neuroscientist* 1997;3:251–262.

51. Rizzo JF, Wyatt J, Loewenstein J, et al. Acute intraocular retinal stimulation in normal and blind humans. *Invest Ophthalmol* Vis Sci 2000;41(102):S532.

52. Rizzo JF, Wyatt J, Loewenstein J, et al. Accuracy and reproducibility of perpepts elicited by electrical stimulation of the retinas of blind and normal subjects. *Invest Ophthalmol* 2001;42:S942.

53. Weiland J. Epiretinal implant experience (update on human experimentation). Paper presented at The Eye and the Chip 2002: World Congress on Artificial Vision, Detroit, Michigan, 2002.

54. Yanai D, Weiland J, Mahadevappa M, et al. Visual perception in blind subjects with microelectronic retinal prothesis. Fort Lauderdale: ARVO, 2003.

55. Potts A, Inoue J. The electrically evoked response (EER) of the visual system. *Invest Ophthalmol* 1968;7:269–278.

56. Potts A, Inoue J. The electrically evoked response (EER) of the visual system. II Effect of adaptation and retinitis pigmentosa. *Invest Ophthalmol* 1969;8:605–612.

57. Kato S. Response of the visual system evoked by an alternating current. *Med Biol Eng Comput* 1983;21:47–50.

58. Rizzo JF, Wyatt J, Loewenstein J, et al. Perceptual efficacy of electrical stimulation of human retina with a microelectrode array during acute surgical trials. *Invest Ophthalmol Vis Sci (in press)*.

59. Eckmiller RE, Baruth O, Neumann D. Retina encoder tuning tests in humans with normal vision. Fort Lauderdale: ARVO, 2003.

60. Chow AY, Packo KH, Pollack JS, et al. Subretinal artificial silicon retina microchip implantation in retinitis pigmentosa patients: long term follow-up. Fort Lauderdale: ARVO, 2003.

61. Chow AY, Peyman GA, Pollack JS, et al. Safety, feasibility and efficacy of subretinal artificial silicon retina prosthesis for the treatment of patients with retinitis pigmentosa. Fort Lauderdale: ARVO, 2002.

62. Pardue MT, Ball SL, Yin H, et al. Neuroprotective effect of the subretinal artificial silicon retina. Fort Lauderdale: ARVO, 2003.

B. RETINAL TRANSPLANTATION

SVEN CRAFOORD
PEEP V. ALGVERE

CLINICAL IMPLICATIONS

The concept of cell transplantation to replace photoreceptors or retinal pigment epithelial cells emerged from the fact that lost visual function in some macular diseases or retinal dystrophies appears secondary to or related to retinal pigment epithelial cell degeneration. The most common disorder affecting the retinal pigment epithelial layer is age-related macular degeneration (ARMD), which has become the leading cause of visual deterioration and social blindness in the western world. Approximately 2% to 3% of the patients with ARMD, namely those with extra or juxtafoveal choroidal neovascularization, can be treated with laser photocoagulation. Although new treatment modalities have been introduced, such as photodynamic therapy and macular relocation surgery, only selected cases of neovascular ARMD are eligible for treatment at the present time.

Retinal dystrophies involving the retinal pigment epithelium (RPE) can reduce visual function in humans. Sorsby's fundus dystrophy, two forms of autosomal recessive retinitis pigmentosa (RP), and, to some extent, Stargardt's disease (1) appear to be due to defects unique to the RPE (2). In addition, in more generalized retinal degenerations, such as Usher syndrome (type 1B) with X-linked retinitis pigmentosa, the defective gene is expressed strongly in the RPE and weakly in the neural retina (3–5). Macular degeneration in vitelliform macular degeneration (Best's disease) is caused by a gene mutation affecting the RPE (6,7). Mutations in the *RPE65* gene, which is expressed almost exclusively in the RPE, underlie Leber congenital amaurosis and early-onset retinal dystrophy (8). Genetic generalized defects, such as choroideremia and gyrate atrophy, also involve the RPE and might be candidates for RPE, iris pigment epithelial (IPE), or stem cell transplantation.

EXPERIMENTAL AND SURGICAL EXPERIENCE

Several research groups around the world have postulated the possibility of RPE transplantation to replace the diseased cells to treat or minimize tissue damage in certain retinal disorders. A number of achievements have supported this postulate and, since the 1980s, several animal experiments and some human trials with RPE transplantation have been performed. One achievement was the successful experiments on the Royal of College Surgeons (RCS) rat showing for the first time that the grafted cells survived and rescued photoreceptors for a period of time (9). The introduction of gene therapy for some retinal dystrophies was another great achievement. Following subretinal injection of recombinant adeno-associated virus (rAAV) containing specific cDNA, a photoreceptor cell rescue was achieved in retinal degeneration (rd) mice (10,11). Using a rAAV for gene transfer, functional and structural recovery of the retina in the *RPE65*-null mutation dog was demonstrated (12).

A prerequisite for a successful transplantation is a precise and nontraumatizing surgical technique. For perfection of the procedure the following criteria are important: (a) creation of a small controlled lesion and subsequent detachment of the neural retina, (b) precise injection or implantation of the RPE or IPE cells into the subretinal space with minimal damage to the host retina, (c) avoidance of hemorrhage and damage to Bruch's membrane, and (d) reattachment of the host retina (13). Today two surgical approaches for RPE or IPE cell transplantation are used. The pars plana (transvitreous) method has been adopted for animal experiments (14–16). This technique is similar to the clinical procedures of vitrectomy that have been used in humans for almost 30 years. The transscleral approach has been used particularly in animals with small eyes and large crystalline lenses, such as mice and rats. An incision is made through the posterior sclera and choroid with a thin needle to permit injection of transplanted cells into the subretinal space. A major disadvantage of this technique is breakdown of the outer blood–retina barrier (BRB) with penetration of the choroid that is believed to create a pathway for the invasion of inflammatory and immunologically active cells as a part of the wound-healing process.

Several investigators have used rabbits as hosts for experimental transplantation of RPE and IPE cells (14,16–22).

The rabbit is an ideal surgical model because of the large size of the eye and good transpupillary visualization with an operating microscope. However, rabbits serve only as a normal animal model and have neither retinal vasculature nor macular anatomy similar to humans. Experiments with monkeys receiving xenografts (transplant from another species) of human fetal RPE cells have been reported (18,23). In addition, human trials with allografts (transplant from same species) of fetal RPE cells transplanted to ARMD patients with choroidal neovascularization or geographic atrophy have been performed (24–26).

Different techniques of transplantation have been performed. Cell suspensions can be successfully injected through a small retinotomy to create a bleb beneath the neurosensory retina in the subretinal space. Alternatively, implantation of a monolayer of RPE or IPE cells on a suitable substrate (e.g., anterior lens capsule, amniotic membrane, ultrathin collagen sheets) would assure the correct polarity and cellular contacts but technical difficulties have to be overcome, such as avoiding the folding or curling of the patch graft.

RETINAL PIGMENT EPITHELIUM

Structure

The retina consists of the neurosensory retina, which contains the photoreceptors, and the RPE (Fig. 12-6). The RPE consists of a monolayer of hexagonal cells on Bruch's membrane. The RPE differs from other epithelia in that the cells originate from the neural ectoderm. The RPE consists of postmitotic cells, which do not divide under normal condi-

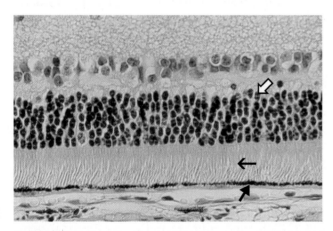

FIGURE 12-6. Normal neurosensory retina and retinal pigment epithelium in rabbit. There is an even contour and apical pigmentation of the regular RPE layer (hematoxylin-eosin, ×540). The *black bold arrow* indicates RPE, the *thin arrow* indicates photoreceptor outer segments, and the *white arrow* indicates the photoreceptor nuclear layer. (From Crafoord S, Geng L, Seregard S, et al. Experimental transplantation of autologous iris pigment epithelial cells to the subretinal space. *Acta Ophthalmol Scand* 2001;79:509–514, with permission.)

tions. However, in response to pathological stimuli, such as retinal detachment, the RPE can proliferate, detach from Bruch's membrane, migrate, and participate in the development of proliferative vitreoretinopathy (27). Under various pathological conditions, RPE cells may dedifferentiate into macrophagic or fibroblastic phenotypes.

Retinal pigment epithelial cells form a monolayer with a distinct apical domain, which have many microvilli in contact with photoreceptor outer segments but do not have anatomic or synaptic connections to the neural retina. The tight junctions (zonula occludens) between the apical sides of the RPE cells establish the BRB that prevents free passage of water and ions. The inner barrier is formed by the capillary endothelium of the intrinsic retinal vessels. The apical side of the RPE cell has numerous long microvilli, which extend upward to partially surround the photoreceptor outer segments. The apical cytoplasm contains microfilaments and microtubules, and the greatest concentration of melanin granules. The midportion contains the nucleus, synthetic machinery, and lysosomes (digestive vesicles). The basal membrane has increased surface area for absorption and secretion created by convoluted infoldings.

Functional Features

The concept of RPE transplantation evolved from successful culturing of RPE. Retinal pigment epithelial cells easily grow in tissue culture and form sheets of confluent monolayers. Much of our understanding of RPE functions has evolved from experiments with cultured RPE cells. Phagocytic capacity and accumulation of lipofuscin, for instance, can be investigated by feeding RPE cells photoreceptor outer segments (28). The RPE plays a central role in regulating the microenvironment surrounding the photoreceptors in the retina, where the events of phototransduction take place.

The physiologic workload of the RPE is impressive. It includes (a) environment and metabolic control (including BRB), transport (of water, nutrients and ions), dehydration (of the subretinal space), synthesis (of enzymes, growth factors, pigments), interaction with metabolic factors (endocrine, vascular and proliferative) (29); (b) visual pigment cycle including vitamin A transport and metabolism (30); (c) outer segment phagocytosis (31) with digestion and recycling of membrane material; (d) interphotoreceptor matrix and retinal adhesion as seen in specialized matrix ensheathment of rods and cones, and metabolic control of adhesion; (e) electrical activity such as the response to light-induced ionic changes; (f) light-induced chemical signals and nonphotic response to chemical agents; (g) repair and reactivity in regeneration and repair, immunologic interactions, scarring and pigment migration, and modulation of fibrovascular proliferation.

The maintenance of RPE polarity is an important issue. The RPE apical–basal polarity seems to be modifiable (32).

With age, lipofuscin gradually accumulates in the RPE, presumably due to insufficient digestion of outer segment material in the RPE lysosomes. Evidence exists that excessive accumulation of lipofuscin is harmful to RPE cells, causing a deterioration in their function, an increased sensitivity to blue light and other noxious stimuli, and eventually leading to alterations in Bruch's membrane. Such events have been proposed in ARMD (33). Involvement of oxidative mechanisms are implicated in blue light-induced damage to lipofuscin (A2E)-laden RPE leading to apoptotic death of RPE cells (34).

Immunologic Aspects

The RPE cells express major histocompatibility complex (MHC) class I and class II antigens. The fetal human RPE cells express class I antigens from the sixth gestational week and class II antigens beginning at week 10 to12 and continuing onward (35). Generally, these antigens are likely to induce immunologic rejection of xenografts and allografts. Fetal RPE cells do not express co-stimulatory molecules (CD 40, 80, 86); however, adhesion molecules (CD 54, 58) are expressed very early in development. Fetal RPE cells appear unable to directly activate purified T-cells, although in the presence of antigen-presenting cells, lymphocyte proliferation is observed (36).

The anterior chamber, as well as the subretinal space, is considered to be an immunologically privileged area (37–40). This privileged status appears to depend completely or in part upon an active process that promotes tolerance. In the anterior chamber, this active process has been called anterior chamber associated immune deviation (ACAID) (37,41–46). This response includes (a) suppressed delayed hypersensitivity, (b) preserved humoral immunity, and (c) primed cytotoxic T-cell responses. ACAID is regarded as an evolutionary adaptation that favors immune effectors to eliminate ocular pathogens with minimal risk of destroying vision. The immunologic privilege of the subretinal space, however, is not considered static or permanent (40,47,48).

To maintain the immune privilege of the eye, an intact BRB and blood–aqueous barrier are crucial, as is the blood–brain barrier for the central nervous system (49). It was observed in eyes with breakdown of the outer BRB that RPE allografts to the subretinal space were disrupted within 3 months but persisted much longer when the BRB remained intact (26). This notion is supported by experiments in tissue culture showing that RPE cells suppress T-lymphocytes (50,51). RPE may constitute an immunologic barrier by inducing apoptosis of T-cells (52). In addition, the RPE is capable of producing transforming growth factor-β, which is believed to be involved in the maintenance of the immunosuppressive ocular environment, secretion of prostaglandin E2 and nitric oxide, which also inhibit lymphocytic proliferation (53).

The surgical technique for minimizing operative trauma and the postoperative cellular response after grafting cells into the subretinal space was discussed by Al-Amro et al.(54). The authors concluded that destruction of Bruch's membrane, the BRB, and choroid, as occurs in the transscleral approach, might induce adverse effects on graft survival by enhancing immunologic effects.

Experimental RPE Transplantation

The RCS rat has been extensively used as host for RPE and IPE cell transplantation. This is an animal model of retinal dystrophy exhibiting RPE dysfunction. In the RCS rat, the RPE is incapable of phagocytosing photoreceptor outer segments, which accumulate in the subretinal space and secondarily cause photoreceptor degeneration. Thus, the RCS rat has served as a most useful experimental model for assessing the effect after RPE, IPE, photoreceptor, and stem cell transplantation on photoreceptor survival. After RPE or IPE cell grafting in the RCS rat (40,55–64), several investigators have demonstrated a transient and beneficial effect on photoreceptor rescue.

The RPE allografts transplanted into the subretinal space of rabbits are tolerated for up to 3 months (16,17,22), as was also found in studies using immunosuppressive therapy (17,65). Recently, this scenario was confirmed by experiments using triple immune suppression when transplanting porcine RPE (xenografts) to the rabbit subretinal space; by 12 weeks after surgery, there was no statistically significant difference in the number of grafted cells in the immune-suppressed versus immune-competent group of rabbits (65a). We observed that transplanted cells in the rabbit could survive for 6 months, but frequently there was local disruption of the grafted RPE cells. This was interpreted as immunogenic graft rejection (22). However, it is possible that the microenvironment in the subretinal space also limits the survival of grafted cells.

The classic acute graft rejection is characterized by invasion of mononuclear cells, such as plasma cells, macrophages, and immature lymphocytes, particularly T-lymphocytes (66). We did not observe these cells in experiments with RPE allografts. There was no invasion of T-lymphocytes, but macrophages were commonly seen after 6 months. However, it is conceivable, that ACAID or similar mechanisms modified the immunologic response. ACAID is associated with the active suppression or downregulation of the systemic delayed-type of hypersensitivity (43,67–70). Short-term experiments indicate that transplantation of RPE into the subretinal space also induces a deviant immune response at postimplantation day 12 in contrast to subconjunctival RPE allografts that rapidly undergo rejection (39,71,72). Embryonic retinal allografts, which are tolerated in the subretinal space, were found to be rejected within 1 month when transplanted into the choroid (73). Our results corroborate those of other investigators that the subretinal space is likely an immunologically privileged site, not displaying the characteristic T-cell response occurring in classic host versus graft rejection.

Photoreceptors appeared normal on light microscopy at 3 months, but at 6 months the photoreceptors overlying the transplants generally exhibited pathological changes. A conspicuous finding was the focal invasion of macrophages into the transplanted area with cell death as demonstrated by positive TUNEL staining. These cells were identified as macrophages using monoclonal antibodies (RAM 11), a marker for rabbit macrophages. Such macrophages were encountered at 3 months, but were common at 6 months, and were generally associated with focal photoreceptor damage of varying degree of severity.

It is conceivable that the release of foreign substances triggers a phagocytic response to remove the allogeneic material. Macrophages and retinal microglia (74,75) have the capability to act as antigen-presenting cells and take up allogeneic MHC peptides from the transplanted RPE and present the foreign material to the host's T-cells. Macrophage responses are also known to be common in retinal diseases (76). In ARMD, giant cells were found in areas of RPE atrophy (77), and blood-borne macrophages are abundant in disciform scar tissue (78). In addition, it is well known that RPE cells dedifferentiate and develop macrophagelike phenotypes (79).

A phagocytic response could be induced to remove foreign or superfluous cells from the subretinal space and from those that are unable to survive over time. Treatment of retinal allografts transplanted to the rabbit subretinal space with cyclosporin A did not change the extent of the macrophage response or the associated photoreceptor damage (65).

It is possible that the survival of the grafted cells is limited. A possible reason is that grafted cells could not settle down onto Bruch's membrane because of the host's native RPE layer. The autologous transplant would then be disrupted and cellular debris could induce a macrophage response. The cellular response after grafted IPE cells is not regarded as a host versus graft rejection of immunogenic origin.

Clinical Experience

Clinical studies on humans transplanted with fetal RPE allografts to the subretinal space suggested two different phenomena. The RPE allograft demonstrated clinical signs of rejection at 3 months in cases where breakdown of the BRB occurred following surgical removal of subfoveal fibrovascular membranes. However, patch transplants of RPE remained virtually unchanged for 24 months when the BRB was intact in nonexudative ARMD, such as geographic atrophy (24–26).

In a clinical pilot study, Binder et al. (80) demonstrated good tolerance and improved vision in patients with submacular membrane removal and transposition of autologous RPE cells from the peripheral retina to the subfoveal region, a procedure excluding immunogenic responses.

IRIS PIGMENT EPITHELIUM

The iris pigment epithelium is anatomically continuous with the ciliary epithelium and RPE. IPE and RPE cells have the same embryologic origin, a similar structure and morphology but there are some major differences. IPE cells are arranged in a double layer. The posterior IPE layer is heavily pigmented with numerous melanin granules and borders the posterior iris surface. The anterior IPE layer has a basal muscular portion, the myofibrils of which constitute part of the iris musculature (81). The two layers seem to have the capacity to maintain a physiological blood–aqueous barrier. In IPE cells, vimentin was consistently detected but these cells do not express cytokeratins (82).

Whereas RPE cells continuously phagocytose photoreceptor outer segments, the IPE probably does not execute any phagocytosis *in situ*. Recently, however, it has been shown that porcine IPE cells (83) and rat IPE cells (84,85) can successfully be cultured and that these cells acquire the ability to phagocytose rod outer segments in culture (86). Because IPE cells are phenotypically plastic, have many properties in common with RPE cells (87), and have the same embryologic origin, it is reasonable to hypothesize that IPE cells transplanted into the subretinal space could execute several RPE activities and, possibly, transdifferentiate into RPE-like cells (88).

Iris Pigment Epithelium Transplantation Results

The main advantage of transplanting autologous IPE cells is to exclude immunologic reactions in the interpretation of the results. However, the question remains if IPE can perform the same tasks as the RPE.

Subretinal transplants of autologous IPE cells were found to survive for at least 3 months (88). However, in a study using rabbits, the autologous IPE grafts usually persisted for 6 months and were not destroyed to the same extent as were the RPE grafts (89,90). *In vitro* experiments indicate that IPE cells acquire the ability to phagocytose photoreceptor outer segments (83,85,86,91). When exposed to photoreceptor outer segments in tissue culture, IPE cells develop a lipofuscin-specific fluorescence identical to that emitted by RPE cells (28). IPE cells in tissue culture also demonstrate a functional barrier against macromolecules like RPE (92). Little is known of the retinoid metabolism of transplanted IPE cells in the subretinal space. IPE cells in culture did not show any retinoid metabolism (93), but the presence of mRNA for cellular retinaldehyde binding protein (CRALBP) and for other related substances suggests the possibility that IPE cells could metabolize retinol in the proper microenvironment (94).

The grafted IPE cells in our experiments in rabbits seemed to form a compound layer with host RPE (Fig. 12-7) and the adjacent photoreceptors were preserved and

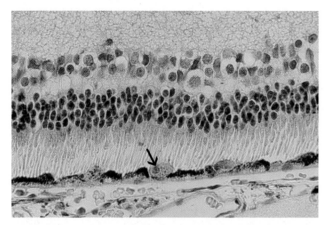

FIGURE 12-7. Presumed transplanted IPE cells form a composite cellular layer in the subretinal space, showing cells of different shape, size and pigmentation (*arrow*) on top of native RPE. Photoreceptors appear normal, exhibiting long outer segments at 6 months after transplantation (hematoxylin-eosin, ×540). (From Crafoord S, Geng L, Seregard S, et al. Photoreceptor survival in transplantation of autologous iris pigment epithelial cells to the subretinal space. *Acta Ophthalmol Scand* 2002;80:387–394, with permission.)

displayed normal morphology. Transplanted cells phagocytosed outer segments in the host retina (Fig. 12-8). Photoreceptors overlying the transplanted IPE generally survived provided the grafted cells formed a monolayer or had integrated with the RPE forming only a few cellular layers. This suggests that most physiologic mechanisms normally performed by the RPE can be executed by the grafted IPE.

Our experimental studies indicate that autologous IPE grafts are not associated with as severe adverse effects on photoreceptors as are RPE allografts. It is most probable that autologous IPE cells do not induce an immunogenic response whereas RPE allografts are likely to provoke graft rejection. Cultured autologous IPE cells incubated with low-density lipoprotein with DiL complex (Molecular Probe, Leiden, The Netherlands) are detected in the microscope using a fluorescein filter. These cells were transplanted into the submacular region of monkeys (95). After 6 months, transplanted cells could still be identified and some cells were observed to engulf photoreceptor outer segments.

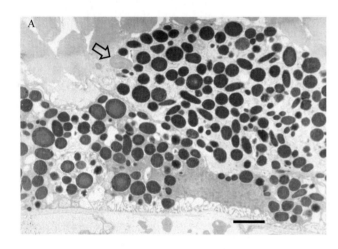

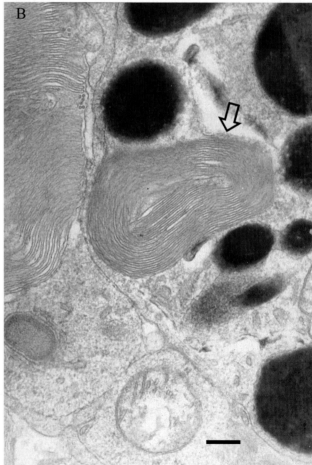

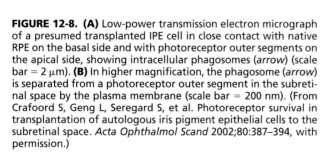

FIGURE 12-8. (A) Low-power transmission electron micrograph of a presumed transplanted IPE cell in close contact with native RPE on the basal side and with photoreceptor outer segments on the apical side, showing intracellular phagosomes (*arrow*) (scale bar = 2 μm). **(B)** In higher magnification, the phagosome (*arrow*) is separated from a photoreceptor outer segment in the subretinal space by the plasma membrane (scale bar = 200 nm). (From Crafoord S, Geng L, Seregard S, et al. Photoreceptor survival in transplantation of autologous iris pigment epithelial cells to the subretinal space. *Acta Ophthalmol Scand* 2002;80:387–394, with permission.)

Clinical Experience

Clinical observations have been reported on patients with ARMD in whom the subfoveal membranes were removed and an autologous IPE cell suspension was injected into the subretinal space (96–98). No rejection or serious adverse effect could be noted. However, no significant improvement in macular function could be detected.

PHOTORECEPTOR TRANSPLANTATION

Background

RP is caused by a multitude of genetic defects, all leading to a degeneration of the rod and, subsequently, cone photoreceptors. More than 100 different mutations involving the photoreceptor structure, RPE, and phototransduction cascade have been identified in RP patients. RP patients suffer from night blindness, loss of the peripheral visual field and, in later stages, loss of central vision. These symptoms correlate well with electroretinographic findings. To replace malfunctioning photoreceptors in this disease, experiments have been performed to transplant neurosensory retina (48,99).

Experimental Studies

Pure sheets of rods, isolated from normal mice, were transplanted into the subretinal space of mice lacking rods but possessing about 30% of the normal number of cones. In this model, the transplanted rod sheets were able to rescue about 40% of the remaining cones otherwise destined to die during the 2-week observation period. This study provided support that cone survival depends specifically on rods (100). A study on long-term survival of retinal cell transplants indicated that cells of the grafted inner retina survived for up to 583 days, whereas photoreceptor cells appeared to require the support of the host RPE for survival (101). Then, in 1998, two research groups independently showed that full-thickness sheets could be transplanted into different animals. These grafts developed normal photoreceptors and survived for extended time periods without the need for immunosuppression (102,103,104). Additionally, Seiler and Aramant demonstrated that visual evoked responses could be measured from the superior colliculus corresponding to the placement of the transplant in the retina in two different rat retinal degeneration models. Their study suggested that transplants could form synaptic connections with the host retina (105). In addition, recovery of retinotectal visual function was demonstrated (106). Finally, Zhang et al. (107) concluded that the host photoreceptor layer appeared to play a role in limiting graft-host anatomical integration. Only in areas where the host photoreceptor layer was discontinuous or completely missing was bridging of neuronal fibers between the graft and the host retina observed.

To study the functional results of neural retinal transplantation, Radner et al. (108) measured the ganglion cell response directly from the retinal surface over the transplant using a differential bipolar surface electrode. Increased spontaneous ganglion cell activity at the subretinal transplantation site was recorded but it wasn't certain if this response was secondary to neurochemically active substances. No light response was recorded. However, this technique may be useful to assess functional results of future transplantation.

Immunology

The host immune response seems to be different when fragmented embryonic cells are used instead of full-thickness retinal transplants (109). Rabbits transplanted with full-thickness allogeneic embryonic retina had no immune response, whereas those grafted with fragmented neurosensory retina demonstrated MHC class I- and II-labeled cells, indicating an immune response.

Xenogeneic and adult neuronal retinal grafts were shown to survive and develop in the immune-privileged subretinal space, if carefully handled and if the integrity of the transplant was kept intact (110,111). When neonatal neuronal retinal cells were placed beneath the kidney capsule they accommodated and even differentiated in the non–immune-privileged space, implying that they possessed inherent immune privilege. However, privilege was only partial and temporary (112).

Clinical Experience

The results of clinical experiments so far have been disappointing. Transplantation trials involving fetal full-thickness neurosensory retina have not verified any improvement in vision in patients with late stages of RP. The clinical experience suggests that transplantation of photoreceptor cell sheets is feasible and not associated with significant adverse effects, but patients with advanced RP disease do not seem to benefit from the procedure (48,113). Del Cerro and coworkers (114) describe the histologic findings in a 94-year-old patient with ARMD who 3 years earlier underwent subretinal transplantation of both a fetal neural retinal sheet and a retinal microaggregate suspension. They observed that a long-term survival of transplanted retinal tissue could be achieved in patients without immunosuppression. They concluded that extensive degeneration of the RPE in this patient prevented development of the transplanted photoreceptors and thus prevented visual improvement.

In another study, transplantation of a fetal retinal photoreceptor suspension into the subretinal space was achieved with a safe surgical technique in nine patients (115). There was no definitive improvement in vision, although a high tolerance for the grafted tissue was reported.

STEM CELLS

Background

Previously, the mature mammalian retina was considered unable to regenerate. In 2000, Tropepe et al. (116) identified retinal stem cells located in the pigmented ciliary margin of the adult mouse. These cells clonally proliferated *in vitro* to form sphere colonies of cells that appeared capable of differentiating into rod photoreceptors, bipolar neurons, and Müller glia. Transplantation of embryonic retinal cells has been more promising because the graft differentiates and integrates into the host retina (117). Thus arose the idea of transplanting stem cells from one individual to patients with retinal heredodegenerative diseases or malfunctioning neurosensory retina or RPE.

Different donor stem cells have been isolated and prepared *in vitro*. These include bone marrow cells (118), embryonic stem cells from mouse blastocysts (119), hippocampus-derived progenitor cells from the adult rat (120), and immortalized brain-derived rat medullary raphe progenitor cells (121).

Transplantation of xenogenic retinal progenitor cells to pig subretinal space was recently reported by Warfvinge et al. (122). The retinal progenitor cells survived, integrated, and differentiated in the xenogeneic pig retina for a shorter period, but did not differentiate into mature RPE or retinal cells.

To achieve integration and incorporation of transplanted stem cells, retinal injury appears to be required (118,120,123). Stem cells do not incorporate into normal retina. Chacko et al. (123) isolated stem cell/progenitor populations, which were transplanted into the eyes of rats with retinal injury. The proportion of cells observed to incorporate into the inner retina was consistently higher than those in the outer retina. These findings suggested that cues for specific differentiation were localized within the inner and outer retina. It is reasonable to conclude that these findings demonstrate that injury-induced cues or factors play a role in promoting the incorporation of ocular stem cells or progenitors regardless of their origin or differentiation.

Warfvinge et al. (121) used brain-derived precursor cell lines, which were implanted with a subretinal transplantation technique in adult normal rat eyes. The grafted cells survived for at least 4 weeks and the implanted cells gradually integrated into all major retinal cell layers including the RPE. Wojciechowski et al. (64) demonstrated that the brain-derived precursor cell lines could survive at least 4 months after transplantation in adult normal immunosuppressed rats. They also observed that the implanted cells integrated into the RPE and inner retinal layers, and migrated over long distances within the host.

When successfully transplanted into the subretinal space of RCS rats, embryonic stem cells from mouse blastocysts delayed photoreceptor cell degeneration as determined by the increased number of photoreceptor nuclei preserved compared to control (119). Wojciechowski et al. (64) also observed a promotion of photoreceptor survival extending over more than two-thirds of the superior hemisphere in the retina of the RCS rat transplanted with an immortalized brain-derived precursor cell line.

Clinical Experience

Although several experimental studies have been published, no clinical treatment modality to restore vision through stem cell transplantation is available today.

SUMMARY

Retinal Pigment Epithelium and Iris Pigment Epithelium

Transplantation of suspensions of fresh-pigmented RPE cells to the subretinal space in rabbits is feasible and induces virtually no complications when an atraumatic surgical procedure is used. The allograft forms a monolayer in conjunction with the native RPE and persists almost intact up to 3 months. At 6 months after transplantation, there was a cellular response exhibiting multilayers of cells, such as RPE and macrophages. Damage to adjacent photoreceptors in combination with melanin granules in the subretinal space indicates graft failure. No infiltration of lymphocytes was seen.

To evaluate the impact of nonimmunologic mechanisms, a technique of transplanting fresh autologous IPE cells to the subretinal space of the same eye was developed. Grafted IPE cells were seen to survive for 6 months. There was a remodeling of the cellular layers in the subretinal space over time where grafted IPE cells formed a compound layer with the native RPE cells. The cellular response that developed exhibited macrophages, but no lymphocytes, and was in this respect similar to that observed following RPE transplantation.

In RPE allografts, the photoreceptors overlying the transplants appeared normal on light microscopy at 3 months, but at 6 months the photoreceptors overlying the transplants generally exhibited pathological changes. On the other hand, the photoreceptors displayed normal outer segment length and normal outer nuclear layers above grafted autologous IPE cells at 6 months. Focally, multilayers of grafted IPE and RPE cells together with macrophages were associated with damage to adjacent photoreceptor cells. Thus, cellular multilayers in the subretinal space, irrespective of genesis, may eventually induce adverse effects on photoreceptors. The experiments show that suspensions of allogeneic RPE cells into the subretinal space are likely to cause an immunogenic response that autologous IPE cells do not. It cannot be ruled out that nonimmunogenic mechanisms also play a decisive role on the outcome.

In patients with ARMD in whom subfoveal membranes were surgically removed and autologous IPE cell suspension injected, no rejection or serious adverse effects were observed, but no visual improvement could be demonstrated in these cases (96–98). There were clinical signs of rejection in RPE allografts to patients with ARMD at 3 months after transplantation when there was a prior breakdown of the BRB, whereas patch transplants of RPE remained virtually unchanged for 24 months when the BRB was intact (24–26). Autologous RPE cells from the peripheral retina to the subfoveal region, however, seemed to survive, and a certain improvement of vision was detected (80).

Photoreceptors

It has been shown that photoreceptor degeneration can be limited in experimental animals by transplantation of fresh RPE cells with or without neurosensory retina to the subretinal space. Retinal cell transplants seem to reconstruct retinal circuitry in dystrophic animals. However, additional work is needed before clinical trials can be performed in humans (99).

Stem Cells

Different stem cells or cell progenitors survive, integrate, and migrate into the host retina at different locations within the retina when transplanted into the subretinal space. Retinal injury appears necessary for stem cells to incorporate into normal retina. No clinical method to restore vision by transplanting stem cells is available today.

PART B REFERENCES

1. Allikmets R, Shroyer NF, Singh N, et al. Mutation of the Stargardt disease gene (ABCR) in age-related macular degeneration [comment]. *Science* 1997;277(5333):1805–1807.
2. Gouras P. Transplantation of retinal pigment epithelium. In: Marmor MF, Wolfensberger TJ, eds. *The retinal pigment epithelium: function and disease.* New York: Oxford University Press, 1998:492–507.
3. Hasson T, Heintzelman MB, Santos-Sacchi J, et al. Expression in cochlea and retina of myosin VIIa, the gene product defective in Usher syndrome type 1B. *Proc Natl Acad Sci U S A* 1995; 92:9815–9819.
4. Weil D, Blanchard S, Kaplan J, et al. Defective myosin VIIA gene responsible for Usher syndrome type 1B. *Nature* 1995; 374(6517):60–61.
5. Dryja KL, Manson FD, Edgar AJ, et al. Identification and characterization of the gene for X-linked retinitis pigmentosa. *Am J Hum Genet* 1996;59(Suppl):A256.
6. Bakall B, Marknell T, Ingvast S, et al. The mutation spectrum of the bestrophin protein—functional implications. *Hum Genet* 1999;104:383–389.
7. Petrukhin K, Koisti MJ, Bakall B, et al. Identification of the gene responsible for Best macular dystrophy. *Nat Genet* 1998;19:241–247.
8. Thompson DA, Gyurus P, Fleischer LL, et al. Genetics and phenotypes of RPE65 mutations in inherited retinal degeneration. *Invest Ophthalmol Vis Sci* 2000;41:4293–4299.
9. Li LX, Turner JE. Inherited retinal dystrophy in the RCS rat: prevention of photoreceptor degeneration by pigment epithelial cell transplantation. *Exp Eye Res* 1988;47:911–917.
10. Bennett J, Tanabe T, Sun D, et al. Photoreceptor cell rescue in retinal degeneration (rd) mice by in vivo gene therapy. *Nat Med* 1996;2:649–654.
11. Bennett J, Zeng Y, Bajwa R, et al. Adenovirus-mediated delivery of rhodopsin-promoted bcl-2 results in a delay in photoreceptor cell death in the rd/rd mouse. *Gene Ther* 1998;5:1156–1164.
12. Narfstrom K, Katz ML, Bragadottir R, et al. Functional and structural recovery of the retina after gene therapy in the RPE65 null mutation dog. *Invest Ophthalmol Vis Sci* 2003;44:1663–1672.
13. Lahiri-Munir D. *Retinal pigment epithelial transplantation.* New York: Springer, 1995.
14. Lopez R, Gouras P, Brittis M, et al. Transplantation of cultured rabbit retinal epithelium to rabbit retina using a closed-eye method. *Invest Ophthalmol Vis Sci* 1987;28:1131–1137.
15. Lane C, Boulton M, Marshall J. Transplantation of retinal pigment epithelium using a pars plana approach. *Eye* 1989;3(Pt 1):27–32.
16. el Dirini AA, Wang HM, Ogden TE, et al. Retinal pigment epithelium implantation in the rabbit: technique and morphology. *Graefes Arch Clin Exp Ophthalmol* 1992;230:292–300.
17. Gouras P, Lopez R, Brittis M, et al. The ultrastructure of transplanted rabbit retinal epithelium. *Graefes Arch Clin Exp Ophthalmol* 1992;230:468–475.
18. Sheng Y, Gouras P, Cao H, et al. Patch transplants of human fetal retinal pigment epithelium in rabbit and monkey retina. *Invest Ophthalmol Vis Sci* 1995;36:381–390.
19. Durlu YK, Tamai M. Transplantation of retinal pigment epithelium using viable cryopreserved cells. *Cell Transplant* 1997;6:149–162.
20. He S, Wang HM, Ogden TE, et al. Transplantation of cultured human retinal pigment epithelium into rabbit subretina. *Graefes Arch Clin Exp Ophthalmol* 1993;231:737–742.
21. Seiler MJ, Aramant RB, Bergstrom A. Co-transplantation of embryonic retina and retinal pigment epithelial cells to rabbit retina. *Curr Eye Res* 1995;14:199–207.
22. Crafoord S, Algvere PV, Seregard S, et al. Long-term outcome of RPE allografts to the subretinal space of rabbits. *Acta Ophthalmol Scand* 1999;77:247–254.
23. Berglin L, Gouras P, Sheng Y, et al. Tolerance of human fetal retinal pigment epithelium xenografts in monkey retina. *Graefes Arch Clin Exp Ophthalmol* 1997;235:103–110.
24. Algvere PV, Berglin L, Gouras P, et al. Transplantation of fetal retinal pigment epithelium in age-related macular degeneration with subfoveal neovascularization [comment]. *Graefes Arch Clin Exp Ophthalmol* 1994;232:707–716.
25. Algvere PV, Berglin L, Gouras P, et al. Transplantation of RPE in age-related macular degeneration: observations in disciform lesions and dry RPE atrophy. *Graefes Arch Clin Exp Ophthalmol* 1997;235:149–158.
26. Algvere PV, Gouras P, Dafgard Kopp E. Long-term outcome of RPE allografts in non-immunosuppressed patients with AMD. *Eur J Ophthalmol* 1999;9:217–230.
27. Machemer R, Laqua H. Pigment epithelium proliferation in retinal detachment (massive periretinal proliferation). *Am J Ophthalmol* 1975;80:1–23.
28. Geng L, Wihlmark U, Algvere PV. Lipofuscin accumulation in iris pigment epithelial cells exposed to photoreceptor outer segments. *Exp Eye Res* 1999;69:539–546.

29. Kenyon E, Yu K, La Cour M, et al. Lactate transport mechanisms at apical and basolateral membranes of bovine retinal pigment epithelium. *Am J Physiol* 1994;267(6 Pt 1):C1561–C1573.

30. Rando RR. Molecular mechanisms in visual pigment regeneration. *Photochem Photobiol* 1992;56:1145–1156.

31. Bok D. Retinal photoreceptors disc shedding and pigment epithelium phagocytosis. In: Ryan S, ed. *Retina*. Vol 1. St Louis: Mosby, 1994:81–94.

32. Cao H, Sheng Y, Gouras P, et al. Patch culturing and polarity independence of human fetal RPE. *Invest Ophthalmol Vis Sci* 1994;35(Suppl):1761.

33. Wihlmark U, Wrigstad A, Roberg K, et al. Lipofuscin accumulation in cultured retinal pigment epithelial cells causes enhanced sensitivity to blue light irradiation. *Free Radic Biol Med* 1997;22:1229–1234.

34. Sparrow JR, Zhou J, Ben-Shabat S, et al. Involvement of oxidative mechanisms in blue-light-induced damage to A2E-laden RPE. *Invest Ophthalmol Vis Sci* 2002;43:1222–1227.

35. Dafgard Kopp E, Winter-Vernersson A, Algvere PV. Expression of HLA class I and class II antigens in human fetal RPE cells. *Invest Ophthalmol Vis Sci* 1997;38:947.

36. Dafgard Kopp E, Wilson J. Immunological properties of human fetal RPE during development. *Invest Ophthalmol Vis Sci* 1999; 40:3839.

37. Streilein JW. Anterior chamber associated immune deviation: the privilege of immunity in the eye. *Surv Ophthalmol* 1990; 35:67–73.

38. Jiang LQ, Jorquera M, Streilein JW. Subretinal space and vitreous cavity as immunologically privileged sites for retinal allografts. *Invest Ophthalmol Vis Sci* 1993;34:3347–3354.

39. Kohen L, Enzmann V, Faude F, et al. Mechanisms of graft rejection in the transplantation of retinal pigment epithelial cells. *Ophthalmic Res* 1997;29:298–304.

40. Zhang X, Bok D. Transplantation of retinal pigment epithelial cells and immune response in the subretinal space.[comment]. *Invest Ophthalmol Vis Sci* 1998;39:1021–1027.

41. Kaplan HJ, Streilein JW. Immune response to immunization via the anterior chamber of the eye. I. F. lymphocyte-induced immune deviation. *J Immunol* 1977;118:809–814.

42. Streilein JW, Wilbanks GA, Cousins SW. Immunoregulatory mechanisms of the eye. *J Neuroimmunol* 1992;39:185–200.

43. Streilein JW, Takeuchi M, Taylor AW. Immune privilege, T-cell tolerance, and tissue-restricted autoimmunity. *Hum Immunol* 1997;52:138–143.

44. Wilbanks GA, Streilein JW. Studies on the induction of anterior chamber-associated immune deviation (ACAID). 1. Evidence that an antigen-specific, ACAID-inducing, cell-associated signal exists in the peripheral blood. *J Immunol* 1991;146:2610–2617.

45. Wilbanks GA, Mammolenti M, Streilein JW. Studies on the induction of anterior chamber-associated immune deviation (ACAID). III. Induction of ACAID depends upon intraocular transforming growth factor-beta. *Eur J Immunol* 1992;22:165–173.

46. Wilbanks GA, Mammolenti M, Streilein JW. Studies on the induction of anterior chamber-associated immune deviation (ACAID). II. Eye-derived cells participate in generating blood-borne signals that induce ACAID. *J Immunol* 1991;146:3018–3024.

47. Jiang LQ, Jorquera M, Streilein JW. Immunologic consequences of intraocular implantation of retinal pigment epithelial allografts. *Exp Eye Res* 1994;58:719–728.

48. Berger AS, Tezel TH, Del Priore LV, et al. Photoreceptor transplantation in retinitis pigmentosa: short-term follow-up. *Ophthalmology* 2003;110:383–391.

49. Medawar PB. Immunity to homologous grafted skin: the fate of skin homografts transplanted to the brain, to subcutaneous tissue, and to the anterior chamber of the eye. *Br J Exp Pathol* 1948;29:58–69.

50. Liversidge J, McKay D, Mullen G, et al. Retinal pigment epithelial cells modulate lymphocyte function at the blood-retina barrier by autocrine PGE2 and membrane-bound mechanisms. *Cell Immunol* 1993;149:315–330.

51. Liversidge J, Grabowski P, Ralston S, et al. Rat retinal pigment epithelial cells express an inducible form of nitric oxide synthase and produce nitric oxide in response to inflammatory cytokines and activated T cells. *Immunology* 1994;83:404–409.

52. Jorgensen A, Wiencke AK, la Cour M, et al. Human retinal pigment epithelial cell-induced apoptosis in activated T cells. *Invest Ophthalmol Vis Sci* 1998;39:1590–1599.

53. Liversidge J, Forrester JV. Regulation of immune responses by the retinal pigment epithelium. In: Marmor MF, Wolfensberger TJ, eds. *The retinal pigment epithelium: function and disease.* New York: Oxford University Press, 1998:511–527.

54. Al-Amro S, Tang L, Kaplan HJ. Limitations in the study of immune privilege in the subretinal space of the rodent [comment]. *Invest Ophthalmol Vis Sci* 1999;40:3067–3069.

55. Li LX, Sheedlo HJ, Turner JE. Long-term rescue of photoreceptor cells in the retinas of RCS dystrophic rats by RPE transplants. *Prog Brain Res* 1990;82:179–185.

56. Lin N, Fan W, Sheedlo HJ, et al. Photoreceptor repair in response to RPE transplants in RCS rats: outer segment regeneration. *Curr Eye Res* 1996;15:1069–1077.

57. Sheedlo HJ, Li L, Turner JE. Photoreceptor cell rescue in the RCS rat by RPE transplantation: a therapeutic approach in a model of inherited retinal dystrophy. *Prog Clin Biol Res* 1989;314:645–658.

58. Seaton AD, Sheedlo HJ, Turner JE. A primary role for RPE transplants in the inhibition and regression of neovascularization in the RCS rat. *Invest Ophthalmol Vis Sci* 1994;35:162–169.

59. Gaur V, Agarwal N, Li L, et al. Maintenance of opsin and S-antigen gene expression in RCS dystrophic rats following RPE transplantation. *Exp Eye Res* 1992;54:91–101.

60. Yamamoto S, Du J, Gouras P, et al. Retinal pigment epithelial transplants and retinal function in RCS rats. *Invest Ophthalmol Vis Sci* 1993;34:3068–3075.

61. Lavail MM, Li L, Turner JE, et al. Retinal pigment epithelial cell transplantation in RCS rats: normal metabolism in rescued photoreceptors. *Exp Eye Res* 1992;55:555–562.

62. Roque RS, Imperial CJ, Caldwell RB. Microglial cells invade the outer retina as photoreceptors degenerate in Royal College of Surgeons rats. *Invest Ophthalmol Vis Sci* 1996;37:196–203.

63. Sauve Y, Girman SV, Wang S, et al. Preservation of visual responsiveness in the superior colliculus of RCS rats after retinal pigment epithelium cell transplantation. *Neuroscience* 2002; 114:389–401.

64. Wojciechowski AB, Englund U, Lundberg C, et al. Subretinal transplantation of brain-derived precursor cells to young RCS rats promotes photoreceptor cell survival. *Exp Eye Res* 2002;75: 23–37.

65. Crafoord S, Algvere PV, Kopp ED, et al. Cyclosporine treatment of RPE allografts in the rabbit subretinal space. *Acta Ophthalmol Scand* 2000;78:122–129.

65a. Del Priore L, Ishida O, Johnson E, et al. Triple immune suppression of porcine fetal retinal pigment epithelium xenografts. *Invest Ophthalmol Vis Sci* 2003;44:4044–4053.

66. Hall BM, Bishop GA, Farnsworth A, et al. Identification of the cellular subpopulations infiltrating rejecting cadaver renal allografts. Preponderance of the T4 subset of T cells. *Transplantation* 1984;37:564–570.

67. Grierson I, Hiscott P, Hogg P, et al. Development, repair and regeneration of the retinal pigment epithelium. *Eye* 1994;8(Pt 2):255–262.

68. Niederkorn J, Streilein JW, Shadduck JA. Deviant immune responses to allogeneic tumors injected intracamerally and subcutaneously in mice. *Invest Ophthalmol Vis Sci* 1981;20:355–363.

69. Niederkorn JY, Streilein JW. Alloantigens placed into the anterior chamber of the eye induce specific suppression of delayed-type hypersensitivity but normal cytotoxic T lymphocyte and helper T lymphocyte responses. *J Immunol* 1983;131:2670–2674.

70. Niederkorn JY, Mayhew E. Role of splenic B cells in the immune privilege of the anterior chamber of the eye. European *J Immunol* 1995;25:2783–2787.

71. Grisanti S, Ishioka M, Kosiewicz M, et al. Immunity and immune privilege elicited by cultured retinal pigment epithelial cell transplants. *Invest Ophthalmol Vis Sci* 1997;38:1619–1626.

72. Hoffman LM, Maguire AM, Bennett J. Cell-mediated immune response and stability of intraocular transgene expression after adenovirus-mediated delivery. *Invest Ophthalmol Vis Sci* 1997;38:2224–2233.

73. Larsson J, Juliusson B, Ehinger B. Survival and MHC-expression of embryonic retinal transplants in the choroid. *Acta Ophthalmol Scand* 1998;76:417–421.

74. Kirchhof B, Kirchhof E, Ryan SJ, et al. Macrophage modulation of retinal pigment epithelial cell migration and proliferation. *Graefes Arch Clin Exp Ophthalmol* 1989;227:60–66.

75. Provis JM, Diaz CM, Penfold PL. Microglia in human retina: a heterogeneous population with distinct ontogenies. *Perspect Dev Neurobiol*1996;3:213–222.

76. Nicolai U, Eckardt C. The occurrence of macrophages in the retina and periretinal tissues in ocular diseases. *Ger J Ophthalmol* 1993;2:195–201.

77. Penfold PL, Killingsworth MC, Sarks SH. Senile macular degeneration. The involvement of giant cells in atrophy of the retinal pigment epithelium. *Invest Ophthalmol Vis Sci* 1986;27:364–371.

78. Seregard S, Algvere PV, Berglin L. Immunohistochemical characterization of surgically removed subfoveal fibrovascular membranes. *Graefes Arch Clin Exp Ophthalmol* 1994;232:325–329.

79. Boulton M. Melanin and the retinal pigment epithelium. In: Marmor MF, Wolfensberger TJ, eds. *The retinal pigment epithelium: function and disease.* New York: Oxford University Press, 1998:68–85.

80. Binder S, Stolba U, Krebs I, et al. Transplantation of autologous retinal pigment epithelium in eyes with foveal neovascularization resulting from age-related macular degeneration: a pilot study. *Am J Ophthalmol* 2002;133:215–225.

81. Hogan MJ, Alvarado JA, Weddell JE. *Histology of the human eye: an atlas and textbook.* Philadelphia: Saunders, 1971.

82. Kivela T, Fuchs U, Tarkkanen A. Cytoskeleton in neuroectodermally derived epithelial and muscle cells of the human iris and ciliary body. *J Histochem Cytochem* 1992;40:1517–1526.

83. Schraermeyer U, Enzmann V, Kohen L, et al. Porcine iris pigment epithelial cells can take up retinal outer segments. *Exp Eye Res* 1997;65:277–287.

84. Schraermeyer U, Kociok N, Heimann K. Rescue effects of IPE transplants in RCS rats: short-term results. *Invest Ophthalmol Vis Sci* 1999;40:1545–1556.

85. Rezai KA, Lappas A, Farrokh-siar L, et al. Iris pigment epithelial cells of Long Evans rats demonstrate phagocytic activity. *Exp Eye Res* 1997;65:23–29.

86. Thumann G, Bartz-Schmidt KU, Heimann K, et al. Phagocytosis of rod outer segments by human iris pigment epithelial cells in vitro. *Graefes Arch Clin Exp Ophthalmol* 1998;236:753–757.

87. Rezai KA, Kohen L, Wiedemann P, et al. Iris pigment epithelium transplantation. *Graefes Arch Clin Exp Ophthalmol* 1997;235:558–562.

88. Thumann G, Bartz-Schmidt KU, El Bakri H, et al. Transplantation of autologous iris pigment epithelium to the subretinal space in rabbits [comment]. *Transplantation* 1999;68:195–201.

89. Crafoord S, Geng L, Seregard S, et al. Experimental transplantation of autologous iris pigment epithelial cells to the subretinal space. *Acta Ophthalmol Scand* 2001;79:509–514.

90. Crafoord S, Geng L, Seregard S, et al. Photoreceptor survival in transplantation of autologous iris pigment epithelial cells to the subretinal space. *Acta Ophthalmol Scand* 2002;80:387–394.

91. Dintelmann TS, Heimann K, Kayatz P, et al. Comparative study of ROS degradation by IPE and RPE cells in vitro. *Graefes Arch Clin Exp Ophthalmol* 1999;237:830–839.

92. Rezai KA, Lappas A, Kohen L, et al. Comparison of tight junction permeability for albumin in iris pigment epithelium and retinal pigment epithelium in vitro. *Graefes Arch Clin Exp Ophthalmol* 1997;235:48–55.

93. von Recum HA, Okano T, Kim SW, et al. Maintenance of retinoid metabolism in human retinal pigment epithelium cell culture. *Exp Eye Res* 1999;69:97–107.

94. Thumann G, Kociok N, Bartz-Schmidt KU, et al. Detection of mRNA for proteins involved in retinol metabolism in iris pigment epithelium. *Graefes Arch Clin Exp Ophthalmol* 1999;237:1046–1051.

95. Abe T, Tomita H, Kano T, et al. Autologous iris pigment epithelial cell transplantation in monkey subretinal region. *Curr Eye Res* 2000;20:268–275.

96. Abe T, Yoshida M, Tomita H, et al. Auto iris pigment epithelial cell transplantation in patients with age-related macular degeneration: short-term results. *Tohoku J Exp Med* 2000;191:7–20.

97. Thumann G, Aisenbrey S, Schraermeyer U, et al. Transplantation of autologous iris pigment epithelium after removal of choroidal neovascular membranes. *Arch Ophthalmol* 2000;118:1350–1355.

98. Lappas A, Weinberger AW, Foerster AM, et al. Iris pigment epithelial cell translocation in exudative age-related macular degeneration. A pilot study in patients. *Graefes Arch Clin Exp Ophthalmol* 2000;238:631–641.

99. Lund RD, Kwan AS, Keegan DJ, et al. Cell transplantation as a treatment for retinal disease. *Prog Retin Eye Res* 2001;20:415–449.

100. Mohand-Said S, Hicks D, Dreyfus H, et al. Selective transplantation of rods delays cone loss in a retinitis pigmentosa model. *Arch Ophthalmol* 2000;118:807–811.

101. Sharma RK, Bergstrom A, Zucker CL, et al. Survival of long-term retinal cell transplants. *Acta Ophthalmol Scand* 2000;78:396–402.

102. Ghosh F, Arner K, Ehinger B. Transplant of full-thickness embryonic rabbit retina using pars plana vitrectomy. *Retina* 1998;18:136–142.

103. Seiler MJ, Aramant RB. Intact sheets of fetal retina transplanted to restore damaged rat retinas. *Invest Ophthalmol Vis Sci* 1998;39:2121–2131.

104. Aramant RB, Seiler MJ. Transplanted sheets of human retina and retinal pigment epithelium develop normally in nude rats. [Published erratum appears in *Exp Eye Res* 2003;76:135.]. *Exp Eye Res* 2002;75:115–125.

105. Aramant RB, Seiler MJ. Retinal transplantation: advantages of intact fetal sheets. *Prog Retin Eye Res* 2002;21:57–73.

106. Sagdullaev BT, Aramant RB, Seiler MJ, et al. Retinal transplantation-induced recovery of retinotectal visual function in a rodent model of retinitis pigmentosa. *Invest Ophthalmol Vis Sci* 2003;44:1686–1695.

107. Zhang Y, Arner K, Ehinger B, et al. Limitation of anatomical integration between subretinal transplants and the host retina. *Invest Ophthalmol Vis Sci* 2003;44:324–331.

108. Radner W, Sadda SR, Humayun MS, et al. Increased spontaneous retinal ganglion cell activity in rd mice after neural retinal transplantation. *Invest Ophthalmol Vis Sci* 2002;43:3053–3058.

109. Ghosh F, Larsson J, Wilke K. MHC expression in fragment and full-thickness allogeneic embryonic retinal transplants. *Graefes Arch Clin Exp Ophthalmol* 2000;238:589–598.

110. Rauer O, Ghosh F. Survival of full-thickness retinal xenotransplants without immunosuppression. *Graefes Arch Clin Exp Ophthalmol* 2001;239:145–151.

111. Wasselius J, Ghosh F. Adult rabbit retinal transplants. *Invest Ophthalmol Vis Sci* 2001;42:2632–2638.

112. Ng TF, Osawa H, Hori J, et al. Allogeneic neonatal neuronal retina grafts display partial immune privilege in the subcapsular space of the kidney. *J Immunol* 2002;169:5601–5606.

113. Radtke ND, Seiler MJ, Aramant RB, et al. Transplantation of intact sheets of fetal neural retina with its retinal pigment epithelium in retinitis pigmentosa patients. *Am J Ophthalmol* 2002;133:544–550.

114. del Cerro M, Humayun MS, Sadda SR, et al. Histologic correlation of human neural retinal transplantation. *Invest Ophthalmol Vis Sci* 2000;41:3142–3148.

115. Humayun MS, de Juan E Jr, del Cerro M, et al. Human neural retinal transplantation. *Invest Ophthalmol Vis Sci* 2000;41:3100–3106.

116. Tropepe V, Coles BL, Chiasson BJ, et al. Retinal stem cells in the adult mammalian eye. *Science* 2000;287(5460):2032–2036.

117. Chacko DM, Rogers JA, Turner JE, et al. Survival and differentiation of cultured retinal progenitors transplanted in the subretinal space of the rat. *Biochem Biophys Res Commun* 2000;268:842–846.

118. Tomita M, Adachi Y, Yamada H, et al. Bone marrow-derived stem cells can differentiate into retinal cells in injured rat retina. *Stem Cells* 2002;20:279–283.

119. Schraermeyer U, Thumann G, Luther T, et al. Subretinally transplanted embryonic stem cells rescue photoreceptor cells from degeneration in the RCS rats. *Cell Transplant* 2001;10:673–680.

120. Nishida A, Takahashi M, Tanihara H, et al. Incorporation and differentiation of hippocampus-derived neural stem cells transplanted in injured adult rat retina. *Invest Ophthalmol Vis Sci* 2000;41:4268–4274.

121. Warfvinge K, Kamme C, Englund U, et al. Retinal integration of grafts of brain-derived precursor cell lines implanted subretinally into adult, normal rats. *Exp Neurol* 2001;169:1–12.

122. Warfvinge KKJ, Lavik E, Klassen H, et al. Survival, integration and differentiation of retinal progenitor cells from GFP transgenic mice transplanted subretinally to adult, normal pigs. *Invest Ophthalmol Vis Sci* 2003;224:483.

123. Chacko DM, Das AV, Zhao X, et al. Transplantation of ocular stem cells: the role of injury in incorporation and differentiation of grafted cells in the retina. *Vision Res* 2003;43:937–946.

GENE THERAPY FOR PEDIATRIC RETINAL DISEASES

ALBERT M. MAGUIRE
JEAN BENNETT

Gene therapy is a pharmacologic approach whereby exogenous genes or nucleic acids are introduced into host cells to effect local production of a therapeutic product. This product can be a protein (enzyme, structural protein, etc.) or ribonucleic acid (RNA). The RNA can be designed to bind in antisense (antisense RNA), interfere with RNA processing (RNAi), or have an enzymatic function (ribozyme). Gene therapy takes advantage of the normal transcriptional and translational apparatus of the host cells to produce the pharmacologic compound coded by the exogenous genetic material. Gene therapy therefore requires two events: (i) uptake of the template genetic material and transport to the target cell nucleus, and (ii) expression of the exogenous gene by the host tissue. In theory, it can be used to replace an essential gene product in a disease that is caused by a gene mutation. It also could be used to modulate the production of a substance to positively effect the outcome of a disease that has a complicated pathogenesis, i.e., a combination of genetic and environmental insults. Gene therapy is beneficial in such diseases because it minimizes the number of drug administrations and may more specifically target affected cells or tissues.

Although the spectrum of therapeutic molecules that can be produced through gene therapy is limited to peptides, proteins, and RNAs, this does not limit the types of diseases that can be treated. Genes can produce growth factors or neurotrophic factors that have a nonspecific effect applicable to a variety of disease processes. For example, pigment epithelium-derived growth factor (PEDF) has a potent antiangiogenic effect, and its expression can be efficacious in a variety of conditions characterized by neovascular complications, such as retinopathy of prematurity (ROP), diabetic retinopathy, or age-related macular degeneration (1–7). Likewise, the use of gene therapy techniques to induce the local production of ciliary-derived neurotrophic factor might help prevent progressive photoreceptor loss in a number of retinal degenerative diseases (8–10).Therapy can also be highly specific, with replacement or augmentation of defective gene products in genetic diseases caused by lack-of-function gene mutations. For example, gene therapy with replacement of a functional RPE65-encoding gene can provide specific treatment for some types of Leber congenital amaurosis (LCA) caused by mutations resulting in a nonfunctional *RPE65* gene product (11–13).

Treatment of pediatric retinal diseases presents special issues not encountered with adult disease. The biology of many pediatric retinal conditions either involves or impacts normal development of the retina and the visual system. Changes that occur prenatally, such as in ocular albinism or LCA caused by mutations in the *CRX* gene, are fully manifest at birth (14,15). Treatment performed after birth would be expected to have little impact on these conditions because the biologic effects are irreversible. *In utero* treatment would provide an opportunity to correct the defects before the signs of disease become manifest and thereby allow the development of an anatomically normal and functional retina. However, in diseases that develop pathologic changes postnatally, such as ROP or familial exudative vitreoretinopathy (FEVR), there can be a window of time for intervention after birth to prevent permanent loss of foveal fixation and abnormal development of central visual pathways with amblyopia.

Although the technical demands of *in utero* intervention would present major challenges, there would be distinct advantages. Prenatal application of an exogenous gene or gene product would help induce immune tolerance to the foreign antigen. Transduction efficiency would likely be enhanced because a larger area of the outer retina could be targeted with one injection. This is not only because of the greater number of cells present per unit area in the fetal retina but also because there are no attachments between the neural retina and the retinal pigment epithelium (RPE) in early development. This permits free diffusion of subretinally administered drug. Correction of the defect at an early stage would also reduce the occurrence of later tissue damage. This is important in early-onset retinal degenerations because photoreceptors, which die in these diseases, are terminally differentiated cells after birth and cannot regenerate. Finally, early application of the therapeutic gene would take advantage of the plasticity of the developing retinal to central nervous system (CNS) axonal connections present early in life. If treatment were performed too late in development, higher-order CNS neurons might already have established synapses from other sensory systems, and cortical areas for vision would no longer exist.

Several retinal diseases exhibit a short, well-defined period of biologic activity in the early postnatal period and early childhood. Intervention would need to occur during or before infancy in order to arrest the disease process and salvage retinal function. For example, threshold ROP occurs on average about 37 weeks' postgestational age. Retinal detachment as stage 4 ROP typically occurs about the time of what would have been a full-term delivery, 40 weeks' gestation. The window of opportunity for treatment in ROP is thus limited to a period of a few weeks. In inherited retinoblastoma, tumor appearance usually occurs within the first year of life, sometimes presenting at birth. Effective treatment for retinoblastoma would require intervention within a narrow time period of active tumorigenesis. In LCA, visual deficits are present at birth or in early childhood. The retina undergoes progressive degeneration through childhood and adult life. Intervention with gene therapy would need to occur within a defined time period before histologic degeneration of the photoreceptors and retina developed. This also is true with other early-onset retinal degenerative diseases that manifest a rapid time course for photoreceptor loss.

GENERAL PRINCIPLES OF GENE THERAPY

Gene transfer can be achieved by several different methods. Ultimately, the optimal technique will achieve the gene expression profile required for the specific application with the minimum of toxicity. Naked deoxyribonucleic acid (DNA) does not penetrate cell membranes readily; however, transient expression with modest transduction efficiency can be achieved by a variety of physicochemical techniques. In some instances, electroporation can be used to deliver DNA to target cells (16). Transfer to deep tissue layers (of the cornea) can be achieved by ballistic injection of DNA bound to gold particles (gene gun) (17). Cationic lipids that interact with cell membranes can enhance transfer efficiency (18,19). However, with all of these physicochemical techniques, efficiency of transfer to many cell types and duration of gene expression are quite limited.

Viruses are used to take advantage of their ability to transfer exogenous nucleic acids into host cells. Viral vectors have been considered ideally suited for treatment of many diseases because of their superior gene transfer efficiency and stability of gene expression. Using recombinant DNA engineering techniques, viruses are designed so that their ability to replicate is eliminated and their pathogenic properties are minimized. Different viruses demonstrate distinctly different characteristics with regard to cargo capacity, cell tropism, immune response, and stability of transgene expression (Table 13-1). Of the 636 human gene therapy clinical trials that have been approved, 70.3% used recombinant viruses as gene delivery vectors *(http://www.wiley.co.uk/genetherapy/clinical/)*. Of these human gene therapy trials using recombinant viruses, retrovirus has been used in the most protocols (217) and in the highest number of patients (1,757). Adenovirus is second in these categories, having been used in 171 different protocols and 644 patients. In comparison, adeno-associated virus (AAV) has been used in only 15 different protocols and 36 different patients *(http://www.wiley.co.uk/genetherapy/clinical/)*. To date, there are only two approved human gene therapy clinical trials involving the eye. Both trials—one aimed at choroidal neovascularization and the other at retinoblastoma—involve the use of adenovirus (see later). AAV is under consideration for future human gene therapy clinical trials *(http://crisp.cit.nih.gov/crisp; see grant number 5U10EY013729-02)*.

Recombinant adenovirus is highly efficient at transducing RPE cells and Muller cells (20,21). Onset of gene expression is rapid, occurring within 24 to 48 hours of vector administration compared to physicochemical techniques. However, transduction efficiency with adenovirus of retinal cell types such as photoreceptors is poor. In addition, the duration of gene expression is limited by the lack of integration of the transgene and by the host immune response to the vector (22,23). Nevertheless, the ease of generating recombinant adenovirus vectors and the rapid and high levels of gene expression make this vector a good choice for gene therapy studies. This virus presently is being used to deliver a gene that inhibits neovascularization in patients with choroidal neovascularization secondary to age-related macular degeneration (24).

A significant improvement in gene transfer technology involves generation of "gutted" adenoviruses, viruses in which all viral open reading frames have been removed. These viruses have a large (~38 kb) cargo capacity and also have reduced immunogenicity, as evidenced by the fact that transgene expression persists longer than is observed with earlier-generation adenoviruses (25). It is possible to modify the cellular targeting characteristics of such viruses by changing envelope components (26). Widespread evaluation of gutted adenoviruses remains to be done because these viruses are very difficult to grow and often are contaminated with wild-type virus.

Inflammation from systemic delivery of a viral vector can result in severe toxicity. The most dramatic example, which occurred during a human gene therapy trial, resulted in the death of a human subject (27). Injection of the early-generation (E1-deleted and E3-deleted) recombinant adenoviral vectors into the vitreous also can induce profound inflammatory responses. After high-dose recombinant adenovirus delivery to the eyes of rodents, inflammatory panophthalmitis is seen. The degree of inflammation is markedly less when a vector is administered into the subretinal space.

TABLE 13-1. RECOMBINANT VIRUSES UNDER CONSIDERATION FOR HUMAN GENE THERAPY: TRANSDUCTION CHARACTERISTICS AND POTENTIAL FOR USE IN PEDIATRIC RETINAL DISEASES

Recombinant Virus	Cargo Capacity (kb)	Target Cells: Intravitreal Injection	Target Cells: Subretinal Injection	Stability	Limitations	Clinical Trial (Yes/No) [Disease]
AAV2/2	4.8	Ganglion cells ++; Müller cells	Photoreceptors ++; RPE cells; Müller cells	++++	4.8 Kb cargo capacity [trans-splicing with dual vectors can increase the capacity to 8 kb, but efficiency is reduced	Yes [hemophilia, (96) cystic fibrosis (108, 109)], muscular
AAV2/1	4.8	Ganglion cells +/−	RPE cells	++++	Cargo capacity [trans-splicing with dual vectors can increase the capacity to 8 kb, but efficiency is reduced (62)]	No
AAV2/5	4.8	—	Photoreceptors ++++	++++	Cargo capacity {trans-splicing with dual vectors can increase the capacity to 8 kb, but efficiency is reduced (62)]	No
Lentivirus-VSVG	7.8	—	RPE cells ++++	++++	Virus preparations can be contaminated with cellular proteins	Yes: *Ex vivo* therapy for HIV (111)
Lentivirus-Mokola	7.8	—	RPE cells +++; photoreceptors	++++	Virus preparations can be contaminated with cellular proteins	No
Adenovirus (E1-deleted, E3-deleted)	7.8	Müller cells +; anterior segment structures [corneal endothelium, iris epithelium, trabecular meshwork (112)]	RPE cells +++; Müller cells +	+/−	Immune response (intravitreal >> subretinal (23))	Yes [see: *(http://www.wiley.co.uk/gene-therapy/clinical/)*; cancer, metabolic disease (OTC deficiency), cystic fibrosis, familial hypercholesterolemia, coronary artery disease, AMD (24) retinoblastoma (28)
Gutted adenovirus (Ad5)	37	NR	RPE; photoreceptors (25,113)	++	Difficult to generate; potential contamination with wild-type adenovirus	No
Gutted adenovirus (Ad37)	37	Ciliary body	Photoreceptors +++ (114)	++	Difficult to generate; potential contamination with wild-type adenovirus	No

Only viruses that are capable of transducing postnatal retinal cells are listed. Viruses that have been or are being used in approved human clinical trials are indicated under column entitled "Clinical Trial." Only representative trials are listed. For a complete listing, see the *Journal of Gene Medicine Clinical Trial* Web site *(http://www.wiley.co.uk/genetherapy/clinical/)* or the Office of Biotechnology Activities (OBA) Web site of the National Institutes of Health (NIH) *(http://www4.od.nih.gov/rac/clinicaltrial.htm).*
AMD, Age-related macular degeneration; HIV, human immunodeficiency virus; kb, kilobases; NR, not reported; RPE, retinal pigment epithelium.

This difference in immune response has been attributed to the suppression of the inflammatory response when the vector is placed in the immunologically privileged environment of the subretinal space (23). In addition, injection into the subretinal space reduces the exposure of viral vector to uveal tract structures that are in contact with the vitreous space (e.g. ciliary body, iris). In the human ocular gene therapy trial involving retinoblastoma, the recombinant adenovirus is used to deliver the cDNA encoding thymidine kinase of the herpes simplex virus to humans with retinoblastoma. Treatment with ganciclovir is then used to kill the tumor cells (28). Immune response directed at the adenoviral vector might contribute to the therapeutic effect in this study.

Retroviruses have long been available for use in gene therapy applications. Many retroviral vectors appear to have limited application in retinal gene therapy due to their inability to efficiently target nonreplicating, terminally differentiated cells, such as those in the neural retina. However, one class of retroviruses, lentiviruses, shows similar transduction profiles as adenoviral vectors. The majority of the recombinant lentiviruses that have been evaluated are derived from the human immunodeficiency virus. Multiple safeguards are in place to minimize the risk of producing a wild-type (replication competent) virus in development of recombinant lentiviral vectors. Recombinant lentiviral vectors also have been generated using nonhuman parental strains, such as those derived from the cow, cat, and horse. Onset of expression of human-derived lentivirus occurs within 24 to 48 hours of administration and is seen primarily in the RPE (29–31). Chimeric lentiviral vectors have been engineered by packaging the genetic material from the lentivirus in the envelope of another virus (e.g., the rabies virus Mokola envelope). Altering the envelope can modify the tropism of the vector, altering the range of cell types that the vector will efficiently transduce (31). Lentiviral vectors induce significantly less inflammation than recombinant adenovirus (30). Stability of gene expression is greater, presumably related, in part, to the reduction in the immune response characteristic of this viral species (32). Stability of gene expression also can be related to the fact that retroviral vectors, including lentiviral ones, integrate into the host DNA. Although this might be an advantage, it also poses a risk of insertional mutagenesis. This risk was realized recently in a human gene therapy trial for X-linked severe combined immune deficiency (SCID), in which children whose disease had been "cured" by retroviral treatment developed a leukemialike syndrome (33).

There has been great interest in the development of AAV as a vector for gene therapy. AAV is a parvovirus and has minimal pathogenetic effects in humans or other animals. Although wild-type AAV can integrate into genomic DNA, integration has not been reported after delivery of recombinant AAV to the retina. Instead, the AAV-delivered transgenes appear to remain stable as episomes in the host nucleus, thereby providing stable gene expression over time. AAV has expression profiles that appear particularly favorable for applications to retinal disease. At least eight different AAV serotypes have been identified (34), and several of these serotypes transduce photoreceptor cells with extremely high efficiency (31,35–38). Several AAV serotypes also have a strong tropism for the RPE (31,35). When injected into the vitreous, some AAV vectors are capable of transducing retinal ganglion cells (Fig. 13-1) (39). Although AAV does

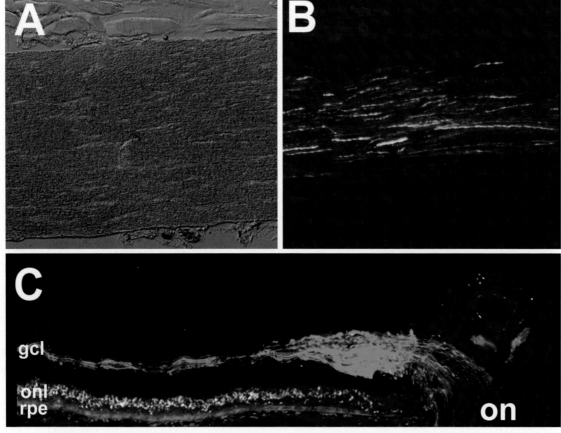

FIGURE 13-1. AAV2/2 targets ganglion cells after intravitreous injection. An AAV vector carrying the gene encoding green fluorescent protein (GFP) was delivered into the vitreous of mice. **A, B:** Optic nerve is shown, without and with GFP-exciting blue excitation light, respectively. **C:** GFP-positive ganglion cells (gcl) leading to the optic nerve (on) are shown. onl, outer nuclear layer; rpe, retinal pigment epithelium. A similar photo to that seen in panel C is presented in Liang et al. (117).

induce an inflammatory response, the response is relatively mild even after injection into the vitreous (40). The most significant limitation to the use of AAV is the limited cargo capacity of the vector. Whereas recombinant adenoviral vectors can accommodate transgenes up to 7.8 kb in size, AAV can package a maximum of 4.8 kb (41,42). Use of dual AAV vectors can overcome this limitation to some extent (see later). Another potential limitation of AAV in therapeutic applications is the prolonged latency period prior to onset of gene expression that is seen with some AAV serotypes (31,35–37). Depending on the animal species treated, the delay to peak levels of transgene expression after vector administration can be up to 8 weeks (43). This is especially true of vectors demonstrating tropism predominant for photoreceptor cells. A corresponding delay in the expression of the transgene can miss the therapeutic window because the active pharmacologic product is absent during the peak period of disease activity. This situation has proven to be important in treating one animal model of early-onset retinitis pigmentosa (RP) caused by a mutation in the PDEβ gene. In *rd1* mice, defects in the PDEβ gene cause complete photoreceptor degeneration within 3 weeks of birth. Photoreceptor loss is therefore complete before the onset of gene expression in some AAV serotypes.

ANIMAL MODELS

Retinopathy of Prematurity Mouse

Numerous animal models exist for various pediatric retinal conditions, thus providing the opportunity to test gene therapy approaches for these diseases (Table 13-2). One well-established model for oxygen-induced retinopathy and ROP is the hyperoxia-hypoxia rodent model (44) (see also Chapter 26 for a discussion on animal models of oxygen-induced retinopathy). In this model, neonatal mice are exposed to a very high oxygen tension for several days and then returned to normal oxygen levels. Neovascularization develops transiently at the junction of vascularized and avascular retina. The degree of neovascularization can be quantified, thus providing measures of retinopathy in these animals.

Several experiments have used this model to test antiangiogenic strategies in retinal neovascularization. AAV vectors containing different antiangiogenic compounds were injected in the early neonatal period, prior to exposing animals to high oxygen (Fig. 13-2). Some studies used adenovirus or AAV serotype 2 vectors (AAV2/2); others used AAV serotype 2 vectors packaged within an AAV serotype 1 capsid (AAV2/1) (Table 13-2) (4,5,7,45–47). Transgene expression occurred relatively soon after intraocular injection, especially after delivery of AAV2/1 vectors, thus exposing areas of potential neovascularization to antiangiogenic transgene products. When delivered in this fashion, several compounds, including pigment epithelium-derived growth factor, angiostatin, endostatin, TIMP3, and soluble

vascular endothelial growth factor receptor-1 (sFlt-1), displayed significant antiangiogenic activity (Fig. 13-2) (4,5,7,45–47). The neovascularization that occurred in these eyes with retinopathy was reduced, often dramatically, without apparent deleterious effects to the native retinal vasculature (48). Using this model, gene therapy-mediated delivery of antiangiogenic compounds thus appears to be a viable approach for primary or adjuvant treatment of oxygen-induced retinopathy.

Spontaneous and Genetically Engineered Animal Models of Retinal Degeneration

RPE65 Mutant Animals

Several animal models exist for inherited retinal degenerations caused by specific gene mutations. Some of these diseases manifest at or soon after birth, whereas others result in early-onset retinopathies that are rapidly progressive. Abnormalities in the gene encoding the RPE-specific RPE65 protein can result in lack of photoreceptor function that is evident at birth. In humans, *RPE65* mutations are responsible for approximately one-fifth of all cases of LCA. LCA can also be caused by mutations in other genes. Likewise, *RPE65* mutations can lead to other human phenotypes. A naturally occurring homolog of lack-of-function *RPE65* mutations occurs in Swedish Briard dogs in which an LCA-like syndrome of congenital nystagmus, blindness, and significantly depressed photoreceptor function occurs (49). A genetically engineered *RPE65* knockout has been developed in mice (50). These animals (*Rpe65⁻/⁻* mice) suffer from a similar LCA-like syndrome.

Gene therapy using AAV carrying a functional *RPE65* transgene has been used successfully to treat the canine and murine models of LCA caused by lack of RPE65 (11–13,51). In the canine disease, when the AAV vector is injected into the subretinal space (Figs. 13-3 and 13-4), animals with abnormal electroretinogram (ERG) responses from birth develop a normal-appearing ERG with amplitudes corresponding to the area of the retina treated (11). Dogs display visual behavior not previously present, and nystagmus eye movements are significantly reduced (11,12,52). Intravitreous injection of vector results in no expression of *RPE65* in the outer retina and no corresponding development of ERG or visual response (11). Successful treatment has been achieved in animals older than age 1 year (53). Histologic degeneration in RPE65 disease is somewhat slow, suggesting that treatment is possible, at least in early childhood (49,54). Recent evidence from human studies, however, indicates that earlier rather than later intervention may be more likely to restore vision. Retinal histologic abnormalities were present in an aborted fetus with an *RPE65* mutation (55), and retinal thinning has been documented in 12- and 13-year-old LCA patients with *RPE65* mutations (56). It may be that *in utero* treatment could potentially rescue as yet unidentified developmental components of the

TABLE 13-2. NONSYNDROMIC PEDIATRIC CONDITIONS THAT MAY BE CANDIDATES FOR GENE THERAPY

Pediatric Retinal Disease	Molecular Target(s)	Strategies Under Consideration	Potential Target Cells	Candidate Virus	Animal Model (Yes/No)
ROP	VEGF; angiogenesis (inhibitors and stimulators)	Delivery of anti-angiogenic molecule (e.g., PEDF, endostatin, etc.)(1,7); 115 inhibition of proangiogenic genes (e.g., VEGF, Hiflα) via ribozymes or RNA; *in utero* vs early postnatal	Ganglion cells Muller cells RPE cells	AAV2/2 AAV2/2 AAV2/1; lentvirus	Yes
Leber congenital amaurosis	RPE65, CRX, GC1, TULP1,	Gene delivery: *in utero* vs early childhood	RPE cells (RPE65) Photoreceptors (CRX, GC1, TULP1, AIPL1, RPGRIP1)	RPE65: AAV2/2; AAV2/1; lentivirus CRX; GC1; TULP1; AIPL1; RPGRIP1: AAV2/2; AAV2/1; AAV2/5	Yes
Autosomal recessive RP	PDEβ	Gene delivery: *in utero* vs early postnatal through early childhood	Rod photoreceptors	AAV2/5	Yes
Stargardt disease (fundus flavimaculatus)	ABCR (=ABCA4)	Gene delivery; postnatal	Rod photoreceptors	AAV2/5 (trans-splicing (62); gutted (sialic acid-pseudotyped) adenovirus	Yes
X-linked RP	RPGR	Gene delivery: early postnatal	Rod photoreceptors	AAV2/5 (trans-splicing (62); gutted (sialic acid-pseudotyped) adenovirus	Yes
Choroideremia	REP-1	Gene delivery: early postnatal	Rod photoreceptors and RPE	AAV2/5	No
Mucopolysaccharidosis (MPS) VI, VII	MPS VI: arylsulfatase B; MPS VII: β-glucuronidase	Gene delivery: early postnatal	RPE (retinal disease) Ganglion cells (CNS disease)	AAV2/1, lentivirus AAV2/2	Yes
Juvenile Batten disease (ceroid lipofuscinosis, neuronal 3)	CLN3 (116)	Gene delivery: early postnatal	RPE (retinal disease) Ganglion cells (CNS disease)	AAV2/1, lentivirus AAV2/2	Yes
Retinoblastoma	HStk	Early postnatal	Tumor cells	Adenovirus (early generations acceptable because inflammatory response may contribute to therapeutic effect)	Yes
Ocular albinism	OA1	*In utero*	RPE cells	AAV2/1; AAV2/2; lentivirus	Yes
Retinal dysgenesis	CRX	*In utero*	Retinal progenitor cells	AAV2/2; AAV2/5	Yes
Retinal dysgenesis	NR2E3	*In utero*	Retinal progenitor cells	AAV2/2;AAV2/5	Yes
Retinal dygenesis/LCA/Coats-like exudative vasculopathy	CRB1	*In utero*	Retinal progenitor cells	AAV2/2; AAV2/5	Yes

(continued)

TABLE 13-2. (CONTINUED)

Pediatric Retinal Disease	Molecular Target(s)	Strategies Under Consideration	Potential Target Cells	Candidate Virus	Animal Model (Yes/No)
Achromatopsia	CNGA3	*In utero*	Retinal progenitor cells	AAV2/2; AAV2/5	Yes
X-linked juvenile retinoschisis	XLRS1	*In utero; postnatal*	Retinal progenitor cells	AAV2/2; AAV2/5	Yes
Enhanced S-cone syndrome	NRL	*In utero*	Retinal progenitor cells	AAV2/2; AAV2/5	Yes
Norrie disease	ND (86)	*In utero*	Ganglion cells; photoreceptors; other?	AAV2/2; AAV2/5; other?	Yes

Listed are the diseases, the strategies presently under consideration, and the optimal virus given the current understanding of target cell type/stability/inflammatory response. See text for details. As the technology improves, gutted adenovirus pseudotyped to target photoreceptor-rich sialic acid sequences may become choice vectors for targeting photoreceptor disease. At present, it is easier and there is less chance of contamination to generate AAV vectors. In cases were the cargo capacity of AAV vectors is exceeded, however, gutted adenoviral vectors may play an important role. The only alternative, at present, is to use dual (trans-splicing) AAV vectors.

CNS, central nervous system; LCA, Leber congenital amaurosis; PEDF, pigment epithelium-derived growth factor; ROP, retinopathy of prematurity; RP, retinitis pigmentosa; RPGR, retinitis pigmentosa GTPase regulator; VEGF, vascular endothelial growth factor.

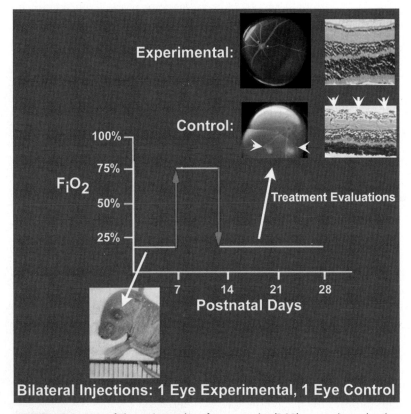

FIGURE 13-2. Use of the retinopathy of prematurity (ROP) mouse in evaluation of gene-based strategies to block retinal neovascularization. Paradigm for evaluating effects of gene therapy in the ROP mouse. The experimental agent is injected into one eye and the control agent is injected in the contralateral eye shortly after birth. The pups (and their mothers) are placed in a high oxygen (75% O_2) for 5 days starting on postnatal day 7 and then are returned to normoxia. Assays performed several days after return to normoxia reveal neovascularization in the control eye and effect of the treatment in the contralateral experimental eye. In this particular example, fluorescein angiography and histologic sections reveal inner retinal neovascularization *(arrowheads)* in the control eye but not in the experimental (AAV2/1.CMV.PEDF-treated) eye (7). Scale bars under the mouse pup are in millimeters.

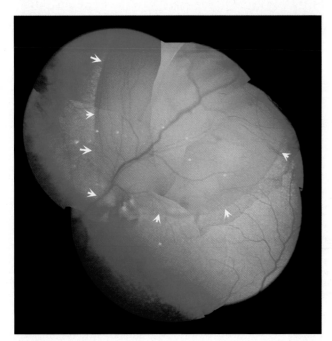

FIGURE 13-3. Appearance of retina of a dog immediately after subretinal injection with a recombinant AAV. Montage of fundus photos taken with a red-free filter. *Arrows* indicate borders of the bleb (the region of retina detached by the injection). This area reattached within 2 hours of injection. The injection site was in the superior (tapetal) retina.

disease process that may be initiated during gestation. Dejneka et al. (13) recently showed that *in utero* treatment of $Rpe65^{-/-}$ mice can result in functional and biochemical recovery identical to that seen in postnatally treated mice and postnatally treated *RPE65* mutant dogs.

Other Early-Onset/Rapidly Progressive Retinal Degeneration Animal Models

Animal models are available for the study of a variety of early-onset and aggressive human retinal degenerative diseases (Table 13-2). A particularly aggressive form of autosomal recessive RP is caused by lack-of-function mutations in the β-subunit of cGMP rod photoreceptor-specific phosphodiesterase (PDEβ). Similar to models for RPE65-based LCA, there are both mouse and dog models for this disease. In both species, lack of PDEβ impedes the differentiation of rod photoreceptors and leads to their early demise (see earlier). Rod photoreceptors in the *rd1* mouse die by postnatal age 3 weeks and in the *rcd1* dog by age 6 months. A second mouse model of PDEβ-based disease has recently been identified: the *rd10* mouse (57). Early-onset and rapid retinal degeneration also occurs in these animals, but it is slightly slower than in the *rd1* mouse.

There have been several reports of successful slowing of the disease process in the murine models of PDEβ-based disease. Success has been achieved through the delivery of

wild-type PDEβ cDNA in a variety of viral vectors, including a first-generation adenoviral vector, AAV, gutted adenovirus, and a lentivirus (25,58–60). Unfortunately, rescue in all of these reports was transient, apparently due to the overwhelming apoptotic cell death that takes place in this disease. It might be that studies in the *rcd1* dog, which has a longer window of opportunity for treatment, will lead to a longer period of rescue. Alternatively, *in utero* treatment of the murine models could be successful.

There is a murine model of Stargardt disease, which is a juvenile-onset macular degeneration. This *abcr^{-/-}* mouse models many features of Stargardt disease, except that macular structure cannot be assessed because the mouse lacks a macula (61). Treatment of Stargardt disease by gene replacement therapy presents several problems. The *ABCR* (Stargardt, *ABCA4*) cDNA is quite large, on the order of 8 kb. This poses limitations as to the type of vector that can be used to carry this gene in one piece (Table 13-1). Only lentivirus or gutted adenovirus can accommodate this gene. Another possible strategy would involve splitting the cDNA in two at a natural splicing site, and each piece would be car-

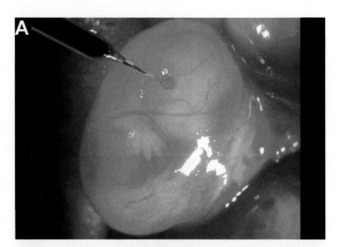

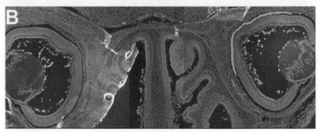

FIGURE 13-4. Delivery of the reporter gene green fluorescent protein (GFP) to the retina of a mouse fetus. **A:** AAV2/1.CMV.EGFP was injected subretinally in one eye of a fetal mouse on embryonic day 14. **B:** This resulted in transgene expression in the retinal pigment epithelium (RPE), apparent at birth through analysis of histologic sections. (From Surace E, Auricchio A, Reich S, et al. Delivery of adeno-associated viral vectors to the fetal retina: impact of viral capsid proteins on retinal neuronal progenitor transduction. *J Virol* 2003;77:7957–7963, with permission.)

ried in by two different AAV vectors. This approach has been demonstrated using the reporter gene *lacZ* (62). Gene therapy studies are in progress with this animal model (Bennett et al, unpublished data).

Both murine and canine animal models are also available for study of another severe and early-onset form of RP: X-linked RP due to mutations in retinitis pigmentosa GTPase regulator (RPGR) (63,64). As yet there are no reports of gene-based corrections in these animal models. For development of treatment of other early-onset retinal degenerations, we must await generation or identification of the appropriate animal model. Gene-based treatments exist, for example, for choroideremia, but they cannot be tested yet *in vivo* due to a lack of a model (65).

Lysosomal Storage Diseases

A variety of storage diseases exist in which there is an abnormal accumulation of substrate in a variety of tissues leading to multisystem disease, including retinal disease. The mucopolysaccharidoses (MPSs) are a group of such diseases characterized by the abnormal accumulation of glycosaminoglycans (heparan sulfate, dermatan sulfate, keratan sulfate) in the lysosomes of various tissues as a result of defects in carbohydrate metabolism (66). Ocular abnormalities include corneal clouding up to retinal degeneration, optic atrophy, and glaucoma.

Multiple animal models of MPSs exist and include (i) a feline model of MPS VI (deficiency of arylsulfatase B), and (ii) murine, feline, and canine models of MPS VII (deficiency of β-glucuronidase) (67,68). These models share multiple pathologic abnormalities with humans, including those seen in the eye.

Gene therapy has been successful in animal models by treating the ocular manifestations of two diseases: MPS VII and MPS VI. Li and Davidson (69) treated MPS VII mice with gene therapy. These mice develop photoreceptor degeneration secondary to defects in the RPE, and they possess lysosomal storage vacuoles in keratocytes in the corneal stroma, corneal endothelial cells, RPE, and cells in the choroid and sclera (69). Injection into the vitreous of the adenovirus carrying the human β-glucuronidase gene resulted in complete clearance of the storage defect in RPE cells, with partial phenotypic correction in corneal endothelial cells. Similar results were reported by Sands et al. (70). Intravenous administration of a recombinant AAV encoding the human β-glucuronidase cDNA also resulted in nearly complete elimination of lysosomal storage vacuoles in the RPE of these animals (71). Kamata et al. (72) aimed to treat the corneal clouding in the MPS VII mouse by delivering an adenovirus expressing human β-glucuronidase into the corneal stroma following lamellar keratotomy. Histology revealed a rapid and nearly complete elimination of vacuoles in the areas of the cornea examined. Recently, a larger animal model has been used to explore the efficacy of treating MPS VI ocular

disorders via gene therapy. Ho et al. (73) used an AAV to deliver arylsulfatase B to the subretinal space of the MPS VI cat. This model is characterized by the presence of vacuolated inclusions in the RPE, cornea, conjunctiva, sclera, choroid, and stroma of the iris and ciliary body (49). AAV treatment appeared to reverse the disease phenotype in the RPE.

In future studies, it will be interesting to extend the approach to other animal models of storage diseases. Juvenile Batten disease (ceroid lipofuscinosis, neuronal 3) is one such target (Table 13-2). Besides ocular manifestations, this disease manifests severe CNS deterioration. It might be possible to target the CNS disease with gene therapy through treatment of the eye. Delivery of genes to retinal ganglion cells (Fig. 13-1) allows distribution of transgenic proteins along the trajectories of the retinal ganglion cell axons (Fig. 13-3) (39). Such an approach at treating CNS disease has been reported to be successful in a murine model of MPS (74). The recent generation of a murine model of Batten disease will facilitate such studies (75).

Retinoblastoma

Gene therapy studies have focused on developing an effective eye-sparing treatment for retinoblastoma. Current protocols use enucleation to treat large unilateral tumors in patients. This is often used in conjunction with chemotherapy or radiotherapy. Such procedures can be cosmetically destructive for pediatric patients. The goal of gene therapy is to eliminate the need for such drastic treatments and preserve the integrity of the eye. The availability of animal models for retinoblastoma has facilitated such studies (Table 13-2).

Two murine models of human retinoblastoma have been developed: one metastatic and one nonmetastatic. In the first model, cells from the human-derived Y79 retinoblastoma cell line are injected into the vitreous of nude mice. These cells form intraocular tumors in the vitreous cavity, and the tumors progressively invade the retina, subretinal space, choroid, optic nerve head, and anterior chamber of the eye. The tumors progress into the subarachnoid space and focally invade the brain, where they often migrate to the contralateral optic nerve. In the second model, WERI-Rb tumors are injected into the vitreous of nude mice. Tumor cells were localized in the eye with only anterior choroidal invasion at late stages (76).

Hurwitz et al. (77) have used an Ad vector that encodes the herpes simplex virus thymidine kinase gene *(HStk)*. Virus was directly administered to experimental tumors in mice, and animals were subsequently treated with ganciclovir (77). Transduced cells were thus rendered susceptible to ganciclovir cytotoxicity, and tumor growth was inhibited. These results allowed for approval of a phase I clinical trial for the treatment of retinoblastoma. In this trial, ganciclovir is used to ablate the tumors that have been treated with AdV-thymidine kinase. This trial is currently underway, and early results appear promising.

Retinal Dysgenesis

Ocular Albinism: Retinal Dysgenesis and Abnormal Visual Tract Development

All forms of albinism lead to abnormal development of the retina and the visual tracts leading to the brain. In particular, humans with albinism have abnormal foveal development and poor fine visual discrimination. An animal model of albinism has been generated by disrupting the *Oa1* gene (Table 13-2) (78). Mice normally lack foveas (and maculae); therefore, foveal abnormalities cannot be reproduced in this species. Nevertheless, the *Oa1*$^{-/-}$ mouse manifests two features that are present in the human disease and that might be amenable to correction through gene transfer: (i) the presence in the RPE of macromelanosomes, which appear shortly after birth and increase in number until postnatal day 7; and (ii) the misrouting of optic fibers at the chiasm. Because the *Oa1* gene is expressed only in the RPE layer in the eye, it is possible that both the melanosomal and optic chiasm defects can be corrected by transferring the normal *Oa1* cDNA to the RPE early in development (i.e., *in utero*).

Other Gene Defects Affecting Retinal Development

Retinal dysgenesis can result from *CRX, NR2E3,* or *CRB1 lack-of-function* mutations (Table 13-2). Animal models for some of these diseases exist and are amenable to gene therapy studies. The *crx* knockout mouse demonstrates photoreceptor abnormalities early in life and severely impaired ERGs (rod more than cone) (79). The *NR2E3* gene is a nuclear receptor gene. Lack of this gene product causes enhanced S-cone syndrome (see Chapter 10), a disorder of retinal cell fate (80). The phenotype in the *rd7* mouse has been shown to result from an *Nr2E3* mutation (57) and could potentially be used for gene therapy studies.

Although mutations in the neural retina leucine zipper gene *NRL* can result in autosomal dominant RP, lack of function of *Nrl* in a mouse model has been shown to have a dramatic effect on retinal differentiation. *Nrl*$^{-/-}$ mice lack rod photoreceptors and have only "cod" (i.e., cone) mutations (81). This animal is thought to model the enhanced S-cone syndrome in humans (82).

X-linked juvenile retinoschisis is another disease that evolves from abnormal retinal differentiation. Lack of the retinoschisis gene product results in separation of the retina at the level of the nerve fiber and ganglion cell layers. This results in cystic degeneration of the central retina. ERGs of affected males have preserved rod and cone photoreceptor systems but substantially reduced b waves, indicating loss of bipolar cell activity (83,84). There is no therapy available for this disease. Availability of a murine model of this disease would allow gene therapy approaches for treating this disease (85).

Similar to X-linked retinoschisis, Norrie disease can involve retinal schisis. The identification of the involved gene

in, and the generation of, an animal model of this disease will be useful in developing a gene-based therapy (86).

Mutations in the *Crumbs homolog 1 (CRB1)* gene have been shown to result in a variety of early-onset retinal disorders, including defective retinal lamination, LCA, and Coats-like exudative vasculopathy (56,87,88). A spontaneous mouse mutant, the rd8 mouse with this defect was recently identified (89). Finally, achromatopsia can result from mutations in the gene encoding the a-subunit of the cone photoreceptor cGMP-gated cation channels *CNGA3* or *CNGB3* (90). A canine model with CNGB3 mutations has been identified (91).

APPLICATION OF GENE THERAPY TO PEDIATRIC RETINAL DISEASES

Successful treatment of animal models has provided proof of principle for treatment of pediatric retinal diseases. Numerous conditions exist that may be amenable to intervention using a gene therapy approach (Table 13-2). Timing of intervention requires careful consideration if successful therapy is to be achieved. Many pediatric retinal conditions manifest at an early stage of development and therefore would require early postnatal treatment or even *in utero* therapy (Fig. 13-4). Although *in utero* therapy presents substantial technical challenges (Fig. 13-5), certain advantages may be afforded by the timing of intervention. Exposure of antigen at this early stage can induce tolerance to the foreign transgene, thus minimizing the immune response. Efficiency of gene transfer and a reduction in latency for gene expression in actively replicating retinal cells might be increased. In addition, wound healing might be improved because scar formation is minimized with fetal surgery.

Several early-onset retinal diseases will be optimally treated in the early postnatal period when disease activity is maximal. ROP has a predictable course regarding risk for progression that can be determined by certain clinical factors. Treatment could be optimized by intervention at certain time points. Heritable retinoblastoma may likewise be treated at time points most favorable for therapeutic intervention. Conditions such as early-onset RP or Stargardt disease might best be treated when the amblyogenic potential of surgical intervention is minimized, and the early phase of eye growth is largely complete.

In many instances, the continuous production of transgene product might be unnecessary or possibly deleterious to ocular function or viability. Often, disease processes are transient. Expression of the abnormality in heritable retinoblastoma occurs in replicating cells. Thus, after completion of eye growth and development, the disease process in inactive and additional treatment likely is unnecessary. In some cases, regulation of the transgene production could be desirable in order to titer the potential toxic effect related to overproduction of the transgene. For example, it is known that overproduction of wild-type rhodopsin can, itself, cause

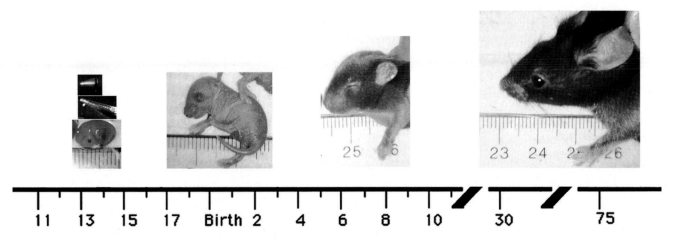

FIGURE 13-5. Only a small amount of vector is needed to target the eye. This amount is even smaller in fetal and early postnatal eyes. Age is presented in days before birth (fetal days) and postnatal (P). For size perspective, globes of C57Bl/6 mice are shown at fetal day 14, P1, P7, and adulthood (2 months). The tips of a ballpoint pen and a pencil are shown in comparison with the fetal day 14 animal.

retinal degeneration in otherwise normal animals (92). Vectors can be made with regulatable promoter systems that control the expression of transgene products. Target cells are coinfected with two vectors, one containing a "transactivator" and the second containing the therapeutic transgene regulated by an upstream promoter (93,94). The first vector will bind a pharmacologic agent such as tetracycline, which can be administered systemically. Binding of this agent induces production of the transactivator, which, in turn, binds to the promoter of the second vector, either turning on expression of the transgene or turning it off. Delivery of the active transgene product is therefore directly controlled by the application or withdrawal of an agent such as tetracycline. Thus, this regulatable system provides a method by which gene expression can be turned on or turned off as required.

UNIQUE CHALLENGES OF GENE THERAPY STUDIES INVOLVING ANIMAL MODELS OF PEDIATRIC RETINAL DISEASES

Gene Therapy: General Concerns

Probably the greatest barrier to the application of gene therapy to pediatric retinal disease is its acceptance by both the regulatory community and the lay public. Although gene therapy is the most logical approach to treatment of some incurable genetic diseases, there has been significant distrust and concern with this discipline. This is largely a result of the untimely death of a participant in a human gene therapy trial for systemic ornithine transcarbamylase (OTC) deficiency. The results of this phase I trial suggested some therapeutic efficacy for the treatment. However, the outcome was completely overshadowed by the death of Jesse Gelsinger, who, although affected with OTC, had been able to survive on a severely restricted low-protein diet. Questions raised concerning the immunogenicity of the vector and foreknowledge of its potential toxicity have rightly emphasized safety concerns and have raised the threshold for approval of new human gene therapy clinical trials (27). Nevertheless, over the past few years, there have been undisputed gene therapy successes. A retrovirus-mediated gene therapy treatment for X-linked SCID has allowed children, who would otherwise have succumbed to their disease, to lead normal lives (95). The recent finding that two of the treated children had developed a leukemialike syndrome was a setback for this project. However, the SCID clinical trials have been allowed to continue now that this risk has been identified. In the second human gene therapy success, patients treated with gene therapy for hemophilia have been able to significantly reduce their dependence on clotting factor medication (37,96). Modifications of the delivery method of the vector will likely further improve its therapeutic effect. Finally, there have been remarkable successes of gene therapy in animal models. Dogs with a crippling arthropathy due to a naturally occurring lysosomal storage disease display protection after retroviral delivery of the missing enzyme and preserve the ability to locomote (97). Other canine breeds that are born blind as a result of lack of an enzyme involved in vitamin A metabolism have restoration of vision after AAV-mediated delivery of the missing gene (11). Extrapolations of these and other remarkable successes provide reasonable hope for treatment of these incurable human conditions and certainly merit testing in future human clinical trials.

One challenge in the development of human gene therapy clinical trials is that the prerequisite preclinical safety studies are time consuming and expensive. Often by the time these are completed, technologic improvements in viral vectors have been made. The investigators are "locked in" to using the earlier generation vectors, however, because of the time and monetary investments in the preclinical studies. With more experience with particular recombinant viruses, however, it is likely that there will be faster transition from one vector to the next. The expense of the preclinical studies and the human trials is another potential barrier to the development of new treatments. Although some preclinical and early phase clinical studies can be covered by research grants, the expense becomes prohibitive during progression to phase II and higher trials. It will be critical that links among basic scientists, physician scientists, and industry be fostered so that promising results can be brought to fruition. Many pediatric retinal diseases are considered "orphan" diseases" in that there are fewer than 200,000 patients in the country known to have each disease. Development of treatment for orphan diseases will need special support because few pharmaceutical companies are willing to shoulder the costs of a trial that is not likely to bring profit.

Pediatric/Fetal Concerns

The greatest barrier to successful development of gene therapy treatment for pediatric retinal disease will be to provide a convincing demonstration of safety. This is especially true in ophthalmic applications because the diseases involved, with the one exception of retinoblastoma, have no risk of mortality. The potential benefits will have to far outweigh the potential risks. In addition, many of the conditions, most notably early-onset RP(s) and Stargardt disease, are slowly progressive, lifelong afflictions. Thus, delivery of therapy for these conditions must not only lack toxicity over a prolonged period of time but must maintain efficacy over several decades if treatment is to be of value.

Fortunately, ophthalmic application for gene therapy has distinct advantages over systemic applications. First, toxicity is lower with ophthalmic applications. The retina, measured in milligrams of mass, requires only a fraction (1/1,000th) of the amount of vector typically used in systemic applications (Fig. 13-5), e.g., for the liver measured in kilograms of mass. Second, unlike the liver, bone marrow, or other organ systems, the eye is not essential for viability. Failure of retinal physiology or destruction of the eye will lead to blindness but not to death. There is a concern, however, that retrograde transport of transgene product along ganglion cell axons to the CNS could be a potential source of extraocular toxicity. Although it is conceivable that a transgene product would have unanticipated deleterious effects in the CNS, the axons could be effectively and permanently interrupted if such toxicity required intervention. Third, the eye provides an immune privileged environment that dramatically reduces the inflammatory response of administered vectors (32).

Finally, although *in utero* gene transfer is a fascinating and promising field, much work needs to be done before this method can be considered seriously for treatment of any disease, let alone retinal disease. Direct *in utero* gene therapy has not been performed in humans, although several successful studies have been reported in animals. Successful *in utero* reporter gene transfer has been accomplished in lung, skeletal muscle, peritoneum, blood vessels, retina (Fig. 13-4), and brain in animals ranging from mice to monkeys (98–102). *In utero* somatic gene therapy was deemed therapeutically successful in animal models of hemophilia (both factor VIII and factor IX deficiency), mucopolysaccharidosis (type I), epilepsy, and LCA (13,100,103–107). In an LCA study, treatment effects were, in some cases, better after gene delivery to fetuses than after delivery to adult animals. The treated fetuses developed normally and matured into healthy adult animals with normal fertility. None of their offspring carried the therapeutic transgene, an important finding because germline transmission is a concern of the Food and Drug Administration (FDA). Nevertheless, *in utero* gene therapy poses special challenges to informed consent. Little is known about the long-term impact of *in utero* treatment on the fetus or on the mother. The parents often have an overlay of desperation that might interfere with rational decision making in context of the informed consent for their infants or children. Selecting blinding diseases with no good alternatives might make the risks tolerable.

There are many reasons for considering *in utero* therapy for particular pediatric retinal diseases. For these diseases, it makes sense to intervene as early as possible in order to prevent the onset of disease symptoms. Obviously, this approach is far from the stage of implementation, and it will likely not be considered unless a number of pediatric retinal gene therapy trials are successful. In the next decade, it is likely that a number of retinal gene therapy trials will be performed in adult patients, and some of these will be extended to pediatric patients. If these trials are successful, it will not be long until *in utero* retinal gene therapy is considered seriously for human application.

Acknowledgment: This work was supported in part by NIH U10EY013729, R01 EY10820, and EY12156, the Foundation Fighting Blindness, the Lois Pope LIFE Foundation, The William and Mary Greve International Research Scholar Award, Research to Prevent Blindness, Inc, the Ruth and Milton Steinbach Fund, the Paul and Evanina Mackall Trust, the Sam B. and Barbara G. Williams fund of the Cleveland Foundation, and the F.M. Kirby Foundation.

REFERENCES

1. Mori K, Duh E, Gehlbach P, et al. Pigment epithelium-derived factor inhibits retinal and choroidal neovascularization. *J Cell Physiol* 2001;188:253–263.
2. Mori K, Gehlbach P, Ando A, et al. Regression of ocular neovascularization in response to increased expression of pigment epithelium-derived factor. *Invest Ophthalmol Vis Sci* 2002;43: 2428–2434.

3. Mori K, Gehlbach P, Ando, A, et al. Intraocular adenoviral vector-mediated gene transfer in proliferative retinopathies. *Invest Ophthalmol Vis Sci* 2002;43:1610–1615.

4. Mori K, Gehlbach P, Yamamoto S, et al. AAV-mediated gene transfer of pigment epithelium-derived factor inhibits choroidal neovascularization. *Invest Ophthalmol Vis Sci* 2002;43:1994–2000.

5. Raisler BJ, Berns KI, Grant MB, et al. Adeno-associated virus type-2 expression of pigmented epithelium-derived factor or Kringles 1–3 of angiostatin reduce retinal neovascularization. *Proc Natl Acad Sci USA* 2002;99:8909–8914.

6. Stellmach VV, Crawford S, Zhou W, et al. Prevention of ischemia-induced retinopathy by the natural ocular antiangiogenic agent pigment epithelium-derived factor. *Proc Natl Acad Sci USA* 2001;98:2593–2597.

7. Auricchio A, Behling KC, Maguire AM, et al. Inhibition of retinal neovascularization by intraocular viral-mediated delivery of anti-angiogenic agents. *Mol Ther* 2002;6:490–494.

8. Cayouette M, Gravel C. Adenovirus-mediated gene transfer of ciliary neurotrophic factor can prevent photoreceptor degeneration in the retinal degeneration (rd) mouse. *Hum Gene Ther* 1997;8:423–430.

9. Liang FQ, Dejneka NS, Cohen DR, et al. AAV-mediated delivery of ciliary neurotrophic factor prolongs photoreceptor survival in the rhodopsin knockout mouse. *Mol Ther* 2001;3:241–248.

10. Peterson WM, Flannery JG, Hauswirth WW, et al. Enhanced survival of photoreceptors in P23H mutant rhodopsin transgenic rats by adeno-associated virus (AAV)-mediated delivery of neurotrophic genes. *Invest Ophthalmol Vis Sci* 1998;39:S1117.

11. Acland GM, Aguirre GD, Ray J, et al. Gene therapy restores vision in a canine model of childhood blindness. *Nat Genet* 2001;28:92–95.

12. Narfstrom K, Katz ML, Bragadottir R, et al. Functional and structural recovery of the retina after gene therapy in the RPE65 Null mutation dog. *Invest Ophthalmol Vis Sci* 2003;44:1663–1672.

13. Dejneka N, Surace E, Aleman T, et al. In utero gene therapy rescues vision in a murine model of congenital blindness. *Mol Ther* 2004;9:182.

14. Cremers FP, Van Den Hurk JA, Den Hollander AI. Molecular genetics of Leber congenital amaurosis. *Hum Mol Genet* 2002;11:1169–1176.

15. Kinnear P, Jay B, Witkop C Jr. Albinism. *Surv Ophthalmol* 1985;30:75–101.

16. Mo X, Yokoyama A, Oshitari T, et al. Rescue of axotomized retinal ganglion cells by *BDNF* gene electroporation in adult rats. *Invest Ophthalmol Vis Sci* 2002;43:2401–2405.

17. Tanelian D, Barry M, Johnston S, et al. Controlled gene gun delivery and expression of DNA within the cornea. *Biotechniques* 1997;23:484–488.

18. Maguire AM, Sun D, Zack DJ, Bennett J. In vivo gene transfer into adult mammalian retina. *Invest Ophthalmol Vis Sci* 1993;34:1455.

19. Hangai M, Kaneda Y, Tanihara H, et al. In vivo gene transfer into the retina mediated by a novel liposome system. *Invest Ophthalmol Vis Sci* 1996;37:2678–2685.

20. Bennett J, Wilson J, Sun D, et al. Adenovirus vector-mediated in vivo gene transfer into adult murine retina. *Invest Ophthalmol Vis Sci* 1994;35:2535–2542.

21. Li T, Adamian M, Roof DJ, et al. In vivo transfer of a reporter gene to the retina mediated by an adenoviral vector. *Invest Ophthalmol Vis Sci* 1994;35:2543–2549.

22. Reichel M, Ali R, Thrasher A, et al. Immune responses limit adenovirally mediated gene expression in the adult mouse eye. *Gene Ther* 1998;5:1038–1046.

23. Hoffman LM, Maguire AM, et al. Cell-mediated immune response and stability of intraocular transgene expression after adenovirus-mediated delivery. *Invest Ophthalmol Vis Sci* 1997;38:2224–2233.

24. Rasmussen H, Chu KW, Campochiaro P, et al. Clinical protocol. An open-label, phase I, single administration, dose-escalation study of ADGVPEDF.11D (ADPEDF) in neovascular-age-related macular degeneration (AMD). *Hum Gene Ther* 2001;12:2029–2032.

25. Kumar-Singh R, Yamashita C, Tran K, et al. Construction of encapsidated (gutted) adenovirus minichromosomes and their application to rescue of photoreceptor degeneration. *Meth Enzymol* 2000;316:724–743.

26. Von Seggern DJ, Aguilar E, Kinder K, et al. In vivo transduction of photoreceptors or ciliary body by intravitreal injection of pseudotyped adenoviral vectors. *Mol Ther* 2003;7:27–34.

27. Wade N. Patient dies while undergoing gene therapy. *New York Times.* Sept. 29, 1999; pg 1.

28. Hurwitz R, Brenner M, Poplack D, et al. Retinoblastoma treatment. *Science* 1999;284:2066.

29. Lai C, Gouras P, Doi K, et al. Tracking RPE transplants labeled by retroviral gene transfer with green fluorescent protein. *Invest Ophthalmol Vis Sci* 1999;40:2141–2146.

30. Karakousis P, Anand V, Wakefield J, et al. Favorable immune response following subretinal administration of lentivirus. (submitted).

31. Auricchio A, Kobinger G, Anand V, et al. Exchange of surface proteins impacts on viral vector cellular specificity and transduction characteristics: the retina as a model. *Hum Mol Genet* 2001;10:3075–3081.

32. Bennett J. Immune response following intraocular delivery of recombinant viral vectors. *Gene Ther* 2003;10:977–982.

33. Stolberg SG. Trials are halted on a gene therapy. *New York Times.* Oct. 4, 2002; pg 1.

34. Gao G-P, AlviraM, Wang L, et al. Novel adeno-associated viruses from rhesus monkeys as vectors for human gene therapy. *Proc Natl Acad Sci USA* 2002;99:11854–11859.

35. Rabinowitz J, Rolling F, Li C, et al. Cross-packaging of a single adeno-associated virus (AAV) type 2 vector genome into multiple AAV serotypes enables transduction with broad specificity. *J Virol* 2002;76:791–801.

36. Bennett J, Duan D, Engelhardt JF, et al. Real-time, noninvasive in vivo assessment of adeno-associated virus-mediated retinal transduction. *Invest Ophthalmol Vis Sci* 1997;38:2857–2863.

37. Bennett J, Maguire AM, Cideciyan AV, et al. Recombinant adeno-associated virus-mediated gene transfer to the monkey retina. *Proc Natl Acad Sci USA* 1999;96:9920–9925.

38. Flannery J, Zolotukin S, Vaquero M, et al. Efficient photoreceptor-targeted gene expression in vivo by recombinant-adeno-associated virus. *Proc Natl Acad Sci USA* 1997;94:6916–6921.

39. Dudus L, Anand V, Acland GM, et al. Persistent transgene product in retina, optic nerve and brain after intraocular injection of rAAV. *Vision Res* 1999;39:2545–2553.

40. Anand V, Duffy B, Yang Z, et al. A deviant immune response to viral proteins and transgene product is generated on subretinal administration of adenovirus and adeno-associated virus. *Mol Ther* 2002;5:125–132.

41. Carter BJ. The promise of adeno-associated virus vectors. *Nat Biotech* 1996;14:1725–1726.

42. Kozarsky KF, Wilson JM. Gene therapy: adenovirus vectors. *Curr Opin Genet Dev* 1993;3:499–503.

43. Bennett J, Anand V, Acland GM, et al. Cross-species comparison of in vivo reporter gene expression after rAAV-mediated retinal transduction. *Meth Enzymol* 2000;316:777–789.

44. Smith LE, Wesolowski E, McLellan A, et al. Oxygen-induced retinopathy in the mouse. *Invest Ophthalmol Vis Sci* 1994; 35:101–111.

45. Lai YK, Shen WY, Brankov M, et al. Potential long-term inhibition of ocular neovascularisation by recombinant adeno-associated virus-mediated secretion gene therapy. *Gene Ther* 2002; 9:804–13.

46. Lai CC, Wu WC, Chen SL, et al. Suppression of choroidal neovascularization by adeno-associated virus vector expressing angiostatin. *Invest Ophthalmol Vis Sci* 2001;42:2401–407.

47. Bainbridge JW, Mistry A, De Alwis M, et al. Inhibition of retinal neovascularisation by gene transfer of soluble VEGF receptor sFlt-1. *Gene Ther* 2002;9:320–326.

48. Wong W, Auricchio A, Maguire A, et al. Effect of over-expression of pigment epithelium-derived factor (PEDF) on developing retinal vasculature in the mouse eye. *Invest Ophthalmol Vis Sci* 2003;ARVO abstract 4593.

49. Aguirre G, Baldwin V, Pearce-Kelling S, et al. Congenital stationary night blindness in the dog: common mutation in the RPE65 gene indicates founder effect. *Mol Vis* 1998;4:23.

50. Redmond TM, Yu S, Lee E, et al. Rpe65 is necessary for production of 11-cis-vitamin A in the retinal visual cycle. *Nat Genet* 1998;20:344–351.

51. Narfstrom K, Katz ML, Ford M, et al. In vivo gene therapy in young and adult RPE65-/- dogs produces long-term visual improvement. *J Hered* 2003;94:31–37.

52. Jacobs J, Dell'Osso L, Hertle R, et al. Gene therapy to abolish congenital nystagmus in RPE65-deficient canines. *Invest Ophthalmol Vis Sci* 2003;ARVO abstract 4249.

53. Acland G, Aguirre G, Aleman T, et al. Continuing evaluation of gene therapy in the RPE65 mutant dog. *Invest Ophthalmol Vis Sci* 2002;ARVO abstract 4593.

54. Van Hooser JP, Aleman TS, He YG, et al. Rapid restoration of visual pigment and function with oral retinoid in a mouse model of childhood blindness. *Proc Natl Acad Sci USA* 2000;97: 8623–8628.

55. Porto FBO, Perrault I, Hicks D, et al. Prenatal human ocular degeneration occurs in Leber's congenital amaurosis (LCA2). *J Gene Med* 2002;4:390–396.

56. Jacobson S, Cideciyan A, Aleman T, et al. *Crumbs homologue 1 (CRB1)* mutations result in a thick human retina with abnormal lamination. *Hum Mol Genet* 2003;12:1073–1078.

57. Chang B, Hawes N, Hurd R, et al. Retinal degeneration mutants in the mouse. *Vision Res* 2002;42:517–525.

58. Jomary C, Vincent K, Grist J, et al. Rescue of photoreceptor function by AAV-mediated gene transfer in a mouse model of inherited retinal degeneration. *Gene Ther* 1997;4:683–690.

59. Bennett J, Tanabe T, Sun D, et al. Photoreceptor cell rescue in retinal degeneration (*rd*) mice by in vivo gene therapy. *Nat Med* 1996;2:649–654.

60. Takahashi M, Miyoshi H, Verma IM, et al. Rescue from photoreceptor degeneration in the rd mouse by human immunodeficiency virus vector-mediated gene transfer. *J Virol* 1999;73: 7812–7816.

61. Weng J, Mata N, Azarian S, et al. Insights into the function of rim protein in photoreceptors and etiology of Stargardt's disease from the phenotype in abcr knockout mice. *Cell* 1999;98: 13–23.

62. Reich S, Maguire A, Auricchio A, et al. Efficient trans-splicing in the retina expands the utility of adeno-associated virus as a vector for gene therapy. *Hum Gene Ther* 2003;14:37–44.

63. Gerber S, Perrault I, Hanein S, et al. Complete exon-intron structure of the RPGR-interacting protein (RPGRIP1) gene allows the identification of mutations underlying Leber congenital amaurosis. *Eur J Hum Genet* 2001;9:561–571.

64. Zeiss C, Ray K, Acland G, et al. Mapping of X-linked progressive retinal atrophy (XLPRA), the canine homolog of retinitis pigmentosa 3 (RP3). *Hum Mol Genet* 2000;9:531–537.

65. Anand V, Duarte B, Brunsmann F, et al. Gene therapy for choroideremia: in vitro rescue mediated by recombinant adenovirus. *Vision Res* 2003;43:919–926.

66. Neufeld EF, Munezer J. The mucopolysaccharidoses. In: Scriver CR, Beaudet CR, Sly WS. et al. *The metabolic and molecular bases of inherited disease*. New York: McGraw-Hill, 2001:3421–3452.

67. Haskins M, Aguirre G, Jezyk P, et al. The pathology of the feline model of mucopolysaccharidosis I. *Am J Pathol* 1983;112: 27–36.

68. Ray J, Wolfe J, Aguirre G, et al. Retroviral vector mediated β-glucuronidase cDNA transfer to the retinal pigment epithelium: stable expression and modification of metabolism in normal and diseased cells. *Invest Ophthalmol Vis Sci* 1998;39:1658–1666.

69. Li T, Davidson BL. Phenotype correction in retinal pigment epithelium in murine mucopolysaccharidosis VII by adenovirus-mediated gene transfer. *Proc Natl Acad Sci USA* 1995;92: 7700–7704.

70. Sands MS, Wolfe JH, Birkenmeier EH, et al. Gene therapy for murine mucopolysaccharidosis type VII. *Neuromuscul Disord* 1997;7:352–360.

71. Daly TM, Vogler C, Levy B, et al. Neonatal gene transfer leads to widespread correction of pathology in a murine model of lysosomal storage disease. *Proc Natl Acad Sci USA* 1999;96:2296–2300.

72. Kamata Y, Okuyama T, Kosuga M, et al. Adenovirus-mediated gene therapy for corneal clouding in mice with mucopolysaccharidosis Type VII. *Mol Ther* 2001;4:307–312.

73. Ho T, Maguire A, Aguirre G, et al. Phenotypic rescue after adeno-associated virus (AAV)-mediated delivery of arylsulfatase B (ASB) to the retinal pigment epithelium (RPE) of feline mucopolysaccharidosis VI (MPS VI). *J Gene Med* 2002;4:613–621.

74. Hennig A, Levy B, Ogilvie J, et al. Intravitreal gene therapy reduces lysosomal storage in specific areas of the CNS in mucopolysaccharidosis VII mice. *J Neurosci* 2003;23:3302–3307.

75. Seigel G, Lotery AJ, Kummer A, et al. Retinal pathology and function in a Cln3 knockout mouse model of juvenile neuronal ceroid lipofuscinosis (batten disease). *Mol Cell Neurosci* 2002;19:515–527.

76. Chevez-Barrios P, Hurwitz M, Louie K, et al. Metastatic and nonmetastatic models of retinoblastoma. *Am J Pathol* 2000;157:1405–1412.

77. Hurwitz RL, Marcus KT, Chevez-Barrios P, et al. Suicide gene therapy of retinoblastoma in a murine model. *Invest Ophthalmol Vis Sci* 1998;39:S1118.

78. Incerti B, Cortese K, Pizzigoni A, et al. Oa1 knock-out: new insights on the pathogenesis of ocular albinism type 1. *Hum Mol Genet* 2000;9:2781–2788.

79. Furukawa R, Morrow E, Li T, et al. Retinopathy and attenuated circadian entrainment in Crx-deficient mice. *Nat Genet* 1999;23:466–470.

80. Haider NB, Jacobson SG, Cideciyan AV, et al. Mutation of a nuclear receptor gene, NR2E3, causes enhanced S cone syndrome, a disorder of retinal cell fate. *Nat Genet* 2000;24: 127–131.

81. Bessant D, Papyne A, Mitton K, et al. A mutation in *NRL* is associated with autosomal dominant retinitis pigmentosa. *Nat Genet* 1999;21:355–356.

82. Mears A, Kondo M, Swain P, et al. Nrl is required for rod photoreceptor development. *Nat Genet* 2001;29:447–452.

83. Robson J, Frishman L. Dissecting the dark-adapted electroretinogram. *Doc Ophthalmol* 1998;95:187–215.

84. Sauer CG, Gehrig A, Warneke-Wittstock R, et al. Positional cloning of the gene associated with X-linked juvenile retinoschisis. *Nat Genet* 1997;17:164–170.

85. Weber B, Schrewe H, Molday L, et al. Inactivation of the murine X-linked juvenile retinoschisis gene, Rs1h, suggests a role of retinoschisin in retinal cell layer organization and synaptic structure. *Proc Natl Acad Sci USA* 2002;99:6222–6227.

86. Meindl A, Berger W, Meitinger T, et al. Norrie disease is caused by mutations in an extracellular protein resembling C-terminal globular domain of Mucins. *Nat Genet* 1992;2:139–143.

87. Lotery AJ, Jacobson SG, Fishman GA, et al. Mutations in the CRB1 gene cause Leber congenital amaurosis. *Arch Ophthalmol* 2001;119:415–420.

88. den Hollander AI, Heckenlively JR, van den Born LI, et al. Leber congenital amaurosis and retinitis pigmentosa with Coats-like exudative vasculopathy are associated with mutations in the crumbs homologue 1 (CRB1) gene. *Am J Hum Genet* 2001;69:198–203.

89. Mehalow A, Kameya S, Smith R, NL, et al. CRB1 is essential for external limiting membrane integrity and photoreceptor morphogenesis in the mammalian retina. *Hum Mol Genet* 2003;12:2179–2189.

90. Kohl S, Marx T, Giddings I, et al. Total colour blindness is caused by mutations in the gene encoding the a-subunit of the cone photoreceptor cGMP-gated cation channel. *Nat Genet* 1998;19:257–259.

91. Sidjanin D, Lowe J, McElwee J, et al. Canine CNGB3 mutations establish cone degeneration as orthologous to the human achromatopsia locus ACHM3. *Hum Mol Genet* 2002;11:1823–1833.

92. Olsson J, Gordon J, Pawlyk B, et al. Transgenic mice with a rhodopsin mutation (Pro23His): a mouse model of autosomal dominant retinitis pigmentosa. *Neuron* 1992;9:815–830.

93. Dejneka NS, Auricchio A, Maguire AM, et al. Pharmacologically regulated gene expression in the retina following transduction with viral vectors. *Gene Ther* 2001;8:442–446.

94. McGee LH, Rendahl KG, Quiroz D, et al. AAV-mediated delivery of a tet-inducible reporter gene to the rat retina. *Invest Ophthalmol Vis Sci* 2000;41:S396.

95. Cavazzana-Calvo M, Hacein-Bey S, de Saint Basile G, et al. Gene therapy of human severe combined immunodeficiency (SCID)-X1 disease. *Science* 2000;288:669–672.

96. Kay MA, Manno CS, Ragni MV, et al. Evidence for gene transfer and expression of factor IX in haemophilia B patients treated with an AAV vector. *Nat Genet* 2000;24:257–261.

97. Ponder KP, Melniczek JR, Xu L, et al. Therapeutic neonatal hepatic gene therapy in mucopolysaccharidosis VII dogs. *Proc Natl Acad Sci USA* 2002;20:13102–13107.

98. Surace E, Auricchio A, Reich S, et al. Delivery of adeno-associated viral vectors to the fetal retina: impact of viral capsid proteins on retinal neuronal progenitor transduction. *J Virol* 2003;77:7957–7963.

99. Sekhon H, Larson J. In utero gene transfer into the pulmonary epithelium. *Nat Med* 1995;1:1201–1203.

100. Schneider H, Muhle C, Douar A, et al. Sustained delivery of therapeutic concentrations of human clotting factor IX: a comparison of adenoviral and AAV vectors administered in utero. *J Gene Med* 2002;4:46–53.

101. Tarantal A, Lee C, Ekert J, et al. Lentiviral vector gene transfer into fetal rhesus monkeys *(Macaca mulatta)*: lung-targeting approaches. *Mol Ther* 2001;4:614–621.

102. Porada C, Tran N, Eglitis M, et al. In utero gene therapy: transfer and long-term expression of the bacterial neo(r) gene in sheep after direct injection of retroviral vectors into preimmune fetuses. *Hum Gene Ther* 1998;9:1571–1585.

103. David A, Cook T, Waddington S, et al. Ultrasound-guided percutaneous delivery of adenoviral vectors encoding the beta-galactosidase and human factor IX genes to early gestation fetal sheep in utero. *Hum Gene Ther* 2003;14:353–364.

104. Waddington S, Buckley S, Nivsarkar M, et al. In utero gene transfer of human factor IX to fetal mice can induce postnatal tolerance of the exogenous clotting factor. *Blood* 2003;15:1359–1366.

105. Ogawara M, Takahashi M, Shimizu T, et al. Adenoviral expression of protein-L-isoaspartyl methyltransferase (PIMT) partially attenuates the biochemical changes in PIMT-deficient mice. *J Neurosci Res* 2002;69:353–361.

106. Lipshutz G, Sarkar R, Flebbe-Rehwaldt L, et al. Short-term correction of factor VIII deficiency in a murine model of hemophilia A after delivery of adenovirus murine factor VIII in utero. *Proc Natl Acad Sci USA* 1999;96:13324–13329.

107. Meertens L, Zhao Y, Rosic-Kablar S, et al. In utero injection of alpha-L-iduronidase-carrying retrovirus in canine mucopolysaccharidosis type I: infection of multiple tissues and neonatal gene expression. *Hum Gene Ther* 2002;13:1809–1820.

108. Wagner J, Nepomuceno I, Messner, A, et al. A phase II, double-blind, randomized, placebo-controlled clinical trial of tgAAVCF using maxillary sinus delivery in patients with cystic fibrosis with antrostomies. *Hum Gene Ther* 2002;13:1349–1359.

109. Flotte T, Zeitlin P, Reynolds T, et al. Phase 1 clinical trial of intranasal and endobronchial administration of a recombinant adeno-associated virus serotype 2 (rAAV2)-CFTR vector in adult cystic fibrosis patients: a two-part clinical study. *Hum Gene Ther* 2003;14:1079–1088.

110. Stedman H, Wilson J, Finke R, et al. Phase I clinical trial utilizing gene therapy for limb girdle muscular dystrophy: alpha-, bet-, gamma-, or delta-sarcoglycan gene delivered with intramuscular instillations of adeno-associated vectors. *Hum Gene Ther* 2000;11:777–790.

111. MacGregor R. Clinical protocol. A phase 1 open-label clinical trial of the safety and tolerability of single escalating doses of autologous CD4 T cells transduced with VRX496 in HIV-positive subjects. *Hum Gene Ther* 2001;12:2028–2029.

112. Budenz D, Bennett J, Alonso L, et al. In vivo gene transfer into murine trabecular meshwork and corneal endothelial cells. *Invest Ophthalmol Vis Sci* 1995;36:2211–2215.

113. Kumar-Singh R, Farber D. Encapsidated adenovirus mini-chromosome-mediated delivery of genes to the retina: application to the rescue of photoreceptor degeneration. *Hum Mol Genet* 1998;7:1893–1900.

114. Von Seggern DJ, Aguilar E, Kinder K, et al. In vivo transduction of photoreceptors or ciliary body by intravitreal injection of pseudotyped adenoviral vectors. *Mol Ther* 2003;7:27–34.

115. Reich S, Fosnot J, Kuroki A, et al. Small interfering RNA targeting VEGF effectively inhibits ocular neovascularization in a mouse model. *Mol Vis* 2003;9:210–216.

116. Kremmidiotis G, Lensink I, Bilton R, et al. The Batten disease gene product (CLN3p) is a Golgi integral membrane protein. *Hum Mol Genet* 1999;8:523–531.

117. Liang F-Q, Aleman TS, Dejneka NS, et al. Long-term protection of retinal structure but not function using rAAV.CNTF in animal models of retinitis pigmentosa. *Mol Ther* 2001;4:461–472.

14

RETINOBLASTOMA

R. MAX CONWAY
THOMAS M. AABERG, JR.
G. BAKER HUBBARD III
JOAN M. O'BRIEN

Retinoblastoma (RB) is a disease that has advanced our understanding of the management of pediatric solid tumors and our fundamental understanding of the etiology of cancer. With steady advances in knowledge of the natural history, epidemiology, pathogenesis, cellular biology, and therapeutics for RB, in western societies more than 90% of children are treated at an early stage while the tumor is still confined to the globe, with excellent prospects for life (1). Morbidity today has also been dramatically reduced, and a large majority of children affected by RB can look forward to good vision and excellent cosmesis (2). Concomitant with these clinical advances, isolation of the RB gene has provided insight into the genetic basis for malignant transformation. Although our understanding of the genetics and molecular biology of RB has undoubtedly had an impact on diagnosis and screening for the disease, surprisingly to date, this knowledge has had little direct influence on therapy, which has advanced empirically.

HISTORICAL CONTEXT

The foundations for modern understanding of RB can be traced back to the early nineteenth century, when the Scottish surgeon James Wardrop first recognized RB as a distinct pathologic entity and published detailed descriptions of this condition (3). Through his meticulous work, Wardrop identified the retinal origin of the tumor, characterized the clinical course of advanced disease, described optic nerve invasion, and proposed that enucleation could be curative. His observations and clinical predications have proved to be remarkably accurate, and they remain of clinical relevance today. It was not until the development of the ophthalmoscope by Helmholtz in 1851 that Wardrop's ideas regarding treatment could be tested. The ophthalmoscope allowed diagnosis of intraocular disease, and enucleation was accomplished before the tumor had spread outside the globe (4). The work of von Graefe and others improved surgical techniques for enucleation (5–7). By isolating the rectus muscles, von Graefe achieved proptosis of the globe and ob-

tained a longer section of optic nerve, thereby reducing the risk of unresected tumor remaining at the surgical margin of the optic nerve. This technique improved survival from 5% in 1869 to 57% by the turn of the century (8,9).

Subsequent decades witnessed advances in understanding the pathology of RB. In 1864, Virchow proposed the term *retinal glioma* for this tumor, reflecting his now rejected hypothesis that the tumor arose from cells of glial origin (10). Later, Flexner (11) and Wintersteiner (12) proposed a neuroepithelial origin for RB and interpreted the rosettes that bear their names as attempts at photoreceptor differentiation. Verhoeff and others stressed the embryonic nature of RB and suggested that the tumor was derived from undifferentiated embryonic retinal cells or retinoblasts. He proposed the term *retinoblastoma* to reflect this cell of origin (13). In recent decades, more differentiated tumors displaying benign characteristics have been recognized and called *retinocytoma* or, more recently, *retinoma* (14,15). The histogenesis of RB continues to be a subject of considerable research interest and debate.

Hilgartner (16), followed by Schoenberg (17), first advocated the use of radiotherapy to treat RB. Radiotherapy provided a successful alternative to enucleation and had particular application in bilaterally affected patients. In the last decade, systemic chemotherapy used in conjunction with local therapy has minimized the requirement for enucleation and for external beam radiotherapy, with its attendant complications in pediatric patients (18,19).

In parallel with progress in clinical understanding, significant progress has been made in understanding the genetics of RB. From RB pedigree studies in 1971, Knudson concluded that RB could be caused by a germinal or a somatic mutation and proposed his "two-hit hypothesis." In this hypothesis, Knudson proposed that two "hits" or mutations were required to produce RB. Knudson also collated information regarding clinical characteristics of patients, including patterns of disease, age of onset, and family history, which would pave the way for precise localization and eventual cloning of the RB tumor susceptibility gene (20–23).

The identification and cloning of the RB gene *(RB1)* in 1987 produced a quantum leap in our understanding of the etiology of cancer (21–23). Prior to the identification of *RB1,* it was widely believed that cancer was caused by activation of oncogenes. Even in the 1980s, however, studies involving the fusion of normal cells with cancer cells in culture suggested the existence of elements within normal cells that could suppress the malignant phenotype. These elements remained enigmatic until cloning of *RB1* in 1987 provided the first unequivocal proof of the existence of a tumor suppressor element. Since the identification of *RB1,* many other tumor suppressor genes have been identified. The protein products of these genes appear to be important in regulating cellular growth and differentiation. When the function of these proteins is reduced through mutation or deletion in the germline, malignancy may develop.

Abnormalities in *RB1* have been detected in many common malignancies, such as breast, lung, and prostate cancer (24). These observations suggested that *RB1* dysfunction or pathway deregulation could play a central role in the development of many cancers.

Basic science understanding of the *RB1* gene and its protein product pRB has so far preceded our ability to apply this knowledge to the human disease in the form of new therapies. It is likely that in the new millennium, these and other advances in our understanding of this disease at the molecular level will yield dramatic improvements in the lives of RB patients and their families.

EPIDEMIOLOGY

RB is the most common eye cancer of childhood. The disease affects approximately 1 in 20,000 children in the United States and accounts for 12% of infant cancers (1,25–27). In other developed countries, the reported incidence of RB ranges between 1 in 17,000 and 1 in 29,000 individuals (28–31). Analysis of these incidences has suggested that the large reported variation is more likely due to incomplete diagnosis and reporting than to true differences in the frequency of the disease. Recently, an increasing incidence of RB and other pediatric cancers has been reported in the developed world; the basis for this increase is not currently understood (32). Patients in developing regions present with RB at a much later stage in the course of their disease and have a considerably worsened outcome (33), suggesting a need for strategies to improve diagnosis and treatment of this disease in the developing world.

All cases of RB arise from mutations in both copies of the *RB1* gene. The first mutation may either involve the germline or may be confined to the tumor itself. This distinction produces two fundamentally different forms of the disease: heritable RB and nonheritable RB. Heritable and nonheritable RB have quite distinct epidemiologic and clinical features. In brief, approximately 40% of patients have heritable or germline RB. Children of these patients are at nearly 50% risk for the development of RB because the trait is transmitted in an autosomal dominant fashion. Patients with heritable RB have an 80% to 90% risk of developing bilateral eye disease in infancy, and these patients have a lifetime predisposition to develop other nonocular cancers (34,35). Approximately 8% of germline RB patients will develop a second primary intracranial malignancy in childhood, termed *trilateral RB* (36). These tumors represent primitive neuroectodermal malignancies for which treatment is minimally effective. Thirty percent of heritable RB patients will develop a nonocular neoplasm by age 40 years (37).

The remaining 60% of RB patients have the nonheritable or somatic form of the disease. In these patients, both *RB1* mutations have occurred within a single retinal cell, resulting in unilateral, unifocal eye disease. The ocular disease remains unilateral in these patients, and the cancer syndrome is not transmissible. No predisposition to develop later nonocular malignancies is observed in these somatic RB patients.

The mean age at diagnosis for RB patients is 13 months for bilateral RB and 24 months for unilateral cases (38,39). Patients diagnosed as a result of family screening are considerably younger, and many cases are detected near birth. More than two thirds of RB cases develop in children younger than 2 years, and 95% occur in children younger than 5 years (27,39). The onset of new tumors after age 7 years is unusual, although rare cases presenting in adolescence or adulthood have been reported (40–50). Patients diagnosed with RB must be very closely monitored for the development of new retinal tumors, which are likely to occur in early childhood in those patients with heritable disease (38,39).

ENVIRONMENTAL FACTORS

New germline mutations in the human RB gene are known to arise preferentially on paternally derived chromosomes. Some studies have suggested an increased parental age in sporadic hereditary RB (51,52). Approximately 80% of heritable RB cases have a paternally derived mutant allele, although no differences in paternal age between paternally and maternally derived mutations have been observed (53). We do not yet understand what environmental factors, if any, influence the development of initial mutations in the *RB1* gene. Environmental factors, however, likely have a role in the predisposition to second cancers observed in adults with the heritable form of RB, because the distribution of second cancers in these patients is influenced by previous exposure to radiotherapy.

PATHOLOGY OF RETINOBLASTOMA

Thorough understanding of pathologic features, including growth patterns and mode of tumor extension, is critical for diagnosis, staging, and management decisions in RB patients. RB is composed of a solid well-vascularized tumor mass with regions of viable tumor cells surrounding vessels and interspersed zones of necrosis and calcification. Additionally, apoptotic cells, cells of the mononuclear phagocyte series, lymphocytes, and reactive glial cells have been observed in these tumors (54–57).

RB represents a malignant tumor of neuroectodermal origin arising from the nucleated layers of the retina. Malignant cells usually are poorly differentiated, rounded cells of variable size and shape with a high nuclear-to-cytoplasmic ratio and numerous mitoses. RB may display variable cellular differentiation, although most cases encountered are relatively undifferentiated (54). Photoreceptor differentiation is suggested by tumor cell rosette and fleurette formation; the morphologic features of these structures have been meticulously demonstrated by a number of histopathologic and ultrastructural studies (Fig. 14-1) (11,12,54,58,59). The Flexner-Wintersteiner rosette is not specific for RB, but it does represent a characteristic pathologic feature. These rosettes have also been observed in pineoblastoma and medulloepithelioma (54). The Homer-Wright rosette is less frequently observed in RB and is less specific; this rosette is found in a variety of other neuroblastic tumors (54). Glial differentiation may be observed in RB (60). Although true glial differentiation is difficult to distinguish from reactive gliosis, studies in tissue culture have demonstrated the biopotential of RB cells to differentiate along a neuronal or glial cell lineage (56,57,60).

Cell death usually is very prominent in RB specimens, and extensive areas of cell death are interspersed with zones of viable tumor cells surrounding blood vessels. A number of investigations suggest that tumor cells displaced from feeder vessels by more than 100 μm undergo ischemic necrosis. This observation has been attributed to the metabolic demands of this highly active tumor outstripping the supply of nutrients (61). Although necrotic portions of RB tumors do not characteristically provoke an inflammatory response, massive necrosis in large tumors may occasionally become clinically relevant by producing marked inflammation that involves surrounding tissues and simulates orbital cellulitis (62).

Apoptosis plays a critical role in growth regulation of many tumor types. This form of cell death has been reported in RB primary tumors and in cell lines and has been recognized as the primary mechanism of RB cell death in response to radiation, cytotoxic chemotherapy, and other therapeutic approaches (63,64). Cell death in RB is frequently accompanied by dystrophic calcification. In one clinical series, more than 80% of RB tumors showed calcification, and the degree of calcification appeared to be related to tumor size, with small tumors tending to be less calcified. Extraocular RB tumor does not typically demonstrate calcification (65,66).

Tumor vasculature is another critical histopathologic feature of RB. The development of an intrinsic tumor blood supply, termed *tumor angiogenesis,* is critical to the growth of primary tumors and also influences metastatic extension by providing access to the systemic vasculature. One significant mechanism promoting angiogenesis in tumors is the production of vascular endothelial growth factor (VEGF). VEGF mRNA and protein have been demonstrated in RB cells, and the expression of VEGF is increased by hypoxia (67–70). Vascular endothelia at intraocular sites distant from the tumor may respond to high intraocular levels of VEGF by increasing expression of VEGF receptors. An increase in VEGF receptors could have relevance for neoplasm-related ocular angiogenesis, such as iris neovascularization, which is occasionally observed in RB patients (69). Leukocytes, particularly cells of the mononuclear phagocyte

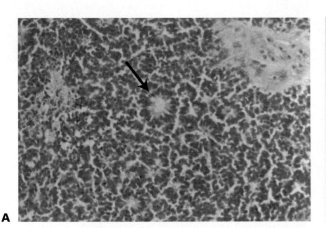
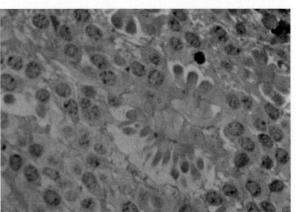

A   B

FIGURE 14-1. A: Hematoxylin and eosin stained section from a retinoblastoma specimen. Region of viable tumor cells demonstrating rosette formation. A prominent Flexner Wintersteiner rosette is indicated. A tumor vascular complex is present at the *top right-hand corner* (×25). **B:** Toluidine blue stained section from a retinoblastoma specimen showing fleurette formation, an expression of photoreceptor differentiation (×100).

series, have been observed in RB primary specimens in association with tumor vasculature. The role of these cells in immune surveillance, tumor development, and angiogenesis remains to be determined (56,57).

Left untreated, RB grows relentlessly, filling the ocular cavity and eventually spreading extraocularly. Four primary patterns of intraocular RB growth have been described (54). The endophytic growth pattern is characterized by growth of tumor toward the vitreous space; in this case, the tumor mass may be directly visualized with the ophthalmoscope (Fig. 14-2). In the exophytic growth pattern, tumor grows from the outer retina toward the choroid, elevating the retina and presenting as serous retinal detachment (Fig. 14-2). In practice, most RB patients display a combination of these two growth patterns; this is termed a *mixed growth pattern.* A fourth pattern, known as *diffuse RB,* is clinically significant. Although this form is rare, accounting for only 1% to 2% of all RB cases, the tumor insidiously infiltrates the retina, producing plaquelike thickening. The clinical signs in this form are subtle, with consequent delays in diagnosis (71–73).

RB cells are poorly cohesive; they readily disseminate throughout the globe. One mechanism underlying loss of cellular cohesion in RB may include deranged expression of intercellular adhesion molecules such as N-cadherin (74,75). RB cells are shed into the vitreous as small spheroids called *vitreous seeds* (from endophytic growth) or into the subretinal space (from exophytic lesions). RB tumor cells frequently disseminate away from the main tumor mass, involving ocular structures such as distant retina, lens capsule, or anterior chamber. This dissemination can result in secondary ocular complications such as glaucoma or pseudouveitis (54). Retinal seeding can occasionally mimic multicentric RB, leading to the inaccurate diagnosis of germinal mutation. In large tumors with extensive vitreous and subretinal seeding, the distinction between unifocal and multifocal disease may be virtually impossible to determine clinically.

RISK OF METASTASIS

RB may spread extraocularly and can extend outside the eye by a number of routes. The most frequently observed route of extension is through invasion of the central nervous system (CNS) down the optic nerve, followed by direct extraocular spread and involvement of the orbit. Tumor cells may invade the optic nerve directly or may invade the leptomeninges, gaining access to the orbital

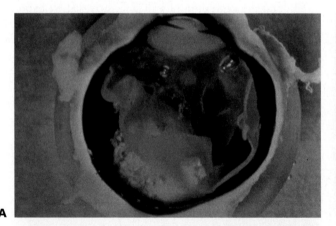

A

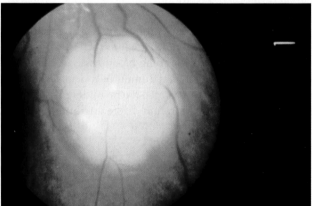

B

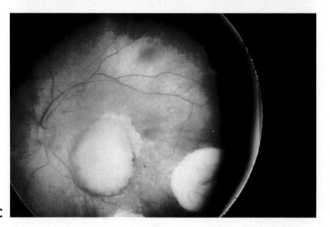

C

FIGURE 14-2. A: Gross pathology specimen demonstrating the exophytic pattern of retinoblastoma tumor growth. The chalky white tumor mass at the posterior pole had prominent calcification, arose from the retina, and grew in a scleral direction. Such tumors have a tendency to spread in the subretinal space. **B:** Clinical ophthalmoscopic appearance of an exophytic retinoblastoma. The tumor demonstrates a pale yellow color and is covered by the overlying retina, which often has a serous detachment. The retinal vessels overlying the tumor tend to be dilated and tortuous. **C:** Multiple endophytic tumors in a patient with heritable retinoblastoma. These tumors appear as pale chalky masses due to prominent calcification.

apex, optic chiasm, base of the brain, and subarachnoid space (54). Extension of RB cells into the optic nerve is considered a major histopathologic risk factor for the development of metastases, particularly when the tumor extends beyond the lamina cribrosa. If the optic nerve is involved posterior to the line of surgical transection at the time of enucleation, patients demonstrate a dramatically worsened clinical course (76–81). RB tumor cells may also invade the retinal pigment epithelium, Bruch membrane, and choroid. Exposure to the rich choroidal vasculature provides tumor cells access to emissary vascular channels and ultimately to the systemic circulation. The sclera may also be directly invaded by tumor cells. It has been suggested that the exophytic growth pattern is associated with increased risk for choroidal or orbital involvement and metastases, although this hypothesis remains clinically unproved (54,76). It has also been suggested that massive invasion of the choroid is an independent risk factor for disease dissemination (77–84). Tumor cells that spread hematogenously produce widespread metastases to lungs, brain, bone, and other viscera. Lymphatic dissemination of RB may occasionally occur in cases that extend anteriorly and allow tumor cells access to the bulbar conjunctiva and to the eyelid lymphatics (54).

The complex molecular interactions among tumor cells, parenchymal tissue, and extracellular matrix are currently not fully understood. Recent research suggests that a growth and invasion advantage may be conferred on subgroups of tumor cells that become independent of normal mechanisms for cell death or apoptosis and avoid tissue constraints, allowing spread to distant sites. These clones of more aggressive cells arise through ongoing mutagenic and epigenetic phenomena within the tumor. Some molecular mechanisms identified in RB and other tumors that could facilitate these changes include up-regulation of telomerase activity, N-*myc* oncogene amplification, p53 inactivation, changes in cell adhesion molecules (e.g., cadherins), altered expression of integrin subunits by tumor cells, and increased expression of angiogenic factors (85–88). Greater understanding of these critical molecular processes is likely to yield better and more specific therapies for this disease in future.

OVERVIEW OF RETINOBLASTOMA GENETICS

Retinoblastoma Gene and Protein Product

RB is one of very few cancers in which a single genetic mutation predicts disease development at very high penetrance. The presence of an underlying genetic mutation in RB was predicted by Knudson in 1971, and this prediction led to identification of the RB susceptibility gene locus, with subsequent cloning of this tumor suppressor gene in 1987. Identification of the *RB1* gene provided definitive evidence

that loss of tumor suppressor gene function is important in the etiology of cancer. Although it has recently been proposed that other genes may be involved in the development of RB, in order for RB to arise, a mutation on both alleles of the *RB1* gene is required (15).

The *RB1* gene encompasses 180,000 bases on chromosome 13q14 and contains 27 exons. The gene encodes a 4.7-kDa message that results in a 105-kDa nuclear phosphoprotein. The RB protein, known as pRB, is a transcriptional modulator expressed throughout development in all cells of adult humans (89,90). The protein has two conserved regions where important functional domains reside and which also represent sites for viral oncogene binding (e.g., SV40 T-antigen, adenovirus E1A, and human papilloma virus E7). Oncogenic viruses are capable of inactivating pRB through binding, thereby inducing malignant transformation. Many of the clinically relevant mutations that have been observed in *RB1* affect these conserved regions of the protein (34,91–93). Mutations have also been observed in the promoter region of the gene; these mutations affect recognition sequences for transcription factors (e.g., ATF and SP-1) (94).

Mutations affecting the *RB1* locus appear to be very heterogeneous. Few preferential sites for mutation, or "hot spots," have been identified (34,95). Only 3% to 5% of constitutional mutations in *RB1* are cytogenetically recognizable; these include interstitial deletions or translocations involving 13q. The remainder of mutations are submicroscopic, including point mutations, microdeletions, and duplications. In more than 90% of *RB1* mutations, deoxyribonucleic acid (DNA) alterations result in a truncated mRNA product (34,89). The second mutation that occurs in the retinal cell of origin of the tumor is a result of chromosomal abnormalities, such as nondisjunction, loss of heterozygosity due to mitotic recombination, or large deletion (89,96). This second event may be more influenced by environmental factors, including ionizing radiation. Therapeutic radiation exposure influences the distribution of nonocular tumors.

The RB protein has a critical and complex role in the regulation of cellular growth and differentiation. pRB binds to more than 30 separate cellular proteins, including transcription factors, nuclear matrix proteins, growth regulators, protein phosphatases, and protein kinases (97). One of the best understood functions of pRB involves regulation of the cell cycle through inhibition of the transcription factor E2F (98,99). In this role, the active hypophosphorylated form of pRB acts at a restriction point in late G1 of the cell cycle to inhibit the E2F family of transcription factors. These factors in turn regulate expression of a large set of genes, including, among others, c-*myc*, b-*myb*, cdc2, E2F-1, and the dihydrofolate reductase gene associated with cell division in S phase (98,99). The phosphorylation and dephosphorylation of pRB itself are controlled by a complex series of cell cycle–dependent and cell cycle–independent enzymes,

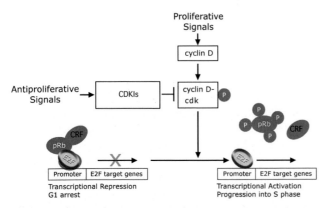

FIGURE 14-3. Schematic representation of pRB function in the regulation of the cell cycle. Active hypophosphorylated pRB blocks cell cycle progression by repressing E2F target genes through binding promoter bound E2F and by recruiting chromatin remodeling factors (CRF) including histone deacetylase. Phosphorylation of pRB is controlled by cyclin cyclin–dependent kinase (cyclin-cdk) complexes resulting in inactivation of pRB, allowing transcriptional activation of E2F target genes. Cyclin-dependent kinase inhibitors (CDKI) positively regulate pRB by inhibiting the negative regulators, the cyclin-cdk complexes.

including cyclin cyclin–dependent kinase complexes (cyclin-cdk) and cyclin-dependent kinase inhibitors (CDKIs) (100,101) (Fig. 14-3).

In addition to its role in cell cycle regulation, pRB has important effects on cellular differentiation. These effects include cell cycle arrest, suppression of apoptosis, and transcriptional activation of tissue-specific genes (90). These effects may be particularly important in tissues such as muscle, bone, fat, and nerve (102–106).

Despite the ubiquitous expression of pRB in all dividing cells, germline mutations in humans appear very specifically to cause RB and tumors of mesenchymal origin. These mesenchymal tumors include osteosarcoma, leiomyosarcoma, and malignant fibrous histiocytoma (107). In contrast, somatic alterations in pRB, which occur mainly through functional inactivation of upstream regulators, are involved in the progression of many common cancers. These include carcinoma of the breast, bladder, and prostate; small cell lung cancer; leukemia; and glioblastoma (100). For example, mutation of p16^{Ink4a} (a CDKI) and amplification of cyclin D, both upstream regulators of pRB, are frequently observed in these malignancies (108,109). The vulnerability of *RB1*-deficient cells in the retina and certain connective tissues to tumor development in the presence of *RB1* germline mutation has never been adequately explained. It is possible that this vulnerability arises from a critical requirement for pRb in terminal differentiation of these tissues.

Although mutation in both *RB1* alleles initiates RB, other chromosomal abnormalities and mutations have also been consistently observed. These other consistent genetic abnormalities include trisomy 1p, loss of heterozygosity for chromosome 17, and isochromosome formation at 6p

(110–112). These abnormalities could represent secondary changes due to genetic instability and could play a role in mediating malignant progression, allowing clones of malignant cells to acquire selective growth advantage. Interestingly, reconstitution of RB cells, RB-null carcinoma cells, or sarcoma cells with functional pRB only partially modulates the malignant phenotype (113). This suggests that other consistent genetic alterations may be important for development of the full tumor phenotype.

Clinical Genetics

Heritable Retinoblastoma

Although only 10% of RB patients have a family history of this disease, new germline mutations account for an additional 30%, meaning that 40% of RB patients have a heritable form of RB. Patients with heritable disease have a mutation (or first "hit," according to Knudson's hypothesis) involving *RB1* in every cell of their bodies. This is termed a *germline mutation* because the mutation either was inherited from a parent or, more commonly, developed at the one-cell stage of embryonic development in the affected individual. Individuals with germline mutations in *RB1* are capable of passing on the mutation to their offspring. Mutation in the other copy of *RB1* (the second "hit" described by Knudson) occurs in a pluripotent retinal cell that gives rise to the malignant tumor. In this heritable form of RB, patients demonstrate bilateral, multifocal retinal tumors, which are pathognomonic for heritable disease. Although the RB gene at the cellular level is recessive (i.e., both RB alleles must be abnormal in order for the tumor phenotype to be expressed) at the level of the individual, the mutation behaves in an autosomal dominant manner, with 80% to 90% penetrance (114) (Table 14-1).

TABLE 14.1. CLINICAL AND GENETIC FORMS OF RETINOBLASTOMA

Family History	Frequency	Phenotype
Clinical Forms of Retinoblastoma		
Sporadic	90%	Unilateral Bilateral^a
Familial	10%	Bilateral (unilateral)^b

Type of Mutation	Frequency	Hereditary
Genetic Forms of Retinoblastoma		
Somatic	60%	Nonheritable
New germline mutation^a	30%	Heritable
Transmitted germline mutation	10%	Heritable

^{a} Some of these cases may represent parental mosaicism.
^{b} Fifteen percent of total germline mutations present as unilateral diseases.

Nonheritable Retinoblastoma

The remaining 60% of RB cases represent nonheritable or somatic disease. In this nonheritable form, mutations in both *RB1* alleles (i.e., both the first and the second "hits") occur within a single retinal cell of origin for the tumor. Such events are rare; therefore, these patients demonstrate a single unilateral, unifocal tumor. Unilateral disease presents, on average, at a later age than does bilateral disease.

It should be recognized that approximately 15% of patients who present with unilateral RB have the heritable form of this disease, but by chance they have developed a tumor in only one eye (115–117). The relationship between the clinical and the genetic forms of RB is summarized in Table 14-1.

Second Tumor Predisposition

As a consequence of germline mutation in *RB1*, patients with heritable RB should be regarded as having a genetic cancer predisposition syndrome. The clinical consequences of this syndrome are that these patients develop not only multiple, bilateral retinal tumors, but they also demonstrate a several-fold increased risk for developing second malignancies in later life, including osteogenic sarcoma, fibrosarcoma, and melanoma (34,35). These second nonocular tumors may occur anywhere throughout the body, although their distribution appears to be increased within the radiation field following radiotherapy (34,35,37,118,119). By age 40 years, 30% of heritable RB patients will have developed a second nonocular cancer (37). Additionally, approximately 8% of hereditary RB patients will develop midline intracranial primitive neuroectodermal tumors (PNETs, formerly called *trilateral RB*), which frequently occur in the pineal region (36). These tumors usually occur in conjunction with bilateral disease, although PNETs have also been described in patients with unilateral retinal tumors (120).

Genetic Mosaicism

It recently has been recognized that 10% of RB families demonstrate germline or somatic mosaicism (121,122). *Mosaicism* refers to the presence of two or more cell lineages differing in genotype in an individual. If a mutation develops at the *RB1* locus during later stages of embryonic development, the lineage of cells derived from this original mutation-bearing cell will carry an identical *RB1* mutation. In contrast, cells derived from unaffected lineages will carry normal copies of *RB1*. If the mutant *RB1* is carried in the gametes but not in the eye, the affected individual could pass the mutation to offspring without personally demonstrating clinical evidence of RB. The practical significance of mosaicism in one of a proband's parents is that siblings of this proband would be at higher risk for developing the disease

than previously believed (123). Therefore, siblings should receive early and regular screening for development of this disease (123). Parents who are mosaic for mutant *RB1* may also be at personal risk to develop malignancies in cell lineages that carry the mutant gene. These individuals should receive prompt referral to an oncologist if systemic complaints suggestive of malignancy develop.

Low-Penetrance Retinoblastoma

Forms of RB have been described in families where a proportion of *RB1* mutation carriers do not develop eye tumors. This clinical circumstance is termed *low-penetrance RB*. In other families, *RB1* mutation carriers either develop unilateral disease or demonstrate a benign variant of RB called *retinoma*. This clinical circumstance is described as *low-expressivity* RB. Low-penetrance and low-expressivity forms of RB have been associated with *RB1* mutations that either partially inactivate the protein or reduce protein expression (124,125). Recognition of these kindreds is important because they allow more accurate genetic counseling for affected families (96,114,126).

Current Status of Genetic Counseling and DNA Testing

It is important that all ophthalmologists who treat patients with RB inform patients and families of the potential heritable nature of this disease. Families also should be made aware that germline mutation in *RB1* confers a lifetime second tumor predisposition. Referral to a pediatric oncologist for second tumor surveillance is indicated.

Genetic counseling is often performed by the ophthalmologist in conjunction with a clinical genetics service. A careful and complete family history should be taken at the time of the initial referral. Examination of relatives for retinoma or regressed RB can be very helpful in some cases, as this suggests carrier status for the affected relative.

Traditionally, when genetic testing was undertaken in patients with a family history of RB, testing was accomplished by genetic linkage analysis using informative polymorphisms to identify affected family members. Polymorphisms are neutral DNA sequence alterations that occur frequently in populations and allow tracking of gene loci and associated regions in a pedigree. These polymorphisms provide a straightforward way to perform genetic screening in large affected kindreds.

In the majority of patients with RB, tissue from only one individual is available for analysis, and the testing procedure becomes more complex. Cytogenetic testing can be performed, but this approach demonstrates chromosomal abnormalities at the RB locus in only 7% to 8% of patients with bilateral RB (127). DNA fragment analysis techniques are fairly rapid and can detect smaller DNA rearrangements. However, these techniques detect mutations in only 16% of germline patients because the vast majority have small deletions, insertions, and point mutations without evident "hot spots"(34,95). To detect these submicroscopic changes, sophisticated techniques have been developed, including single-strand conformational polymorphism analysis, multiplex polymerase chain reaction, and automated direct DNA sequencing. Although these techniques are very sensitive, they are time consuming for routine clinical practice and for RB screening (89).

One new approach that shows promise exploits the fact that more than 90% of *RB1* mutations result in a truncated protein product due to the introduction of premature stop codons (34,89). The test, called a *protein truncation test,* utilizes the technique of *in vitro* transcription and translation to test for these premature stop signals. This technique has been used successfully to detect mutations in other diseases, including neurofibromatosis I, adenomatous polyposis coli, and breast cancer (128). In this approach, *RB1* mRNA is isolated from peripheral blood leukocytes, and templates of overlapping subsets of the *RB1* gene are generated by reverse transcriptase-polymerase chain reaction. These templates are then translated by *in vitro* transcription and translation technique into protein products, which then are screened for truncation by gel electrophoresis. This technique is relatively rapid, detecting mutations within 7 days of blood collection. In preliminary testing, it has been found to be 70% sensitive in detecting mutations (129).

The process of genetic counseling necessarily involves carrying out genetic testing and providing specific information about disease risk. Many other issues may need to be explored, including issues of family guilt, anxieties about the future, and misconceptions regarding the disease or its sequelae. The genetic counselor should recognize that many ethical issues are raised by genetic counseling, including issues of confidentiality, questions of paternity, and concerns surrounding third party interests (e.g., insurance). Counselors should remain open to explore fully these issues with families and refer to other experts as appropriate.

CLINICAL PRESENTATION AND DIFFERENTIAL DIAGNOSIS

When there is a family history of RB, most cases in the United States are detected as part of RB screening programs. In these siblings or offspring of RB patients, the diagnosis usually is made at a very early stage in infancy when the tumors are small, offering the best opportunity for treatment aimed at preserving the eye and the vision.

In unaffected families, RB presents either incidentally or following referral by a family physician or pediatrician. Often the first sign of the disease is a white pupil (leukocoria) or strabismus, usually noticed initially by a patient's parent or relative. White pupil, or leukocoria, was first described as a presentation for RB by Hayes in 1767 and unfortunately

remains the most common presenting sign of this disease today (in approximately 60% of cases) (Fig. 14-4) (130–133). Strabismus is the second most frequent presentation of RB (in approximately 20% of cases), and this observation reinforces the need to perform a dilated retinal examination in all new patients who present with strabismus. Other less frequent presentations for RB include intraocular inflammation, iris neovascularization, hyphema, pseudohypopyon, preseptal/orbital cellulitis, and glaucoma (Fig. 14-4). With increased awareness and the advent of early screening programs, some patients may be found at a very early stage with no signs apart from the presence of a small retinal lesion.

The clinical presentations of RB that simulate inflammation are associated with the greatest diagnostic difficulty. True inflammation may arise in an eye with RB due to extensive tumor cell necrosis. This situation frequently occurs with larger tumors, and the accompanying inflammation may simulate preseptal or orbital cellulitis. If RB is suspected, identifying the apparent cellulitis as a masquerade syndrome is often straightforward. Children with true orbital cellulitis exhibit fever, leukocytosis, and sinusitis. These findings are generally absent in patients with RB. The presence of normal sinuses and evidence for an intraocular mass are easily documented with computed tomography (CT) imaging (Fig. 14-4).

Another less straightforward clinical presentation for RB involves friable tumor cells that detach from the main tumor mass and subsequently spread throughout the eye. These tumor cells may simulate the white blood cells of a hypopyon and may suggest uveitis as an initial diagnosis (Fig. 14-4). Secondary glaucoma, due to mass effect from the tumor producing angle closure or due to secondary iris neovascularization, occasionally may produce a diagnostic challenge.

Rarely in the developed world, patients may present with evidence of extraocular spread, metastatic disease, or CNS symptoms due to a PNET. Proptosis, although rare as a presenting sign of RB in industrialized societies, unfortunately is a common presentation in less-developed countries. Proptosis was the most common presentation of RB (65% of cases) in one study from India (33). This presentation carries a poor prognosis because it is frequently associated with advanced disease and extraocular spread into the orbit.

RB occasionally may occur in association with other congenital abnormalities, including cleft palate, cardiovascular defects, infantile cortical hyperostosis, dentinogenesis imperfecta, incontinentia pigmenti, or familial congenital cataracts. Patients also may demonstrate features of 13q–syndrome, associated with deletions in the distal part of chromosome 13q. These patients demonstrate mental retardation, broad nasal bridge, hypertelorism, microphthalmia, micrognathia, cleft palate, or foot and toe abnormalities (134,135).

Clinically, an endophytic tumor appears as a white- or cream-colored mass that penetrates the internal limiting membrane of the retina and demonstrates prominent white

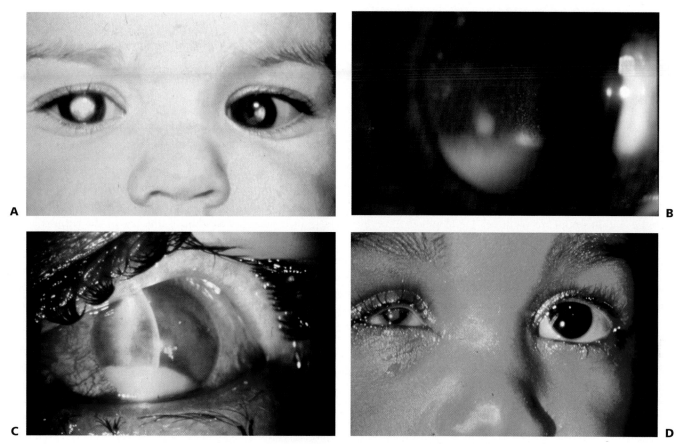

FIGURE 14-4. A: Heritable retinoblastoma patient presenting with bilateral leukocoria, the most commonly reported presenting sign of this condition. **B:** Retinoblastoma cells have a propensity to detach from the primary tumor mass and spread throughout the eye, as illustrated by a patient with endophytic retinoblastoma who developed marked tumors cells in the vitreous, resembling a vitritis. **C:** Occasionally tumor necrosis may produce an inflammatory response associated with a red eye and conjunctival injection as seen in this patient. The patient also has a tumor hypopyon. **D:** Massive tumor necrosis in a phthisical eye of a patient with retinoblastoma has resulted in marked inflammation involving the orbit, simulating an orbital cellulitis with lid swelling and pain on eye movement.

chalky areas that represent intrinsic calcification. The vessels associated with endophytic RB usually are small, irregular tumor vessels that stand in marked contrast to the dilated or aneurysmal blood vessels observed in Coats disease. Endophytic RB may be associated with seeding of tumor cells into the vitreous space. These clumps of cells present as snow-ball-like spheroids within the vitreous cavity with intervening clear spaces. Occasionally, vitreous seeding from RB may be so extensive that the anterior chamber is involved. This presentation with a tumor hypopyon can resemble endophthalmitis (Fig. 14-4).

In its exophytic form, RB tumors usually are yellow to white in coloration and are observed deep to the overlying retina, which is often serously detached. The retinal vessels overlying the tumor may be dilated and tortuous. In contrast to serous detachments from other causes, an underlying mass with characteristic features usually can be demonstrated by ultrasound, CT, or magnetic resonance (MR) imaging. Occasionally intraretinal and subretinal exudation

may mimic Coats disease, making diagnosis difficult (Fig. 14-2) (136).

Detached tumor cells in the vitreous or subretinal space have the capacity to implant and to grow at other retinal sites, producing multiple tumor foci. Most large tumors have both exophytic and endophytic features. Very small RBs may appear as pale grayish masses confined to the retina.

The diffuse form of RB is the most difficult form to accurately diagnose. Diffuse RB often presents in older children as a resistant uveitis with mild conjunctival hyperemia and pseudohypopyon. Ophthalmoscopy may reveal a diffuse gray-white opacification and retinal thickening with vitreous seeds. Frequently this form of RB is situated in a more anterior location, underscoring the importance of dilated fundus examination with scleral indentation. In the absence of a well-defined mass with a lower incidence of intrinsic calcification, ultrasound, CT, and MR imaging may be less informative in establishing the diagnosis of diffuse RB (71–73).

The clinical diagnosis of RB always requires that this malignant tumor be distinguished from other simulating disease processes. In a study of 500 patients referred to the Wills Eye Hospital for suspected RB, only 58% of referred patients were found to have RB on clinical evaluation. The remaining 212 patients received diagnoses of 23 different forms of pseudoretinoblastoma (133,136). The most common simulating lesions were persistent hyperplastic primary vitreous (PHPV) (28%), Coats disease (16%), and presumed ocular toxocariasis (16%), followed by retinopathy of prematurity and retinal hamartoma. Other simulating lesions included hereditary conditions, such as familial exudative vitreoretinopathy, congenital retinoschisis, Norrie disease, and incontinentia pigmenti. Developmental conditions that were mistaken for RB included retinal or optic nerve coloboma, retinal dysplasia, congenital retinal folds, and myelinated nerve fibers. Inflammatory or infectious conditions, including congenital toxoplasmosis or toxocariasis, or cytomegalovirus or herpesvirus retinitis, also can simulate RB. Tumors such as medulloepithelioma, choroidal hemangioma, glioneuroma, capillary hemangioma, and ocular infiltrates from leukemia occasionally can present initially as RB. It should always be recalled in the setting of media opacities, such as hyphema, cataract, or vitreous hemorrhage, that the diagnosis of RB is not excluded until the retina has been thoroughly examined or imaged to exclude a concomitant tumor. RB coexisting with other conditions, such as PHPV or cataract, has been reported (137). In practice, most clinical cases of RB can be diagnosed by careful clinical evaluation by an experienced examiner and the judicious application of supplemental investigations. Table 14-2 summarizes the salient diagnostic features of the more common lesions that simulate RB.

Whenever RB is suspected, a detailed medical history should be taken at initial examination, including a prenatal and birth history. Historical features suggesting a pseudoretinoblastoma should be specifically investigated (Table 14-2). A family history should be obtained, and a detailed family tree should be diagrammed in the medical record. A history of RB or other forms of cancer, as well as a history of ocular malformations, blindness, or enucleation in other family members, should be questioned. Enucleations occurring within a family are often better remembered than the precise diagnosis of RB. The family tree should document the ages and health status of all siblings and near relatives.

In every child with suspected RB, a complete physical examination is required. Specific features associated with simulating lesions and/or RB syndromes or systemic metastases should be evaluated. For example, the child should be examined for evidence of tuberous sclerosis (e.g., ash leaf spots) or dysmorphic features suggesting a 13q–deletion syndrome. Evidence for underlying systemic disease or metastases, such as cachexia, wasting, or developmental delay, should be investigated. Clinical features of PNETs associated with trilateral RB include abnormal eye movements, vomiting, seizure, headache, and changes in cognition. We routinely refer all patients with suspected RB to a knowledgeable pediatric oncologist for a complete history and physical examination.

The ophthalmologic evaluation of a child with suspected RB should be detailed and complete. Visual acuity and visual function should be assessed with each eye patched. The visual potential of each eye is an important determinant for future therapy. External examination of the patient should evaluate for dysmorphic features, lymphadenopathy, or proptosis. Pupils and eye movements should be evaluated for evidence of a concomitant intracranial disease process. Careful anterior segment examination is necessary to evaluate the size of the corneas and the clinical appearance of anterior segment structures. For example, a unilateral small corneal diameter may suggest PHPV rather than RB. Signs of intraocular inflammation should be sought on slitlamp evaluation. Although RB may rarely produce a pseudouveitis or tumor hypopyon, signs of intraocular inflammation are more often associated with granulomatous uveitis, such as toxocariasis, or with other pediatric uveitis syndromes. Intraocular pressures for each eye should be recorded, and the cause of any pressure elevation should be investigated.

Bilateral dilated fundus examination with scleral depression is performed under general anesthesia. Scleral indentation must be performed for 360 degrees of the globe in order to inspect the entire surface of the retina to detect anteriorly located tumors (138). In one series, RB in the periphery of the fundus was detected using scleral indentation in 65% of cases (138). Color fundus photos with a wide-angle contact camera and retinal drawings should be performed to document the size and location of all retinal tumors. This documentation is essential to plan treatment and to monitor subsequent treatment response.

Supplementary investigations are frequently used to aid in the diagnosis and staging of patients referred with RB. Ultrasound is a useful tool, particularly for confirming the initial diagnosis and for evaluating features of intraocular disease. In larger tumors, A-scan echography typically demonstrates high-intensity echoes within the tumor that correspond to areas of tumor calcification. The tumor surface nearest the sclera may be anechoic. B scan often demonstrates an intraocular mass with scattered highly reflective echoes within the tumor and with attenuation of normal soft tissue signals posterior to the tumor. In patients with advanced disease, exudative retinal detachment, vitreous seeding, and subretinal seeding also may be demonstrated by ultrasound (Fig. 14-5) (139).

CT and MR imaging are used to confirm the diagnosis of RB and to evaluate for extraocular extension of disease. CT imaging is sensitive for detecting the intrinsic tumor calcification characteristic of RB and evaluating for extraocular extension, as well as for evaluating the orbit and surrounding bony structures. MR imaging is particularly valuable for

TABLE 14-2. DIAGNOSTIC FEATURES OF MOST COMMON LESIONS SIMULATING RETINOBLASTOMA

Simulating Lesion	Clinical Features	Imaging Features (US/CT)	Special Investigation
Persistent hyperplastic primary vitreous	Dx within weeks of birth	Retrolental mass present	MRI: No retinal mass
	Unilateral Small corneal diameter, microphthalmia HA remnants, elongated ciliary processes	HA remnants No retinal masses	
Coats' disease	Dx at 4–10 years of age, male > female Retinal unilateral telangiectasia Yellow intraretinal exudation and exudative RD Cholesterol clefts, retinal refractile particles	No distinct retinal tumor[a] Moderate MI particles on A scan[b]	FA: Retinal telangiectasia with leakage
Ocular Toxocariasis	Hx of exposure to puppies or eating earth Subretinal granuloma or retinal inflammatory mass Intraocular inflammation or cicatrization (+/−/+++)	Mass without HI particles No calcification	*Toxocara canis* serology
Retinopathy of prematurity	Bilateral, asymmetric Hx of prematurity/LBW/ oxygen therapy Vitreoretinal tractional and pigmentary changes	No distinct retinal tumor	FA: Demarcation line or ridge between vascularized and nonvascularized retina
Combined hamartoma	Unilateral, gray tumor, ILM contraction	US: Mass involving all levels (RPE, retina, vitreous)	FA: Vascular tortuosity, retinal traction
Astrocytic hamartoma	Associated with tuberous sclerosis (AD) Pale multinodular tumors Lesions at/near optic disc	Calcification may occur[c]	MRI: Associated intracranial and systemic lesions

[a] RB can produce a Coats-like reaction with a large amount of retinal exudation. In these eyes, US can usually detect the retinal tumor beneath the exudate.
[b] Correspond to the refractile cholesterol particles seen clinically. These particles are much less reflective than the calcium particles seen with retinoblastoma (Shields et al. *Retina* 1991;11:232–243).
[c] Calcification is not specific to RB, although it is very characteristic. The calcification in astrocytomas appears clinically as refractile yellow areas vs the chalky white appearance in RB.
CT, computed tomography imaging; Dx, diagnosis; FA, fluorescein angiography; HA, hyaloid artery; HI, high intensity; Hx, history; ILM, internal limiting membrane; LBW, low birth weight; MI, medium intensity; MRI, magnetic resonance imaging; RD, retinal detachment; RPE, retinal pigment epithelium; US, ultrasound imaging; AD, autosomal dominant.

evaluating optic nerve extension or CNS disease. RB is hyperintense on T1-weighted images and hypointense on T2-weighted images (Fig. 14-5) (140).

Bone marrow aspiration and lumbar puncture may be obtained to evaluate for systemic spread, although routine requirement for these studies has recently been questioned. Other investigations, such as bone scans, are performed based on the overall clinical assessment of the patient. In most cases, complete metastatic evaluation is reserved for patients who present with features of advanced disease.

Families with a new diagnosis of RB require considerable psychological and emotional support during this period of initial diagnosis. The attending ophthalmologist, pediatrician, pediatric oncologist, and other health professionals need to demonstrate a caring attitude and should be responsive to the needs of the patient, the parents, and other family members with regard to emotional support and information. The attending ophthalmologist needs to be available to spend considerable time with the family of a child with newly diagnosed RB. Showing the parents CT scans or other images of the tumor will frequently assist in the process of enabling them to accept the recommended treatment plan. Support, information, and visual documentation of the disease are particularly helpful when

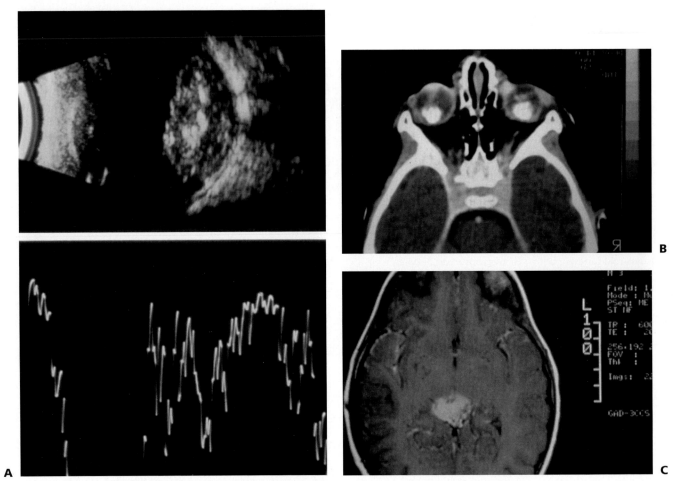

FIGURE 14-5. A: Ultrasound scan of retinoblastoma showing a retinal mass located at the posterior pole. Both A and B scans demonstrate that the mass has areas of high internal reflectivity due to intrinsic calcification. Intrinsic tumor calcium may produce a shadowing of the soft tissues behind the tumor. **B:** Computed tomographic scanning performed with contrast demonstrates bilateral retinoblastoma tumors involving the posterior poles with dense calcium deposits. **C:** T1-weighted magnetic resonance imaging scan with gadolinium enhancement demonstrating an enhancing primitive neuroectodermal tumor (PNET) in a patient with heritable retinoblastoma.

enucleation is being considered. Parents need to be given time to deal with a new diagnosis of RB. Often parents are surprised by the initial diagnosis, and little information from the first consultation is assimilated. The attending ophthalmologist needs to be prepared to repeat information according to the needs and emotional state of the family. Discussion of the child's case at a multidisciplinary pediatric tumor board with consensus on appropriate treatment is frequently reassuring to families. We have found that many families obtain benefit by referral to a multidisciplinary RB follow-up clinic, where it is apparent that older children with this diagnosis are leading full and healthy lives after successful treatment. An inordinate delay in proceeding to treatment should be discouraged, however, because delay of a number of weeks can make a difference between an eye with visual potential and one without.

TREATMENT

A treatment plan should be individualized for each patient and will be determined by many factors, including the size and location of ocular tumors, visual potential of the affected eye, and the presence of optic nerve, orbital, or metastatic disease.

In recent years, significant changes have occurred in initial approaches to the therapy of RB. Chemoreduction with local therapy is frequently the first-line management for patients with bilateral RB. As the therapy for this disease is complex and involves expertise across a variety of specialties, management usually is performed through a multidisciplinary approach at centers of expertise in pediatric and ocular cancer. Treatment modalities, including surgery, local therapies (laser ablation, diode hyperthermia, or cryotherapy), chemotherapy, and brachytherapy or external beam radiotherapy may be used. Also important are psychological and social support for the child and family, visual rehabilitation, achievement of best cosmesis involving experts in prosthetics, and finally the scheduling of ongoing examinations for the patient, genetic counseling for the family, and screening for other at-risk pediatric family members.

The majority of children with unilateral RB present with leukocoria. This presentation usually represents advanced local disease, with greater than 60% involvement of the globe, and these patients rarely demonstrate visual potential in the affected eye. Enucleation should certainly be considered in these children because it spares them the toxicity of systemic chemotherapy or radiation and provides an acceptable cosmetic outcome (141–145). Other clinical indications for enucleation include advanced neovascular glaucoma producing pain or RB in an eye that is devoid of visual potential.

The surgical approach to enucleation in children with RB should facilitate obtaining a long section of optic nerve and should avoid inadvertent globe penetration. Any tumor at the surgical margin is an undesirable outcome that is associated with a significantly increased risk for the development of metastatic disease, and this situation mandates further therapy (76). If RB is confined to the globe, an orbital prosthesis is routinely placed at the time of enucleation; therefore, it is important to preserve conjunctiva, Tenon capsule, and extraocular muscles for integration of the implant. It also is important to completely cover the prosthesis with Tenon capsule and conjunctiva; we use a meticulous three-level closure to minimize extrusion and to provide the best cosmesis.

Unilateral cases detected at an early stage with visual potential may be successfully managed by modalities that preserve the globe and maintain useful vision. These approaches include use of local therapies alone or in conjunction with brachytherapy. Serial application of laser ablation, diode hyperthermia, and cryotherapy may occasionally be sufficient in this subgroup of patients. In the presence of vitreous seeding, however, other modalities must be considered. For larger localized tumors located more than 2 mm away from the macula and optic nerve or in patients with focal relapse after local therapy, good responses to brachytherapy may be obtained, including successful control of mild-to-moderate vitreous seeding (146–148). Tumors considered for brachytherapy should ideally be smaller than 15 mm in basal diameter and less than 8 mm in thickness (146,149). Complications associated with plaque placement include radiation retinopathy and papillopathy, and early cataract formation (146,149). Patients who have had previous chemotherapy have an increased risk for development of neovascular complications following brachytherapy, and dose reduction should be considered (149).

Although external beam radiation therapy (EBRT) effectively treats RB, it is associated with significant complica-

tions, including cataract; midfacial hypoplasia, especially if radiation is administered at age less than 1 year; growth hormone deficiency; radiation retinopathy, vasculopathy, and optic neuropathy; neovascular glaucoma; and dry eye (150–155). A major problem in management following radiation is the high incidence of cataract (approximately 10%), especially when an anterior approach for therapy is used (153). Although these cataracts can be successfully removed later in life, an eye with RB cannot undergo intraocular surgery when any concern exists regarding disease activity because tumor cells could be disseminated by an intraocular procedure. Delaying cataract extraction results in visual deprivation during the critical period and has produced amblyopia in these RB patients. The presence of cataract can make small intraocular tumor recurrences that would be amenable to local therapy difficult to detect.

Radiation therapy in RB patients has been associated with increased frequency of second primary malignancies within the radiation field (35,37,118,119,156–168). The original studies describing this problem reviewed patient outcomes following treatment with older radiotherapy techniques, such as orthovoltage sources and single-port delivery systems. Newer radiation techniques have considerably reduced the dose received by surrounding tissues during the treatment of RB (169). RB patients who receive EBRT after age 1 year may show a lower rate of second tumor development, suggesting that EBRT may still have a role if therapy is delayed (118).

Chemoreduction using systemic chemotherapy combined with local therapy (photoablation, cryotherapy, or thermotherapy) is a mainstay of therapy for bilateral disease and has replaced enucleation and EBRT in many patients with heritable RB. The goal of chemoreduction is to reduce the volume of retinal tumors in order to allow ablation of residual disease with local therapy. This approach frequently preserves the eye and the visual potential (170,171). In many cases enucleation can be avoided, and radiotherapy is frequently not required. Most centers using this approach employ serial aggressive local therapy (SALT) (170–175). A SALT treatment plan consists of a number of cycles of chemotherapy during which patients also receive local therapy. A number of studies suggest that local therapy acts synergistically with chemotherapy, possibly by increasing the uptake of the chemotherapeutic agents into the eye (176–178). The agents currently used for systemic chemotherapy include carboplatin, vincristine, etoposide (VP-16), and sometimes cyclosporin A. The dosage range varies across centers, although standard regimens are under consideration by the Children's Oncology Group of the National Institutes of Health. In general, higher-dose regimens are used for patients with larger tumors associated with vitreous and subretinal seeding. Children with smaller tumors may respond well to lower-dose protocols.

All chemotherapeutic agents are associated with potential toxicity. Carboplatin may produce otologic toxicity and high-frequency hearing loss that is unacceptable in children who already may have reduced vision. Pretreatment audiologic testing and ongoing surveillance for the development of hearing loss is very important (179). Long-term mutagenesis and reduced fertility have also been reported. Vincristine may have major neurologic toxicities, including numbness and tingling in the extremities and loss of deep tendon reflexes, which may be reversible with dose reduction or cessation of therapy (180). Severe constipation may also be observed with this agent. The dose-limiting toxicity for VP-16 is leukopenia that occurs during treatment. The risk also exists for development of nonlymphocytic leukemia associated with a translocation at chromosome 11q23. This disease appears a short time interval (usually between 1 and 3 years) after cessation of VP-16 chemotherapy. Fortunately, it appears that the standard doses used for chemoreduction in RB are associated with a low risk for the development of this devastating complication. Additionally, nausea, vomiting, diarrhea, and stomatitis are observed in 15% of patients receiving VP-16 intravenously (180).

Systemic chemotherapy may be associated with other problems. Multiple anesthetics are needed, both for application of local treatment and for increased surveillance required to detect new tumors following completion of the treatment. Chemotherapy remains less effective against very large tumors and vitreous and subretinal seeding. In advanced cases, enucleation may be required for the worse eye in bilateral disease. Finally, for the heritable form of RB, we do not know the effect the potential mutagenicity of various chemotherapeutic agents will have upon the incidence of second cancers in later life.

Patients who relapse with intraocular disease that cannot be controlled by standard SALT therapy have a number of treatment options still available to them. Such patients may be candidates for increased dose chemotherapy with the addition of subconjunctival carboplatin. Cyclosporin A is another agent that may be added to the chemotherapeutic regimen to increase efficacy, and the addition of this agent has been shown to be effective in managing advanced intraocular disease, including vitreous and subretinal seeding (171,174). Cyclosporin A competitively inhibits the p glycoprotein (pGp) pump. Up-regulation of this pump reduces the concentration of some chemotherapeutic agents in cancer cells by pumping agents out of the cell into the extracellular space. The expression of pGp appears to be up-regulated on tumor cells by prior exposure to chemotherapeutic agents and may be a source of resistance to chemotherapy. Unfortunately, cyclosporin A is associated with increased toxicity, including renal dysfunction, tremor, hypertension, hyperlipidemia, hirsutism, and gum hyperplasia (180). Radiation remains an effective option in the treatment of RB, and ERBT may have a role in salvaging an only eye that has not responded to other therapies when the only alternative is enucleation.

Metastatic RB has traditionally been associated with a poor prognosis. However, encouraging results have been reported with the use of high-dose systemic and intrathecal chemotherapy and total body irradiation with bone marrow rescue, resulting in disease-free survival up to 80 months after diagnosis (181). Other studies have demonstrated effective treatment of orbital disease with a combination of surgery and high-dose chemotherapy (182,183). Despite attempts at aggressive treatments for PNET with systemic and intrathecal chemotherapy and craniospinal irradiation, outcomes for this condition remain disappointing (36,38,133).

Beyond the life- and sight-threatening implications, the diagnosis of RB has many far-reaching and long-term consequences for the lives of the affected individual and family members. Issues surrounding cosmesis and body image, visual rehabilitation, special educational needs, and success at mastery of knowledge and tasks will have an impact on the patient's psychosocial adaptation and integration. Psychological effects on other members of the family may also play a role in how successfully the entire family copes with the patient's disease process. Because RB involves accepting a very serious diagnosis, an often difficult treatment process, and many years of follow-up examinations, the developmental, social, and psychological health of the patient and family should be considered throughout their experience with this disease.

FOLLOW-UP AND MONITORING OF CHILDREN WITH RETINOBLASTOMA

In the heritable form of RB, significant risk for the development of further retinal tumors exists throughout childhood, and children should be closely and serially monitored during this period. Close follow-up is particularly necessary with chemoreduction and associated serial local treatment. The frequency of examination depends upon the age of the patient, stage of treatment, and estimated risk for further tumors in that individual. Children with sporadic unilateral RB should also be examined under anesthesia serially, as 15% of unilateral cases represent heritable disease. These patients remain at risk to develop disease in their remaining normal eye. We also screen heritable patients for development of PNETs with MR imaging every 6 months under the same anesthesia.

Heritable RB is a lifelong illness, potentially familial, which confers an increased risk for the development of other malignancies. For this reason, we follow all children with RB in a multidisciplinary clinic composed of experts with different perspectives and unique areas of expertise. As a group, these physicians monitor, evaluate, and intervene in a timely fashion to minimize adverse consequences of RB as a diagnosis. After age 7 years, we see RB patients annually and schedule siblings on the same day to reduce the number of required visits for the family.

In the ocular oncology unit, the patient's vision and refraction are checked. A complete ophthalmologic examination is undertaken to exclude reactivations in the primary tumor(s) and to look for evidence of treatment complications, including radiation- or chemotherapy-related retinopathy or vasculopathy. In many cases, visual rehabilitation is undertaken. An ocularist is available to optimize the fitting of the prosthesis over the orbital implant to maximize cosmesis. A pediatric oncologist and a school specialist perform a complete medical history and physical examination to evaluate general health and to exclude problems related to previous therapy. Detailed review of systems and physical examination are undertaken to exclude the development of second malignancies. We have not found that routine bone scans used to detect osteogenic sarcoma yield any earlier diagnoses. It is important to recognize that the 15% of patients with sporadic unilateral RB and an underlying germline mutation at the *RB1* locus remain at risk for developing primary intracranial midline tumors, as well as second malignancies.

Patients are also monitored for endocrine deficiencies, as well as for problems with midfacial hypoplasia that can develop in the setting of radiation therapy. Educational and nursing specialists evaluate the children to identify behavioral or learning difficulties. The multidisciplinary environment also fosters strong support between RB families. Newly diagnosed families are often relieved to see healthy older children who carry the RB diagnosis. Information on support services, visual devices, braille books, and other practical considerations are provided by clinic personnel, as well as by discussion between families. Long-term friendships between RB families emerge in this setting.

Retinoblastoma Screening

When the RB mutation is detected in a family, precise individualized genetic counseling is provided. However, in many cases, the RB gene mutation is not identified, usually because of lack of access to genetic testing. In this situation, even if the proband has unilateral RB, offspring and siblings born into a family with RB are examined first at birth and then again within the first weeks of life in order to detect intraretinal tumors while they are small and amenable to local therapies. Periodic dilated indentation ophthalmoscopy is continued throughout infancy and childhood as siblings with initially normal examinations occasionally can develop tumors months after the initial normal examination (123). We now recognize that germline mosaicism for *RB1* mutations occurs in at least 10% of RB kindreds (122). This finding, along with recognition of low-penetrance kindreds, suggests that a significant minority of patients exists who have inherited a mutant *RB1* gene from an asymptomatic carrier. Without definitive genetic testing available for the majority of our families, at the present time we regard all RB patients as potentially heritable cases. Until genetic testing is widely available, we believe the financial cost and minimal morbidity associated with serial examinations under anesthesia are justified in order to detect this significant minority of patients with heritable disease before symptoms arise.

PROGNOSIS

With steady advances in the diagnosis and treatment of RB, children with this disease now have an excellent prognosis for life with decreased ocular and visual morbidity. In developed countries, the mortality rate associated with RB has fallen to less than 10% (1,184,185). Although the risk for metastatic disease in children with bilateral RB appears to be higher than for individuals with unilateral RB, the survival from metastatic disease is similar for both groups (185). Survivors with heritable RB have a worse long-term prognosis than patients with nonheritable RB because germline *RB1* mutation confers a predisposition for the development of second nonocular cancers (37). A 50% overall mortality has been observed 25 years after the diagnosis of bilateral RB (184). This statistic emphasizes the need to counsel patients with heritable RB that careful follow-up for second tumor development is required and that annual second tumor screening should be a family priority.

The outlook for vision in RB has improved with the development of treatments that preserve vision and avoid enucleation. In one recent series of 74 children, the enucleation rate was 62%, and 58% of patients had a visual acuity in the better eye between 20/20 and 20/40. Only 9% of patients demonstrated visual acuity of 20/400 or worse. The final visual acuity in this series was influenced by multiple factors, most notably tumor location. The final visual outcome could not be predicted by the disease stage at initial presentation (2).

Management of metastatic RB remains a difficult clinical problem. One factor that improves the prognosis for survival in patients with metastatic disease is early detection. A number of studies have examined risk factors for the development of metastatic disease. Early recognition of these risk factors and prompt treatment may help to reduce mortality associated with disease dissemination (76). Major clinical risk factors for the development of metastatic RB include advanced intraocular disease at diagnosis, delays in diagnosis, or history of prior intraocular surgery (76,184–187). Accepted histopathologic risk factors include tumor cells extending to the surgical margin of the optic nerve and microscopic extraocular involvement by tumor cells (79,80). Minor degrees of choroidal involvement or retrolaminar optic nerve invasion with a free transection margin are more questionable risk factors. The outlook for patients who develop PNETs remains poor, with mortality approaching 100% at 5 years. Research into better treatments for this condition is urgently needed (36).

SUMMARY AND FUTURE DIRECTIONS

Despite significant advances in our understanding and management of RB, challenges remain ahead. A better understanding is needed of the molecular events surrounding RB cell death, angiogenesis, and metastasis. Rapid, cost-effective methods of genetic testing for RB need to be developed and made widely available. An immediate and ongoing priority is the discovery of new therapeutic options with better efficacy and lower toxicity, as well as a clearer definition of which treatments should be applied for different stages of disease. Finally, more effective clinical screening is needed. Education of primary care physicians and the community should become a priority for ophthalmologists.

Acknowledgment: This work is supported in part by NIH/NEI 5RO1EY013812-02, Research to Prevent Blindness, The Sand Hill Foundation, That Man May See Foundation, and Neil Hamilton Fairley Fellowship, National Health & Medical Research Council, Canberra, ACT, Australia.

REFERENCES

1. Tamboli PA, Podgor MJ, Horm JW. The incidence of retinoblastoma in the United States: 1974–1985. *Arch Ophthalmol* 1990;108:128–132.
2. Hall LS, Ceisler E, Abramson DH. Visual outcomes in children with bilateral retinoblastoma. *J AAPOS* 1999;3:138–142.
3. Wardrop J. *Observations on the fungus haematodes or soft cancer.* Edinburgh: George Ramsay and Co., 1809.
4. Helmholtz H. *Berschreibung eines Augen-Spiegels zur Unter-suchung der Netzhaut im lebenden Auge.* Berlin: A Förstner'schne Verlagsbuchhandlung, 1851.
5. Ferrall JM. Fungoid tumor of the orbit: operation. *Dublin Med Press* 1841;5:281.
6. Bonnet A. Cancer mélanique de l'oeil; structure du cancer; disposition de ses vaisseaux. *Bull Soc Anat Paris* 1846;21:73, 76.
7. Lagrange F (citing Von Graefe). *Traité des tumeurs de l'oeil, de l'orbiteet et des annexes. Tome Premier: Tumeurs de l'oeil.* Paris: Steinhiel; 1901.
8. Hirschberg J. *Der Markschwamm der Netzhaut; eine monographie.* Berlin: Hirschwald, 1869.
9. Leber T. Beirträge zur Kenntnis der Struktur des Netzhaut-glioms. *Albrecht von Graefes Arch Ophthalmol* 1911;78:381–411.
10. Virchow R. *Die Drankhaften Geschwulste.* Berlin, Germany: Harshwald, 1864.
11. Flexner S. A peculiar glioma (neuroepithelioma) of the retina. *Bull Johns Hopkins Hosp* 1891;2.
12. Wintersteiner H. *Die Neuroepithelioma Retinae: Eine Anatomiche and Klinische Studie.* Leipzig, Germany: Dentisae, 1897.
13. Verhoeff FH, Jackson E. Minutes of the proceedings of the 62nd annual meeting. *Trans Am Ophthalmol Soc* 1926;24:38–43.
14. Margo C, Hidayat A, Kopelman J, et al. Retinocytoma. A benign variant of retinoblastoma. *Arch Ophthalmol* 1983;101:1519–1531.
15. Gallie BL, Ellsworth RM, Abramson DH, et al. Retinoma: spontaneous regression of retinoblastoma or benign manifestation of the mutation? *Br J Cancer* 1982;45:513–521.
16. Hilgartner HL. Report of a case of double glioma treated with x-ray. *Med Insurance* 1902–1903;18:322.
17. Schoenberg MJ. A case of bilateral glioma of the retina apparently arrested in the non-enucleated eye by radium treatment. *Arch Ophthalmol* 1919;48:485–488.
18. Gallie BL, Budning A, DeBoer G, et al. Chemotherapy with focal therapy can cure intraocular retinoblastoma without radio-therapy. *Arch Ophthalmol* 1996;114:1321–1328.
19. O'Brien JM, Smith BJ. Chemotherapy in the treatment of retinoblastoma. *Int Ophthalmol Clin* 1996;36:11–24.
20. Knudson AG Jr. Mutation and cancer: statistical study of retinoblastoma. *Proc Natl Acad Sci USA* 1971;68:820–823.
21. Friend SH, Bernards R, Rogelj S, et al. A human DNA segment with properties of the gene that predisposes to retinoblastoma and osteosarcoma. *Nature* 1986;323:643–646.
22. Lee W-H, Bookstein R, Hong F, et al. Human retinoblastoma susceptibility gene: cloning, identification, and sequence. *Science* 1987;235:1394–1399.
23. Fung Y-KT, Murphree AL, T'Ang A, et al. Structural evidence for the authenticity of the human retinoblastoma gene. *Science* 1987;236:1657–1661.
24. Sherr CJ. Cancer cell cycles. *Science* 1996;274:1672–1677.
25. Devesa SS. The incidence of retinoblastoma. *Am J Ophthalmol* 1975;80:263–265.
26. Bishop JO, Madson EC. Retinoblastoma. Review of current status. *Surv Ophthalmol* 1975;19:342–66.
27. SEER Program (National Cancer Institute (U.S.)), National Cancer Institute (U.S.). *Cancer incidence and survival among children and adolescents: United States SEER Program, 1975–1995.* Bethesda, MD: National Cancer Institute, 1999.
28. Suckling RD, Fitzgerald PH, Stewart J, et al. The incidence and epidemiology of retinoblastoma in New Zealand: A 30 year survey. *Br J Cancer* 1982;46:729–736.
29. Kock E, Naeser P. Retinoblastoma in Sweden 1958–1971: a clinical and histopathological study. *Acta Ophthal K* 1979;57:344–350.
30. O'Day J, Billson FA, Hoyt CS. Retinoblastoma in Victoria. *Med J Aust* 1977;2:428–432.
31. Czeizel A, Gardonyi J. Retinoblastoma in Hungary, 1960–1968. *Humangenetik* 1974;22:153–158.
32. Gurney JG, Ross JA, Wall DA, et al. Infant cancer in the U.S.: histology-specific incidence and trends, 1973 to 1992. *J Pediatr Hematol Oncol* 1997;19:428–432.
33. Chakrabati AK, Biswas G, Das S. Malignant orbital tumors: observation in North Bengal. *J Ind Med Assoc* 1993;91:154–155.
34. Harbour JW. Overview of RB gene mutations in patients with retinoblastoma. Implications for clinical genetic screening. *Ophthalmology* 1998;105:1442–1447.
35. Wong FL, Boice JD Jr, Abramson DH, et al. Cancer incidence after retinoblastoma. Radiation dose and sarcoma risk. *JAMA* 1997;278:1262–1267.
36. DePotter PV, Shields CL, Shields JA. Clinical variations of trilateral retinoblastoma: a report of 13 cases. *J Pediatr Ophthalmol Strabismus* 1994;31:26–31.
37. Eng C, Li FP, Abramson DH, et al. Mortality from second tumors among long-term survivors of retinoblastoma. *J Natl Cancer Inst* 1993;85:1121–1128.
38. Shields CL, Shields JA. *Intraocular tumors: a text and atlas.* Philadelphia, PA: WB Saunders, 1992: 305–319.
39. Rubenfeld M, Abramson DH, Ellsworth RM, et al. Unilateral versus bilateral retinoblastoma: correlation between age at diagnosis and stage of ocular disease. *Ophthalmology* 1986;27:1016–1019.
40. Park JJ, Gole GA, Finnigan S, et al. Late presentation of a unilateral sporadic retinoblastoma in a 16-year-old girl. *Aust N Z J Ophthalmol* 1999;27:365–368.

41. Shields CL, Shields JA, Shah P. Retinoblastoma in older children. *Ophthalmology* 1991;27:395–399.

42. Mietz H, Hutton WL, Font RL. Unilateral retinoblastoma in an adult. Report of a case and review of the literature. *Ophthalmology* 1997;27:43–47.

43. Zakka KA, Yee RD, Foos RY. Retinoblastoma in a 12-year-old girl. *Ann Ophthalmol* 1983;27:88–91.

44. Shields JA, Michelson JB, Leonard BC, et al. Retinoblastoma in an eighteen-year-old male. *J Pediatr Ophthalmol* 1976;27:274–277.

45. Bovenmyer SD. Retinoblastoma in a female aged seventeen years. *Surv Ophthalmol* 1967;27:479–485.

46. Takahashi T, Tamura S, Inoue M, et al. Retinoblastoma in a 26-year-old adult. *Ophthalmology* 1983;27:179–183.

47. Berkeley JS, Kalita BC. Retinoblastoma in an adult. *Lancet* 1977;27:508–509.

48. Makley TA. Retinoblastoma in a 52-year-old man. *Arch Ophthalmol* 1963;27:325–327.

49. Mehra KS, Hamid S. Retinoblastoma in an adult. *Am J Ophthalmol* 1961;27:405–406.

50. Verhoeff FH. Retinoblastoma: report of a case of a man aged forty-eight. *Arch Ophthalmol* 1929;27:643–650.

51. Moll AC, Imhof SM, Kuik DJ, et al. High parental age is associated with sporadic hereditary retinoblastoma: the Dutch retinoblastoma register 1862–1994. *Hum Genet* 1996;98:109–112.

52. DerKinderen DJ, Koten JW, Tan KE, et al. Parental age in sporadic hereditary retinoblastoma. *Am J Ophthalmol* 1990;110:605–609.

53. Dryja TP, Morrow JF, Rapaport JM. Quantification of the paternal allele bias for new germline mutations in the retinoblastoma gene. *Hum Genet* 1997;100:446–449.

54. Spencer WH. *Ophthalmic pathology: an atlas and textbook,* 4th ed. Philadelphia: WB Saunders, 1996L1332–1380.

55. McLean I. *Retinoblastoma, retinocytomas and pseudoretinoblastomas.* Philadelphia, PA: WB Saunders, 1996.

56. Madigan MC, Penfold PL. Human retinoblastoma: a morphological study of apoptotic, leukocytic, and vascular elements. *Ultrastruct Pathol* 1997;21:95–107.

57. Madigan MC, Penfold PL, King NJ, et al. Immunoglobulin superfamily expression in primary retinoblastoma and retinoblastoma cell lines. *Oncol Res* 2002;13:103–111.

58. Tso MO, Zimmerman LE, Fine BS. The nature of retinoblastoma, I: photoreceptor differentiation: a clinical and histopathological study. *Am J Ophthalmol* 1970;69:339–349.

59. Tso MO, Fine BS, Zimmerman LE. The nature of retinoblastoma. II: Photoreceptor differentiation: an electron microscope study. *Am J Ophthalmol* 1970;69:350–359.

60. Nork TM, Schwartz TL, Doshi HM, et al. Retinoblastoma. Cell of origin. *Arch Ophthalmol* 1995;113:791–802.

61. Burnier MN, McLean IW, Zimmerman LE, et al. Retinoblastoma. The relationship of proliferating cells to blood vessels. *Invest Ophthalmol Vis Sci* 1990;31:2037–2040.

62. Foster BS, Mukai S. Intraocular retinoblastoma presenting as ocular and orbital inflammation. *Int Ophthalmol Clin* 1996;36:153–160.

63. Conway RM, Madigan MC, Billson FA, et al. Vincristine- and cisplatin-induced apoptosis in human retinoblastoma. Potentiation by sodium butyrate. *Eur J Cancer* 1998;34:1741–1748.

64. Zhang M, Stevens G, Madigan MC. In vitro effects of radiation on human retinoblastoma cells. *Int J Cancer* 2001;96[Suppl]:7–14.

65. Bullock J, Campbell RJ, Waller RRD. Calcification in retinoblastoma. *Invest Ophthalmol Vis Sci* 1977;16:252–255.

66. Char DH, Hedges TR 3rd, Norman D. Retinoblastoma. CT diagnosis. *Ophthalmology* 1984;91:1347–1350.

67. Stitt AW, Simpson DA, Boocock C, et al. Expression of vascular endothelial growth factor (VEGF) and its receptors is regulated in eyes with intra-ocular tumours. *J Pathol* 1998;186:306–312.

68. Pe'er J, Shweiki D, Itin A, et al. Hypoxia-induced expression of vascular endothelial growth factor by retinal cells is a common factor in neovascularizing ocular diseases. *Lab Invest* 1995;72:638–645.

69. Pe'er J, Neufeld M, Baras M, et al. Rubeosis iridis in retinoblastoma. Histologic findings and the possible role of vascular endothelial growth factor in its induction. *Ophthalmology* 1997;104:1251–1258.

70. Kvanta A, Steen B, Seregard S. Expression of vascular endothelial growth factor (VEGF) in retinoblastoma but not in posterior uveal melanoma. *Exp Eye Res* 1996;63:511–518.

71. Morgan G. Diffuse infiltrating retinoblastoma. *Br J Ophthalmol* 1971;55:600–606.

72. Nicholson DH, Norton EW. Diffuse infiltrating retinoblastoma. *Trans Am Ophthalmol Soc* 1980;78:265–289.

73. Materin MA, Shields CL, Shields JA, et al. Diffuse infiltrating retinoblastoma simulating uveitis in a 7-year-old boy. *Arch Ophthalmol* 2000;118:442–443.

74. Van Aken EH, Papeleu P, De Potter P, et al. Structure and function of the N-cadherin/catenin complex in retinoblastoma. *Invest Ophthalmol Vis Sci* 2002;43:595–602.

75. Schiffman JS, Grunwald GB. Differential cell adhesion and expression of N-cadherin among retinoblastoma cell lines. *Invest Ophthalmol Vis Sci* 1992;33:1568–1574.

76. Finger PT, Harbour JW, Karcioglu ZA. Risk factors for metastasis in retinoblastoma. *Surv Ophthalmol* 2002;47:1–16.

77. Rubin CM, Robison LL, Cameron JD, et al. Intraocular retinoblastoma group V: an analysis of prognostic factors. *J Clin Oncol* 1985;3:680–685.

78. Karcioglu ZA, Haik BG. *Tissue diagnosis: intraocular tumors.* New York: McMillan, 1987.

79. Kopelman JE, McLean IW, Rosenberg SH. Multivariate analysis of risk factors for metastasis in retinoblastoma treated by enucleation. *Ophthalmology* 1987;94:371–377.

80. Messmer EP, Heinrich T, Hopping W, et al. Risk factors for metastases in patients with retinoblastoma. *Ophthalmology* 1991;98:136–141.

81. Shields CL, Shields JA, Baez K, et al. Optic nerve invasion of retinoblastoma. Metastatic potential and clinical risk factors. *Cancer* 1994;73:692–698.

82. Hungerford J. Factors influencing metastasis in retinoblastoma. *Br J Ophthalmol* 1993;77:541.

83. Stannard D, Lipper S, Sealy R, et al. Retinoblastoma: correlation of invasion of the optic nerve and choroid with prognosis and metastases. *Br J Ophthalmol* 1979;63:560–570.

84. McLean IW, Rosenberg SH, Messmer EP, et al. Prognostic factors in cases of retinoblastoma: analysis of 974 patients from Germany and the United States treated by enucleation. In: Bornfeld N, Gragoudas ES, Hopping W, eds. *Tumors of the eye.* Amsterdam, The Netherlands: Kugler, 1991: 69–72.

85. Gupta J, Han LP, Wang P, et al. Development of retinoblastoma in the absence of telomerase activity. *J Natl Cancer Inst* 1996;88:1152–1157.

86. Doz F, Peter M, Schleiermacher G, et al. N-myc amplification, loss of heterozygosity on the short arm of chromosome 1 and DNA ploidy in retinoblastoma. *Eur J Cancer* 1996;32A:645–649.

87. Schiffman JS, Grunwald GB. Differential cell adhesion and expression of N-cadherin among retinoblastoma cell lines. *Invest Ophthalmol Vis Sci* 1992;33:1568–1574.

88. Skubitz AP, Grossman MD, McCarthy JB, et al. The decreased adhesion of Y79 retinoblastoma cells to extracellular matrix

proteins is due to a deficit of integrin receptors. *Invest Ophthalmol Vis Sci* 1994;35:2820–2833.

89. Lohmann DR. RB1 gene mutations in retinoblastoma. *Hum Mutat* 1999;14:283–288.

90. Lipinski MM, Jacks T. The retinoblastoma gene family in differentiation and development. *Oncogene* 1999;18:7873–7882.

91. Whyte P, Buchkovich KJ, Horowitz JM, et al. Association between an oncogene and an anti-oncogene: the adenovirus E1A proteins bind to the retinoblastoma gene product. *Nature* 1988;334:124–129.

92. DeCaprio JA, Ludlow JW, Figge J, et al. SV40 large tumor antigen forms a specific complex with the product of the retinoblastoma susceptibility gene. *Cell* 1988;54:275–283.

93. Dyson N, Howley PM, Munger K, et al. The human papilloma virus-16 E7 oncoprotein is able to bind to the retinoblastoma gene product. *Science* 1989;243:934–937.

94. Fujita T, Ohtani-Fujita N, Sakai T, et al. Low frequency of oncogenic mutations in the core promoter region of the RB1 gene. *Hum Mutat* 1999;13:410–411.

95. Zhang K, Wang MX, Munier F, et al. Molecular genetics of retinoblastoma. *Int Ophthalmol Clin* 1993;33:53–65.

96. Bremner R, Du DC, Connolly-Wilson MJ, et al. Deletion of RB exons 24 and 25 causes low-penetrance retinoblastoma. *Am J Hum Genet* 1997;61:556–570.

97. Morris EJ, Dyson NJ. Retinoblastoma protein partners. *Adv Cancer Res* 2001;82:1–54.

98. Weinberg RA. The retinoblastoma protein and cell cycle control. *Cell* 1995;81:323–330.

99. Dyson N. The regulation of E2F by pRB-family proteins. *Genes Dev* 1998;12:2245–2262.

100. Sherr CJ. Cancer cell cycles. *Science* 1996;274:1672–1677.

101. Sherr CJ, Roberts JM. CDK inhibitors: positive and negative regulators of G1-phase progression. *Genes Dev* 1999;13:1501–1512.

102. Lee EY, Chang CY, Hu N, et al. Mice deficient for Rb are nonviable and show defects in neurogenesis and haematopoiesis. *Nature* 1992;359:288–294.

103. Jacks T, Fazeli A, Schmitt EM, et al. Effects of an Rb mutation in the mouse. *Nature* 1992;359:295–300.

104. Clarke AR, Maandag ER, van Roon M, et al. Requirement for a functional Rb-1 gene in murine development. *Nature* 1992;359:328–330.

105. Zacksenhaus E, Jiang Z, Chung D, et al. pRb controls proliferation, differentiation, and death of skeletal muscle cells and other lineages during embryogenesis. *Genes Dev* 1996;10:3051–3064.

106. Thomas DM, Carty SA, Piscopo DM, et al. The retinoblastoma protein acts as a transcriptional coactivator required for osteogenic differentiation. *Mol Cell* 2001;8:303–316.

107. Sellers WR, Kaelin WG Jr. Role of the retinoblastoma protein in the pathogenesis of human cancer. *J Clin Oncol* 1997;15:3301–3312.

108. Ruas M, Peters G. The p16INK4a/CDKN2A tumor suppressor and its relatives. *Biochim Biophys Acta* 1998;1378:F115–F177.

109. Hall M, Peters G. Genetic alterations of cyclins, cyclin-dependent kinases, and Cdk inhibitors in human cancer. *Adv Cancer Res* 1996;68:67–108.

110. Kato MV, Shimizu T, Ishizaki K, et al. Loss of heterozygosity on chromosome 17 and mutation of the p53 gene in retinoblastoma. *Cancer Lett* 1996;106:75–82.

111. Oliveros O, Yunis E. Chromosome evolution in retinoblastoma. *Cancer Genet Cytogenet* 1995;82:155–160.

112. Cano J, Oliveros O, Yunis E. Phenotype variants, malignancy, and additional copies of 6p in retinoblastoma. *Cancer Genet Cytogenet* 1994;76:112–115.

113. Muncaster MM, Cohen BL, Phillips RA, et al. Failure of RB1 to reverse the malignant phenotype of human tumor cell lines. *Cancer Res* 1992;52:654–661.

114. Dryja TP, Rapaport J, McGee TL, et al. Molecular etiology of low-penetrance retinoblastoma in two pedigrees. *Am J Hum Genet* 1993;52:1122–1128.

115. Pendergrass TW, Davis S. Incidence of retinoblastoma in the United States. *Arch Ophthalmol* 1980;98:1204–1210.

116. Wiggs JL, Dryja TP. Predicting the risk of hereditary retinoblastoma. *Am J Ophthalmol* 1988:106:346–351.

117. Vogel, F. Genetics of retinoblastoma. *Hum Genet* 1979;52:1–54.

118. Abramson DH, Frank CM. Second nonocular tumors in survivors of bilateral retinoblastoma, a possible age effect on radiation-related risk. *Ophthalmology* 1998;105:573–580.

119. Mohney BG, Robertson DM, Schomberg PJ, et al. Second nonocular tumors in survivors of heritable retinoblastoma and prior radiation therapy. *Am J Ophthalmol* 1998:126:230–237.

120. Ibarra MS, O'Brien JM. Is screening for primitive neuroectodermal tumors in patients with unilateral retinoblastoma necessary? *J Am Assoc Pediatr Ophthalmol Strabismus* 2000;4:54–56.

121. Munier FL, Thonney F, Girardet A, et al. Evidence of somatic and germinal mosaicism in pseudo-low-penetrant hereditary retinoblastoma, by constitutional and single-sperm mutation analysis. *Am J Hum Genet* 1998;63:1903–1908.

122. Sippel KC, Fraioli RE, Smith GD, et al. Frequency of somatic and germ-line mosaicism in retinoblastoma: implications for genetic counseling. *Am J Hum Genet* 1998;62:610–619.

123. Smith JH, Murray TG, Fulton L, et al. Siblings of retinoblastoma patients: are we underestimating their risk? *Am J Ophthalmol* 2000;129:396–398.

124. Harbour JW. Molecular basis of low-penetrance retinoblastoma. *Arch Ophthalmol* 2001;119:1699–1704.

125. Singh AD, Santos CM, Shields CL, et al. Observations on 17 patients with retinocytoma. *Arch Ophthalmol* 2000;118:199–205.

126. Ohtani-Fujita N, Dryja TP, Rapaport J, et al. Hypermethylation in the retinoblastoma gene is associated with unilateral, sporadic retinoblastoma. *Cancer Genet Cytogenet* 1997;98:43–49.

127. Bunin GR, Emanuel BS, Meadows AT, et al. Frequency of 13q abnormalities among 203 patients with retinoblastoma. *J Natl Cancer Inst* 1989;81:370–374.

128. DenDunnen JT, Van Ommen G-JB. The protein truncation test: a review. *Hum Mutat* 1999;14:95–102.

129. Tsai T, Fulton L, Smith BJ, et al. Rapid identification of germline mutations in retinoblastoma by protein truncation testing. *Arch Ophthalmol* 2004;122:239–248.

130. Albert DM. Historic review of retinoblastoma. *Ophthalmology* 1987;94:654–662.

131. Ellsworth RM. The practical management of retinoblastoma. *Trans Am Ophthalmol Soc* 1969;67:463–534.

132. Shields JA, Augsburger JJ. Current approaches to the diagnosis and management of retinoblastoma. *Surv Ophthalmol* 1981;25:347–372.

133. Petersen RA. Retinoblastoma. In: Albert DM, Jakobiec FA, eds. *Principles and practice of ophthalmology*, 2nd ed. Philadelphia, PA: WB Saunders, 2000: 5095–5102.

134. Motegi T, Kaga M, Kadowaki H, et al. A recognizable pattern of the midface of retinoblastoma patients with interstitial deletion of 13q. *Hum Genet* 1983;64:160–162.

135. Baud O, Cormier-Daire V, Lyonnet S, et al. Dysmorphic phenotype and neurological impairment in 22 retinoblastoma patients with constitutional cytogenetic 13q deletion. *Clin Genet* 1999;55:478–482.

136. Shields JA, Shields CL, Parsons HM. Differential diagnosis of retinoblastoma. *Retina* 1991;11:232–243.
137. Liang JC, Augsburger JJ, Shields JA. Diffuse infiltrating retinoblastoma associated with persistent primary vitreous. *J Pediatr Ophthalmol Strabismus* 1985;22:31–33.
138. Howard GM, Ellsworth RM. Findings in the peripheral fundi of patients with retinoblastoma. *Am J Ophthalmol* 1966;62:243–250.
139. Roth DB, Scott IU, Murray TG, et al. Echography of retinoblastoma: histopathologic correlation and serial evaluation after globe-conserving radiotherapy or chemotherapy. *J Pediatr Ophthalmol Strabismus* 2001;38:136–143.
140. Potter PD, Shields CL, Shields JA, et al. The role of magnetic resonance imaging in children with intraocular tumors and simulating lesions. *Ophthalmology* 1996;103:1774–1783.
141. Christmas NJ, Van Quill K, Murray TG, et al. Evaluation of efficacy and complications: primary pediatric orbital implants after enucleation. *Arch Ophthalmol* 2000;118:503–506.
142. Gigantelli JW. Enucleation and retinoblastoma: to what lengths must we go? *Arch Ophthalmol* 2001;119:144–145.
143. Tawfik HA, Zico OM. Orbital implants in postenucleation retinoblastoma. *Ophthalmology* 2001;108:639–640.
144. Lee V, Subak-Sharpe I, Hungerford JL, et al. Exposure of primary orbital implants in postenucleation retinoblastoma patients. *Ophthalmology* 2000;107:940–945; discussion 946.
145. Kaltreider SA, Peake LR, Carter BT. Pediatric enucleation: analysis of volume replacement. *Arch Ophthalmol* 2001;119:379–384.
146. Shields CA, Shields JA, De Potter P. New treatment modalities for retinoblastoma. *Curr Opinion Ophthalmol* 1996;7:20–26.
147. Chan MF, Fung AY, Hu YC, et al. The measurement of three dimensional dose distribution of a ruthenium-106 ophthalmological applicator using magnetic resonance imaging of BANG polymer gels. *J Appl Clin Med Phys* 2001;2:85–89.
148. Stannard C, Sealy R, Hering E, et al. Localized whole eye radiotherapy for retinoblastoma using a (125)I applicator, "claws." *Int J Radiat Oncol Biol Phys* 2001;51:399–409.
149. Shields CL, Shields JA, Cater J, et al. Plaque radiotherapy for retinoblastoma: long-term tumor control and treatment complications in 208 tumors. *Ophthalmology* 2001;108:2116–2121.
150. Scott IU, O'Brien JM, Murray TG. Retinoblastoma: a review emphasizing genetics and management strategies. *Semin Ophthalmol* 1997;12:59–71.
151. Hernadez, JC, Brady LW, Shields JA, et al. External beam radiation for retinoblastoma: results, patterns of failure, and a proposal for treatment guidelines. *Int J Radiat Oncol Biol Phys* 1996;35:125–132.
152. Foote RL, Garretson BR, Schomberg PJ, et al. External beam irradiation for retinoblastoma: patterns of failure and dose-response analysis. *Int J Radiat Oncol Biol Phys* 1989;16:823–830.
153. Scott IU, Murray TG, Feuer WJ, et al. External beam radiotherapy in retinoblastoma: a comparison of two techniques. *Arch Ophthalmol* 1999;117:766–770.
154. Peylan-Ramu N, Bin-Nun A, Skleir-Levy M, et al. Orbital growth retardation in retinoblastoma survivors: work in progress. *Med Pediatr Oncol* 2001;37:465–470.
155. Adan L, Trivin C, Sainte-Rose C, et al. GH deficiency caused by cranial irradiation during childhood: factors and markers in young adults. *J Clin Endocrinol Metab* 2001;86:5245–5251.
156. Draper GJ, Sanders BM, Kingston JE. Second primary neoplasms in patients with retinoblastoma. *Br J Cancer* 1986;53:661–671.
157. Roarty JD, McLean IW, Zimmerman LE. Incidence of second neoplasms in patients with bilateral retinoblastoma. *Ophthalmology* 1988;95:1583–1587.
158. Traboulsi EI, Zimmerman LE, Manz HJ. Cutaneous malignant melanoma in survivors of heritable retinoblastoma. *Arch Ophthalmol* 1988;106:1059–1061.
159. Moppett J, Oakhill A, Duncan AW. Second malignancies in children: the usual suspects? *Eur J Radiol* 2001;38:235–248.
160. Chauveinc L, Mosseri V, Quintana E, et al. Osteosarcoma following retinoblastoma: age at onset and latency period. *Ophthalmic Genet* 2001;22:77–88.
161. Ragusa R, Russo S, Villari L, et al. Hodgkin's disease as a second malignant neoplasm in childhood: report of a case and review of the literature. *Pediatr Hematol Oncol* 2001;18:407–414.
162. Moll AC, Imhof SM, Schouten-Van Meeteren AY, et al. Second primary tumors in hereditary retinoblastoma: a register-based study, 1945–1997: is there an age effect on radiation-related risk? *Ophthalmology* 2001;108:1109–1114.
163. Kivela T, Asko-Seljavaara S, Pihkala U, et al. Sebaceous carcinoma of the eyelid associated with retinoblastoma. *Ophthalmology* 2001;108:1124–1128.
164. Wenzel CT, Halperin EC, Fisher SR. Second malignant neoplasms of the head and neck in survivors of retinoblastoma. *Ear Nose Throat J* 2001;80:106,109–112.
165. Shields JA, Husson M, Shields CL, et al. Orbital malignant fibrous histiocytoma following irradiation for retinoblastoma. *Ophthalmic Plast Reconstr Surg* 2001;17:58–61.
166. Singh AD, Shields CL, Shields JA, et al. Occurrence of retinoblastoma and uveal melanoma in same patient. *Retina* 2000;20:305–306.
167. Marta U, Zsuzsanna S, Jozsef B, et al. Rare incidence of three consecutive primary tumors in the maxillofacial region: retinoblastoma, leiomyosarcoma, and choriocarcinoma: case report. *J Carniofac Surg* 2001;12:464–468.
168. Abramson DH, Melson MR, Dunkel IJ, et al. Third (fourth and fifth) nonocular tumors in survivors of retinoblastoma. *Ophthalmology* 2001;108:1868–1876.
169. Abramson DH, Ellsworth RM, Kitchin FD, et al. Second nonocular tumors in retinoblastoma survivors. Are they radiation-induced? *Ophthalmology* 1984;91:1351–1355.
170. Uusitalo M, Wheeler S, O'Brien JM. New approaches in the clinical management of retinoblastoma. *Ophthalmol Clin N Am* 1999;12:255–264.
171. Chan HSL, DeBoer G, Thiessen JJ, et al. Combining cyclosporin with chemotherapy controls intraocular retinoblastoma without requiring radiation. *Clin Cancer Res* 1996;2:1499–1508.
172. Shields CL, DePotter P, Himelstein BP, et al. Chemoreduction in the initial management of intraocular retinoblastoma. *Arch Ophthalmol* 1996;114:1330–1338.
173. Shields CL, Shields JA, Needle M, et al. Combined chemoreduction and adjuvant treatment for intraocular retinoblastoma. *Ophthalmology* 1997;104:2101–2111.
174. Gallie BL, Budning A, DeBoer G, et al. Chemotherapy with focal therapy can cure intraocular retinoblastoma without radiotherapy. *Arch Ophthalmol* 1996;114:1321–1328.
175. Bornfeld N, Schuler A, Bechrakis N, et al. Preliminary results of primary chemotherapy in retinoblastoma. *Klin Padiatr* 1997;209:216–221.
176. Wilson TW, Chan HS, Moselhy GM, et al. Penetration of chemotherapy into vitreous is increased by cryotherapy and cyclosporine in rabbits. *Arch Ophthalmol* 1996;114:1390–1395.
177. Pfeffer MR, Teicher BA, Holden SA, et al. The interaction of cisplatinum plus etoposide with radiation + hyperthermia. *Int J Radiat Oncol Biol Phys* 1990;19:1439–1447.
178. Murray TG, Cicciarelli N, McCabe CM, et al. In vitro efficacy of carboplatin and hyperthermia in a murine retinoblastoma cell line. *Invest Ophthalmol Vis Sci* 1997;38:2516–2522.

179. Doz F. Carboplatin in pediatrics. *Bull Cancer* 2000;87(Spec No):25–29.

180. Hardman JG, Limbirds LE, eds. *Goodman & Gilman's: the pharmacological basis of therapeutics,* 10th ed. New York: McGraw Hill Medical Publishing Division, 2001:1417, 1421–1422, 1466–1469.

181. Dunkel IJ, Aledo A, Kernan NA, et al. Successful treatment of metastatic retinoblastoma. *Cancer* 2000;89:2117–2121.

182. Goble RR, McKenzie J, Kingston JE, et al. Orbital recurrence of retinoblastoma successfully treated by combined therapy. *Br J Ophthalmol* 1990;74:97–98.

183. Pratt CB, Crom DB, Howarth CC. The use of chemotherapy for extraocular retinoblastoma. *Med Pediatr Oncol* 1985;13:330–333.

184. Abramson DH, Ellsworth RM, Grumbach N, et al. Retinoblastoma: survival, age at detection and comparison 1914–1958, 1958–1983. *J Pediatr Ophthalmol Strabismus* 1985;22:246–250.

185. Abramson DH, Ellsworth RM, Grumbach N, et al. Retinoblastoma: correlation between age at diagnosis and survival. *J Pediatr Ophthalmol Strabismus* 1986;23:174–177.

186. Goddard AG, Kinston JE, Hungerford JL. Delay in diagnosis of retinoblastoma: risk factors and treatment outcome. *Br J Ophthalmol* 1999;83:1320–1323.

187. Stevenson KE, Hungerford JL, Garner A. Local extraocular extension of retinoblastoma following intraocular surgery. *Br J Ophthalmol* 1989;73:739–742.

OTHER TUMORS IN INFANTS AND CHILDREN

MARSHA C. CHEUNG
JOAN M. O'BRIEN
THOMAS M. AABERG, JR.
G. BAKER HUBBARD III

CIRCUMSCRIBED CHOROIDAL HEMANGIOMA

Definition and Prevalence

Choroidal hemangioma is a benign vascular tumor classified into two types, diffuse and circumscribed, based on the degree of choroidal involvement (1–4). The diffuse process occurs in Sturge-Weber syndrome (discussed later in this chapter), whereas the circumscribed form is usually not associated with cutaneous lesions or other systemic findings. In 1976, Witschel and Font (5) reported the clinicopathologic characteristics of 71 choroidal hemangiomas. In their study, 37% represented the diffuse type and 63% were circumscribed.

Choroidal hemangioma represents the most common vascular tumor of the choroid. The exact incidence of these tumors is unknown, but choroidal hemangioma is diagnosed in approximately 1 case per 40 cases of posterior uveal melanoma (3). Because these lesions are often asymptomatic and may remain undiagnosed, their prevalence may be much higher.

Genetics and Environmental Associations

No known environmental factors contribute to the development of choroidal hemangioma. No genetic associations have been identified to date.

Pathology and Pathophysiology

Choroidal hemangioma contains microscopically congested vessels. The histologic appearance of these tumors demonstrates complete absence of cellular proliferation in the blood vessel walls, suggesting that these lesions are nonproliferative in origin (5). Histopathologically, choroidal hemangioma has been described as a circumscribed tumor with sharply demarcated margins, leading to compression of surrounding melanocytes and choroidal lamellae (5).

Choroidal hemangioma is thought to be a congenital hamartomatous tumor. The exact cause and pathophysiology are unknown, although some have suggested that the underlying process involves arteriovenous shunts that are present in embryogenesis and subsequently disappear during normal development (6).

Clinical Features

Patients with choroidal hemangioma often present with ocular symptoms in adulthood, in contrast to those who present with Sturge-Weber–associated hemangioma in childhood. Both types of choroidal hemangioma are likely present at birth, with the circumscribed variant frequently remaining undetected until adulthood. The circumscribed form should be included in the differential diagnosis of a pediatric intraocular tumor. These tumors typically present with blurry vision, metamorphopsia due to serous fluid, or hyperopia due to retinal elevation by the tumor (7).

Choroidal hemangioma lesions are typically nonpigmented elevated masses with a characteristic orange-red color (Fig. 15-1). Irregular pigmentation may be present at the tumor surface or on its edges. These tumors are almost always unilateral and solitary.

Most circumscribed choroidal hemangiomas are located in the postequatorial fundus (5,8). The posterior margin of the majority of these circumscribed lesions is located within two disc diameters of the optic disc or the fovea (8). Most of these lesions are less than 19 mm in diameter and have a mean elevation of 3 mm (8). Choroidal hemangiomas do not grow significantly over time, although a few cases of such tumor growth have been documented (9,10).

Subretinal fluid is commonly associated with this tumor and is responsible for the most common presenting symptoms (7). Circumscribed choroidal hemangiomas have been associated with choroidal neovascularization (11). These lesions have also been reported in rare instances to resolve spontaneously, leaving only a chorioretinal scar.

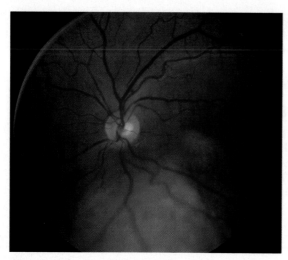

FIGURE 15-1. The orange-red elevated mass demonstrates the characteristic appearance of choroidal hemangiomas.

Visual acuity in patients with choroidal hemangioma can be completely normal or may be decreased from a number of mechanisms. Vision loss and visual field defects associated with choroidal hemangioma may result from exudative retinal detachment, induced hyperopia, macular edema, retinal degeneration, loss of photoreceptors, chorioretinal adhesions, and cystoid degeneration. '

Diagnostic Studies

The diagnosis of choroidal hemangioma is usually made based on ophthalmoscopic findings, although several ancillary studies can be used to help confirm the diagnosis. Ultrasonography shows high internal reflectivity on A-scan, and acoustic solidity on B-scan images. Fluorescein angiography demonstrates early filling within large vascular channels comprising the tumor. Late frames show diffuse hyperfluorescence due to leakage of dye from the tumor surface (12a). Indocyanine green angiography shows accumulation of dye early with subsequent washout later in the study (12b).

Differential Diagnosis

Despite the characteristic clinical features of choroidal hemangioma, this tumor can be challenging to distinguish from other choroidal tumors including amelanotic melanoma, choroidal osteoma, choroidal metastasis, or retinoblastoma. In addition, these lesions can mimic posterior scleritis or other inflammatory conditions.

Management

Treatment of choroidal hemangiomas is generally limited to those that are vision threatening, and treatment planning depends upon tumor size and location (13). Hemangiomas that do not affect vision and are not associated with subretinal fluid are followed by observation. These lesions are characteristically nonprogressive in nature.

Laser photocoagulation remains an important treatment and is indicated when the tumor causes loss of vision secondary to serous retinal detachment (8,13). Historically, focal lesions were treated with laser to cause resorption of subretinal fluid and readhesion of the neurosensory retina and retinal pigment epithelium. Subretinal fluid has been reported to resolve in 62% to 100% of cases following laser therapy (7).

Radiation therapy is frequently used in the treatment of choroidal hemangioma, including external beam radiation, plaque radiotherapy, or proton-beam irradiation. Numerous reports have indicated that these treatments offer good results in terms of successful resolution of subretinal fluid (14–18). Shields and colleagues (7) concluded that plaque radiotherapy should be considered early in the treatment of choroidal hemangioma lesions that are resistant to laser treatment before chronic macular edema develops. They recommended that patients with the greatest risk for poor visual acuity be treated aggressively with external beam radiation or low-dose plaque radiotherapy.

Recent advances in treatment provide additional alternatives including photodynamic therapy (PDT) and transpupillary thermotherapy. Both of these methods have been reported to reduce subretinal fluid associated with choroidal hemangioma (19–26). PDT has been proposed as an especially efficacious, safe, noninvasive option for tumors located at the fovea (20–26).

Outcomes

Because choroidal hemangioma is a benign tumor that does not undergo malignant transformation, patients with this lesion have an excellent prognosis for life. Visual prognosis, however, is significantly less positive. Despite the benign nature of these tumors, approximately 50% of affected patients have long-term visual acuity of 20/200 or worse (7). Final visual acuity is dependent upon numerous factors including initial visual acuity, failure of previous laser treatment, multiple quadrants of subretinal fluid, chronic submacular fluid, chronic cystoid macular edema, or chronic retinal pigment epithelial changes (7).

Children with choroidal hemangiomas face the additional problem of amblyopia in the affected eye. Amblyopia can result from refractive changes and induced hyperopia due to undetected tumors. Because early intervention can be effective in achieving resolution of subretinal fluid and restoration of visual function, prompt referral to an ophthalmologist with experience treating circumscribed choroidal hemangioma is especially important in children suspected of having this lesion.

MEDULLOEPITHELIOMA

Definition and Prevalence

Medulloepithelioma is a rare embryonal tumor that arises from the medullary epithelium on the inner layer of the developing optic cup (27). Verhoeff (28) first described this tumor histopathologically as a teratoneuroma in 1904. Medulloepithelioma is classified into teratoid and nonteratoid forms. The nonteratoid form, otherwise known as a diktyoma, represents only medullary epithelial cells. In contrast, teratoid forms of this tumor contain heterotopic tissues including cartilage, skeletal muscle, and brainlike tissue (29). Either form can be benign or malignant (27,30,31). In terms of epidemiology, medulloepithelioma is a very rare tumor, the exact prevalence of which is unknown.

Intraocular medulloepithelioma often has a malignant histologic appearance. Extraocular extension with distant metastasis to the lungs, mediastinum, and lymph nodes has been documented (30,32). Broughton and Zimmerman (30) reported in their study of 56 cases, that 66% were malignant, and that of those, 30% were teratoid. Shields and colleagues (33) reported in their series that 90% were malignant, and of those 56% were teratoid. Despite a malignant histologic appearance, the Broughton series, as well as others (31,33,34), suggest that distant metastases are rarely if ever seen in the absence of local extraocular extension.

Genetics and Environmental Factors

No reported environmental or genetic factors have been associated with medulloepithelioma.

Pathology and Pathophysiology

Differentiation of the medullary epithelium that lines the optic cup normally produces the retina photoreceptors, glial and neuronal tissues, nonpigmented ciliary epithelium, pigmented epithelium of the iris, muscles of the iris, and components of the vitreous.

Histopathologic studies demonstrate that medulloepithelioma contains elements that resemble the medullary epithelium, the optic cup and/or vessel, pigmented and nonpigmented ciliary epithelium, vitreous, or neuroglia (30). Medulloepitheliomas often contain heterotopic tissues such as cartilage, rhabdomyoblasts, skeletal muscle, and brainlike tissues (29). This feature results from the capacity of the primitive medullary epithelium to differentiate into a variety of neural and mesenchymal tissues types.

Clinical Features

Medulloepithelioma characteristically presents in early childhood, at a mean age of 4 years, but these tumors can also be diagnosed in adults. This lesion can present as a ciliary body mass, or more rarely as a tumor of the optic nerve or retina (34–36). Steinkuller and Font (37) concluded that medulloepithelioma should be considered a neoplasm of the eye and of the orbit.

Medulloepithelioma frequently presents with decreased vision and pain. Other common signs include leukocoria, and a mass in the anterior chamber, iris, or ciliary body (30). One of the earliest signs may be a notch in the lens, "a lens coloboma," in the quadrant of the tumor (38). This coloboma occurs because the embryonal tumor prevents normal zonular development in the associated lens quadrant.

Medulloepithelioma has the capacity to progress and to become locally invasive and destructive to surrounding intraocular tissues. Loss of vision occurs secondary to cataract, subluxed lens, neoplastic cyclitic membrane formation, or glaucoma (33). Other findings associated with this tumor include uveitis and retinal detachment (30). Iris neovascularization has also been reported as a manifestation of medulloepithelioma (33,39). Neovascular glaucoma discovered in a child with a normal fundus examination should raise suspicion for occult medulloepithelioma.

The presence of cysts within a tumor is highly suggestive of medulloepithelioma (33). Foci of cartilage, appearing as whitish opacities within the tumor, are also a characteristic finding in the teratoid form of medulloepithelioma (33).

Diagnostic Studies

The diagnosis of medulloepithelioma is primarily a clinical one, and the role of additional studies to confirm the diagnosis is not well established. A-scan ultrasonography has been reported to show irregular high internal reflectivity with areas of moderate reflectivity and B-scan can demonstrate characteristic cysts within the tumor (40). Shields et al. (41) described dense echogenic areas in a medulloepithelioma that are similar in appearance to calcifications in retinoblastoma. These authors also described the tumor's vascular pattern, demonstrating numerous leaking vessels, on fluorescein angiography (41).

Magnetic resonance imaging (MRI) of medulloepithelioma is hyperintense on T1-weighted images and hypointense on T2-weighted images, a result similar to that for malignant melanoma (42). Ultrasound biomicroscopy has recently emerged as a helpful diagnostic tool for evaluating tumors involving the anterior uveal tract; this approach may be particularly useful in demonstrating the multicystic appearance of medulloepithelioma (41,43).

Differential Diagnosis

Given the wide variety of presentations and possible locations for medulloepithelioma, the differential diagnosis is broad. Diagnoses that should be considered include congenital and inflammatory conditions such as persistent hyperplastic primary vitreous, pars planitis, or vascular malformations, and numerous tumors including retinoblastoma, melanoma, melanocytoma, iridociliary cyst, rhabdomyosarcoma, neuroblastoma, or teratoma.

Management

Treatment of medulloepithelioma is surgical and usually requires enucleation. Medulloepithelioma frequently recurs following local resection (31,41). Furthermore, these tumors are friable and, therefore, very difficult to remove surgically. Small, anteriorly located tumors may occasionally be followed by observation and/or treated with local resection. Given the tumor's high risk for recurrence and the subsequent necessity for enucleation, as well as the difficulty of local resection, most authors recommend primary enucleation (31,33). Cases involving known extrascleral extension may require exenteration.

Neither local radiation nor chemotherapy has an established role in the primary treatment of medulloepithelioma. In cases involving risk for recurrence of the tumor, however, these methods may be used as adjunctive therapy.

Outcomes

The visual outcome in patients diagnosed with medulloepithelioma is poor, and most patients with this disease lose the affected eye. Life expectancy, however, for patients with medulloepithelioma is surprisingly good, despite the malignant nature of the tumor. In the largest series of 56 patients with medulloepithelioma, four known tumor-associated deaths were reported. The most important prognostic feature was extraocular extension (30).

As with other intraocular tumors, early diagnosis is important in determining final clinical outcome. Unfortunately, diagnosis is often delayed in patients with medulloepithelioma; most of these patients experience a delay in surgical treatment for more than 1 year after the initial onset of symptoms (30).

CHOROIDAL OSTEOMA

Definition and Prevalence

Choroidal osteoma is a benign choroidal tumor consisting of mature bone. This disease was first described clinically by Gass et al. (44) in 1978. Choroidal osteoma is likely a congenital lesion, and it often presents in infants, although the diagnosis may not be made until adulthood. Lesions of choroidal osteomas are more common in females and most often found adjacent to the optic nerve or located within the macula.

The exact incidence and prevalence of choroidal osteoma are unknown, although it has been suggested that these tumors frequently are asymptomatic, often are initially misdiagnosed, and are not rare (45).

Genetics and Environmental Factors

Choroidal osteoma has no known association with environmental factors. No genetic associations have been identified.

Pathology and Pathophysiology

Choroidal osteoma is composed of bony trabeculae with osteoblasts, osteocytes, and osteoclasts (44,46). Large, endothelial-lined, cavernous spaces are covered with small capillary blood vessels. The choriocapillaris can be altered and even destroyed in the involved areas. Overlying retinal pigment epithelium (RPE) can undergo degeneration.

The pathogenesis of choroidal osteoma is not known. One suggested mechanism is that a focal choroiditis may lead to calcification near the optic nerve (47). Another possibility is that the choroidal osteoma represents an osseous choristoma, wherein normal tissue is absent at the affected site (48). The lesion's peripapillary location is typical of other developmental tumors described in this chapter, such as astrocytic hamartoma, combined retinal hamartoma, and retinal capillary hemangioma.

Intraocular calcification can be associated with trauma, long-standing retinal detachment, inflammation, abnormalities in calcium and phosphorus levels, and phthisis bulbi. Choroidal osteoma has been reported following intraocular inflammation (47,49). Serum calcium, phosphorus, and alkaline phosphatase levels are, however, found to be within the normal range in patients with choroidal osteoma.

Because females are more frequently diagnosed with choroidal osteoma than males, a hormonal role may be suggested in the pathogenesis; however, endocrine abnormalities have not been documented in these patients. A hereditary component in the pathogenesis is evident in some cases (50). Noble (50) speculated that a congenital, possibly inherited, defect in the choroid remains undetectable until osseous calcification is initiated through the influence of additional factors.

Clinical Features

The location of choroidal osteoma dictates the patient's presenting symptoms. Although this lesion may be diagnosed at any age, it is likely present at birth. Choroidal osteoma frequently remains asymptomatic and undetected, especially in the community setting (45). Once the fovea is involved by the tumor, with associated neovascularization and exudative retinal detachment, the patient can present with decreased vision, visual field defects, and metamorphopsia.

Choroidal osteoma lesions are characteristically elevated, yellow-orange masses. The tumors can appear mottled or spotted due to clumping of orange or brown pigment on their surface (51). Frequently, choroidal osteomas are solitary, although they occasionally occur as multiple lesions. Small distinctive tufts of vessels are often found on the tumor surface. These feeder vessels are best visualized on fluorescein angiography, and characteristically, they demonstrate no leakage (52).

Choroidal osteoma presents posteriorly, usually within the macula or adjacent to the optic nerve. Approximately 75% of cases are unilateral, with tumor dimensions of up to 22 mm in diameter and up to 2.5 mm in height (46).

Subretinal fluid can be present overlying choroidal osteoma. This presentation raises the suspicion of choroidal neovascularization with subsequent formation of subretinal fluid and/or hemorrhage (44,52). Choroidal neovascularization can occur in approximately one third of patients with choroidal osteoma (52).

Slow growth of choroidal osteoma occurs in approximately 50% of patients with these tumors. Growth is demonstrated either in an overall increase in size, or in the formation of pseudopod projections extending out from the tumor's central mass (53). Rapid growth in choroidal osteoma has been reported (54). Spontaneous involution of the tumor has also been documented (55).

Diagnostic Studies

Choroidal osteoma can be diagnosed clinically. Although the characteristic appearance of this lesion often serves to differentiate it from other tumors, diagnostic studies are frequently helpful.

Ultrasonography is particularly useful in differentiating choroidal osteoma from other lesions. A-scan ultrasonography demonstrates a high-intensity echo spike from the inner surface of the tumor, with decreased amplitudes of orbital soft tissue echoes posterior to the tumor. B-scan indicates a highly reflective choroidal mass with acoustic shadowing posterior to the tumor (46,52).

Fluorescein angiography demonstrates early diffuse, irregular hyperfluorescence, with hyperfluorescence of the vascular tufts, and late staining. In the late frames, the spiderlike vascular tufts may stand out in negative relief as hypofluorescent lines against a bright background (46,52). Choroidal neovascular membranes exhibit an early lacy pattern of hyperfluorescence with early leakage.

On computed tomography (CT) scan, choroidal osteoma demonstrates the same density as bone. On MRI, these tumors exhibit characteristics similar to ocular melanoma: hyperintense to vitreous on T1-weighted imaging and hypointense on T2-weighted imaging (56).

Differential Diagnosis

The differential diagnosis of choroidal osteoma includes other intraocular tumors, such as amelanotic choroidal nevi, choroidal melanoma, choroidal metastasis, and circumscribed choroidal hemangioma. Choroidal osteoma may appear similar to osseous metaplasia that can occur in other tumors, and this lesion should also be carefully distinguished from posterior scleritis or subretinal hemorrhage. Idiopathic sclerochoroidal calcifications should be included in the differential diagnosis for choroidal osteoma; however, the former are more often multiple, often bilateral, and are found typically along the superotemporal vascular arcades (51).

Linear nevus sebaceous syndrome presents with osseous choroidal choristoma, which should be carefully distinguished from choroidal hemangioma. This syndrome, however, also presents with characteristic systemic findings: midline facial linear nevus of Jadassohn, seizures, cognitive developmental deficits, and multiple eye findings including lipodermoids; colobomas of the lids, iris, and choroid; and choroidal calcification (57).

Management

Choroidal osteoma is typically not treated when the patient is asymptomatic. Periodic dilated fundus examinations and self-monitoring with the use of an Amsler grid can facilitate timely diagnosis in patients who develop choroidal neovascular membranes.

Regression of choroidal osteoma by argon laser photoablation has been described (58). Laser photocoagulation has been shown to have some success when used for treatment of a subfoveal neovascularization membrane when vision is threatened (45,59). Laser treatment can cause retinal anastomosis with both arteriolar and venular vessels within the tumor (45). Successful treatment of a RPE leak by focal laser has been reported (45). Use of photodynamic therapy for choroidal neovascularization (CNV) in choroidal osteoma has also been described with successful closure of the CNV in a patient who refused laser treatment (60).

Because the etiology of choroidal osteoma is unknown at this time, no preventive measures have been suggested.

Outcomes

Visual loss to 20/200 or worse has been reported to occur by 20 years past diagnosis in approximately 60% of patients with choroidal osteoma (53). The major cause of vision loss is CNV. At 20 years from diagnosis, the risk of developing CNV is more than 50%. In one study, successful treatment of these membranes was reported in only 25% of patients (53). Hemorrhage associated with choroidal osteoma typically resolves but can cause a subretinal, vision-limiting disciform scar. The prognosis for life in these patients is the same as for the general population.

CONGENITAL HYPERTROPHY OF THE RETINAL PIGMENT EPITHELIUM

Definition and Prevalence

Congenital hypertrophy of the retinal pigment epithelium (CHRPE) was first described by Buettner (61) in 1975. Although this tumor is congenital, the diagnosis may be made at any age. CHRPE presents as solitary or multifocal lesions. Isolated CHRPE lesions are seen in the normal population. These hyperpigmented, isolated lesions are flat and circumscribed, and represent congenital hypertrophy of the pigment epithelium with no primary involvement of the overlying retina. Multifocal lesions appear in two forms. One form of multifocal disease is unilateral and consists of lesions grouped to resemble animal footprints. These lesions are typically demonstrated in only one sector of the fundus and are sometimes referred to as "bear tracks," or congenital grouped pigmentation of the retina (62). The second multifocal form of CHRPE is bilateral. The multifocal lesions in the bilateral form assume a more random distribution and are not grouped together in a single sector of the fundus (62,63) (Fig. 15-2) Bilateral multifocal CHRPE is associated with familial adenomatous polyposis (FAP) (64–73).

Familial adenomatous polyposis is a genetically inherited, autosomal dominant disease characterized by more than 100 polyps of the colon and rectum, predisposing these patients to colon cancer. Gardner's syndrome involves the development of extracolonic manifestations of FAP, and consists of intestinal polyps, characteristic patches of CHRPE, skeletal hamartoma, and soft tissue tumors. Both intracolonic and extracolonic presentations are now recognized as phenotypic variations of the same disease. CHRPE is the most common extraintestinal manifestation associated with familial adenomatous polyposis (74).

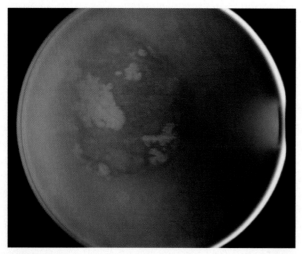

FIGURE 15-2. Congenital hypertrophy of the retinal pigment epithelium, demonstrating characteristic lacunae.

Because many CHRPE lesions may remain undiagnosed, the exact prevalence of this disease is unknown. FAP accounts for approximately 1% of all colon cancers, affecting 1 in 7,500 to 10,000 individuals (74).

Genetics and Environmental Factors

The gene responsible for FAP, designated the adenomatous polyposis coli (APC) gene, was cloned in 1991, and mapped to chromosome 5 (75,76). APC is a tumor-suppressor gene, with a demonstrated involvement in the carcinogenesis of colon cancer (77). More than 250 APC mutations have already been identified (78).

This oncogene plays a role in tumor formation in the gastrointestinal tract, soft tissue, and bone. One study suggests that APC gene alterations may lead to defects in RPE melanogenesis and to focal RPE lesions (79).

Mutation analysis of APC is now an option for many families affected by familial adenomatous polyposis. A direct correlation has been demonstrated between the locus of the APC mutation and the retinal phenotypic disease expression. Careful delineation of the phenotype of the CHRPE lesions allows focused investigation of the APC mutation within certain coding regions. CHRPE lesions are only demonstrated when the mutation is located between codons 464 to 1,387 of the APC gene (80).

No environmental factors have been reported in association with CHRPE.

Pathology and Pathophysiology

Idiopathic solitary CHRPE histopathologically exhibits a monolayer of hypertrophied RPE cells with large pigment granules and photoreceptor degeneration overlying the RPE (61).

The histopathology described in Gardner's syndrome demonstrates a more pervasive melanogenesis of the RPE (79). Several different configurations are described: a monolayer of hypertrophied cells; a mound of pigmented RPE cells between the RPE basement membrane and Bruch's membrane; or a multilayered mound of hyperplastic RPE in a nodular or mushroom-shaped configuration (79,81). All of these conformations show cellular hyperplasia of the RPE. Although the fundus lesions in Gardner's syndrome are referred to as CHRPE, this distinctive feature of cellular hyperplasia corresponds to a hamartomatous malformation of the RPE, not hypertrophy alone.

Electron microscopy has shown absence of autofluorescent lipofuscin granules in CHRPE lesions suggesting that RPE cells in CHRPE lack the catabolic functions of normal RPE cells (82).

Clinical Symptoms and Signs

Congenital hypertrophy of the RPE can present as a solitary lesion or as a collection of multiple lesions. Although some investigators classify these two disease forms differently, both forms are included in this discussion due to their similarities. Several of their clinical and histopathologic differences have previously been described in this section.

Congenital hypertrophy of the retinal pigment epithelium lesions are congenital and have been observed in newborns. Solitary CHRPE lesions are demonstrated in the normal population as a benign incidental finding. A patient presenting with CHRPE typically has normal vision and normal anterior segments. Fundus examination reveals a flat, circumscribed, nonprogressive lesion. Size, shape, and degree of pigmentation of the lesions are quite variable (83) CHRPE lesions can be oval or round, with areas of pigmentation and depigmentation, and are often surrounded by a characteristic halo of depigmentation. CHRPE can present anywhere in the fundus; approximately 70% of these lesions are located in the temporal quadrant (84).

While CHRPE lesions are typically flat and nonprogressive, five patients were reported to have a nodular lesion arising from CHRPE (85). In each case, the nodular growth slowly progressed, fed by its own vasculature, causing exudative retinal detachment and chronic cystoid macular edema (85). This presentation may represent secondary reactive RPE proliferation or an acquired adenoma from CHRPE (85). One case of adenocarcinoma was reported to arise from CHRPE, suggesting that CHRPE lesions should be observed for neoplastic development, although this disease course is unusual (86).

The Association of Congenital Hypertrophy of the Retinal Pigment Epithelium with Gardner's Syndrome and Familial Adenomatous Polyposis

Familial adenomatous polyposis, Gardner's syndrome, and CHRPE are all closely related. The ocular lesions in FAP have been reported to be bilateral in 86% of cases (83). Ocular lesions are observed in the presence or absence of other systemic manifestations of Gardner's syndrome. The presence of multiple fundus lesions (more than four) or bilateral lesions has been reported to be a highly specific and sensitive phenotypic marker for Gardner's syndrome (87). CHRPE lesions have been reported to be present in about two thirds of families with FAP (83).

Families with FAP can differ in the presenting number and type of RPE lesions, although studies have demonstrated that affected individuals within a single family have similar pigmented lesions (88). In families with known FAP, the presence of retinal lesions revealed by fundus examination is highly predictive for the development of intestinal polyps; however, a negative examination cannot exclude risk for polyp formation (88).

Diagnostic Studies

Congenital hypertrophy of the retinal pigment epithelium lesions are very distinctive and are generally diagnosed clinically. Studies, however, can support the diagnosis. Fluorescein angiography demonstrates blockage of choroidal fluorescence in the hyperpigmented areas of the lesions in all phases of the study. Hypopigmented areas can exhibit hyperfluorescence, both early and late (window defect). CHRPE lesions do not leak on fluorescein angiography (FA), as the overlying retinal vasculature and choriocapillaris are normal.

Visual field testing can indicate scotomas that correspond to the lesions, presumably representing progressive degeneration of the overlying photoreceptors (61). Because CHRPE lesions are flat, ultrasound studies lack diagnostic utility.

Differential Diagnosis

The differential diagnosis of a solitary CHRPE lesion should include choroidal nevus or choroidal melanoma. Multiple bilateral CHRPE lesions indicate greater suspicion of an underlying polyposis syndrome. Chorioretinal scars from toxoplasmosis, secondary hyperplasia of the RPE, sickle cell disease (sunburst lesions), sector retinitis pigmentosa, and pigmented retinopathies should also be considered in the differential diagnosis of CHRPE lesions.

Management

Treatment is not indicated for either solitary or multifocal CHRPE lesions. These lesions should be observed routinely, and if the patient's medical history is suggestive, FAP or Gardner's syndrome should be investigated.

Outcomes

The prognoses for vision and for life are very good with solitary CHRPE lesions. In patients with FAP or Gardner's syndrome, however, the prognosis for life is altered by the risk of malignant transformation of the colonic polyps. Ophthalmologic examinations revealing multiple bilateral CHRPE lesions may identify children and families at risk for developing polyposis and colon cancer.

COMBINED HAMARTOMA OF THE RETINA AND RETINAL PIGMENT EPITHELIUM

Definition and Prevalence

Combined hamartoma of the retina and of the RPE was first described by Gass (89) in 1973. Gass organized these lesions into categories based on location within the fundus: on the disc, next to the disc, in the macula, and in the periphery.

A hamartoma is a benign proliferation of cells that normally are found in the affected area. This ocular hamartomatous malformation involves the sensory retina, the retinal pigment epithelium, the retinal vasculature, and the overlying vitreous. Combined hamartoma of the retina and RPE is a rare lesion, and its exact prevalence is unknown.

Genetics and Environmental Factors

No known environmental factors or genetic associations have been identified for combined hamartoma of the retina and RPE.

Pathology and Pathophysiology

Combined hamartoma of the retina and RPE appears histopathologically with disorganized retina and retinal vascular tortuosity (90). Hyperplastic cells of the RPE migrate into the retina (91). Gliosis is present at the retinal surface leading to retinal distortion and folding. The vitreoretinal interface is altered with associated traction on the sensory retina.

These ocular hamartomatous lesions are characterized by benign growth of glial, vascular, or pigmented tissue from the RPE. Some lesions contain prominent vascular tissue while others are composed predominantly of glial tissue, which can lead to formation of preretinal or epiretinal membranes.

The pathogenesis of combined hamartoma of the RPE and retina is uncertain. Although the majority of patients with combined hamartoma do not present with other systemic diseases, these lesions have been reported in association with neurofibromatosis, tuberous sclerosis, ncontinentia pigmenti, bilateral colobomas of the optic disc, optic nerve head drusen, juvenile retinoschisis, juvenile nasopharyngeal angiofibroma, Gorlin syndrome, and sickle cell anemia (89,92–96). These associations may indicate a developmental etiology, as suggested by Gass (92).

Clinical Features

Combined hamartoma of the retina and RPE presents most frequently as painless loss of vision. Other presenting symptoms include metamorphopsia, floaters, strabismus, leukocoria, and occasionally ocular pain (92). Combined hamartoma may also be discovered as an incidental finding on routine ophthalmologic examination. Changes in vision associated with these lesions occur due to a variety of factors: involvement of the optic nerve or fovea, alterations at the vitreoretinal surface with epiretinal membrane formation and subsequent macular traction, or subretinal and intraretinal exudation.

On ophthalmologic examination, combined hamartoma of the retina and RPE appears pigmented and elevated,

often with distortion of the retina and tortuous overlying vessels (Fig. 15-3). Because the pigmentation in these lesions is variable, the diagnosis is challenging in some cases. The location of the lesion, either juxtapapillary or peripheral, may also have an affect on its appearance (89). A juxtapapillary lesion characteristically appears as a solitary elevated mass adjacent to or immediately overlying the optic disc. In these lesions, contraction of overlying glial tissues often results in striae and distortion of the retina. Peripheral lesions can resemble an elevated ridge with accompanying traction of the vessels toward the lesion (97).

Combined retina and RPE hamartoma is typically unilateral, although bilateral cases have been described (94,98). When bilateral, combined hamartoma is frequently associated with type 1 or type 2 neurofibromatosis (62,99–104). Ocular combined hamartoma is a congenital lesion. The diagnosis can be made at any age, including infancy and most frequently in childhood (89,92,105). Combined hamartoma of the retina and RPE is characteristically nonprogressive, although cases involving growth have been reported (106,107). Complications associated with combined retina and RPE hamartoma include retinoschisis, retinal holes, vitreous hemorrhage, choroidal neovascularization, retinal hemorrhages, and exudative retinal detachment (92,108,109).

Diagnostic Studies

Fluorescein angiography is a useful tool in evaluating ocular combined hamartoma. Early FA phases demonstrate large tortuous vessels within the tumor, abnormal retinal capillaries, and late leakage of tumor vessels.

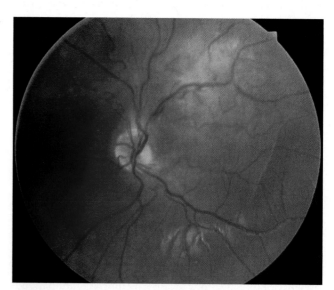

FIGURE 15-3. Combined hamartomas of the retina and retinal pigment epithelium are pigmented elevated masses which are frequently associated with overlying glial tissues which produce retina distortion and striae.

Ultrasound studies are not frequently useful in evaluating these lesions. Optical coherence tomography demonstrated an elevated hyperreflective mass, hyporeflective shadowing of the underlying tissues, and cystoid macular edema (110).

Differential Diagnosis

Combined hamartoma can be challenging to distinguish from an epiretinal membrane, particularly when the hamartoma is minimally pigmented and minimally elevated. Both hamartoma and membrane involve vitreo-retinal interface changes associated with vascular tortuosity. Pigmentation and elevation are clues that the presentation is a hamartoma. Elevated and pigmented lesions can resemble choroidal melanoma, although the latter lesion does not have vitreoretinal interface changes or vascular tortuosity. Retinoblastoma or *Toxocara canis* may be considered initially in the differential diagnosis of lightly pigmented combined hamartomatous lesions in young children (111).

Peripapillary combined hamartoma has a presentation similar to morning glory disc anomaly, although the latter condition does not exhibit the characteristic elevation of combined hamartoma. With their tractional distortion of the retina, peripheral hamartomatous lesions can mimic retinopathy of prematurity.

Management

No well-established treatment plan has been developed for combined hamartoma of the retina and RPE. Therapy for this lesion has included treatment for amblyopia, which has demonstrated utility in selected patients (92). Vitreous surgery with epiretinal membrane removal is another treatment with reported success (112–114). Other patients with combined hamartoma have been treated with pars plana vitrectomy and membrane peeling without any subsequent improvement in their visual acuity (92,115).

Outcomes

Patients with combined hamartoma of the retina and RPE demonstrate a wide spectrum of visual acuity. In one study, approximately one-quarter of the patients lost at least two lines of visual acuity; approximately one-third of patients exhibited vision of 20/200 or worse (92). A patient affected with the characteristically unilateral form of this disease typically experiences normal vision in the unaffected eye. No report has been made of malignant transformation of combined hamartoma of the retina and RPE lesions. The prognosis for life in these patients is normal.

PHAKOMATOSES

The phakomatoses are a group of syndromes characterized by multiple associated lesions in multiple organ systems. Characteristically, patients with phakomatoses demonstrate hamartomatous malformations, which are abnormal proliferations of tissues that are normally found in the affected organ system. All these syndromes demonstrate ocular manifestations upon fundus examination. Phakomatoses discussed individually in this chapter include Von Hippel-Lindau syndrome, tuberous sclerosis, neurofibromatosis, Wyburn-Mason syndrome, and Sturge-Weber syndrome.

Von Hippel-Lindau Syndrome

Definition and Prevalence

Von Hippel-Lindau (VHL) syndrome is an autosomal dominant condition characterized by angiomas of the retina, cerebellum, brain stem, and spine, accompanied by adenomas, angiomas, and cysts of the kidney, liver, and pancreas. Renal cell carcinoma occurs in approximately 25% of VHL patients, and pheochromocytoma occurs in approximately 10% (62). Incidence of VHL is estimated at 1 in 36,000 births (116).

Pathology and Pathophysiology

Histopathologically, the retinal lesions of VHL are hemangioblastomas identical to the lesions also found in the central nervous system (CNS) (117). These vascular masses are composed of retinal capillaries exhibiting normal endothelium, basement membrane, and pericytes. Capillaries within the lesion may demonstrate abnormal fenestrations (118,119). Plump vacuolated interstitial cells with foamy cytoplasm, which are likely of glial origin, separate the capillary channels (117,120,121). Growth of these retinal lesions can extend inward toward the vitreous (endophytic type) or outward toward the choroid (exophytic type) (122,123).

Genetics and Environmental Factors

The pathogenesis of VHL disease is associated with a mutation in the VHL tumor suppressor gene (124). This syndrome follows an autosomal-dominant inheritance pattern with variable penetrance. The VHL gene was mapped to chromosome 3p25 in 1988, and was cloned in 1993 (125,126). Recent studies have suggested that tumor formation in VHL disease follows the "two-hit" model initially hypothesized by Knudson (116,126–128) for retinoblastoma. According to this model, germline transmission of one mutation (first hit) is followed by a genetic alteration of the second allele in specific somatic tissues (second hit) (129). Loss of both normal functioning alleles of the VHL gene results in subsequent loss of functional VHL protein. Normal VHL protein appears to down-regulate production of vascular endothelial growth factor (VEGF) (130,131). Both the absence of functioning VHL gene product, and the expected upregulation of VEGF have been demonstrated in retinal capillary hemangioma (127). Mutations in the VHL gene are highly variable and include large deletions, small deletions or insertions, and nonsense or missense point mutations (124). Genetic diagnosis by direct mutation analysis may be possible in up to 75% of families with VHL (132–134). DNA testing is a valuable tool in patients with retinal findings suggestive of VHL, particularly in families having no known history of the disease (135).

No specific environmental factors have been associated with VHL.

Clinical Features

Retinal hemangioblastoma is observed in approximately two-thirds of patients with VHL disease (136,137). Of reported VHL patients with retinal tumors, 25% will demonstrate associated cerebellar hemangioblastoma. Many other organs are affected by cysts, including the pancreas, kidneys, liver, adrenal glands, and epididymis. VHL is also characterized by renal cell carcinoma (22%), and pheochromocytoma is a less common but serious association (137). Although patients with VHL demonstrate brain and CNS tumor involvement, they exhibit normal cognitive capacity.

A patient with VHL disease may present with decreased visual acuity, or may be asymptomatic with retinal tumors discovered as an incidental finding upon routine ophthalmologic examination. Alternatively, a patient may become symptomatic when retinal lesions cause a visual field defect associated with subretinal fluid, or retinal detachment; these lesions may also cause metamorphopsia from a macular pucker. Retinal lesions in VHL may become visible upon ophthalmologic examination during childhood. Because patients are frequently asymptomatic, however, they may be diagnosed at any time throughout adulthood.

In VHL disease, retinal capillary hemangioma appears as globular red-orange masses in the fundus. A characteristic feature of these retinal tumors is a pair of dilated, tortuous feeding and draining vessels traveling between the lesion and the optic nerve (Fig. 15-4). Angiomas may form anywhere in the fundus: rarely at the posterior pole (1%), more commonly at the optic disc (8%), and most frequently in the temporal peripheral retina (136).

Patients with VHL disease demonstrate retinal masses that are solitary or multiple, with the mean number of these lesions in genetic carriers of the disease reported as 1.85 (range of 0 to 15) (136). Lesions may present either unilaterally or bilaterally. Solitary unilateral lesions are less likely to be associated with VHL disease, whereas multiple bilateral lesions are invariably indicative of VHL syndrome. The size of these lesions varies, ranging from small vascular tufts to large masses. Retinal tumors in VHL demonstrate limited ability to proliferate; however, leakage of thin vessels with subsequent fluid buildup may result in

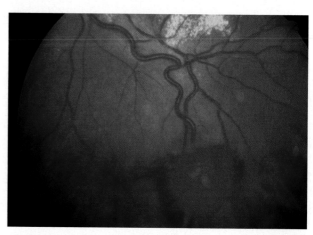

FIGURE 15-4. Retinal capillary hemangioma in Von Hippel-Lindau syndrome has a striking appearance. This example demonstrates a pair of tortuous feeder vessels.

the appearance of tumor growth. Lipid exudate in the macula is a common cause of decreased visual acuity in these patients.

Complications of retinal angioma in VHL include exudation of fluid into the subretinal space and subsequent retinal detachment. Preretinal membranes may form causing traction on the retina. Patients who develop retinal detachments are at significant risk for secondary glaucoma, cataract, or vitreous hemorrhage. Disc and retinal neovascularization may also occur.

Differential Diagnosis

The differential diagnosis of retinal capillary hemangioma associated with VHL disease varies with the location of the lesions. Peripheral lesions with dilated feeding and draining vessels are highly characteristic and are frequently diagnosed based on ophthalmoscopic appearance. In the presence of massive subretinal exudation with retinal detachment, however, the lesion may resemble other entities. In children, the differential diagnosis should primarily include Coats' disease, familial exudative vitreoretinopathy, and retinoblastoma. Additional lesions considered in the differential may include racemose hemangioma, retinal cavernous hemangioma, sickle cell retinopathy, retinal astrocytoma, and nematode endophthalmitis (138).

The differential diagnosis for juxtapapillary capillary hemangioma, particularly the exophytic form, involves entities distinct from those considered in the diagnosis of peripheral lesions. Exophytic juxtapapillary hemangioma may obscure the disc margin, making this lesion challenging to distinguish from other causes of disc edema. The swollen disc appearance in juxtapapillary capillary hemangioma is more frequently unilateral, although bilateral cases have been reported. Papilledema subsequent to increased intracranial pressure may be a diagnostic consideration in patients presenting with intracranial VHL lesions. Choroidal neovascularization and choroidal hemangioma may also enter the differential diagnosis in VHL (132,138).

Diagnostic Studies

Diagnosis of peripheral capillary hemangioma is frequently made prior to performing any ancillary studies because of the characteristic appearance of the lesion on ophthalmoscopy. Standard fundus photography is helpful to document lesion growth, stability, or response to treatment. FA shows rapid filling of the tumor by the feeding artery in early phases. Midphase photographs show intense staining of the tumor, and late frames show leakage of dye from the tumor into the vitreous (62,138). Fluorescein angiography may be particularly useful in distinguishing juxtapapillary capillary hemangioma from other causes of disc edema.

A detailed family history should be taken in all patients diagnosed with retinal hemangioblastoma, with suspicion of VHL disease. In addition, patients presenting with retinal hemangioblastoma should be screened for other manifestations of VHL, with an MRI of head and spine, as well as a CT scan of the abdomen.

Management

Whether in patients with solitary non-VHL lesions or in individuals in whom VHL disease is diagnosed, management of retinal capillary hemangioma is oriented toward reducing the destructive exudation associated with these lesions. Various methods for ablating retinal capillary hemangioma have been previously reported; mainstays of recent treatment, however, have included laser photocoagulation and cryotherapy (126,139–149). Small asymptomatic lesions may remain stable for many years, and observation on regular follow-up is an option in these patients (142). For symptomatic patients, laser photocoagulation is effective in treating smaller and more posterior lesions not associated with significant retinal detachment. Cryotherapy is efficacious in larger and more anterior lesions. In a recent large series, laser photocoagulation effectively controlled 18 of 18 (100%) extrapapillary hemangiomas measuring 1.5 mm or smaller in diameter, and 8 of 17 (47%) larger lesions (142). Seven of eight juxtapapillary lesions were controlled with laser. Extrapapillary lesions larger than 1.5 mm were successfully controlled with cryotherapy in 28 of 39 (72%) cases (142). More than one session of cryotherapy or laser treatment may be required for control of the exudative process. For lesions larger than 3.5 to 4 mm, treatment with plaque radiotherapy has been demonstrated to be more effective than cryotherapy (142,150). In cases involving large exudative detachments, rhegmatogenous detachments, or tractional detachments of the macula, operative intervention with scleral buckling or vitrectomy may be beneficial (151–154).

Treatment of retinal capillary hemangioma with transpupillary thermotherapy and photodynamic therapy has been recently reported (142,155–159). The role for these modalities in the treatment of capillary hemangioma remains unclear. Photodynamic therapy may demonstrate theoretical advantages over other treatments, and patients treated with this modality to date have reportedly done well (158,159).

Recent studies have also reported rapid and significant improvement in visual acuity in patients with VHL hemangioblastoma following systemic treatment with the VEGF receptor inhibitor SU5416 (160,161). Although lesion size remained unchanged by treatment in these studies, associated cystoid macular edema was significantly decreased (160,161). In patients with VHL-associated or solitary non-VHL angiomas, long-term follow-up is important to promptly detect, and if necessary to treat any further development of symptoms, growth of lesions, or new retinal tumors.

Outcomes

Untreated, retinal hemangioblastoma typically has a poor prognosis. Severe vision loss has been associated with presentation of retinal lesions at an early age (136). In one study, the prognosis for vision in patients presenting with retinal hemangioblastoma was reported as better in those individuals whose diagnosis did not include VHL disease than in those who were diagnosed with the VHL syndrome (162). Another study found equal visual outcome in both these groups (163).

In patients with VHL disease, associated nonocular malignancies, particularly renal cell carcinoma, indicate a worse prognosis. The most common causes of mortality in patients with VHL are cerebellar hemangioblastoma and renal cell carcinoma (137).

Future Treatments

Discovery of the VHL protein targeting hypoxia-inducible factors and the protein's role in angiogenesis may facilitate the development of new treatments. Development of drugs specifically active on hypoxia inducible factors and VEGF may play a role in future in treating VHL disease (164).

Tuberous Sclerosis
Definition and Prevalence

Tuberous sclerosis (TS) is a rare, hereditary phakomatosis first described by Bourneville (165) in 1880. The disorder has been characterized classically by a triad of presenting symptoms: seizures, cognitive developmental deficits, and adenoma sebaceum of the skin (166). Clinical expression of

TS, however, is highly variable. The National Tuberous Sclerosis Association has established a more complex set of diagnostic criteria based on the presence of one or more of the following features: adenoma sebaceum, ungual fibroma, cortical tubers, subependymal nodules, retinal astrocytic hamartoma, cardiac rhabdomyoma, hypopigmented (ash-leaf) skin patches, and infantile spasms, among other features (167). The incidence of TS has been estimated at 1 in 15,000 live births. Retinal astrocytic hamartoma develops in approximately 50% of patients with TS (168,169).

Genetics and Environmental Factors

Tuberous sclerosis is an autosomal dominant syndrome, demonstrating incomplete penetrance and variable expression. It is estimated that up to 80% of cases represent new mutations. Two genetic loci, 9q34 and 16p13.3, have been identified in association with TS. The TSC2 gene was identified in 1993; its protein product is called tuberin (170,171). Tuberin is a tumor suppressor, high levels of which are found in the brain, kidney, heart, skin, and vessels. The protein product of TSC1, hamartin, is also thought to function as a tumor suppressor. Hamartin and tuberin are believed to act in synergy to regulate cell growth and differentiation (170,171).

No specific environmental associations are known in TS.

Pathology and Pathophysiology

Histologically, retinal astrocytic hamartoma in TS is composed of spindle-shaped fibrous astrocytes containing small oval nuclei arising from the nerve fiber layer of the retina (172,173). Larger lesions may have areas of calcific degeneration and may contain cystoid spaces filled with serous exudate or blood (62). A rare histopathologic variant, giant cell astrocytoma has also been reported (174).

Clinical Features

Although the most common ocular manifestation of TS is the retinal astrocytic hamartoma, this lesion is not pathognomonic for the syndrome. Retinal astrocytoma is a benign lesion that can also occur in patients with neurofibromatosis, and rarely in the normal population. These retinal lesions are most commonly located near the macula, and, more rarely, may involve the optic disc, although they typically do not significantly affect vision. When associated with TS (or neurofibromatosis), retinal astrocytoma is more likely to be found in multiple lesions than when not associated with an underlying systemic condition (175).

Retinal astrocytoma can vary in appearance, and three basic types have been described (176). The first type, often found in young children, is flat with a smooth, translucent appearance. Frequently observed in older patients, the second type is nodular and elevated with a calcified

appearance. Although age associations with the type of lesion are observed, either of these two types may be demonstrated in patients of any age. Translucent retinal astrocytoma is more challenging to detect clinically, and in some presentations only the obscuration of the retinal vessels is observed. The nodular lesions are frequently more easily visualized, having a characteristic yellow-to-white coloration and a clusterlike appearance (Fig. 15-5). The third type of these astrocytic lesions exhibits characteristics of both of the other two forms. These mixed-type lesions may result from the translucent hamartoma form evolving over time into the mulberry cluster, calcified form, although this process has not been completely elucidated.

Retinal astrocytic hamartoma is frequently congenital and nonprogressive. These lesions have been reported in infancy, diagnosed within the first few weeks of life (177). In some cases, however, these retinal tumors have been reported to progress (175), and some have been observed to calcify over time (178). New lesions may arise from retina that appeared normal on presentation in some patients with TS, suggesting that not all retinal astrocytomas are congenital (178). Spontaneous regression of these retinal lesions in the setting of TS has been reported (179).

Complications of retinal astrocytic tumors reported in rare cases include vitreous seeding, vitreous hemorrhage, and vitreoretinal traction at the tumor surface (176,180,181). A rare invasive giant cell astrocytoma of the retina was reported in one patient presenting in infancy with TS. The tumor's steadily aggressive growth was associated

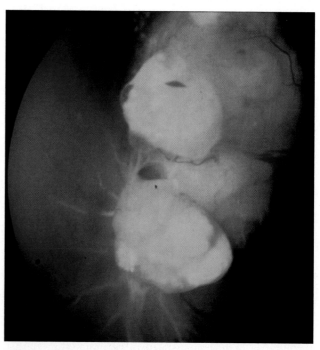

FIGURE 15-5. Astrocytic hamartomas in tuberous sclerosis vary greatly in appearance, but some of these tumors demonstrate this nodular, elevated, clusterlike configuration.

with subsequent development of neovascular glaucoma and spontaneous perforation of the sclera. Because the eye became blind and painful, enucleation was performed when the patient was 12 years of age (182).

Other ocular manifestations described in association with TS include fundus depigmentation, iris depigmentation, subconjunctival nodules, eyelid angiofibroma, hamartoma of the iris and ciliary epithelium, and ocular coloboma (176,177,183,184).

Nonophthalmologic features of TS include facial angiofibroma, ungular fibroma, benign lesions of the CNS (cortical tubers and cerebral astrocytoma), and hamartomatous tumors of virtually any organ in the body, including the kidneys, heart, liver, and lungs (185). Patients may demonstrate skin lesions such as hypopigmented macules ("ash-leaf spots"), which are characteristic of TS and are sometimes present at birth (Fig. 15-6). Also characteristic of TS are shagreen patches, which are thickened skin lesions commonly found on the back. Facial angiofibroma, referred to as adenoma sebaceum, is a condition associated with TS that presents in childhood and must be carefully distinguished from acne. Tuberous cortical lesions and nodular lesions in the basal ganglia and periventricular area are also presentations in TS. Seizures are frequently observed in patients with TS, and cognitive deficits or developmental delay are present in approximately half of TS patients. Malignant astrocytoma may present in TS, although this lesion is observed infrequently in this syndrome.

Diagnostic Studies

In patients with TS, retinal astrocytoma demonstrates early hypofluorescence on fluorescein angiography with late staining. A-scan ultrasound indicates a mass of medium reflectivity, while B-scan may demonstrate focal calcifications

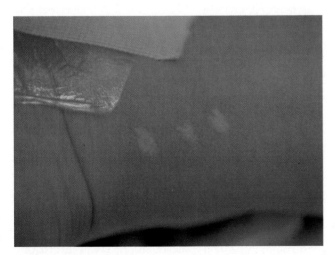

FIGURE 15-6. Hypopigmented macules, known as "ash leaf spots," are most often present at birth in patients with tuberous sclerosis. These cutaneous lesions can be useful in making the clinical diagnosis.

similar to those observed in retinoblastoma. The ultrasound pattern may closely correspond to that associated with choroidal osteoma and some cases of retinoblastoma (172). Diagnostic studies are frequently selected to distinguish TS from neurofibromatosis. Neuroimaging is helpful in demonstrating the subependymal nodules of TS, as well as in distinguishing the sphenoid dysplasia, meningioma, or vestibular schwannoma of neurofibromatosis.

Differential Diagnosis

Retinoblastoma is an important consideration in the differential diagnosis of retinal astrocytic hamartoma in TS, due to the frequent characteristic presence of focal areas of calcification in both types of lesions. Other entities within the differential diagnosis include amelanotic choroidal melanoma, Coats' disease, myelinated nerve fiber layer, and choroiditis. In patients with TS, systemic findings of the disease, such as the various skin lesions and intracranial findings, provide specific clues to aid in diagnosis.

Management

Except in rare cases, retinal astrocytic hamartoma of TS requires no treatment. Current treatments for this syndrome are supportive rather than curative. One complication of TS requiring long-term care is seizure, necessitating neurologic consultation and management. Antiepileptic drugs, dermatology treatments, and occupational therapy for developmental deficits are commonly employed in treating TS patients.

Outcomes

In patients with ocular lesions associated with TS, the prognosis for vision is good, because visual acuity is frequently unaffected unless retinal tumors involve the fovea. The most common causes of morbidity in patients with TS are neurologic complications of intractable seizures and hydrocephalus. Renal hamartoma in TS patients may also be associated with significant complications. Cardiac or pulmonary complications may arise in the presence of lesions in the heart or lungs.

Neurofibromatosis

Definition and Prevalence

Neurofibromatosis (NF) is a heritable phakomatosis characterized by lesions composed of melanocytes or neuroglial cells (187). Initial signs of the disease may be present at birth, or develop throughout childhood and adolescence as the disease progresses. NF-1 and NF-2 are two distinct forms of neurofibromatosis, each demonstrating different clinical and genetic features. The primary retinal lesions in NF-1 are astrocytic hamartomas, which can be identical to those found in TS. NF-1, the much more common form, affects approximately 1 in 4,000, while NF-2 affects approximately 1 in 50,000.

Genetics and Environmental Factors

Neurofibromatosis 1 and 2 are both autosomal dominant diseases with high penetrance. Nearly 50% of cases of NF-1 are sporadic, and the other half of cases is transmitted genetically. The gene for NF-1 is located on chromosome 17; the gene for NF-2 is on chromosome 22 (187).

Neurofibromin has been identified as the protein product of the NF-1 gene; this protein is believed to play a role in the regulation of cellular proliferation and tumor suppression. Mutation of the NF-1 gene leads to subsequent formation of the many different tumors of this syndrome. Pathogenesis of the tumors is believed to involve the Ras pathways (187). No known environmental factors are associated with NF.

Pathology and Pathophysiology

Neurofibromatosis is a disorder of the neuroectodermal cell line. NF tumors originate from neural crest cells, such as sensory neurons, Schwann cells, and melanocytes.

Clinical Features

Neurofibromatosis 1 is a progressive disease with numerous and variable manifestations affecting multiple organ systems including the eye, skin, and CNS. Retinal tumors associated with NF-1 include retinal astrocytic hamartoma (most common), retinal capillary hemangioma, and combined hamartoma of the RPE and retina. These lesions may all cause vision loss in these patients (188).

Similar to the retinal astrocytic lesions in TS, retinal astrocytic hamartomas in NF-1 are benign and are often located near the optic disc. One series reported 42 cases of astrocytic retinal tumors. Of these patients, 14% had neurofibromatosis, and their tumors were more frequently located adjacent to or on the disc (189). These lesions demonstrate the white, mulberry-cluster appearance of astrocytic hamartoma also observed in TS. Involvement of the retina by tumor is extensive with subsequent neovascular glaucoma and retinal detachment (188).

Combined hamartoma of the retina and RPE in neurofibromatosis has been reported (188,190,191). Retinal capillary hemangioma has also been described in association with NF (188,192). Optic nerve glioma is another characteristic tumor in NF-1, which can cause significant vision loss or proptosis. These lesions may be unilateral or bilateral and may also affect the optic chiasm. Optic nerve glioma typically presents symptomatically in young children. Nonocular complications of this tumor include pituitary dysfunction and hydrocephalus. Optic nerve sheath meningioma may also be associated with NF-1, although this lesion is less common in childhood.

Neurofibromatosis 1 is characterized by uveal masses of the iris and choroid. On dark irides, the iris lesions, termed "Lisch nodules," may appear hypopigmented, whereas on light irides the masses demonstrate darker pigmentation. The iris lesions increase in number with age and are observed nearly universally in adults with NF-1 (193). Choroidal lesions in NF-1 are less common than those in the iris, but are still demonstrated in approximately one-third of these patients as flat masses, ranging in coloration from white to yellow to darkly pigmented. Patients with NF-1 are also believed to have an increased risk for development of uveal melanoma.

Numerous nonocular findings are demonstrated in neurofibromatosis-1. Flat, hyperpigmented macules (café-au-lait spots) are the most common cutaneous presentation in this disease. The number and size of these cutaneous macules vary, and they become larger and more numerous with increasing age. Other distinctive findings in NF-1 include nodular cutaneous and subcutaneous neurofibroma, plexiform neurofibroma, and bony lesions. Plexiform neurofibroma in NF-1 may involve the eyelid, giving it an S-shaped appearance. These eyelid lesions may cause ptosis and may be challenging to resect.

Pheochromocytoma, other soft tissue tumors, and benign and malignant CNS tumors have also been reported in association with neurofibromatosis-1. Patients with CNS abnormalities may demonstrate hydrocephalus, seizures, cognitive deficits, and developmental delay. Other more occult findings of NF-1 include visceral tumors such as gastrointestinal neurofibromas, enlarged corneal nerves, choroidal ovoid bodies, and orbital neurofibromas.

Neurofibromatosis 2 presents significantly more rarely than neurofibromatosis-1. Briefly, NF-2 is characterized by acoustic neuroma, neurofibroma, meningioma, glioma, and/or schwannoma. The most common eye finding in NF-2 is either cortical or posterior subcapsular cataract (194). NF-2 patients often have a keratopathy secondary to facial palsies. As in NF-1, retinal hamartoma and Lisch nodules may be present, although these lesions are much less common in NF-2. Complications of both NF-1 and NF-2 arise primarily due to progression of the hamartomatous tumors in the eye, skin, and CNS.

Association of Neurofibromatosis 1 and Glaucoma

Neurofibromatosis 1 is associated with glaucoma, which is most commonly found ipsilateral to the eyelid involved by plexiform neurofibroma. In infancy, glaucoma in patients with NF-1 is associated with buphthalmos. NF-1 patients with glaucoma may demonstrate abnormalities of the trabecular meshwork, whereas others may exhibit angle closure due to progression of lesions infiltrating the angle.

Diagnostic Studies

Patients demonstrating any findings suggestive of neurofibromatosis-1 should have a complete ophthalmological examination to evaluate optic nerve function, iris, disc appearance, choroid, and intraocular pressure. On fluorescein angiography, retinal astrocytoma, the most common retinal lesion in NF-1, is hypofluorescent on early phases with late staining. B-scan ultrasonography may reveal focal calcifications in these lesions. CT scanning and MRI are helpful in evaluating extension of optic nerve or optic chiasm glioma, although routine screening with MRI in the absence of nerve abnormalities on ophthalmologic examination has not been suggested for all cases.

Differential Diagnosis

When neurofibromatosis 1 or 2 is suspected, the differential diagnosis of a retinal mass resembling an astrocytic hamartoma in a child or teenager should also include retinoblastoma, Coats' disease, toxoplasmosis, toxocariasis, and choroidal melanoma. Presentation with other associated manifestations of neurofibromatosis, including cutaneous lesions, is also diagnostically helpful.

Management

Treatment of retinal astrocytomas associated with neurofibromatosis is typically observational follow-up. In one series of patients with NF-1, however, these retinal lesions were threatening to vision in some cases, requiring surgical intervention including retinal detachment repair, photocoagulation, or cryopexy (188).

Treatment of optic nerve glioma is challenging due to this lesion's variable and sometimes unpredictable course. Optic nerve tumors in NF-1 frequently do not progress in the years immediately following diagnosis (195). Unless these lesions exhibit aggressive growth, they are often followed by observation. Surgical excision of optic nerve glioma can be globe-preserving, although resection frequently does not preserve vision in the affected eye. Radiation and chemotherapy have been employed as treatments in optic nerve glioma with varying degrees of success (196–198). Optic nerve glioma has also been reported to exhibit spontaneous regression (199).

A medical regimen is typically the initial treatment for NF-1 associated glaucoma, although this condition may prove intractable to medical therapy. Surgical intervention is frequently required including goniotomy, trabeculotomy, trabeculectomy, and installation of an aqueous shunt.

Treatment of cutaneous manifestations of NF includes possible resection of the neurofibroma tumors. These lesions often recur, however, and they are only excised in cases in which the patient is experiencing pain or significant impairment. Pigmentation defects in neurofibromatosis are not treated. CNS manifestations of this disease may require treatment with anticonvulsants, and, in the setting of hydrocephalus, neurosurgical treatment may be necessary. Visceral tumors may also require surgical resection.

Outcomes

Visual acuity in NF-1 patients with optic nerve abnormalities is often reduced, particularly in patients demonstrating concurrent amblyopia in the affected eye. Patients may have increased morbidity and mortality when they exhibit more severe presentations of neurofibromatosis, such as CNS tumors, severe seizures, or other aggressive malignancies.

Future Treatments

Knowledge of the role in tumorigenesis of the Ras protein pathway in neurofibromatosis has led to the evaluation of the utility of Ras inhibitors in treatment of these patients (200,201).

Wyburn-Mason Syndrome

Definition and Prevalence

Initially described and named after its discoverer in 1943, Wyburn-Mason syndrome (WMS) is a rare, nonheritable disorder characterized by arteriovenous (AV) malformations of the eye and CNS (202). Congenital AV malformations in WMS primarily involve the retina, optic disc, and midbrain; the retinal lesion is known as racemose hemangioma. AV malformations may also occur elsewhere in the body in WMS, including the skin, nasopharynx, orbit, lung, and spine. Although the exact incidence is unreported, WMS is considered a rare condition worldwide.

Genetics and Environmental Factors

Wyburn-Mason syndrome is nonheritable, and no known genetic associations or environmental factors have been found.

Pathology and Pathophysiology

Although it has been determined that WMS is a congenital, nonheritable disorder, the pathogenesis has not otherwise been delineated (203,204). Vessel walls demonstrate fibromuscular medial coats of variable thickness and acellular fibrohyalin adventitial coverings. Dilated vascular channels may occupy the entire thickness of the retina. Cystoid changes may be observed, as well as loss of ganglion cell bodies and axons (205,206). Further details of the histopathology of racemose hemangioma in WMS remain to be discovered.

Clinical Features

Most patients with racemose hemangioma in WMS experience reduced visual acuity. The extent of the vascular malformation varies widely, and the lesions have been divided into three groups with clinicopathologic characteristics ranging from least to most severe (205). Group I is comprised of patients demonstrating interposition of an abnormal capillary plexus between a major communicating artery and vein. These patients are typically asymptomatic, and retinal lesions in this group are rarely associated with cerebrovascular malformations. Group II patients demonstrate direct arteriovenous communications without the interposition of capillary elements. Microvasculature adjacent to AV lesions may be altered, and beading and multiple fusiform dilations of the large vessel walls may be observed. Group III patients demonstrate many anastomosing channels of large caliber. These channels are so intertwined and convoluted that separation into their arterial and venous components may be difficult. Perivascular sheathing, exudation, and pigmentary degeneration may also be observed. Fundus changes in group III patients are similar to those originally described by Wyburn-Mason (138,202,203), and visual acuity in this group is frequently poor. Group III patients also demonstrate a high incidence of CNS lesions (138,203). One study suggests that group I and II retinal vascular lesions are typically isolated. If patients in these first two groups are asymptomatic, systemic work-up is not indicated (207). More severe cases may be associated with retinal vascular occlusion, retinal ischemia, and focal exudation, which can lead to progressive vision loss (207–210). Racemose hemangioma manifests unilaterally and is typically nonprogressive although the pattern of vascular tortuosity may alter over time.

Central nervous system AV malformations in WMS are more frequently observed ipsilateral to the retinal lesions. In one series of 80 cases of retinal AV malformations, 30% of these patients also demonstrated CNS malformations (211). Retinal lesions in WMS may extend from an intracranial AV malformation, traveling along the optic nerve to the retinal vasculature.

Visual acuity in WMS patients with retinal AV malformations depends upon the size and extent of the defective vasculature, and ranges from normal to severely reduced. Patients with diffuse, large, markedly dilated, and tortuous vessels are frequently severely impaired, and are consequently often diagnosed earlier than asymptomatic patients with milder forms of WMS. Reported visual field defects in patients with this syndrome indicate scotoma associated with retinal arteriovenous malformations (212). Complications of the retinal AV malformations reported in WMS include intraocular hemorrhage, secondary neovascular glaucoma, macular hole, central retinal vein obstruction, macroaneurysm, retinal hemorrhage, and vitreous hemorrhage (213). Extensive exudation and retinal detachment are not typical in racemose hemangioma.

Neurologic symptoms in WMS depend on the location and size of the CNS lesions. Patients demonstrating these lesions may develop headaches, cranial nerve palsies, visual field abnormalities, seizures, weakness, mental status changes, and papilledema. CNS lesions in WMS are commonly hemorrhagic.

Diagnostic Studies

In most cases, the diagnosis of racemose hemangioma in WMS may be determined upon examination by indirect ophthalmoscopy. FA demonstrates rapid filling of the vascular malformation and provides dramatic documentation of the lesion. MRI of the brain is indicated to delineate CNS manifestations in patients with more severe forms of WMS.

Differential Diagnosis

Other retinal vascular abnormalities, such as retinal arterial and venous collaterals and retinal telangiectasis, should be included in the differential diagnosis of racemose hemangioma in WMS.

Management

No treatment is indicated for the primary lesions in WMS. The utility of laser photocoagulation or cryotherapy for these lesions has yet to be clearly defined.

Outcomes

Visual prognosis for patients with ocular AV malformations in WMS varies widely depending upon the extent of retinal or optic nerve involvement. In patients demonstrating less severe forms of this disease, the prognosis for vision and quality of life is typically good. For patients with more severe manifestations of WMS, associated CNS vascular malformations can lead to cerebral hemorrhage with potentially devastating consequences.

Sturge-Weber Syndrome

Definition and Prevalence

Sturge-Weber syndrome (SWS) is a nonhereditary phakomatosis manifesting in a range of symptoms from partial to complete expression of the disease. In its complete form, SWS is characterized by ipsilateral angiomatous malformations involving the face, brain, and eye. Patients frequently demonstrate seizures and intracranial calcifications (204,214). Characteristic ocular findings of SWS include diffuse choroidal hemangioma and glaucoma (215,216). The exact incidence and prevalence of SWS are not known.

Pathology and Pathophysiology

In contrast to circumscribed choroidal hemangioma, the diffuse type observed in SWS demonstrates a gradual transition at the margin of the lesion with progressively less engorgement of the vessels as observed on light microscopy (216). In one large histopathologic series, diffuse choroidal hemangiomas were classified as mixed cavernous and capillary type tumors exhibiting both large and small blood vessels (216).

The pathogenesis of SWS is poorly understood. SWS is believed to be associated with a defect in neural crest cell migration and differentiation (217). These precursor cells give rise to ocular tissues, meninges, and the dermis. Over-production of angiogenic factors may play a role in the pathogenesis of this disease.

Genetics and Environmental Factors

Sturge-Weber syndrome is associated with no known environmental or genetic factors.

Clinical Features

Patients with SWS are usually diagnosed at birth or in early infancy when the presence of a facial hemangioma (port wine stain or nevus flammeus) prompts evaluation. Choroidal thickening associated with diffuse choroidal hemangioma may produce prominent hyperopia with associated anisometropic amblyopia. Glaucoma may result from iris neovascularization or from episcleral vascular changes associated with SWS. On fundus examination of patients with choroidal hemangioma, a diffuse red or orange thickening of the choroid is observed posteriorly. In some cases, the fundus of the affected eye demonstrates a dramatically deeper red coloration than that of the opposite eye, and the term "tomato-catsup fundus" has been used to describe this appearance (218). Diffuse choroidal hemangioma in SWS is usually thickest in the macular region, and then blends imperceptibly into the normal choroid anteriorly.

Dilated and tortuous retinal vessels are commonly observed in eyes with diffuse choroidal hemangioma. Patients with SWS may also demonstrate exudative retinal detachment with cystoid degeneration of the macula. These exudative detachments are associated with subretinal fluid that shifts with movement of the patient's head. Total retinal detachment with secondary cataract and leukocoria may be observed (204,214,219). Development of choroidal neovascularization associated with choroidal hemangioma has also been described (220).

Glaucoma is the most common and most serious ocular manifestation in SWS, presenting in approximately 70% of SWS patients (215). Intraocular pressure may be elevated at birth as a form of congenital glaucoma, or glaucoma may become symptomatic later during childhood. Intraocular pressure in patients with SWS may be elevated secondary to increased episcleral venous pressure or a developmental defect in the angle. Additional ocular manifestations in patients with SWS include vascular malformations of the eyelids, episclera, conjunctiva, retina, and choroid. Patients with SWS may demonstrate retinal vascular tortuosity, iris heterochromia, and strabismus (215). SWS with bilateral optic neuropathy has been reported (221).

Cutaneous and CNS lesions of SWS are also congenital. Cutaneous lesions, or nevus flammeus, present ipsilaterally to brain vascular malformations. Characteristically, SWS patients demonstrate a sharply demarcated port-wine--colored lesion that may involve the scalp, forehead, eyelids, and lower face. These cutaneous lesions may undergo thickening over time, with hypertrophy of underlying bone and soft tissues. CNS angiomatosis in SWS may lead to calcium deposition in the brain. Decreased cerebral volume with venous abnormalities and enlargement of the choroid plexus may also be observed. Clinically, these lesions may present in SWS patients as seizures, cognitive developmental deficits, hemiplegia, and other focal neurologic deficits.

Diagnostic Studies

Sturge-Weber syndrome is frequently diagnosed clinically based upon the presence of a port-wine stain and choroidal thickening due to diffuse choroidal hemangioma, as well as upon other characteristic ocular and CNS symptoms. Ultrasonography and fluorescein angiography may be useful diagnostic aids in some cases. B-scan ultrasonography demonstrates marked thickening of the choroid, often with overlying retinal detachment, while A-scan ultrasound demonstrates high internal reflectivity. On fluorescein angiography, widespread early filling of the tumor with late leakage is observed (204,219). Although not commonly utilized in SWS, CT and MRI scans can be helpful because CT scan can demonstrate abnormal thickening of the choroid with enhancement of the globe, while MRI exhibits a distinctive high signal on T1-weighted images (222).

Differential Diagnosis

The differential diagnosis of choroidal hemangioma in SWS includes circumscribed choroidal hemangioma unassociated with SWS, amelanotic choroidal nevus or melanoma, choroidal osteoma, retinal pigment epithelial detachment, scleritis, and retinal capillary hemangioma.

Management and Outcomes

In SWS, children with diffuse choroidal hemangioma may demonstrate associated hyperopic shift, glaucoma, and exudative retinal detachment. Refraction, corrective lenses, and amblyopia therapy are indicated for hyperopia and anisometropic amblyopia. Port-wine lesions may be treated with laser to decrease vascularity for improved cosmesis. When glaucoma is treated with filtering surgery, subretinal exudation may worsen in the early postoperative period. Visual acuity in patients with SWS-associated glaucoma has been reported to be 20/40 or better in two-thirds of patients (215).

Several modalities have been described in the treatment of exudative retinal detachment associated with diffuse choroidal hemangioma. Because hemangioma and associated retinal detachment are more extensive in SWS, treatment for diffuse choroidal hemangioma in this syndrome has not been as successful as in the circumscribed variety. Xenon- and argon-laser photocoagulation have been employed in treating these lesions although achieving resolution of subretinal fluid may be challenging (204,214,219). Radiation treatment in diffuse choroidal hemangioma has been used with some success (223–226). In a series of five patients with SWS, treatment of diffuse choroidal hemangioma with lens-sparing external beam radiotherapy was examined. A total dose ranging from 1,200 to 4,000 cGy in fraction sizes from 150 to 200 cGy was used (223). Radiation treatment resulted in complete resolution of retinal detachment in all five cases. With a mean follow-up of 40 months, two patients had significant improvement in visual acuity, and the other three had no change. No recurrence of subretinal fluid or cataract formation was reported during the follow-up period in any of the five patients (223).

REFERENCES

1. Gass JD. *Stereoscopic atlas of macular diseases.* St Louis: CV Mosby, 1997:208–212.
2. Shields JA, Shields CL. *Atlas of intraocular tumors.* Philadelphia: Lippincott Williams & Wilkins, 1999:170–179.
3. Shields JA, Shields CL. *Intraocular tumors. A text and atlas.* Philadelphia: WB Saunders, 1992:252–255.
4. Char DH. *Tumors of the eye and ocular adnexa.* Lewiston, NY: BC Decker, 2001:107–108.
5. Witschel H, Font RL. Hemangioma of the choroid. A clinicopathologic study of 71 cases and a review of the literature. *Surv Ophthalmol* 1976;20:415–431.
6. Heimann K. The development of the choroid in man. *Ophthalmol Res* 1972:257–273.
7. Shields CL, Honavar SG, Shields JA, Cater J, Demirici H. Circumscribed choroidal hemangioma: clinical manifestations and factors predictive of visual outcome in 200 consecutive cases. *Ophthalmology* 2001;108:2237–2248.
8. Anand R, Augsburger JJ, Shields JA. Circumscribed choroidal hemangiomas. *Arch Ophthalmol* 1989;107:1338–1342.
9. Medlock RD, Augsburger JJ, Wilkinson CP, et al. Enlargement of circumscribed choroidal hemangiomas. *Retina* 1991;11:385–388.
10. Shields JA, Stephens RF, Eagle RC Jr, et al. Progressive enlargement of a circumscribed choroidal hemangioma. A clinicopathologic correlation. *Arch Ophthalmol* 1992;110:1276–1278.
11. Ruby AJ, Jampol LM, Goldberg MF, et al. Choroidal neovascularization associated with choroidal hemangiomas. *Arch Ophthalmol* 1992;110:658–661.

12a. Norton EWD, Gutman F. Fluorescein angiography and hemangiomas of the choroid. *Arch Ophthalmol* 1967;78:121–125.
12b. Shields CL, Shields JA, De Potter P. Patterns of indocyanine green videoangiography of choroidal tumors. *Br J Ophthalmol* 1995;79:237–245.
13. Sanborn GE, Augsburger JJ, Shields JA. Treatment of circumscribed choroidal hemangiomas. *Ophthalmology* 1982;89:1374–1380.
14. Zografos L, Bercher L, Chamot L, et al. Cobalt-60 treatment of choroidal hemangiomas. *Am J Ophthalmol* 1996;121:190–199.
15. Shields JA. Radiotherapy of circumscribed choroidal hemangiomas. *Ophthalmology* 1997;104:1784.
16. Schilling H, Bornfeld N. Long-term results after low-dose ocular irradiation for choroidal hemangiomas. *Curr Opin Ophthalmol* 1998;9:51–55.
17. Hannouche D, Frau E, Desjardins L, et al. Efficacy of proton therapy in circumscribed choroidal hemangiomas associated with serous retinal detachment. *Ophthalmology* 1997;104:100–103.
18. Zografos L, Egger E, Bercher L, et al. Proton beam irradiation of choroidal hemangiomas. *Am J Ophthalmol* 1998;126:261–268.
19. Othmane IS, Shields CL, Shields JA, et al. Circumscribed choroidal hemangioma managed by transpupillary thermotherapy. *Arch Ophthalmol* 1999;117:136–137.
20. Porrini G, Giovannini A, Amato G, et al. Photodynamic therapy of circumscribed choroidal hemangioma. *Ophthalmology* 2003;110:674–680.
21. Schmidt-Erfurth UM, Michels S, Kusserow C, et al. Photodynamic therapy for symptomatic choroidal hemangioma: visual and anatomic results. *Ophthalmology* 2002;109:2284–2294.
22. Barbazetto I., Schmidt-Erfurth U. Photodynamic therapy of choroidal hemangioma: two case reports. *Graefes Arch Clin Exp Ophthalmol* 2000;238:214–221.
23. Madreperla SA. Choroidal hemangioma treated with photodynamic therapy using verteporfin. *Arch Ophthalmol* 2001;119:1606–1610.
24. Robertson DM. Photodynamic therapy for choroidal hemangioma associated with serous retinal detachment. *Arch Ophthalmol* 2002;120:1155–1161.
25. Sheidow TG, Harbour JW. Photodynamic therapy for circumscribed choroidal hemangioma. *Can J Ophthalmol* 2002;37:314–317.
26. Jurklies B, Anastassiou G, Ortmans S, et al. Photodynamic therapy using verteporfin in circumscribed choroidal haemangioma. *Br J Ophthalmol* 2003;87:84–89.
27. Shields JA, Shields CL. *Intraocular tumors: A text and atlas.* Philadelphia: WB Saunders, 1992:465–481.
28. Verhoeff FH. A rare tumor arising from the pars ciliaris retinae (teratoneuroma), of a nature hitherto unrecognized and its relation to the so-called glioma retinae. *Trans Am Ophthalmol Soc* 1904;10:351–377.
29. Yanko L, Behar A. Teratoid intraocular medulloepithelioma. *Am J Ophthalmol* 1978;85:850–853.
30. Broughton WC, Zimmerman LE. A clinicopathologic study of 56 cases of intraocular medulloepithelioma. *Am J Ophthalmol* 1978;85:407–418.
31. Canning CR, McCartney AC, Hungerford J. Medulloepithelioma (diktyoma). *Br J Ophthalmol* 1988;72:764–767.
32. Hennis HL, Saunders RA, Shields JA. Malignant teratoid medulloepithelioma of the ciliary body. *J Clin Neuroophthalmol* 1990;10:291–292.
33. Shields JA, Eagle RC Jr, Shields CL, Potter PD. Congenital neoplasms of the nonpigmented ciliary epithelium (medulloepithelioma). *Ophthalmology* 1996;103:1998–2006.
34. Anderson SR. Medulloepithelioma of the retina. *Int Ophthalmol Clin* 1962;483–506.

35. O'Keefe M, Fulcher T, Kelly P, et al. Medulloepithelioma of the optic nerve head. *Arch Ophthalmol* 1997;115:1325–1327.

36. Mullaney J. Primary malignant medulloepithelioma of the retina stalk. *Am J Ophthalmol* 1974;77:499–504.

37. Steinkuller PG, Font RL. Congenital malignant teratoid neoplasm of the eye and orbit: case report and review of the literature. *Ophthalmology* 1997;104:38–42.

38. Brownstein S, Barsoum-Homsy M, Conway VH, et al. Nonteratoid medulloepithelioma of the ciliary body. *Ophthalmology* 1984;91:1118–1122.

39. Singh A, Singh AD, Shields CL, et al. Iris neovascularization in children as a manifestation of underlying medulloepithelioma. *J Pediatr Ophthalmol Strabismus* 2001;38:224–228.

40. Foster RE, Murray RG, Byrne SF, et al. Echographic features of medulloepithelioma. *Am J Ophthalmol* 2000;130:364–366.

41. Shields JA, Eagle RC Jr, Shields CL, et al. Fluorescein angiography and ultrasonography of malignant intraocular medulloepithelioma. *J Pediatr Ophthalmol Strabismus* 1996;33:193–196.

42. Husain SE, Husain N, Boniuk M, et al. Malignant nonteratoid medulloepithelioma of the ciliary body in an adult. *Ophthalmology* 1998;105:596–599.

43. Orellana J, Moura RA, Font RL, et al. Medulloepithelioma diagnosed by ultrasound and vitreous aspirate. Electron microscopic observations. *Ophthalmology* 1983;90:1531–1539.

44. Gass JD, Guerry RK, Jack RL, et al. Choroidal osteoma. *Arch Ophthalmol* 1978;96:428–435.

45. Browning DJ. Choroidal osteoma: observations from a community setting. *Ophthalmology* 2003;110:1327–1334.

46. Shields CL, Shields JA, Augsburger JJ. Choroidal osteoma. *Surv Ophthalmol* 1988;33:17–27.

47. Trimble SN, Schatz H. Choroidal osteoma after intraocular inflammation. *Am J Ophthalmol* 1983;96:759–764.

48. Williams AT, Font RL, Van Dyk HJ, et al. Osseous choristoma of the choroid simulating a choroidal melanoma. Association with a positive 32P test. *Arch Ophthalmol* 1978;96: 1874–1877.

49. Katz RS, Gass JD. Multiple choroidal osteomas developing in association with recurrent orbital inflammatory pseudotumor. *Arch Ophthalmol* 1983;101:1724–1727.

50. Noble KG. Bilateral choroidal osteoma in three siblings. *Am J Ophthalmol* 1990;109:656–660.

51. Kadrmas EF, Weiter JJ. Choroidal osteoma. *Int Ophthalmol Clin* 1997;37:171–182.

52. Gass JDM. New observations concerning choroidal osteomas. *Int Ophthalmol* 1979;1:71–84.

53. Aylward GW, Chang TS, Pautler SE, et al. A long-term follow-up of choroidal osteoma. *Arch Ophthalmol* 1998;116: 1337–1341.

54. Zsuzsanna P, Balint K. A case of a fast-growing bilateral choroidal osteoma. *Retina* 2001;21:657–659.

55. Buettner H. Spontaneous involution of a choroidal osteoma. *Arch Ophthalmol* 1990;108:1517–1518.

56. De Potter P, Shields, JA, Shields CL. Magnetic resonance imaging in choroidal osteoma. *Retina* 1991;11:221–223.

57. Lambert HM, Sipperley JO, Shore JW, et al. Linear nevus sebaceous syndrome. *Ophthalmology* 1987;94:278–282.

58. Rose SJ, Burke JF, Brockhurst RJ. Argon laser photoablation of a choroidal osteoma. *Retina* 1991;11:224–228.

59. Morrison DL, Magargal LE, Ehrlich DR, et al. Review of choroidal osteoma: successful krypton red laser photocoagulation of an associated subretinal neovascular membrane involving the fovea. *Ophthalmic Surg* 1987;18:299–303.

60. Battaglia Parodi M, Da Pozzo S, et al. Photodynamic therapy for choroidal neovascularization associated with choroidal osteoma. *Retina* 2001;21:660–661.

61. Buettner H. Congenital hypertrophy of the retinal pigment epithelium. *Am J Ophthalmol* 1975;79:177–189.

62. Gass JM. Developmental tumors of the retinal pigment epithelium and retina. In: Gass JM, ed. *Stereoscopic atlas of macular diseases*. St. Louis: Mosby-Year Book, 1997:809–865.

63. Shields JA, Shields CL. Tumors and related lesions of the pigment epithelium. In: Zorab R, ed. *Intraocular tumors: a text and atlas*. Philadelphia: WB Saunders, 1992:437–444.

64. Blair NP, Trempe CL. Hypertrophy of the retinal pigment epithelium associated with Gardner's syndrome. *Am J Ophthalmol* 1980;90:661–667.

65. Aiello LP, Traboulsi E. Pigmented fundus lesions in a preterm infant with familial adenomatous polyposis. *Arch Ophthalmol* 1993;111:302–303.

66. Pang CP, Fan DS, Keung JW, et al. Congenital hypertrophy of the retinal pigment epithelium and APC mutations in Chinese with familial adenomatous polyposis. *Ophthalmologica* 2001;215:408–411.

67. Romania A. Congenital hypertrophy of the retinal pigment epithelium in familial adenomatous polyposis. *Ophthalmology* 1989;96:879–884.

68. Berk T, Cohen Z, McLeod RS, Parker JA. Congenital hypertrophy of the retinal pigment epithelium as a marker for familial adenomatous polyposis. *Dis Colon Rectum* 1988; 31:253–257.

69. Diaz-Llopis M, Menezo JL. Congenital hypertrophy of the retinal pigment epithelium and familial polyposis of the colon. *Am J Ophthalmol* 1987;103:235–236.

70. Diaz-Llopis M, Menezo JL. Congenital hypertrophy of the retinal pigment epithelium in familial adenomatous polyposis. *Arch Ophthalmol* 1988;106:412–413.

71. Traboulsi EI, Maumenee IH, Krush AJ, et al. Pigmented ocular fundus lesions in the inherited gastrointestinal polyposis syndromes and in hereditary nonpolyposis colorectal cancer. *Ophthalmology* 1988;95:964–969.

72. Lynch HT, Priluck I, Fitzsimmons ML. Congenital hypertrophy of retinal pigment epithelium in non-Gardner's polyposis kindreds. *Lancet* 1987;2:333.

73. Buettner H. Congenital hypertrophy of the retinal pigment epithelium in familial polyposis coli. *Int Ophthalmol* 1987; 10:109–110.

74. Tiret A, Parc C. Fundus lesions of adenomatous polyposis. *Curr Opin Ophthalmol* 1999;10:168–172.

75. Groden J, Thliveris A, Samowitz M, et al. Identification and characterization of the familial adenomatous polyposis coli gene. *Cell* 1991;66:589–600.

76. Kinzler KW, Nilbert MC, Vogelstein B, et al. Identification of a gene located at chromosome 5q21 that is mutated in colorectal cancers. *Science* 1991;251:1366–1370.

77. Kartheuser A, West S, Walon C, et al. The genetic background of familial adenomatous polyposis. Linkage analysis, the APC gene identification and mutation screening. *Acta Gastroenterol Belg* 1995;58:433–451.

78. Olschwang S, Tiret A, Laurent-Puig P, et al. Restriction of ocular fundus lesions to a specific subgroup of APC mutations in adenomatous polyposis coli patients. *Cell* 1993;75: 959–968.

79. Traboulsi EI, Murphy SF, de la Cruz ZC, et al. A clinicopathologic study of the eyes in familial adenomatous polyposis with extracolonic manifestations (Gardner's syndrome). *Am J Ophthalmol* 1990;110:550–561.

80. Caspari R, Olschwang S, Friedl W, et al. Familial adenomatous polyposis: desmoid tumours and lack of ophthalmic lesions (CHRPE) associated with APC mutations beyond codon 1444. *Human Mol Genet* 1995;4:337–340.

81. Kasner L, Traboulsi EI, Delacruz Z, et al. A histopathologic study of the pigmented fundus lesions in familial adenomatous polyposis. *Retina* 1992;12:35–42.

82. Lloyd WC III, Eagle RC Jr, Shields JA, et al. Congenital hypertrophy of the retinal pigment epithelium: Electron microscopic and morphometric observations. *Ophthalmology* 1990;97:1052–1060.

83. Tiret A, Taiel-Sartral M, Tiret E, et al. Diagnostic value of fundus examination in familial adenomatous polyposis. *Br J Ophthalmol* 1997;81:755–758.

84. Purcell JJ, Shields JA. Hypertrophy with hyperpigmentation of the retinal pigment epithelium. *Arch Ophthalmol* 1975;93:1122–1126.

85. Shields JA, Shields CL, Singh AD. Acquired tumors arising from congenital hypertrophy of the retinal pigment epithelium. *Arch Ophthalmol* 2000;118:637–641.

86. Shields JA, Shields CL, Eagle RC, et al. Adenocarcinoma arising from congenital hypertrophy of the retinal pigment epithelium. *Arch Ophthalmol* 2001;119:597–602.

87. Traboulsi EI, Krush AJ, Gardner EJ, et al. Prevalence and importance of pigmented ocular fundus lesions in Gardner's syndrome. *N Engl J Med* 1987;316:661–667.

88. Parker JA, Berk T, Bapat BV. Familial variation in retinal pigmentation in adenomatous polyposis. *Can J Ophthalmol* 1995;30:138–141.

89. Gass JDM. An unusual hamartoma of the pigment epithelium and retina simulating choroidal melanoma and retinoblastoma. *Trans Am Ophthalmol Soc* 1973;71:171–183.

90. Laqua H, Wessing A. Congenital retino-pigment epithelial malformation, previously described as hamartoma. *Am J Ophthalmol* 1979;87:34–42.

91. Vogel MH, Zimmerman LE, Gass JDM. Proliferation of the juxtapapillary retinal pigment epithelium simulating malignant melanoma. *Doc Ophthalmol* 1969;26:461–481.

92. Schachat AP, Shields JA, Fine SL, et al. Combined hamartomas of the retina and retinal pigment epithelium. *Ophthalmology* 1984;91:1609–1615.

93. Wang CL, Brucker AJ. Vitreous hemorrhage secondary to juxtapapillary vascular hamartoma of the retina. *Retina* 1984;4:44–47.

94. Palmer ML, Carney MD, Combs JL. Combined hamartomas of the retinal pigment epithelium and retina. *Retina* 1990;10:33–36.

95. Fonseca RA, Dantas MA, Kaga T, et al. Combined hamartoma of the retina and retinal pigment epithelium associated with juvenile nasopharyngeal angiofibroma. *Am J Ophthalmol* 2001;132:131–132.

96. De Potter P, Stanescu D, Caspers-Velu L, et al. Photo essay: combined hamartoma of the retina and retinal pigment epithelium in Gorlin syndrome. *Arch Ophthalmol* 2000;118: 1004–1005.

97. Shields JA, Shields CL. *Intraocular tumors.* A text and atlas. Philadelphia: WB Saunders, 1992:446–449.

98. Blumenthal EZ, Papmichael G, Merin S. Combined hamartoma of the retina and retinal pigment epithelium: a bilateral presentation. *Retina* 1998;18:557–559.

99. Good WV, Erodsky MC, Edwards MS, Hoyt WF. Bilateral retinal hamartomas in neurofibromatosis type 2. *Br J Ophthalmol* 1991;75:190.

100. Sivalingam A, Augsburger J, Perilongo G, et al. Combined hamartoma of the retina and retinal pigment epithelium in a patient with neurofibromatosis type 2. *J Pediatr Ophthalmol Strabismus* 1991;28:320–322.

101. Bouzas EA, Parry DM, Eldridge R, et al. Familial occurrence of combined pigment epithelial and retinal hamartomas associated with neurofibromatosis 2. *Retina* 1992;12:103–107.

102. Destro M, D'Amico DJ, Gragoudas ES, et al. Retinal manifestations of neurofibromatosis. Diagnosis and management. *Arch Ophthalmol* 1991;109:662–666.

103. Cotlier E. Cafe-au-lait spots of the fundus in neurofibromatosis. *Arch Ophthalmol* 1977;95:1990–1992.

104. Landau K, Dossetor FM, Hoyt WF, et al. Retinal hamartoma in neurofibromatosis 2. *Arch Ophthalmol* 1990;108:328–329.

105. McLean EB. Hamartoma of the retinal pigment epithelium. *Am J Ophthalmol* 1976;82:227–231.

106. Rosenberg PR, Walsh JB. Retinal pigment epithelial hamartoma—unusual manifestations. *Br J Ophthalmol* 1984;68:439–442.

107. Font RL, Moura RA, Shetlar DJ, et al. Combined hamartoma of sensory retina and retinal pigment epithelium. *Retina* 1989;9:302–311.

108. Schachat AP, Glaser BM. Retinal hamartoma, acquired retinoschisis, and retinal hole. *Am J Ophthalmol* 1985;99:604–605.

109. Kahn D, Goldberg MF, Jednock N. Combined retinal–retina pigment epithelial hamartoma presenting as a vitreous hemorrhage. *Retina* 1984;4:40–43.

110. Ting TD, McCuen BW II, Fekrat S. Combined hamartoma of the retina and retinal pigment epithelium: optical coherence tomography. *Retina* 2002;22:98–101.

111. Eliott D, Schachat AP. Combined hamartoma of the retina and retinal pigment epithelium. In: Ryan SJ, ed. *Retina.* St. Louis: Mosby, 2001:640–646.

112. Sappenfield DL, Gitter KA. Surgical intervention for combined retinal–retinal pigment epithelial hamartoma. *Retina* 1990;10:119–124.

113. Mason JO III. Visual improvement after pars plana vitrectomy and membrane peeling for vitreoretinal traction associated with combined hamartoma of the retina and retinal pigment epithelium. *Retina* 2002;22:824–825.

114. Stallman JB. Visual improvement after pars plana vitrectomy and membrane peeling for vitreoretinal traction associated with combined hamartoma of the retina and retinal pigment epithelium. *Retina* 2002;22:101–104.

115. McDonald HR, Abrams GW, Burke JM, et al. Clinicopathologic results of vitreous surgery for epiretinal membranes in patients with combined retinal and retinal pigment epithelial hamartomas. *Am J Ophthalmol* 1985;100:806–813.

116. Maher ER, Iselius L, Yates JR, et al. Von Hippel-Lindau disease: a genetic study. *J Med Genet* 1991;28:443–447.

117. Grossniklaus HE, Thomas JW, Vigneswaran N. Retinal hemangioblastoma. A histologic, immunohistochemical, and ultrastructural evaluation. *Ophthalmology* 1992;99:140–145.

118. Mottow-Lippa L, Tso MO, Peyman GA, et al. von Hippel angiomatosis. A light, electron microscopic, and immunoperoxidase characterization. *Ophthalmology* 1983;90:848–855.

119. Jakobiec FA, Font RL, Johnson FB. Angiomatosis retinae: an ultrastructural study and lipid analysis. *Cancer* 1976;38:2042–2056.

120. Nicholson DH, Green WR, Kenyon KR. Light and electron microscopic study of early lesions in angiomatosis retinae. *Am J Ophthalmol* 1976;82:193–204.

121. Whitson JT, Welch RB, Green WR. Von Hippel-Lindau disease: case report of a patient with spontaneous regression of a retinal angioma. *Retina* 1986;6:253–259.

122. Nicholson DH, Anderson LS, Blodi C. Rhegmatogenous retinal detachment in angiomatosis retinae. *Am J Ophthalmol* 1986;101:187–189.

123. Gass JD, Braunstein R. Sessile and exophytic capillary angiomas of the juxtapapillary retina and optic nerve head. *Arch Ophthalmol* 1980;98:1790–1797.

124. MacDonald IM, Bech-Hansen NT, Britton WA Jr, et al. The phakomatoses: recent advances in genetics. *Can J Ophthalmol* 1997;32:4–11.

125. Seizinger BR, Rouleau GA, Ozelius LJ. Von Hippel-Lindau disease maps to the region of chromosome 3 associated with renal cell carcinoma. *Nature* 1988;332:268–269.

126. Latif F, Tory K, Gnarra J, et al. Identification of the von Hippel-Lindau disease tumor suppressor gene. *Science* 1993; 260:1317–1320.

127. Chan CC, Vortmeyer AO, Chew EY, et al. VHL gene deletion and enhanced VEGF gene expression detected in the stromal cells of retinal angioma. *Arch Ophthalmol* 1999;117:625–630.

128. Chang JH, Spraul CW, Lynn ML, et al. The two-stage mutation model in retinal hemangioblastoma. *Ophthalmic Genet* 1998;19:123–130.

129. Knudson AG Jr. Mutation and cancer: statistical study of retinoblastoma. *Proc Nat Acad Sci U S A* 1971;68:820–882.

130. Iliopoulos O, Levy AP, Jiang C, et al. Negative regulation of hypoxia-inducible genes by the von Hippel-Lindau protein. *Proc Nat Acad Sci U S A* 1996;93:10595–10599.

131. Siemeister G, Weindel K, Mohrs K, et al. Reversion of deregulated expression of vascular endothelial growth factor in human renal carcinoma cells by von Hippel-Lindau tumor suppressor protein. *Cancer Res* 1996;56:2299–2301.

132. Hinz BJ, Schachat AP. Capillary hemangioma of the retina and von Hippel-Lindau disease. In: Ryan SJ, ed. *Retina*. St. Louis: Mosby, 2001:576–587.

133. Crossey PA, Richards FM, Foster K, et al. Identification of intragenic mutations in the von Hippel-Lindau disease tumour suppressor gene and correlation with disease phenotype. *Hum Mol Genet* 1994;3:1303–1308.

134. Richards FM, Crossey PA, Phipps ME, et al. Detailed mapping of germline deletions of the von Hippel-Lindau disease tumour suppressor gene. *Hum Mol Genet* 1994;3:595–598.

135. Patel RJ, Appukuttan B, Ott S, et al. DNA-based diagnosis of the von Hippel-Lindau syndrome. *Am J Ophthalmol* 2000; 129:258–260.

136. Webster AR, Maher ER, Moore AT. Clinical characteristics of ocular angiomatosis in von Hippel-Lindau disease and correlation with germline mutation. *Arch Ophthalmol* 1999; 117:371–378.

137. Hardwig P, Robertson DM. Von Hippel-Lindau disease: a familial, often lethal, multi-system phakomatosis. *Ophthalmology* 1984;91:263–270.

138. Shields JA, Shields CL. Vascular tumors of the retina and optic disc. In: Zorab R, ed. *Intraocular tumors: a text and atlas.* Philadelphia: WB Saunders, 1992:394–406.

139. Annesley WH Jr, Leonard BC, Shields JA, et al. Fifteen-year review of treated cases of retinal angiomatosis. *Trans Am Acad Ophthalmol Otolaryngol* 1977;83:446–453.

140. Cardoso RD, Brockhurst RJ. Perforating diathermy coagulation for retinal angiomas. *Arch Ophthalmol* 1976;94:1702–1715.

141. Peyman GA, Rednam KR, Mottow-Lippa L, et al. Treatment of large von Hippel tumors by eye wall resection. *Ophthalmology* 1983;90:840–847.

142. Singh AD, Nouri M, Shields CL, et al. Treatment of retinal capillary hemangioma. *Ophthalmology* 2002;109:1799–1806.

143. Blodi CF, Russell SR, Pulido JS, et al. Direct and feeder vessel photocoagulation of retinal angiomas with dye yellow laser. *Ophthalmology* 1990;97:791–797.

144. Goldberg MF, Koenig S. Argon laser treatment of von Hippel-Lindau retinal angiomas. I. Clinical and angiography findings. *Arch Ophthalmol* 1974;92:121–125.

145. Lane CM, Turner G, Gregor ZJ, et al. Laser treatment of retinal angiomatosis. *Eye* 1989;3:33–38.

146. Schmidt D, Natt E, Neumann HP. Long-term results of laser treatment for retinal angiomatosis in von Hippel-Lindau disease. *Eur J Med Res* 2000;5:47–58.

147. Watzke RC. Cryotherapy for retinal angiomatosis. A clinico-pathologic report. *Arch Ophthalmol* 1974;92:399–401.

148. Welch RB. Von Hippel-Lindau disease: the recognition and treatment of early angiomatosis retinae and the use of cryosurgery as an adjunct to therapy. *Trans Am Ophthalmol Soc* 1970;68:367–424.

149. Amoils SP, Smith TR. Cryotherapy of angiomatosis retinae. *Arch Ophthalmol* 1969;81:689–691.

150. Kreusel KM, Bornfeld N, Lommatzsch A, et al. Ruthenium-106 brachytherapy for peripheral retinal capillary hemangioma. *Ophthalmology* 1998;105:1386–1392.

151. Johnson MW, Flynn HW, Gass JM. Pars plana vitrectomy and direct diathermy for complications of multiple retinal angiomas. *Ophthalmic Surg Lasers* 1992;23:47–50.

152. Machemer R, Williams J. Pathogenesis and therapy of traction detachment in various retinal vascular diseases. *Am J Ophthalmol* 1988;105:170–181.

153. McDonald HR, Schatz H, Johnson RN, et al. Vitrectomy in eyes with peripheral retinal angioma associated with traction macular detachment. *Ophthalmology* 1996;103:329–335.

154. Majji AB. Paramacular Von Hippel angioma with tractional macular detachment. *Ophthalmic Surg Lasers* 2002;33:145–147.

155. Kamal A, Watts AR, Rennie IG. Indocyanine green enhanced transpupillary thermotherapy of circumscribed choroidal haemangioma. *Eye* 2000;14:701–705.

156. Parmer DN, Mireskandari K, McHugh D. Transpupillary thermotherapy for retinal capillary hemangioma in von Hippel-Lindau disease. *Ophthalmic Surg Lasers* 2000;31:334–336.

157. Costa RA, Meirelles RL, Cardillo JA, et al. Retinal capillary hemangioma treatment by indocyanine green-mediated photothrombosis. *Am J Ophthalmol* 2003;135:395–398.

158. Atebara NH. Retinal capillary hemangioma treated with verteporfin photodynamic therapy. *Am J Ophthalmol* 2002; 134:788–790.

159. Rodriguez-Coleman H, Spaide RF, Yannuzzi LA. Treatment of angiomatous lesions of the retina with photodynamic therapy. *Retina* 2002;22:228–232.

160. Girmens JF, Erginay A, Massin P. Treatment of von Hippel-Lindau retinal hemangioblastoma by the vascular endothelial growth factor receptor inhibitor SU5416 is more effective for associated macular edema than for hemangioblastomas. *Am J Ophthalmol* 2003;136:194–196.

161. Aiello LP, George DJ, Cahill MT. Rapid and durable recovery of visual function in a patient with von Hippel-Lindau syndrome after systemic therapy with vascular endothelial growth factor receptor inhibitor su5416. *Ophthalmology* 2002;109:1745–1751.

162. Niemela M, Lemeta S, Sainio M, et al. Hemangioblastomas of the retina: impact of von Hippel-Lindau disease. *Invest Ophthalmol Vis Sci* 2000;41:1909–1915.

163. Webster AR, Maher ER, Bird AC, et al. A clinical and molecular genetic analysis of solitary ocular angioma. *Ophthalmology* 1999;106:623–629.

164. Na X, Wu G, Ryan CK, et al. Overproduction of vascular endothelial growth factor related to von Hippel-Lindau tumor suppressor gene mutations and hypoxia-inducible factor-1 alpha expression in renal cell carcinomas. *J Urol* 2003;170:593–594.

165. Bourneville DM. Sclerose tubereuse de circonvolutions cerebrales: idiotie et epilesie hemiplegique. *Arch Neurol* 1880; 1:81–91.

166. Vogt H. Zur Diagnostic der turberosen Sclerose. *Z Erforschung Behandlung Jugendl Schwachsinns* 1908;2:1–16.

167. Roach ES, Smith M, Huttenlocher P, et al. Diagnostic criteria: tuberous sclerosis complex: report of the Diagnostic Criteria Committee of the National Tuberous Sclerosis Association. *J Child Neurol* 1992;7:221–224.

168. Hunt A, Lindenbaum RH. Tuberous sclerosis: a new estimate of prevalence within the Oxford region. *J Med Genet* 1984; 21:272–277.

169. Lagos JC, Gomez MC. Tuberous sclerosis: reappraisal of a clinical entity. *Mayo Clin Proc* 1967;42:26–49.

170. Sampson JR. TSC1 and TSC2: genes that are mutated in the human genetic disorder tuberous sclerosis. *Biochem Soc Trans* 2003;31:592–596.

171. Tee AR, Manning BD, Roux PP. Tuberous sclerosis complex gene products, tuberin and hamartin, control mTOR signaling by acting as a GTPase-activating protein complex toward Rheb. *Curr Biol* 2003;13:1259–1268.

172. Shields JA, Shields CL. Glial tumors of the retina and optic disc. In: Zorab R, ed. *Intraocular tumors: a text and atlas.* Philadelphia: WB Saunders, 1992:421–435.

173. McLean IW. Tumors of the retina. In: Rosai J, ed. *Tumors of the eye and ocular adnexa.* Washington, DC: Armed Forces Institute of Pathology, 1994:97–154.

174. Jakobiec FA, Brodie SE, Haik B, Iwamoto T. Giant cell astrocytoma of the retina. A tumor of possible Mueller cell origin. *Ophthalmology* 1983;90:1565–1576.

175. Nyboer JH, Robertson DM, Gomez MR. Retinal lesions in tuberous sclerosis. *Arch Ophthalmol* 1976;94:1277–1280.

176. Robertson DM. Ophthalmic findings. In: Gomez MR, ed. *Tuberous sclerosis,* 2nd ed. New York: Raven Press, 1988: 88–109.

177. Mullaney PB, Jacquemin C, Abboud E, et al. Tuberous sclerosis in infancy. *J Pediatr Ophthalmol Strabismus* 1997;34: 372–375.

178. Zimmer-Galler IE, Robertson DM. Long-term observation of retinal lesions in tuberous sclerosis. *Am J Ophthalmol* 1995;119:318–324.

179. Kiratli H, Bilgic S. Spontaneous regression of retinal astrocytic hamartoma in a patient with tuberous sclerosis. *Am J Ophthalmol* 2002;133:715–716.

180. Kroll AJ, Ricker DP, Robb RM, et al. Vitreous hemorrhage complicating retinal astrocytic hamartoma. *Surv Ophthalmol* 1981;26:31–38.

181. de Juan E Jr, Green WR, Gupta PK, et al. Vitreous seeding by retinal astrocytic hamartoma in a patient with tuberous sclerosis. *Retina* 1984;4:100–102.

182. Gunduz K, Eagle RC Jr, Shields CL, et al. Invasive giant cell astrocytoma of the retina in a patient with tuberous sclerosis. *Ophthalmology* 1999;106:639–642.

183. Lucchese NJ, Goldberg MF. Iris and fundus pigmentary changes in tuberous sclerosis. *J Pediatr Ophthalmol Strabismus* 1981;18:45–48.

184. Eagle RC Jr, Shields JA, Shields CL. Hamartomas of the iris and ciliary epithelium in tuberous sclerosis complex. *Arch Ophthalmol* 2000;118:711–715.

185. Gomez MR. Phenotypes of the tuberous sclerosis complex with a revision of diagnostic criteria. *Ann NY Acad Sci* 1991; 615:1–7.

187. Reynolds RM, Browning GG, Nawroz I, et al. Von Recklinghausen's neurofibromatosis: neurofibromatosis type 1. *Lancet* 2003;361:1552–1554.

188. Destro M, D'Amico DJ, Gragoudas ES, et al. Retinal manifestations of neurofibromatosis. Diagnosis and management. *Arch Ophthalmol* 1991;109:662–666.

189. Ulbright TM, Fulling KH, Helveston EM. Astrocytic tumors of the retina. Differentiation of sporadic tumors from phakomatosis-associated tumors. *Arch Pathol Lab Med* 1984;108: 160–163.

190. Gass JDM. An unusual hamartoma of the pigment epithelium and retina simulating choroidal melanoma and retinoblastoma. *Trans Am Ophthalmol Soc* 1973;71:171–185.

191. Vianna RN, Pacheco DF, Vasconcelos MM, et al. Combined hamartoma of the retina and retinal pigment epithelium associated with neurofibromatosis type-1. *Int Ophthalmol* 2001; 24:63–66.

192. Frenkel M. Retinal angiomatosis in a patient with neurofibromatosis. *Am J Ophthalmol* 1967;63:804–808.

193. Lewis RA, Riccardi VM. Von Recklinghausen neurofibromatosis. Incidence of iris hamartomata. *Ophthalmology* 1981;88: 348–354.

194. Bouzas EA, Freidlin V, Parry DM, et al. Lens opacities in neurofibromatosis 2: further significant correlations. *Br J Ophthalmol* 1993;77:354–357.

195. Listernick R, Charrow J, Greenwald M, et al. Natural history of optic pathway tumors in children with neurofibromatosis type 1: a longitudinal study. *J Pediatr* 1994;125:63–66.

196. Glaser JS, Hoyt WF, Corbett J. Visual morbidity with chiasmal glioma. Long-term studies of visual fields in untreated and irradiated cases. *Arch Ophthalmol* 1971;85:3–12.

197. Miller NR, Iliff WJ, Green WR. Evaluation and management of gliomas of the anterior visual pathways. *Brain* 1974;97: 743–754.

198. Khafaga Y, Hassounah M, Kandil A, et al. Optic gliomas: a retrospective analysis of 50 cases. *Int J Radiat Oncol Biol Phys* 2003;56:807–812.

199. Parsa CF, Hoyt CS, Lesser RL, et al. Spontaneous regression of optic gliomas: thirteen cases documented by serial neuroimaging. *Arch Ophthalmol* 2001;119:516–529.

200. Guha A. Ras activation in astrocytomas and neurofibromas. *Can J Neurol* 1998;25:267–281.

201. Evans JJ, Lee JH, Park YS, et al. Future treatment modalities for meningiomas: targeting of neurofibromatosis type 2 and Ras-regulated pathways. *Neurosurg Clin N Am* 2000;11: 717–733.

202. Wyburn-Mason R. Arteriovenous aneurysm of midbrain and retina, facial nevi, and mental changes. *Brain* 1943;66: 163–203.

203. Shields JA, Shields CL. Systemic hamartomatoses ("Phakomatoses"). In: Zorab R, ed. *Intraocular tumors: a text and atlas.* Philadelphia: WB Saunders, 1992:513–539.

204. Ferry AP. Other phakomatoses. In: Ryan SJ, ed. *Retina.* St. Louis: Mosby, 2001:596–607.

205. Archer DB, Deutman A, Ernest JT, et al. Arteriovenous communications of the retina. *Am J Ophthalmol* 1973;75: 224–241.

206. Cameron ME, Greer CH. Congenital arterio-venous aneurysm of the retina: a postmortem report. *Br J Ophthalmol* 1968; 52:768–772.

207. Mansour AM, Walsh JB, Henkind P. Arteriovenous anastomoses of the retina. *Ophthalmology* 1987;94:35–40.

208. Bloom PA, Laidlaw A, Easty DL. Spontaneous development of retinal ischaemia and rubeosis in eyes with retinal racemose angioma. *Br J Ophthalmol* 1993;77:124–125.

209. Schatz H, Chang LF, Ober RR, et al. Central retinal vein occlusion associated with retinal arteriovenous malformation. *Ophthalmology* 1993;100:24–30.

210. Tilanus MD, Hoyng C, Deutman AF, et al. Congenital arteriovenous communications and the development of two types of leaking retinal macroaneurysms. *Am J Ophthalmol* 1991; 112:31–33.

211. Theron J, Newton TH, Hoyt WF. Unilateral retinocephalic vascular malformations. *Neuroradiology* 1974;7:185–196.

212. Williams TD. Retinal arteriovenous communication. *Optometry* 2001;72:309–314.

213. Mansour AM, Wells CG, Jampol LM. Ocular complications of arteriovenous communications of the retina. *Arch Ophthalmol* 1989;107:232–236.

214. Gass JDM. Choroidal tumors. In: Gass JDM, ed. *Stereoscopic atlas of macular diseases.* St. Louis: Mosby-Year Book, 1997: 208–221.

215. Sullivan TJ, Clarke MP, Morin JD. The ocular manifestations of Sturge-Weber syndrome. *J Pediatr Ophthalmol Strabismus* 1992:29:349–356.

216. Witschel H, Font RL. Hemangioma of the choroid: a clinicopathologic study of 71 cases and a review of the literature. *Surv Ophthalmol* 1976;20:415–431.

217. Tripathi BJ, Tripathi RC. Neural crest origin of human trabecular meshwork and its implications for the pathogenesis of glaucoma. *Am J Ophthalmol* 1989;107:583–590.

218. Susac JO, Smith JL, Scelfo RJ. The "tomato-catsup" fundus in Sturge-Weber syndrome. *Arch Ophthalmol* 1974;92:69–70.

219. Shields JA, Shields CL. Vascular tumors of the uvea. In: Zorab R, ed. *Intraocular tumors: a text and atlas.* Philadelphia: WB Saunders, 1992:239–259.

220. Ruby AJ, Jampol LM, Goldberg MF, et al. Choroidal neovascularization associated with choroidal hemangiomas. *Arch Ophthalmol* 1992;110:658–661.

221. Sadda SR, Miller NR, Tamargo R, et al. Bilateral optic neuropathy associated with diffuse cerebral angiomatosis in Sturge-Weber syndrome. *J Neuroophthalmol* 2000;20:28–31.

222. Griffiths PD, Boodram MB, Blaser S, et al. Abnormal ocular enhancement in Sturge-Weber syndrome: correlation of ocular MR and CT findings with clinical and intracranial imaging findings. *Am J Neuroradiol* 1996;17:749–754.

223. Madreperla SA, Hungerford JL, Plowman PN, et al. Choroidal hemangiomas: visual and anatomic results of treatment by photocoagulation or radiation therapy. *Ophthalmology* 1997; 104:1773–1778.

224. Zografos L, Egger E, Bercher L, et al. Proton beam irradiation of choroidal hemangiomas. *Am J Ophthalmol* 1998;126:261–268.

225. Scott TA, Augsburger JJ, Brady LW, et al. Low dose ocular irradiation for diffuse choroidal hemangiomas associated with bullous nonrhegmatogenous retinal detachment. *Retina* 1991; 11:389–393.

226. Plowman PN, Harnett AN. Radiotherapy in benign orbital disease. I: Complicated ocular angiomas. *Br J Ophthalmol* 1988; 72:286–288.

16

UVEITIS AFFECTING INFANTS AND CHILDREN: INFECTIOUS CAUSES

ALBERT T. VITALE
C. STEPHEN FOSTER

INTRODUCTION

Uveitis arising in children, as with that in adults, encompasses a broad and disparate group of inflammatory and infectious disease entities that may occur as an isolated ocular condition or as a manifestation of an underlying systemic disease. There are distinct features of childhood uveitis, which require special consideration and present unique diagnostic and therapeutic challenges (1–11).

Uveitis is less common in children than in adults. Thus, less information is available in the literature to guide management. Complete ocular examinations are difficult and frequently require general anesthesia. Unique endogenous uveitic syndromes appear, such as juvenile idiopathic arthritis–associated iridocyclitis (JIA) (formally known as juvenile rheumatoid arthritis or JRA) and Kawasaki's disease. Also, children may present with distinct clinical symptoms and signs when they do present with uveitic conditions that also affect adults. For example, in young children with sarcoidosis, skin and articular stigmata are more common than pulmonary disease. The interpretation of laboratory data and the choice of assay must be modified to reflect differences in the normative values of certain tests, such as the physiologically elevated serum angiotensin-converting enzyme (ACE) levels in children. Also, the differential diagnosis varies considerably with the age of the child. This is particularly important with respect to unique masquerade syndromes occurring in children, such as retinoblastoma, leukemia, juvenile xanthogranuloma, and retinitis pigmentosa, all of which can present as posterior uveitis. Approximately 40% of uveitis cases affect the posterior segment in children, compared to about 20% in adults, and children have a disproportionately higher percentage of infectious etiologies, both acquired and congenital (12), compared to adults. The overall prognosis is worse in children than in adults, in part, due to frequent delay in the diagnosis and institution of appropriate treatment. Children can be either unable or reticent to provide accurate histories or descriptions of their visual complaints. Their uveitis is of-

ten chronic, recurrent, and difficult to control. As a consequence of chronic inflammation and corticosteroid therapy, vision-robbing complications arise, such as cataract, maculopathy, glaucoma, and band keratopathy. Tolerance of even low-grade inflammation may promote ongoing, cumulative, and frequently irreversible damage to vital ocular structures. The risk of amblyopia is a unique concern in children under the age of 10 years with uveitis and significantly influences medical treatment and the timing of surgical intervention. The prognosis for visual rehabilitation through ocular surgery of all types is guarded in children. This is true because the inflammatory response to surgical trauma is greater than in adults. Thus, a proportionately greater number of children with uveitis are blinded by their disease compared to adults. Routine annual vision screening examinations need be emphasized to parents, school personnel, and other medical colleagues, especially pediatricians.

This chapter presents the epidemiology and classification of common causes of uveitis in children; the differential diagnosis by anatomical location, age of presentation, and unique aspects of the ophthalmic assessment; diagnostic testing; and therapy. Specific infectious uveitic entities will be presented. Specific uveitic entities of autoimmune or idiopathic origin, masquerade syndromes, and unique aspects of immunomodulatory therapy in children will be presented in Chapter 17.

The goal is to provide a systematic and practical diagnostic approach and effect a shift to more aggressive treatment to reduce the prevalence of blindness caused by pediatric uveitis. The stakes of suboptimal treatment are incredibly high, not only for these children and their parents, but also for society at large, both in terms of the cost of visual debility and the loss of untapped human potential.

EPIDEMIOLOGY AND CLASSIFICATION

The incidence of uveitis in the United States and in developed countries in the West has been estimated at between

14 and 17 cases per 100,000, with 38,000 new cases per year and a prevalence of approximately 38 per 100,000 (13–17). In urban southern India, active or past uveitis was reported in one of every 140 people, a higher overall disease prevalence (18). It has been estimated that uveitis causes 10% of legal blindness in the United States, and upwards of 24% in West Africa and other regions of the developing world where onchocerciasis is endemic (19–21).

Pediatric uveitis is a relatively rare disease, comprising between 5% and 10% of patients treated at tertiary uveitis referral centers (Table 16-1) (7,11,12, 22–32). It is less common than adult uveitis. Several population based studies in the United States, United Kingdom, and Finland reported the incidence of pediatric uveitis to be 4.3 to 6 per 100,000 (22,33,34) in contrast to adult uveitis with estimates of 27.2 per 100,000 (34).

The International Uveitis Study Group (IUSG) proposed a unified classification system for the diagnosis of uveitis (35) based on (i) the anatomical location of the inflammation, (ii) its time course as acute or chronic (less than or greater than 12 weeks duration), (iii) its laterality (involving one or both eyes, simultaneously or sequentially), (iv) as granulomatous ("mutton fat" keratic precipitates, iris nodules or chorioretinal granulomata) or nongranulomatous, and (v) by its association with systemic disease. In this classification, the anatomical location of the intraocular inflammation is grouped as follows: anterior uveitis (involving the iris or pars plicata), intermediate uveitis (involving any combination of the pars plana, anterior vitreous, or adjacent retina), posterior uveitis (involving any combination of the retina, choroid or overlying vitreous), and panuveitis (diffuse inflammation encompassing both anterior and posterior compartments of the eye). We have found it useful to include inflammation of adjacent "nonuveal" structures such as the cornea, sclera, optic nerve, and retinal vasculature, which may provide additional insight into the diagnosis (36) (Table 16-2).

Although the anatomical breakdown and prevalence of pediatric uveitis varies with geographic and demographic differences (18,34,35) and referral bias (22), the following general patterns have emerged: (i) approximately 30% to 40% of children with uveitis have anterior uveitis (mostly JIA, if associated with systemic disease); (ii) 10% to 20% have intermediate uveitis (mostly idiopathic); (iii) 5% to 10% have panuveitis (mostly idiopathic); and (iv) posterior uveitis accounts for 40% to 50% of uveitis in children (toxoplasmic retinochoroiditis being the most common pathogen) (7) (Table 16-1). However, geographic variance in types of uveitic presentations exists (22,32,34).

DIFFERENTIAL DIAGNOSIS OF CHILDHOOD UVEITIS

The differential diagnosis of childhood uveitis classically can be divided into three categories: *inflammatory conditions of infectious etiology, endogenous uveitis of autoimmune or idiopathic origin*, and *masquerade syndromes*. The most common anterior *infectious uveitis* is from herpes simplex virus (HSV) or varicella zoster virus (VZV), whereas toxoplasmosis is the most common cause of posterior *infectious uveitis*. Other infectious etiologies include (i) parasitic infection from ocular toxocariasis, diffuse unilateral subacute neuroretinitis (DUSN); (ii) viral retinitis from human immunodeficiency virus (HIV), HSV, VZV, cytomegalovirus (CMV), measles, mumps, rubella, lymphotrophic choriomeningitis virus, Epstein-Barr virus (EBV); (iii) spirochetes causing syphilis, Lyme disease (LD); and (iv) bacterial infections causing cat-scratch disease, endophthalmitis, and tuberculosis. The most common form of *noninfectious, endogenous uveitis* in childhood is JIA. Kawasaki's disease, tubulointerstitial nephritis and uveitis syndrome (TINU), and postviral uveitis are rare forms of endogenous uveitis that predominate in the pediatric, compared to the adult, age group. Seronegative spondyloarthropathies (ankylosing spondylitis, reactive arthritis, inflammatory bowel disease, and psoriatic arthritis), Fuchs' heterochromic iridocyclitis, pars planitis, ocular sarcoidosis, Vogt-Koyanagi-Harada disease, sympathetic ophthalmia, and Adamantiades-Behçet disease (ABD) also occur less commonly in children than adults. *Pediatric masquerade syndromes* in childhood include intraocular neoplasms (such as retinoblastoma), ocular manifestations of systemic malignancies (including leukemia and lymphoma), juvenile xanthogranuloma, inherited retinal degenerations (such as retinitis pigmentosa), congenital vascular abnormalities (such as Coats' disease), endophthalmitis and the sequelae of ocular trauma (including retained intraocular foreign body).

The expanded IUSG guidelines (Table 16-2) account for the character of the inflammation, involvement of the retinal vasculature (Tables 16-3–16-5), and the age of the patient at presentation (Table 16-6).

DIAGNOSTIC APPROACH

The most important step in approaching pediatric uveitis is a comprehensive medical history and review of systems. When a child is unable or unwilling to provide historical details or accurate descriptions of their ocular complaint, the parents or caregivers must be queried as to the onset and character of signs and symptoms such as pain, redness, epiphora, photophobia, decreased vision, or metamorphopsia. Subtle behavioral changes at home or difficulties at school can be important pieces of history that herald the beginning of a visual problem. In the setting of established pathology (leukocoria), examination of old photographs is useful in establishing the onset of disease. The age of onset can influence the differential diagnosis. Posterior uveitis in an infant raises the specter of a neoplastic masquerade syndrome, which would be less likely in an older child.

TABLE 16-1. POPULATION AND CLINIC-BASED STUDIES UVEITIS IN CHILDREN

Citation	Location	Age (yr)	Sample Size	Children	F:M	Anterior	Intermediate	Posterior	Diffuse	Idiopathic	Toxoplasm	JIA	Toxocara
Kimura and Hogan (23)	San Francisco, CA	<17	251	13.2%	1.2:10	31.5%	17.5%	49.0%	2.0%	35.5%	39.4%	5.6%	80.0%
Cross (24)	London	<16	59			17.0%		22.0%	61.0%	59.0%	13.5%	5.1%	0.0%
Perkins (12)	London	<16	150	5.0%	1.3:1	49.2%		39.3%	11.3%	43.3%	20.6%	5.3%	10.0%
Kazdan et al. (25)	Toronto	<16	117			47.0%	17.9%	50.4%	2.6%	35.0%	23.0%	12.0%	0.0%
Makley et al. (26)	Ohio	<17	75	12.5%		10.8%	20.0%	67.7%	1.5%	46.7%	29.2%		3.1%
Kanski and Shun-Shin (27)	London	<16	340			100.0%				6.2%		81.5%	
Tugal-Tutkun et al. (28)	Boston, MA	<17	130		1.5:1	58.4%	20.0%	13.8%	7.6%	36.8%	7.7%	41.5%	3.1%
Pivetti-Pezzi (29)	Rome	<16	267		1:1	33.3%	25.1%	26.6%	15.0%	54.3%	11.6%	9.4%	2.6%
Soylu et al. (30)	Adana, Turkey	<17	90		1.1:1	33.3%	8.9%	23.3%	34.4%	34.4%	25.6%	3.3%	1.1%
Paivonsalo-Hirtanen et al.	Turku, Finland	<16	1122	4.9%	1.6:1	90.9%	1.8%	5.5%	1.8%	40.0%	7.3%	36.3%	0.0%
Stoffel et al. (31)	Bern, Switzerland	<17	70	33.6%	1.4:1	57.0%		14.0%	29.0%			46.0%	
Bonezra et al. (32)	Jerusalem	<19	821	33.6%	1.01:1	13.4%	41.7%	14.1%	30.8%		72.0%	74.9%	9.4%
Edelsten et al. (22)	London	<20	249		1.8:1	70.0%		30.0%		44.0%	2.4%	47.0%	
de Boer et al. (11)	Netherlands	<16	123		1:03:01	36.0%	24.0%	29.0%	21.0%		10.0%	20.0%	

F:M, female:male ratio; JIA, juvenile idiopathic arthritis.
* Paivonsalo-Hirtanen T, Tuominen J, Saari KM. Uveitis in children: population-based study in Finland. *Acta Ophthalmol Scand* 2000;78:84–88.

TABLE 16-2. EXPANDED CLASSIFICATION OF UVEITIS

Type	Clinical description
Anterior uveitis	Iritis

Intermediate uveitis	Iridocyclitis
	Cyclitis
	  Phacogenic uveitis
	  Pars planitis
	Vitreitis
	Fuchs' heterochromic iridocyclitis
	Peripheral uveitis

Posterior uveitis	Choroiditis Retinochoroiditis Retinal vasculitis Neuroretinitis
Panuveitis	Inflammation involving all anatomic segments of the uvea
Keratouveitis	Uveal inflammation with associated corneal involvement
Sclerouveitis	Uveal inflammation with associated scleritis

TABLE 16-4. DIFFERENTIAL DIAGNOSIS OF CHILDHOOD UVEITIS: ANATOMIC LOCATION

Intermediate Uveitis	Panuveitis
Pars planitis	Adamantiades-Behçets disease
Juvenile idiopathic arthritis	Sympathetic ophthalmia
Multiple sclerosis	Orbital pseudotumor
Lyme disease	Vogt-Koyanagi-Harada syndrome
Cat-scratch disease	Lyme disease
Toxocariasis	Cat scratch disease
Masquerades	Masquerades
Sarcoidosis	Sarcoidosis
	Syphilis
	Familial juvenile systemic granulomatosis

TABLE 16-3. DIFFERENTIAL DIAGNOSIS OF CHILDHOOD UVEITIS: ANATOMICAL LOCATION

Anterior Non Granulomatous Uveitis	Anterior Granulomatous Uveitis
Juvenile idiopathic arthritis	Sarcoidosis
Herpetic disease	Herpetic disease
HLA-B27–associated disease	Inflammatory bowel disease
Systemic lupus erythematosus	Syphilis
Fuch's heterochromic iridocyclitis	Lyme disease
Kawasaki's disease	Leprosy
Tubulointerstitial nephritis and uveitis	Tuberculosis
Trauma	Trauma
Viral syndromes	Sympathetic ophthalmia
Postbacterial infection (*Yersinia, streptococcal*)	Fungal disease
Adamantiades-Behçet's disease	Multiple sclerosis
Human immunodeficiency virus	
Leukemia	
Drug induced	
Chronic infantile neurologic cutaneous and articular/ neonatal-onset multisystem inflammatory disease syndrome	

TABLE 16-5. DIFFERENTIAL DIAGNOSIS OF CHILDHOOD UVEITIS: ANATOMICAL LOCATION

Posterior Uveitis without Vasculitis	Posterior Uveitis with Vasculitis
Toxocariasis	Toxoplasmosis
Leukemia	Sarcoidosis
Tuberculosis	Syphilis
Vogt-Koyanagi syndrome	Lyme disease
Trauma (intraocular foreign body)	Acute retinal necrosis (HSV/VZV)
Rubella	CMV retinitis
DUSN	HIV
Endophthalmitis	Multiple sclerosis
POHS	Paraviral syndrome
Masquerades	Inflammatory bowel disease
	Kawasaki's disease
	Adamantiades-Behçet's disease
	Polyarteritis nodosa
	Wegener's granulomatosis
	Systemic lupus erythematosus
	Masquerades

CMV, cytomegalovirus; DUSN, diffuse subacute unilateral neuroretinitis; HIV, human immunodeficiency virus; HSV, herpes simplex virus, POHS, presumed ocular histoplasmosis syndrome; VZV, varicella zoster virus.

TABLE 16-6. DIFFERENTIAL DIAGNOSIS OF INTERMEDIATE AND POSTERIOR PEDIATRIC UVEITIS: AGE AT PRESENTATION

Infants (0–2 yr)	**Adolescents (10–20 yr) [cont.]**
HSV retinitis	APMPPE
Toxocariasis	POHS
Retinoblastoma	DUSN
Rubella	Leukemia
Congenital syphilis	JIA
Children (2–10 yr)	**Any childhood age**
Toxoplasmosis	HIV retinopathy
Toxocariasis	CMV retinitis
Leukemia	Acute retinal necrosis (VZV/HSV)
JIA	Endophthalmitis
SSPE	Sarcoidosis
Lyme disease	Lyme disease[†]
Cat-scratch disease	Cat-scratch disease
CINCA/NOMID*	TINU[‡]
Familial juvenile	Tuberculosis
systemic granulomatosis	Vogt-Koyanagi-Harada syndrome[§]
	Sympathetic ophthalmia
Adolescents (10–20 yr)	ABD
Toxoplasmosis	Traumatic (intraocular foreign body)
Pars planitis	
HLA-B27–associated disease	

ABD, Adamantiades-Behçet's disease; APPMPE, Acute posterior multifocal placoid pigment epitheliopathy; CMV, cytomegalovirus; DUSN, diffuse subacute unilateral neuroretinitis; HIV, human immunodeficiency virus; HSV, herpes simplex virus; JIA, juvenile idiopathic arthritis; POHS, presumed ocular histoplasmosis syndrome; SSPE, subacute sclerosing panencephalitis; TINU, tubulointerstitial nephritis and uveitis syndrome; VZV, varicella zoster virus.
* Chronic infantile neurologic cutaneous and articular neonatal-onset multisystem inflammatory disease syndrome.
[†] Highest incidence in those <15 years of age or between 30 and 59 years of age (38).
[‡] Typically occurs in childhood and adolescence with a marked female preponderance (39).
[§] Occurs at all ages, youngest age reported was 4 years (40).

Historical details should be obtained regarding the past medical histories of both the child (birth weight, vaccinations, developmental milestones, systemic disease associations) and the parents (sexually transmitted diseases, intravenous drug use, HIV status, dietary and exposure history to animals during pregnancy, intrapartum viral infections, tuberculosis exposure, history of connective tissue diseases) to formulate a differential diagnosis and guide further diagnostic investigations (4).

The ocular examination can provide important objective clues to the diagnosis in an otherwise nonverbal child, but obtaining this information can be extremely challenging, particularly in infants and toddlers. Although information can be obtained in the office setting, even with the aid of a papoose and portable slitlamp, a complete evaluation almost always requires examination under anesthesia, especially to exclude the possibility of retinoblastoma. Certain findings alert the clinician. Strabismus might be secondary to severe inflammation or retinitis (such as with JIA or CMV), whereas inattention from a hearing disability in the setting of pigmentary retinopathy might indicate congenital rubella or syphilis.

Laboratory tests are used in most cases to confirm the clinical impression or to exclude diagnostic possibilities rather than serve as a "diagnostic battery". Rosenbaum and Wernick (37) found that routine screening of all uveitis patients for antinuclear antibodies (ANA) resulted in approximately 100 false-positive results for every one positive test result in patients with systemic lupus erythematosus. Therefore, disease-specific testing should be performed in those patients in whom there is a relatively high degree of suspicion for particular diagnoses as suggested by history and examination.

A basic diagnostic stepladder algorithm for pediatric uveitis is as follows. For recurrent, nongranulomatous anterior uveitis, obtain a (i) complete blood count (CBC), (ii) urinalysis (UA), (iii) ANA, and (iv) human leukocyte antigen (HLA)-B27 testing, depending on the review of systems. In cases of anterior granulomatous uveitis, whether first time or recurrent, obtain a (i) CBC, (ii) UA, (iii) fluorescent treponemal antibody absorption test (FTA-ABS), (iv) Lyme disease (LD) antibody titers and Western blot, (v) purified protein derivative (PPD) skin testing, (vi) chest x-ray, (vii) ANA, (viii) angiotensin converting enzyme (ACE) and serum lysozyme analysis within the appropriate clinical context. For patients with intermediate uveitis, obtain a (i) CBC, (ii) UA, (iii) chest x-ray, (iv) FTA-ABS, (v) ACE and serum lysozyme analysis, and (vi) Lyme, (vii) *Bartonella*, and (viii) ANA titers. If a diagnosis of sarcoidosis is strongly suspected, thin-cut spiral computed tomography (CT) of the chest and/or gallium scanning can be fruitful. In children presenting with posterior uveitis and vitreitis, especially with retinal vasculitis or retinal granulomata, obtain a (i) CBC, (ii) UA, (iii) ACE and serum lysozyme analysis, (iv) FTA-ABS, (v) PPD, (vi) chest x-ray, and (vii) *Toxoplasma gondii*, (viii) *Toxocara canis, (ix)* Lyme and (x) *Bartonella* serologies. An audiogram or lumbar puncture would be warranted if tinnitus or meningeal signs or symptoms emerged as positives on review of systems. Finally, diagnostic vitrectomy is used in cases in which all noninvasive studies are unrevealing and in which divergent therapeutic alternatives are being considered.

THERAPY

Medical therapy of uveitis is a double-edged sword. The ultimate goal is to achieve complete and sustained inflammatory suppression to reduce visually debilitating complications of the disease and minimize ocular morbidity or systemic toxicity from therapy. We suggest a stepladder algorithm that is both steroid-sparing to reduce cataract formation and growth retardation (38) and titrated to the clinical picture (39). Initial use of corticosteroids is advocated by all routes (topical, periocular, systemic), followed by nonsteroidal antiinflammatory drugs (NSAID) systemically, peripheral retinal cryopexy or indirect laser photocoagulation in selected patients with intermediate uveitis, systemic immunomodulatory chemotherapy, and finally pars plana vitrectomy (PPV) with intraocular steroid injection.

In the child with *chronic nongranulomatous or granulomatous anterior uveitis*, an approach involving topical steroids, followed by an examination under anesthesia as necessary, and, finally, periocular steroid injections, is used. If this fails, systemic steroids are given with clear goals as to desired outcome and duration of therapy. If the uveitis recurs as steroids are tapered, chronic oral NSAIDs such as naproxen or tolmetin are recommended. (6) Although we have not found topical NSAIDs to be of particular value in the treatment of anterior uveitis, our experience suggests that long-term (2 years), daily, oral NSAID therapy can be extremely successful in approximately 70% of children with recurrent nongranulomatous anterior uveitis.

In *granulomatous anterior uveitis*, topical steroids are frequently insufficient, and systemic therapy, particularly with NSAIDs, may be used earlier. If unsuccessful, then systemic immunomodulatory chemotherapy is considered, beginning with once-weekly low-dose methotrexate or daily cyclosporine. Immunomodulatory therapy (corticosteroids, antimetabolites, alkylating agents, T-cell inhibitors, and biological agents) can be used in patients with inflammatory ocular disease (9,38).

Topical steroids penetrate poorly into the anterior vitreous and posterior segment. Consequently, for *intermediate uveitis*, particularly when complicated by cystoid macular edema (CME), the first step in our therapeutic stepladder is periocular steroid injection, with adjunctive topical steroids for anterior chamber "spillover" reaction. We prefer to inject through the preorbital septum, through the lower lid, elevating the globe slightly with the nondominant index finger, in a manner similar to that for peribulbar anesthesia. Steroid (1 mL of 40-mg/mL triamcinolone acetonide) is drawn into a 3-mL syringe with a 27-gauge, 5/8-in needle. This is then introduced between the globe and the lateral third of the orbital margin, advanced to the hub, and with a quick wiggle of the syringe to assure nonengagement of the sclera, the drug is injected swiftly to avoid precipitation. This method appears to have almost no risk of ocular penetration and has excellent antiinflammatory efficacy, particularly for CME. It is rarely associated with an intraocular pressure rise in patients with intermediate uveitis who have had no previous steroid response. Finally, the transseptal approach, particularly in the pediatric age group, is accepted and can be done without the need for general anesthesia.

Additional potential complications of periocular steroid administration include not only the promotion of cataract and glaucoma, but also ptosis, strabismus due to extraocular muscle fibrosis, and orbital fat herniation through the lower lid following multiple injections (40). Should a series of six transseptal steroid injections, each separated by at least 2 weeks, fail to achieve inflammatory control, a systemic NSAID is then added. Pars plana cryopexy or indirect laser photocoagulation, especially in the presence of peripheral neovascularization, may be necessary for patients in whom periocular and/or NSAID therapy fails.

The final rung in our stepladder algorithm in the treatment of intermediate uveitis varies according to the patient's age, sex, underlying disease, and lens status. Should immunosuppressive therapy be commenced, our first choices would include once-weekly, low-dose methotrexate or daily, low-dose cyclosporine alone or in combination with a short course of systemic steroids. PPV, with or without pars plana lensectomy (PPL), cataract extraction and intraocular lens implantation, or in the setting of established pseudophakia, may positively affect the natural course of pars planitis, with improved visual acuity, reduction in the frequency and severity of inflammatory recurrences, reversal of hypotony (39–42), and regression of CME (41–43). In addition, PPV together with microbiological, cytological, and molecular biological examination of vitreous biopsy specimens provides an essential diagnostic tool in the management of atypical cases. Finally, PPV is the only modality for the treatment of certain posterior segment complications of inflammatory disease, including tractional and rhegmatogenous retinal detachment, epiretinal membrane formation, vitreous opacification, and hemorrhage.

Patients with *posterior uveitis*, depending on the diagnosis, usually require specific antimicrobial therapy, systemic steroids or immunomodulatory therapy early in their disease. The medical therapy for specific infectious and non-infectious posterior uveitic entities will be presented below and in Chapter 17.

Short-acting mydriatic agents are commonly used in the setting of anterior chamber inflammation, irrespective of the primary anatomical location of the disease, to relieve pain associated with pupillary sphincter and ciliary muscle spasm, and to prevent the formation of posterior synechiae. During episodes of acute inflammation, cyclopentolate 1% and tropicamide 1% (0.5% concentrations in infants) are used twice daily. For chronic anterior uveitis, once-daily administration at bedtime is used to prevent amblyopia. Several different mydriatic regimens and "cocktails" containing mixtures of dilating agents, applied topically or injected subconjunctivally, have been used with varying degrees of success in an effort to break established synechiae (44–46). We have had success using a mixture of equal parts of cocaine 4%, epinephrine 1:1,000, and atropine 1% soaked on a cotton pledget, applied topically for 15 minutes, to an anesthetized eye in proximity to the area of the synechiae.

The subject of cataract extraction and lens implantation in children with uveitis is complex, and a comprehensive discussion of the matter is beyond the scope of this presentation. Although successful cataract extraction with lens implantation has been reported in nearly every form of pediatric uveitis (47–49), it is, nonetheless, especially challenging because of the more exuberant inflammatory response in children to surgical trauma and to alterations in ocular tissues and physiology as a consequence of chronic, relapsing inflammation as seen in JIA. A successful outcome strongly depends on the establishment of a definitive diagnosis, proper case selection, preoperative inflammatory control for a minimum of 3 months, and intensive, vigilant perioperative and postoperative antiinflammatory therapy (50–52), and less so on surgical technique chosen. Unless contraindicated, we recommend supplemental, perioperative antiinflammatory therapy with prednisone (1 mg/kg daily), one drop of 1% prednisolone acetate eight times a day beginning 2 days before surgery, an oral NSAID such as naproxen 125 mg twice daily, and a topical NSAID such as flurbiprofen (Ocufen) four times daily. The relative benefits of lens implantation in children, including reduced risk of amblyopia and lack of need for contact lens or aphakic spectacle correction, must be balanced against well-documented possible surgical complications. Risk factors associated with poor outcomes following intraocular lens (IOL) implantation in 19 uveitic eyes (53) included pars planitis and panuveitis, chronic smoldering inflammation despite aggressive medical therapy (e.g., sarcoidosis), and JIA (the highest risk because of young age at onset and chronic intraocular inflammation). Although IOL implantation remains unresolved, experience (54–58) suggests that, with rare exceptions, a conservative approach consisting of PPV and PPL, without lens implantation, should be pursued in the setting of severe, chronic childhood uveitis, including JIA.

TOXOPLASMOSIS

Prevalence and Epidemiology

Toxoplasmosis is the leading cause of posterior uveitis in all age groups (59,60), being more common in children than adults (7) and accounting for 70% of pediatric posterior and panuveitis (3).

Etiology and Pathogenesis

Toxoplasmosis may be either acquired or congenitally transmitted with ocular disease resulting from the proliferation of the obligate intracellular protozoan, *Toxoplasma gondii*. Once in the retinal tissue, it proliferates and causes hypersensitivity reactions and inflammation of the adjacent tissue, vessels, vitreous, and choroid. The organism has trophism for cardiac, muscular, and neural tissue. Cats are the definitive host and the organisms may exist in three forms: the trophozoite (actively replicating), the tissue cyst (latent), and the oocyst (soil form), seen only in the intestinal mucosa of the feline host (61). Transmission to humans may occur by all three forms of the organism through ingestion of oocysts or tissue cysts, vertical transplacental spread, or inadvertent direct inoculation.

The major sources of infection in humans include tissue cysts, contained in raw or undercooked meats, and less commonly, oocysts in contaminated fruit, vegetables, water, and soil (litter boxes). Uncommon modes of *T. gondii* transmission include infection following organ transplantation (62), transfusion of blood products (63), and accidental autoinnoculation of tachyzoites among laboratory personnel (64).

Maternal transmission to the fetus may occur following primary *T. gondii* infection acquired during pregnancy. It has been estimated that between 70% and 80% of women of childbearing age in the United States are at risk for contracting the disease (65); however, the incidence of acquiring toxoplasmosis during pregnancy is only 0.2% to 1% (66). The risk of congenital transmission among immunocompetent women infected prior to pregnancy is exceedingly small, in distinction to chronically infected, immunocompromised women in whom vertical transmission to their fetuses may occur. Overall, 40% of primary maternal infections result in congenital infection (67), with a transplacental transmission rate of *T. gondii* of 10% to 15% in the first trimester, 30% in the second, and 60% in the third among untreated women (66). Treatment during pregnancy reduces these rates. The higher rate in the third trimester is thought to be due to the greater vascularity of the placenta during this time. By contrast, the risk of severe disease developing in the fetus is inversely proportional to gestational age. Disease acquired early in pregnancy often results in spontaneous abortion, stillbirth, or severe congenital disease, whereas that acquired later in gestation may produce an asymptomatic, normal-appearing infant with a latent infection. Manifestations of congenital infection in the perinatal period vary widely, ranging from the presence of peripheral retinal scars, low birth weight, or persistent jaundice to the classical triad of signs including convulsions, cerebral calcifications, and chorioretinitis (68). Most cases of congenital toxoplasmosis present as subclinical or chronic infection, with ocular and central nervous system sequelae appearing months to years later. Long-term follow-up of congenitally infected children has shown that one or more episodes of chorioretinitis will develop in up to 85% after a mean of 3.7 years, resulting in significant visual impairment and blindness (69,70).

Congenital infection with toxoplasmosis is estimated to affect 3,000 infants born in the United States each year (71) with estimates of the prevalence varying widely, in parallel with the rates of seropositivity throughout the world (72). Recent epidemiologic data have provided new insights into the pathogenesis of ocular toxoplasmosis and have challenged the classic teaching that the vast majority of active toxoplasmic inflammatory foci arise from the reactivation of congenital retinochoroidal scars (73,74). Population-based studies performed in southern Brazil (Rio Grande do Sul), where the infection rates with *T. gondii* are very high, reported an exceptionally high rate of ocular toxoplasmosis (75). Seropositivity as demonstrated by immunoglobulin G (IgG) antibody was nearly universal, whereas immunoglobulin M (IgM) antibodies against *T. gondii* were detected in less that 1% of newborns, indicating the rarity of congenital disease. Furthermore, families with multiple, nontwin siblings with ocular toxoplasmosis were observed. Finally, the prevalence of ocular disease increased with age, suggesting that ocular infections could be attributed to postnatally acquired infections.

The true incidence of acquired ocular disease has been difficult to establish given the fact that infection is frequently asymptomatic. In a study of 154 patients with active ocular toxoplasmosis, congenital disease occurred in 13 (8%), postnatal infection in 17 (11%), and the exact time of infection being indeterminate for 124 (81%) patients (76). However, data are accumulating to suggest that at least two-thirds of ocular toxoplasmosis is caused by acquired, postnatal infection (74). In acquired disease, inflammatory foci in the retina may arise in the absence of a preexisting retinochoroidal scar. Recurrent toxoplasmic retinochoroiditis may then be seen to arise from remotely acquired infection rather than from a congenital source, with retinal lesions associated with a well-documented acquired infection reactivating in a manner similar to that seen with congenital infection (73,77,78). Primary preventative strategies now encompass children and adults as well as pregnant women at risk for developing ocular disease as a result of postnatal infection.

A variety of host and parasitic factors may increase the severity of disease presentation, including: immunosuppression, presence of HLA-Bw62 (79), and possibly lineage determined by major surface antigens of the parasite (SAG-1 and SAG-2) (80).

Symptoms and Signs

Clinically, ocular toxoplasmosis presents as a focal, necrotizing retinochoroiditis. Reactivation typically occurs adjacent to an old chorioretinal scar (satellite formation), producing an oval or circular yellow-white, raised retinal lesion with varying degrees of overlying vitreitis, choroiditis, and vasculitis. The retinal vasculitis may be an arteritis or phlebitis, proximate or remote from the inflammatory focus. Not infrequently, nongranulomatous anterior uveitis and elevated intraocular pressure present. Inflammation is self-limited in immunocompetent patients, lasting approximately 6 weeks. Recurrent inflammation is common, occurring in 79% of 154 patients followed-up for more than 5 years (76). Bilateral involvement varies between 22% and 40% (76,81–83) and is more frequently observed (65% to 97%) in patients with congenital toxoplasmosis (71,76,84,85). Macular lesions (Fig. 16-1) were found in 58% of patients with congenital toxoplasmosis (retrospective review) (76), whereas peripheral lesions were seen in 64% of patients (prospectively reported) (71). This difference may be attributable to an underestimation of asymptomatic peripheral lesions.

Atypical presentations of toxoplasmosis are uncommon and include (86) those mimicking acute retinal necrosis (particularly in the immunosuppressed or elderly), neuroretinitis, punctuate outer retinal necrosis, occlusive retinal vasculitis, retinal and subretinal neovascularization, rhegmatogenous and serous retinal detachment, a pigmentary retinopathy mimicking retinitis pigmentosa, scleritis, and a dubious association with Fuchs' heterochromic iridocyclitis and various optic nerve pathologies.

Diagnosis

In most cases, the diagnosis is made based on the characteristic findings of the ocular exam. Serologic testing for spe-

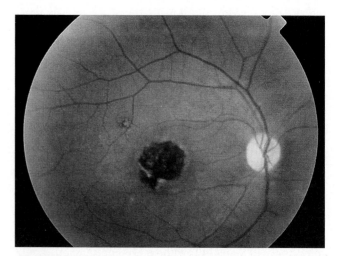

FIGURE 16-1. Central macular retinochoroidal hyperpigmented scar typical of congenital toxoplasmosis. A smaller inactive retinochoroidal scar is seen in the supratemporal macula.

cific anti–*T. gondii* antibodies is helpful to support the clinical impression, particularly when the ophthalmic findings are atypical. IgG antibodies can cross the placenta, whereas IgM antibodies cannot. Detection of IgM and immunoglobulin A (IgA) antibodies in the first year of life or the persistence of IgG beyond 1 year is indicative of prenatal infection. IgM and IgA antibodies usually decline to undectable levels in the first year of life, and so the presence of IgG in later childhood may be due to prenatal or postnatal infection (87). Thus, most patients with stigmata of *T. gondii* infection have detectable IgG antibodies only, which may persist at variable titers after an acute infection and fail to confirm recent or active infection. The demonstration of local, ocular anti-*Toxoplasma* antibody production using the Witmer-Desmonts coefficient has been employed mostly by European investigators to establish the diagnosis of active ocular toxoplasmosis (88). The ratio of anti-*Toxoplasma* IgG antibody levels in the serum is compared to that in the aqueous humor, after correcting for total protein concentration, producing this coefficient, which, if greater than four, is indicative of local antibody production and a diagnosis of ocular toxoplasmosis. Polymerase chain reaction (PCR)-based assays of aqueous and vitreous samples are highly sensitive and specific in establishing the diagnosis (89,90). Finally, tissue culture techniques with vitreous humor samples from patients have been successfully employed in the detection and growth of tachyzoites *in vitro* (91).

Management

Treatment is almost always indicated for newborns, children with any active-appearing lesion irrespective of location, immunosuppressed patients, or pregnant women with acquired disease.

Early and prolonged antibiotic therapy throughout the first year of life may be advisable as it has been shown to reduce the recurrence rate from 85% in untreated or undertreated infants (69,70) to 4% to 13% (71,92). A favorable visual outcome was reported (93) in all but 1 of 18 children born to mothers infected with toxoplasmosis before 25 weeks gestation who had been treated prenatally with a regimen of alternating pyrimethamine, sulfonamides, and spiramycin, and in whom treatment was continued from birth to 1 year of age. However, diagnosis requires PCR analysis of amniotic fluid, and amniocentesis creates other fetal risks.

Relative indications for treatment in older children include large or multiple active lesions, macular lesions abutting the optic nerve or a large blood vessel, lesions associated with moderate to severe vitreitis or hemorrhage, and those producing moderate decrease in visual acuity. Suggested treatment regimens for infants and children usually involve the combination of pyrimethamine, sulfadiazine and folinic acid (Table 16-7). Folinic acid is routinely added to prevent the leukopenia and thrombocytopenia associated with pyrimethamine therapy. Clindamycin is a reasonable alter-

native to pyrimethamine as is trimethoprim-sulfamethoxazole (Bactrim) for sulfadiazine. Atovaquone (Mepron) is also active against both tachyzoites and cystic forms of *T. gondii* and has been successfully used in HIV patients (94) and immunocompetent individuals (95). Systemic prednisone (1 mg/kg daily) can be added within 24 to 48 hours following the commencement of antibiotic therapy for vision-threatening lesions. Topical steroids and cycloplegia are used to treat anterior segment inflammation. Periocular corticosteroids are contraindicated as uncontrolled proliferation of the organism might result from local ocular immunosuppression produced by the depot. PPV may be required diagnostically in atypical cases and therapeutically to address inflammatory complications, such as vitreous opacification, retinal detachment, epiretinal membranes, or retinal neovascularization.

Overall, the prognosis of ocular toxoplasmosis is good for immunocompetent patients with extramacular lesions. In a review of 154 patients (76), 24% eventually became blind in one or both eyes, and bilateral blindness, was more frequent among patients with congenital ocular disease.

TOXOCARIASIS

Prevalence

Parasitic infections of the eye are a major cause of blindness worldwide. The genus *Toxocara* is one of the most commonly recognized etiologies in the United States, South America, Canada, and Europe (96). Ocular toxocariasis (OT) accounted for 37% of childhood retinal disease diagnoses (97), while *Toxocara* and other visceral larvae migrans were the cause of intraocular inflammation in 28.3% of all uveitis cases and 9.4% of all pediatric uveitis cases (32). OT has also been reported in young adults and in individuals up to the age of 50 years (98).

Etiology and Pathogenesis

Human toxocariasis results from tissue invasion by the second stage larvae of *Toxocara canis* or *Toxocara cati,* roundworm parasites which complete their life cycles in the small intestines of dogs and cats respectively. Transmission to humans occurs through geophagia, the oral-fecal route, or ingestion of contaminated foods (99). A history of pica and contact with dogs, especially puppies, is common in children with toxocariasis. Following ingestion of the ova, organisms grow into second stage larvae in the small intestine, enter the portal circulation, disseminate throughout the body by hematogenous and lymphatic routes and ultimately encyst in the target tissue (100). Organisms reach the eye through the choroidal, ciliary, or retinal arteries. Further development of *T. canis* into a sexually mature adult worm does not occur in humans, and so its ova are not shed in the alimentary tract, rendering stool analysis for larvae unproductive.

TABLE 16-7. DRUGS USED IN THE TREATMENT OF NEONATAL AND CHILDHOOD OCULAR TOXOPLASMOSIS

Drug	Dosage	Notes
Pyrimethamine	Children: 4-mg/kg loading dose followed by 1-mg/kg per day divided in two doses	Reversible dose-related bone marrow suppression Simultaneous administration of folinic acid
	Follow weekly with CBC	Contraindicated in the first trimester of pregnancy (potential teratogenicity)
	Newborns should be treated daily for the first 6 mo and then three times/wk for their first year of life. Dosage 1 mg/kg per day divided into two doses	Minimizes the size of retinochoroidal scar
Sulfadiazine	Children: 100 mg/kg per d divided every 6 h	Adverse effects: photosensitivity, Stevens-Johnson syndrome, crystalluria, and hematologic problems
	Newborns should be treated daily for their first years of life. Dosage: 100 mg/kg per d divided into two doses	Contraindicated in the third trimester of pregnancy (kernicterus) and during breast feeding
		Hemolytic anemia if G6PD deficient
		Synergistic with pyrimethamine
Folinic acid	5–20 mg/day during pyrimethamine therapy, depending on neutrophil count	Prevents bone marrow suppression when administered as an adjuvant of pyrimethamine therapy
Clindamycin	Children: 16–20 mg/kg per d divided every 6 h	Adverse effects: skin rashes, diarrhea and pseudomembranous colitis
		Synergistic with pyrimethamine and sulfonamides
Spiramycin	Pregnancy: 500 mg every 6 h for 3 wk; regiment may be repeated after 21 d	Drug of choice during pregnancy
	Children: 100 mg/kg per d divided every 6h	Reduces the incidence of congenital transmission
		In utero treatment of infected fetus improved visual outcome
		Not FDA approved
Prednisone	Children: 1–2 mg/kg per d	Indicated in active disease involving the posterior pole or optic nerve or if there is severe vitreous inflammation
		Start at the same time or within 48 h of initiating antimicrobial therapy, and taper off before discontinuation

CBC, Complete blood count; G6PD, glucose-6-posphate dehydrogenase; FDA, US Food and Drug Administration
Modified from Da Mata AP, Orfice F. Toxoplasmosis. In: Foster CS, Vitale AT, eds. *Diagnosis and treatment of uveitis.* Philadelphia: WB Saunders, 2001;403, with permission.

The nature and severity of human disease is dependent on the parasitic burden, site of infection, migratory behavior, and host inflammatory response and is manifested as one of two forms: visceral larval migrans (VML) or OT. While fulminant cases have been reported (101), VML is typically a mild, self-limited condition occurring in younger children, aged 2 to 4 years, and is characterized by fever, pulmonary symptoms, hepatosplenomegaly, and pronounced eosinophilia (102). There is a direct relationship between the degree of peripheral eosinophilia and the level of exposure to *Toxocara* larvae (103). VML and OT rarely present contemporaneously or at later times in the same individual. In a study of 245 patients with VML, only 5% had any evidence of ocular involvement (104). Furthermore, OT first appears in older children with an average of 7.5 (104) to 8.6 (105) years, whereas the age at presentation for VML is con-siderably younger, with a mean of 15 to 30 months (104). Finally, peripheral eosinophilia is not a feature of OT.

Symptoms and Signs

Patients with OT present with painless, unilateral decreased vision, strabismus, or leukocoria. Bilateral disease is exceedingly rare (106), with both eyes affected with equal frequency and a delay, of up to a year (117). The anterior segment is white and quiet and the posterior segment findings vary as follows: (i) peripheral granuloma, (ii) posterior pole granuloma, (iii) chronic endophthalmitis, or (iv) atypical features. Of these presentations, the peripheral retinal location is the most common. The localized forms (peripheral and posterior pole granulomata) are thought to arise as later, cicatricial manifestations *Toxocara* infection after resolution of the acute inflammatory phase (99). Tractional forces may produce retinal detachment (tractional, rhegmatogenous, or combined), macular distortion, or optic nerve dysfunction and consequent visual loss.

An uncommon variant of this form is that of unilateral pars planitis with diffuse peripheral inflammatory exudates (107). As the ocular media clear, a discrete intraretinal or subretinal mass with overlying vessels can present in the posterior pole (Fig. 16-2) or temporal to the optic disc (108). Patients with endophthalmitis present at an earlier age than those with peripheral or posterior pole granulomata, typically with a painless, quiet external eye, despite signs of considerable intraocular inflammation (109), including granulomatous anterior uveitis, hypopyon, a severe vitreitis, and a poorly defined retinal or vitreous abscess, sometimes contributing to leukocoria. The visual prognosis is dependent on the location of the inflammatory foci and the development of membrane formation with cicatricial and tractional sequelae in the vitreous cavity, retina, and ciliary body. Atypical presentations of sometimes presumed OT have been described (99) and include inflammatory iris mass and intracorneal larvae (110), lens involvement (111), optic disc granuloma (112), papillitis (113), and motile larvae in the retina (114) and vitreous (115).

Diagnosis

The diagnosis of OT is essentially clinical, based on characteristic lesion morphology, supportive laboratory data, and imaging studies. The serum enzyme-linked immunosorbent assay (ELISA) for *T. canis* is both a highly sensitive and specific indicator of prior exposure to the organism. The cutoff titer chosen for a positive serum ELISA titer is 1:8 providing 91% sensitivity and 90% specificity when combined

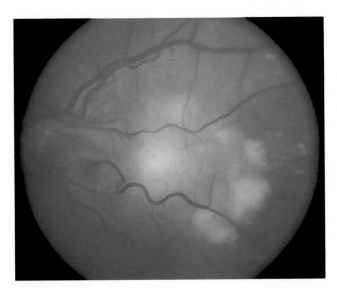

FIGURE 16-2. Macular, posterior granuloma in a patient with toxocara chorioretinitis.

with findings on the clinical examination (116). A 32% false-positive rate (117) and false-negative results in patients with retinoblastoma (RB) have been reported (116). Serum titers decrease over time (118), so any positive titer is regarded as significant in the appropriate clinical context.

Imaging studies, particularly ultrasound examination and CT, are useful. Three echographic patterns in 11 patients with OT were reported (119): (i) a solid, highly reflective peripheral mass (located in the temporal periphery in 91% of patients); (ii) a vitreous membrane extending between the posterior pole and the mass; and (iii) traction retinal detachment or fold from the posterior pole to the mass. Also described was pseudocystic transformation of the peripheral vitreous on ultrasound biomicroscopy (120). Intraocular calcification is not uniformly present, but may be seen in eyes with OT with significant ocular disruption or phthisis.

Cytological evaluation of aqueous fluid for eosinophils or malignant cells is indicative of OT and RB, respectively (121). As previously discussed with regard to the diagnosis of toxoplasmosis, intraocular fluids may also be sampled for specific *T. canis* antibodies to provide evidence of primary ocular involvement by calculating the Witmer-Desmonts coefficient (122,123). Toxocara larvae were recovered during PPV (124).

Differential Diagnosis

As RB is the most common malignant intraocular neoplasm of childhood, it is critically important to distinguish it, particularly the sporadic, unilateral variant, from OT. Factors which may be helpful in making this distinction include the following: (i) mean age at presentation for OT 7.5 to 8.9 years versus for RB 22 to 23 months (104,105), (ii) paucity of inflammatory stigmata in RB, and (iii) growth of RB lesions. Furthermore, normal levels of aqueous humor lactate dehydrogenase and phosphoglucose isomerase, the demonstration of eosinophils in vitreous or aqueous aspirates, and the absence of malignant cells favor a diagnosis of OT (125).

Infectious endophthalmitis is distinguished by a history of recent trauma or ocular surgery, immune deficiency or recent sepsis in the setting of painful visual loss together with conspicuous signs of external inflammation. Other entities considered include: toxoplasmic retinochoroiditis, pars planitis, retinopathy of prematurity, familial exudative vitreoretinopathy, persistent fetal vasculature, and Coats' disease.

Management

The management of VML includes the use of anthelminthic agents, antibiotics, and steroids (126). There is no uniformly satisfactory treatment for OT, with medical therapy aimed at reducing the inflammatory response in an effort to prevent the formation of membranes and secondary structural ocular damage. Periocular and systemic steroids (0.5 to 1.0 mg/kg prednisone daily) are the mainstays for eyes with active vitreitis. In contrast to active toxoplasmic retinochoroiditis, it is unlikely that corticosteroid-induced immune suppression leads to inflammatory exacerbation as *T. canis* larvae do not replicate in humans. Thiabendazole (50 mg/kg per day for 7 days) has been suggested (126) should there be no response to systemic steroids, and there are reports of clinical improvement of OT treated with thiabendazole (25 mg/kg twice daily for 5 days with a maximum of 3 g/day), albendazole (800 mg twice daily for 6 days), or mebendazole (100 to 200 mg twice daily for 5 days) (125). Although it has been suggested that anthelminthic therapy may provoke intraocular inflammation due a hypersensitivity response to dead larvae (115), clinical and experimental evidence indicate that this is not the case (127–129). Severe inflammation with abscess is associated with live motile organisms (127). The ultimate utility of anthelminthic therapy remains an open question (111).

Vitreoretinal surgical techniques have been successfully used to address postinflammatory complications: vitreous opacification, retinal detachment, and epiretinal membrane formation with vitreomacular or optic nerve traction (130–134). Laser photocoagulation of live, motile larvae may be considered if identified on clinical examination (98,114,135,136) and in the treatment of the rare occurrence of choroidal neovascular membranes arising in association with inactive *Toxocara* granulomata (137).

DIFFUSE UNILATERAL SUBACUTE NEURORETINITIS

Prevalence

Diffuse unilateral subacute neuroretinitis (DUSN) is an uncommon but important nematode ocular infection to consider in the differential diagnosis of pediatric posterior uveitis, as early recognition and treatment may preserve vision.

Initially described in 1978 (138), most reported cases are from North America, being most prevalent in the southeastern and northern Midwest regions of the United States and in the Caribbean islands. Cases of DUSN have since been reported in northwestern Europe (139) and South America, particularly in Brazil, where it is considered an important cause of posterior uveitis in children and young adults (140,141). Males are affected more frequently than females, most often during the second and third decades of life with a range in age of 8 to 65 years (142,143).

Etiology and Pathogenesis

Evidence to date suggests that DUSN is caused by a solitary nematode of two different sizes that migrates through the subretinal space (143). The smaller worm, proposed to be *Ancylostoma canium* or *T. canis* (134,144,145), measures 400 to 1,000 μm in length and appears to be endemic to the southeastern United States, Caribbean islands, and Brazil.

The larger worm, proposed to be *Baylisascaris procyonis* (146), is 1,500 to 2,000 μm in length and has been described in the northern Midwest United States and Canada (147).

Symptoms and Signs

The clinical course of DUSN is characterized by the insidious onset of unilateral visual loss from recurrent episodes of focal, multifocal, and diffuse inflammation of the retina, retinal pigment epithelium (RPE), and optic nerve in otherwise healthy young subjects. Patients may complain of unilateral paracentral or central scotomata, mild ocular discomfort, or transient obscurations of vision in the early stages of the disease or with profound visual loss at late presentation (142). The early stage of the disease is characterized by unilateral, moderate to severe vitreitis, optic disc swelling, and multiple, focal, gray-white lesions, varying in size from 1,200 to 1,500 μm, in the peripapillary and juxtamacular outer retina. These lesions are evanescent and occasionally have associated overlying serous retinal detachment. It is at this stage that subretinal worms are most readily visualized. Only two cases of bilateral DUSN were reported with neurological disease (neural larva migrans) (148).

Diagnosis

The diagnosis of DUSN is clinical, supported by the observation of a subretinal worm. Laboratory evaluations are typically negative. Electroretinographic (ERG) abnormalities include mild to moderate decrease in rod and cone function, with the b wave more affected than the a wave even early in the disease course. The ERG is rarely extinguished, even late in the disease course, distinguishing it from tapetoretinal degenerations (142).

Differential Diagnosis

Considerations during early presentation include sarcoid-associated uveitis, an outer retinal pigment epithelial disorder such as multifocal choroiditis and panuveitis, acute multifocal posterior placoid pigment epitheliopathy, multiple evanescent white-dot syndrome, serpiginous choroidopathy, ABD, toxoplasmosis, presumed ocular histoplasmosis syndrome, and nonspecific optic neuritis or papillitis (149).

The later stages are typified by retinal arterial narrowing, optic atrophy, diffuse pigment epithelial degeneration, and an abnormal electroretinogram. These findings might be confused with posttraumatic chorioretinopathy, occlusive vascular disease, toxic retinopathy, and retinitis pigmentosa (150).

Management

If the worm is visualized, direct laser treatment of the subretinal worm is highly effective in halting the progression of the disease and in improving visual acuity (143,151,152). The worm shows a tropism toward light and may be lured away for the macula by directing a bright examining light on the organism prior to treatment (153). Medical therapy with corticosteroids has shown an initial transient improvement in inflammatory control followed by recurrence of symptoms and progression of visual loss (142). Successful treatment with oral thiabendazole (22 mg/kg twice daily for 2 to 4 days with a maximum daily dose of 3 g) was reported in patients with DUSN and moderate to severe vitreous inflammation (154). Therapeutic response was determined by (i) death of the worm with fading of retinal lesions and the appearance of a single active focus within 1 week of treatment, (ii) resolution of vitreitis with a chorioretinal scar at the site of the nematode by 4 months, or (iii) inactivity and absence of new lesions by 6 months. Ivermectin as a single dose of 0.15 to 2.0 mg/kg in adults appears to be larvicidal for the nematodes causing DUSN, with a marked reduction in intraocular filaria (155).

HIV/AIDS: SYSTEMIC CONSIDERATIONS

Prevalence

In the United States, the number of AIDS cases reported annually among children less than 13 years of age has declined from a peak of 949 in 1992 to 105 cases in 2000 (156). In sharp contrast, it has been recently estimated that there are 1.3 million children worldwide under the age of 15 with HIV/AIDS, 90% of whom reside in the developing world, and that among these children, 3.8 million have died since the beginning of the epidemic (157). Equally devastating is the estimate that 8 million children worldwide have been orphaned by HIV (158).

HIV in Children

HIV infection in children occurs almost exclusively from perinatal transmission. The fetus can be infected in utero, but more commonly, children are exposed to the virus intrapartum, or from breastfeeding. The median survival time of HIV infected children ranges from between 5 and 8 years (159—162). There appears to be a bimodal distribution of clinical progression: children presenting with symptoms in the first few months of life have a rapid downhill course with a precipitous decline in CD4+ T-lymphocyte count, the early development of an AIDS-defining illnesses (ADI) (particularly *Pneumocystis carinii* pneumonia), and high mortality (163). In addition to early onset of HIV-related symptoms, predictors of rapid progression include evidence of *in utero* transmission, hepatosplenomegaly at birth, and failure to thrive and high viral loads after 1 month of life (164–166). Those who present later tend to have a more chronic course.

Although *P. carinii* pneumonia is the most common systemic opportunistic infection in both adults and children, recurrent bacterial infections are more common in HIV-infected children, including bacteremia secondary to *Streptococcus pneumoniae, Haemophilus influenza,* and *Salmonella* species, genitourinary tract infections with *Escherichia coli,* and skin and soft tissue infection with *Staphylococcus aureus* and *Streptococcus viridans* (167–169). Kaposi's sarcoma, and certain other opportunistic pathogens found in adults, such as toxoplasmosis, tuberculosis, and cryptococcosis are uncommon in children. On the other hand, certain clinical entities, such as encephalitis and lymphocytic interstitial pneumopathy, a syndrome characterized by progressive bilateral reticulonodular infiltrates, are typical of children with AIDS (170).

The viral loads are higher and incubation period shorter in children infected with HIV as compared to adults. Infants and children normally have higher CD4+ T-lymphocyte counts than adults, and these numbers normally decline with age (171). The Centers for Disease Control and Prevention (CDC) has provided a classification based on CD4+ T-lymphocyte counts (Table 16-8) and severity of symptoms (Table 16-9). Severe immune suppression is defined as less than 750 cells/μL (<15%) for children less than 1 year of age, less than 500 cells/μL (<15%) for children aged 1 to 5

TABLE 16-8. 1994 REVISED HIV PEDIATRIC CLASSIFICATION SYSTEM: IMMUNE CATEGORIES BASED ON AGE-SPECIFIC CD4+ T-LYMPHOCYTE COUNT AND PERCENT

Immune Category	CD4+ T-lymphocyte Count/mL (%)		
	<12 mo	1–5 yr	6-12 yrs
1. No suppression	>1500 (>25)	>1000 (>25)	>500 (>25)
2. Moderate suppression	750-1499 (15-24)	500-999 (15-24)	200-499 (15-24)
3. Severe suppression	<750 (<15)	<500 <(15)	<200 (<15)

Modified from Centers for Disease Control and Prevention. 1994 revised classification system for human immunodeficiency virus in children less than 13 years of age. *MMWR Morb Mortal Wkly Rep* 1994;43(RR-12):1, with permission.

TABLE 16-9. CENTERS FOR DISEASE CONTROL AND PREVENTION 1994 REVISED HIV PEDIATRIC CLASSIFICATION SYSTEM: CLINICAL CATEGORIES BASED ON SIGNS AND SYMPTOMS

Clinical Category	Diagnoses	Clinical Category	Diagnoses
N	Asymptomatic	C	Multiple, recurrent severe bacterial infections
	Single category-A event		Esophageal or pulmonary candidiasis
			Disseminated coccidioidomycosis
A	Mildly symptomatic with		Extrapulmonary cryptococcosis
	two or more of the following:		Cryptosporidoisis or isosporiasis
	Lymphadenopathy		CMV disease at >1 mo of age
	Hepatomegaly		Encephalopathy
	Splenomegaly		Herpes simplex virus infection >1 mo of age
	Dermatitis		Disseminated histoplasmosis
	Parotitis		Kaposi's sarcoma
	Recurrent URI sinusitis, otitis media		Primary lymphoma of the brain
B	Moderately symptomatic		Burkitt's or immunoblastic lymphoma
	includes but not limited to:		Disseminated or extrapulmonary mycobacterial tuberculosis
	Anemia		
	Neutropenia		Disseminated other or unspecified mycobacterium sp.
	Thrombocytopenia		Disseminated *Mycobacterium avium*
	Cardiomyopathy		*Pneumocystitis carinii* pneumonia
	CMV infection, <1 month of age		Progressive multifocal leukoencephalopathy
	Hepatitis		Recurrent salmonella (nontyphoid) septicemia
	Pneumonia		Toxoplasmosis of the brain (>1 mo of age)
	Lymphoid interstitial pneumonia		Wasting syndrome

HIV, human immunodeficiency virus; URI, upper respiratory infection; CMV, cytomegalovirus.
Modified from Centers for Disease Control and Prevention. 1994 revised classification system for human immunodeficiency virus infection in children less than 13 years of age. *MMWR Morb Moral Wkly Rep* 1994;43(RR-12):1–10, with permission.

years, and less than 200 cells/μL (<15%) for children older than 6 years (adult criterion) (Table 16-9). Declining CD4+ T-lymphocyte counts and CD4 percentages are the hallmarks of disease progression in children (172).

Diagnosis

Early serologic diagnosis of HIV infection in infants and children is complicated by the presence and persistence of maternal anti-HIV antibodies for months in the newborn. At the present time, however, the diagnosis can be made in most infants by 1 month of age using direct viral detection techniques, including peripheral blood mononuclear cell (PBMC) co-culture, DNA PCR of the infant's PBMCs, or HIV RNA in the plasma. DNA PCR is the method of choice for the diagnosis of HIV in infants with early presumptive detection of infection always being confirmed by later repeat testing (173,174).

HIV/AIDS: OCULAR COMPLICATIONS

Prevalence

Ocular disease in children with HIV/AIDS is far less common than in adults with only 8 of 40 (20%) reported ocular findings related to AIDS (175) as compared to published reports of 50% to 73% for adults during the same time period.

Etiology and Pathogenesis

Cytomegalovirus retinitis and cotton wool spots, as in adults, are the most common ocular complications of HIV/AIDS infection, reported between 1.6% to 5% (167,175,176). The prevalence of CMV retinitis is higher in children with CD4+ T-lymphocyte counts below 100 cells/μL. Of those pediatric patients with CMV retinitis, more than one-third eventually developed retinal detachments. Other infections include toxoplasmosis (175,177), herpes keratitis, herpes zoster ophthalmicus, and periocular molluscum (177,178). Peripheral retinal perivasculitis has been reported in HIV-positive African children and has not been associated with CMV retinitis routinely (170), but believed to be part of diffuse infiltrative lymphocytosis syndrome (179).

The question as to why CMV retinitis develops less frequently in children than in adults remains unanswered. One possibility is that children are less likely to have been exposed to CMV. However, CMV retinitis developed in only 5% of 149 children with current or prior elevation of CMV immunoglobulin levels (180).

Symptoms and Signs

The most common manifestation of HIV retinal microvasculopathy is the cotton-wool spot, although intraretinal hemorrhages, white-centered hemorrhages (Roth spots), microaneurysms, and retinal ischemia also occur. Peripheral retinal microvasculopathy has also been reported (181).

Cytomegalovirus retinitis can present as (i) classic or fulminant retinitis with retinal hemorrhage in the distribution of the nerve fiber layer (Fig. 16-3); (ii) granular form found more often in the periphery, with less retinal edema and hemorrhage and active retinitis appearing at the borders of the lesion; or (iii) perivascular CMV, described as a variant of frosted branch angiitis, a retinal perivasculitis initially described in immunocompetent children. (Fig. 16-4)

It has been suggested that HIV-positive children with severe immunosuppression (CD4+ lymphocyte counts within category 3), evidence of systemic CMV infection, or exposure of the development of some other form of advanced HIV disease be examined every 3 or 4 months (167,168). In children with chronic disease, complete ocular examinations are conducted annually.

Diagnosis

Diagnosis of individual infections is often clinical, although PCR analysis of ocular fluid and occasionally chorioretinal biopsy and histopathology are required.

Management

Ocular drug toxicity has been reported in 5% to 10% of children with HIV/AIDS treated with high doses of didanosine (2′, 3′-dideoxyinosine) and is manifested by focal peripheral atrophy of the retinal pigment epithelium with

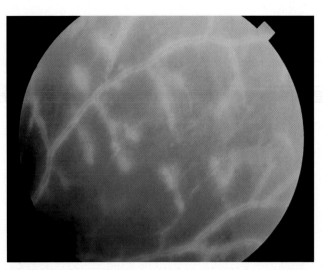

FIGURE 16-4. Peripheral frosted branch angiitis associated with cytomegalovirus retinitis.

accompanying electroretinographic and electrooculographic abnormalities (182,183). Toxicity is related to both the peak and cumulative doses and the electrophysiologic abnormalities appear to be reversible. In addition, bilateral, stellate, corneal endothelial deposits have been reported in 6 of 25 HIV-positive children receiving rifabutin prophylaxis for *Mycobacterium avium* complex bacteremia (184).

The optimal treatment for CMV retinitis in children has yet to be established. Present therapeutic regimens with ganciclovir and foscarnet are similar to those used in adults, with the drug dosages adjusted for body weight (185–189). Recovery of immune function in patients treated with HAART for HIV/ AIDS or discontinuation of immunosuppressive drugs in children requiring this therapy may allow discontinuation of maintenance antiviral therapy (190,191). Oral preparations of ganciclovir (30 mg/kg of ganciclovir administered every 8 hours) have only recently shown promise in the pediatric population (192).

Finally, while intravitreous therapy with ganciclovir, foscarnet, cidofovir, or fomivirsen is theoretically available for the treatment of CMV retinitis in children, the need for frequent injections, most likely under general anesthesia, may make this an impractical option. The safety and efficacy of intravitreal sustained- release devices awaits further evaluation in children.

HERPES SIMPLEX VIRUS

Prevalence

Herpes simplex virus (HSV) infections in the perinatal period are becoming increasingly common with an incidence of approximately 1 in 2,000 to 1 in 5,000 births per year in the United States (193), of which 4% are congenital, 86% natal, and 10% postnatal (194).

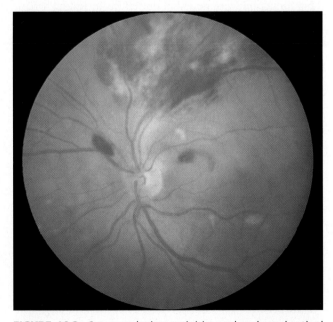

FIGURE 16-3. Cytomegalovirus retinitis: wedge-shaped retinal infiltrate with accompanying intraretinal hemorrhage following the nerve fiber layer distribution in the superotemporal arcade, multiple intraretinal hemorrhages, and multiple cotton wool spots.

Etiology and Pathogenesis

Herpes simplex virus belongs to the herpes family of viruses that include CMV, VZV, and EBV. HSV occurs as two antigenic types: HSV-1, usually associated with oral-facial infection and encephalitis; and HSV-2, which causes genital infections and is sexually transmitted (195). Both viruses establish latency in sensory neurons and are capable of producing pathologic lesions upon reactivation at sites both near to and distant from the point of entry into the body.

The overwhelming majority of perinatal HSV cases are due to HSV-2 infection as the result of contact with infected genital secretions at the time of delivery. Infection rates vary from 33% to 50% for infants delivered vaginally to mothers with primary genital herpes, 3% to 5% for mothers with recurrent lesions, and less than 3% with recurrent asymptomatic shedding at the time of delivery (196). Perinatal HSV-1 infections are usually acquired postnatally through contact with immediate family members who have symptomatic or asymptomatic oral-labial HSV infection, or from nosocomial transmission (195). Congenital infection is thought to occur transplacentally, during maternal leukocyte-associated viremia (197).

Symptoms and Signs

Systemic manifestations of both antigenic subtypes of congenital HSV infection include intrauterine growth retardation, low birth weight, microcephaly, hydranencephaly, intracranial calcifications, encephalitis, seizures, psychomotor retardation, pneumonitis, hepatomegaly, and recurrent, grouped, cutaneous vesicles (198,199). There is a higher rate of spontaneous abortion and prematurity among HSV-infected fetuses (200). Infants with natal or postnatal herpes usually present with a clinical picture resembling that of bacterial sepsis with cyanosis, vomiting, anorexia, respiratory distress, lethargy, and alterations in temperature (196). Approximately 75% of all neonates present with skin lesions consisting of vesicles, occurring singly or in clusters, found predominantly on the eyelids, perioral area, and the trunk. Untreated neonatal HSV infection carries a high overall mortality (49%) (201), and only 26% of survivors develop normally (202).

Approximately 13% of infants with perinatal HSV infection have ocular involvement with disease being limited to the eye in one-third of these (202). Ophthalmic findings from *in utero* herpetic infection include active chorioretinitis (198–200,203) or inactive chorioretinal scars (204), keratitis and vitreitis (203), and congenital malformations (microphthalmia, retrocorneal masses, lenticular opacity, optic atrophy, and retinal dysplasia) (198,205,206). Infection during the first trimester is believed associated with teratogenic malformations; second trimester disease with inactive chorioretinal scarring without malformation; and third trimester infection within a clinical pattern identical to that

of active neonatally acquired infection (204). Typical ocular findings in neonatally acquired HSV include corneal ulceration, anterior uveitis, cataract formation, vitreitis, chorioretinitis, and optic atrophy (207). A prolonged latency of the virus within retinal tissues is suggested by the relatively high incidence of chorioretinal scars in this long-term study of children examined from 1 to 15 years after infection (208).

Diagnosis

The diagnosis of perinatal herpetic infection is made in the appropriate clinical context and by isolation of the virus from vesicular fluid, nasal secretions, conjunctiva secretions, buffy coat of whole blood, or spinal fluid of the infant (196).

Differential Diagnosis

It is important to note that the signs of quiescent or active herpetic ocular disease may be present at birth or later in the neonatal period, and so, must be differentiated from non-herpetic infectious diseases such as *Toxoplasma*, rubella, and CMV infections.

Management

The drug of choice for disseminated HSV infections in neonates, including herpes simplex retinitis, is acyclovir (30 mg/kg daily for 10 days to 4 weeks intravenously) (209). The major side effect of systemically administered acyclovir is nephrotoxicity. Vidarabine may also be administered as a single intravenous infusion, 15 to 30 mg/kg per day, over a 12-hour period, with potential side effects including hepatic toxicity and bone marrow suppression (196).

VARICELLA-ZOSTER VIRUS

Varicella-zoster virus produces two distinct disease syndromes: primary infection presents as varicella (chickenpox), a highly contagious and usually benign illness of childhood; and subsequent reactivation, usually later in adult life, of latent varicella-zoster virus in dorsal-root ganglia, resulting in a dermatomal cutaneous eruption known as "herpes-zoster" or "shingles" (210). Likewise, VZV retinitis may occur, uncommonly, during the course of primary infection, either following "chickenpox" or as a feature of congenital VZV infection, or as a reactivation of the infection later in life in patients with a history of varicella in childhood. While the retinitis is necrotizing in all cases, its presentation may vary in severity, due to both host and viral factors.

Prevalence

Congenital varicella infection is rare with a 2% risk of embryopathy due to maternal varicella during the first 20 weeks of pregnancy (196). Should maternal disease develop within 5 days before delivery or 48 hours postpartum, infant mortality can be as high as 50% due to fulminant systemic disease in an immature newborn immune system and lack of protective transplacental maternal antibodies (195,211,212).

Signs and Symptoms

Systemic manifestations of the congenital varicella syndrome include cutaneous scars, limb hypoplasia, low birth weight, cerebral atrophy, seizures, psychomotor retardation, developmental delay, and neuropathic bladder (212). Ocular findings consist of chorioretinal scarring, atrophy and hypoplasia of the optic nerve, congenital cataract, Horner's syndrome, and bulbar palsy (212–214). The chorioretinal scars are typically unilateral, occurring in either the macula or retinal periphery, and vary in size. The scars themselves show chorioretinal atrophy with central pigmentation and surrounding depigmentation or a depigmented center, mimicking those of congenital rubella, syphilis, and inactive toxoplasmosis, particularly when present in the posterior pole. The unaffected retina between the scars appears normal. Presumably, the chorioretinitis resolves by the time of delivery as active retinitis has yet to be reported during the neonatal period.

Diagnosis

The diagnosis of congenital varicella syndrome is essentially clinical with the recognition of the characteristic defects in the neonate and a history of maternal varicella.

Differential Diagnosis

The inactive chorioretinal scars must be differentiated from other infectious agents producing congenital infections, commonly known by the pneumonic TORCH (toxoplasmosis, others [syphilis, VZV, EBV, HIV, and lymphocytic choriomeningitis virus], rubella, CMV, and HSV). This differential diagnosis is made by the clinical history and serologic testing of both the infant and mother.

ACUTE RETINAL NECROSIS SYNDROME

The acute retinal necrosis syndrome, initially described by Urayama and colleagues in 1971 (215), is a part of a spectrum of necrotizing herpetic retinopathies whose clinical expression is largely determined by the immune status of the host (216). Originally described in otherwise healthy adults, ARN has been shown to be caused by reactivated herpes infection due to HSV-1, HSV-2, VZV, or CMV, usually appearing years after primary infection from chickenpox or herpes simplex mucocutaneous disease (217) Rarely, ARN may occur as a primary necrotizing retinitis associated with

chickenpox (218). ARN and its variants, most notably progressive outer retinal necrosis (219), have been described in patients with AIDS. Necrotizing herpetic retinitis may also be acquired in the immunocompromised patient, often with accompanying viral encephalitis (220).

Prevalence

Acute retinal necrosis syndrome remains largely a disease of adults despite the fact that chickenpox and herpetic infection are largely acquired during childhood. The literature of ARN in the pediatric population is scant (218,221–226), with the youngest case report being in a child of 4 years (227).

Symptoms and Signs

The classical clinical triad of ARN consists of unilateral moderate to severe anterior uveitis and vitreitis, severe, occlusive retinal arteritis, and progressive peripheral retinal necrosis (217). Optic nerve inflammation and atrophy are commonly seen. The peripheral retinitis produces areas of whitening, or "thumbprints" which may coalesce into broad geographic areas with pseudopodlike projections over a period of days, progressing centrifugally toward the posterior pole. Retinitis is frequently associated with arteritis (Fig. 16-5). Full-thickness retinal necrosis develops, leaving thin, atrophic retina with multiple full-thickness holes in its wake. These holes, together with consequent vitreous condensation, fibrosis, and traction, are responsible for the increased frequency of

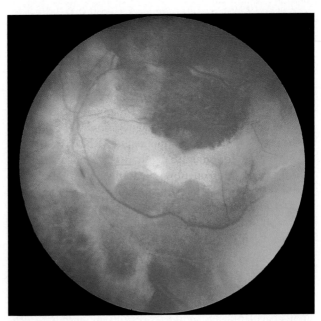

FIGURE 16-5. Acute retinal necrosis: 360-degree confluent peripheral retinitis proceeding towards the posterior pole associated with retinal vasculitis, intraretinal hemorrhage, subhyaloid hemorrhage, and optic disc swelling.

rhegmatogenous retinal detachment seen in between 24% to 80% of these eyes (217). The contralateral eye becomes involved in approximately one-third of cases, usually between 4 and 6 weeks of disease onset. The long-term visual prognosis of ARN, despite successful retinal reattachment, is guarded, with approximately one-third of patients left with 20/200 acuity or worse (228).

Etiology

Previous reports (218,229) have suggested that ARN associated with primary chickenpox infection may represent a "mild type" of disease; however, a 4-year-old boy with ARN following uncomplicated chickenpox infection (227) had unusually severe retinitis eventuating in a total retinal detachment and poor visual outcome. It has been demonstrated that VZV and HSV-1 seem to occur predominantly in patients older than 25 years while HSV-2 is found in those younger than 25 years of age (225,230). In addition, the retinitis has been associated with preexisting chorioretinal scars and intraocular disease associated with other nonocular stigmata of HSV infection.

Diagnosis

The diagnosis is most often made clinically on the basis of the history and findings on the ocular exam. PCR analysis of the aqueous humor or vitreous biopsy specimens in patients with features of necrotizing viral retinitis can provide specific etiological confirmation and is both safe and highly sensitive (231). Prompt recognition and immediate treatment are essential to reduce the risk of severe visual loss.

Management

Medical therapy of ARN consists of intravenous acyclovir, 1,500 mg/m^2 daily, in three divided doses, for 10 to 14 days (228). Antithrombotic therapy with heparin or aspirin (125 to 650 mg/day) has been suggested as adjunctive therapy as it is thought that platelet hyperaggregation may contribute to the occlusive vascular component of ARN. Systemic corticosteroids (prednisone 1.0 mg/kg per day and tapered over 2 to 6 weeks) are frequently added under antiviral cover to suppress the considerable inflammatory component of this disease. Following parenteral acyclovir therapy, oral acyclovir (800 mg five times daily for an adult) is given for 3 months. Palay and colleagues (232) demonstrated a reduction in disease onset in the fellow eye from 75% to 35% in patients given oral acyclovir following intravenous therapy for acute ARN.

Surgical therapy for ARN includes prophylactic laser photocoagulation (as soon as media clarity permits) to the posterior border of necrotic retina to prevent retinal detachment. Retinal detachment repair almost always requires PPV, membrane removal, endolaser photocoagulation, gas or oil tamponade, with or without the addition of a scleral buckle due to the multiplicity and posterior location of the retinal breaks.

RUBELLA

Reported cases of rubella and congenital rubella syndrome (CRS) have fallen precipitously in the United States since the introduction of a vaccine in 1969 (233). The peak age incidence has also shifted from 5 to 9 years in the prevaccine era, to older children (15 to 19 years) and young adults (20 to 24 years) (195,196,234). Approximately 5% to 25% of women of childbearing age who lack rubella antibody are susceptible to primary infection (196) as are certain at risk groups including religious communities who refuse vaccination, immigrant women, and persons in institutions (235,236).

Congenital Infection

The fetus is infected with rubella virus transplacentally secondary to maternal viremia during the course of primary infection. The frequency of fetal infection and congenital defects vary with the gestational age at the time of maternal infection. Fetal infection rates are 81% to 100% during the first 10 weeks, 50% between weeks 11 and 20, 37% from 20 to 25 weeks, and 100% during the last month of pregnancy. The rate of congenital defects varies inversely with gestational age as follows: 90% from weeks 2 to 10, 34% in weeks 11 to 12, 17% in weeks 13 to 16, 3% in weeks 17 to 18, and none thereafter (237,238). While obvious maternal infection during the first trimester of pregnancy may end in spontaneous abortion, stillbirth, or severe fetal malformations, seropositive, asymptomatic maternal rubella may also result in severe fetal disease.

Pathophysiology

Although the mechanism of rubella embryopathy is not known at a cellular level, it is thought that the virus inhibits cellular multiplication together with the establishment of chronic, persistent infection during organogenesis (239). Persistence of viral replication after birth, with ongoing tissue damage, is central to the pathogenesis of CRS and may explain the appearance of hearing, neurological, or ocular deficits long after birth (240,241).

Symptoms and Signs

The classic features of the CRS include cardiac malformations (patent ductus arteriosus, interventricular septal defects, or pulmonic stenosis), ocular lesions (chorioretinitis, cataract, corneal clouding, and microphthalmia) and deafness. Hearing loss is the most common systemic finding, occurring in 44% of cases (242). Other systemic manifestations of the CRS include intrauterine growth retardation, microcephaly, mental retardation, hepatosplenomegaly, thrombocytopenic purpura, interstitial pneumonia, myocarditis or myocardial necrosis, and metaphyseal bone lesions (195). Patients with congenital rubella are at greater risk for developing diabetes mellitus and subsequent diabetic retinopathy (243).

Prevalence

The overall incidence of ocular anomalies in CRS varies between 30% and 78% (244–246). Cataract and glaucoma follow viral infection during the first 2 months of gestation while pigmentary retinopathy follows exposure during the first 5 months (247,248). Pigmentary retinopathy, often described as "salt and pepper," is the most common ocular finding occurring in 60% of cases of CRS, although its true incidence is difficult to establish due to difficulty in visualization of the retina posed by the frequent presence of concomitant cataract and nystagmus (244,249,250). It can be stationary or progressive (251). The appearance of this pigmentary disturbance can vary from small, black irregular masses, finely stippled, bone spiculelike changes to gross pigmentary irregularities with coarse, blotchy mottling (Fig. 16-6). Choroidal neovascularization with subretinal hemorrhage is a rare complication but may reduce vision (250,252–257). Unless otherwise compromised by glaucoma, the optic nerve and the retinal vessels are typically normal in appearance.

Congenital (nuclear) cataracts and microphthalmia are the most frequent causes of poor visual acuity (244). An exuberant inflammatory response can follow lens extraction most likely due to the persistence of virus in the cataractous lens (241). Glaucoma is found in about 10% of patients with CRS and may be due to multiple causes, including abnormal development of the angle, chronic iridocyclitis, and

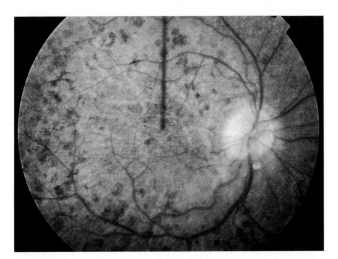

FIGURE 16-6. Congenital rubella: diffuse retinal pigment epithelial mottling with "salt-and-pepper" appearance.

secondary angle-closure due to an enlarged cataract (258). The diagnosis should be suspected in patients with bilateral disease and corneal edema. Less common ocular abnormalities include iris hypoplasia and chronic, granulomatous iridocyclitis.

Diagnosis

The diagnosis of congenital rubella is made by the presence of maternal rubella infection together with the observation of congenital anomalies. Given that a significant proportion of maternal rubella infection is subclinical, definitive diagnosis in the mother depends on laboratory confirmation of virus cultured from the nasopharynx or serologic testing with hemagglutination inhibition, ELISA, or fluorescent assay. Diagnostic criteria for rubella infection include a fourfold increase in rubella-specific IgG in paired sera 1 to 2 weeks apart, or the new appearance of rubella specific IgM (249). As the fetus is capable of mounting an immune response to rubella virus, specific IgM or IgA antibody to rubella in cord blood confirms the diagnosis.

Differential Diagnosis

The differential diagnosis of congenital rubella retinitis consists of the TORCH syndrome, viral infections such as mumps, roseola, and vaccinoencephalitis (195), and syphilis, which can produce a "salt and pepper" funduscopic appearance.

Management

There is no specific antiviral therapy for congenital rubella and treatment is supportive.

Acquired Infection

The incubation period for acquired infection is 14 to 21 days with a prodrome of 1 to 5 days in adolescents and adults prior to the onset of the rubella exanthem (259). An erythematous, maculopapular rash appears first on the face, spreads towards the hands and feet, involves the entire body within 24 hours, and disappears by the third day. The rash is not always present and the occurrence of fever is variable. Lymphadenopathy is invariably present. Arthritis, encephalitis, and thrombocytopenic purpura sometimes complicate the course.

Signs and Symptoms

The most frequent ocular complication of acquired rubella infection is conjunctivitis (70%), followed by the infrequent occurrence of epithelial keratitis (7.6%), and retinitis (260,261). Acquired rubella retinitis has been described in only two case reports, both of which involved adults

(262,263). Patients presented with acute onset of decreased vision and disseminated chorioretinitis with multiple large areas of bullous neurosensory detachment, underlying pigment epithelial detachments involving the entire posterior pole, anterior chamber and preretinal vitreous cells, dark gray atrophic lesions of the retinal pigment epithelium, normal retinal vessels and optic nerve, and the absence of retinal hemorrhage. The neurosensory detachments resolved spontaneously and visual acuity returned to normal.

Diagnosis

Diagnostic criteria for rubella infection include a fourfold increase in rubella-specific IgG in paired sera 1 to 2 weeks apart, or the new appearance of rubella-specific IgM (249).

Management

Uncomplicated acquired rubella does not require specific therapy. Acquired rubella retinitis and postvaccination optic neuritis respond well to systemic steroids (263,264).

LYMPHOCYTIC CHORIOMENINGITIS VIRUS

Lymphocytic choriomeningitis virus (LCMV) is an underrecognized fetal teratogen, the vertical transmission of which can cause intrauterine death, hydrocephalus, and chorioretinitis. It should be included in the TORCH group of congenital infections (265).

Etiology and Pathogenesis

The LCMV belongs to the Arenaviridae family of single-stranded RNA viruses with rodent reservoirs (266,267). Chronically infected common house mice (*Mus musculus*) and hamsters serve as the primary host and reservoir for the virus, which are transferred vertically within these populations by intrauterine infection during maternal viremia (268,269). The virus is shed in nasal secretions, saliva, milk, semen, urine, and feces with human acquisition resulting from contamination of food or fomites, aerosolization of the virus, and possibly from the bites of infected rodents. Acquired LCMV infection is asymptomatic or mild in one-third of cases while CNS disease, predominantly aseptic meningitis or meningoencephalitis, develops in approximately half of cases (265). Fatalities are rare and recovery is generally complete, although this may take months.

Signs and Symptoms

Systemic findings included macrocephaly and microcephaly (270), hydrocephalus or intracranial calcifications (265,271), mild mental retardation, seizures, and visual impairment (271).

The most common ocular finding is chorioretinal scars mainly in the retinal periphery as reported in 47 of 52 infants (272). These scars can involve the macula and consist of alternating patches of pigmentary migration and atrophy, resembling most closely those seen in congenital toxoplasmosis (272). Other less common ocular findings include bilateral optic atrophy, nystagmus, esotropia, exotropia, cataract, and microphthalmia. Ocular findings in the absence of neurological findings are rare (273).

Diagnosis

The diagnosis is made by serologic testing of the mother and the infant. The immunofluorescent antibody (IFA) test and Western blot assays are sensitive, detect both IGM and IgG antibody, and are commercially available (274,275). An ELISA through the CDC and PCR to detect LCMV RNA are diagnostic (276).

Differential Diagnosis

The differential diagnosis of congenital LCMV includes: the TORCH syndrome, especially congenital toxoplasmosis. The intracerebral calcifications of congenital toxoplasmosis tend to be diffuse, whereas those with congenital LCMV are associated with a more periventricular location (265). Ultimately, the differential diagnostic possibilities are excluded by the absence of cultures that are positive for CMV, HSV and serologic testing negative for rubella, *T. pallidum*, or *T. gondii*. Congenital LCMV should be strongly considered in unexplained hydrocephalus, micro- or macrocephaly, intracranial calcifications, chorioretinal scars, and nonimmune hydrops (265).

Management

Treatment of congenital LCMV is largely supportive. However, ribavirin, which is used successfully in other arenavirus infections, and immunomodulatory agents are potential therapeutic alternatives (277).

EPSTEIN-BARR VIRUS
Etiology and Pathogenesis

Epstein-Barr virus is a ubiquitous double-stranded DNA virus with a complex capsid and envelope belonging to the group of gamma herpes viruses (195). It is the viral agent commonly associated with infectious mononucleosis (IM), a systemic syndrome predominantly affecting adolescents between the ages of 14 and 18 years (278). Transmission is primarily through saliva, although it can be transmitted by blood transfusions. EBV has a B-lymphocyte tropism as these are the only cells known to have surface receptors for the virus (195). EBV has been implicated in the pathogenesis of Burkitt's lymphoma, especially among African children, and in the development of nasopharyngeal carcinoma.

Symptoms and Signs

Ocular manifestations of EBV may arise from congenital infection, or much more commonly, during primary infection in the context of infectious mononucleosis (IM). Congenital cataracts have been reported with congenital EBV infection (279). Ocular manifestations of acquired IM include, most commonly, a mild, self-limited follicular conjunctivitis early in the course of the disease; epithelial or stromal keratitis; episcleritis; bilateral granulomatous iritis and iridocyclitis (280); and less frequent complications such as dacryoadenitis, cranial nerve palsies, and Parinaud's oculoglandular syndrome (281). Isolated optic disc edema or optic neuritis (282), macular edema, retinal hemorrhages, retinitis (Fig. 16-7), choroiditis, vitreitis (283,284), "punctate outer retinitis" (284), progressive subretinal fibrosis and uveitis, and secondary choroidal neovascularization have been reported with EBV and IM (285). Anterior and posterior uveitis associated with EBV infection, in the absence of clinical IM, has also been reported, although mostly in adults (286–289).

Diagnosis

The diagnosis is made clinically and based on serologic evidence of antibodies against a variety of EBV-specific capsid antigens. During IM, the EBV viral capsid antigen (VCA) IgM antibody, followed by the VCA IgG titers, rise in a parallel fashion during viral incubation, 4 to 5 weeks following exposure to the virus. The early antigen (EA) rises with the onset of clinical disease, usually within 5 to 10 weeks of exposure, rises to a maximum, and then falls to undetectable

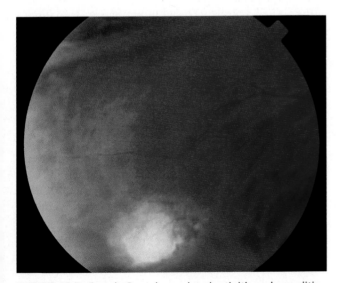

FIGURE 16-7. Epstein-Barr virus–related retinitis and vasculitis.

levels 6 to 12 months after resolution of the infection. The EBV nuclear antigen antibody appears slowly, within 2 months, and persists for life, whereas the VCA IgM titer falls to undetectable levels after resolution of the infection. The diagnosis of chronic EBV infection is best supported by abnormally elevated anti-VCA IgM and anti-EA antibody levels (290,291).

Management

Most ocular disease is self-limited and does not require treatment. However, iridocyclitis may be treated with topical corticosteroids and cycloplegia and posterior uveitis with systemic steroids. The role of antiviral therapy is unknown.

MEASLES VIRUS
Prevalence

Measles is typically a disease of childhood and despite the existence of a safe, effective, and inexpensive vaccine for over 40 years, it remains the fifth leading cause of mortality among children under five years of age worldwide, with an estimated 77,000 deaths in the year 2000 (292) (see also Chapter 18). In contrast, a total of 116 confirmed cases of measles were reported to the United States in 2001 (293).

Etiology and Pathogenesis

Congenital and acquired measles infection is caused by a single-stranded RNA virus of the genus *Morbillivirus* in the Paramyxoviridae family and may affect multiple ocular structures or result in devastating neurological disease. Humans and monkeys are the only natural hosts. The virus is highly contagious and is transmitted directly or via aerosolization of nasopharyngeal secretions to mucus membranes of the conjunctiva or respiratory tract of susceptible individuals. Infected individuals may transmit the virus from 5 days after exposure to 5 days following the skin rash, which may appear 14 days after initial exposure (294). Congenital measles is transmitted through the placenta.

Symptoms and Signs
Congenital Measles

Prenatal transmission during the first trimester results in spontaneous abortion in approximately 20% of cases while congenital infection later in gestation may result in premature birth (195). Congenital measles may produce the following systemic anomalies: cardiomyopathy, pyloric stenosis, genu valgum, deafness, mongolism, vertebral abnormalities, cleft lip, cleft palate, rudimentary ear (295).

Ocular manifestations of congenital measles infection include: cataract, optic nerve head drusen, and bilateral diffuse pigmentary retinopathy involving both the posterior pole and retinal periphery (295) with normal or attenuated retinal vessels, retinal edema, or macular star formation (296). The ERG and visual acuity are usually normal. The differential diagnosis includes entities comprising the TORCH syndrome, atypical retinitis pigmentosa, Leber's idiopathic stellate neuroretinitis, and maternal infection from the influenza virus during the third, fourth, or sixth months of pregnancy (195).

Acquired Measles

The initial systemic manifestations of acquired measles arise 9 to 19 days following exposure. One to two days before the appearance of a red, maculopapular rash that spreads from head downwards, Koplik's spots (blue-white dots surrounded by a red areola) appear typically on the buccal mucosa opposite the lower molars or occasionally on the conjunctiva, where they are called Hirschberg's spots (297). The rash resolves in the order in which it appeared, usually within 6 days.

The most common ocular complications of measles are keratitis and mild, papillary, nonpurulent conjunctivitis. Bilateral epithelial keratitis is seen in 76% of patients (298). Both keratitis and conjunctivitis usually resolve without sequelae; however, postmeasles blindness from corneal complications is a significant problem worldwide.

Measles retinopathy is more common in acquired than congenital measles and may occur in the presence or absence of encephalitis. An acute and often profound loss of vision develops 6 to 12 days after the appearance of exanthema and is characterized by attenuated arterioles, diffuse retinal edema, macular star, scattered retinal hemorrhages, blurred disc margins, and a clear media (299). With resolution of systemic symptoms and of the acute retinopathy, arteriolar attenuation with or without perivascular sheathing, optic disc pallor, and a secondary pigmentary retinopathy appearing as "bone spicule," "salt and pepper," or paravenous retinochoroidal atrophy (300) can arise.

The ERG is usually extinguished during the acute phase of measles retinopathy but may show a return of activity as the inflammation resolves and vision improves (299,300). Visual field testing may reveal severe constriction, ring scotomas, or small peripheral islands of vision. Resolution of acquired measles retinopathy over a period of weeks to months is usually associated with a return of useful vision; however, the extended visual prognosis is guarded due to the possibility of permanent visual field constriction.

Diagnosis

The diagnosis of measles and attendant ocular sequelae is made clinically by observation of the sequence of symptoms. The virus may be recovered from the nasopharynx, conjunctiva, lymphoid tissues, respiratory mucus membranes, urine and blood for a few days prior to and several days after the rash (294). Leukopenia is observed during the prodrome and serologic confirmation includes: complement fixation, ELISA, immunofluorescent and hemagglutination inhibition assays.

Differential Diagnosis

Acquired measles retinopathy is differentiated from central serous chorioretinopathy, Vogt-Koyanagi-Harada disease, toxoplasmic retinochoroiditis, retinitis pigmentosa, Leber's stellate idiopathic neuroretinitis, and other viral retinopathies.

Management

Supportive treatment of the systemic manifestations of measles is usually sufficient as the disease is self-limiting. In high-risk populations (e.g., pregnant women, children under 1 year of age, and immunosuppressed individuals), infection may be prevented by prophylactic treatment with gamma-globulin, 0.25 mL/kg of body weight, administered within 5 days of exposure (294). Likewise, the ocular manifestations of measles are treated symptomatically with topical antiviral or antibiotics to prevent secondary infections in patients with keratitis or conjunctivitis. Consideration should be given to the use of systemic corticosteroids for cases of acute measles retinopathy. In developing nations, vitamin A deficiency is corrected (Chapter 18).

SUBACUTE SCLEROSING PANENCEPHALITIS
Prevalence

Encephalomyelitis and subacute sclerosing panencephalitis (SSPE) can be late complications of measles infection. SSPE is rare, estimated to occur in 8.5 per 1,000,000 measles cases in the United States (301), and most often arises in unvaccinated children, 6 to 8 years following primary infection.

Symptoms and Signs

Onset is usually in late childhood or adolescence and is characterized by the insidious onset visual impairment, behavioral disturbances, and memory impairment, followed by myoclonus and progression to spastic quadriparesis, dementia, and death within 1 to 3 years. Ocular findings are reported in 10% to 50% of patients and may precede the neurologic manifestations by several weeks to 2 years (302,303). The most frequent ocular finding is a maculopathy, consisting of focal retinitis and RPE changes, occurring in 36% of patients (304–311). Retinitis may progress within several days to involve the posterior pole and peripheral retina. Other ophthalmoscopic findings include optic disc swelling and papilledema, optic atrophy, macular edema, macular pigment epithelial disturbances, small intraretinal hemorrhages, gliotic scar, whitish retinal infiltrates, serous macular detachment, drusen, preretinal membranes, macular hole, cortical blindness, hemianopsia, horizontal nystagmus, and ptosis (304,306,306,310,312–317). Characteristically, there is little, if any vitreitis, with mottling and scarring of the RPE as the retinitis resolves.

Diagnosis

The diagnosis is made based on the clinical manifestations, the presence of characteristic, periodic electroencephalographic discharges, a demonstration of raised IgG antibody titer against measles in the plasma and cerebrospinal fluid (CSF), and histopathology suggestive of panencephalitis on brain biopsy (318).

Differential Diagnosis

The differential diagnosis of the posterior segment findings associated with SSPE include those seen with necrotizing viral retinitis due to HSV, VZV, and CMV as well as those with multiple sclerosis (MS). In contrast to SSPE, MS is not a panencephalitis and magnetic resonance imaging reveal focal periventricular white matter lesions.

Management

Definitive treatment of SSPE is undetermined. A combination of oral isoprinosine (Inosiplex) and intraventricular interferon alpha appear to be the most effective treatments (318).

SYPHILIS

Syphilis is an uncommon cause of uveitis in the pediatric age group with ocular involvement occurring in both the acquired and congenital forms of the disease as a result of infection with the spirochete, *Treponema pallidum*. Congenital syphilis usually results from transplacental infection of the developing fetus (although the newborn may occasionally become infected by direct contact with a chancre in the birth canal), while acquired syphilis is a sexually transmitted disease. Most syphilitic disease described in children is congenital; however, the presence of acquired disease should raise the possibility of sexual precocity or child sexual abuse. Similarly, children who may have acquired HIV through sexual abuse should be evaluated for syphilis (319).

Congenital Syphilis

In 2001, a total of 441 cases of congenital syphilis were reported (rate: 11.1 per 100,000 live births), reflecting a similarly sharp decline in primary and secondary syphilis among women over the past decade (293). Congenital syphilis persists in the United States largely because a substantial number of women do not receive serologic testing until late in pregnancy, if at all, which is in turn related to absent or late prenatal care (320). In general, the longer the interval between maternal infection and pregnancy, the more benign the outcome in the infant (Kassowitz's law) (321).

Acquired Syphilis

The progression of untreated, acquired syphilis has been well described. *Primary syphilis* is characterized by the chancre, a painless, solitary lesion that originates at the inoculation site following exposure, transmission, and an incubation period of approximately 3 weeks. It resolves spontaneously in 3 to 12 weeks irrespective of treatment. The central nervous system may be seeded with treponemes at this time without neurological findings (321). *Secondary syphilis* occurs 6 to 8 weeks later and is characterized by lymphadenopathy and a generalized maculopapular rash, which may be prominent on the palms and soles. Uveitis occurs in approximately 10% of cases (322). Following this is a latency period ranging from one year (early latency) to decades (late latency). One third of untreated patients progress to *tertiary syphilis*, which is classified as: benign tertiary syphilis (the characteristic lesion, the gumma), cardiovascular syphilis, and neurosyphilis. Uveitis can occur at all stages of the infection, including primary syphilis (323). As the eye is considered an extension of the central nervous system, ocular syphilis is best conceived as a variant of neurosyphilis. This notion has important implications with respect to diagnostic testing and treatment.

Diagnosis

A confirmed case of congenital syphilis is one in which *T. pallidum* is identified by darkfield microscopy, fluorescent antibody, or other specific stains in specimens from cutaneous lesions, the placenta, umbilical cord, or autopsy material of an affected infant. A presumptive case of congenital syphilis is made in an infant whose mother was inadequately treated or received no treatment by time of delivery, regardless of findings in the infant, or who had a positive serologic test result for syphilis in addition to physical findings and evidence of cell, protein, or Venereal Disease Research Laboratory (VDRL) in the CSF (CDC) (324).

Primary syphilis can be diagnosed by direct visualization of spirochetes. Otherwise, positive serology within the appropriate clinical context, is required. Serologic tests are the nontreponemal antigen tests (rapid plasma regain or VDRL) and the treponemal antigen test (the fluorescent treponemal antigen absorption test [FTA-ABS] being the most common). Nontreponemal antibody titers are generally high during active infection, as in primary or secondary syphilis, and drop when the spirochetes are not active, such as during latent syphilis, or after adequate treatment. They are useful barometers in monitoring therapy with respect to both systemic and ocular disease. The FTA-ABS test result becomes positive during the secondary stage of syphilis, and with few exceptions (325), remains positive for the patient's lifetime, irrespective of treatment status. Although nontreponemal tests are appropriate for screening large populations with a relatively lower risk for syphilis, specific treponemal tests (i.e., FTA-ABS) have a higher predictive value in the setting of uveitis and should be employed in conjunction with nontreponemal tests in the diagnosis and treatment of ocular syphilis (325–327). Testing for HIV should be performed in all patients with ocular syphilis.

Examination of the CSF for syphilis is warranted in every case of syphilitic uveitis (326a,327b,328). Finally, full neurosyphilis regimes should be employed in both acquired and congenital disease, irrespective of when uveitis occurred after primary infection (Table 16-10). Reinfection is possible following adequate treatment and acquired syphilis may occur in individuals who have had the congenital form of the disease.

Symptoms and Signs

The most commonly reported systemic findings in early (<2 years of age) congenital syphilis are hepatosplenomegaly, characteristic changes of the long bones on radiographic examination, distended abdomen, desquamative skin rash, low birth weight, pneumonia, and severe anemia (319). Late (>2 years) manifestations of congenital syphilis are the result of scarring from the early systemic disease and include Hutchison teeth, mulberry molars, abnormal facies, eighth nerve deafness, bone changes such as saber shins and perforation of the hard palate, cutaneous lesions especially rhagades, and neurosyphilis. Unlike acquired syphilis, cardiovascular complications are an unusual complication of late congenital syphilis.

TABLE 16-10. ANTIBIOTIC THERAPY FOR CONGENITAL AND ACQUIRED OCULAR SYPHILIS

Congenital syphilis, newborns
Aqueous crystalline penicillin G 50,000 U/kg per dose intravenously every 12 hr during the first 7 d of life and every 8 hr thereafter for 10 to 14 d, or procaine penicillin G, 50,000 U/kg per dose intramuscularly in a single daily dose for 10 to 14 d

Congenital syphilis in older infants and children
Aqueous crystalline penicillin G, 200,000 to 300,000 U/kg per d administered as 50,000 U/kg every 4 to 6 hr intravenously for 10 to 14 d

Acquired ocular syphilis
Aqueous crystalline penicillin G, 12–24 million U intravenously per d for 10 to 14 d administered as 3–4 million U intravenously every 4 hr or as a continuous infusion; thereafter, patients can be supplemented with intramuscular benzathine penicillin G at a dose of 2.4 million U/wk for 3 wk

Ocular inflammatory disease may present at birth or years later, including uveitis, interstitial keratitis, optic neuritis, glaucoma, and congenital cataract. Multifocal chorioretinitis and less commonly, retinal vasculitis, are the most frequent form of uveitis in early congenital infection (329), producing the "salt and pepper" fundus. Nonulcerative stromal keratitis, often accompanied by anterior uveitis, is the most common inflammatory sign of untreated late congenital syphilis, occurring in 20% to 50% of cases, more commonly in girls (329). The constellation of interstitial keratitis, eighth nerve deafness, and Hutchison teeth is called Hutchinson's triad.

Acquired syphilitic uveitis may present as an isolated anterior uveitis, intermediate uveitis, and a wide variety of posterior uveitides, including panuveitis. Posterior segment findings in acquired syphilis include vitritis, chorioretinitis, necrotizing retinitis, retinal vasculitis, optic papillitis, and neuroretinitis, and "syphilitic posterior placoid chorioretinitis" (330). Optic neuritis, optic atrophy, cranial nerve palsies, and pupillary abnormalities are suggestive of neurosyphilis.

Management

The recommended treatment regimens for congenital, acquired and HIV coinfected ocular syphilis are listed in Table 16-10. Penicillin allergy requires either desensitization or alternative therapy. In adults, doxycycline (200 mg orally once daily) or tetracycline (500 mg orally four times daily) for 30 days has been traditionally used (327b). Clarithromycin, ceftriaxone, and chloramphenicol have been used with success (331–333). Two to 12 hours after treatment with penicillin, an acute systemic (Jarisch-Herxheimer) reaction consisting of headache, malaise, tachypnea, tachycardia, leukocytosis, and fever, which usually resolves within a day, may develop in a variable number of patients, including newborns. Prednisone may be used to mitigate symptoms but treatment with penicillin should not be discontinued.

LYME DISEASE
Prevalence

Lyme borreliosis is a multisystemic disorder with protean ocular manifestations caused by the spirochete *Borrelia burgdorferi* sensu lato. It is the most common tick-borne infection in Germany (334) and in the United States, concentrated in the Northeast, Mid-Atlantic, and upper Midwest regions. In the year 2000, the incidence of LD in the US was 6.3 per 100,000 population, nearly double that in 1991 (335). In 2001, there were 17,029 cases reported to the CDC, the largest proportion being among children aged 5 to 9 and adults of 50 to 59 years (267). This may be due to a greater exposure risk to infected ticks among these age groups, less frequent use of personal protective measures, or differential use of health care services.

Etiology and Pathogenesis

B. burgdorferi sensu lato is transmitted to humans by infected *Ixodes scapularis* in the Northeast, Mid-Atlantic, and Midwest and by *Ixodes pacificus* in the Western United States, the preferred hosts of which include the white-footed mouse and the white-tailed deer for *I. scapularis* and lizards for *I. pacificus*. Chronic arthritis has been associated with HLA-DR-4 and HLA-DR2 haplotypes in North American patients with a poorer response to antibiotics noted in HLA-DR4 individuals (336). In Europe, *Ixodes ricinus* is the primary tick vector. *Borrelia afzelii* and *Borrelia garnii* are the two genospecies identified as the infectious agents in Europe, where acrodermatitis and neurological symptoms are more commonly recognized than joint symptoms (337). No consistent HLA associations have been identified among European patients.

Symptoms and Signs

The clinical course of LD has been divided into three stages. Early disease has a characteristic macular rash known as erythema migrans, which appears at the site of the tick bite within 2 to 28 days, enlarges, and becomes papular. The paracentral area may clear, forming a "bull's eye," with the site of the bite marking the center (Fig. 16-8). Constitutional symptoms include fever, malaise, fatigue, myalgias, and arthralgias. Positive identification of erythema migrans is diagnostic of LD; however, between 20% to 40% of patients never develop the rash (338,339).

Disseminated disease occurs several weeks after exposure, with hematogenous spread of the spirochete to the skin, CNS, joints, heart, and eyes. A secondary rash known as erythema chronicum migrans may occur at sites remote from the site of the tick inoculation. If left untreated, up to 80% of erythema migrans patients in the United States develop joint manifestations, most commonly a monoarthritis or oligoarthritis involving the large joints, typically the knee (340). Joint manifestations may be the only clinical feature of LD, especially in children. Meningitis or radiculitis (more common in Europe) (341) and cardiac findings, especially atrioventricular block (342), can occur in treated patients (343).

The most frequent manifestation of persistent disease is Lyme arthritis presenting as episodic arthritis, which may become chronic. Acrodermatitis chronica atrophicans occurs predominantly among European women between the age of 40 and 70 years (344). Chronic neurological syndromes may develop in some patients and include neuropsychiatric disease, radiculopathy, chronic fatigue, peripheral neuropathy, or memory loss (345).

The spectrum of ocular findings of Lyme borreliosis is expanding. The most common ocular manifestation of the

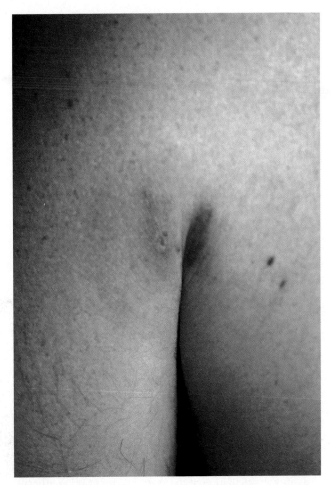

FIGURE 16-8. Erythema migrans: target-shaped skin lesion centered on the tick bite.

early stage is a follicular conjunctivitis (11% of patients (346) and. episcleritis (347), which can also occur during the disseminated and late stages. Disseminated disease is accompanied by cranial nerve involvement (CNII, III, IV, V, VI, and most commonly VII), Bell's palsy (346), optic neuritis, papilledema in association with meningitis, papillitis often associated with Lyme uveitis (348), and Horner's syndrome (349). Intraocular inflammation may manifest as anterior uveitis, intermediate uveitis, posterior uveitis (including vitreitis, retinal vasculitis, choroiditis, and neuroretinitis) and panuveitis. Intermediate uveitis is the most common intraocular presentation (337) and is frequently accompanied by a severe vitreitis, granulomatous anterior chamber reaction, papillitis, neurosensory retinitis, choroiditis, or panuveitis (348,350). Choroidal involvement may lead to pigment epithelial clumping which may resemble inflammatory syndromes such as those produced by syphilis or rubella. Keratitis occurring months to years after the onset of infection is the most common ocular manifestation of the persistent disease. The keratitis is thought to represent an immune phenomenon rather than an infectious process as it responds to topical steroids alone.

Ocular manifestations of LD have rarely been described in children (348,350, 351–355,356) and included late keratitis (351), anterior uveitis (350,353), and intermediate uveitis (less common than in adults) (348,353,354). Visual loss was usually symptomatic in children with arthritic LD, suggesting that regular screening examinations were likely unnecessary (356).

Diagnosis

The diagnosis of LD is made based on the history, clinical presentation, and supportive laboratory data. Erythema migrans (Fig. 16-8) is the most specific clinical marker for LD and, if present, is diagnostic of the disease in the appropriate clinical context, obviating the need for serologic testing (339,357). ELISA is the most commonly employed serologic test. The interpretation of test results is fraught with problems arising from a lack of standardization of values for which a positive test result is defined, cross-reactivity with other spirochetes (syphilis), and so, the not infrequent occurrence of false-positive and false-negative test results. For cases in which initial screening with ELISA is equivocal, Western immunoblotting should be used to corroborate the result (357). Lyme titers should not be routinely included in the laboratory workup of patients with uveitis who are not from endemic areas or fail to exhibit signs of symptoms suggestive of LD on examination or review of systems. In these patients, a positive result is more likely to represent a false-positive result (358). As previously described for ocular toxoplasmosis, calculation of the Witmer-Desmonts coefficient may be indicative of local (intraocular) antibody production and active infection. PCR has been successfully used as a diagnostic tool to amplify both genomic and plasmid *B. burgdorferi* DNA from a variety of tissues, including the ocular fluids (359), with the highest yields obtained for the skin (360).

Management

Patients with LD associated intraocular inflammation are best regarded as having CNS infection, and so, require neurological or neuroophthalmic dosing regimens. For children, ceftriaxone (75 to 100 mg/kg daily, in a single daily intravenous dose, maximum 2g) or cefotaxime (150 to 200 mg/kg daily, divided into three or four intravenous doses, maximum, 6 g daily) for 14 to 28 days is recommended (361). An alternative is intravenous penicillin G (200,000 to 400,000 U/kg daily, maximum of 18 to 24 million units daily) divided into doses administered every four hours for those with normal renal function. In adults, ceftriaxone (2 g administered intravenously, once daily for 14 to 28 days) is recommended for neurological disease (361). Intravenous penicillin G at a dose of 18 to 24 million units daily, divided into doses given every 4 hours, may be a satisfactory alternative. For adults intolerant of both penicillin and cephalosporins, doxycycline (200 to 400 mg daily) in two divided doses given orally or intravenously for 14 to 28 days may be adequate. After systemic therapy has been initiated, anterior segment inflammation may be treated with topical corticosteroids and mydriatics. The use of systemic corticosteroids has been described as part of the management of LD; however, its routine use is controversial as it has been associated with an increase in antibiotic treatment failures (350). As with syphilis, Jarisch-Herxheimer reaction may complicate antibiotic therapy for LD.

Patients may be reinfected with *B. burgdorferi* following successful antibiotic therapy (362,363). Patients with severe or chronic systemic or ocular manifestations of LD should also be tested for human granulocytic ehrlichiosis (HGE) and babesiosis (362,363). The best treatment of LD is prevention, which can be successfully accomplished by avoiding tick-infested habitats, using repellents, and wearing protective outer garments, promptly removing ticks, reducing tick populations, and by vaccination. LYMErix, the Lyme vaccine produced by GlaxoSmith Kline pharmaceuticals, was removed from the market in February 2002 and is no longer available (267).

ENDOPHTHALMITIS

Endophthalmitis is broadly divided into exogenous and endogenous categories. Exogenous endophthalmitis occurs as a result of the inadvertent inoculation of microbes into the eye following intraocular surgery or penetrating trauma. Endogenous endophthalmitis (metastatic) is intraocular infection resulting from hematogenous spread of organisms to the eye. Endophthalmitis arising among infants and children is most often posttraumatic or endogenous where, in the latter case, it may masquerade as noninfectious inflammatory disease or intraocular malignancy.

Posttraumatic Endophthalmitis: Etiology

Posttraumatic endophthalmitis in children is a rare complication of penetrating ocular injury and may be caused by bacteria or fungi (364). Exogenous bacterial endophthalmitis presents within days of the traumatic insult, with the possible exception of infection due to anaerobic organisms such as *Propionibacterium acnes* or fungi, which may not become evident for weeks or months after surgery. The microbiologic spectrum of pediatric posttraumatic endophthalmitis differs from that in adults in whom *Staphylococcus epidermidis* and *Bacillus cereus* are the predominant pathogens. Among 12 pediatric patients with posttraumatic endophthalmitis ranging in age from 18 months to 13 years (mean 8 years of age), *Streptococcal* species were found in 55.6% of cases that were culture positive while both *S. epidermidis* and *B. cereus* were noted in only 12.5% of eyes (365).

Posttraumatic Endophthalmitis: Diagnosis and Management

The successful management of both postoperative and post-traumatic endophthalmitis requires prompt diagnosis, with both aqueous and vitreous tap or diagnostic vitrectomy for microbiologic identification of the causative organisms, and treatment with intravitreous, broad spectrum antibiotics, such as vancomycin (1 mg in 0.1 mL), ceftazidime (2.25 mg in 0.1 mL), and in cases where infection with fungus is unlikely, dexamethasone (0.4 mg in 0.1 mL). In addition, subconjunctival vancomycin (25 mg) and gentamicin (20 mg) may be administered. For cases of suspected fungal endophthalmitis, intravitreous amphotericin B (5 to 10 μg) is the drug of choice. In contrast to the management of postoperative endophthalmitis, broad-spectrum systemic antibiotic coverage with vancomycin and ceftazidime, or fourth-generation quinolones, such as gatifloxacin, are frequently used for posttraumatic, bacterial endophthalmitis (366).

Endogenous Endophthalmitis: Prevalence

Endogenous endophthalmitis is an uncommon entity, comprising between 8% and 10% of all forms of endophthalmitis (367,368). Neonates and children, however, are at particular risk for endogenous infections, accounting for a third of the patients with metastatic bacterial infections (369).

Endogenous Endophthalmitis: Etiology

Endogenous endophthalmitis occurs most often in the setting of systemic immunosuppression and in hospitalized patients requiring prolonged venous access, respiratory support, or those undergoing nonocular surgical procedures. It is an important consideration in neonates in whom the immune system may not fully mature for up to 1 year (370).

The microbiological spectrum of endogenous bacterial endophthalmitis encompasses a broad range of Gram-positive and Gram-negative organisms. Geographic variance occurs (371). Neonatal endophthalmitis occurs from *Pseudomonas aeruginosa*, *S. pneumoniae*, and group B streptococci (372), whereas in children it is more often from *Haemophilus influenza*, *Staphylococcus aureus*, and *Neisseria meningitidis* (369). Endogenous *N. meningitidis* endophthalmitis occurs much less frequently than it had in the past, prior to the introduction of effective treatment for meningococcal meningitis. Unlike other patients with metastatic endophthalmitis, patients with meningococcal endophthalmitis are not typically immunocompromised, but may present with a variety of nonocular manifestations including, rashes in 50% of cases, joint involvement, pericarditis, and cranial nerve palsies (373).

Candida species are an important cause of nosocomial infections and are the most common fungal organisms found in endogenous endophthalmitis in neonates (372), and in pediatric and adult populations (Fig. 16-9). *Aspergillus* species is the second most common culprit with a host of other organisms much less frequently causing endogenous fungal endophthalmitis including *Cryptococcus neoformans*, *Coccidioides immitis*, *Sporothrix schenckii*, *Blastomyces dermatitidis*, *Histoplasma capsulatum*, *Fusarium* species, and *Mucor* species. In patients with candidemia, the prevalence rates of fungal endophthalmitis have ranged between 28% and 45% (374–376). However, in children with candidemia, neither endophthalmitis nor chorioretinitis was identified (377,378). Despite this very low prevalence, ocular involvement with *Candida* species may still occur in children (379,380). Over a 10-year period, two were found to have bilateral chorioretinitis and one had chorioretinitis with secondary endophthalmitis (381). It is likely that the early treatment of candidemic patients using amphotericin, fluconazole, or other systemic antifungals prevents severe ocular involvement (382,377).

Fungal disease may have an insidious onset. Typically, symptoms include reduced vision, photophobia, and sometimes pain (383). Hypopyon, corneal edema, elevated intraocular pressure, and periorbital edema may be observed. When the latter is seen in conjunction with proptosis, it is suggestive of a concomitant orbital cellulitis (384).

Symptoms and Signs

Symptoms include reduced vision and varying degrees of pain. Concurrent or prior inflammation include: prominent epibulbar vascular injection, layered hypopyon (may appear as an anterior capsular opacity or a circular infiltrate surrounding the pupil), posterior synechiae, gray and diffuse vitreous cells as opposed to white, soft clumps typical of retinoblastoma (385).

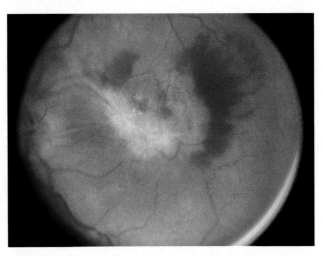

FIGURE 16-9. Candida retinitis involving the macula with accompanying intraretinal hemorrhage.

Diagnosis

Vitreous "fluff balls" or a "string of pearls" are usually associated with a fungal infection, the same findings may be seen in patients with active intermediate uveitis. Roth spots are seen in both bacterial and fungal infections. Endogenous endophthalmitis is unlikely to be confused with other conditions given the typical clinical context, however, when it presents as an isolated, posterior, focal endophthalmitis, the differential diagnosis includes toxoplasmosis, toxocariasis, retinoblastoma, pars planitis, and necrotizing viral retinitis.

Management

Intraocular fluid is obtained for microbiological analysis, usually in the form of vitreous biopsy. Identification of organisms from infected systemic sites may prove invaluable in making the diagnosis. The mainstay of therapy consists of intravitreous antibiotics, with or without PPV, with broadspectrum, empiric antibiotic coverage with vancomycin, ceftazidime, and corticosteroids (Decadron) in cases of bacterial disease, or with specific antibiotics directed against a suspected or known pathogen. Intravitreous steroid has not been associated with an exacerbation of fungal endophthalmitis when injected with intravitreous amphotericin (386,387). Patients with endogenous bacterial endophthalmitis should be on systemic antibiotics. Systemic antifungal therapy in fungemic patients may be instrumental in preventing serious ocular infection. Intravenous amphotericin B, however, not only has very poor ocular penetration, but also carries a significant renal toxic risk. When used, the dosage of systemic amphotericin B is 0.5 to 1.0 mg/kg daily. Less toxic imidazole compounds such as fluconazole, with an average dosage of 200 to 400 mg/day for *Candida* endophthalmitis, with or without PPV, are excellent supplements to intravitreous therapy (388).

The role of PPV in the management of endogenous endophthalmitis is unclear. Systemic therapy alone has been reported to achieve vitreous clearance with excellent visual acuity in some patients (383). Perhaps this approach may be preferred in eyes with focal posterior segment disease or mild vitreitis and certainly in those confined to intensive care units or otherwise too ill to undergo a surgical procedure. Vitrectomy is preferred in cases of diffuse vitreous involvement, particularly with virulent organisms such as Gram-negative bacteria of fungi, when the fundus cannot be visualized, and the visual acuity is significantly reduced.

TUBERCULOSIS

Prevalence

Tuberculosis (TB) is an uncommon cause of uveitis both among children and adults in developed nations; however, it remains the most important systemic infectious disease worldwide with respect to morbidity and mortality. In the United States, following many years of annual decline in the number of cases, the annual incidence of TB increased 14% between 1985 and 1993, coincident with the AIDS epidemic and increased immigration from regions of the world where TB is endemic (11).

Etiology

Tuberculosis is caused by *Mycobacterium tuberculosis*, an acid-fast–staining obligate aerobe, and is most commonly transmitted by aerosolized droplets. Only 10% of infected individuals become symptomatic; the vast majority remains infected without manifesting overt disease. Usually, it is asymptomatic, but symptomatic disease, classically manifested by fever, night sweats, and weight loss, may present with both pulmonary and extrapulmonary infection. This is important to keep in mind when conducting a review of systems in uveitis patients with signs suggestive of a tuberculous etiology as histopathologically proven intraocular TB has been shown to occur in patients with both asymptomatic disease and in those with extrapulmonary TB.

Symptoms and Signs

Primary ocular TB is defined as that in which the eye is the primary portal of entry, manifesting mainly as conjunctival, corneal and scleral disease. Secondary ocular TB often causes uveitis and occurs as a result of hematogenous dissemination from the primary source of infection. Intraocular TB has been described in children as young as 1 year of age (389) and recently, among adolescents of immigrant families (390). The most common presentation is that of a disseminated choroiditis, and is characterized by deep, multiple, discrete, yellow lesions from between 0.5 to 3.0 mm in diameter, numbering from five to several hundred (391–393). Lesions are seen mostly in the posterior pole and may be accompanied by disc edema, nerve fiber layer hemorrhages, varying degrees of vitreitis, and granulomatous anterior uveitis (Fig. 16-10). Alternatively, a focal choroiditis presenting as a single large, elevated choroidal mass, varying in size from 4 to 14 mm, often with overlying serous retinal detachment, may be seen (394–395). These must be distinguished from retinoblastoma, choroidal melanoma, or focal choroidal granulomata arising in sarcoid uveitis or toxocaral infection. Other posterior segment findings include subretinal abscess, retinal vasculitis, retinal detachment, choroidal neovascularization, and optic neuritis (396). In some cases, the disease is fulminant, progressing to panophthalmitis. External ocular and anterior segment findings include scleritis, phlyctenulosis, interstitial keratitis, corneal infiltrates, anterior chamber mass, and chronic granulomatous anterior uveitis (397). The uveitis was thought to be a hypersensitivity reaction to tuberculoprotein.

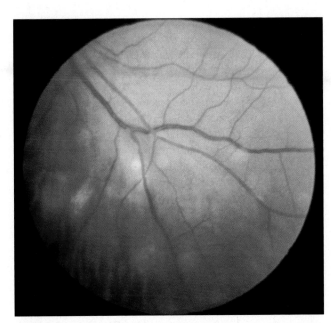

FIGURE 16-10. Multiple discrete yellowish choroidal lesions in a patient with pulmonary tuberculosis.

Diagnosis

The diagnosis of ocular TB is difficult and most often presumptive. A positive PPD indicates prior exposure to TB, not necessarily active systemic disease. It is recommended that PPD testing may be helpful when the index of suspicion is high given the history or examination or in areas where prevalence is high (398) and the bacilli Calmette-Guerin vaccination is not routinely given. Chest radiography or microbiological analysis of sputum, urine, gastric aspirates, or cervical lymph node biopsy for acid-fast bacilli may yield the diagnosis of systemic disease. However, failure to demonstrate systemic disease does not exclude the possibility of intraocular infection (399). In some cases of ocular disease with remote infection, definitive diagnosis may rely on the demonstration of intraocular infection by analysis of intraocular fluids or tissue biopsy. Nucleic acid amplification techniques, with transcription-mediated amplification of the 16S rRNA or the PCR amplification of unique DNA sequences of *M. tuberculosis* can be used (400). Chorioretinal biopsy, used in conjunction with nucleic acid amplification techniques and routine histopathology may be necessary in atypical cases. Detection of antibodies against purified cord factor (trehalose-6,6'-dimycolate), the most antigenic and most abundant cell wall component of tubercle bacilli, is useful for rapid serodiagnosis of pulmonary TB and may well be useful to support the diagnosis of ocular infection (401).

Differential Diagnosis

Sarcoid and toxocara granulomata, primary ocular neoplasms such as retinoblastoma and choroidal melanoma,

and metastatic disease, especially endophthalmitis, are considered. Fluorescein angiography reveals early hypofluorescence followed by late hyperfluorescence with leakage in the presence of a choroidal tubercle and may be useful in differentiating these from other lesions, including choroidal melanoma (394).

Management

It is important for the ophthalmologist to be familiar with the current treatment guidelines for TB even though the specifics of therapy may be deferred to a pediatric infectious disease specialist (402). In brief, treatment entails systemic, multidrug therapy for 6 to 9 months, beginning with an initial 2-month induction course of isoniazid (INH), rifampin, and pyrazinamide, administered daily. Should the possibility of drug resistance arise, another agent such as ethambutol or streptomycin, is added to the initial triple drug regimen, followed by a 4-month continuation of INH and rifampin. More than 95% of immunocompetent patients can be successfully treated with a full course of therapy provided compliance. Direct observed therapy plays a critical role in assuring this success and is now the standard of care in the treatment of tuberculosis. Drug resistance, especially among HIV-infected patients, has emerged as a significant problem in recent years (403).

BARTONELLA (CAT-SCRATCH DISEASE)

Prevalence

Cat-scratch disease (CSD) is a feline-associated zoonotic disease with an estimated annual incidence in the United States of 22,000 cases (404). It has worldwide distribution and occurs in immunocompetent individuals of all ages; however, the highest age-specific incidence is among children less than 10 years of age (405). Cats are the primary mammalian reservoir for *Bartonella henselae* (406). CSD occurs predominantly in the fall and winter, either due to seasonal fluctuations in zoonotic transmission between felines or temporal changes in animal behavior and reproduction (407). The disease is most prevalent in the southern states, California, and Hawaii, reflecting the distribution of cat fleas, *B. henselae* antibodies, and positive blood cultures among cats in these regions (408). Important risk factors for infection include scratches, licks, and bites from domestic cats, particularly kittens. Not surprisingly, children and young adults, who are more likely to be in contact with these animals, are at increased risk. Human to human transmission has not been described and the role of cat fleas or other arthropods in the transmission of *B. henselae* to humans is unknown. Recurrent CSD among immunocompetent individuals is rare as infection confers lasting immunity (409).

In immunosuppressed patients, *B. henselae* infection induces a vasoproliferative response, producing a vascular lesion similar to Kaposi's sarcoma in those with AIDS, whereas in the immunocompetent host with CSD, the response is necrotizing, often with microabscess formation (410,411).

Etiology

Among the 14 currently recognized species of the genus *Bartonella*, five are known to cause disease in humans, the most well known being *B. henselae*, the etiologic agent in CSD (412).

Symptoms and Signs

The most common systemic manifestation of *B. henselae infection* is CSD, which presents as a mild to moderate flulike illness associated with regional adenopathy (407). These usually precede the ocular manifestations of CSD (413). In most patients, an erythematous papule forms at the site of primary cutaneous injury 3 to 10 days following primary inoculation and 1 to 2 weeks before the onset of lymphadenopathy and constitutional symptoms. The patient may complain of headache, anorexia, nausea, vomiting, sore throat, and tender lymphadenopathy. Less common systemic manifestations of CSD include encephalitis, osteomyelitis, and hepatosplenic disease.

Ocular involvement occurs in 5% to 10% of patients with CSD (407). A follicular conjunctivitis affecting the bulbar and palpebral conjunctiva may be observed 1 to 2 weeks following exposure. Should the conjunctiva be the primary site of inoculation, a conjunctival granuloma may appear. The combination of a unilateral, granulomatous conjunctivitis and regional lymphadenopathy defines the clinical entity known as Parinaud's oculoglandular syndrome and is the most common ocular manifestation of CSD, affecting approximately 5% of patients (407). Other entities to be considered in the differential diagnosis of Parinaud's oculoglandular syndrome include tularemia, tuberculosis, syphilis, sporotrichosis, and acute *Chlamydia trachomatis* infection (414).

The most common posterior segment complication of *B. henselae* infection is neuroretinitis, a clinical syndrome characterized by abrupt visual loss, unilateral optic disc swelling, and macular star formation, occurring in 1% to 2% of patients with CSD (407,414,415). This syndrome was also called idiopathic stellate maculopathy (417) and renamed *Leber's idiopathic stellate neuroretinitis* (416) Over the years, evidence has accumulated (416,418–421) to suggest that *B. henselae* infection is the most common cause of this syndrome.

Visual loss (ranging from 20/25 to 20/200) follows the onset of constitutional symptoms by approximately 2 to 3 weeks (413). Although neuroretinitis most frequently occurs unilaterally, bilateral, often asymmetric, cases have been reported (422). Optic disc edema, associated with peripapillary serous retinal detachment, usually occurs 2 to 4

weeks prior to the appearance of the macular star, and may be an early sign of systemic *B. henselae* infection (423). The development of a macular star is variable: it may be partial or incomplete; lipid exudates may extend well outside the macula or nasal to the disc in severe cases (424) or not appear at all (423). When incomplete, a partial macular star is usually seen in the nasal macula (Fig. 16-11). The macular star resolves in approximately 8 to 12 weeks.

Most patients with neuroretinitis associated with *Bartonella* infection have some degree of anterior chamber inflammation and vitreitis (425). Multiple foci (50 to 300 μm) of retinitis or choroiditis may be observed (415,420,427,546), and when present, provide strong support for the diagnosis of *B. henselae* infection (427,428). Branch retinal artery (415,427,429), venous occlusive events (427), neurosensory macular detachments (430), epiretinal membranes (431), inflammatory mass of the optic nerve head (424), peripapillary angiomatosis (432), intermediate uveitis (433), retinal white dot syndrome (427), orbital abscess (434), panuveitis (435,436), optic disc swelling, or focal retinochoroiditis (433,436) have also been described.

Diagnosis

The diagnosis of CSD is made based on the characteristic clinical features together with confirmatory serologic testing. The IFA assay for the detection of serum anti–*B. henselae* antibodies is 88% sensitive and 94% specific (409), with titers greater than 1:64 being considered positive. Enzyme immunoassays (EIA) and Western blot procedures have also been developed, with the EIA having an IgG sensitivity of 86% to 95% and a specificity of 96% compared with IFA (437,438). A single positive IFA or EIA titer for IgG or IgM antibodies is generally sufficient to confirm CSD. IgG levels

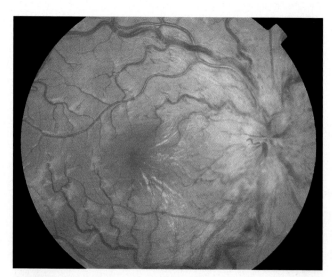

FIGURE 16-11. Optic disc swelling, moderate vascular engorgement, and partial macular star in a patient with cat-scratch disease.

rise during the first 2 months after disease onset, followed by a gradual decline (406). Other diagnostic assays include bacterial culture, which may require 12 to 45 days for colonies to become apparent (439), and PCR-based techniques, which target the bacterial 16S rRNA gene (440) or *B. henselae* DNA (441).

Differential Diagnosis

The differential diagnosis of neuroretinitis includes (i) infectious etiologies such as syphilis, LD, tuberculosis, DUSN, toxoplasmosis, toxocariasis, leptospirosis, mumps, varicella, and herpes simplex (416); (ii) noninfectious inflammatory conditions such as sarcoidosis; and (iii) other conditions such as acute systemic hypertension, diabetes mellitus, increased intracranial pressure (pseudotumor cerebri), anterior ischemic optic neuropathy, and leukemic infiltration of the optic nerve (442).

Management

Definitive treatment recommendations for CSD and its ocular complications have not emerged. In most cases, it is a self-limited illness with an overall excellent visual prognosis. In several studies (420,427,421), a good visual prognosis extended to both treated and untreated patients. Severe systemic or ocular complications of *Bartonella* infection are usually treated for 2 to 4 weeks with systemic antibiotics despite the fact that their efficacy has not been proven in randomized controlled trials. Antibiotics used include doxycycline, erythromycin, rifampin, trimethoprim-sulfamethoxazole, ciprofloxacin and intramuscular gentamicin (443). The effect of oral corticosteroids on the course of the systemic and ocular manifestations of *B. henselae* infection is unknown. Recent experience with azithromycin suggests that this antibiotic may hasten the resolution of adenopathy of CSD (444). For patients with severe disease, doxycycline (100 mg given twice daily) in combination with rifampin (300 mg orally twice daily) or rifampin alone, have been successful (445). While doxycycline has better intraocular penetration than erythromycin, it should be avoided in children less than 9 years of age due to the risk of permanent teeth discoloration (446). Furthermore, the safety of ciprofloxacin in individuals younger than the age of 18 has not been established. The specifics of antibiotic therapy in children with CSD and the ocular complications should be managed in consultation with a pediatric infectious disease specialist.

UVEITIS AND OTHER SYSTEMIC BACTERIAL INFECTIONS

The poststreptococcal syndrome classically includes acute rheumatic fever, poststreptococcal reactive arthritis, and acute glomerulonephritis; however, there is evidence that uveitis should be included as a manifestation of this disease (447–451).

Symptoms and Signs

Ocular findings have included bilateral conjunctival injection with mild to severe anterior chamber cell and flare, mild bilateral vitreous cellular reaction with clusters of cells near the inferior vitreous base, retinal vascular sheathing, scleritis, and glaucoma (447–451).

Typically, the inciting streptococcal infection (pharyngitis or rheumatic fever) precedes the onset of systemic symptoms, including uveitis, by 1 to 3 weeks. The uveitis is thought to be an immunological reaction to exogenous and endogenous antigens. An autoimmune reaction to host tissues, which possess epitopes similar to streptococcal antigens, is thought to arise by the activation of sensitized lymphocytes as a result of streptococcal infection (450).

Diagnosis

The diagnosis is made within the appropriate clinical context and by the demonstration of elevated antistreptolysin O titers, positive throat smears, and cultures. The uveitis usually responds to topical corticosteroids, however, inflammation may recur with recurrent streptococcal infections. The frequency and severity of recurrent attacks may be reduced by penicillin prophylaxis and tonsillectomy (450).

Differential Diagnosis

A similar uveitic syndrome, thought to be of autoimmune origin, has been described in association with systemic *Yersinia* infection. Acute anterior uveitis, conjunctivitis, arthritis, and other autoimmune sequelae may arise weeks to months following *Yersinia* infection, usually occurring in children older than 10 years of age (452). Systemic manifestations typically include fever, abdominal pain, and diarrhea. The diagnosis is made by the demonstration of anti-*Yersinia* antibodies on serologic testing.

Management

The anterior uveitis responds to treatment with topical steroids.

REFERENCES

1. Giles CL. Uveitis in childhood: part I. Anterior. *Ann Ophthalmol* 1989;21:13–19.
2. Giles CL. Uveitis in childhood: part II. Intermediate. *Ann Ophthalmol* 1989;21:20–22.
3. Giles CL. Uveitis in childhood: part III. Posterior. *Ann Ophthalmol* 1989;21:23–28.
4. Okada AA, Foster CS. Posterior uveitis in the pediatric population. *Int Ophthalmol Clin* 1992;32(I):121–125.

5. Dunn JP. Uveitis in children. Focal points. *Am Acad Ophthalmol* 1995;XIII:1–14.

6. Nguyen OD, Foster CS. Saving the vision of children with juvenile rheumatoid arthritis-associated uveitis. *JAMA* 1998; 280:1133–1134.

7. Cunningham ET. Uveitis in children. *Ocul Immunol Inflamm* 2000;8:251–261.

8. Samson CM, Ekong A, Foster CS. Uveitis in children: diagnosis and management. *Int Ophthalmol Clin* 2001;41: 199–216.

9. Smith JR. Management of uveitis in pediatric patients: special considerations. *Pediatr Drugs* 2002;4:183–189.

10. Holland GN, Steihm ER. Special considerations in the evaluation and management of uveitis in children. *Am J Ophthalmol* 2003;135:867–878.

11. de Boer J, Wulffraat N, Rothova A. Visual loss in uveitis of childhood. *Br J Ophthalmol* 2003;87: 879–884.

12. Perkins ES. Pattern of uveitis in children. *Br J Ophthalmol* 1966;50:169–185.

13. Silverstein A. Changing trends in the etiological diagnosis of uveitis. *Doc Ophthalmol* 1997;94:25–37.

14. Baarsma GS. The epidemiology and genetics of endogenous uveitis: a review. *Curr Eye Res* 1992;11(Suppl):1–9.

15. Vadot E, Barth E, Billet P. Epidemiology of uveitis-preliminary results of a prospective study in Savoy. In: Saari KM, ed. *Uveitis update.* Amsterdam: Elsevier, 1984:13–16.

16. Tran VT, Auer C, Guex-Crosier. Epidemiology of uvetis in Switzerland. *Ocul Immunol Inflamm* 1994;2:169–176.

17. Miettinen R. Incidence of uveitis in northern Finland. *Acta Ophthalmol* 1977;55:252–260.

18. Dandona L, Dandona R, John RK. Population based assessment of uveitis in an urban population in Southern India. *Br J Ophthalmol* 2000;84:706–709.

19. Nussenblatt RB. The natural course of uveitis. *Int Ophthalmol* 1990;141:303–308.

20. Ronday MJH, Stilma JS, Barbe RF, et al. Blindness from uveitis in a hospital population in Sierra Leone. *Br J Ophthalmol* 1994;78:690–693.

21. Suttorp-Schulten MSA, Rothova A. The possible impact of uveitis in blindness: a literature survey. *Br J Ophthalmol* 1996; 80:844–848.

22. Edelsten C, Ashwin R, Stanford MR, et al. Visual loss associated with pediatric uveitis in English primary and referral centers. *Am J Ophthalmol* 2003;135:676–680.

23. Kimura SJ, Hogan MJ. Uveitis in children: analysis of 274 cases. *Trans Am Ophthalmol Soc* 1964;62:173–192.

24. Cross AG. Uveitis in children. *Trans Ophthalmol Soc UK* 1965;85:409–419.

25. Kazdan JJ, McCulloch JC, Crawford JS. Uveitis in children. *CMAJ* 1967;96:385–391.

26. Mackley TA Jr, Long J, Suie T. Uveitis in children. *J Pediatr Ophthalmol* 1969;6:136–139.

27. Kanski JJ, Shun-Shin GA. Systemic uveitis syndromes in childhood: an analysis of 340 cases. *Ophthalmology* 1983;91: 1247–1252.

28. Tugal-Tutkun I, Havrlikova K, Power WJ. Changing patterns of uveitis in childhood. *Ophthalmology* 1996;103:375–383.

29. Pivetti-Pezzi P. Uveitis in children. *Eur J Ophthalmol* 1996;6: 293–298.

30. Soylu M, Ozdemir G, Anli A. Pediatric uveitis in Southern Turkey. *Ocul Immunol Inflamm* 1997;5:197–202.

31. Stoffel PB, Sauvain MJ, Von Vigier RO. Non-infectious causes of uveitis in 70 Swiss children. *Acta Paediatr* 2000; 89:955–958.

32. BenEzra D, Cohen E, Maftzir G. Patterns of Inflammation in children. *Bull Soc Belg Ophthalmol* 2001;279:35–38.

33. Darrell RW, Wagener HP, Kurland LT. Epidemiology of uveitis: incidence and prevalence in a small urban community. *Arch Ophthalmol* 1962;68:503–514.

34. Paivonsalo-Hietanen T, Tuominen J, et al. Uveitis in children: population-based study in Finland. *Acta Ophthalmol Scand* 2000;78;84–88.

35. Bolch-Michel E, Nussenblatt RB. International uveitis study group recommendations for the evaluation of intraocular inflammatory disease. *Am J Ophthalmol* 1987;103:234–235.

36. Harper SL, Chorich LJ, Foster CS. Diagnosis of uveitis. In: Foster CS, Vitale AT, eds. *Diagnosis and treatment of uveitis.* Philadelphia: WB Saunders, 2001:81–82.

37. Rosenbaum JT, Wernick R. The utility of routine screening for systemic lupus erythematosis or tuberculosis. *Arch Ophthalmol* 1990;108:1291.

38. Jabs DA, Rosenbaum JT, Foster CS. Guidelines for the use of immunosuppressive drugs in patients with ocular inflammatory disorders: recommendations of an expert panel. *Am J Ophthalmol* 2000;130:492–513.

39. Foster CS. General principles and philosophy. In: Foster CS, Vitale AT, eds. *Diagnosis and treatment of uveitis.* Philadelphia: WB Saunders, 2001:27–33.

40. Smith JR, George RK, Rosenbaum JT. Lower lid herniation of orbital fat may complicate periocular corticosteroid injection. *Am J Ophthalmol*

41. Meiler WR, Will BR, Lewis H. Vitrectomy in the management of peripheral uveitis. *Ophthalmology* 1988;95:859–864.

42. Heimann K, Schmanke L, Brunner R. Pars plana vitrectomy in the treatment of chronic uveitis. *Dev Ophthalmol* 1992;23:196–203.

43. Eckardt C, Bacskulin A. Vitrectomy in intermediate uveitis. *Dev Ophthalmol* 1992;23:232–238.

44. Heiligenhaus A, Bornfeld N, Foerster MH. Long term results of pars plana vitrectomy in the management of complicated uveitis. *Br J Ophthalmol* 1994;78:549–554.

45. Dugel PU, Rao NA, Ozler S. Pars plana vitrectomy for intraocular inflammation related to cystoid macular edema unresponsive to corticosteroids: A preliminary study. *Ophthalmology* 1992;99:1535–1541.

46. Vitale AT. Mydriatic and cycloplegic agents. In: Foster CS, Vitale AT, eds. *Diagnosis and treatment of uveitis.* Philadelphia: WB Saunders, 2001:159–166.

47. Probst LE, Holland EJ. Intraocular lens implantation in patients with juvenile rheumatoid arthritis. *Am J Ophthalmol* 1996;122: 161–170.

48. Lundvall A, Zetterstrom C. Cataract extraction and intraocular lens implantation in children with uveitis. *Br J Ophthalmol* 2000;84:791–793.

49. Ben Ezra D, Cohen E. Cataract surgery in children with chronic uveitis. *Ophthalmology* 2000;107:1255–1260.

50. Foster CS, Fong LP, Singh G. Cataract surgery and intraocular lens implantation in patients with uveitis. *Ophthalmology* 1989;96;281–288.

51. Kaufman AH, Foster CS. Cataract extraction in patients with pars planitis. *Ophthalmology* 1993;100:1210–1217.

52. Akova YA, Foster CS. Cataract surgery in patients with sarcoidosis-associated uveitis. *Ophthalmology* 1994;1 01:473–479.

53. Foster CS, Stavrou P, Zafirakis P. Intraocular lens explanation in patients with uveitis. *Am J Ophthalmol* 1999;128:31–37.

54. Foster CS, Barrett F. Cataract development and cataract surgery in patients with juvenile rheumatoid arthritis- associated iridocyclitis. *Ophthalmology* 1993;100:809–817.

55. Dana MR, Merayo Lloves J, Schaumberg DA, et al. Visual outcomes prognosticators in juvenile rheumatoid arthritis-associated uveitis. *Ophthalmology* 1997;104:236–244.

56. Kanski JJ. Juvenile arthritis and uveitis. *Surv Ophthalmol* 1990;34:253–267.

57. Fox GM, Flynn HW, Davis JL. Causes of reduced visual acuity on long term follow-up after cataract extraction in patients with uveitis and juvenile rheumatoid arthritis. *Am J Ophthalmol* 1992;114:708–714.

58. Holland GN. Intraocular lens implantation in patients with juvenile rheumatoid arthritis-associated uveitis: an unresolved management issue. *Am J Ophthalmol* 1996;12:255–257.

59. Holland GN, O'Connor GR, Belfort R Jr. Toxoplasmosis. In: Pepose JS, Holland GN, Wilhelmus KR, eds. *Ocular infection and immunity*. St Louis: Mosby-Year Book, 1996:1183–1223.

60. Rodruguez A, Calonge M, Pedroza-Seres M, et al. Referral patterns of uveitis in a tertiary eye care center. *Arch Ophthalmol* 1996;114:593–599.

61. Nussenblatt RB, Belfort R Jr. Ocular toxoplasmosis: an old disease revisited. *JAMA* 1994;271:304–307.

62. Britt RH, Enzmann DR, Remingon JS. Intracranial infection in cardiac transplant recipients. *Ann Neurol* 1981;9:107–119.

63. Siegel SE, Lunde MN, Gelderman AH, et al. Transmission of toxoplasmosis by leukocyte transfusion. *Blood* 1971;37:388–394.

64. Ramadan AM, Nussenblatt RB. Toxoplasmosis. In: Guyer DR, Yannuzzi LA, Chang S, et al, eds. *Retina-vitreous-macula*. Philadelphia: WB Saunders, 1999:671–696

65. Kimball AC, Kean BH, Fuchs F. Congenital toxoplasmosis: a prospective study of 4,048 obstetric patients. *Am J Obstet Gynecol* 1971;11:211–218.

66. Wong SY, Remington JS. Toxoplasmosis in pregnancy. *Clin Infect Dis* 1994;18:853–862.

67. Desmonts G, Couvreur J. Congenital toxoplasmosis. *N Engl J Med* 1974;290:1110–1116.

68. Couvreur J, Desmonts G, Tournier G. A study of a homogeneous series of 210 cases of congenital toxoplasmosis in 0 to 11 months detected prospectively. *Ann Pediatr (Paris)* 1984;31:815–819.

69. Koppe, JG, Kloosterman GJ. Congenital toxoplasmosis: long-term follow-up. *Pediatr Padol* 1982;17:171–179.

70. Wilson CB, Remington JS, Stagno S. Development of adverse sequelae in children born with subclinical congenital Toxoplasma infection. *Pediatrics* 1980;66:767–774.

71. Mets MD, Holfels E, Boyer KM, et al. Eye manifestations of congenital toxoplasmosis. *Am J Ophthalmol* 1996;122:309–324.

72. Da Mata AP, Orefice F. Toxoplasmosis. In: Foster CS, Vitale AT, eds. *Diagnosis and treatment of uveitis*. Philadelphia: WB Saunders, 2001:385–410.

73. Holland GN. Reconsidering the pathogenesis of ocular toxoplasmosis. *Am J Ophthalmol* 1999;128:502–505.

74. Gilbert RE, Stanford MR. Is ocular toxoplasmosis caused by prenatal or post-natal infection? *Br J Ophthalmol* 2000;84:224–226.

75. Glasner PD, Silveira C, Kruszon-Moran D, et al. An unusually high prevalence of ocular toxoplasmosis in southern Brazil. *Am J Ophthalmol* 1992;114:136–144.

76. Bosch-Driessen LE, Berendschot TT, Ongkosuwito JV. Ocular toxoplasmosis: clinical features and prognosis in 154 patients. *Ophthalmology* 2002;109:869–878.

77. Burnett, Shortt SG, Isaac-Renton J. Multiple cases of acquired toxoplasmosis retinitis presenting in an outbreak. *Ophthalmology* 1998;105:1032–1037.

78. Couvreur J, Thulliez PH. Acquired toxoplasmosis with ocular or neurologic involvement. *Presse Med* 1996;25:438–442.

79. Meenken C, Rothova A, de Waal LP. HLA typing in congenital toxoplasmosis. *Br J Ophthalmol* 1995;79:494–497.

80. Howe KD, Silbey LD. *Toxoplasma gondii* comprises three clonal lineages: correlation of parasite genotype with human disease. *J Infect Dis* 1995;172:1561–1566.

81. Hogan MJ. Ocular toxoplasmosis in adults. *Surv Ophthalmol* 1961: 6:935–951.

82. Freidmann CT, Knox DL. Variations in recurrent active toxoplasmic retinochroiditis. *Arch Ophthalmol* 1969;81:481–493.

83. Rothova A. Ocular involvement in toxoplasmosis. *Br J Ophthalmol* 1993;77:371–377.

84. O'Connor GR. Manifestations and management of ocular toxoplasmosis. *Bull NY Acad Med* 1974;50:192–210.

85. Meenken C, Assies J, van Nieuwenhuizen O. Long term ocular and neurological involvement in severe congenital toxoplasmosis. *Br J Ophthalmol* 1995;79:581–584.

86. Smith JR, Cunningham ET. Atypical presentations of ocular toxoplasmosis. *Curr Opin Ophthalmol* 2002;13:387–392.

87. Remington JS, McLeod R, Desmonts G. Toxoplasmosis. In: Remington JS, Klein J, eds. *Infectious disease of the fetus and newborn*. Philadelphia: WB Saunders, 1995;4:140–267.

88. Desmont G. Definitive serological diagnosis of ocular toxoplasmosis. *Arch Ophthalmol* 1996;76:839–851.

89. Verbraak FD, Galema M, van den Horn GH, et al. Serological and polymerase chain reaction-based analysis of aqueous humor samples in patients with AIDS and necrotizing retinitis. *AIDS* 1996;10:1091–1099.

90. Montoya JG, Parmley, Lisenfeld O. Use of the polymerase chain reaction for diagnosis or ocular toxoplasmosis. *Ophthalmology* 1999;106:1554–1563.

91. Miller D, Davais J, Rosa R. Utility of tissue culture for detection of *Toxoplasma gondii* in vitreous humor of patients diagnosed with toxoplasmic retinochoroiditis. *J Clin Microbiol* 2000;38:3840–3842.

92. McAuley J, Boyer KM, Patel D. Early and longitudinal evaluations of treated infants and children and untreated historical patients with congenital toxoplasmosis: the Chicago Collaborative Treatment Trial. *Clin Infect Dis* 1994;18:38–72.

93. Brezin AP, Thulliez P, Couvreur J. Ophthalmic outcomes after prenatal and postnatal treatment of congenital toxoplasmosis. *Am J Ophthalmol* 2003;135:779–784.

94. Lopez JS, De Smet MD, Masur H. Orally administered 566C80 for treatment of ocular toxoplasmosis in a patient with the acquired immunodeficiency syndrome. *Am J Ophthalmol* 1992;113:331–333.

95. Pearson PA, Piracha AR, Sen HA. Atovaquone for the treatment of toxoplasma retinochoroiditis in immunocompetent patients. *Ophthalmology* 1999;160:148–153.

96. Parke DW II, Shaver RP. Toxocariasis. In: Pepose JS, Holland GN, Wilhemus KR, eds. *Ocular infection and immunity*. St. Louis: Mosby–Year Book, 1966:1225–1235.

97. Schantz PM, Weis PE, Pollard ZS, et al. Risk factors for toxocaral ocular larva migrans: a case-control study. *Am J Public Health* 1980;70:1269–1272.

98. Raistrick ER, Hart JCD. Adult toxocaral infection with focal retinal lesion. *BMJ* 1975;3:416.

99. Maguire AM. Ocular Toxocariasis. In: Guyer DR, Yannuzzi LA, Chang S, et al, eds. *Retina-vitreous-macula*. Philadelphia: WB Saunders, 1999:697–708.

100. Sprent JSA. The life cycles of nematodes in the family Ascaridea blanchard 1896. *J Parasitol* 1954;40:608–617.

101. Beaver PC, Snyder CH, Carrerra GM. Chronic eosinophilia due to visceral larva migrans: report of three cases. *Pediatrics* 1952;9:7–19.

102. Schantz PM, Glickman LT. Current concepts in parasitology: toxocaral visceral larva migrans. *N Engl J Med* 1978;298:436–439.

103. Glickman LT, Schantz PM. Epidemiology and Pathogenesis of Zoonotic Toxocariasis. *Epidemiol Rev* 1981;3:230–250.

104. Brown DH. Ocular *Toxocara canis* II. Clinical review. *J Pediatr Ophthalmol* 1970;7:182–191.

105. Schantz PM, Meyer D, Glickman LT. Clinical, serologic, and epidemiologic characteristics of ocular toxocariasis. *Am J Trop Med Hyg* 1980;70:1269–1272.

106. Benitez del Castillo JM, Herreros G, Guillen JL. Bilateral ocular toxocariasis demonstrated by aqueous humor enzyme-linked immunosorbent assay. *Am J Ophthalmol* 1995;119:514–516.

107. Hogan MJ, Kimura SJ, Spencer WH. Visceral larva migrans and peripheral retinitis. *JAMA* 1965;194:1345–1347.

108. Ashton N. Larval granulomatosis of the retina due to toxocara. *Br J Ophthalmol* 1960;44:129–148.

109. Wilder HC. Nematode endophthalmitis. *Trans Am Acad Ophthalmol Otolaryngol* 1950;55:99–109.

110. Baldone JA, Clark WB, Jung RC. Nematode ophthalmitis: report of two cases. *Am J Ophthalmol* 1964;57:763–766.

111. Shields JA. Ocular toxocariasis: a review. *Surv Ophthalmol* 1984;28:361–381.

112. Bird AC, Smith JL, Curtin VT. Nematode optic neuritis. *Am J Ophthalmol* 1970;69:72–77.

113. Phillips CI, Mackenzie AD. Toxocara larva papillitis. *BMJ* 1973;1:154–155.

114. Sorr EM. Meandering ocular toxocariasis. *Retina* 1984;4:90–96.

115. Byers B, Kimura SJ. Uveitis after death of larva in the vitreous cavity. *Am J Ophthalmol* 1974;77:63–66.

116. Pollard ZF, Jarrett WH, Hagler WF. ELISA for diagnosis of ocular toxocariasis. *Ophthalmology* 1979;86:743–749.

117. Ellis GS Jr, Pakalnis VA, Worley G, et al. *Toxocara canis* infestation: clinical and epidemiological associations with zero positivity in kindergarten children. *Ophthalmology* 1986;93:1032–1037.

118. Searl FS, Moazed K, Albert DN. Ocular toxocariasis presenting as leukocoria in a patient with low ELISA titer to *Toxocara canis*. *Ophthalmology* 1981;88:1302–1306.

119. Wan WL, Cano MR, Prince KJ. Echographic characteristics of ocular toxocariasis. *Ophthalmology* 1991;98:28–32.

120. Tran VT, Lumbroso L, LeHoang P. Ultrasound biomicroscopy in peripheral retinovitreal toxocariasis. *Am J Ophthalmol* 1999;127:607–609.

121. Shields JA, Lerner HA, Felberg NT. Aqueous cytology and enzymes in nematode endophthalmitis. *Am J Ophthalmol* 1977;84:319–322.

122. Biglan AW, Glickman LT, Lobes LA Jr. Serum and vitreous Toxocara antibody in nematode endophthalmitis. *Am J Ophthalmol* 1979;88:898–901.

123. Felberg NT, Shields JA, Federman JL. Antibody to *Toxocara canis* in the aqueous humor. *Arch Ophthalmol* 1981;99:1563–1564.

124. Maguire AM, Green WR, Michels RG. Recovery of intraocular *Toxocara canis* by pars plana vitrectomy. *Ophthalmology* 1990;97:675–680.

125. Romero-Rangel T, Foster CS. Ocular toxocariasis. In: Foster CS, Vitale AT, eds. *Diagnosis and treatment of uveitis*. Philadelphia: WB Saunders, 2001:428–436.

126. Dinning WJ, Gillespie SH, Cooling RJ. Toxocariasis: a practical approach to management of ocular disease. *Eye* 1988;2:580–582.

127. Nichols RL. The etiology of visceral larva migrans. I. Diagnostic morphology of infective second-stage Toxocara larvae. *J Parasitol* 1956;42:349–362.

128. Watzke RC, Oaks JA, Folk JC. *Toxocara canis* infection in the eye: correlation of clinical observations with developing pathology in the primate model. *Arch Ophthalmol* 1984;102:282–291.

129. Luxenberg MW. An experimental approach to the study of intraocular *Toxocara canis*. *Trans Am Ophthalmol Soc* 1979;77:542–601.

130. Belmont JB, Irvine A, Benson W. Vitrectomy in ocular toxocariasis. *Arch Ophthalmol* 1982;100:1912–1915.

131. Small KW, McCuen BW, deJuan E. Surgical management of retinal traction caused by toxocariasis. *Am J Ophthalmol* 1989;108:10–14.

132. Hagler WS, Pollard ZF, Jarrett WH. Results of surgery for *Toxocara canis*. *Ophthalmology* 1981;88:1081–1086.

133. Rodriguez A. Early pars plana vitrectomy in chronic endophthalmitis of toxocariasis. *Graefes Arch Clin Exp Ophthalmol* 1986;224:218–220.

134. Amin HI, McDonald HR, Han DP, et al. Vitrectomy update for macular traction in ocular toxocariasis. *Retina* 2000;20:80–85.

135. Siam A-L. Toxocaral chorio-retinitis. Treatment of early cases with photocoagulation. *Br J Ophthalmol* 1973;57:700–703.

136. Fitzgerald CR, Rubin ML. Intraocular parasite destroyed by photocoagulation. *Arch Ophthalmol* 1974;91:162–164.

137. Monshizadeh R, Ashrafzadeh M, Rumelt S. Choroidal neovascular membrane: a late complication of inactive Toxocara chorioretinitis. *Retina* 2000;20:219–220.

138. Gass JDM, Scelso R. Diffuse unilateral subacute neuroretinitis. *J R Soc Med* 1978;71:95–111.

139. Harto MA, Rodriguez-Salvador V, Aviñó JA. Diffuse unilateral sub acute neuroretinitis in Europe. *Eur J Ophthalmol* 1999;9:58–62.

140. de Souza EC, da Cunha SL, Gass JDM. Diffuse unilateral sub acute neuroretinitis in South America. *Arch Ophthalmol* 1992;110:1261–1263.

141. Cialdini, AP, de Souza EC, Avila MP. The first South American case of unilateral sub acute neuroretinitis caused by a large nematode. *Arch Ophthalmol* 1999;117:1431–1432.

142. Gass JDM, Gilbert WR, Guerry RK. Diffuse unilateral subacute neuroretinitis. *Ophthalmology* 1978;85:521–545.

143. Gass JDM, Braunstein RA. Further observation concerning the diffuse unilateral subacute neuroretinitis syndrome. *Arch Ophthalmol* 1983;101:1689–1697.

144. Cassella AMB, Bonomo PP, Farah ME. Diffuse unilateral sub acute neuroretinitis (DUSN): 3 cases in Paraná State. *Arq Bras Oftalmol* 1994;57:77–79.

145. de Souza EC, Nakashima Y. Diffuse unilateral sub acute neuroretinitis: report of transvitreal surgical removal of a sub retinal nematode. *Ophthalmology* 1995;102:1183–1186.

146. Kazakos EA. Diffuse unilateral neuroretinitis syndrome: probable cause. *Arch Ophthalmol* 1984;102:967–968.

147. Yuen VH, Chang TS, Hooper PL. Diffuse unilateral sub acute neuroretinitis syndrome in Canada. *Arch Ophthalmol* 1996;114:1279–1282.

148. Mets MB, Noble GA, Basti S, et al. *Eye* findings of diffuse subacute neuroretinitis and multiple choroidal infiltrates associated with neural larva migrans due to Baylisascaris procyonis. *Am J Ophthalmol* 2003;135:888–890.

149. Slakter JS, Ciardella AP. Diffuse unilateral subacute neuroretinitis. In: Guyer DR, Yannuzzi LA, Chang S, Shields JA, Green WR, eds. *Retina-vitreous-macula*. Philadelphia: WB Saunders, 1999:806–812.

150. Barney NP. Diffuse unilateral subacute neuroretinitis. In: Foster CF, Vitale AT, eds. *Diagnosis and treatment of uveitis*. Philadelphia: WB Saunders, 2001:475–479.

151. Gass JDM. *Stereoscopic atlas of macular disease: diagnosis and treatment*, 3rd ed. St. Louis: CB Mosby, 1983, pp. 470–479, 510, 511.

152. Raymond LA, Guitierrez Y, Strong LE. Living retinal nematodes (filarial like) destroyed with photocoagulation. *Ophthalmology* 1978;85:944–949.

153. Sabrosa NA, de Souza EC. Nematode infections of the eye: toxocariasis and diffuse unilateral subacute neuroretinitis. *Curr Opin Ophthalmol* 2001;12:450–454.

154. Gass JDM, Callanan DG, Bowman CB. Oral therapy in diffuse unilateral subacute neuroretinitis. *Arch Ophthalmol* 1992;110: 675–680.

155. Davis JL, Gass JDM. Diffuse unilateral subacute neuroretinitis. In: Pepose JS, Holland GN, Wilhelmus KR, eds. *Ocular infection and immunity.* St. Louis: Mosby-Year Book, 1966:1243–1247.

156. Centers for Disease Control and Prevention. *HIV/AIDS surveillance report.* Atlanta: US Department of Health and Human Services, CDC, 2001:13.

157. http://www.unaids.org/epidemic_update/report/EPI_report.htm.

158. Joint United Nations Programme on HIV/AIDS. *Report on the global HIV/AIDS epidemic, June 1998.* Geneva: Joint United Nations Programme on HIV/AIDS, 1998.

159. Blanche S, Newell ML, Mayaux MJ, et al. Morbidity and mortality in European children vertically infected by HIV–I. The French Pediatric HIV Infection Study Group and European Collaborative Study. *J Acquir Immune Defic Syndr Hum Retrovirol* 1997;14:442–450.

160. Natural history of vertically acquired immunodeficiency virus-I infection. The European Collaborative Study. *Pediatrics* 1994; 94:815–819.

161. Wei X, Ghosh SK, Taylor ME, et al. Viral dynamics in human immunodeficiency virus type I infection. *Nature* 1995;373: 117–122.

162. Pizzo PA, Wilfert CM. Markers and determinants of disease progression in children with HIV infection. The Pediatric AIDS Siena Workshop II. *J Acquir Immune Defic Syndr Hum Retrovirol* 1995;8:30–44.

163. Turner BJ, Denison M, Eppes SC. Survival experience of 789 children with acquired immunodeficiency syndrome. *Paediatr Infect Dis J* 1993;12:310–320.

164. Kuhn L, Abrams EJ, Weedon J, et al. Disease progression and early viral dynamics in human immunodeficiency virus-infected children exposed to zidovudine during prenatal and perinatal periods. *J Infect Dis* 2000;182:104–111.

165. Dickover RE, Dillon M, Leung KM, et al. Early prognostic indicators in primary perinatal human immunodeficiency virus type I infection: importance of viral RNA and the timing of transmission on long-term outcome. *J Infect Dis* 1998;178: 375–387.

166. Shearer WT, Quinn TC, LaRussa P, et al. Viral load and disease progression in infants infected with human immunodeficiency virus type 1. Women and Infants Transmission Study Group. *N Engl J Med* 1997;336:1337–1342.

167. Cunningham ET Jr, Belfort R Jr. *HIV/AIDS and the eye: a global perspective.* San Francisco: American Academy of Ophthalmology, 2002.

168. Abrams EJ. Opportunistic infections and other clinical manifestations of HIV disease in children. *Pediatr Clin North Am* 2000;47:79–108.

169. Nicholas SW. The opportunistic and bacterial infections associated with pediatric human immunodeficiency virus disease. *Acta Paeditr Suppl* 1994;400:46–50.

170. Kestelyn P, Lepage P, Karita E. Ocular manifestations of infection with the human immunodeficiency virus in an African pediatric population. *Ocular Immunol Inflamm* 2000;8:263–273.

171. Cervia J. HIV/AIDS rounds: HIV in children. *AIDS Patient Care STDS* 1999;13:165–173.

172. Pavia AT, Christenson JC. Pediatric AIDS. In: Sande MA, Volberding PA, eds. *The medical management of AIDS*, 6th ed. Philadelphia: WB Saunders, 1999:525–535.

173. Luzuriaga K, Sullivan JL. DNA polymerase chain reaction for the diagnosis of vertical HIV infection. *JAMA* 1996;275: 1360–1361.

174. Paul MO, Tetali S, Lesser ML, et al. Laboratory diagnosis of infection status in infants perinatally exposed to human immunodeficiency virus type I. *J Infect Dis* 1996;173:68–76.

175. Dennehey PJ, Warman R, Flynn JT. Ocular manifestations in pediatric patients with acquired immunodeficiency syndrome. *Arch Ophthalmol* 1989;107:978–982.

176. De Smet MD, Nussenblatt RB. Ocular manifestations of HIV in the pediatric population. In: Pizzo PA, Wilfert CM, eds. *Pediatric AIDS: the challenge of HIV infection in infants, children and adolescents.* 2nd ed. Baltimore: Williams & Wilkins, 1994:457–466.

177. Girard B, Prevost-Moravia G, Courpotin C. Ophthalmologic manifestations observed in a pediatric HIV-seropositive population. *J Fr Ophthalmol* 1997;20:49–60.

178. Livingston PG, Kerr NC, Sullivan JL. Ocular disease in children with vertically acquired human immunodeficiency virus infection. *J AAPOS* 1998;2:177–181.

179. Kestelyn P, Lepage P, Van de Perre P. Perivasculitis of the retinal vessels as an important sign in children with AIDS-related complex. *Am J Ophthalmol* 1995;100:614–615.

180. Baumal CR, Levin AV, Kavalec CC. Screening from cytomegalovirus retinitis in children. *Arch Pediatr Adolesc Med* 1996;150:1186–1192.

181. Tejada P, Sarminto B, Ramos JR. Retinal microvasculopathy in human immunodeficiency type I (HIV) infected children. *Int Ophthalmol* 1997–98;21:319–321.

182. Whitcup SM, Butler KM, Caruso R, et al. Retinal toxicity in human immunodeficiency virus infected children treated with 2'-, 3'- dideoxyinosine. *Am J Ophthalmol* 1992;113:1–7.

183. Whitcup SM, Dastgheib K, Nussenblatt RB. A clinicopathologic report of the retinal lesions associated with didanosine. *Arch Ophthalmol* 1994;112:1594–1598.

184. Smith JA, Mueller BU, Nussenblatt RB. Corneal endothelial deposits in children positive for human immunodeficiency virus receiving rifabutin prophylaxis for Mycobacterium avium complex bacteremia. *Am J Ophthalmol* 1999;127:164–169.

185. Buhles WC Jr, Mastre BJ, Tinker AJ. Ganciclovir treatment of life- or sight-threatening cytomegalovirus infection: experience in 314 immunocompromised patients. *Rev Infect Dis* 1998; 10(Suppl 3):S495–S506.

186. Fanning MM, Read SE, Benson M, et al. Foscarnet therapy of cytomegalovirus retinitis in AIDS. *J Acquir Immune Defic Syndr* 1990;3:472–479.

187. Walmsley SL, Chew E, Read SE, et al. Treatment of cytomegalovirus retinitis with trisodium phosphonoformate hexahydrate (foscarnet). *J Infect Dis* 1998;157:569–572.

188. Walton RC, Whitcup SM, Mueller BU. Combined intravenous ganciclovir and foscarnet for children with recurrent cytomegalovirus retinitis. *Ophthalmology* 1995;102:1865–1870.

189. Bartlett JG. *The Johns Hopkins Hospital 1997 guide to medical care of patients with HIV infection.* Baltimore: Williams & Wilkins;1997:107–109.

190. Baumal CR, Levin AV, Read SE. Cytomegalovirus retinitis in immunosuppressed children. *Am J Ophthalmol* 1999;127: 550–558.

191. Whitley RJ, Jacobson MA, Friedberg DM, et al. Guidelines for the treatment of cytomegalovirus diseases in patients with AIDS in the era of potent antiretroviral therapy: recommendations of an international panel. International AIDS Society—USA. *Arch Intern Med* 1998;158:957–969.

192. Frenkel LM, Capparelli EV, Dankner WM, et al. Oral ganciclovir in children: pharmacokinetics, safety, tolerance, and antiviral effects. *J Infect Dis* 2000;182:1616–1624.

193. Whitley RJ, Roizman B. Herpes simplex virus infections. *Lancet* 2001;357:1513–1518.

194. Whitley RJ, Kinderlin DW, Roizman B. Herpes simplex virus. *Clin Infect Dis* 98;26:541–555.

195. Yoser SI, Forster DJ, Rao NA. Systemic viral infections and their retinal and choroidal manifestations. *Surv Ophthalmol* 1993;37:313–352.

196. Overhall JC, Jr. Viral infections of the fetus and neonate. In: Feigin RD, Cherry JD, eds. *Textbook of pediatric infectious disease*, vol 1, ed 4. Philadelphia: WB Saunders, 1998:856–892.

197. Mets MB. I: manifestations of intrauterine infections. *Ophthalmol Clin North Am* 2001;14:521–531.

198. Komorous JM, Wheeler CE, Birggaman RA. Intrauterine herpes simplex infections. *Arch Dermatol* 1997;113:918–922.

199. Hutto C, Arvin A, Jacob R, et al. Intrauterine herpes simplex virus infections. *J Pediatr* 1997;110:97–101.

200. Nahmias AJ, Hagler WS. Ocular manifestations of herpes simplex in the newborn (neonatal ocular herpes). *Int Ophthalmol Clin* 1972;12:191–213.

201. Whitley R, Arvin A, Prober C, et al. A controlled trial comparing vidarabine with acyclovir in neonatal herpes simplex virus infection. Infectious Diseases Collaborative Antiviral Study Group. *N Engl J Med* 1991;324:444–49.

202. Nahmias AJ, Keyserling HL, Kerrick GM. Herpes simplex. In: Remington JS, Klein JO, eds. *Infectious diseases of the fetus and newborn infant*. II md ed. Philadelphia: WB Saunders, 1983:636–78.

203. Hagler WS, Walters PV, Nahmais AJ. Ocular involvement in neonatal herpes simplex virus infections. *Arch Ophthalmol* 1969;82:169–176.

204. Reynolds JD, Griebel M, Mallory S. Congenital herpes simplex retinitis. *Am J Ophthalmol* 1986;102:33–36.

205. Montgomery JR, Flanders RW, Yow MD. Congenital anomalies in herpes virus infections. *Am J Dis Child* 1973;126:364–366.

206. South MA, Tompkins WA, Morris CR. Congenital malformation of the central nervous system associated with genital (type 2) herpes virus. *J Pediatr* 1969;75:13–18.

207. Nas AJ, Visintine AM, Caldwell DR. Infections with herpes simplex virus in neonate. *Surv Ophthalmol* 1976;21:100–105.

208. El Azazi M, Malm G, Forsgren M. Late ophthalmologic manifestations of neonatal herpes simplex virus infections. *Am J Ophthalmol* 1990;109:1–7.

209. Margolis TP, Atherton FS. Herpes simplex virus diseases: posterior segment of the eye. In: Pepose JS, Holland GN, Wilhelmus KR, eds. *Ocular infection & immunity*. St. Louis: Mosby, 1996:1155–1167.

210. Gnann JW, Whitley RJ. Herpes zoster. *N Engl J Med* 2002;347:340–346.

211. Rappersberger K. Infections with herpes simplex and varicella zoster virus in pregnancy: clinical manifestations in mother, fetus and newborn—therapeutic options. *Hautarzt* 1999;50:706–714.

212. De Nicola LK, Hanshaw JB. Congenital and neonatal varicella. *J Pediatr* 1979;94:175–176.

213. Lambert SR, Taylor D, Kriss A. Ocular manifestations of the congenital varicella syndrome. *Arch Ophthalmol* 1989;107:52–56.

214. Mendivil A, Mendivil MP, Cuartero V. Ocular manifestations of the congenital–zoster syndrome. *Ophthalmologica* 1992;205:191–193.

215. Urayama A, Yamada N, Sasaki T. Unilateral acute uveitis with retinal periarteritis and detachment. *Jpn J Clin Ophthalmol* 1971;25:607–619.

216. Holland GN, Executive Committee of American Uveitis Society. Standard diagnostic criteria for acute retinal necrosis. *Am J Ophthalmol* 1994;117:663–667.

217. Culbertson WW, Dix RD. Varicella-zoster virus diseases: Posterior segment of the eye. In: Pepose JS, Holland GN, Wilhelmus KR, eds. *Ocular infection & immunity*. St. Louis: Mosby;1996. p. 1131–1154.

218. Culbertson WW, Broad RD, Flynn HW Jr, et al. Chicken pox-associated acute retinal necrosis syndrome. *Ophthalmology* 1991;98:1641–1645.

219. Engstrom RE Jr, Holland GN, Margolis TP, et al. The progressive outer retinal necrosis syndrome. A variant of necrotising herpetic retinopathy in patients with AIDS. *Ophthalmology* 1994;101:1488–1502.

220. Uninsky E, Jampol LM, Kaufman S, et al. Disseminated herpes simplex infection with retinitis in a renal allograft recipient. *Ophthalmology* 1983;90:175–178.

221. Falcone PM, Brockhurst RJ. Delayed onset of bilateral acute retinal necrosis: A 34–year interval. *Ann Ophthalmol* 1993;25:373–374.

222. Thompson WS, Culbertson WW, Smiddy WE. Acute retinal necrosis caused by reactivation of herpes simplex virus type 2. *Am J Ophthalmol* 1994;118:205–211.

223. Ganatra JB, Chandler D, Santos C. Viral causes of the acute retinal necrosis syndrome. *Am J Ophthalmol* 2000;129:166–172.

224. Smith JR, Chee SP. Acute retinal necrosis syndrome complicating chicken pox. *Singapore Med J* 2000;41:602–603.

225. Tan JCH, Byles D, Stanford MR. Acute retinal necrosis in children caused by herpes simplex virus. *Retina* 2001;21:344–347.

226. Chen S, Weinberg GA. Acute retinal necrosis syndrome in a child. *Pediatr Infect Dis J* 2002;21:78–80.

227. Lee WH, Charles SJ. Acute retinal necrosis following chicken pox in a healthy 4-year-old patient. *Br J Ophthalmol* 2000;84:667–668.

228. Blumenkranz MF, Culbertson WW, Clarkson JG. Treatment of the acute retinal necrosis syndrome with intravenous acyclovir. *Ophthalmology* 1986;93:296–300.

229. Matsuo T, Nakayama T, Koyama T. A proposed mild type of acute retinal necrosis syndrome. *Am J Ophthalmol* 1998;105:579–583.

230. Van Gelder RN, Willig JL, Holland GN. Herpes simplex virus type 2 as a cause of acute retinal necrosis syndrome in young patients. *Ophthalmology* 2001;108:869–876.

231. Tran THC, Rozenberg F, Cassoux N. Polymerase chain reaction analysis of aqueous humor samples in necrotising retinitis. *Br J Ophthalmol* 2003;87:79–83.

232. Palay DA, Sternberg P Jr, Davis J, et al. Decrease in the risk of bilateral acute retinal necrosis by acyclovir therapy. *Am J Ophthalmol* 1991;112:250–255.

233. Bart KJ, Orenstein WA, Hinman AR. The virtual elimination of rubella and mumps from the United States and the use of combined measles, mumps and rubella vaccines (MMR) to elimination measles. *Dev Biol Stand* 1986;65:45–52.

234. Lee SF, Lueder GT. Measles, mumps and rubella. In: Pepose JS, Holland GN, Wilhelmus KR, eds. *Ocular infection and symbol immunity*. St. Louis: Mosby, 1996:237–265.

235. Lindergren ML, Fehrs LJ, Hadler SC. Update: Rubella and congenital rubella syndrome, 1980–1990. *Epidemiol Rev* 1991;13:341–348.

236. Lee SH, Ewert DP, Frederick PD. Resurgence of congenital rubella syndrome in the 1990s: Report on missed opportunities and failed prevention policies among women of childbearing age. *JAMA* 1992;267:2616–2620.

237. Miller E. Rubella in the United Kingdom. *Epidemiology* 1991;107:31–42.

238. Grillner L, Forsgren M, Barr, B. Outcome of rubella during pregnancy with special reference to the 17th–24th weeks of gestation. *Scand J Infect Dis* 1983;15:321–325.

239. Letko E, Foster CS. Rubella. In: Foster CS, Vitale AT, eds. *Diagnosis and treatment of uveitis.* Philadelphia: W.B. Saunders & Company;2001. p. 343–347.

240. South NA, Sever JL. Teratogen update: the congenital rubella syndrome. *Teratology* 1985;31:297–307.

241. Boger WP. Late ocular manifestation in congenital rubella syndrome. *Ophthalmology* 1980;87:1244—12–52.

242. Keir E. Results of rubella in pregnancy. II. Hearing deficits. *Med J Aust* 1965;2:691–698.

243. McEvoy RC, Fedun B, Cooper LZ, et al. Children at high risk of diabetes mellitus: New York studies of families with diabetes and of children with congenital rubella syndrome. *Adv Exp Med Biol* 1998;246:221–227.

244. Givens KT, Lee DA, Jones T. Congenital rubella syndrome: Ophthalmic manifestations and associated systemic disorders. *Br J Ophthalmol* 1993;77:358–363.

245. Boniuk M. Glaucoma in the congenital rubella syndrome. *Int Ophthalmol Clin* 1992;12:121–136.

246. Harley RD. Discussion, comments. In: Boniuk M. The prevalence of Phthisis Bulbi as a complication of cataract surgery in the congenital rubella syndrome. *Trans Am Acad Ophthalmol Otolaryngol* 1970;74:360–368.

247. Miller E, Cradock-Watson JE, Pollack TM. Consequences of confirmed maternal rubella at successive stages of pregnancy. *Lancet* 1982;II:781–784.

248. Nishida Y, Oshima K. Congenital rubella syndrome: Correlation of gestational age at time of maternal rubella with type of defect. *J Pediatr* 1979;94:763–765.

249. Arnold J. Ocular manifestations of congenital rubella. *Curr Opin Ophthalmol* 1995;6:45–50.

250. Arnold J, McIntosh EDG, Martin FJ. A 50-year follow-up of ocular defects in congenital rubella: Late ocular manifestations. *Aust NZ J Ophthalmol* 1994;22:1–6.

251. Collis WJ, Cohen DN. Rubella retinopathy: A progressive disorder. *Arch Ophthalmol* 1970;84:33–35.

252. Deutman AF, Grizzard WS. Rubella retinopathy and subretinal neovascularization. *Am J Ophthalmol* 1978;85:82–87.

253. Frank KE, Purnell EW. Subretinal neovascularization following rubella retinopathy. *Am J Ophthalmol* 1978;86:462–466.

254. Orth DH, Fishman GA, Segall M. Rubella maculopathy. *Br J Ophthalmol* 1980;64:201–205.

255. Slusher NM, Tyler NE. Rubella retinopathy and subretinal neovascularization. *Am J Ophthalmol* 1982;14:292–294.

256. Bonomo PP. Involution without disciform scarring of subretinal neovascularization in presumed rubella retinopathy. A report. *Acta Ophthalmol (Copenh)* 1982;60:141–146.

257. Grever SL, Helveston VN. Subretinal neovascularization in a 10-year-old child. *J Pediatr Ophthalmol Strabismus* 1992;29:250–251.

258. Wolff, SM. The ocular manifestations of congenital rubella. *Trans Am Ophthalmol Soc* 1972;70:577–614.

259. Gross PA, Portnoy D, Mathies AW Jr. A rubella outbreak among adolescent boys. *Am J Dis Child* 1970;119:329–331.

260. Zimmerman LE. Histopathologic basis for ocular manifestations of congenital rubella syndrome. *Am J Ophthalmol* 1968;65:837–862.

261. Matoba A. Ocular viral infections. *Pediatr Infect Dis* 1984;3:358–368.

262. Gerstle C, Zinn KM. Rubella-associated retinitis in adult. Report of a case. *Mt. Sinai J Med* 1976;43:303–308.

263. Hayashi M, Yoshimura N, Kondo T. Acute rubella retinal pigment epithelitis in an adult. *Am J Ophthalmol* 1982;93:285–288.

264. Kazarian EL, Gager WE. Optic neuritis complicating measles, mumps, and rubella vaccination. *Am J Ophthalmol* 1978;86:544–547.

265. Barton LL, Mets MB. Congenital lymphocytic choriomeningitis virus infection: decade of rediscovery. *Clin Infect Dis* 2001;33:370–374.

266. Armstrong C, Lillie R. Experimental lymphocytic choriomeningitis of monkeys and mice produced by a virus encountered in studies of the 1933 St. Louis encephalitis epidemic. *Public Health Rep* 1934;49:1019–1027.

267. Rowe W, Murphy P, Bergold G, et al. Arenoviruses: proposed name for a newly defined virus group. *J Virol* 1970;5:651–652.

268. Childs J, Glass G, Korch G. Lymphocytic choriomeningitis virus infection and house mouse (MUS musclus) distribution in urban Baltimore. *Am J Trop Med Hyg* 1992;47:27–34.

269. Hirsch M, Moellering R, Pope H. Lymphocytic-choriomeningitis-virus infection traced to a pet hamster. *N Engl J Med* 1974;291:610–612.

270. Wright R, Johnson D, Neuman M, et al. Congenital lymphocytic choriomeningitis virus syndrome: a disease that mimics congenital toxoplasmosis or Cytomegalovirus infection. *Pediatrics* 1997;100:E9–E14.

272. Mets MB, Barton LL, Kahn AS. Lymphocytic choriomeningitis virus: an underdiagnosed cause of congenital chorioretinitis. *Am J Ophthalmol* 2000;130:209–215.

276. Enders G, Varho-Göbel N, Löhler J. Congenital lymphocytic choriomeningitis virus infection: an underdiagnosed disease. *Pediatr Infect Dis J* 1999;18:652–655.

273. Brezin AP, Thulliez P, Cisneros B. Lymphocytic choriomeningitis virus chorioretinitis mimicking ocular toxoplasmosis in two otherwise normal children. *Am J Ophthalmol* 2000;130:245–247.

271. Barton LL, Mets MB, Beauchamp CL. Lymphocytic choriomeningitis virus: emerging fetal teratogen. *Am J Obstet Gynecol* 2002;187:1715–1716.

274. Lewis DJ, Walter PD, Thacker WL. Comparison of three tests for the serological diagnosis of lymphocytic choriomeningitis virus infection. *J Clin Microbiol* 1975;2:193–197.

275. Lehmann-Grube F, Kallay M, Ibscher B. Serologic diagnosis of human infections with lymphocytic choriomeningitis virus: comparative evaluation of seven methods. *J Med Virol* 1979;4;125–136.

277. Gessner A, Lother H. Homologous interference of lymphocytic choriomeningitis virus involving a Ribazirin-susceptible block in virus replication. *J Virol* 1989;63:1827–1832.

278. Henle W, Henle G. Epstein-Barr virus and infectious mononucleosis. *N Engl J Med* 1973;288:263–264.

281. Matoba AY. Ocular disease associated with Epstein-Barr virus infection. *Surv Ophthalmol* 1990;35:145–149.

279. Goldberg GM, Xulginiti VA, Ray CG, et al. In utero Epstein-Barr virus (infectious mononucleosis) infection. *JAMA* 1981;246:1579–1581.

280. Morishima N, Miyakawa S, Akazawa Y. A case of uveitis associated with chronic active Epstein-Barr virus infection. *Ophthalmologica* 1996;210:186–188.

282. Karpe G, Wising P. Retinal changes with acute reduction of vision as initial symptoms of infectious mononucleosis. *Acta Ophthalmol* 1948;26:19–24.

283. Kelly ST, Rosenthal AR, Micholson KG. Retinochoroiditis in acute Epstein-Barr virus infection. *Br J Ophthalmol* 1989;73:1002–1003.

284. Raymond LA, Wilson CA, Linnemann Jr CC. Punctate outer retinitis in acute Epstein-Barr virus infection. *Am J Ophthalmol* 1987;104:427–426.

285. Palestine AG, Nussenblatt RB, Chan CC. Histopathology of the subretinal fibrosis and uveitis syndrome. *Ophthalmology* 1985;92:838–844.

286. Wong KW, D'Amico DJ, Hedges TR III. Ocular involvement associated with chronic Epstein-Barr virus disease. *Arch Ophthalmol* 1987;105:788–792.

287. Usui M, Sakai J. Three cases of EB virus-associated uveitis. *Int Ophthalmol* 1990;14:371–376.

288. Tiedeman JS. Epstein-Barr viral antibodies in multifocal choroiditis and panuveitis. *Am J Ophthalmol* 1987;103:659–663.

289. Zierhut M, Foster CS. Multiple sclerosis, sarcoidosis and other diseases in patients with pars planitis. *Dev Ophthalmol* 1992;23:41–47.

290. Tosato G. The Epstein-Barr virus and the immune system. *Adv Cancer Res* 1987;49:75–125.

291. Thorley-Lawson DA. Epstein-Barr virus: exploiting the immune system. *Nat Rev Immunol* 2001;1:75–82.

294. Cherry JD. Measles virus. In: Feigan RD, Cherry, JD, eds. *Textbook of pediatric infectious disease*, vol. 1, ed. 4. Philadelphia: WB Saunders, 1998:2054–2074.

292. Centers for Disease Control and Prevention. Update: global measles control and mortality reduction—worldwide, 1991–2001. *MMWR* 2003;52:471–75.

293. Centers for Disease Control and Prevention. Summary of notifiable diseases—United States, 2001. *MMWR* 2003;50:1–108.

295. Metz HS, Harkey ME. Pigmentary retinopathy following maternal measles (morbilli) infection. *Am J Ophthalmol* 1968;66:1107–1110.

296. Guzzinati GC. Sulla possizilitá di lesioni oculari congenita da morbillo e da etatite epidemica. *Boll Ocul (Italia)* 1954;12:833–841.

297. Letko E, Foster CS. Measles. In: Foster CS, Vitale AT, eds. *Diagnosis and treatment of uveitis*. Philadelphia: WB Saunders, 2001:336–341.

298. Dekkers NWHM. The cornea in measles. In: Darrell RW, ed. *Viral diseases of the eye*. Philadelphia: Lea & Febiger, 1985:239.

299. Scheie HD, Morse PH. Rubeola retinopathy. *Arch Ophthalmol* 1972;88:341–344.

300. Foxman SG, Heckenlively JR, Sinclair SH. Rubeola retinopathy and pigmented paravenous retinochoroidal atrophy. *Am J Ophthalmol* 1985;99:605606.

301. Centers for Disease Control and Prevention. Subacute sclerosing panencephalitis surveillance—United States. *MMWR* 1982;31:585–588.

302. Green SH, Wirtschafter J. Ophthalmic findings in subacute sclerosing panencephalitis. *Br J Ophthalmol* 1973;57:780–777.

303. Caruso JM, Robbins-Tien D, Brown W. Atypical chorioretinitis as an early presentation of subacute sclerosing panencephalitis. *J Pediatr Ophthalmol Strabismus* 2000;37:119–122.

304. Robb RM, Watters GV. Ophthalmic manifestation of subacute sclerosing panencephalitis. *Arch Ophthalmol* 1970;83:426–435.

305. Zagami AS, Lethlean AK. Chorioretinitis as a possible very early manifestation of subacute sclerosing panencephalitis. *Aust J Med* 1991;21:350–352.

306. De Laey JJ, Hanssens N, Colette P. Subacute sclerosing panencephalitis: fundus changes and histopathologic correlation. *Doc Ophthalmol* 1983;56:11–21.

307. Kovacs D, Bastag O. Fluoroangiographic picture of the acute stage of the retinal lesion in subacute sclerosing panencephalitis. *Ophthalmologica* 1978;177:264–269.

308. Landers MD, Klintworth GK. Subacute sclerosing panencephalitis (SSPE). A clinicopathologic study of the retinal lesions. *Arch Ophthalmol* 1971;86:156–163.

309. Meyers E, Mailin M, Zonis S. Subacute sclerosing panencephalitis: clinicopathological study of the eyes. *J Pediatr Ophthalmol Strabismus* 1978;15:19–23.

310. Nelson DA, Weiner A, Yanoff M. Retinal lesions in subacute sclerosing panencephalitis. *Arch Ophthalmol* 1970;84:613–621.

311. Otradovec J. The clinical picture of chorioretinal changes in subacute sclerosing leukoencephalitis. *Sb Lek* 1968;70:229–236.

312. Salmon JS, Tan EL, Murray AND. Visual loss with dancing extremities and mental disturbances. *Surv Ophthalmol* 1991;35:299–306.

313. Morgan B, Cohen DN, Rothner AD. Ocular manifestations of subacute sclerosing panencephalitis. *Am J Dis Child* 1976;130:1019–1021.

314. Hiatt RL, Grizzard HT, McNeer P. Ophthalmic manifestations of subacute sclerosing panencephalitis (Dawson's encephalitis). *Trans Am Acad Ophthalmol Otolaryngol* 1971;75:344–350.

315. Gravina RF, Nakanishi AS, Faden A. Subacute sclerosing panencephalitis. *Am J Ophthalmol* 1978;86:106–109.

316. Font RO, Jenis EH, Tuck KD. Measles maculopathy associated with subacute sclerosing panencephalitis. Immunofluorescent and immuno-ultrastructural studies. *Arch Pathol* 1973;96:168–174.

317. Raymond LA, Kersteine RS, Shelburne SA Jr. Preretinal vitreous membrane in subacute sclerosing panencephalitis. *Arch Ophthalmol* 1976;94:1412–1413.

318. Garg RG. Subacute sclerosing panencephalitis. *Postgrad Med J* 2002;78:63–70.

319. Gutman LT. Syphilis. In: Feigin R, Cherry JD, eds. *Textbook of pediatric infectious disease*, vol 1, ed 4. Philadelphia: W.B. Saunders Company. 1998:1543–1556.

320. Centers for Disease Control and Prevention. Congenital syphilis—United States, 2000. *MMWR* 2001;50:573–577.

321. Evans HE, Frenkel LD. Congenital syphilis. *Clin Perinatol* 1994;21:149–162.

322. Crouch ER, Goldberg MF. Retinal periarteritis secondary to syphilis. *Arch Ophthalmol* 1997;93:384–387.

323. Spoor TC, Ramocki JM, Mesi FA. Osler syphilis 1986. *J Clin Neuroophthalmol* 1997;7:191–195.

324. Centers for Disease Control and Prevention. Guidelines for the prevention and control of congenital syphilis. *MMWR* 1988;37(Suppl 1):1–13.

325. Margo CE, Hamed LM. Ocular syphilis. *Surv Ophthalmol* 1992;37:203–220.

326a. Browning DJ. Posterior segment manifestations of active ocular syphilis, their response to a neurosyphilis regimen of penicillin therapy, and the influence of human immunodeficiency virus status on response. *Ophthalmology* 2000;107:215–223.

326b. Tamesis R, Foster CS. Ocular syphilis. *Ophthalmology* 1990;97:1281–1287.

327a. Schlaegel TF, O'Connor GR. Metastatic nonsuppurative uveitis. *Int Ophthalmol Clin* 1977;17:87–108.

327b. Samson MC, Foster CS. Syphilis. In: Foster CS, Vitale AT, eds. *Diagnosis and treatment of uveitis*. Philadelphia: W.B. Saunders Company;2001. p. 237–244.

328. Katz DA, Berger JR, Duncan RC. Neurosyphilis. *Arch Neurol* 1993;50:243–249.

329. Wilhelmus KR, Lukehart SA. Syphilis. In: Pepose JS, Holland GN, Wilhelmus KR, eds. *Ocular infections & immunity*. St. Louis: Mosby;1996. p. 1437–1466.

330. Gass JDM, Braunstein RA, Chenoweth RG. Acute syphilitic posterior placoid chorioretinitis. *Ophthalmology* 1990;97:1288–1297.

331. Shalaby IA, Dunn JT, Sem BA. Syphilitic uveitis in human immunodeficiency virus-infected patients. *Arch Ophthalmol* 1997;115:469–473.

332. Dowell ME, Ross PG, Musher DM. Response of latent syphilis or neurosyphilis to ceftriaxone therapy in persons infected with human immunodeficiency virus. *Am J Med* 1992;93:481–488.

333. Passo NS, Rosenbaum JT. Ocular syphilis in patients with human immunodeficiency virus infection. *Am J Ophthalmol* 1988; 106:1–6.
334. Huppertz HI, Bohme M, Stamdaert SM. Incidents of Lyme borreliosis in the Wurzburg region of Germany. *Eur J Clin Microbiol Infect Dis* 1999;18:697–703.
335. Centers for Disease Control and Prevention. Lyme disease–United States, 2000. *MMWR* 2002;51:29–31.
336. Steere AC, Dwyer E, Winchester R. Association of chronic Lyme arthritis with HLA-DR4 and HAA-DR2 alleles. *N Engl J Med* 1990;323:219–223.
337. Baer JC. Borrieliosis. In: Foster CS, Vitale AT, eds. *Diagnosis and treatment of uveitis.* Philadelphia: W.B. Saunders Company;2001. p. 345–359.
338. Centers for Disease Control and Prevention. Case definitions for infectious conditions under public health surveillance. *MMWR* 1997;46(RR-10):20–21.
339. American College of Physicians: Guidelines for laboratory evaluation in the diagnosis of Lyme disease. *Ann Intern Med* 1997;127:1106–1108.
340. Steere AC, Schoen RT, Taylor E. The clinical evolution of Lyme arthritis. *Ann Intern Med* 1987;107:725–731.
341. Haass A. Lyme neuroborreliosis. *Curr Opin Neurol* 1998;11: 253–258.
342. Paparone PW. Cardiovascular manifestations of Lyme disease. *J Am Osteopath Assoc* 1997;97:156–161.
343. Nadelman RB, Wormser GP. Lyme borreliosis. *Lancet* 1998; 352:557–565.
344. Berger DW, Johnson RC, Kodner C. Cultivation of Borrelia burgdorferi from the blood of two patients with erythema migrans lesions lacking extracutaneous signs and symptoms of Lyme disease. *J Acad Dermatol* 1994;30:48–51.
345. Winterkorn JNS. Lyme disease: Neurologic and ophthalmic manifestations. *Surv Ophthalmol* 1990;35:191–304.
346. Steere AC, Malawista SE, Snydman DR, et al. Lyme arthritis: an epidemic of oligoarticular in children and adults in three Connecticut communities. *Arthritis Rheum* 1997;20:7–17.
347. Mikkilä HO, Seppälä IJT, Viljanen MK. The expanding clinical spectrum of ocular Lyme borreliosis. *Ophthalmology* 2000;107:581–587.
348. Karma A, Seppälä I, Mikkilä. Diagnosis and clinical characteristics of ocular Lyme borreliosis. *Am J Ophthalmol* 1995; 119:127–135.
349. Glauser TA, Brennan PJ, Galetta SL. Reversible Horner's syndrome and Lyme disease. *J Clin Neurophathomol* 1989;9: 225–228.
350. Winward KE, Smith JL, Culbertson WW. Ocular Lyme borreliosis. *Am J Ophthalmol* 1989;108:651–657.
351. Szer IS, Taylor E, Steere AC. The long-term course of Lyme arthritis in children. *N Eng J Med* 1991;325:159–163.
352. Monbaerts IM, Naudgal PC, Knockaert DC. Bilateral follicular conjunctivitis in a manifestation of Lyme disease. *Am J Ophthalmol* 1991;112:96–97.
353. Reim H, Reim M. Ocular findings in infection with Borrelia burgdorseri. *Klin Monatsbl Augenheilkd* 1992;201:83–91.
354. Gues-Crosier Y, Herbort CP. Lyme disease in Switzerland: ocular involvement. *Klin Monatsbl Augenheilkd* 1992;200:545–546.
355. Karma A, Pirttila TA, Viljanen MK. Secondary retinitis pigmentosa and cerebral demyelination in Lyme borreliosis. *Br J Ophthalmol* 1993;77:120–122.
356. Huppertz HI, Nunchmeier D, Lieb W. Ocular manifestations in children and adolescents with Lyme arthritis. *Br J Ophthalmol* 1999;83:1149–1152.
357. Tugwell D, Weinstein A, Welos G, et al. Laboratory evaluations in the diagnosis of Lyme disease. *Ann Intern Med* 1997;127: 1109–1123.
358. Rosenbaum JT. Prevalence of Lyme disease among patients with uveitis. *Am J Ophthalmol* 1991;112:462–463.
359. Hilton E, Smith C, Sood F. Ocular Lyme borreliosis diagnosed by polymerase chain reaction on vitreous fluid. *Ann Intern Med* 1996;1125:424–425.
360. Coyle PK. *Borrelia burgdorseri* infection: Clinical diagnostic techniques. *Immunol Invest* 1997;26:117–128.
361. Wormser GP, Nadelman RB, Dattwyler RJ, et al. Practical guidelines for the treatment of Lyme disease. The Infectious Diseases Society of America. *Clin Infect Dis* 2000;31:1–14.
362. Sweeney CJ, Ghassemi M, Agger WA. Coinfection with Babesia microti and Borrelia burgdorseri in a western Wisconsin residence. *Mayo Clin Proc* 1998;73:338–341.
363. Walker DH, Darbour AG, Oliver JH, et al. Emerging bacterial zonotic and vector-borne diseases. Ecological and epidemiological factors. *JAMA* 1996;275:463–469.
364. Puliafito CAS, Haas J. Infectious endophthalmitis. Review of 36 cases. *Ophthalmology* 1982;89:921–929.
365. Alfaro DZ, Roth DB, Laughlin RM. Paediatric post-traumatic endophthalmitis. *Br J Ophthalmol* 1995;79:888–891.
366. Hariprasad SM, Mieler WF, Holz ER. Vitreous and aqueous penetration of orally administered gatifloxacin in humans. *Arch Ophthalmol* 2003;121:345–350.
367. Okada AA, Johnson RP, Liles WC. Endogenous bacterial endophthalmitis: Report of a ten-year retrospective study. *Ophthalmology* 1994;101:832–838.
368. Shrader SK, Band JD, Lauter CB. The clinical spectrum of endophthalmitis: incidents, predisposing factors, and features influencing outcome. *J Infect Dis* 1990;162:115–120.
369. Greenwald NJ, Wohl LD, Sell CH. Metastatic endophthalmitis: a contemporary reappraisal. *Surv Ophthalmol* 1986;31: 81–101.
370. Samson CM, Foster, CS. Masquerade syndromes: endophthalmitis. In: Foster CS, Vitale AT, eds. *Diagnosis and treatment of uveitis.* Philadelphia: W.B. Saunders Company;2001. p. 528–536.
371. Wong JS, Chan TK, Lee HM. Endogenous bacterial endophthalmitis: an east Asian experience and a reappraisal of a severe ocular affliction. *Ophthalmology* 2000;107:1483–1491.
372. Persaud D, Moss WJ, Muñoz JL. Serious eye infections in children. *Pediatr Ann* 1993;22:379–383.
373. Wong JS, Balakrishnan V. Neisseria meningitidis endogenous endophthalmitis: case report and literature review. *J Pediatr Ophthalmol Strabismus* 1999;36:145–152.
374. Park DW II, Jones DB, Gentry LO. Endogenous endophthalmitis among patients with candidemia. *Ophthalmology* 1982;89:789–796.
375. Bross J, Talbot GH, Maislin G. Risk factors for nosocomial candidemia: a case-controlled study in adults without leukemia. *Am J Med* 1989;87:614–620.
376. Brooks RG. Prospective study of *Candida* endophthalmitis in hospitalized patients with candidemia. *Arch Intern Med* 1989;149:2226–2228.
377. Donahue SP, Hein E, Sinatra RB. Ocular involvement in children with candidemia. *Am J Ophthalmol* 2003;135:886–887.
378. Makhoul IR, Kassis I, Smolkin T. Review of 49 neonates with acquired fungal sepsis: further characterization. *Pediatrics* 2001;107:61–66.
379. Shah JK, Vander J, Eagle RC. Intralenticular *Candida* species abscess in a premature infant. *Am J Ophthalmol* 2000;129:390–391.
380. Stern JH, Calvano C, Simon JW. Recurrent endogenous candidal endophthalmitis in a premature infant. *J AATOS* 2001;5:50–51.
381. Noyola DE, Fernandez M, Moylett EH. Ophthalmologic, visceral and cardiac involvement in neonates with candidemia. *Clin Infect Dis* 2001;32:1018–1023.

382. Donahue SP, Greven CM, Zuravleff JJ, et al. Intraocular candidiasis in patients with candidemia. *Ophthalmology* 1994; 101:1302–1309.

383. Luttrull JK, Wan WL, Kubak BN. Treatment of ocular fungal infections with oral fluconazole. *Am J Ophthalmol* 1995; 419:477–481.

384. Patel AS, Hemady RK, Rodrigues M. Endogenous Fusarium endophthalmitis in a patient with acute lymphocytic leukemia. *Am J Ophthalmol* 1994;117:363–368.

385. Shields JA, Shields CL, Eagle RC Jr. Endogenous endophthalmitis simulating retinoblastoma. The 1993 David and Mary Seslen Endowment Lecture. *Retina* 1995;15:213–219.

386. Gottlieb JL, McAllister IL, Guttman FA. Choroidal blastomycosis. A report of two cases. *Retina* 1995;15:248–252.

387. Coats ML, Peyman GA. Intravitreal corticosteroids in the treatment of exogenous fungal endophthalmitis. *Retina* 1992;12: 46–51.

388. Christmas NJ, Smiddy WE. Vitrectomy and systemic fluconazole for treatment of endogenous fungal endophthalmitis. *Ophthalmic Surg Lasers* 1996;27:1012–1018.

389. McMoli TE, Mordi VP, Grange A. Tuberculosis panophthalmitis. *J Pediatr Ophthalmol Strabismus* 1978;15:383–385.

390. Waheeb S, Al-Saadi M, Quinn AG. Tuberculosis chorioretinitis. *Can J Ophthalmol* 2001;36:344–346.

391. Grewal A, Kim RY, Cunningham ET. Miliary tuberculosis. *Arch Ophthalmol* 1998;116:953–954.

392. Barondes MJ, Sponsel WE, Stevens TS. Tuberculosis choroiditis diagnosed by chorioretinal endobiopsy. *Am J Ophthalmol* 1991;112:460–461.

393. Mansour AM, Haymond R. Choroidal tuberculosis without evidence of extraocular tuberculosis. *Graefe's Arch Clin Exp Ophthalmol* 1990;228: 382–385.

394. Cangemi FE, Freidman AH, Josphberg R. Tuberculoma of the choroid. *Ophthalmology* 1980;87:252–258.

395. Lyon CE, Grimson BS, Pfeiffer RLL. Clinopathological correlation of a solitary choroidal tuberculoma. *Ophthalmology* 1985; 92:845–850.

396. Rosen PH, Spalton DJ, Grahan EM. Intraocular tuberculosis. *I* 1990;4:486–492.

397. Helm CJ, Holland GN. Ocular tuberculosis. *Surv Ophthalmol* 1993;38:229–256.

398. Morinura Y, Okada AA, Kawahara S, et al. Tuberculin skin testing in uveitis patients and treatment of presumed intraocular tuberculosis in Japan. *Ophthalmology* 2002;109: 851–857.

399. Ni C, Papale JJ, Robinson NL. Uveal tuberculosis. *Int Ophthalmol Clin* 1982;22:103–124.

400. Samson MC, Foster CS. Tuberculosis. In: Foster CS, Vitale AT, eds. *Diagnosis and treatment of uveitis*. Philadelphia: W.B. Saunders Company;2001. p. 264–271.

401. Fakai J, Matsuwawa S, Usui M. New diagnostic approach for ocular tuberculosis by ELISA using the cord factor as antigen. *Br J Ophthalmol* 2001;85:130–133.

402. Centers for Disease Control and Prevention. Treatment of tuberculosis. American Thoracic Society, CDC, and Infectious Diseases Society of America. *MMWR* 2003;52 (RR11):1–77.

403. Edlin BR, Tokars JI, Grieco MH, et al. An outbreak of multidrug-resistant tuberculosis among hospitalized patients with the acquired immunodeficiency syndrome. *N Eng J Med* 1992;326:1514–1521.

404. Jackson FLA, Perkins BA, Wenger JD. Cat-scratch disease in the United States: an analysis of three national databases. *Am J Public Health* 1993;83:1707–1711.

405. Hamilton DH, Zangwill KM, Hadler JL. Cat-scratch disease—Connecticut, 1992–1993. *J Infect Dis* 1995;172:570–573.

406. Dalton MJ, Robinson LE, Cooper J. Use of *Bartonella* antigens for the serologic diagnosis of cat-scratch disease at a national referral center. *Arch Intern Med* 1995;155:1670–1676.

407. Carithers HA, Cat scratch disease: an overview based on a study of 1,200 patients. *Am J Dis Child* 1985;139:1124–1133.

408. Jameson P, Green C, Regnery R, et al. Prevalence of *Bartonella henselae* antibodies in pet cats throughout regions of North America. *J Infect Dis* 1995;172:1145–1149.

409. Regnery RL, Olson JG, Perkins BA. Serological response to "Rochalimaea henselae" antigen in suspected cat-scratch disease. *Lancet* 1992;339:1443–1445.

410. LeBoit PE, Berger TG, Egbert BM, et al. Epitheloid haemangioma-like vascular proliferation in AIDS; manifestation of cat scratch disease bacillus infection? *Lancet* 1988;1(8592): 960–963.

411. Adal KA, Cockerell CJ, Petri WA Jr. Cat-scratch disease, bacillary angiomatosis, and other infections due to Rochalimaea. *N Engl J Med* 1994;330:1509–1515.

412. Regnery R, Pappero J. Unraveling the mysteries associated with cat-scratch disease, Bacillary angiomatosis, and related syndromes. *Emerg Infect Dis* 1995;1:16–21.

413. Chorich LJ III. Bartonella. In: Foster CS, Vitale AT, eds. *Diagnosis and treatment of uveitis*. Philadelphia: W.B. Saunders Company;2001. p. 260–263.

414. Jones DB. Cat-scratch disease. In: Pepose JS, Holland GN, Wilhelmus KR, eds. *Ocular infection and immunity*. St. Louis: Mosby-Year Book;1996. p. 1389–1397.

415. Ormerod LD, Skolnick KA, Menosky NM. Retinal and choroidal manifestations of cat-scratch disease. *Ophthalmology* 1998;105:1024–1031.

416. Dreyer RF, Hopen G, Gass JDM. Leber's idiopathic stellate neuroretinitis. *Arch Ophthalmol* 1984;102:1140–1145.

417. Leber T. Die pseudonephritischen Netzhauterkrankunden die Retinitis steolata: die Turtschersche Netzhauteffektion nach schwerer Schadelzerletzung. In: Graefe AC, Saemisch T, eds. *Graefe-Saemisch Handbuch der der Augerheilkunde, ed. 2.* Leipzig, East Germany: Englemann;1916: vol. 7, Pt. 2, Ch. 10.

418. Golnick KC, Marotto ME, Fanous NM, et al. Ophthalmic manifestations of Rochalimaea species. *Am J Ophthalmol* 1994;118:145–151.

419. Gass JD. Diseases of the optic nerve that may simulate macular disease. *Trans Am Acad Ophthalmol Otolaryngol* 1977;83: 763–770.

420. Reed JB, Scales DK, Wong MT. *Bartonella henselae* neuroretinitis in cat-scratch disease. Diagnosis, management and sequellae. *Ophthalmology* 1998;105:459–466.

421. Suhler ED, Lauer AK, Rosenbaum, JT. Prevalence of serologic evidence of cat scratch disease in patients with neuroretinitis. *Ophthalmology* 2000;107:871–876.

422. Wade MK, Po S, Wong IG. Bilateral *Bartonella*-associated neuroretinitis. *Retina* 1999;19:355–356.

423. Wade MK, Levi L, Jones MR. Optic disc edema associated with peripapillary serous retinal detachment: an early sign of systemic *Bartonella henselae* infection. *Am J Ophthalmol* 2000;130: 321–328.

424. Cunningham ET Jr, McDonald HR, Schatz H. Inflammatory mass of the optic nerve head associated with systemic Bartonella henselae infection. *Arch Ophthalmol* 1997;115:1596–1597.

425. Omerod LD, Dailey JP. Ocular manifestations of cat-scratch disease. *Curr Opin Ophthalmol* 1999;10:209–216.

426. Pollock SC, Kristinsson J. Cat-scratch disease manifesting as a unifocal helioid choroiditis. *Arch Ophthalmol* 1998;116: 1249–1250.

427. Solley WA, Martin DF, Newman NJ, et al. Cat scratch disease: posterior segment manifestations. *Ophthalmology* 1999;106: 1546–1553.

428. Cunningham ET Jr, Koehler JE. Ocular bartonellosis. *Am J Ophthalmol* 2000;130:340–349.

429. Cohen SN, Davis JL, Gass JDM. Branch retinal arterial occlusions in multifocal retinitis with optic nerve edema. *Arch Ophthalmol* 1995;113:1271–1276.

430. Zacchei AC, Newman NJ, Sternberg P. Serous retinal detachment of the macula which is associated with cat scratch disease. *Am J Ophthalmol* 1995;120:796–797.

431. Canzano JC, Lim JI. Pars plana vitrectomy for epiretinal membrane secondary to cat scratch neuroretinitis. *Retina* 2001;21:272–273.

432. Fish RH, Hogan RN, Nightingale SD. Peripapillary angiomatosis associated with cat-scratch neuroretinitis. *Arch Ophthalmol* 1992;110:323.

433. Soheilian M, Markomichelakis N, Foster CS. Intermediate uveitis and retinal vasculitis as manifestations of cat scratch disease. *Am J Ophthalmol* 1996;122:582–584.

434. Gaebler JW, Burgett RA, Caldneyer KS. Subacute orbital abscess in a four-year-old with a new kitten. *Pediatr Infect Dis J* 1998;17:844–846.

435. Rothova A, Kerkhoff F, Hooft HJ. Bartonella serology for patients with intraocular inflammatory disease. *Retina* 1998;18:348–355.

436. Kerkhoff FT, Offewaarde JM, de Loos WS, et al. Presumed ocular bartonellosis. *Br J Ophthalmol* 1999;83:270–275.

437. Litwin CM, Martins TB, Hill HRR. Immunologic response to *Bartonella henselae* as determined by enzyme immunoassay and Western blot analysis. *Am J Clin Pathol* 1997;108:202–209.

438. Barka NE, Hadfield T, Patnaik M. EIA for detection of Rochalimaea henselae-reactive IgG, IgM and IgA antibodies in patients with suspected cat-scratch disease. *J Infect Dis* 1993;167:1503–1504.

439. Maurin N, Birtles R, Raoult D. Current knowledge of *Bartonella* species. *Eur J Clin Microbiol Infect Dis* 1997;16:487–506.

440. Relman DA, Loutit JS, Schmidt TM. The agent of bacillary angiomatosis. An approach to the identification of uncultured pathogens. *N Eng J Med* 1990;323:1573–1580.

441. Labalette P, Bermond D, Dedes Z. Cat-scratch disease neuroretinitis diagnosed by polymerase chain reaction approach. *Am J Ophthalmol* 2001;132:575–576.

442. McDonald HR. Diagnostic and therapeutic challenges. *Retina* 2003;23:224–229.

443. Margileth AM. Antibiotic therapy for cat-scratch disease. Clinical study of therapeutic outcome in 268 patients and a review of the literature. *Pediatr Infect Dis J* 1992;11:474–478.

444. Bass JW, Freitas BC, Freitas AD, et al. Prospective randomized double blind placebo-controlled evaluation of azithromycin for the treatment of cat-scratch disease. *Pediatr Infect Dis J* 1998;17:447–452.

445. Sprach DH, Koehler JE. *Bartonella*-associated infection. *Infect Dis Clin North Am* 1998;12:137–155.

446. Arisoy EF, Correa AG, Wagner ML. Hepatosplenic cat-scratch disease in children: selected clinical features and treatment. *Clin Infect Dis* 1999;28:778–784.

447. Cokingtin CD, Han DP. Bilateral nongranulomatous uveitis and a poststreptococcal syndrome. *Am J Ophthalmol* 1991;112:595–596.

448. Ortiz JM, Kamerling JM, Fischer D. Scleritis, uveitis, and glaucoma in a patient with rheumatic fever. *Am J Ophthalmol* 1995;120:538–539.

449. Hall AJ, Barton K, Watson PG. Scleritis in association with poststreptococcal vasculitis. *Arch Ophthalmol* 1993;111:1324–1325.

450. Leiba H, Barash J, Pollack A. Poststreptococcal uveitis. *Am J Ophthalmol* 1998;126:317–318.

451. Benjamin A, Tufail A, Holland GN. Uveitis as the only clinical manifestation of poststreptococcal syndrome. *Am J Ophthalmol* 1997;123:258–260.

452. Saari KM, Maki M, Paivonsalo T. Acute anterior uveitis and conjunctivitis following Yersinia infection in children. *Int Ophthalmol* 1986;9:237–241.

UVEITIS AFFECTING INFANTS AND CHILDREN: NONINFECTIOUS CAUSES

C. STEPHEN FOSTER
ALBERT T. VITALE
LEILA KUMP
ZEIN GHASSAN

Children account for approximately 10% of uveitis cases cared for in tertiary uveitis referral centers, yet among children, an extraordinarily high percentage experience recurrent or chronic disease, and 40% have posterior segment involvement. Infectious etiologies account for approximately 20% of the cases. The uveitis associated with juvenile idiopathic arthritis (juvenile rheumatoid arthritis) accounts for approximately 37% of the noninfectious uveitis cases. The epidemiologic characteristics of pediatric uveitis have been addressed in the introductory section of the preceding chapter. It is the noninfectious uveitis entities to which this chapter is devoted.

NONINFECTIOUS UVEITIS SYNDROMES IN CHILDREN

Juvenile Idiopathic Arthritis–Associated Iridocyclitis

Prevalence

Juvenile idiopathic arthritis (JIA) is a systemic autoimmune disease that affects approximately 70,000 children in the United States.

Pathogenesis and Etiology

Like most autoimmune diseases, its pathogenesis appears to be multifactorial, with some identified genetic predispositions, and the onset possibly triggered by microbial contact.

Clinical Signs and Symptoms

The peak age of onset of JIA is between ages 6 months and 4 years, and the onset can be subcategorized into three broad modes of onset: systemic; polyarticular; and oligoarticular. Uveitis almost never develops in the systemic onset patients, whereas uveitis develops in 20% of children with oligoarticular onset JIA (four or fewer joints involved at disease onset). Uveitis may also develop in about 5% of polyarticular onset JIA patients.

The uveitis associated with JIA is typically silent; that is, the patient is unaware that he or she has intraocular inflammation. This is an unusual aspect of JIA, because most individuals with other forms of uveitis experience pain, ocular redness, light sensitivity, or diminished vision. The uveitis may develop before articular manifestations of JIA become manifest. Therefore, intraocular inflammation may have been present for long periods of time before the patient seeks medical care. Some of the poorer visual outcomes occur in children in whom the uveitis onset preceded the development of arthritis. Other markers of poor prognosis include positive human leukocyte antigen (HLA)-DR5 haplotype, positive antinuclear antibody (ANA), female gender, young age at onset, presence of posterior synechiae at first slit-lamp biomicroscopic examination, and delayed referral to an ocular immunologist experienced in the use of nonsteroidal antiinflammatory/immunomodulatory medications (1–5).

Regrettably, even with ophthalmologists and rheumatologists following the recommendations of the American Academy of Pediatrics (6) for biomicroscopic screening of children with JIA, significant visual impairment develops in as many as 25% of children with JIA, and in some regions, as many as 12% become blind in at least one eye (7). In a publication of 18 patients with JIA, the final visual acuity was imperfect in 40%, quite poor in 20%, and completely lost in 10 eyes (8). The authors concluded that 70% of the eyes of the patients that they observed were either visually handicapped or totally blind, and emphasized that some of the publications reporting a more favorable ocular prognosis in children with JIA-associated uveitis might suffer from case selection bias and inadequate longitudinal follow-up. Thus, whereas others (9–11) reported poor outcomes in their JIA populations 15 years ago, recent reports that indicate that the prevalence of uveitis has been steadily decreasing as a consequence of better JIA management by rheumatologists (12–15) may have some bias. In this study of 18 adult patients with long-standing JIA-associated uveitis (mean duration of uveitis, 20.5 years) and ocular complications at the time of first evaluation at a specialty clinic, visual acuity was less than 20/150 in 30% of the patients, and three eyes were phthisical (8). The authors concluded that the long-term prognosis of ocular involvement in patients with JIA-associated uveitis was still poor, with final visual acuity of 20/50 or worse in 70% of the eyes. They believed that outcomes would be improved with earlier disease detection and more vigorous therapy by physicians skilled in the use of immunomodulatory agents. We share this view. Often children have suffered irreversible damage to ocular structures before they are even evaluated by an ophthalmologist (6). We believe that at least two critical changes must occur to reduce blindness secondary to JIA-associated uveitis. One is legislation that would require vision testing of very young children. Such legislation would mandate annual testing of visual acuity in preschool and elementary school children, and referral to an ophthalmologist of any child with visual acuity less than 20/40 in either eye. It would also provide support for the development of effective programs to deal with the logistical and challenging aspects of special vision testing required for younger children (e.g., Allen cards). The other change would be to emphasize the importance of training in ocular immunology in all schools of medicine and support experts in ocular immunology. One may wonder if these reported case series are representative of outcomes for patients with JIA-associated uveitis or, alternatively, reflect "outlier" aberrant experiences. However, when year after year, series of such patient collections are reported from many areas around the globe, all with the same depressing statistics, one can draw but a single logical conclusion from the data: too many children with JIA-associated uveitis lose vision to the point of being permanently visually handicapped as a consequence of delayed diagnosis and inadequate treatment. Even as this chapter is being written, yet another such report, accepted for presentation at the 2003 Annual Meeting of the American Academy of Ophthalmology, illustrates this phenomenon. Rosenberg and associates, from the Bascom Palmer Eye Institute, University of Miami, reported 34 patients in a group of 149 pediatric uveitis cases followed for up to 10 years, reporting band keratopathy, glaucoma, cataract, macular edema, and hypotony in many, finding that the cumulative proportion of patients with complications continued to rise through time, with substantial numbers of eyes and patients with visual acuity of 20/200 or less in the better eye (16).

Management

We typically treat JIA-associated uveitis in exactly the same way we typically treat all noninfectious uveitis,; i.e., initially with aggressive topical steroid. Regional steroid injections (generally requiring anesthesia) are added to the program if the uveitis is not abolished through the frequent application of topical steroids. Brief (no longer than 3 months) systemic steroid therapy may also be employed. We use a stepladder

paradigm in the care of patients with JIA-associated uveitis. Steroid therapy represents the first step and chronic oral nonsteroidal antiinflammatory drug (NSAID) therapy the second step, used for cases in which the uveitis recurs with every attempt to taper topical steroids. A variety of oral NSAIDs could be used, but the two with the longest track record in the hands of pediatric rheumatologists are naproxen and tolmetin. Tolmetin is the NSAID that has been formally studied and shown effective for prolonged remission of JIA-associated uveitis (17). The therapy should be coordinated with the patient's pediatrician or pediatric rheumatologist.

Some patients with JIA-associated uveitis have recurrences of the uveitis despite the chronic use of an oral NSAID. These patients must be advanced to the third step of therapy: immunomodulatory therapy. A great number of immunomodulatory agents have been used in this context, but methotrexate, by far, has the longest efficacy and safety track record. For this reason, it is typically our next choice in patients who have JIA-associated uveitis which recurs as topical steroids are withdrawn, despite the chronic use of an oral NSAID. We typically begin at a dosage of 0.15 mg/kg body weight once weekly administered orally and ask that the child also take 1 mg of folic acid per day, a strategy that has been clearly shown to reduce the likelihood of hepatotoxicity in patients receiving methotrexate (18). We advance the dose of methotrexate, as needed and tolerated, to achieve the goal of complete freedom of all recurrences of all inflammation at all times off all steroids, making the dose changes approximately every 6 to 8 weeks. The uveitis associated with JIA often requires much higher doses of methotrexate to induce a durable remission of the uveitis than does the arthritis associated with JIA, but children tolerate such doses of this medication quite well. The bioavailability of the medication is variable after oral administration. Therefore, we will switch patients to subcutaneous administration if the uveitis persists despite multiple increases in the orally administered dose.

Potential side effects of methotrexate include hepatotoxicity, bone marrow suppression, interstitial pneumonitis, mucositis, nausea, fatigue, and alopecia. Most of these potential side effects are medically trivial, but hepatotoxicity, interstitial pneumonitis, and bone marrow suppression are not. Therefore, it is mandatory that the patient be regularly monitored by an expert and experienced in prescribing and monitoring of immunomodulatory therapy in general, and methotrexate in particular. Patients are reexamined monthly and undergo blood drawing for assay of liver function, blood urea nitrogen (BUN), creatinine, and complete blood count. Suppression of the bone marrow, in our experience, is extraordinarily rare. Rising liver enzymes is an indication of hepatotoxicity, and although rheumatologists, in general, tolerate a 30% rise above the upper limits of normal before reducing the methotrexate dose by 50%, our tolerance for rising liver enzymes is less, and we typically back off on the dose of the medication if the patient has elevated enzymes on two occasions separated by 2 weeks. Interstitial pneumonitis is characterized by diminished exercise tolerance and by development of cough. It, like chemical hepatitis, is reversible if detected early in the course of its development and the drug is discontinued.

Patients with JIA-associated uveitis on methotrexate are usually treated for a minimum of 2 years after the uveitis has vanished while off all steroids. We find that approximately 60% of our JIA patients experience a durable remission, allowing withdrawal and discontinuation of methotrexate after 2 years of freedom from uveitis activity (19). This means, of course, that 40% of our patients do not succeed with methotrexate as monotherapy. For them, alternative agents are explored, until the agent or combination of agents is found that accomplishes the goal: no inflammation, off all steroids. This is a trial and error exercise that can be extremely frustrating for patient, family, and doctor. But to give up on the quest for disease remission is, in our view, an enormous mistake. It is important to persist, to not give up on the patient, and to ultimately prevail over the problem. The other medications that we use include cyclosporin (up to 5 mg/kg daily), azathioprine (3 mg/kg daily), chlorambucil (0.1 mg/kg daily), intravenous cyclophosphamide (1 g/m^2 once monthly), intravenous immunoglobulin (2 g/kg per cycle, once monthly), and daclizumab (1 mg/kg per infusion, once every 2 weeks).

The complications of JIA-associated iridocyclitis may require surgical management. Cataract and glaucoma, in particular, occur in many patients with JIA, and the glaucoma that develops, is frequently resistant to adequate medical control. Approximately 40% of patients referred to us with JIA-associated uveitis already have glaucoma and often cataract at the time of first referral. Questions arise regarding whether to consider surgery, what type of surgery (cataract extraction, intraocular lens [IOL] implantation, possible trabeculectomy, use of mitomycin-C, and valve tube shunts), and the timing of possible surgery. The timing of surgery is particularly important in the child because of the added concern of amblyopia. However, operating on the inflamed eye, particularly for cataract surgery, is notorious for poor outcomes (20–22). Therefore, the urgency of prevailing over the active uveitis is even more palpable.

The experience of most uveitis specialists has been that children with JIA-associated iridocyclitis are poor candidates for IOL placement (23–25). The formation of inflammatory membranes behind or around the implant, with membrane contraction and progressive hypotony can lead to phthisis. In most instances, we do not recommend IOL placement in the child with JIA-associated uveitis. Outcomes published in the medical literature support cataract removal, the performance of a total vitrectomy, and visual rehabilitation with an aphakic soft contact lens (26–28). With coexistent glaucoma, we favor the use of an Ahmed valve tube shunt (29) rather than a trabeculectomy, which brings the additional risk of endophthalmitis in a contact lens wearer with a filtering bleb.

Differential Diagnosis

The differential diagnosis of pediatric uveitis is relatively broad, yet JIA-associated uveitis is often the only entity (aside from "idiopathic") which comes to mind when one is faced with a child with panuveitis. Chapter 16, Table 16-6 lists many of the entities which can cause or at least be associated with uveitis in children, and it also attempts to list most likely causes by age group. The rest of this chapter will be devoted to a discussion of the types and causes of uveitis that are either most common or most potentially devastating to the eye or other systems. The most rare entities, such as, for example, the uveitis found in 50% of the 60 children reported in the world's literature with the Chronic Infantile Neurological Cutaneous and Articular/Neonatal Onset Multisystem Inflammatory Disease Syndrome (CINCA-NOMID) are referenced for the interested readers' further study (30).

Seronegative Spondyloarthropathies

The seronegative spondyloarthropathies include disorders that share many clinical features, including a predisposition to sacroiliitis and uveitis. A substantial number of patients with seronegative spondyloarthropathies also have the *HLA-B27* gene. Several hypotheses have evolved to explain why patients who are HLA-B27 positive might be overrepresented in groups of patients with various inflammatory diseases, including ankylosing spondylitis, reactive arthritis, psoriasis, inflammatory bowel disease, and uncharacterized anterior uveitis. One compelling hypothesis is that of "molecular mimicry". Inappropriate, autoimmune inflammation develops after the HLA-B27–positive individual mounts an immune response against a microbe, such as *Klebsiella*, *Chlamydia*, *Salmonella*, or *Yersinia*, which has proteins with amino acid sequences and conformational characteristics identical to those of the HLA-B27 protein on the surface of all nucleated cells of patients who are HLA-B27 positive. Although the seronegative spondyloarthropathies are most common in adults, they each can occur in children.

Ankylosing Spondylitis

Epidemiology

Pediatric ankylosing spondylitis (AS) is a well-characterized syndrome, and in children, just as in the adult form of AS, HLA-B27–positive males predominate over females. Juvenile-onset spondyloarthropathies occur in children under the age of 16 years. AS typically begins after the age of 10 years. Seronegative implies that the patients are rheumatoid factor negative. Chronic iridocyclitis can develop in as many as 15% of children with juvenile AS.

Clinical Signs and Symptoms

The problem begins insidiously, generally with morning low-back stiffness and, eventually, the evolution of dull low-back pain that improves throughout the course of the day. Direct pressure over the sacroiliac joints often elicits pain, and the patient is found to have limited lower-spine flexibility, with inability to touch his or her toes without bending the knees. Peripheral arthritis can also occur, usually affecting the knees, shoulders, or hips, and, as in JIA, the temporomandibular joint (TMJ) may be involved. It may be the single peripheral joint involved in AS, and one must avoid ascribing TMJ symptoms to "TMJ syndrome" rather than to true arthritis. Enthesopathy or inflammation of the tendons, particularly at their points of insertion into bone, is highly typical of AS, with exquisite tenderness in the areas of tendon inflammation.

The anterior uveitis is generally acute, unilateral, and recurrent, but eventually becomes bilateral or alternating. Unlike JIA associated uveitis, the uveitis associated with the seronegative spondyloarthropathies is often obvious to the patient, with red eye, ocular discomfort, and photophobia.

Management

Therapy typically should include aggressive topical steroids (every 30 to 60 minutes while awake) and cycloplegia. In instances in which this does not result in a significant reduction in the intensity of the anterior chamber reaction, a short burst of systemic steroid (1.5 mg/kg daily) is appropriate, with a relatively rapid taper (reducing the dose every 5 to 7 days). More stubborn cases will require regional steroid injection, often requiring brief general anesthesia.

HLA-B27–associated uveitis tends to be nongranulomatous and recurrent, and we and others (31) have found that the long-term use of an oral NSAID may be effective in preventing recurrences in those patients who are experiencing multiple recurrences. Specifically, chronic use of an oral NSAID is prescribed in patients without contraindications and who have had their third episode of recurrent uveitis. Approximately 70% of such patients have no further recurrences after steroid taper and discontinuation. The choice and dosing of the NSAID is made in conjunction with the child's rheumatologist.

Diagnosis

The modified New York criteria for diagnosing AS are shown in Table 17-1. Notice that HLA-B27 positivity is not required for the diagnosis; 5% to 10% of patients with AS are HLA-B27 negative.

TABLE 17-1. NEW YORK CLINICAL CRITERIA FOR ANKYLOSING SPONDYLITIS

1. Limitation of motion of the lumbar spine in all three planes (anterior, flexion, lateral flexion and extension).

2. A history of pain or the presence of pain at the dorsolumbar junction or in the lumbar spine.

3. Limitation of chest expansion to 1 in. (2.5 cm) or less, measured at the level of the fourth intercostals space.

Definite ankylosing spondylitis if (i) grade 3 or 4 bilateral sacroiliitis associated with at least one clinical criterion; or (ii) grade 3 or 4 unilateral or grade 2 bilateral sacroiliitis associated with clinical criterion 1 or both clinical criteria 2 and 3. Probable ankylosing spondylitis if grade 3 or 4 bilateral sacroiliitis exists without any signs or symptoms satisfying the clinical criteria.

Reactive Arthritis

Reactive arthritis, previously designated as "Reiter's syndrome," was originally defined as the triad of arthritis, conjunctivitis, and noninfectious urethritis, but uveitis may substitute for or be present along with conjunctivitis in patients with reactive arthritis. Stoll was probably the first to describe the relationship of eye, urethra, and joint inflammation following epidemic dysentery (32), and Brodie (33) described the triad following venereal infection in 1818. Hans Reiter (34), in 1916, described a lieutenant in the Prussian army in whom urethritis and conjunctivitis developed following an episode of dysentery, with subsequent onset of arthritis. However, Reiter also engaged in crimes against humanity, performing many experiments on prisoners of war in 1939 to 1945, and recent efforts and recommendations (appropriate, in our view) to remove his eponymic relationship with the disorder previously described by others have been published (35).

Prevalence

Reactive arthritis may occur in children. Although it is not terribly rare in adults, it certainly is rare in children.

Diagnosis

Approximately 75% of adults in whom reactive arthritis develops are HLA-B27 positive, while 90% of children are HLA-B27 positive. Uveitis develops in about 2% of pediatric patients with reactive arthritis.

Clinical Signs and Symptoms

The uveitis associated with this syndrome is identical to that associated with AS. Uveitis will develop in approximately 12% of patients with reactive arthritis, and the initial attack is typically unilateral and acute. As in AS, the inflammation in reactive arthritis is generally recurrent, nongranulomatous, and may be associated with a hypopyon.

Management

Therapy most appropriately is with intensive topical steroid administration, with additional steroids through additional routes of administration as needed for treatment resistance.

Psoriasis

Children may develop psoriasis, and whether or not the arthritis that can be associated with psoriasis emerges, uveitis may be associated with the development of psoriasis.

Prevalence and Epidemiology

Psoriasis is slightly more likely to develop in girls than in boys (3:2), and the mean age of onset is approximately 9 years. The prevalence of uveitis in patients with psoriasis is unknown. However, in psoriatic arthritis, uveitis may occur in up to 20% of all patients and 15% of pediatric patients.

Clinical Signs and Symptoms

The uveitis associated with psoriasis without arthritis has some differences from the uveitis associated with psoriatic arthritis (36). The skin lesions of psoriasis typically precede the development of either joint or eye inflammation, but we have seen numerous cases in which the patient had psoriasis, and the diagnosis was made upon subsequent dermatologic consultation as a consequence of our examination of the skin during the patient's evaluation for his or her uveitis. Small hidden patches of itchy, scaly dermatitis may come and go in the axilla, on the umbilicus, on the genitalia, on the back, or on the scalp.

The uveitis is nongranulomatous, acute and unilateral, but eventually both eyes are involved nonsimultaneously. It is more severe and stubborn in those patients who are HLA-B27 positive. About 80% of patients with psoriatic arthritis in whom uveitis develops are also commonly antinuclear antibody positive. Oligoarticular arthritis can be present as long as 10 years before the onset of the dermatologic manifestations of psoriasis; hence, the diagnosis of JIA has often erroneously been made earlier in these children.

Management

Therapy is with aggressive topical steroid and cycloplegic, and chronic oral NSAIDs may also be helpful in reducing the likelihood of recurrent inflammation. Treatment-resistant cases respond well to low-dose once-weekly methotrexate, daily cyclosporin, and possibly to tumor necrosis factor α (TNF-α) antagonist therapy.

Enteropathic Arthritis

Prevalence

Enteropathic arthritis associated uveitis may occur in patients with either Crohn's disease or with ulcerative colitis. These disorders are associated with peripheral arthritis (20% of patients with Crohn's disease and 10% of patients with ulcerative colitis), and with sacroiliitis (10% of patients with either Crohn's disease or ulcerative colitis). Uveitis occurs in upwards of 10% of patients with inflammatory bowel disease, and is more common in patients with Crohn's disease than with ulcerative colitis.

Diagnostic Studies

Enteropathic arthritis is also associated with HLA-B27–associated haplotypy, but uveitis may occur in patients without enteropathic arthritis, but simply with inflammatory bowel disease, and in patients who have inflammatory bowel disease who are HLA-B27 negative.

Clinical Signs and Symptoms

Its behavior is similar to that of patients with the other seronegative spondyloarthropathy–associated uveitides, and appropriate treatment is the same as well.

Management

Surgical excision of the inflamed bowel may be beneficial in management of the extraintestinal symptoms, including peripheral arthritis and uveitis (37). Immunomodulatory medication (especially with 6-mercaptopurine), and anticytokine therapy (especially with anti–TNF-α agents) may be critical elements in the eventual successful control of the patient's intestinal and extraintestinal problems.

Cervical spondylitis

Cervical spondylitis can occur in young girls, with cervical apophyseal joint fusion and symmetric destructive polyarthritis involving small joints in the hands and wrists. Although patients can be HLA-B27 positive or negative, 65% are negative for the rheumatoid factor and ANA negative. Chronic iridocyclitis quite indistinguishable from that of JIA develops in patients who are positive for HLA-B27 and ANA. However, recurrent acute uveitis indistinguishable from that of patients with AS or other "typical" seronegative spondyloarthropathies typically develops in patients positive for HLA-B27 but negative for ANA.

Sarcoidosis

Sarcoidosis is a chronic multisystem noncaseating granulomatous disease of unknown cause. There are two types of sarcoidosis in children. Late-onset sarcoidosis occurs in children between 8 and 15 years old, and early-onset sarcoidosis develops in children less then 4 years old (38,39). Early-onset patients are primarily white, and pulmonary involvement is less common (35%), making it more difficult to make the correct diagnosis, especially because articular involvement may mimic JIA (40,41).

In contrast, the older children and adolescents usually present with multi system disease similar to adults with sarcoidosis. There is generally no familial history of sarcoidosis, and bilateral hilar lymphadenopathy or pulmonary involvement is visible on chest radiographs in 90% of cases. Eye and skin lesions occur in 30% of late-onset juvenile sarcoidosis. Because other diseases, including mycobacterial or fungal infection and berylliosis, can also produce noncaseating (hard) granulomas, the histologic diagnosis of sarcoidosis is made by exclusion. Vasculitis is a relatively unique complication associated with juvenile sarcoidosis.

Blau's syndrome (familial juvenile systemic granulomatosis) is an autosomal dominant granulomatous disease of childhood, with clinical features almost identical to early-onset sarcoidosis (42,43). The disease susceptibility locus is on the pericentromeric region of chromosome 16 (44). Renal and hepatic granuloma have recently been described in this disease (45,46). The granulomas of the skin and synovial biopsy from the patient with Blau syndrome are identical to those seen in sarcoidosis (47).

Prevalence and Epidemiology

Sarcoidosis is rare in children, but the youngest reported patient was 2 months old (6), and another was 3 months old (48). A recent study from Denmark estimated an annual incidence of two or three cases of sarcoidosis per million children (49). The prevalence of sarcoidosis is higher in women than in men, but the majority of reported pediatric cases emphasizes the frequency of sarcoidosis is similar in the two genders (50). The distribution is widely different between countries and regions. The prevalence of sarcoidosis in the United States is highest in the southeast, and it is 10 to 20 times more common in African-Americans than in whites. The disorder is especially common in Irish and Swedish women. In contrast, the disease is rare in India, Southeast Asia, New Zealand, and in mainland China (51).

Etiology and Pathogenesis

The etiology of sarcoidosis is unknown. The disease may be secondary to an altered immune response to unknown agents. Numerous immunologic abnormalities are present, including activated CD4+ lymphocytes in involved organs, such as lung, secreting IL-2, IL-6, gamma-interferon, and other mediators. CD4+ T lymphocytes in the blood, by contrast, are reduced in number and are not activated. Alveolar macrophages are also activated with increased class II HLA expression and increased antigen-presenting capacity. The cytokines and factors secreted by these cells may account for the characteristic features of pulmonary sarcoidosis: influx of monocytes, alveolitis, noncaseating granuloma formation in the lung, and the resulting progressive fibrosis (52). Similar to other T-cell responses to antigen, the T-cell proliferation in the sarcoid lung is oligoclonal, rather than a generalized nonspecific response (53).

Systemic Manifestations

Early-onset juvenile sarcoidosis is characterized by the triad of skin eruptions, arthritis, and uveitis. This may mimic JIA without bilateral hilar lymphadenopathy. Intermittent fever and synovial swelling can be present in both conditions (40). Early differentiation of sarcoidosis from JIA is important in planning treatment strategies and in counseling patients and families. Skin changes may help differentiate between the two diseases at their onset. The rash seen in JIA is transient and comprised of pink macules, whereas the rash seen in sarcoidosis presents with variable erythema, papules, plaques, and ichthyosiform lesions (54). The cutaneous manifestations may be the earliest sign, occurring before joint or eye involvement and include papules, plaques, nodules, erythema nodosum, and hypopigmented or hyperpigmented areas. Lupus pernio is frequent in adults but rare in children (55). A skin biopsy should be performed to confirm the diagnosis. Sarcoid arthritis in children is characterized by painless, boggy synovial and tendon sheath effusions with mild limitation of motion, whereas in JIA there is pain, limitation of movement, and destructive changes found on radiographs. Two Japanese cases of early onset of sarcoidosis mimicking JIA emphasize the importance of tissue biopsy for early diagnosis (41).

Late-onset juvenile sarcoidosis in children between 8 and 15 years is similar to that of adults. It usually presents with multisystem disease with lymphadenopathy, hepatosplenomegaly, parotid fullness, and pulmonary involvement, as well as generalized constitutional signs and symptoms, such as fever, anorexia, and malaise (56,57).

A wide spectrum of vasculitis in pediatric sarcoidosis has been reported, including leukocytoclastic vasculitis (58), vasculitis of small- to medium-sized vessels (59), and large-vessel vasculitis (60,61). Early-onset juvenile sarcoidosis patients should be carefully followed for the development of vasculitis (62).

Neurologic dysfunction secondary to sarcoidosis is rare in children (63–65). Granulomas are the most common manifestation, and when in the basal area of the meninges and brain cause seventh nerve palsy and hydrocephalus (66). Growth deficiency has been reported in association with brain magnetic resonance imaging (MRI) abnormalities, and hypothalamic infiltration can manifest as diabetes insipidus (67,68).

Renal disease can manifest as granulomas in the renal parenchyma, or as hypercalciuria with nephrocalcinosis (69–73). Biopsy-proven renal granulomatous sarcoidosis has been described in 11 children, 9 of whom developed renal failure (74). A review of published series of 328 children with sarcoidosis estimated the prevalence of hypercreatinemia to be 26%, proteinuria or abnormalities in urinary sediment 31%, hypercalciuria 47%, and hypercalcemia 21%. Kidney stones were reported in eight cases. Therefore, renal involvement could be more common than currently thought. The urogenital tract can be involved (75,76).

The liver may contain scattered granulomas in up to 90% of patients, more commonly in the portal triads than in the lobular parenchyma. Liver enzymes are then often mildly elevated. A needle biopsy can be helpful in obtaining the diagnosis (77).

Bone marrow involvement is rare. The localization is typically in the distal ends of the phalangeal bones of the hands and feet creating small circumscribed areas of bone resorption within the marrow cavity, a diffuse reticulated pattern throughout the cavity, and widening of the long shafts or new bone formation on the outer surfaces.

Myositis with granulomas in the muscles has also been described (78–81). One 11-year-old boy had sarcoidosis with generalized brawny induration of muscle, arthritis, and renal involvement, as evidenced by nephrocalcinosis and nephrolithiasis. The muscle fibers had been compressed and gradually replaced by an increase of connective tissue containing sarcoid granulomas (82).

Ocular Signs and Symptoms

The ocular manifestations of sarcoidosis in children are similar to those seen in adults. Anterior uveitis is the most common ocular manifestation in both the younger (81%) and the older pediatric groups (21% to 48%) (83).The inflammation may be chronic and granulomatous, with minimal pain and photophobia. Multiple areas of interstitial keratitis, corneal limbal nodules, mutton fat keratic precipitates, and iris nodules may be observed. Bilateral lower motor neuron facial palsy and bilateral hearing loss have also been reported (84,85). An acute, nongranulomatous type of uveitis can also occur, typically characterized by pain, redness, and photophobia. Posterior segment involvement is the most vision-threatening manifestation, with vitreitis, pars planitis, papillitis, chorioretinal granulomas (appearing sometimes as multifocal choroiditis), macular edema, branch retinal vein occlusion (86), retinal periphlebitis, subretinal neovascular membranes, and optic nerve granulomas.

Lacrimal gland involvement, commonly found in adult patients with sarcoidosis, rarely occurs in children (87).

Diagnosis

Angiotensin-converting enzyme (ACE), which is produced by macrophages and by the epithelioid cells of the sarcoid granuloma, reflects the total body granuloma load. ACE levels are commonly higher in children than in adults. The ACE is not specific for sarcoidosis and can be elevated in several other systemic diseases that affect the lungs or the liver. When ACE levels are compared to age-matched controls (88), 80% of children with pediatric sarcoidosis have elevated ACE. Hilar adenopathy may be seen, with or without parenchymal involvement. Gallium scanning and thin-cut spiral computed tomography (CT) scanning are more sensitive to detect early lung involvement, and MRI to diagnose sarcoidosis in children who present with fever of unknown origin by demonstrating multifocal nodular lesions in the bone marrow of the lower extremities (89). Fine needle aspiration biopsy cytology of the lung has been suggested as an adjunct in the diagnosis of children with suspected sarcoidosis, through a demonstration of epithelioid histocytes and multinucleated foreign body type giant cells without accompanying necrosis or acute inflammation (91). Biopsy of easy to reach areas, such as skin, lymph nodes, and conjunctiva, especially when conjunctival nodules are present, is highly recommended in the diagnostic effort (92).

Prognosis

The course of sarcoidosis is unpredictable, and the prognosis of childhood sarcoidosis is not significantly different from that in adults. The disease is characterized by (i) progressive chronicity or (ii) periods of activity interspersed with remissions, sometimes permanent and spontaneous or initiated by steroid therapy. Overall, 65% to 70% of affected patients recover with minimal or no residual manifestations, whereas 20% have some lung dysfunction or permanent visual impairment. Some patients die of cardiac or central nervous system damage. Patients who present with hilar lymphadenopathy (stage I) have the best prognosis, followed by those with adenopathy and pulmonary infiltration (stage II). Patients with stage III pulmonary disease and adenopathy have few spontaneous remissions and are most likely to develop chronic pulmonary disease.

Management

The current therapy of choice for sarcoidosis in children with multisystem involvement is oral corticosteroids. Corticosteroids produce rapid symptomatic improvement, but may not affect the long-term prognosis. Steroid treatment should be instituted in the presence of respiratory symptoms, such as dyspnea, cough, or chest pain, or in the presence of severe impairment of pulmonary function tests. Steroids are also the primary treatment for the ocular manifestations of sarcoidosis. Low-dose oral methotrexate is effective and safe for treatment of childhood sarcoidosis and has steroid sparing properties (92,93).

Other immunosuppressive medications have been reported with successful results in the care of adults with sarcoidosis; these include azathioprine, cyclosporine, and cyclophosphamide (94–96).

Tubulointerstitial Nephritis and Uveitis

Prevalence and Epidemiology

Uveitis can occur in patients with tubulointerstitial nephritis (97). Approximately 135 cases of tubulointerstitial nephritis and uveitis (TINU) have been reported. Three-fourths of the patients have been female, and the median age has been 15 years (range, 9 to 74 years). The uveitis has been bilateral 75% of the time, and has been anterior 80% of the time. There is no racial or geographic predilection.

Clinical Signs and Symptoms

Tubulointerstitial nephritis typically develops acutely, usually provoked by medication or a microbe, and begins with fever and malaise, followed by flank tenderness, and pyuria. Although the nephritis in patients with TINU generally resolves without producing permanent renal deficit, the uveitis associated with TINU can be especially stubborn and recurrent or chronic. The uveitis can be anterior, intermediate, posterior, or a panuveitis, and it may be simultaneously bilateral, alternatingly bilateral, or unilateral. It may be nongranulomatous or granulomatous, and may include the presence of frank retinal vasculitis, with intraretinal hemorrhages and exudates. In a 2001 review (98), 15% of cases identified in the literature had a "prolonged course of uveitis with multiple exacerbations." Patients younger than 20 years of age were more likely to have a chronic course of uveitis than older patients. Complications were reported in 21% of the patients analyzed and included macular edema, macular pucker, and chorioretinal scarring. Complications from steroid therapy included cataract, glaucoma, and iatrogenic Cushing's syndrome.

Diagnosis

Proteinuria, hematuria, rising BUN and creatinine levels, and biopsy-proven TINU with edema and inflammatory cells in the renal interstitium are the hallmarks of this usually self-limited disorder. We (99) and others (100) have identified apparent HLA associations, supporting HLA as a risk factor for TINU and the concept that the syndrome develops in genetically predisposed individuals upon contact with a triggering drug or microbe. The diagnosis of TINU is generally straight forward, but diagnostic challenges can exist. Thus, diagnostic criteria have been proposed categorizing cases as (i) "definite" if interstitial nephritis has been diagnosed by biopsy, (ii) "probable" if the nephritis has been diagnosed clinically, and (iii) "possible" if the nephritis has been diagnosed clinically and the uveitis is "atypical."

Management

The nephritis generally resolves without permanent renal deficit, either spontaneously or after the prescribing of systemic steroid therapy. Immunomodulatory agents, such as methotrexate, azathioprine, cyclosporin, and mycophenolate mofetil, have been used in the care of 11 patients with TINU who were inadequately responsive to steroids or in whom steroid-associated toxicity developed (101).

Pars Planitis

The International Uveitis Study Group has defined "idiopathic intermediate uveitis" as an inflammatory syndrome affecting anterior vitreous, peripheral retina, and ciliary body with no or minimal involvement of the anterior segment or choroid. There is often a peripheral perivasculitis (102). The term pars planitis is quite frequently used instead of intermediate uveitis. Many ophthalmologists, including our group, reserve it for cases with inflammation centered in pars plana; i.e., with pars planitis as one specific form of intermediate uveitis.

Many terms have been used to describe this disease. The first description was probably chronic cyclitis termed by Fuchs (103) in 1908. Schepens (104) used the term peripheral uveitis in 1950 and, in 1960, Welch (105) coined the term pars planitis. Other names previously utilized, like chronic cyclitis, vitreitis, cyclochorioretinitis, chronic posterior cyclitis, and peripheral uveoretinitis, are rarely used today.

Prevalence and Epidemiology

Intermediate uveitis is estimated to represent one-fifth of all cases of pediatric uveitis (106). There appears to be no specific predilection for race or gender. The prevalence of pars planitis peaks between childhood and the fourth decade, but older people can also be affected. Seventy to ninety percent of cases are bilateral (107). About one-third of patients with unilateral involvement at the time of presentation develop bilateral involvement during the following years (106). No inheritance pattern has been defined, but random reports of familial cases support the idea that this disease may have genetic links (108–117).

Clinical Signs and Symptoms

Patients with pars planitis generally present with complaints of floaters and blurred vision. They typically have a quiet and white eye. In some children, intermediate uveitis is found accidentally on routine screening. Pain, redness, tearing, and photophobia are less common, and present when the anterior segment is involved. Anterior segment inflammation is seen more commonly in children with pars planitis than in adults. Moderate to severe cells and flare, keratic precipitates, band keratopathy, and even posterior synechiae can be found (118). Children presenting with idiopathic pars planitis have a worse visual acuity at initial diagnosis and follow-up than do adults (119). Posterior subcapsular cataracts are frequently found at presentation (120).

Vitreous cells are the most important diagnostic finding in patients with intermediate uveitis. Cellular exudates in the vitreous and on the pars plana are seen on depressed peripheral examination of retina in patients with active pars planitis, whereas old cellular debris, crenated residua of prior vitreous exudates, and a collagen band or "snow-bank" are generally present in the patient with inactive pars planitis. Snowbanks can extend from a few clock hours inferiorly to 360 degrees of the retinal periphery. The distinction between active and inactive pars planitis is not always apparent, but the distinction is important to avoid unnecessary treatment and implement therapy appropriately when inflammation is active. The feature indicative of inactive pars planitis is a sharp-edged, white band at the pars plana in the absence of vitreous cells or exudates. However, if vitreous cells surround this snow-bank or there are collections of exudates, appearing as fluffy snowballs on the pars plana or in the vitreous, pars planitis is considered active. The collagen snowbank reflects the consequences of inflammation involving peripheral retina and the vitreous base (121). The presence of snowbanks or snowballs is not required to diagnose intermediate uveitis, but is the major clinical feature defining pars planitis. The presence of snowbanks is associated with worse visual outcome (122,123).

Other signs of the disease include peripheral retinal vasculitis with sheathing of both venules and arterioles. Vasculitis can lead to occlusion and neovascularization of the peripheral retina and optic nerve. Vasculitis was found in 10% to 32% of cases (124–126).

Autoimmune endotheliopathy is a rare finding in the anterior segment associated with intermediate uveitis. Peripheral corneal edema evolves, with keratic precipitates lying in a linear fashion and marking the border of edematous cornea from normal cornea. This transplant rejectionlike appearance signifies an autoimmune etiology of intermediate uveitis (127–129).

The higher prevalence of complications in children compared to adults is likely explained by the more asymptomatic course of intermediate uveitis in children, later referral, and greater degree of irreparable damage on initial presentation. Complications of pars planitis in children include cataract, macular edema, secondary glaucoma, band keratopathy, retinal detachment, optic neuropathy, neovascularization of the peripheral retina or optic nerve, vitreous hemorrhage, and formation of inflammatory membranes. Secondary amblyopia can also occur.

Cataract develops in about 50% of patients with intermediate uveitis (107). It is associated with both uncontrolled inflammation and corticosteroid use. Posterior subcapsular cataract is the most commonly observed type (120), in part secondary to steroid treatment. Cataract formation is less common in patients who were treated with immunosuppressive medications early in the course of disease rather than in patients treated for prolonged periods of time with corticosteroids (122,130,131).

Cystoid macular edema, in 12% to 50% of cases (107), and maculopathy from macular hole and epiretinal membrane are the most common causes of severe visual impairment in patients with intermediate uveitis. Secondary glaucoma occurs predominantly as a result of topical corticosteroid therapy (132). In most studies, ocular hypertension has not been reported in association with intermediate uveitis (133).

Band keratopathy is considered a hallmark of uveitis that began in childhood. It can be severe, especially in younger children (134), and is seen with anterior segment involvement, which is more common in children than adults. Severe band keratopathy may preclude successful visual rehabilitation with aphakic contact lenses in some uveitic children.

Exudative retinal detachment occurs in 5% to 17% of patients with intermediate uveitis (124,130,135,136). Except for the Vogt-Koyanagi-Harada syndrome and intermediate uveitis, exudative retinal detachment is uncommonly seen in other uveitic entities. Patients with pars planitis may present with bullous retinoschisis, mostly in the inferior periphery. Both exudative retinal detachments and retinoschisis may be related to a Coats-like vascular response secondary to chronic inflammation (137).

Vitreoretinal traction is reported in 3% to 22% of intermediate uveitis patients and can cause retinal tears, and combined rhegmatogenous-tractional retinal detachments (138). Rhegmatogenous retinal detachment due to uveitis in children has been reported in up to 15% of cases (139).

Rhegmatogenous retinal detachments in intermediate uveitis were classified by Brockhurst and Schepens (140) into four types. Type I retinal detachments occurred secondary to small breaks near the ora serrata associated with exudate, were low lying, chronic, with demarcation lines, and often resolved spontaneously. These patients typically had a benign course. Type II detachments were associated with a large dialysis at the posterior edge of the pars plana exudates. They were slowly progressive and could resolve spontaneously if vitreoretinal exudates occluded the break. Type II detachments were observed in patients with mild chronic inflammation. Type III detachments occurred due to large breaks secondary to neovascularization of the vitreous base and extensive pars plana exudation. These detachments had a rapidly progressive course and were associated with severe, chronic uveitis. Type IV retinal detachments occurred in patients with anterior proliferative vitreoretinopathy associated with vascular cicatricial tissue, which produced circumferential traction, fixed retinal folds from periphery to the optic nerve, and total retinal detachments. There was extensive pars plana exudation that obscured the view of the breaks. This type of retinal detachment was due to a fulminant, explosive course of intermediate uveitis and had a poor prognosis.

Optic nerve involvement in intermediate uveitis is observed more commonly in children than in adults (106,113,114,135,136,141). Disc edema is present in 3% to 50% of eyes (114,134–136,142) and can lead to optic nerve atrophy when long-standing. Optic neuritis in pars planitis patients occurs in association with multiple sclerosis (MS) in up to 38.5% of cases (143,144). Even though MS is exceptionally rare in children, one may consider a systemic workup for a pediatric patient if a patient is a female, has a bilateral intermediate uveitis, and especially if she is HLA-DR15 positive.

Profound retinal ischemia can result in optic disc neovascularization, but peripheral retinal neovascularization is more common. Secondary vitreous hemorrhages can occur and if nonclearing may require surgical intervention (145). Children with pars planitis are more likely than adults to have vitreous hemorrhage (131). Peripheral retinal neovascularization may lead to vascular cyclitic membranes. Epiretinal membranes can also occur in pars planitis but are rarely considered visually significant.

Etiology and Pathogenesis

The etiology and pathogenesis of intermediate uveitis are unclear. It is widely accepted that in some cases intermediate uveitis represents an autoimmune disorder of the eye, such as in association with MS and sarcoidosis. It also appears to be a T-cell–mediated disease and can be reproduced in experimental models in animals. It responds well to immunosuppressive therapy. Lymphocytes from patients with intermediate uveitis but not from patients with any other type of uveitis respond to exposure to type II collagen *in vitro* with proliferation and cytokine production. This suggests that type II collagen, which is richly present in vitreous, may act as an autoantigen (146).

Intermediate uveitis has been linked to various HLA antigens. The association of HLA-DR15, pars planitis, and MS is well documented (147–151). Associations of HLA-B8, B51 and MS, and pars planitis have also been described (151). There is one report about a possible association of HLA-A28 with pars planitis (152). A circulating 36-kd protein was identified in the serum of patients with active pars planitis that may serve as a marker and even play a particular role in the etiology (153,154). These associations require further investigation.

There are few histologic studies on patients with pars planitis. Active vitreous inflammatory cell exudates, or "snowballs," were found to be composed of epithelioid cells and multinucleated giant cells (155). Exudative material of pars plana, or a snowbank, was found to be acellular in one of the latest studies, except on the uveal side, where there were cytokeratin-positive retinal pigment epithelial cells. The extracellular matrix of the "snowbank" contained tenascin and collagen types I, II, and III. There was no immunoreactivity for laminin and fibronectin (156). In previous studies, fibrous astrocytes producing larger-diameter collagen fibrils were noticed (121,155). Eyes showed prominent lymphocytic cuffing and mural infiltration of retinal veins, with sparing of the arterioles. Choroidal involvement has been demonstrated only in severe cases. These findings clearly demonstrate that intermediate uveitis is not primarily a chorioretinal disease.

Diagnosis

The diagnosis of intermediate uveitis is clinical, based on the absence of choroidal involvement, no or minimal anterior segment inflammation, and the presence of vitreous exudates and pars plana exudates, which are pathognomonic for pars planitis.

A careful history and review of systems is necessary and should be sought from the patient, parents, or caregivers. Possible exposure to ticks, rash, or arthritis may suggest Lyme disease, whereas contact with cats may point to a possible diagnosis of Bartonella. Fevers, night sweats, and fatigue may be associated with tuberculosis or sarcoidosis. In these cases, chest x-rays may be diagnostic. Gallium scan or chest CT in patients with equivocal or negative results of chest x-rays can reveal subclinical sarcoidosis. Serologic testing for sarcoidosis should include an ACE level. In children, ACE levels are higher than in adults. Children previously treated with steroids may have suppressed ACE levels, thus an ACE level may be normal in the presence of sarcoidosis. Elevated serum lysozyme levels can occur in granulomatous disorders like sarcoid, tuberculosis, and leprosy. It is extremely important to exclude infectious causes of intermediate uveitis. Serologic tests for Lyme disease, cat-scratch disease (Bartonella), and syphilis should be considered. Other infectious entities include toxocariasis, Whipple's disease, human T-cell leukemia virus type1, and Epstein-Barr virus.

Previously treated severe anterior uveitis can create confusion due to spillover of inflammatory cells into the anterior vitreous, and present a picture of an intermediate uveitis. In such cases, if the history is not typical for acute anterior uveitis, a clinician may choose to observe the course of the disease. Inflammatory cellular aggregates in the vitreous are found rarely in iridocyclitis and never in iritis.

The association between MS and pars planitis has been well documented (157–166). The diagnosis of pars planitis may precede the diagnosis of MS, be made concurrently, or follow it years later. Patients are usually white females with bilateral disease. The incidence of uveitis in MS varies from 1% to 33%, and pars planitis is the most common subtype of uveitis (144,155,157).

Vascular sheathing can vary from 2% to 44% and averages 20% (158,159). Periphlebitis at the time of diagnosis of pars planitis is associated with an increased risk for developing MS or optic neuritis, or both (130). The severity of MS has been correlated with the presence of vascular sheathing (160). Although MS is extremely rare in patients younger than 25 years of age, cases have been reported in children. Considering the frequency of demyelinating lesions of the brain in patients with pars planitis, an MRI in patients with pars planitis who are HLA-DR15 positive or who have any, even subtle, neurologic signs or symptoms should be considered.

Sarcoidosis has been described in association with intermediate uveitis (166–169). Pulmonary sarcoidosis may precede, follow, or be diagnosed concurrently with pars planitis. Ocular findings in intermediate uveitis seen in pars planitis, such as CME, optic nerve swelling, periphlebitis, and retrobulbar optic neuritis are no different whether sarcoidosis is also present.

Management

Although intermediate uveitis is often considered one of the most benign forms of uveitis, accurate statistics about the overall prognosis of patients with this disease are not available. The severity of intermediate uveitis that occurs in the chronic phase of inflammation leads to significant visual impairment. Four groups were described by Brockhurst and Schepens (138) according to the clinical course. Severe disease was present in two groups, comprising 25% of all patients. Others reported 42% of patients with intermediate uveitis (124) to have moderate and 39% severe inflammation, and 20% of the patients lost vision to 20/40 or worse.

We recommend early and aggressive treatment of intermediate uveitis to preserve visual function, rather than waiting until visual acuity falls. A significant number of patients with intermediate uveitis (20%) who started on treatment when visual acuity dropped to 20/40 never recovered normal vision despite aggressive therapy (124). We use a stepladder approach to treatment of intermediate uveitis. After treatable infectious and noninfectious entities have been ruled out, we use the following regimen. The first step is administration of topical corticosteroids in the presence of anterior segment inflammation, together with regional corticosteroid injections (triamcinolone, 40 mg every 3 to 5 weeks). Periocular injections may be safely performed in the office in children as young as 10 years old with good cooperation. We limit the number of periocular steroid injections to no more than six. Step two is oral NSAIDs, if inflammation recurs following the third steroid injection, and topical NSAIDs in the presence of CME. Step three is a short course of systemic corticosteroids for persistent inflammation. Prednisone is prescribed at a dosage of 1 mg/kg per day orally, and is tapered after 2 weeks of treatment, as guided by the clinical response. Oral steroid therapy is limited to 3 months of tapering regimen. Step four is peripheral retinal cryopexy or indirect laser photocoagulation should pars planitis recur following the sixth regional steroid injection. Step five is therapeutic pars plana vitrectomy or immunosuppressive chemotherapy in case of recalcitrant inflammation.

Immunosuppressive drugs used in our practice include cyclosporine, methotrexate, or mycophenolate mofetil as a first choice. Azathioprine is the second choice, and cyclophosphamide and chlorambucil are the drugs of last resort.

OTHER NONINFECTIOUS DISORDERS AFFECTING INFANTS AND CHILDREN

Several disorders of considerably less epidemiologic importance include Adamantiades-Behçet's disease, Vogt-Koyanagi-Harada syndrome, Fuchs' heterochromic iridocyclitis, and Kawasaki disease.

Vogt-Koyanagi-Harada Syndrome

Epidemiology

Vogt-Koyanagi-Harada syndrome (VKH) is extraordinarily uncommon in children, but has been reported (170).

Clinical Signs and Symptoms

The disorder is characterized by bilateral panuveitis with exudative retinal detachment, dysacusis, meningismus, vitiligo, alopecia, and poliosis. Not all of these features occur in every patient, and the uveitis can precede the evolution of the extraocular manifestations, making diagnosis difficult and delayed. The disorder is chronic and can severely impair vision.

Management

Acute care is treatment with high-dose systemic corticosteroids. Relapse with steroid tapering is common, prompting the International Uveitis Study Group to recommend routinely steroid-sparing immunomodulatory agents in VKH. The visual outcomes in patients treated with steroids alone are quite poor, with vision-limiting posterior segment pathology as a consequence of chorioretinal scarring or subretinal neovascularization.

Fuchs' Heterochromic Iridocyclitis

Epidemiology

Although rare, Fuchs' heterochromic iridocyclitis (FHI) has also been reported in children (171).

Clinical Signs and Symptoms

The disorder is commonly asymptomatic, and may be first detected as a lighter colored iris (heterochromia) and a cataract in the affected eye. The keratic precipitates, characteristic of FHI, are dispersed throughout the entire extent of the endothelium, are gray-white, and are typically star-shaped. The most vision-robbing characteristic of FHI, however, is glaucoma.

Management

Glaucoma of FHI patients should be treated aggressively and often evolves to require surgery.

Kawasaki Disease

Kawasaki disease, an acute systemic febrile illness of unknown etiology, generally causes conjunctivitis in conjunction with the oral mucosal lesions and dermatitis, but anterior uveitis also occurs (172). The uveitis resolves with the resolution of the systemic disease.

Adamantiades-Behçet's Disease

Adamantiades-Behçet's disease (ABD) is an idiopathic, multisystem inflammatory vascular disorder that is chronic, recurrent-remitting, and progressive.

History

Benedictos Adamantiades (173), a Greek ophthalmologist, presented and later published a case of a 20-year-old man who suffered from recurrent iritis with hypopyon resulting in blindness and associated with phlebitis, recurrent mouth ulcers, genital ulcers, and knee arthritis (174). Six years later, in 1937, Hulsi Behçet (175), a Turkish professor of dermatology, described three patients with oral and genital ulcers and recurrent iritis. It was suggested that the disease be called Adamantiades-Behçet's disease to reflect the important contribution both these physicians made (176).

Prevalence and Epidemiology

The prevalence of ABD varies greatly among different countries. It is the highest in the East Asian and the Mediterranean countries. The exact incidence, prevalence, and family occurrence of the disease are unknown. Familial cases are uncommon, but isolated instances involving parents with affected children have been described, and a pair of monozygotic brothers concordant for the disease has been confirmed (176–178).

The highest prevalence of ABD is in Turkey with 80 to 300 cases per 100,000 population (179,180). In contrast, 8 to 10 cases per 100,000 exist in Japan, 0.6 per 100,000 in England, and 0.3 per 100,000 in the United States (181). The prevalence of ABD in Greece is 6 cases per 100,000 (177), and in Iran it is 16 to 100 cases in 100,000 (182). ABD has been observed to occur at an earlier age in males than in females. A recent study (183) showed that more females were affected, with a ratio of 1.5:1, in contrast to some reports of a male predominance (184,185) or no sex difference (184–186). The age group distribution of disease onset in 65 children was reviewed: 33 boys and 32 girls from Turkey (187), France (188), Saudi Arabia (189) and Iran (190). Most were white and of Turkish or European decent. The mean age at onset of the disease was 8.4 years (0 to 16 years), and the mean age at diagnosis was 13 years. The follow-up was at least 5 years for 32% (21 of 65) of patients, with a mean period of 3.4 years (0 to 13 years) (186). The mean disease duration was greater in adults than in children (12.9 ± 3.6 years versus 9.6 ± 4.9 years; $p < 0.05$). In another series of 59 patients with ABD, the mean age at disease onset was 8.4 ± 4.5 years in children and 29.8 ± 7.9 years in adults. The age of onset was significantly lower in male versus female patients (188).

Pathophysiology and Immunopathogenesis

The cause of ABD is unknown. Immunologic and genetic factors as well as infections have been studied, and all probably contribute to the development of this disorder (191). ABD is generally considered an autoimmune disease, but there are many ways in which it differs from classic autoimmune diseases. Its male preponderance, the lack of association with other autoimmune diseases, the absence of autoantibodies, the hyperactivity of B cells, and the lack of definite T-cell hypofunction differ from many of the other "classic" autoimmune disorders (175,192).

During the active stage of ABD, T cells are activated, observed by overexpression of CD25, and HLA class II (HLA-DR) expression on T cells is down-regulated. Both helper (CD4) and suppressor or cytotoxic (CD8) T cells have cytophilic immunoglobulin A bound to their surfaces in ABD. In addition, an increased percentage of T-cell receptor has been found in the circulation of patients with ABD (193,194). Proinflammatory cytokines such as interleukin (IL) 1a, IL-6, IL-8, TNF-α, and soluble IL-2 receptors are elevated in the sera of patients with ABD (187,195–197).

The immune system in patients with ABD is characterized by divergent cytokine production profiles of mixed TH1/TH2 (TH0) cell origin. Interferon-γ is critical in modulating the IL-4, IL-10, and IL-12 cytokine network in this disease (198). There is a statically significant association between antiphospholipid antibodies and retinal vascular disease in ABD patients. Antibodies against the endothelium have also been detected in patients with ABD, and may play a role in active thrombophlebitis or retinal vasculitis. Endothelial damage may be induced by increased levels of von Willebrand factor, which is also increased in ABD patients, particularly in those with vasculitis (199).

HLA-B5 phenotype and its subtype, HLA-B51 (200), is overrepresented in patients with ABD compared to the general population. HLA-DR1 and HLA-DQW1 have also been shown to be significantly under-represented in patients with ABD (201). Specific associations are also observed between HLA type and clinical manifestations of ABD. HLA-B5 occurs more frequently in patients with ocular lesions, whereas HLA-B27 is increased in those with arthritis symptoms and HLA-B12 is associated with mucocutaneous lesions (202). The allele *B*5101* is found in 80% of patients with ABD compared with 26% in controls (203) and is found in ABD that occurs at a younger age in the presence of erythema nodosum (204), a lesion consisting of occlusive vasculitis that affects small blood vessels, particularly venules.

Vasculitis can affect large veins and cause thrombophlebitis or larger arteries, and cause gangrene or aneurysm formation. Deposition of C3 and C9 in blood vessels walls and circulating immune complexes also occurs in patients with ABD (204).

Recent studies investigated *MICA* (major histocompatibility complex class I chain-related genes) polymorphisms in an Italian series of patients with juvenile Behçet's disease (JABD) and compared these genetic findings with the high prevalence of inflammatory mucosal disease, which occurs in Western populations. The study of *MICA* gene polymorphisms disclosed an independent association with the genetic risk for JABD. The combination of MICA A6 and HLA–B51 is the strongest genetic marker for this disease. Homozygous A6 patients appear to develop more severe mucosal gut involvement. This finding sheds new light on the role of a receptor for *MICA*, named NKG2D that is usually localized in gut mucosa (205).

In the brain, demyelinization is the most common finding, followed by encephalomalacia, with perivascular infiltration in the brain stem, spinal cord, cerebrum, and cerebellum (206).

The mucocutaneous lesions in ABD are characterized by the presence of neutrophils, fibrinoid necrosis, and perivascular infiltrate (207). Increased number of mast cells has also been reported in recurrent mucocutaneous ulcers (208).

Ocular histopathologic changes show infiltration with neutrophils and later with lymphocytes, monocytes, and mast cells. Veins are more affected than arteries; the retinal vascular endothelial cells become swollen, neutrophils marginate, and thrombus formation begins. Rod and cone areas are destroyed, but retinal pigment epithelium destruction is minimal. Posterior ciliary arteries can also be affected, leading to optic ischemic neuropathy and optic atrophy (175).

Diagnosis

There are no definitive diagnostic laboratory findings for ABD. It is diagnosed clinically (209) (Table 17-2). Several clinical criteria systems exist. The criteria of the International Study Group for Behçet's Disease include recurrent oral aphthous ulcers (three times in 1 year) plus two other manifestations: (i) genital ulcers, (ii) uveitis or retinal vasculitis, (iii) skin lesions (erythema nodosum, papulopustular lesions, or acneiform nodules), or (iv) a positive pathergy test result (181) (Table 17-2). Neurologic, urogenital, vascular, intestinal, and pulmonary lesions are seen in patients with ABD (184), and the diagnostic criteria of the Behçet's Syndrome Research Committee of Japan include minor features of the disease in their diagnostic criteria and a designation of "incomplete Behçet's disease" for patients with two of the four major features of the disease involving skin, eye, mouth, or genitals plus two minor features. A "Behçet's disease suspect" would be a patient with only two of the major features of the disease or one major plus two minor features.

TABLE 17-2. DIAGNOSTIC SYSTEM OF ADAMANTIADES-CLASSIFICATION OF BEHÇET DISEASE SUGGESTED BY THE INTERNATIONAL STUDY GROUP FOR BEHÇET'S DISEASE

Recurrent oral ulceration
  Minor aphthous, major aphthous, or herpetiform ulceration observed by a physician or reported reliably by a patient
  Recurrent at least three times in one 12-month period

Plus **two** of the following:

Recurrent genital ulceration
  Recurrent genital aphthous ulceration or scarring, especially males, observed by a physician or reported reliably by a patient

Eye lesions
  Anterior uveitis
  Posterior uveitis
  Cells in vitreous on slit-lamp examination
  Retinal vasculitis observed by qualified physician (ophthalmologist)

Skin lesions
  Erythema nodosumlike lesions observed by physician or reliably reported by a patient
  Pseudofolliculitis
  Papulopustular lesions
  Acneiform nodules consistent with Behçet's disease observed by a physician and in postadolescent patients not receiving corticosteroids

Positive pathergy test result
  To be read by a physician at 24–48 hr, performed with oblique insertion of a 20-gauge or smaller needle under sterile conditions

---

A transient neonatal form of ABD meeting three criteria for the diagnosis of ABD has been described in infants born to mothers with the syndrome (181). These criteria were stomatitis, genital ulcers, and bullous skin lesions. The occurrence of transient ABD in neonates supports the idea that the disease is immunologic. Neonatal manifestations occur in a number of autoimmune diseases mediated by the trans-placental transfer of maternal immunoglobulin G (IgG). IgG is cleared from the neonatal circulation within 4 months, accounting for the transient nature of the neonatal illness (210,211)

Clinical Course

The onset of ABD is usually after puberty, and it affects predominantly young adults between ages 20 and 40 years, but there are observations of patients with onset before puberty (212,213). Studies are sparse on pediatric cases (190, 214,215) and few compare adult and pediatric cases (185,189,216–218). Most studies defined pediatric ABD as the first disease manifestation appearing before age 16 years (218). Juvenile-onset disease was characterized by an increase in familial cases, a lower incidence of severe complications and a delay of the clinical course. It was less severe than adult-onset disease, especially because the frequency of systemic involvement was higher in adult-onset disease (218–220a).

Clinical Signs and Symptoms

The first manifestation of ABD in children is almost always oral ulcers. Ocular involvement may be unilateral initially, but the disease becomes bilateral in over 90% of patients (190). Several groups recently investigated the features of juvenile ABD. There is no consensus regarding the age at which juvenile disease should be discriminated from adult disease or how the diagnosis should be determined, whether by classical criteria or by the age at the onset of the disease (181). Most recent studies (183,184,218) confirm the following features for children believed to have ABD.

Mucosal Lesions

Buccal aphthosis was present in almost all (96% to 100%) children, and was the presenting symptom in 60% of them. Lesions occurred on the lip, cheek, tongue, palate, tonsil, gingiva, and pharynx, and were discrete, round, or oval white ulcerations 3 to 15 mm in diameter with a red rim. Lesions occurred as seldom as three per year or were present almost constantly. The mean age at onset was 4 years. The ulcers were painful and sometimes were associated with facial edema, compared with those seen in Stevens-Johnson and reactive arthritis syndromes, which are painless, with irregular rims or heaped-up edges. Many older ABD patients have nonoral aphthosis as their first disease manifestation (188).

Genital Ulcers

Genital ulcers occurred in 70% of cases, usually after the buccal aphthosis, and were similar in appearance to oral ulcers. The children with genital lesions were older at disease onset than children without them (8.6 ± 3.7 years versus 6.4 ± 3.2 years). The lesions affected the vulva, scrotum, and penis. Perianal ulceration was also noted in some children, age 3 to 4 years, and was associated with genital ulceration (218,221).

Skin Lesions

Skin lesions were present in 90% of pediatric ABD patients, with similar rates in males and females. The cutaneous lesions included papules, pustules, acneiform lesions, pyoderma gangrenosa-type lesions, palpable purpura, hypopigmented areas, and purulent bullae. Pustular eruptions were the most common type of skin lesion (183). The result of a pathergy test was positive in 80% of the patients.

Ocular Involvement

Eye lesions were present in 60% of ABD children. These included conjunctivitis, scleritis, uveitis, papilledema, retinal vasculitis, and optic atrophy. A recent international collaborative study of 86 cases showed that uveitis was strictly anterior in 8% (5 of 65) of the cases, strictly posterior in 9% (6 of 65), and panuveitic in 28% (18 of 65). The uveitis was bilateral in most (26 of 29) instances.

Eighty-nine percent of patients had severe uveitis, retinal vasculitis, or both. Uveitis or vasculitis was significantly more frequent in boys than in girls (2.25 male:female sex ratio of 27:12) (186).

Joint Involvement

The arthritis of ABD is usually pauciarticular, involving knee, ankle, hip, metatarsophalangeal joints, the shoulder, and the sternoclavicular joint. Low-back pain (without sacroiliitis) also was reported in one patient (186). Arthritis usually becomes gradually generalized.

Neurological Involvement

Neurologic signs are present in 15% of pediatric ABD patients and it is the most serious manifestation of ABD. Signs include headache, meningitis, benign intracranial hypertension, brain stem involvement, neuropsychiatric symptoms, meningoencephalitis (184), hemiparesis or paraparesis with spastic quadriparesis, and seizures. MRI and CT findings include ventricular dilatation and hyperintensity signals in the pons, brainstem, putamen, and upper medulla. Cerebral venous thrombosis may present with ABD (222,223). Dural sinus thrombosis may occur. Cerebral spinal fluid analysis may show elevated protein levels and a sterile hypercellularity, with lymphocytosis. Organic psychiatric disturbances were reported with severe neurologic symptoms. Depression, loss of memory, and personality changes were reported (186).

Gastrointestinal Involvement

The frequency of gastrointestinal involvement in patients with Behçet's disease varies widely, from no reports in 297 patients in Turkey (224) to at least 15% in a series of Japanese patients (225). The most frequent complaints were abdominal pain, vomiting, flatulence, diarrhea, and constipation. Radiologic examinations demonstrate thickened mucosal folds, pseudopolyps, deformity of bowel loops, ulcerations, and fistulae (226). Ulcerations are localized or diffuse, with the majority (76%) occurring in the ileocecal region (227). Rare cases of esophageal involvement have been reported.

The differentiation of Behçet's disease from chronic nonspecific ulcerative colitis and especially Crohn's disease depends on the character of the intestinal endoscopic and radiologic findings as well as the associated extraintestinal manifestations. The correct extraintestinal diagnosis may be obscured by the presence of Behçet's disease and ulcerative colitis or Crohn's disease in the same family (228). Baba and others (225) noted that the ileocecal locations and the depth of the ulcers in Behçet's disease distinguish this disease from chronic ulcerative colitis. In comparison with Crohn's disease there was less inflammation in the area surrounding the ulcer, and granulomas were not seen (225,227). Fistula formation has been reported in Behçet's disease (226,229). The recurrent genital ulcers and central nervous system signs seen in Behçet's disease are rarely found in ulcerative colitis or Crohn's disease (228). Findings on examination may include hepatomegaly and splenomegaly, and on endoscopy, ulcerative colitis, duodenitis, and esophagitis. Gastrointestinal features were significantly more frequent in French children with ABD (186).

Vascular Involvement

The vasculitis process affects both arterial and venous systems. Venous thrombosis has been observed in 15% of children with ABD. The location of thrombosis occurred most often in the lower extremities, but it can occur in the cerebral circulation, including the inferior vena cava and central retinal artery or vein. Arterial complications, including aneurysms and thrombosis, may be fatal.

Pulmonary Involvement

Pulmonary signs included generalized lymphadenopathy, parenchymal infarction related to venous thrombosis, chest pain, and hemoptysis (186). Pulmonary artery involvement can lead to life threatening hemoptysis from pulmonary hemorrhage.

Renal and Urologic Involvement

Renal involvement results in proteinuria and hematuria. Urethritis, orchitis, or epididymitis may occur.

Cardiac Involvement

Myocarditis and arrhythmia may occur in children with ABD.

Comparison of Clinical Manifestations in Juvenile versus Adult ABD

A clinical study of ABD in childhood in comparison to adult-onset disease showed that all patients had recurrent oral ulcers, and similar ocular and skin lesions and positive pathergy test results were found in children and adults. In contrast, genital ulcers were significantly more common in adults than in children. Similar prevalences were found in children and adults for arthritis, vascular involvement, and recurrent headaches. Compared with adults, children with ABD had a tendency towards more nonspecific gastrointestinal symptoms and towards central nervous system (CNS) involvement other than headaches.

It is difficult to establish the diagnosis of ABD in children because of the prolonged interval between the first symptom and the complete manifestations of the disease. Therefore, it is advisable to follow the children with "incomplete" ABD for prolonged periods and observe for development of the complete form of the disease. Although there are no laboratory tests that are specific for the diagnosis of ABD, some may be helpful. The erythrocyte sedimentation rate, C-reactive protein, and other acute phase reactants, such as properdin factor b and $\alpha 1$-acid glycoprotein, may be elevated during the acute phase of ABD. Addition-ally, longitudinal monitoring of soluble CD25 molecules in the serum (soluble IL 2 receptor) along with these acute phase reactants, may be useful, since a rise in these markers often precedes the development of a clinically obvious recurrence, thereby providing the clinician the opportunity for preventative treatment (176). A positive serum HLA-B5 supports the diagnosis.

Management

The choice of medical therapy is based on the severity of the disease. In general, treatment should be more aggressive when the following are present: Complete ABD, vascular involvement, retinal and bilateral involvement, CNS involvement, male sex, and a geographic origin in the Mediterranean basin or Far East (176). The most commonly used agents today are corticosteroids, cytotoxic drugs, colchicine, cyclosporine-A, and thalidomide.

Systemic and topical corticosteroids have a beneficial effect on the acute ocular inflammation. Although corticosteroids alone have failed to prevent vision loss in patients with ABD (177,230), 1 to 1.5 mg/kg of prednisone per day are useful to quickly control acute inflammation. Combined therapy with other immunosuppressive drugs is appropriate for acute posterior segment inflammation while awaiting the full effect of the cytotoxic drugs. Then the corticosteroids are gradually tapered. In anterior segment inflammation, topical corticosteroids, with or without periocular corticosteroids are required (177).

Indicated in severe uveitis with retinal involvement, the immunosuppressive therapy agents that are currently used in treatment of ocular ABD include azathioprine, chlorambucil, cyclophosphamide, cyclosporine, methotrexate, and mycophenolate mofetil.

Azathioprine is an immunosuppressive drug that affects rapidly proliferating cells such as activated lymphocytes. The dosage is 2 or 3 mg/kg per day. Variable results have been achieved for vision preservation (233—236); it is effective in treating oral and genital ulcers and arthritis.

Chlorambucil is a slow-acting alkylating agent. Chlorambucil (0.1 mg/kg per day) produces favorable results in ABD patients. It was effective in two-thirds of patients, with no serious side effects observed (232).

Cyclophosphamide is a fast-acting alkylating agent, and it has been shown to be superior to steroids in suppressing ocular inflammation in patients with ABD (238). Both cyclophosphamide and chlorambucil were superior to cyclosporine-A in management of posterior segment manifestations of ABD (233,234). Others found cyclophosphamide less effective compared with oral cyclosporine-A during the first 6 months (235).

Cyclosporin is superior to colchicine (236) in the prevention of ocular inflammatory recurrence when combined with corticosteroids, and the combination is more effective in improving visual acuity than the higher-dose cyclosporine-A as monotherapy (237–240). The use of 5 mg/kg per day or less, reduces the likelihood of nephrotoxicity from the medication.

Mycophenolate mofetil is a novel immunosuppressive agent that blocks DNA synthesis by inhibiting the enzyme inosine monophosphate dehydrogenase (241). Two ABD patients were successfully treated with mycophenolate mofetil added to their therapeutic regimens (249).

Other treatment modalities have been tried in ocular ABD, including interferon (242–246), plasma pheresis (247,248), penicillin (249), and thalidomide (250). Awareness of the danger of axonal neuropathy and teratogenesis at all times during thalidomide therapy is of course crucial. A low dose is probably as effective as higher dose (251).

Colchicine is both antiinflammatory and antimitotic, mediated mainly through its inhibition of microtubule formation. Because enhanced neutrophil migration is a characteristic feature of ABD, colchicine (0.6 mg per day) is most useful in prophylaxis of recurrent inflammatory episodes or mild unilateral involvement (231).

Masquerade Syndromes

Both malignant and nonmalignant disorders that are not primarily inflammatory may "masquerade" as uveitis. Nonmalignant masquerades include retinal detachment, retinal degenerations, intraocular foreign body, pigment dispersion syndrome, ocular ischemic syndrome, and juvenile xanthogranuloma. Malignant masquerades include intraocular and CNS lymphoma, retinoblastoma, leukemia, malignant melanoma, and metastatic malignancy. Many of these entities, such as melanoma, metastatic malignancy, pigment dispersion syndrome, and ocular ischemia syndrome, are extraordinarily rare in children. However, failure to consider a masquerade in the assessment of the patient with chronic, steroid-resistant uveitis could be fatal.

Intraocular and Central Nervous System Lymphoma

Intraocular-CNS lymphoma, most commonly a diffuse large B-cell lymphoma (rarely T cell in origin) (252,253), is rare. The incidence of this malignancy has trebled over the past 15 years, and although it typically occurs in adults, it can occur in children (254). While states of immunodeficiency pose increased risk for development of intraocular-CNS lymphoma, such states are by no means required for it to develop. The cancer arises multifocally in eye, brain, spinal cord, and leptomeninges. Ocular involvement precedes extraocular manifestations in 50% to 80% of cases reported in the ophthalmic literature; the data, however, are different in those cases reported in the neurologic literature. About 20% of patients with primary CNS lymphoma exhibit ocular manifestations at the time of the diagnosis.

Clinical Signs and Symptoms

Blurred vision and floaters are the most common initial symptoms, and ophthalmologic examination discloses a "quiet" eye with anterior chamber and vitreous cells, with the latter being the most prominent feature of the findings. The vitreous cells tend to aggregate in clumps or sheets, and may be surprisingly numerous by the time ophthalmologic evaluation is performed. Retinal or subretinal lesions may or may not be evident, but such lesions eventually manifest multifocally as yellow, generally round infiltrates of variable size under the retinal pigment epithelium.

The "inflammation" may respond to systemic or periocular steroid injections, but relapse as the effect of the steroid diminishes, and eventually become treatment resistant. Most of the patients have no CNS manifestations, and unless such manifestations are present, even subtly on neurologic review of systems and examination, the likelihood of finding CNS pathology on spinal tapping or neuroimaging studies is quite small. The patient presenting with the ocular manifestations of primary ocular-CNS lymphoma typically feels and looks well, unlike the patient with systemic non-Hodgkin's lymphoma in whom ocular involvement develops. The systemic non-Hodgkin's lymphoma patient has generally had systemic manifestations, with constitutional symptoms and lymphadenopathy before any ocular manifestation evolves. Ocular involvement very often presents with a hypopyon in the "quiet" eye, hyphema, and/or choroidal infiltrates on funduscopic examination. Such infiltrates may be large and may pose some degree of confusion with the possibility of lymphoma.

Lymphoid hyperplasia of the uvea, characterized by well-differentiated lymphocytic infiltration of the uveal tract, may present unilaterally with "uveitis," and mucosal-associated lymphoid tissue lymphoma may also masquerade as ocular inflammation (255).

Diagnosis

Vitreous biopsy is the cornerstone to definitively diagnosing primary intraocular-CNS lymphoma, and a high index of suspicion must precede consideration of vitreous biopsy. The vast majority of cells in the vitreous infiltrate of the patient who has primary intraocular-CNS lymphoma are reactive; i.e., lymphocytes reacting to the presence of a few malignant cells in the eye. Consequently, the cytopathologist has very few frankly malignant lymphocytes available to him or her from the specimen obtained by the vitreoretinal surgeon. Therefore, the diagnosis may be missed by a single vitreous biopsy and multiple biopsies must sometimes be performed to secure the diagnosis. Efforts to obtain an early definitive diagnosis are important, so that life-saving therapy can be instituted early to reduce patient mortality. The 5-year survival rate is less than 5% and the reported median survival is 12 to 26 months.

One of the most important diagnostic advances is polymerase chain reaction technology to investigate the possibility of monoclonality in the cellular infiltrate. In the case of B-cell lymphomas, oligonucleotide primer pairs for immunoglobulin H gene rearrangement analyses provide a relatively new, extremely potent additional diagnostic tool. Additionally, a high IL-10 to IL-6 ratio in the vitreous, supports a diagnosis of lymphoma, whereas a high IL-6 to IL-10 ratio in the vitreous supports the diagnosis of inflammation.

Leukemia

Ocular involvement is more common in acute leukemias than in the chronic ones (256). Uveitis "masquerade" may occur as a consequence of leukemic cell infiltration into the eye producing a pseudohypopyon, "vitreitis", or vascular leukemic exudates mimicking retinal vasculitis. These manifestations are in distinction to the more classic leukemic ophthalmopathy of extensive retinal hemorrhages with or without Roth spots. Nodular retinal infiltrates may also occur (257). The choroid may actually be the area of the eye most routinely infiltrated by leukemia cells (256). A subretinal mass and/or serous retinal detachment may be the presenting manifestation of leukemia.

The pseudohypopyon associated with leukemic infiltration into the anterior chamber is mobile, such that it can shift relative to the patient's position when sitting versus when lying on the side, has a creamy-white color, and shows diagnostic cytopathologic characteristics. Secondary glaucoma is rare as a consequence of leukemic infiltration of the trabecular meshwork. Diffuse infiltration of the iris by leukemic cells can produce heterochromia.

The blood–eye barrier may prevent effective intravenous chemotherapeutic measures. Accordingly, local radiation therapy is commonly required to treat ocular involvement with leukemias. The development of an ocular manifestation of leukemia believed to be in remission is an ominous sign.

Retinoblastoma

Retinoblastoma occurs in approximately 1 in 20,000 infants, typically discovered in children below the age of 5 years, with 40% being familial and 60% sporadic. Seventy percent of the cases are unilateral.

Strabismus and leukocoria are the most common features which stimulate an ophthalmologic evaluation, with discovery of the tumor, but a misdiagnosis of uveitis can occur in 40% (258) and be the presenting manifestation, either because of reactive inflammation to necrosis of some of the tumor or as a consequence of tumor cells managing to make their way into the anterior chamber (259,260). Retinoblastoma is discussed in detail in Chapter 14.

Juvenile Xanthogranuloma

Juvenile xanthogranuloma occurs in infants and young children, with the predominant manifestation being widespread cutaneous papules. Ocular involvement is relatively frequent with iris and ciliary body tumors. The most common ocular manifestation resulting in "uveitis masquerade" is the development of an iris nodule or nodules with cells in the anterior chamber. Glaucoma in the affected eye is also typical, and heterochromia and spontaneous hyphema may also develop. Most patients are under the age of 2 years at first time of presentation (261), and the vast majority of patients (approximately 85%) with ocular involvement present during the first year of life (262). Extraocular sites can be involved and include testes, spleen, lung, pericardium, bone, and gastrointestinal tract. It is discussed in Chapter 15.

Diagnosis

The diagnosis should be considered in the child with "uveitis" who has hyphema, secondary glaucoma, and/or iris nodules, with typical or suspicious skin lesions. The diagnosis is confirmed by skin biopsy. In the absence of skin lesions, aqueous paracentesis with cytologic evaluation can be diagnostic, with the discovery of Touton giant cells and foamy histiocytes (263). But the high frequency of the typical skin manifestations in the disorder emphasizes yet again the importance of the ophthalmologist's careful attention to extraocular features of any patient with ocular inflammatory disease.

The differential diagnosis of an iris mass in a child includes lymphangioma, hemangioma, melanoma, iris leiomyoma, and sarcoidosis.

Management

Treatment for juvenile xanthogranuloma without ocular involvement typically is by observation only. Uveal involvement of disease, however, mandates therapy, without which glaucoma, hyphema, and amblyopia are almost inevitable. Topical steroid therapy is typically the initial step in a stepladder algorithmic approach in aggressiveness to treating intraocular juvenile xanthogranuloma, with ocular hypotensives and systemic acetazolamide as needed for control of elevated intraocular pressure. Systemic steroids and low-dose radiation therapy (300 to 400 cGy) should be employed in the event that steroid therapy does not result in resolution of the intraocular problem (264), and excisional biopsy may be seriously considered if the tumor is smaller than one-fourth of the surface area of the iris (265). We would typically reserve this for cases in which all other therapies have failed. The visual prognosis is variable, depending upon the ocular complications that develop, with poor prognosis in cases involving secondary glaucoma and hyphema with corneal blood staining.

Intraocular Foreign Bodies

Intraocular foreign bodies (IOFBs) can cause intraocular inflammation, and persistent uveitis is one of the most common complications of IOFBs. Additionally, children sustaining a penetrating injury may be unaware that the eye has been injured much less been penetrated, and the child may be unwilling to reveal to his or her parents that an accident has occurred even if he knows that the eye has been injured. Therefore, retained IOFB causing a uveitis masquerade should be considered in all instances of chronic or treatment-resistant uveitis.

The peak age incidence for IOFB is 18 to 25 years, with a male predominance, but both sexes can be affected, and children, even very young children, may experience this potentially blinding problem. Signs on examination that should make the ophthalmologist suspicious for an IOFB uveitic masquerade include hyphema, fluorescein staining defect of the cornea or conjunctiva, iris transillumination defect, irregular pupil secondary to a pupillary sphincter defect, discontinuity in the lens capsule, localized cataract, vitreous hemorrhage, and inordinately low intraocular pressure. Any history of at-risk activity for IOFB prior to the onset of the uveitis is crucial in raising the diagnostic suspicion. X-ray, CT scanning, and ultrasonography are particularly useful for identification and localization of IOFBs. Plain radiographs are useful in the detection of intraocular metallic materials, but because of better resolution, CT scanning has in many instances replaced plain x-rays. Thin-cut spiral CT scanning can identify IOFBs down to the 0.7-mm level. MRI scanning is not appropriate, of course, for assessment of the patient suspected of a metallic IOFB, but is excellent in the patient suspected or known to have an IOFB that is nonmetallic.

Management

Management of the problem typically involves localization of and removal of the IOFB. This may involve the need for cataract extraction along with complete pars plana vitrectomy and even retinotomy with removal of the subretinal foreign bodies. Prophylactic postoperative intraocular antibiotic with or without steroid is often appropriate at the end of the surgical case (see also Chapter 33).

REFERENCES

1. Rothova A, Suttorp-van Schulten MS, Frits Treffers W, et al. Causes and frequency of blindness in patients with intraocular inflammatory disease. *Br J Ophthalmol* 1996;80:332–336.
2. Malagon C, Van Kerckhove C, Giannini EH, et al. The iridocyclitis of early onset pauciarticular juvenile rheumatoid arthritis: outcome in immunogenetically characterized patients. *J Rheumatol* 1992;19:160–163.
3. Dana MR, Merayo-Lloves J, Schaumberg DA, et al. Visual outcomes prognosticators in juvenile rheumatoid arthritis-associated uveitis. *Ophthalmology* 1997;104:236–244.
4. Nguyen QD, Foster CS. Saving the vision of children with juvenile rheumatoid arthritis-associated uveitis. *JAMA* 1998, 280:1133–1134.
5. Ceisler EJ, Foster CS. Juvenile rheumatoid arthritis and uveitis: minimizing the blinding complications. *Int Ophthalmol Clin* 1996;36:91–107.
6. American Academy of Pediatrics. Guidelines for examinations in children with juvenile rheumatoid arthritis (RE9320). *Pediatrics* 1993;92:295–296.
7. Rosenberg AM. Uveitis associated with juvenile rheumatoid arthritis. *Semin Arthritis Rheum* 1987;16:158–173.
8. Özdal PC, Vianna RNG, Deschenes J. Visual outcome of juvenile rheumatoid arthritis associated uveitis in adults. *Ocul Immunol Inflamm* 2004 *(in press)*.
9. Kanski JJ. Uveitis in juvenile chronic arthritis: incidence, clinical features and prognosis. *Eye* 1988;2:641–645.
10. Chylack LT Jr. The ocular manifestations of juvenile rheumatoid arthritis. *Arthritis Rheum* 1977;20:217–223.
11. Wolf MD, Lichter PR, Ragsdale CG. Prognostic factors in the uveitis of juvenile rheumatoid arthritis. *Ophthalmology* 1987; 94:1242–1248.
12. Sherry DD, Mellins ED, Wedgwood RJ. Decreasing severity of chronic uveitis in children with pauciarticular arthritis. *Am J Dis Child* 1991;145:1026–1028.
13. Chalom EC, Goldsmith DP, Koehler MA, et al. Prevalence and outcome of uveitis in a regional cohort of patients with juvenile rheumatoid arthritis. *J Rheumatol* 1997;24:2031–2034.
14. Kotaniemi K, Kautiainen H, Karma A, et al. Occurrence of uveitis in recently diagnosed juvenile chronic arthritis: a prospective study. *Ophthalmology*. 2001;108:2071–2075.
15. Cabral DA, Petty RE, Malleson PN, et al. Visual prognosis in children with chronic anterior uveitis and arthritis. *J Rheumatol* 1994;21:2370–2375.
16. Rosenberg KD, Feuer WJ, Davis JL. Ocular complications of pediatric uveitis. *Ophthalmology* 2004 *(in press)*.
17. Olsen NY, Lindsley CB, Godfrey WA. Nonsteroidal antiinflammatory drug therapy in chronic childhood iridocyclitis. *Am J Dis Child* 1988;142:1289–1292.
18. Hoekstra M, van Ede AE, Haagsma CJ, et al. Factors associated with toxicity, final dose, and efficacy of methotrexate in patients with rheumatoid arthritis. *Ann Rheum Dis* 2003;62:423–426.
19. Samson CM, Waheed N, Baltatzis S, et al. Methotrexate therapy for chronic noninfectious uveitis: analysis of a case series of 160 patients. *Ophthalmology* 2001;108:1134–1139.
20. Hooper PL, Rao NA, Smith RE. Cataract extraction in uveitis patients. *Surv Ophthalmol* 1990;35:120–144.
21. Kanski JJ. Lensectomy for complicated cataract in juvenile chronic iridocyclitis [see comments]. *Br J Ophthalmol* 1992;76:72–75.
22. Smiley WK. The eye in juvenile rheumatoid arthritis. *Trans Ophthalmol Soc U K* 1974;94:817–829.
23. Smith RE, Nozik RA. Surgery in uveitis patients. In: Smith RE, Nozik RA, eds: *Uveitis: a clinical approach to diagnosis and management*. Baltimore: Williams & Wilkins, 1989:113–114.
24. Kanski JJ. Juvenile arthritis and uveitis. *Surv Ophthalmol* 1990;31:253.
25. Holland GN. Intraocular lens implantation in patients with juvenile rheumatoid arthritisi-associated uveitis; an unresolved management issue. *Am J Ophthalmol* 1996;122:161–170.
26. Foster CS, Barrett F. Cataract development and cataract surgery in patients with juvenile rheumatoid arthritis-associated iridocyclitis. *Ophthalmology* 1993;100:809–817.
27. Hooper PL, Rao NA, Smith RE. Cataract extraction in uveitis patients. *Surv Ophthalmol* 1990;35:120–144.
28. Flynn HW, Davis JL, Culbertson WW. Pars plana lensectomy and vitrectomy for complicated cataracts in juvenile rheumatoid arthritis. *Ophthalmology* 1988;95:1114–1119.

29. Da Mata A, Burk SE, Netland PA, et al. Management of uveitic glaucoma with Ahmed glaucoma valve implantation. *Ophthalmology* 1999;106:2168–2172.

30. Dollfus H, Häfner R, Hoffman HM, et al. Chronic infantile neurological cutaneous and articular/neonatal onset multisystem inflammatory disease syndrome: ocular manifestations in recently recognized chronic inflammatory disease of childhood. *Arch Ophthalmol* 2000;118:1386–1392.

31. Lovell DJ, Giannini EW, Brewer EJ. Time course of response to nonsteroidal antiinflammatory drugs in juvenile rheumatoid arthritis. *Arthritis Rheum* 1984;23:1433

32. Stoll M (1776). Cited by Foster CS, Vitale AT. *Diagnosis and treatment of uveitis*, Philadelphia: WB Saunders 2002:584.

33. Brodie BC. Inflammation of the synovial membranes of joints. In: Hurst, Rees, Orme, Brown, eds. *Pathological and surgical observations on diseases of the joints.* London: Longman, 1818: 6–63.

34. Reiter H. Ueber eine bisher unerkannte Spriochaeteninfektion (Spirochaetosis arthritica). Dtsch Med Wochenscher 1916; 42:1535–1536.

35. Panush RS, Paraschiv D, Dorff RE. The tainted legacy of Hans Reiter. *Semin Arthritis Rheum* 2003;32:231–236.

36. Foster CS, Durrani K. Psoriatic uveitis: a distinct clinical entity? 2004 *(in press).*

37. Hopkins OJ, Horan E, Burton IL, et al. Ocular disorders in a series of 332 patients with Crohn's disease. *Br J Ophthalmol* 1974;58:732.

38. Hetherington S. Sarcoidosis in young children. *Am J Dis Child* 1982;136:13–15.

39. Fink CW, Cimaz R. Early onset sarcoidosis: not a benign disease. *J Rheumatol* 1997;24:174–177.

40. Sarigol SS, Hay MH, Wyllie R. Sarcoidosis in preschool children with hepatic involvement mimicking juvenile rheumatoid arthritis. *J Pediatr Gastroenterol* Nutr 1999;28:510–512.

41. Yotsumoto S, Takahashi Y, Takei S, et al. Early onset sarcoidosis masquerading as juvenile rheumatoid arthritis. *J Am Acad Dermatol* 2000;43:969–971.

42. Blau EB. Familial granulomatous arthritis, iritis, and rash. *J Pediatr* 1985;107:689–693.

43. Latkany PA, Jabs DA, Smith JR, et al. Multifocal choroiditis in patients with familial juvenile systemic granulomatosis. *Am J Ophthalmol* 2002;134:897–903.

44. Tromp G, Kuivaniemi H, Raphael S, et al. Genetic linkage of familial granulomatous inflammatory arthritis, skin rash, and uveitis to chromosome 16. *Am J Hum Genet* 1996; 59:1097–1107.

45. Ting SS, Ziegler J, Fischer E. Familial granulomatous arthritis (Blau syndrome) with granulomatous renal lesions. *J Pediatr* 1998;133:450–452.

46. Saini SK, Rose CD. Liver involvement in familial granulomatous arthritis (Blau syndrome). *J Rheumatol* 1996;23:396–399.

47. de Chadarevian JP, Raphael SA, Murphy GF. Histologic, ultrastructural, and immunocytochemical features of the granulomas seen in a child with the syndrome of familial granulomatous arthritis, uveitis, and rash. *Arch Pathol Lab Med* 1993; 117:1050–1052.

48. Roy M, Sharma OP, Chan K. Sarcoidosis presenting in infancy: a rare occurrence. *Sarcoidosis Vasc Diffuse Lung Dis* 1999;16: 224–227.

49. Milman N, Hoffmann AL, Byg KE. Sarcoidosis in children. Epidemiology in Danes, clinical features, diagnosis, treatment and prognosis. *Acta Paediatr* 1998;87:871–878.

50. Shetty AK, Gedalia A. Sarcoidosis: a pediatric perspective. *Clin Pediatr* 1998;37:707–717.

51. Foster CS, Vitale AT. *Diagnosis and treatment of uveitis.* Philadelphia: WB Saunders, 2002.

52. Cotran RS, Kumar V, Collins T. *Robbins pathologic basis of disease.* Philadelphia: Saunders, 1999.

53. Moller DR, Konishi K, Kirby M, et al. Bias toward use of a specific T cell receptor beta-chain variable region in a subgroup of individuals with sarcoidosis. *J Clin Invest* 1988;82:1183–1191.

54. Paller AS, Roenigk AH Jr, Caro WA. Extensive ichthyosiform sarcoidosis in a patient with juvenile rheumatoid arthritis. *Arch Dermatol* 1985;121:171–172

55. Cimaz R, Ansell BM. Sarcoidosis in the pediatric age. *Clin Exp Rheumatol* 2002;20:231–237

56. Shetty AK, Gedalia A. Ediatric sarcoidosis. *J Am Acad Dermatol* 2003;48:150–151

57. Pattishall EN, Kendig EL Jr. Sarcoidosis in children. *Pediatr Pulmonol* 1996;22:195–203

58. Kwong T, Valderrama E, Paley C, et al. Systemic necrotizing vasculitis associated with childhood sarcoidosis. *Semin Arthritis Rheum* 1994;23:388–395

59. Gibson LE, Winkelmann RK. Cutaneous granulomatous vasculitis: its relationship to systemic disease. *J Am Acad Dermatol* 1986;14:492–501.

60. Faye-Petersen O, Frankel SR, Schulman PE, et al. Giant cell vasculitis with extravascular granulomas in an adolescent. *Pediatr Pathol* 1991;11:281–295. Erratum in: *Pediatr Pathol* 1991;11:797.

61. Gedalia A, Shetty AK, Ward K, et al. Abdominal aortic aneurysm associated with childhood sarcoidosis. *J Rheumatol* 1996;23:757–759.

62. Hafner R, Vogel P. Sarcoidosis of early onset. A challenge for the pediatric rheumatologist. *Clin Exp Rheumatol* 1993;11: 685–691

63. Lipnick RN, Hung W, Pandian MR. Neurosarcoidosis presenting as secondary amenorrhea in a teenager. *J Adolesc Health* 1993;14:464–467.

64. Ng KL, McDermott N, Romanowski CA, et al. Neurosarcoidosis masquerading as glioma of the optic chiasm in a child. *Postgrad Med J* 1995;71:265–268.

65. Leiba H, Siatkowski RM, Culbertson WW, et al. Neurosarcoidosis presenting as an intracranial mass in childhood. *J Neuroophthalmol* 1996;16:269–273.

66. Pattishall EN, Kendig EL Jr. Sarcoidosis in children. *Pediatr Pulmonol* 1996;22:195–203

67. Basdemir D, Clarke W, Rogol AD. Growth hormone deficiency in a child with sarcoidosis. *Clin Pediatr* 1999;38:315–316

68. Konrad D, Gartenmann M, Martin E, et al. Central diabetes insipidus as the first manifestation of neurosarcoidosis in a 10-year-old girl. *Horm Res* 2000;54:98–100.

69. Martini A, Serenella Scotta M, Magarini U. Sarcoidose granulomateuse des reins avec insuffisance renale chez une fille de douze ans. *Nephrologie* 1980;1:117–119.

70. Stanworth SJ, Kennedy CT, Chetcuti PA, et al. Hypercalcaemia and sarcoidosis in infancy. *J R Soc Med* 1992;85:177–178.

71. Hoffmann AL, Milman N, Nielsen HE, et al. Childhood sarcoidosis presenting with hypercalcaemic crisis. *Sarcoidosis* 1994;11:141–143.

72. Morris KP, Coulthard MG, Smith PJ, et al. Renovascular and growth effects of childhood sarcoid. *Arch Dis Child* 1996;75: 74–75.

73. Herman TE, Shackelford GD, McAlister WH. Pseudotumoral sarcoid granulomatous nephritis in a child: case presentation with sonographic and CT findings. *Pediatr Radiol* 1997;27: 752–754.

74. Coutant R, Leroy B, Niaudet P, et al. Renal granulomatous sarcoidosis in childhood: a report of 11 cases and a review of the literature. *Eur J Pediatr* 1999;158:154–159.

75. Weinberg A, Ginsburg CM. Epididymal sarcoidosis in a prepubertal child. *Am J Dis Child* 1982;136:71–72.

76. Evans SS, Fisher RG, Scott MA, et al. Sarcoidosis presenting as bilateral testicular masses. *Pediatrics* 1997;100:392–394.

77. Sarigol SS, Hay MH, Wyllie R. Sarcoidosis in preschool children with hepatic involvement mimicking juvenile rheumatoid arthritis. *J Pediatr Gastroenterol Nutr* 1999; 28:510–512.

78. Lanjewar DN, Maheshwari MB, Lakhani SN, et al. Childhood sarcoid myopathy manifesting as joint contractures. *Indian Pediatr* 1996;33:128–130.

79. Celle ME, Veneselli E, Rossi GA, et al. Childhood sarcoidosis presenting with prevalent muscular symptoms: report of a case. *Eur J Pediatr* 1997;156:340–341.

80. Zsolway K, Sinai LN, Magnusson M, et al. Two unusual pediatric presentations of sarcoidosis. *Arch Pediatr Adolesc Med* 1998;152:410–411.

81. Rossi GA, Battistini E, Celle ME, et al. Long-lasting myopathy as a major clinical feature of sarcoidosis in a child: case report with a 7-year follow-up. *Sarcoidosis Vasc Diffuse Lung Dis* 2001;18:196–200.

82. Akiyama M, Wada Y, Ando K, et al. 11-year-old boy with sarcoidosis and generalized brawny induration of muscle. *Pediatr Int* 2002;44:93

83. Wright KW, Spiegel PH. *Pediatric Ophthalmology and strabismus.* New York: Springer, 2003.

84. Hegab SM, al-Mutawa SA, Sheriff SM. Sarcoidosis presenting as multilobular limbal corneal nodules. *J Pediatr Ophthalmol Strabismus* 1998;35:323–326.

85. Lennarson P, Barney NP. Interstitial keratitis as presenting ophthalmic sign of sarcoidosis in a child. *J Pediatr Ophthalmol Strabismus* 1995;32:194.

86. Ohara K, Okubo A, Sasaki H, et al. Branch retinal vein occlusion in a child with ocular sarcoidosis. *Am J Ophthalmol* 1995;119:806–807.

87. Hoover DL, Khan JA, Giangiacomo J. Pediatric ocular sarcoidosis. *Surv Ophthalmol* 1986;30:215–228.

88. Rodriguez GE, Shin BC, Abernathy RS, et al. Serum angiotensin-converting enzyme activity in normal children and in those with sarcoidosis. *J Pediatr* 1981;99:68–72.

89. Gedalia A, Shetty AK, Ward KJ, et al. Role of MRI in diagnosis of childhood sarcoidosis with fever of unknown origin. *J Pediatr Orthop* 1997;17:460–462.

90. Wakely PE Jr, Silverman JF, Holbrook CT, et al. Fine needle aspiration biopsy cytology as an adjunct in the diagnosis of childhood sarcoidosis. *Pediatr Pulmonol* 1992;13:117–120.

91. Weinreb RN, Tessler H. Laboratory diagnosis of ophthalmic sarcoidosis. *Surv Ophthalmol* 1984;28:653–664.

92. Gedalia A, Molina JF, Ellis GS Jr, et al. Low-dose methotrexate therapy for childhood sarcoidosis. *J Pediatr* 1997;130:25–29.

93. Shetty AK, Zganjar BE, Ellis GS Jr, et al. Low-dose methotrexate in the treatment of severe juvenile rheumatoid arthritis and sarcoid iritis. *J Pediatr* Ophthalmol Strabismus 1999; 36:125–128.

94. Akova YA, Foster CS. Cataract surgery in patients with sarcoidosis-associated uveitis. *Ophthalmology.* 1994;101:473–479.

95. Lardenoye CW, Van der Lelij A, de Loos WS, et al. Peripheral multifocal chorioretinitis: a distinct clinical entity. *Ophthalmology.* 1997;104:1820–1826.

96. Dana MR, Merayo-Lloves J, Schaumberg DA, et al. Prognosticators for visual outcome in sarcoid uveitis. *Ophthalmology* 1996;103:1846–1853.

97. Dobrin RS, Vernier RL, Fish AL. Acute eosinophilic interstitial nephritis and renal failure with bone marrow-lymph node granulomas and anterior uveitis. A new syndrome. *Am J Med* 1975;59:325–333.

98. Mandeville JTH, Levinson RD, Holland GN. The tubulointerstitial nephritis and uveitis syndrome. *Surv Ophthalmol* 2001; 46:195–208.

99. Gion N, Stavrou P, Foster CS. Immunomodulatory therapy for chronic tubulointerstitial nephritis-associated uveitis. *Am J Ophthalmol* 2000;129:764–768.

100. Levinson RD, Park MS, Rikkers SM, et al. Strong associations between specific HLA-DQ and HLA-DR alleles and the tubulointerstitial nephritis and uveitis syndrome. *Invest Ophthalmol Vis Sci* 2003;44:653–657.

101. Gion N, Stavrou P, Foster CS. Immunomodulatory therapy for chronic tubulointerstitial nephritis associated uveitis (TINU). *Am J Ophthalmol* 2000;129:764–768.

102. Bloch-Michel E, Nussenblatt RB. International uveitis study group recommendations for the evaluation of intraocular inflammatory disease. *Am J Ophthalmol* 1987;103:234–235.

103. Fuchs E. *Textbook of Ophthalmology.* Duane A, trans. Philadelphia: Lippincott, 1908:381–390.

104. Schepens CL. L'inflammation de la region de l'ora serrata et ses sequelles. *Bull Soc Ophthalmol Fr* 1950;73:113–124.

105. Welch RB, Maumenee AE, Wahlen HR. Peripheral posterior segment inflammation, vitreous opacities and edema of the posterior pole: pars planitis. *Arch Ophthalmol* 1960;64:540–549.

106. Nussenblatt RB, Whitcup SM, Palestine AG. Intermediate uveitis. In: *Uveitis. Fundamentals and clinical practice,* 2nd ed. St. Lois, Mosby, 1996:279–288.

107. Foster CS, Vitale AT. Diagnosis and treatment of uveitis. Philadelphia: W.B. Saunders Company, 2002;844–855.

108. Augsberger JJ, Annesley WH, Sergott RC, et al. Familial pars planitis. *Ann Ophthalmol* 1981;13:553–557.

109. Culbertson WW, Giles CL, West C, et al. Familial pars planitis. *Retina* 1983;3:179–181.

110. Doft BH. Pars planitis in identical twins. *Retina* 1983;3:32–33.

111. Duinkerke-Eorela KU, Pinkers A, Cruysberg JRM. Pars planitis in father and son. *Ophthalmic Pediatr Genet* 1990;11: 305–308

112. Giles CL, Tranton JH. Peripheral uveitis in three children of one family. *J Pediatr Ophthalmol Strabismus* 1980;17:297–299.

113. Hogan MJ, Kimura SJ, O'Connor GR. Peripheral retinitis and chronic cyclitis in children. *Trans Ophthalmol Soc U K* 1965;85:39–51.

114. Kimura SJ, Hogan MJ. Chronic cyclitis. *Trans Am Ophthalmol Soc* 1963;61:397–413.

115. Wetzig RP, Chan CC, Nussenblatt RB, et al. Clinical and immunopathological studies of pars planitis in a family. *Br J Ophthalmol* 1988;72:5–10.

116. Tejada P, Sanz A, Criado D. Pars planitis in a family. *Int Ophthalmol* 1994;18:111–113.

117. Lee AG. Familial pars planitis. *Ophthalmic Genet* 1995; 16:17–19.

118. Weiss MJ, Hofeldt A. Intermediate uveitis. In: Gallin P, ed. *Pediatric ophthalmology. A clinical guide.* New York: Thieme, 2000;223–224.

119. Guest S, Funkhouser E, Lightman S. Pars planitis: a comparison of childhood onset and adult onset disease. *Clin Exp Ophthalmol* 2001;29:81–84.

120. Giles CL. In: Nelson LB, Harley RD, eds. Harley's Pediatric *Ophthalmology.* Philadelphia: WB Saunders, 1998;303–305.

121. Pederson JE, Kenyon KR, Green WR, et al. Pathology of pars planitis. *Am J Ophthalmol* 1978;86:762–764.

122. Deane JS, Rosenthal AR. Course and complications of intermediate uveitis. *Acta Ophthalmol Scand* 1997;75:82–84.

123. Henderly DE, Haymond RS, Rao NS, et al. The significance of the pars plana exudate in pars planitis. *Am J Ophthalmol* 1987;103:669–671.

124. Smith RE, Godfrey WA, Kimura. Complications of chronic cyclitis. *Am J Ophthalmol* 1976;82:277–282.

125. Davis JL, Palestine AG, Nussenblatt RB. Neovascularization in uveitis. *Ophthalmology* 1988;95:171.

126. Lauer AK, Smith JR, Robertson JE, et al. Vitreous hemorrhage is a common complication of pediatric pars planitis. *Ophthalmology* 2002;109:95–98.

127. Khodadoust AA, Attarzadeh A. Presumed autoimmune corneal endotheliopathy. *Am J Ophthalmol* 1982;93:718–722.

128. Pivetti-Pezzi P, Tamburi S. Pars planitis and autoimmune endotheliopathy. *Am J Ophthalmol* 1987;104:311–312.

129. Tessler HH. Pars planitis and autoimmune endotheliopathy. *Am J Ophthalmol* 1987;103:599.

130. Malinowski SM, Pulido JS, Folk JC. Long term visual outcome and complications associated with pars planitis. *Ophthalmology* 1993;100:818–824.

131. Giles CL. Pediatric intermediate uveitis. *J Pediatr Ophthalmol Strabismus* 1989;26:136–139.

132. Godfrey WA, Smith RE, Kimura SJ. Chronic cyclitis: corticosteroid therapy. *Trans Am Ophthalmol Soc* 1976;74:178–188.

133. Schlote T, Zierhut M. Ocular hypertension and glaucoma associated with scleritis and uveitis: aspects of epidemiology, pathogenesis, and therapy. *Dev Ophthalmol* 1999;30:91–109.

134. Perkins ES. Patterns of uveitis in children. *Br J Ophthalmol* 1966;50:169–185.

135. Bec P, Arne JL, Philippot V, et al. L'uveo-retinite basale at les autres inflammations de la peripherie retinienne. *Arch Ophthalmol (Paris)* 1977;37:169–196.

136. Pruett RC, Brockhurst RJ, Letts NF. Fluorescein angiography of peripheral uveitis. *Am J Ophthalmol* 1974;77:448–453.

137. Pollack AL, McDonald HR, Johnson RN, et al. Peripheral retinoschisis and exudative retinal detachment in pars planitis. *Retina* 2002;22:719–724.

138. Brockhurst RJ, Shepens CL, Okamura ID. Uveitis. II Peripheral uveitis: clinical description, complications and differential diagnosis. *Am J Ophthalmol* 1960; 49:1257–1266.

139. Weinberg DV, Lyon AT, Greenwald MJ, et al. Rhegmatogenous retinal detachments in children: risk factors and surgical outcomes. *Ophthalmology* 2003;110:1708–1713.

140. Brockhurst RJ, Schepens CL. Uveitis. IV. Peripheral uveitis: the complications of retinal detachment. *Arch Ophthalmol* 1968;80:747–753.

141. Schenk F, Böke W. Fluorenzenzangiographische Befunde bei intermediäree Uveitis. *Klin Mbl Augenheilkd* 1988;193:261–265.

142. Aaberg TM. The enigma of pars planitis. *Am J Ophthalmol* 1987;828–830.

143. Chester GH, Blach RK, Cleary PE. Inflammation in the region of the vitreous base: pPars planitis. *Trans Ophthalmol Soc U K* 1976;96:151–157.

144. Prieto JF, Dios E, Gutierrez JM, et al. Pars planitis: epidemiology, treatment, and association with multiple sclerosis. *Ocul Immunol Inflamm* 2001;9:93–102.

145. Potter MJ, Myckatyn SO, Maberley AL, et al. Vitrectomy for pars planitis complicated by vitreous hemorrhage: visual outcome and long-term follow-up. *Am J Ophthalmol* 2001; 131:514–515.

146. Opremcak EM, Cowans AB, Orosz CG, et al. Enumeration of autoreactive helper T lymphocytes in uveitis. *Invest Ophthalmol Vis Sci* 1991;32:2561–2567.

147. Tang WM, Pulido JS, Eckels DD, et al. The association of HLA-DR15 and intermediate uveitis. *Am J Ophthalmol* 1997;123:70–75.

148. Raja SC, Jabs DA, Dunn JP, et al. Pars planitis: Clinical features and class II HLA associations. *Ophthalmology* 1999;106:594–599.

149 Fredericksen JL, Madsen HO, Ryder LP, et al. HLA typing in acute optic neuritis. Relation to multiple sclerosis and magnetic resonance imaging findings. *Arch Neurol* 1997;54:76–80.

150. Oruc S, Duffy BF, Mohanakumar T, et al. The association of HLA class II with pars planitis. *Am J Ophthalmol* 2001; 131:657–659.

151. Malinowski SM, Pulido JS, Goeken NE, et al. The association of HLA-B8, B51, DR2, and multiple sclerosis in pars planitis. *Ophthalmology* 1993;100:1199–1205.

152. Martin T, Weber M, Schmitt C, et al. Association of intermediate uveitis with HLA-A28: Definition of a new systemic syndrome? *Graefes Arch Clin Exp Ophthalmol* 1995;233:269–274.

153. Bora NS, Bora PS, Kaplan HJ. Identification, quantification, and purification of a 36 kda circulating protein associated with active pars planitis. *Invest Ophthalmol Vis Sci* 1996; 37:1870–1876.

154. Bora NS, Bora PS, Tandhasetti MT, et al. Molecular cloning, sequencing, and expression of the 36 kda protein present in pars planitis. *Invest Ophthalmol Vis Sci* 1996;37:1877–1883.

155. Green WR, Kincaid MC, Michels RG, et al. Pars planitis. *Trans Am Ophthalmol Soc UK* 1981;101:361–367.

156. Abu El-Asrar AM, Geboes K. An immunohistochemical study of the "snowbank" in a case of pars planitis. *Ocul Immunol Inflamm* 2002;10:117–123.

157. Biousse V, Trichet C, Bloch-Michel E, et al. Multiple sclerosis associated with uveitis in two large clinic-based series. *Neurology* 1999;52:179–181.

158. Towler HM, Lightman S. Symptomatic intraocular inflammation in multiple sclerosis. *Clin Exp Ophthalmol* 2000;28:97–102.

159. Rucker CW. Sheathing of the retinal veins in multiple sclerosis. *Proc Staff Meet Mayo Clin* 1944;19:176–178.

160. Engell T. Neurological disease activity in multiple sclerosis patients with periphlebitis retinae. *Acta Neurol Scand* 1986; 73:168–172.

161. Breger BC, Leopold IH. The incidence of uveitis in multiple sclerosis. *Am J Ophthalmol* 1966;62:540–545.

162. Giles CL. Peripheral uveitis in patients with multiple sclerosis. *Am J Ophthalmol* 1970;70:17–19.

163. Porter R. Uveitis in association with multiple sclerosis. *Br J Ophthalmol* 1972;56:478–481.

164. Bamford CR, Ganley JP, Sibley WA, et al. Uveitis, perivenous sheathing and multiple sclerosis. *Neurology* 1978;28:119–124.

165. Arnold AC, Pepose JS, Helper RS, et al. Retinal periphlebitis and retinitis in multiple sclerosis: pathologic characteristics. *Ophthalmology* 1984;91:255–262.

166. Zierhut M, Foster CS. Multiple sclerosis, sarcoidosis, and other diseases in patients with pars planitis. *Dev Ophthalmol* 1992; 23:41–47.

167. Landers PH. Vitreous lesions in Boeck's sarcoid. *Am J Ophthalmol* 1949;32:1740–1741.

168. Crick RP. Ocular sarcoidosis. *Trans Ophthalmol Soc U K* 1955;75:189–206.

169. Jabs DA, Johns CJ. Ocular involvement in chronic sarcoidosis. *Am J Ophthalmol* 1990;97:1281–1287.

170. Cunningham ET, Demetrius R, Frieden IJ, et al. Vogt-Koyanagi-Harada syndrome in a 4-year-old child. *Am J Ophthalmol* 1995;5:675–677.

171. Perkins ES. Pattern of uveitis in children. *Br J Ophthalmol* 1966;50:169–185.

172. Burke MJ, Rennebohm RM. Eye involvement in Kawasaki disease. *J Pediatr Ophthalmol Strabismus* 1981;18:7–11.

173. Adamantiades B. *A case of recurrent hypopyon iritis.* Medical Society of Athens, 1930:586–593.

174. Adamantiades B. Sur un cas d'iritis a hypopyon recidivante. *Ann Ocul* 1931;168:271–274.

175. Behçet M. Uber reziviriende aphtose, durch ein Virus verursachte Geschwure am Mud, am Auge und an den Genitalien. *Derm Wochenschr* 1937;36:1152–1157.

176. Foster CS, Vitale AT. *Diagnosis and treatment of uveitis.* Philadelphia: WB Saunders, 2002.

177. Hamuryudan V, Yurdakul S, Ozbakir F, et al. Monozygotic twins concordant for Behçet's syndrome. *Arthritis Rheum* 1991;34:1071–1072.

178. Palimeris G, Papakonstantinou P, Mantas M. The Adamantiades-Behçet's syndrome in Greece. In: Saari KM, ed. *Uveitis update.* Amsterdam: Excerpta Medica, 1984:321.

179. Stewart B. Genetic analysis of families of patients with Behçet's syndrome: data incompatible with autosomal recessive inheritance. *Ann Rheum Dis* 1986;45:265–268.

180. Yazici H. Behçet's syndrome. In: Klippel JH, Dieppe PA, eds: *Rheumatology.* London: Mosby, 1994.

181. International Study Group for Behçet's Disease. Criteria for diagnosis of Behçet's disease. *Lancet* 1990;335:1078–1080.

182. Yurdakul S, Gunaydin I, Tuzun Y, et al. The prevalence of Behçet's syndrome in a rural area in northern Turkey. *J Rheumatol* 1988;15:820–822.

183. Davatchi F, Shahram F, Akbarian M, et al. The prevalence of Behçet's disease in Iran. In: Nasution AR, Darmawan J, Isbagio H, eds. *Proceedings of the 7th APLAR Congress of Rheumatology.* Japan: Churchill Livingstone, 1992:95–98.

184. Krause I, Uziel Y, Guedj D, et al. Childhood Behçet's disease: clinical features and comparison with adult-onset disease. *Rheumatology* 1999;38:457–462.

185. Shafaie N, Shahram F, Davatchi F, et al. Behçet's disease in children. In: Wechsler B, Godeau P, Eds. *Behçet's disease. Proceedings of the 6th International Conference on Behçet's Disease.* Amsterdam: Excerpta Medica, 1993:381–383.

186. Kari JA, Shah V, Dillon MJ. Behçet's disease in UK children: clinical features and treatment including thalidomide. *Rheumatology* 2001;40:933–938.

187. Sakane T, Suzuki N, Ueda Y, et al. Analysis of interleukin-2 activity in patients with Behçet's disease. Ability of T cells to produce and respond to interleukin-2. *Arthritis Rheum* 1986;29:371–378.

188. Krause I, Uziel Y, Guedj D, et al. Mode of presentation and multisystem involvement in Behçet's disease: the influence of sex and age of disease onset. *J Rheumatol* 1998;25:1566–1569.

189. Lang BA, Laxer RM, Thorner P, et al. Pediatric onset of Behçet's syndrome with myositis: case report and literature review illustrating unusual features. *Arthritis Rheum* 1990;33:418–425.

190. Kone PI, Bernard JL. Behçet's disease in children in France. *Arch Fr Pediatr* 1993;50:561–565.

191. Kone-Paut I, Yurdakul S, Bahabri SA, et al. Clinical features of Behçet's disease in children: an international collaborative study of 86 cases. *J Pediatr* 1998;132:721–725.

192. James DG. Behçet's syndrome. *N Engl J Med* 1979;301:431–432.

193. Mizuki N, Ohno S, Tanaka H, et al. Association of HLA-B51 and lack of association of class II alleles with Behçet's disease. *Tissue Antigens* 1992;40:22–30.

194. Hasan A, Fortune F, Wilson A, et al. Role of gamma delta T cells in pathogenesis and diagnosis of Behçet's disease. *Lancet* 1996;347:789–794.

195. Suzuki Y, Hoshi K, Matsuda T, et al. Increased peripheral blood gamma delta+ T cells and natural killer cells in Behçet's disease. *J Rheumatol* 1992;19:588–592.

196. Sayinalp N, Ozcebe OI, Ozdemir O, et al. Cytokines in Behçet's disease. *J Rheumatol* 1996;23:321–322.

197. al-Dalaan A, al-Sedairy S, al-Balaa S, et al. Enhanced interleukin 8 secretion in circulation of patients with Behçet's disease. *J Rheumatol* 1995;22:904–907.

198. Hamzaoui K, Hamza M, Ayed K. Production of TNF-alpha and IL-1 in active Behçet's disease. *J Rheumatol* 1990;17:1428–1429.

199. Raziuddin S, al-Dalaan A, Bahabri S, et al. Divergent cytokine production profile in Behçet's disease. Altered Th1/Th2 cell cytokine pattern. *J Rheumatol* 1998;25:329–333.

200. Yazici H, Hekim N, Ozbakir F, et al. Von Willebrand factor in Behçet's syndrome. *J Rheumatol* 1987;14:305–306.

201. Ohno S, Ohguchi M, Hirose S, et al. Close association of HLA-Bw51 with Behçet's disease. *Arch Ophthalmol* 1982;100:1455–1458.

202. Numaga J, Matsuki K, Mochizuki M, et al. An HLA-D region restriction fragment associated with refractory Behçet's disease. *Am J Ophthalmol* 1988;15;105:528–533.

203. Lehner T, Barnes CG. Criteria for diagnosis and classification of Behçet's syndrome. In: Lehner T Barnes CG,eds. *Behçet's syndrome: clinical and immunological features.* London: Academic Press, 1979:1–9.

204. Walker WA, Durie PR, Hamilton JR, et al. *Pediatric gastrointestinal disease*, 3rd ed. New York: BC Decker, 2000.

205. Koumantaki Y, Stavropoulos C, Spyropoulou M, et al. HLA-B*5101 in Greek patients with Behçet's disease. *Hum Immunol* 1998;59:250–255.

206. Picco P, Porfirio B, Gattorno M, et al. MICA gene polymorphisms in an Italian paediatric series of juvenile Behçet's disease. *Int J Mol Med* 2002;10:575–578.

207. Chun SI, Su WP, Lee S, et al. Erythema nodosum-like lesions in Behçet's syndrome: a histopathologic study of 30 cases. *J Cutan Pathol* 1989;16:259–265.

208. Kienbaum S, Zouboulis ChC, Waibel M, et al. Chemotactic neutrophilic vasculitis: a new histopathological pattern of vasculitis found in mucocutaneous lesions of patients with Adamantiades-Behçet's disease. In: Wechsler B, Godeau P (eds) *Behçet's disease.* Amsterdam: Excerpta Medica, 1993: 337–341.

209. Shikano S. Ocular pathology of Behçet's Syndrome. In: Moracelli M, Nazzaro P, eds. *International symposium on Behçet's disease.* Basel: Karger, 1966:111–1136.

210. Taylor PV. Autoimmunity and pregnancy. *Clin Immunol Allergy* 1988;2:665–695.

211. Stark AC, Bhakta B, Chamberlain MA, et al. Life-threatening transient neonatal Behçet's disease. *Br J Rheumatol* 1997 Jun;36:700–702. [Published erratum appears in Br *J Rheumatol* 1997;36:1032].

212. Ammann AJ, Johnson A, Fyfe GA, et al. Behçet's syndrome. *J Pediatr* 1985;107:41–43.

213. Sarica R, Azizlerli G, Kose A, et al. Juvenile Behçet's disease among 1784 Turkish Behçet's patients. *Int J Dermatol* 1996;35:109–111.

214. Mundy TM, Miller JJ III. Behçet's disease presenting as chronic aphthous stomatitis in a child. *Pediatrics* 1978;62:205–208.

215. Rakover Y, Adar H, Tal I, et al. Behçet's disease: long-term follow-up of three children and review of the literature. *Pediatrics* 1989;83:986–992.

216. Shafaie N, Shahram F, Davatchi F, et al. Iran's aspects of Behçet's disease in children: 1996 survey. In: Hamza M, ed. *Behçet's disease. Proceedings of the 7th International Conference on Behçet's Disease.* Tunis: Adhoua, 1997:125–129.

217. Pivetti-Pezzi P, Accorinti M, Abdulaziz MA, et al. Behçet's disease in children. *Jpn J Ophthalmol* 1995;39:309–314.

218. Treudler R, Orfanos CE, Zouboulis CC. Twenty-eight cases of juvenile-onset Adamantiades-Behçet disease in Germany. *Dermatology* 1999;199:15–19.

219. Kim DK, Chang SN, Bang D, et al. Clinical analysis of 40 cases of childhood-onset Behçet's disease. *Pediatr Dermatol* 1994;11:95–101.

220. Uziel Y, Brik R, Padeh S, et al. Juvenile Behçet's disease in Israel. The Pediatric Rheumatology Study Group of Israel. *Clin Exp Rheumatol* 1998;16:502–505.

220a. Lakhanpal S, Tani K, Lie JT, et al. Pathologic features of Behçet's syndrome: a review of Japanese autopsy registry data. *Hum Pathol* 1985;16:790–795.

221. Unal M, Yildirim SV, Akbaba M. A recurrent aphthous stomatitis case due to paediatric Behçet's disease. *J Laryngol Otol* 2001;115:576–577.

222. Conner GH. Idiopathic conditions of the mouth and pharynx. In: Bluestone CD, Stool SE, eds. *Pediatric otolaryngology*, 2nd ed. Philadelphia: WB Saunders, 1990:940–947.

223. Budin C, Ranchin B, Glastre C, et al. [Neurologic signs revealing a Behçet's disease: two pediatric case reports.] *Arch Pediatr* 2002;9:1160–1162.

224. Alper G, Yilmaz Y, Ekinci G, et al. Cerebral vein thrombosis in Behçet's disease. *Pediatr Neurol* 2001;25:332–335.

225. Yazici H, Tuzun Y, Pazarli H, et al. Influence of age of onset and patient's sex on the prevalence and severity of manifestations of Behçet's syndrome. *Ann Rheum Dis* 1984;43:783–789.

226. Baba S, Maruta M, Ando K, et al. Interstinal Behçet's disease: report of five cases. *Dis Colon Rectum* 1976;19:428–440.

227. Stringer DA, Cleghorn GJ, Durie PR, et al. Behçet's syndrome involving the gastrointestinal tract—a diagnostic dilemma in childhood. *Pediatr Radiol* 1986;16:131–134.

228. Kasahara Y, Tanaka S, Nishino M, et al. Intestinal involvement in Behçet's disease: review of 136 surgical cases in the Japanese literature. *Dis Colon Rectum* 1981;24:103–106.

229. Yim CW, White RH. Behçet's syndrome in a family with inflammatory bowel disease. *Arch Intern Med* 1985;145:1047–1050.

230. Nussenblatt RB, Palestine AG. Cyclosporine: immunology, pharmacology and therapeutic uses. *Surv Ophthalmol* 1986;31:159–169.

231. Yazici H, Pazarli H, Barnes CG, et al. A controlled trial of azathioprine in Behçet's syndrome. *N Engl J Med* 1990;322:281–285.

232. Mamo JG. Treatment of Behçet's disease with chlorambucil. *Arch Ophthalmol* 1970;84:446–450.

233. Nussenblatt RB, Palestine AG. *Uveitis: fundamentals and clinical practice.* Chicago: Year Book Medical, 1989:116–144.

234. Oniki S, Kurakazu K, Kawata K. Immunosuppressive treatment of Behçet's disease with cyclophosphamide. *Jpn J Ophthalmol* 1976;20:32–40.

235. Fain O, Du LTH, Wechsler B. Pulse cyclophosphamide in Behçet's disease. In: O Duffy JD, Kokmen E, eds. *Behçet's disease: basic and clinical aspects.* New York: Marcel Dekker, 1991:569–573.

236. Ozyazgan Y, Yurdakul S, Yazici H, et al. Low dose cyclosporin A vs. pulsed cyclophosphamide in Behçet's syndrome: a single masked trial. *Br J Ophthalmol* 1992;76:241–243.

237. Masuda K, Nakajima A, Urayama A, et al. Double-masked trial of cyclosporin versus colchicine and long-term open study of cyclosporin in Behçet's disease. *Lancet* 1989;1:1093–1096.

238. Whitcup SM, Salvo EC Jr, Nussenblatt RB. Combined cyclosporine and corticosteroid therapy for sight-threatening uveitis in Behçet's disease. *Am J Ophthalmol* 1994;118:39–45.

239. Sajjadi H, Soheilian M, Ahmadieh H, et al. Low dose cyclosporin-a therapy in Behçet's disease. *J Ocul Pharmacol* 1994;10:553–560.

240. Atmaca LS, Batioglu F. The efficacy of cyclosporin-a in the treatment of Behçet's disease. *Ophthalmic Surg* 1994;25:321–327.

241. Hayasaka S, Kawamoto K, Noda S, et al. Visual prognosis in patients with Behçet's disease receiving colchicine, systemic corticosteroid or cyclosporin. *Ophthalmologica* 1994;208:210–213.

242. Alison AC, Eugui EM. Mycophenolate mofetil (RS-61443): mode of action and effects on graft rejection. In: Thompson AW, Starzl TE, eds. *Immunosuppressive drugs: developments in anti-rejection therapy.* Boston: Arnold, 1994:141–159.

243. Larkin G, Lightman S. Mycophenolate mofetil. A useful immunosuppressive in inflammatory eye disease. *Ophthalmology* 1999;106:370–374.

244. Alpsoy E, Yilmaz E, Basaran E. Interferon therapy for Behçet's disease. *J Am Acad Dermatol* 1994;31:617–619.

245. O'Duffy JD, Calamia K, Cohen S, et al. Interferon-alpha treatment of Behçet's disease. *J Rheumatol* 1998;25:1938–1944.

246. Zouboulis CC, Orfanos CE. Treatment of Adamantiades-Behçet's disease with systemic interferon alpha. *Arch Dermatol* 1998;134:1010–1016.

247. Kotter I, Eckstein AK, Stubiger N, et al. Treatment of ocular symptoms of Behçet's disease with interferon alpha 2a: a pilot study. *Br J Ophthalmol* 1998;82:488–494.

248. Raizman MB, Foster CS. Plasma exchange in the therapy of Behçet's disease. *Graefes Arch Clin Exp Ophthalmol* 1989;227:360–363.

249. Larkin G, Lightman S. Mycophenolate mofetil: a useful immunosuppressive in inflammatory eye diseases. *Ophthalmology* 1999;106:370–374.

250. Calguneri M, Kiraz S, Ertenli I, et al. The effect of prophylactic penicillin treatment on the course of arthritis episodes in patients with Behçet's disease. A randomized clinical trial. *Arthritis Rheum* 1996;39:2062–2065.

251. Gardner-Medwin JM, Smith NJ, et al. Clinical experience with thalidomide in the management of severe oral and genital ulceration in conditions such as Behçet's disease: use of neurophysiological studies to detect thalidomide neuropathy. *Ann Rheum Dis* 1994;53:828–832.

252. Givner I. Malignant lymphoma with ocular involvement: a clinicopathologic report. *Am J Ophthalmol* 1955;39:29–32.

253. Klingele TG, Hogan MJ. Ocular reticulum cell sarcoma. *Am J Ophthalmol* 1975;79:39–47.

254. Qualman SJ, Mendelsohn G, Mann RB, et al. Intraocular lymphomas: natural history based on a clinicopathologic study of eight cases and review of the literature. *Cancer* 1983;52:878–886.

255. Hoang-Xuan T, Bodaghi B, Toublanc M, et al. Scleritis and mucosal-associated lymphoid tissue lymphoma: a new masquerade syndrome. *Ophthalmology* 1996;103:631–635.

256. Kincaid MC, Green WR. Ocular and orbital involvement in leukemia. *Surv Ophthalmol* 1983;27:211–232.

257. Kuwabara R, Aiello LM. Leukemic military nodules in the retina. *Arch Ophthalmol* 1964;72:494–497.

258. Stafford WR, Yannoff M, Parnell BL. Retinoblastoma initially misdiagnosed as primary ocular inflammation. *Arch Ophthlamol* 1969;82:771–773.

259. Weizenblatt S. Differential difficulties in atypical retinoblastoma, report of a case. *Arch Ophthalmol* 1957;58:699.

260. Ellsworth RM. The practical management of retinoblastoma. *Trans Am Ophthalmol Soc* 1969;67:463–534.

261. Tahan SR, Pastel-Levy C, Bhan AK, et al. Juvenile xanthogranuloma: clinical and pathologic characterization. *Arch Pathol Lab Med* 1989;113:1057–1061.

262. Zimmerman LE. Ocular lesions of juvenile xanthogranuloma. Nevoxanthoendothelioma. *Trans Am Acad Ophthalmol Otolaryngol* 1965;69:412–439.

263. Harley RD, Romayanada N, Chan GH. Juvenile xanthogranuloma. *J Pediatr Ophthalmol Strabismus* 1982;19:33–39.

264. Thieme R, Lukassek B, Keinert K. Problems in xanthogranuloma of the anterior uvea. *Klin Monatsbl Augenheilkd* 1980;176:893–898.

265. Gass JDM. Management of juvenile xanthogranuloma of the iris. *Arch Ophthalmol* 1964;71:344–347.

18

WORLDWIDE CAUSES OF
CHILDHOOD BLINDNESS

CLARE GILBERT

This chapter describes what is currently known about the magnitude, distribution, and causes of blindness in children worldwide. It briefly describes some of the major blinding diseases, concentrating on those that are avoidable and emphasizing control at the population level rather than management of individual children.

DEFINITIONS

The definition of blindness in children used throughout this chapter is as follows: an individual aged 0 to 15 years (United Nations Children's Fund [UNICEF] definition of childhood) who has a visual acuity <6/60 (<20/200) in the better eye or a central visual field <10 degrees [World Health Organization (WHO) categories of severe visual impairment and blindness] (1). Although this definition can be readily applied to adults, it is more difficult to measure visual acuity and assess visual fields in young children, particularly in those with additional disabilities. This poses particular challenges not only for clinicians in the clinical setting but also for ophthalmic epidemiologists, who are interested in determining the prevalence of blind children in a community or in undertaking a clinical trial or longitudinal study. This definition also fails to capture the impact of visual loss on a child's functional abilities or quality of life.

EPIDEMIOLOGY OF BLINDNESS IN CHILDREN

Prevalence and Magnitude of Blindness in Children

Reliable population-based data on the prevalence of blindness in children are difficult to obtain for a variety of reasons. First, blindness in children is relatively rare, and there are many causes of blindness. Therefore, large sample sizes are required in cross-sectional surveys to determine accurate estimates of the prevalence of individual diseases.

Second, some industrialized countries keep registers of the blind, but it is difficult to obtain this information and keep it constantly updated. Third, birth defect registers do not use a functional definition of blindness. Last, information collected from health care facilities, social welfare organizations, or special education programs can miss some unregistered blind children and, therefore, is not always reliable.

In developing countries, these potential sources of data are generally not available. Other approaches that have been adopted include interviewing key informants, e.g., community leaders, kindergarten and school teachers, religious leaders, eye care workers, community based rehabilitation workers, and traditional birth attendants (2), with the advantage that a large population can be covered relatively quickly. Questionnaires to parents and caretakers have also been assessed. However, although this tool has good sensitivity and specificity for identifying children with physical and mental impairments, questionnaires do not reliably identify children with sensory impairments (3).

The available data suggest that the prevalence of blindness in children is closely related to the mortality rates of children younger than 5 years. The prevalence of blindness ranges from approximately 0.3 per 1,000 children in countries with low mortality rates of children younger than 5 years (i.e., <10 per 1,000 live births) to 1.5 per 1,000 in the poorest countries of the world that have mortality rates of children younger than 5 years exceeding 250 per 1,000 live births (4,5). Rates are higher in poor countries because (i) there are potentially blinding conditions, such as vitamin A deficiency, malaria, or use of harmful traditional eye medicines, which are not seen in affluent populations; (ii) there is inadequate control of preventable causes of blindness, such as measles infection, ophthalmia neonatorum, and congenital rubella; and (iii) there is inadequate management of conditions requiring optical or surgical treatment. Inadequate management occurs because children are not identified or referred, parents cannot afford the travel and care, or there are inadequately trained and equipped eye facilities to deal with conditions such as high refractive errors, cataract, and glaucoma.

Globally there are estimated to be 1.4 million blind children, almost three fourths of whom live in low-income countries (Table 18-1) (4). Given the variations in prevalence and population structure in countries, the number of blind children ranges from approximately 60 per million total population in high-income settings to 600 per million in the poorest countries (6).

Incidence of Blindness in Children

The rate at which new cases of blindness develop in the child population over time can be estimated from blind registers using new cases as the numerator and through active surveillance systems, such as that used by the British Ophthalmological Surveillance Unit (7). Active surveillance provides accurate incidence data, particularly when more than one source of ascertainment and capture recapture analysis with adjustment of estimates is used.

Estimates of the incidence of childhood visual impairment are available for only a few countries. Using pooled data from the Scandinavian visual impairment registers, the overall annual incidence of all levels of visual impairment was reported to be 0.8 per 10,000 individuals <19 years old in 1993. A recent national UK study reported the annual age group-specific incidence to be the highest in the first year of life (4.0/10,000), with the cumulative incidence, or lifetime risk, increasing to 5.3 per 10,000 by 5 years and to 5.9 per 10,000 by age 16 years (8). There are no data from developing countries, but a figure of 500,000 new cases annually throughout the world has been suggested (4).

Mortality in Blind Children

Many of the blinding eye diseases of childhood are associated with high child mortality. Some examples are chromosomal abnormalities, congenital rubella, prematurity, vitamin A deficiency, measles infection, malaria, meningitis, tumors of the eye and higher visual pathways, and metabolic diseases. It has been estimated that 50% to 60% of blind children die within a few years of becoming blind. This is particularly true of children who become blind from keratomalacia secondary to acute vitamin A deficiency (4). Even in industrialized countries, blind children have a high mortality rate, reported as 10% in the year following the diagnosis of severe visual impairment or blindness in the United Kingdom (8). This means that the prevalence data markedly underestimate the burden of blindness in children because these figures represent only the children who survive.

CAUSES OF BLINDNESS IN CHILDREN

Classification

In 1993 the WHO adopted a new system for classifying the causes of blindness in children. This system accounted for the major affected region within the visual system, i.e., whole globe, cornea, lens, uvea, retina, optic nerve, glaucoma, higher visual pathways, and underlying cause (9). The underlying cause accounts for the time of onset of the insult leading to blindness. Causes of blindness include (i) factors at conception (chromosomal abnormalities and genetic diseases); (ii) factors during the intrauterine period (i.e., infections, drugs, alcohol); (iii) factors during the

TABLE 18–1. ESTIMATED PREVALENCE AND MAGNITUDE OF CHILDHOOD BLINDNESS BY REGION (WHO/PBL, 1999)

World Bank Groupings	Children (Millions)	Prevalence of Blindness/ 1,000 Children	Estimates of Number Blind	Percentage of Blind Children
Former Socialist Economies (FSE)	78	0.51	40,000	2.9
Established Market Economies (EME)	170	0.30	50,000	3.6
Latin America and Caribbean (LAC)	170	0.62	100,000	7.1
Middle East Crescent (MEC)	240	0.80	190,000	13.6
China	340	0.50	210,000	15.0
India	350	0.80	270,000	19.3
Other Asia and Islands (OAI)	260	0.83	220,000	15.6
Sub-Saharan Africa (SSA)	260	1.24	320,000	22.9
Total:	1868	0.75	1,400,000	100

FSE includes eastern European countries and the former USSR; EME includes USA, UK, Japan, Canada, Australia, and Europe; MEC includes Islamic countries along northern Africa, the Middle East, Turkey, Iran, Iraq, Afghanistan, and Pakistan.
Adapted from World Health Organization. Preventing blindness in children. Report of WHO/IAPB scientific meeting. WHO/PBL/00.77. Geneva: World Health Organization, 2000.

perinatal period (i.e., prematurity, ophthalmia neonatorum); (iv) conditions acquired during childhood (i.e., measles, vitamin A deficiency, harmful traditional eye remedies, malaria); and (v) conditions of indeterminable time of onset. Examples of this last category include microphthalmos, which could have several different causes, and cataract, for which the cause is often unknown. The classification system can be modified to group conditions into those that are definitely prenatal and those that occurred after birth.

The new WHO-adopted system and the modified system both are useful, particularly in developing countries, where there is often limited information on the family history or past medical history and limitations regarding facilities for investigation and definitive diagnoses.

Causes of Blindness in Children

Information on the causes of blindness has been collected over the last 10 years using the WHO system. Almost 9,500 blind children have been examined in 35 countries (Tables 18-2 and 18-3) (10–14). Most of these studies have examined children in special education programs. This setting creates an inherent bias because not all blind children are enrolled in these programs. Nonetheless, in several settings, the causes of blindness in children in special education have been compared to causes in children identified in the community, and the findings are broadly comparable. Children with additional handicaps tend to be underrepresented in special education, leading to an underestimate of visual loss from lesions of the optic nerve and higher visual pathways (2,15).

The data on the causes of blindness in children have been applied to estimates of the magnitude of blindness. Retinal conditions are the single most common group causing blindness, followed by corneal scarring (Table 18-4). Of the estimated 380,000 children blind from retinal disorders (6), 40,000 are blind from retinopathy of prematurity (ROP). Other retinal conditions include hereditary retinal dystrophies and toxoplasmosis.

Regional Variation in Causes

Acquired corneal scarring predominates in poor communities, whereas lesions of the central nervous system (CNS) due a variety of causes are more important in affluent societies. In middle-income countries the picture is mixed; cataract, glaucoma, and ROP are important causes.

Cataract and glaucoma are important causes of blindness in children in all regions, particularly in poorer countries. Children in developing countries usually present late in the course of their diseases, so the outcome is compromised even with universally accepted management. In addition, specialist centers are few and far between, and surgery is often undertaken by general ophthalmologists who are not trained or experienced in the surgical management of children. There are also considerable barriers from the parents'

TABLE 18-2. REGIONAL VARIATION IN THE CAUSES OF BLINDNESS IN CHILDREN; DESCRIPTIVE CLASSIFICATION BY WORLD BANK REGION (%)

Region	Wealthiest Region				Poorest Region			
	EME	FSE	LAC	MEC	China	India	OAI	SSA
Number examined	None[a]	504	1,007	1,423	1,131	2,809	850	1,748
Globe	10	12	11	15	26	25	21	9
Cornea	1	2	8	7	4	27	21	36
Lens	8	11	7	19	19	11	19	10
Uvea	2	5	2	3	1	6	3	4
Retina	25	44	47	38	25	20	21	20
Optic nerve	25	15	12	8	14	7	7	10
Glaucoma	1	3	8	7	9	3	6	6
Other (including Central Nervous System)	28	8	5	3	2	1	2	5
Total	100	100	100	100	100	100	100	100

Data from 10,453 blind children.
[a] Data from published studies reanalyzed using WHO categories (1,683 children).
EME (Established Market Economies) includes USA, UK, Japan, Canada, Australia, and Europe; FSE (Former Socialist Economies) includes eastern European countries and the former USSR; LAC, Latin America and Caribbean; MEC (Middle East Crescent) includes Islamic countries along northern Africa, the Middle East, Turkey, Iran, Iraq, Afghanistan, and Pakistan; OAI, Other Asia and Islands; SSA, Sub-Saharan Africa.
Adapted from childhood blindness database held at the London School of Hygiene and Tropical Medicine from World Health Organization. Preventing blindness in children. WHO/PBL/00.77. Geneva: World Health Organization, 2000.

TABLE 18-3. REGIONAL VARIATION IN THE CAUSES OF BLINDNESS IN CHILDREN; ETIOLOGIC CATEGORIES BY WORLD BANK REGION (%)

Region	⟵ Wealthiest Region				Poorest Region ⟶			
	EME	FSE	LAC	MEC	China	India	OAI	SSA
Number examined	None[a,b]	504	1,007	1,423	1,131	2,809	850	1,748
Hereditary	45	18	22	54	31	23	27	20
Intrauterine	7	6	8	1	0	2	3	3
Perinatal	24	28	28	2	2	2	9	6
Childhood	10	5	10	6	14	28	14	34
Unknown	14	43	32	37	53	45	47	37
Total	100	100	100	100	100	100	100	100

[a] Data from published studies.
[b] Etiologic data not available for 72 children.
EME (Established Market Economies) includes USA, UK, Japan, Canada, Australia, and Europe; FSE (Former Socialist Economies) includes eastern European countries and the former USSR; LAC, Latin America and Caribbean; MEC (Middle East Crescent), includes Islamic countries along northern Africa, the Middle East, Turkey, Iran, Iraq, Afghanistan, and Pakistan; OAI, other Asia and Islands; SSA, sub-Saharan Africa.
Adapted from childhood blindness database held at the London School of Hygiene and Tropical Medicine from World Health Organization. Preventing blindness in children. WHO/PBL/00.77. Geneva: World Health Organization, 2000.

TABLE 18-4. MAJOR CAUSES OF BLINDNESS IN CHILDREN AND ESTIMATES OF NUMBERS AFFECTED BY ANATOMIC SITE

Anatomic Site	No. Affected	Percentage	Important Underlying Causes
Retina	380,000	27	Hereditary dystrophies, ROP, toxoplasmosis
Cornea	228,000	17	VADD, measles, HTEM, Ophthalmia neonatorum
Whole globe	237,000	17	Often unknown, hereditary factors
Lens	174,000	12	Hereditary, congenital rubella, unknown
Optic nerve	163,000	11	Trauma, infections, ischemia, tumors
Glaucoma	71,000	5	Unkown, may be familial
Uvea	52,000	4	Inflammation, hereditary factors
Other	95,000	7	Refractive errors, cortical blindness, trauma
Total	1,400,000	100	

HTEM, harmful traditional eye medicines; ROP, retinopathy of prematurity. VADD, vitamin A deficiency disorders.
Adapted from childhood blindness database held at the London School of Hygiene and Tropical Medicine from World Health Organization. Preventing blindness in children. WHO/PBL/00.77. Geneva: World Health Organization, 2000.

perspective, based on cost, fear, the difficulties of travel, and beliefs concerning the cause of their child's problems.

AVOIDABLE CAUSES OF BLINDNESS IN CHILDREN

The principles of prevention that can be applied to any impairment are given in Table 18-5.

Blind school studies performed in Africa, Asia, and Latin America indicate that 14% to 42% of all blind children have preventable conditions. An additional 16% to 33% of children have conditions that can be treated to prevent blindness or restore function. Overall, more than 40% of children are blind from potentially avoidable causes of blindness (4).

Major Avoidable Causes of Blindness in Developing Countries

The major causes of blindness in children in developing countries, such as sub-Saharan Africa and India, are those that cause corneal scarring: vitamin A deficiency disorders (VADD), measles infection, use of harmful traditional eye remedies, ophthalmia neonatorum, congenital rubella, and malaria.

Vitamin A Deficiency Disorders

The definition of vitamin A deficiency is not entirely straightforward and has recently been revised (16) to avoid the term *subclinically deficient*, which gives the misleading impression that this state is benign. The term *vitamin A deficiency disorders* (VADD) is now being used, reflecting the systemic nature and consequences of the deficiency state. Besides being a frequent cause of blindness in children in developing countries, clinical trials have provided conclusive evidence that VADD is also an important cause of child

TABLE 18-5. PRINCIPLES OF PREVENTION FOR ANY IMPAIRMENT

Primary prevention
- Prevention of disease *occurrence,* leading to a reduction in its incidence (e.g., measles immunization)

Secondary prevention
- Prevention of *impairment* by treating the disease, thus reducing the incidence of impairment (e.g., antibiotic treatment of infections, screening and treatment of threshold retinopathy of prematurity)

Tertiary prevention
- Restore *function,* thus reducing the prevalence of the impairment (e.g., surgery on a cataract blind child, rehabilitation to prevent disability)

mortality even in children who do not manifest characteristic eye signs (17). Current estimates suggest that 140 million preschool-aged children and more than 7 million women are vitamin A deficient and more than 10 million of these individuals have clinical complications (16).

Vitamin A is found as retinol in animal food sources such as breast milk, cheese, fish, liver, and eggs, and as carotenes and carotenoids in plant food sources such as mango, papaya, dark green leafy vegetables, and red palm oil (18). Approximately 95% of total body vitamin A is stored in the liver as retinal palmitate. Liver stores usually are sufficient for 6 months. Vitamin A is released from the liver as retinol bound to retinol binding protein and transthyretin (prealbumin) and is transported to tissues. In the eye, the 11-*cis* isomer of retinal (vitamin A aldehyde) combines with opsin to form rhodopsin in the photoreceptors. In somatic cells, retinol is converted to retinoic acid and is important in regulation of gene expression to maintain epithelial tissues and guide differentiation of a variety of other tissues. Thus, vitamin A is necessary for epithelial cell differentiation and growth, gene expression, immune responses, hematopoiesis, and organogenesis and is an essential component of rhodopsin.

VADD results from a combination of poor dietary intake, malabsorption (usually secondary to diarrhea and malnutrition), and increased tissue demand, such as caused by any illness. It is useful to think of the underlying causes of VADD as those that are distal, that is, the macroenvironment, and those that are proximal, such as household and individual factors. Distal causes include all interrelated factors that lead to poverty, such as inadequate education and health care systems, political instability, poor roads and communication systems, unfavorable climate and soil, lack of private landownership, and low prices for products in the international arena. Under these circumstances, the essential elements of primary health care are either unavailable or inaccessible, and income generation is challenging. Proximal causes of VADD at the household level include poor maternal education, inadequate water supplies and sanitation, overcrowding and large family sizes, and lack of land ownership. Malnutrition, measles, and diarrhea are the main factors that can precipitate a borderline deficient child into acute deficiency.

A low dietary intake of vitamin A–rich foods does not necessarily indicate that affordable vitamin A–rich foods are unavailable. Cultural practices, including inadequate breast feeding, traditional child feeding practices, and reduction of pro-vitamin A content by overcooking or sun-drying foods, can promote vitamin deficiency. Children born to women with low vitamin A status characterized by night blindness are also more likely to be deficient. Infants born to women with adequate vitamin A status will have adequate liver stores, but those born to women with inadequate vitamin A stores are unlikely to receive adequate retinol from breast milk (19).

In VADD, dedifferentiation of conjunctival and corneal epithelia leads to loss of goblet cells, squamous metaplasia, and xerosis of the conjunctiva and cornea (xerophthalmia). Bacterial action on deposits of keratin in the conjunctiva leads to accumulation of material that has a white, foamy, cottage cheeselike appearance. These accumulations, Bitot spots, usually are located at the temporal limbus and are pathognomonic of VADD (Fig. 18-1). Reduced photoreceptor rhodopsin causes night blindness and, occasionally, fundus changes in adults. Acute VADD can lead to corneal ulceration and necrosis called *keratomalacia* (Fig. 18-2). Conjunctival xerosis and Bitot spots are signs of longstanding VADD, found principally in children aged 3 to 8 years. Children most at risk for keratomalacia are those aged 6 months to 4 years, who may not have exhibited other features of xerophthalmia before the onset of corneal ulceration, but who frequently have protein energy malnutrition. Because not all children who are vitamin A deficient develop eye signs, it is important to be able to identify *communities* at risk. Children with xerophthalmia represent only the "tip of the iceberg" in that others in the community without eye signs are also likely to have vitamin A deficiency.

A simple, quick, and inexpensive way of assessing the vitamin A status of a community is to determine the prevalence of the different grades of xerophthalmia, particularly of Bitot spots, in children aged 6 to 72 months. The WHO has suggested minimal prevalence criteria to determine areas with a significant public health problem (Table 18-6) (20). The use of mortality rates of children younger than 5 years ("under 5 mortality rate") as a proxy indicator is now being recommended. Communities having an "under 5 mortality rate" >50 per 1,000 live births are highly likely to have VADD and countries with "under 5 mortality rates" in the range from 20 to 50 per 1,000 live births are considered at risk (16). In 1999, 75 countries

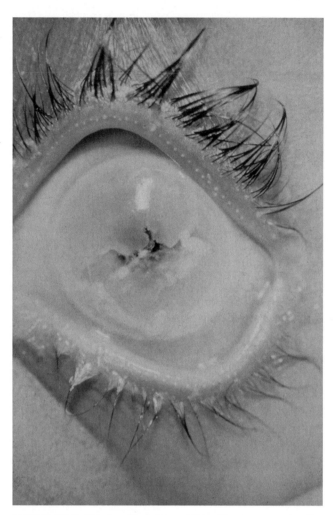

FIGURE 18-2. Keratomalacia in a child with severe, acute vitamin A deficiency disorder. (Courtesy of Allen Foster.)

had "under 5 mortality rates" of >50 per 1,000 live births (Table 18-7).

Corneal grafting in children, particularly penetrating keratoplasty, is always challenging, but in regions of the world where corneal scarring is a major cause of blindness, there are additional obstacles to be overcome. Children often come from the most disadvantaged families in the poorest communities and are unable to afford the surgical, medical, and optical treatments and follow-up care. Children often present late and are already densely amblyopic. Good-quality corneal material is rarely available, and surgeons are generally not trained in the specialized surgical techniques and postoperative care of children. Surgery is complicated by adherent leukomas and secondary cataracts. Corneal scarring often is accompanied by vascularization; therefore, grafting has a high rate of rejection. For all of these reasons, corneal grafting is not recommended as a priority for the control of corneal blindness in children in developing countries (21). However, optical iridectomy, or the creation of a large iridectomy to provide sight through an area of clear

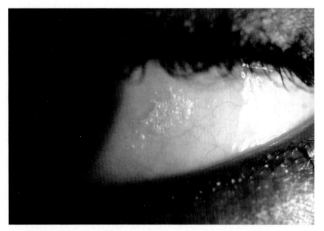

FIGURE 18-1. Bitot spot in a child with longstanding vitamin A deficiency disorder. (Courtesy of Clare Gilbert.)

TABLE 18-6. WORLD HEALTH ORGANIZATION CLASSIFICATION AND MINIMUM PREVALENCE CRITERIA FOR PEDIATRIC XEROPHTHALMIA[a] AND MATERNAL VITAMIN A DEFICIENCY AS A PUBLIC HEALTH PROBLEM

Definition (Code)	Minimum Prevalence (%)
Night blindness (XN)	
Children 2–5 yr	1.0
Pregnant women	5.0
Conjunctival xerosis (X1A)	—
Bitot spots (X1B)	0.5
Corneal xerosis (X2)	0.01
Corneal ulceration/keratomalacia <$^1/_3$ of surface (X3A)	0.01
Corneal ulceration/keratomalacia ≥$^1/_3$ of surface (X3B)	0.01
Xerophthalmic corneal scar (XS)	0.005
Xerophthalmic fundus (XF)	—
Serum retinol >0.70 μmol/L	15.0
Abnormal CIC/RDR/MRDR	20.0[b]

[a] All stages refer to preschool children except where noted.
[b] Provisional cutoffs above which community interventions may be warranted: CIC, conjunctival impression cytology; MRDR, modified relative dose response; RDR, relative dose response. Adapted from Sommer A, Davidson FR. Assessment and control of vitamin A deficiency: the Annecy Accords. J Nutr 2002;132 [9S]:2845S–849S.

cornea, can be very successful, restoring sufficient sight for independent mobility and sometimes for more detailed tasks.

Measles

The measles virus is highly contagious. Despite improved immunization coverage by the Expanded Program of Immunization, measles remains a leading cause of child mortality in developing countries Measles infection accounted for an estimated 850,000 deaths in 1999 or 10% of all childhood deaths (22). Overcrowded living leads to greater viral exposure and is believed to contribute to the severity of disease. This scenario is particularly seen in children in Africa, where the case fatality rate can be as high as 34% (23). African studies show that approximately 1% to 3% of children develop corneal ulceration following measles infections. Approximately one third of children with corneal ulceration had a recent measles infection, and up to 80% of children with corneal scarring reported a history of measles.

The pathogenesis of corneal scarring following measles is complex and is believed to occur from several mechanisms (24): (a) measles keratitis reduces corneal epithelial barrier function; (b) reduced cell-mediated immunity leads to sec-

ondary infections, including bacterial keratitis and herpes simplex keratitis; (c) exposure keratitis; (d) harmful traditional eye medicines, particularly in sub-Saharan Africa where measles infection is severe; and (e) acute vitamin A deficiency leading to corneal ulceration and keratomalacia. Because retinol is required for epithelial differentiation, measles imposes a huge demand on vitamin A stores because all epithelial tissues can be affected. Fever increases metabolic rate and the demand for retinol at a time when the child is ill and anorexic. Stomal herpes ulceration can make eating painful, and in many communities there are customs and taboos regarding diet for sick children. Often sick children are given "soup" made of the local carbohydrate only, without oil, vegetables, protein, or vitamins. Measles infection of the gastrointestinal tract leads to malabsorption and protein-losing enteropathy with loss of retinol blinding protein and retinol in the feces. Retinol is also found in the urine of children with measles. Thus, at a time when the child most needs high levels of retinol, the intake is low, absorption can be reduced, and there is increased loss in the feces and urine. A child who had borderline liver stores of vitamin A as retinal palmitate and normal serum retinol levels can develop severe, acute vitamin A deficiency, corneal ulceration, keratomalacia, and blindness. Clinical

TABLE 18-7. PREVENTION FOR CONTROL OF BLINDNESS DUE TO VITAMIN A DEFICIENCY DISORDERS

Primary prevention
- Poverty alleviation
- Improve water supply and sanitation to prevent diarrhea
- General literacy education of women
- Family planning programs
- Specific education on health and nutrition
  Improve the intake of vitamin A in children and women of childbearing age
  Promote breast feeding
  Appropriate complementary and weaning foods
  Home gardening
  Instruction on the preparation and storage of vitamin A–rich foods
- Fortification of commonly consumed foods
- Measles immunization programs
- Vitamin A prophylaxis of individual children at risk, such as those with measles and severe diarrhea
- Distribution of vitamin A to communities at risk. Vitamin A should be administered at 50,000 IU every month for 3 months for infants aged 0–5 months; 100,000 IU every 4–6 months for infants aged 6–11 months; 200,000 IU every 4–6 months for children aged ≥12 months; two doses of 200,000 at least 1 day apart postpartum (16).

Secondary prevention
- Vitamin A treatment, three doses given over 2 weeks, for all children with signs of xerophthalmia

Tertiary prevention
- Optical iridectomy (?corneal grafting)

TABLE 18-8. PREVENTION FOR CONTROL OF MEASLES-RELATED BLINDNESS

Primary prevention
- Measles immunization.
- Education to reduce the use of harmful traditional eye medicines

Secondary prevention
- Diagnosis and appropriate treatment of corneal ulceration with repeated high-dose vitamin A, antibiotics, and antiviral agents

Tertiary prevention
- Optical iridectomy (corneal grafting)

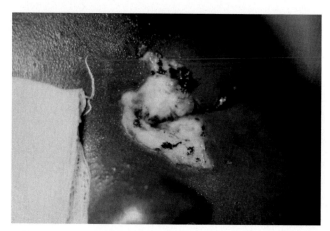

FIGURE 18-3. Lid burn in a Tanzanian child with measles as a result of hot oil administration. (Courtesy of Allen Foster.)

trials have shown that repeated high doses of vitamin A significantly reduce the mortality rate in children with measles. Vitamin A should be given to all children with measles, particularly those who live in areas where VADD is prevalent (Table 18-8) (25).

Harmful Traditional Eye Remedies

Animism is probably one of the oldest religious beliefs, that "a soul or spirit existed in every object, even if it was inanimate. In a future state this soul or spirit would exist as part of an immaterial soul. The spirit, therefore, was thought to be universal" (Alan G. Hefner and Virgilio Guimaraes). In animist societies, disease is believed to have several origins. These may be supernatural, caused by spirits or angered ancestors, result from breaking of taboos, or from the "evil eye" or witchcraft. They may arise as a result of conflict, tension, jealousy, or immoral behavior and can be passed down within the family, believed through the mother. Other origins are believed to come from personal weakness, eating unclean food, or showing disrespect to parents or elders. Remedies are based on these understandings. The WHO has defined traditional healing in the following terms: "the sum total of all the knowledge and practices used in diagnosis, prevention and elimination of physical, mental or social imbalance and relying exclusively on practical experience and observation handed down from generation to generation, whether verbally or in writing. Traditional medicine might be considered a combination of medicine and ancestral experiences. Traditional African medicine might be considered the sum total of practice, ingredients, and procedures that the African has used over time to guard against disease, alleviate suffering, and cure him/herself."

The use of harmful traditional remedies is an important cause of blindness from corneal disease in children in developing countries, particularly in the poorer countries of sub-Saharan Africa (10,24,26,27). These traditional remedies are widespread and can be initiated or used as part of cultural practices within the family or community or administered on the advice of traditional healers. However,

although some traditional practices are harmful, many are benign, (e.g., ritual bathing and dances), and some may even be of benefit, such as direct application of breast milk into the eye, steam baths, and inhalations.

There are several mechanisms whereby traditional remedies can lead to ocular damage and blindness. First, exposure keratitis can result from injury to the adnexa from chemical or thermal burns (Fig. 18-3) or when parents keep the eyes of their children held open, a practice in parts of West Africa believed to prevent blindness in children with measles. Secondary infection can occur. Second, mechanical damage can occur from the insertion of twigs, leaves, ground-up cowrie shells, or sap from plants that are acidic or alkaline. Mechanical damage predisposes to serious infections, including fungi if plant material is inserted. Third, fluids, such as urine or breast milk, can lead to severe infection if they come from an infected individual or a contaminated container. An extreme example is urine from someone infected with gonococcus placed onto a child's cornea (Fig. 18-4). Last, harm-

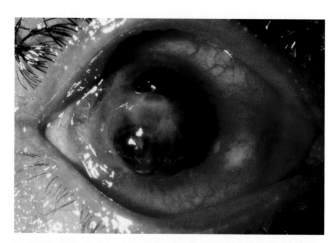

FIGURE 18-4. Gonococcal keratoconjunctivitis in a girl in whom urine was instilled as a treatment for seasonal epidemic conjunctivitis in West Africa. (Courtesy of Clare Gilbert.)

less traditional remedies can lead to corneal blindness indirectly, as a consequence of delay in seeking appropriate treatment.

The practice of traditional healing varies enormously among locales within the same country, and the tradition and remedies often are passed down within the family. Some healers develop and are known for specific areas of expertise. Even in settings where eye care services are available, members of the community often will consult the traditional healer first or even after seeing an eye care worker, because the traditional healer is a respected member of the community who shares local beliefs about the causation of disease (Table 18-9).

Ophthalmia Neonatorum

Ophthalmia neonatorum, defined as conjunctivitis within 28 days of birth, was an important cause of blindness in European children at the turn of the twentieth century. The introduction and widespread use of the Crede method of cleaning the lids immediately after birth, followed by instillation of topical silver nitrate solution, resulted in a dramatic decline in blindness even before antibiotics were available. Based on a few current studies, there are estimated to be several thousand new cases of ophthalmia neonatorum annually, principally in developing countries (29).

Ophthalmia neonatorum can occur from several different organisms, but the most important pathogens are *Chlamydia trachomatis* and *Neisseria gonorrhoeae*. Transmission of these organisms from infected mother to infant is reported to be 18% to 50% for *C. trachomatis* and 28% for *N. gonorrhoeae*. Despite recent public health measures, rates of chlamydial infection, particularly among teenage girls, is increasing in many countries in Europe and North America. Rates of sexually transmitted diseases in Africa, particularly that due to gonorrhea, remain high.

Ophthalmia neonatorum is still principally managed by the Crede method, but other agents have been shown to be effective. Clinical trials, undertaken in different settings,

TABLE 18-9. PREVENTION FOR CONTROL OF BLINDNESS DUE TO HARMFUL TRADITIONAL EYE REMEDIES

Primary prevention
- Good, affordable, accessible primary health and eye care services
- Health education to reduce potentially harmful practices
- Training programs for traditional healers to avoid harmful practices and to become part of the primary eye care system (28)

Secondary prevention
- Early diagnosis and appropriate treatment of corneal ulcers

Tertiary prevention
- Optical iridectomy (?corneal grafting)

TABLE 18-10. PREVENTION OF OPHTHALMIA NEONATORUM

Primary prevention
- Health education to prevent STDs
- Screening and treatment of STDs during pregnancy
- Ocular prophylaxis with 1% silver nitrate solution, 1% tetracycline ointment, 0.5% erythromycin, or 2.5% povidone iodine

Secondary prevention
- Prompt diagnosis and topical or systemic treatment with antibiotics appropriate to the organism and its susceptibility

Tertiary prevention
- None

STD, sexually transmitted disease.

have shown that 1% silver nitrate solution, 1% tetracycline ointment, or 0.5% erythromycin are equally effective against gonococcus. These agents have been recommended by the Canadian Task Force (30). In Africa, 2.5% povidone iodine solution was also reported to be effective (31), and this agent has the advantage of being easy and inexpensive to make in local eye drop production units. Treatment of affected infants requires awareness of specific guidelines on antibiotic susceptibility and availability (29).

The control of gonococcal ophthalmia neonatorum is a challenge in developing countries because the rates of sexually transmitted diseases in general and of penicillinase-producing *N. gonorrhoeae* in particular are high. In addition, most births take place outside health care facilities and are attended by trained or untrained traditional birth attendants or by family members (Table 18-10) (32).

Congenital Rubella Syndrome

Congenital rubella syndrome (CRS) is an unusual cause of blindness in industrialized countries because effective immunization programs are generally in place. However, rubella is still a potentially preventable cause of blindness in many other parts of the world and, for reasons that are explained in the following text, is likely to be underdiagnosed.

In large populations, epidemics of rubella infection occur approximately every 4 years. The frequency of infections is influenced by the number of susceptible individuals in the population, for example, those without protective immunoglobulin G (IgG) antibodies. CRS epidemics are rare and more devastating when they occur in small isolated communities. Factors that affect rates of seroprevalence include population density, geographic location, sex, age (rates increase with increasing age), and social class. The acquired disease is mild and can be subclinical. However, if a woman becomes infected during the first trimester of pregnancy, the developing fetus can be infected, giving rise to intrauterine death, premature birth, perinatal death, and a range of structural and functional abnormalities. CRS includes congenital eye disease, deafness, cardiovascular disease, microcephaly, and developmental delay. When infection occurs during the first 10 weeks of gestation, up to 90% of fetuses are affected, whereas when infection occurs after 17 weeks of gestation, only 3% of fetuses are affected. CRS can be confirmed by isolation of the virus, by polymerase chain reaction detection of viral ribonucleic acid, or by testing for rubella-specific immunoglobulin M (IgM) in the infant's serum or saliva. Because maternal rubella-specific IgG crosses the placenta, IgG cannot be used to confirm the diagnosis of CRS. Rubella-specific IgM antibodies, produced following congenital infection, persist for 3 months after birth in 100% of infants. Detectable levels decline thereafter. Therefore, confirmation of the diagnosis must be made before age 1 year, and antibody testing should be done within the first 6 months of life.

In the United States, an epidemic of rubella in 1963 resulted in an estimated 10,500 infants with moderate-to-severe CRS, 328 infants of whom have had follow-up. Ocular involvement occurred in 42%. Cataract occurred in 54%, microphthalmos in 31%, corneal opacity in 25%, and glaucoma in 15% of subjects (33). However, without a confirmatory test prior to age 1 year, these features cannot be absolutely attributed to CRS. A Jamaican blind school study, performed prior to the introduction of rubella immunization, showed that 39% of children were blind from cataract. CRS was implicated in almost half of these children. Approximately 25% of infants with cataract in Southern India and Bangladesh had positive rubella-specific IgM antibodies using a saliva antibody capture assay (34).

Strategies of immunization include selective targeting of females of childbearing age to protect future mothers. This strategy does not reduce the overall incidence of acquired rubella in children because it does not provide herd immunity. Herd immunity is the protection afforded to non-immunized individuals within a population having an adequate number of immunized individuals within the same population such that the spread of the infecting agent is impeded. Immunization of male and female children, aged 1 to 2 years, can confer herd immunity, providing coverage is sufficiently high. Another strategy is to immunize all infants and women of childbearing age who are seronegative. In the United Kingdom, immunization of girls aged 12 to 13 years was used from 1970 to 1988. This is the current policy in Sri Lanka. In 1988, the UK policy expanded to include immunization for mumps, measles, rubella (MMR) of all infants and selective immunization of seronegative women of childbearing age identified through screening. This approach, together with intermittent "catch-up" mass MMR campaigns, has been highly effective. The number of infants affected has fallen from approximately 200 to 300 per year to 4 to 5 per year, and the majority of cases currently seen is in women who entered the United Kingdom while pregnant.

The best strategy to adopt in individual developing countries warrants careful consideration. Even if infant immunization rates are adequate to prevent epidemics but are still lower than seropositive rates from naturally acquired immunity, the proportion of women of childbearing age who are susceptible to infection can increase. In this situation, more pregnant females would be at risk of infection, and, thus, there would be a greater chance of CRS. This scenario has occurred in Panama and more recently in Greece (35). The WHO has advised that information on the epidemiology of rubella be available prior to implementation of an immunization program in developing countries (36). This information is urgently needed in countries such as India, where MMR is given on an individual basis (Table 18-11).

Malaria

Following severe malaria in children, neurologic sequelae can lead to blindness. This cause of blindness is not encountered outside of the developing world. Malaria due to *Plasmodium falciparum* is the most severe form of malaria, manifested by severe anemia, hemoglobinuria from massive intravascular hemolysis (black water fever), cerebral malaria, and death. The primary burden of cerebral malaria is seen in children in sub-Saharan Africa, where 575,000 children younger than 5 years are estimated to be affected annually. Studies undertaken in Malawi and West Africa showed that children with severe and cerebral malaria can develop characteristic disc and retinal findings. These include papilledema, retinal hemorrhages, Roth spots, cotton wool spots, extensive areas of retinal pallor and edema, and retinal arteriolar and venular changes. Retinal hemorrhages have prognostic significance (37). The retinal features have been attributed to sequestration of red blood cells, often full of late-stage parasites and dehemaglutinized (38). The pathogenesis of cerebral malaria has not been fully elucidated. Findings support immune-mediated mechanisms and hypoxia as causes.

Cerebral malaria has a mortality rate of approximately 19%, even with appropriate medical and supportive treatment. Follow-up studies suggest that between 9,000 and 19,000 annual survivors have neurologic sequelae that persist longer than 6 months (39). If one assumes that

TABLE 18-11. PREVENTION OF CONGENITAL RUBELLA SYNDROME

Primary prevention
- Rubella immunization

Secondary prevention
- Early detection, referral, and management of children with cataracts

Tertiary prevention
- Visual rehabilitation and low-vision services

TABLE 18-12. PREVENTION OF MALARIA

Primary prevention
- Programs to control malaria (bed nets impregnated with insecticides and destruction of mosquito breeding sites)
- Prophylactic agents

Secondary prevention
- Diagnosis and treatment of infected children with effective antimalarial drugs and supportive measures such as blood transfusions

Tertiary prevention
- None possible

approximately 10% of children with neurologic sequelae are cortically blind, this represents between 1,000 and 2,000 new cases annually (40). Many of the children who are cortically blind following cerebral malaria have other serious neurologic problems and in this setting are likely to have a high fatality rate (Table 18-12).

Major Causes in Middle-Income Countries

The blinding eye diseases described earlier do not occur in most middle-income countries because the underlying conditions either are not prevalent or are well controlled. The major causes of potentially avoidable blindness include ROP and toxoplasmosis. In some countries, high rates of autosomal recessive diseases are a consequence of consanguinity.

Retinopathy of Prematurity and Prematurity

There is compelling evidence that blindness in children due to ROP is reaching epidemic proportions in several countries in Latin America and in the Former Socialist Economies (13,41): this has been termed the *third epidemic.* Recent estimates suggest that there are approximately 40,000 children blind from ROP throughout the world, 25,000 of whom live in Latin America. There are several possible reasons for this "epidemic." First, high rates of teenage pregnancy and low attendance at antenatal clinics are believed to increase the rates of premature birth. Second, although neonatal intensive care services are expanding, they are not always staffed by fully trained neonatologists and often have inadequate equipment and personnel for accurate monitoring of infants receiving supplemental oxygen (Fig. 18-5). Third, the population of infants at risk differs from that in western countries in that larger, more mature infants develop threshold ROP. Rates of threshold ROP tend to be higher for any given birth weight than in Europe and North America. Last, there are insufficient screening programs and a shortage of equipment and skilled personnel to treat infants who develop threshold ROP. Taken

together, these factors indicate that the population of infants at risk of threshold ROP is great, whereas resources for screening and treatment are inadequate. It seems likely that ROP will soon become a major cause of blindness in Asian children, particularly in urban settings, unless lessons are learned from the experience of Latin America and Eastern Europe. Indeed, large case series of infants treated for threshold and stage 5 ROP are reported from India (42).

To improve neonatal outcomes, particularly in middle-income countries and in urban settings in developing countries, screening programs need to be structured to suit individual populations of infants at risk. However, there are considerable costs. Decisions to equip and staff neonatal units and provide trained ophthalmologists must be made at the level of the policy makers and politicians and often place demands on scarce resources. Several ophthalmologists in Latin America have already expanded their screening criteria and are examining infants of larger birth weights and older gestational ages than currently screened in Europe and North America (at the same time, there is considerable debate about narrowing the criteria for screening in Europe and North America) (43). As a consequence, the number of infants being examined in Latin America has increased considerably.

In industrialized countries, the neurologic and ocular consequences of prematurity contribute significantly to childhood blindness and disability. However, there is little evidence that prematurity currently is responsible for much blindness in other regions of the world. This may be because survival rates of extremely premature infants, those at risk of ROP, are still relatively low and affected children are likely to have a high mortality rate (Table 18-13).

Toxoplasmosis

Ocular features of congenital toxoplasmosis include chorioretinitis, microphthalmos, cataracts, panuveitis, and optic atrophy (see Chapter 16). Blind school studies suggest that

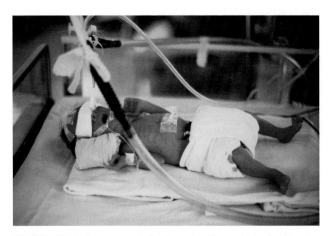

FIGURE 18-5. Premature baby in an incubator in Latin America given unmonitored supplemental oxygen. (Courtesy of Clare Gilbert.)

Primary prevention
- Prevent preterm birth (family planning, antenatal care)
- Provide excellent neonatal care (oxygen monitoring of infants)

Secondary prevention
- Screen all infants at risk (tailor inclusion criteria to the local population at risk)
- Prompt and local treatment of infants with threshold retinopathy of prematurity
- Follow-up and appropriate management of premature infants

Tertiary prevention
- Visual rehabilitation and low-vision services

the proportion of children blind from congenital toxoplasmosis is low, <1.0% in Europe, Asia, and Africa. However, toxoplasmosis is responsible for a significant proportion of blind children in Latin American countries, e.g., toxoplasmosis accounts for 11% in Colombia and Paraguay and 18% in Guatemala (data available on request from C. Gilbert).

Toxoplasmosis is caused by *Toxoplasmosis gondii*. It is similar to rubella infection in that the acquired disease in immunocompetent individuals usually is mild and self-limiting. As the infection resolves, latent cysts remain distributed throughout the body. In 0.3% to 3% of infected individuals, latent cysts in the retina and choroid reactivate and give rise to lesions that can threaten vision. Approximately two thirds of toxoplasmosis chorioretinitis is due to reactivation of acquired infection and one third is due to congenital infection (44).

Rates of infection during pregnancy largely depend on the rates of susceptibility in women of childbearing age. The susceptibility rates vary enormously between and within countries. For example, in Norway, 7% of pregnant women were reported infected, whereas in Brazil, 78% were infected. In France, the incidence of confirmed infection during pregnancy is 8 per 1,000 susceptible pregnancies. The prevalence of infection at birth is 1 per 10,000 live births in the United States and northern Europe, 5 per 10,000 in Poland, and 10 per 10,000 in France. Rates of transmission to the fetus and the risk of subsequent clinical signs such as hydrocephalus, intracranial calcification, and retinochoroiditis are dependent on the timing of infection. At 12 weeks' gestational age, the rate of transmission is 6%, whereas at term it is 80%. However, fetal damage is more likely when infection occurs early in gestation. Taken together, the maximum risk to the fetus occurs when infection occurs at 26 weeks' gestation. At this time point, the risk to the fetus is approximately 10% (45).

Features of congenital infection range from no symptoms to severe disease at birth. Severe complications include growth retardation, hydrocephalus, microcephaly,

intracranial calcification, seizures, jaundice, anemia, and fever. Ocular lesions such as chorioretinitis can be present in 10% to 15% at birth or can develop at any age, with up to 35% occurring by age 8 years. Only a few relatively small longitudinal studies have been undertaken. These suggest that fewer than 20% of infected infants develop chorioretinitis, and, of these, approximately 50% have macular lesions in one or both eyes that lead to unilateral or bilateral visual impairment.

The means to control congenital toxoplasmosis remains controversial. Sources of infection include contaminated soil, water, and food and probably vary from community to community. There is little evidence that health education targeted to women of childbearing age is effective in preventing infection during pregnancy.

Screening and treatment programs for pregnant women and for neonates are in place in several European countries. To assess the risk of postconceptional infection, serial serologic testing of pregnant women has been undertaken to identify women who either seroconvert or are positive at their first antenatal visit. Treatment to prevent mother to fetus transmission and to limit fetal damage depends on the stage of pregnancy at which seroconversion is detected. Generally, spiramycin is given early in pregnancy, and the more potent regimen of pyrimethamine, sulfadiazine, and folinic acid is given when infection occurs later in gestation when the risks of teratogenicity from medications are less. However, no clinical trials have been undertaken to assess the benefits and potential adverse effects of treatment. In addition, follow-up studies have given conflicting results (46), even after accounting for different medications and the gestational period during which the drugs were given. Fetal infection probably occurs within 2 to 3 weeks of infection, during the parasitemia, and before antibodies are detectable. Thus, any treatment might be too late to prevent fetal infection.

Neonatal screening aims to identify neonates with congenital toxoplasmosis, but because the majority of infected neonates have no clinical signs, screening depends on serologic testing. Treatment of infected infants includes pyrimethamine, sulfadiazine, and folinic acid for 6, 12, or 24 months. Although this regimen is potentially harmful, it is justified in infants with clinical disease. However, there is no evidence that treatment is of any benefit for subclinical infection. Therefore, screening healthy infants is of questionable value in the absence of reliable information from well-conducted clinical trials.

Antenatal and neonatal screening programs are costly and require amniocentesis, which has risks. For example, it has been estimated that 18 infants would be lost following amniocentesis for every one confirmed infection that would warrant treatment. Crude estimates of the cost of antenatal screening in France were approximately £32 million in 1992; in Denmark £3 million was spent on neonatal screening (45).

Major Causes in Industrialized Countries

In industrialized countries, lesions of the CNS contribute significantly to blindness, often in association with other impairments and disabilities. Fetal alcohol syndrome (FAS) is emerging as a potential preventable cause.

Lesions of the Central Nervous System

In the United Kingdom, 22% of newly diagnosed children were blind from lesions of the higher visual pathways in 1990, and another 20% were blind from optic atrophy. Studies from other European countries reported 15% to 54% of children were blind from CNS abnormalities. The high figure of 54% was reported from the study from Ireland, which included blind children identified in institutions for the multiply handicapped as well as those registered as blind (47).

In studies from European countries, CNS lesions were attributed to a variety of factors, including metabolic and genetic diseases, the effect of teratogens, intrapartum events associated with birth asphyxia, the consequences of prematurity, and postnatal events including tumors, trauma, and meningitis. Up to 59% of children blind from CNS lesions had additional impairments, most commonly cerebral palsy (CP).

Hypoxia resulting from intrapartum events (during labor) has frequently been recorded as the underlying cause of both CP and blindness. However, there now is considerable evidence suggesting that clinical indicators of birth asphyxia (low Apgar score and low umbilical pH) are poor predictors of neurologic abnormalities (48). In one longitudinal study in Australia, 8% of CP was attributed to intrapartum events (49). Longitudinal population-based studies have shown that the incidence of CP in infants of normal birth weight is relatively stable despite improvements in obstetric care. The underlying cause of CP in children of normal birth weight seems to be ill-defined events or processes occurring before birth that either cause cerebral damage or make the cerebrum more susceptible to damage during delivery.

The incidence of CP and visual loss is higher in children of low birth weight and in those born at or before 32 weeks' gestation (48). Periventricular leukomalacia and paraventricular and intraventricular hemorrhage are found in a higher proportion of preterm infants, particularly those with birth weighs <1,000 g. Infants at the boundaries of survival, i.e., born less than 26 weeks' gestational age, are at the greatest risk. Up to 37% have evidence of CNS injury (50). There is debate concerning the etiologic significance and interrelationships of prenatal, intrapartum, and neonatal events (51). Preterm birth, itself, can be a consequence of adverse intrauterine events and predispose the immature cerebral tissue to damage during birth and the neonatal period. There is some evidence that the survival of extremely low birth weight infants has increased over the last 10 to 15 years, although there also has been an increase in the rates of disability (50).

Fetal Alcohol Syndrome

Alcohol abuse during pregnancy can lead to FAS, which is one of the most common, preventable causes of mental retardation in children in the United States. FAS affects 1.9 of 1,000 live births compared to trisomy 21, which affects 1.6 of 1,000 live births. The diagnostic criteria for FAS are prenatal or postnatal growth retardation, structural or functional CNS abnormalities, and a characteristic facial appearance, which includes microcephaly, short palpebral fissure, poorly developed philtrum, and a flat maxilla. These features can present with varying levels of severity. Up to 90% of children with FAS have ocular signs, including optic nerve abnormalities in 48% (e.g., optic atrophy or optic nerve hypoplasia), tortuous retinal blood vessels in 49% (52), short palpebral fissure, broad telecanthic folds or ptosis in 50%, and strabismus in 40% to 50%. Less common signs include high refractive errors, microphthalmos, nystagmus, cataracts, and corneal opacities (Peter anomaly).

FAS occurs in 30% to 50% of children born to alcoholic women. The safe limit for alcohol consumption during pregnancy has not yet been clarified, but two alcoholic drinks per day is recommended as the upper safe limit. Some effects are caused by binge drinking, which is defined as the consumption of large amounts of alcohol on an erratic basis, whereas others are caused by chronic high intake of alcohol.

CHANGE IN MAJOR CAUSES OVER TIME

The causes of blindness in children reflect levels of development and health care provision. Therefore, it hardly is surprising that the pattern of causes changes over time in response to changes in the wider environment, in medical advances, and in the provision of services. Some notable examples include the increase in blindness from ROP in middle-income countries and the increasingly important contribution of prematurity and FAS in industrialized countries. In developing countries, the marked increase in measles immunizations and multisector initiatives to control micronutrient deficiencies, including vitamin A deficiency, have led to reduced childhood blindness from corneal scarring in many of the poorer regions of the world.

GLOBAL INITIATIVE FOR ELIMINATION OF AVOIDABLE BLINDNESS

The International Agency for the Prevention of Blindness is an umbrella organization of all the agencies, organizations, and professional bodies involved in eye care, prevention of blindness, and services for the blind. Together with the WHO, it has delineated priorities for the control of the major blinding eye disease by the year 2020 in a global initiative called *VISION 2020 the Right to Sight* (53). The control of blindness in children is one of the priorities of this initiative (4). The initiative embodies advocacy, resource mobilization, community participation, human resource development, placement of appropriate infrastructure and equipment, and implementation of cost-effective control strategies. The control of blindness in children is included as a priority not on the basis of the numbers affected, which are small in comparison to the number of blind adults, but because of the long-term impact and consequences of blindness in children (54).

At a recent landmark meeting of the 56th World Health Assembly, the following resolution was endorsed: Member States are urged "to commit themselves to supporting the Global Initiative for the Elimination of Avoidable Blindness by setting up, not later than 2005, a national VISION 2020 plan . . . to establish a national coordinating committee . . . to commence implementation of such plans . . . to include in such action plans effective information systems with standardized indicators and periodic monitoring and evaluation . . . to support the mobilization of resources for the elimination of avoidable blindness" (55). This endorsement of the prevention of blindness should lead to improved planning and effective programs and activities to control blindness in children. If the major avoidable causes of blindness can be controlled, there is a real possibility that the number of blind children in the world could be halved by 2020.

REFERENCES

1. World Health Organization. International classification of impairments, disabilities and handicaps: a manual of classification relating to the consequences of disease. Geneva: World Health Organization, 1980.
2. Bulgan T, Gilbert C. Prevalence and causes of severe visual impairment and blindness in children in Mongolia. *Ophthalmic Epidemiol* 2002;9:271–281.
3. Zaman SS, Khan NZ, Islam S, et al. Validity of the "Ten Questions" for screening serious childhood disability: results from urban Bangladesh. *Int J Epidemiol* 1990;19:613–620.
4. World Health Organization. Preventing blindness in children. Report of WHO/IAPB scientific meeting. Unpublished document WHO/PBL/00.77. Geneva: World Health Organization, 2000.
5. Gilbert CE, Foster A. Childhood blindness in the context of VISION 2020—the Right to Sight. *Bull WHO* 2001;79:227–232.
6. Gilbert C, Rahi J, Quinn G. Visual impairment and blindness in children. In: Johnson G, Minassian D, Weale R, et al., eds. *Epidemiology of eye disease, 2nd ed.* Edward Arnold Ltd.: London, 2003:260–286.
7. Foot B, Stanford M, Rahi J, et al. The British Ophthalmological Surveillance Unit: an evaluation of the first 3 years. The-British-Ophthalmological-Surveillance-Unit-Steering-Committee. *Eye* 2003;17:9–15.
8. Rahi JS, Cable N, British Childhood Visual Impairment Study Group (BCVISG). Severe visual impairment and blindness in children in the UK. *Lancet* 2003;362:1359–1365.
9. Gilbert C, Foster A, Negrel D, et al. Childhood blindness: a new form for recording causes of visual loss in children. *WHO Bull* 1993;71:485–489.
10. Kello AB, Gilbert CE. Causes of severe visual impairment and blindness in children in schools for the blind in Ethiopia. *Br J Ophthalmol* 2003;87:526–530.
11. Steinkuller PG, Du L, Gilbert C, et al. Childhood blindness. J AAPOS 1999;3:26–32.
12. Rahi J, Sripathi S, Gilbert CE, et al. Childhood blindness in India: causes in 1318 blind school students in 9 states. *Eye* 1995;9:545–550.
13. Kocur I, Kuchynka P, Rodny S, et al. Causes of severe visual impairment and blindness in children attending schools for the visually handicapped in the Czech Republic. *Br J Ophthalmol* 2001;85:1149–1152.
14. Reddy SC, Tan BC. Causes of childhood blindness in Malaysia: results from a national study of blind school students. *Int Ophthalmol* 2001;24:53–59.
15. Waddell KM. Childhood blindness and low vision in Uganda. Eye 1998;12:184–192.
16. Sommer A, Davidson FR. Assessment and control of vitamin A deficiency: the Annecy Accords. *J Nutr* 2002;132[9 Suppl]: 2845S–2850S.
17. Glasziou PP, Mackerras DE. Vitamin A supplementation in infectious diseases: a meta-analysis. *Br Med J* 1993;306:366–370.
18. West KP Jr, McLaren D. The epidemiology of vitamin A deficiency disorders (VADD). In: Johnson G, Minassian D, Weale R, et al., *Epidemiology of eye disease, 2nd ed.* Edward Arnold Ltd.: London, 2003:240–259.
19. Underwood BA. Maternal vitamin A status and its importance in infancy and early childhood. *Am J Clin Nutr* 1994;59[2 Suppl]:517S–522S.
20. IVACG Statement. The Annecy Accords to assess and control vitamin A deficiency: summary and clarifications. Washington, DC: International Vitamin A Consultative Group, 2002.
21. Vajpayee RB, Vanathi M, Tandon R, et al. Keratoplasty for keratomalacia in preschool children. *Br J Ophthalmol* 2003; 87:538–542.
22. World Health Organization. Vaccines and biological annual report 2000. *WHO/V&B/01.01*. Geneva: World Health Organization, 2001.
23. Aaby P. Malnutrition and overcrowding/intensive exposure in severe measles infection: review of community studies. *Rev Infect Dis* 1988;10:478–491.
24. Foster A, Sommer A. Corneal ulceration, measles, and childhood blindness in Tanzania. *Br J Ophthalmol* 1987;71:331–343.
25. D'Souza RM, D'Souza R. Vitamin A for treating measles in children. *Cochrane Database Syst Rev* 2002:CD001479.
26. Mselle J. Visual impact of using traditional medicine on the injured eye in Africa. *Acta Trop* 1998;70:185–192.
27. Courtright P, Lewallen S, Kanjaloti S, et al. Traditional eye medicine use among patients with corneal disease in rural Malawi. *Br J Ophthalmol* 1994;78:810–812.
28. Courtright P, Chirambo M, Lewallen S, et al. Collaboration with African traditional healers for the prevention of blindness. *World Scientific:* Singapore, 2000.
29. Moseley J. Ophthalmia neonatorum. In: Wormwald R, Smeeth L, Henshaw K, *Evidence based ophthalmology.* BMJ Books: London, 2004:71–80.
30. Canadian Task Force on the periodic health examination. The periodic health examination, 1992 update: 4. Prophylaxis for gonococcal and chlamydial ophthalmia neonatorum. *Can Med Assoc J* 1992;147:1449–1454.

31. Isenberg SJ, Apt L, Wood M. A controlled trial of povidone-iodine as prophylaxis against ophthalmia neonatorum. *N Engl J Med* 1995;332:562–566.

32. Costello A, Francis V, Byrne A, et al., eds. State of the world's newborns. Save the Children: Washington DC, 2001.

33. Wolff SM. Ocular manifestations of congenital rubella in a prospective study of 328 cases of congenital rubella. *J Paediatr Ophthalmol Strabismus* 1973;10:101–141.

34. Eckstein MB, Brown DWG, Foster A, et al. Congenital rubella in South India: diagnosis using saliva from infants with cataract. *Br Med J* 1996;312:161.

35. Panagiotopoulos T, Antoniadou I, Valassi-Adam E. Incidence of congenital rubella in Greece. *Br Med J* 2000;321:1287.

36. World Health Organization. Report of a meeting on preventing congenital rubella syndrome: immunization strategies, surveillance needs. *WHO/V&B/00.10.* Geneva: World Health Organization, 2000.

37. Lewallen S, Harding SP, Ajewole J, et al. A review of the spectrum of clinical ocular fundus findings in P. falciparum malaria in African children with a proposed classification and grading system. *Trans Royal Soc Trop Med Hyg* 1999;93:619–622.

38. Lewallen S, White VA, Whitten RO, et al. Clinical-histopathological correlation of the abnormal retinal vessels in cerebral malaria. *Arch Ophthalmol* 2000;118:924.

39. Murphy SC, Breman JG. Gaps in the childhood malaria burden in Africa: cerebral malaria, neurological sequelae, anemia, respiratory distress, hypoglycemia, and complications of pregnancy. *Am J Trop Med Hyg* 2001;64:57–67.

40. Brewster DR, Kwiatkowski D, White NJ. Neurological sequelae of cerebral malaria in children. *Lancet* 1990;336:1039–1043.

41. Gilbert C, Rahi J, Eckstein M, et al. Retinopathy of prematurity in middle-income countries. *Lancet* 1997;350:12–14.

42. Gopal L, Sharam T, Shanmugan MP, et al. Surgery for stage 5 retinopathy of prematurity: the learning curve and evolving technique. *Ind J Ophthalmol* 2000;48:101–106.

43. Lee SK, Normand C, McMillan D, et al. Evidence for changing guidelines for routine screening for retinopathy of prematurity. *Arch Pediatr Adolesc Med* 2001;155:387–395.

44. Stanford MS, Gilbert RE. Epidemiology of ocular toxoplasmosis. In: Petersen E, Amboise-Thomas P, eds. *Congenital toxoplasmosis.* Paris: Springer-Verlag, 1999:251–259.

45. Gilbert R. Congenital and perinatal infections: toxoplasmosis. In: Newell ML, McAuley J, eds. *Perinatal infections.* Cambridge: Cambridge University Press, 2000:305–320.

46. Wallon M, Liou C, Garner P, et al. Congenital toxoplasmosis: systematic review of evidence of efficacy of treatment in pregnancy. *Br Med J* 1999;318:1511–1514.

47. Goggin M, O'Keefe M. Childhood blindness in the Republic of Ireland: a national survey. *Br J Ophthalmol* 1991;75:425–429.

48. Paneth N. Birth and the origins of cerebral palsy. N Engl J Med 1986;315:124–126.

49. Blair E, Stanley FJ. Intrapartum asphyxia: a rare cause of cerebral palsy. *J Paediatr* 1988;112:515–519.

50. Hack M, Fanaroff AA. Outcomes of children of extremely low birthweight and gestational age in the 1990s. *Semin Neonatol* 2000;5:89–106.

51. Singha SK, D'Souza SW, Rivlin E, et al. Ischaemic brain lesions at birth in preterm infants: clinical events and developmental outcome. Arch Dis Child 1990;65:1017–1020.

52. Stromland K. Ocular abnormalities in the fetal alcohol syndrome. *Acta Ophthalmol Suppl* 1985;171:7–31.

53. World Health Organization. Global initiative for the elimination of avoidable blindness. *Geneva WHO/PBL/97.61.* Geneva: World Health Organization, 1997.

54. Gilbert C, Foster A. Blindness in children: control priorities and research opportunities. [Editorial] *Br J Ophthal*mol 2001;85:1025–1027.

55. World Health Organization. Report of 56th World Health Assembly. Available at: *http://www.who.int/gb/EB_WHA/PDF/WHA56/ea5626.pdfTables.*

CLINICAL ASSESSMENT AND MANAGEMENT OF RETINAL DISEASES REQUIRING SURGERY IN INFANTS AND CHILDREN

GENERAL SURGICAL CONSIDERATIONS IN INFANTS AND CHILDREN

MICHAEL T. TRESE
ANTONIO CAPONE, JR.

INFORMED CONSENT

Informed consent in the United States constitutes permission from the parent or legal guardian for the physician to perform both examination and surgical therapy. This consent should be obtained prior to any intervention. In the circumstance where parental consent is impossible, a court order can be obtained to perform the needed interventions.

There are many psychological issues that enter into both consent and need for surgical intervention in infants and children. Parents often feel both a responsibility to protect the child and a concern that they somehow may be responsible for whatever problem has affected the child. Most parents of children with known or established medical problems have learned to deal with these issues by the time they reach the vitreoretinal surgeon, but occasionally parents are seen for whom more sensitivity to these issues is necessary. It is rare that parents require psychological counseling, but this should be considered if the family is having difficulty coping with the issues of a child with severe ocular problems.

SURGICAL ANATOMY AND THE VITREORETINAL INTERFACE

The surgical anatomy relative to each vitreoretinal disease is addressed in the respective disease management sections in this textbook. However, some general considerations are important. Customarily, the size of the eye gives some insight into the severity of the intraocular disease. It is often true in bilaterally affected individuals that the smaller eye is the worse eye. Even eyes of 6-mm corneal diameters rarely can achieve visions as good as 20/200. However, it also is possible for small eyes to achieve visual acuities that are unexpected in eyes of that size. It often is helpful to advise parents of the possibility that one eye may be smaller than the other as the child ages. Another issue relative to the anatomy of the pediatric retina is that, in several dis-

eases, the retina is larger than the retinal pigment epithelial area. This anatomic occurrence leads to retinal folds that are radial or circumferential and that can be attached to the lens.

One of the most significant steps in vitreoretinal surgery in infants and children is selecting the location of entry into the eye. In eyes of children younger than 6 months postterm, particularly those with retinopathy of prematurity (ROP), the pars plana ciliaris may not be developed and, therefore, anterior entry is advisable (1). When performing lens-sparing vitrectomy in ROP eyes, we enter approximately 0.5 mm posterior to the limbus. In ROP eyes in which lensectomy is being performed, we enter through the iris root and into the lens anterior to the lens equator to avoid injury to any retinal fold in the posterior chamber. This also is true in diseases, such as persistent fetal vasculature syndrome, where the periphery may not be seen well and peripheral anatomic anomalies are often present. It is wise to err on the side of anterior entry in all surgical interventions involving infants and young children to avoid inadvertent retinal damage. We prefer using two-port vitrectomy in children and entering in the horizontal meridians at 3 and 9 o'clock. This allows good ability to view the retina superiorly and inferiorly, even in very small orbits. Entry into these locations does not cause damage to the long posterior ciliary nerves or vessels.

One of the most challenging parts of vitrectomy in infants and children is management of the vitreoretinal interface. The vitreoretinal interface consists of a very adherent posterior hyaloid that frequently, if not uniformly, cannot be easily peeled or perhaps peeled at all from the anterior retinal surface. Investigational enzymatic materials such as plasmin enzyme might prove useful for cleaving or weakening the vitreoretinal adhesion (2,3).

The vitreous of many dystrophic eyes, as well as eyes with ROP, is different than the solid vitreous of the term infant. The vitreous in ROP and dystrophic eyes is characterized by layers of solid and liquid sheets. These sheets can be separated from each other and frequently give the surgeon the false impression that they have peeled the hyaloid, when in reality the hyaloid remains along the retinal surface, or a schisis of the hyaloid occurs. It often is necessary to leave cortical vitreous along the retinal surface when performing vitreoretinal surgery in children and infants. In one series, it was shown that, after removal of subretinal neovascular membranes in younger individuals, redetachment rates and surgical results were not negatively impacted by leaving the cortical hyaloid in that setting (D. D'Amico, *personal communication, 2003*). In conditions characterized by progressive retinal dragging, such as ROP and familial exudative vitreoretinopathy (FEVR), it is our impression that removing the hyaloid may be desirable to minimize posterior segment distortion. However, hyaloid removal in children has increased risk of retinal tears, which are difficult to treat successfully.

SURGICAL TEAM

In dealing with extremely small infants, who often have young parents and come from poor socioeconomic settings, it is very important to adopt a team approach to their care. This frequently requires not only skilled retinal personnel, but also an anesthesiologist who is comfortable with the care of pediatric patients, particularly with very low birth weight premature infants. It also involves interaction with the pediatrician, neonatologist, social services, the pediatric ophthalmologist, vision therapist, vision teachers, and the school system. These patients are a challenge preoperatively, intraoperatively, and postoperatively, and all of the care must be coordinated in order to realize maximal development of the visual system. It is important to remember that these patients are "learning to see" at the time they are receiving surgical intervention. Care is taken to avoid adding to the amblyogenic issues, particularly with unilaterally affected infants. In addition, it is necessary to document that the patient's family has been told that they must interact with other members of the team caring for the child. This requires the surgeon interacting with the other members of the support staff by providing good communication of the child's structural findings and encouraging aggressive refractive and amblyopic care.

Frequently, the surgeon is asked to predict the visual potential of the child. This is an extremely difficult question to answer and is difficult to predict based on anatomic results alone. We have seen several children with extraordinarily distorted retinas, who had visual acuities between 20/20 and 20/60 (4). Conversely, we have seen children with excellent anatomic outcomes following surgery who have had no light perception vision. This supports the philosophy of aggressive refractive and amblyopic care until the child's visual potential can be determined, at approximately age 4 or 5 years. Working hard for low levels of vision is extremely important to the child and family as the child develops. The child with low levels of vision (20/1900 or less) usually is able to visu-

ally ambulate and functions at a much higher level than the adult with the same level of vision.

EXAMINATION UNDER ANESTHESIA

Evaluation of the child may be very difficult in an office setting. Examination under anesthesia (EUA) is extremely important for complete retinal evaluation of the far periphery or even the posterior pole in a child who cannot be examined adequately in the office setting. This may be due to the child's immaturity, mental status, or combative nature. One also must determine the urgency of evaluation, depending on the tempo of the particular disease. It is best to perform EUAs in the hospital or in an ambulatory surgical center that is comfortable with pediatric anesthesia so that appropriate treatment (cryotherapy, laser, or more sophisticated vitreoretinal surgical interventions) may be applied, if necessary, without the need for a second anesthetic procedure.

INTRAOCULAR GAS AND INHALATION ANESTHESIA, PATIENT POSITION, AND POSTOPERATIVE CARE

The surgeon who cares for infants and children must realize that there are several anesthesia concerns unique to infants and children with vitreoretinal problems that require a different mindset than caring for adults. The use of expanding gases poses a higher risk in children. For that reason, in children, if a sustained gas is needed, we usually use 10% C3F8 well below the isoexpansion percentage of 14% (5). Most often we use air. Nitrous oxide anesthesia is avoided since it can cause unexpected expansion and then shrinkage of the air bubble. This also is true of air travel that allows the bubble to expand as the air atmospheric pressure is reduced. The family should be cautioned in this regard. The child should wear a bracelet indicating whether air or gas is in the eye, and that nitrous oxide anesthesia and air travel should be avoided until all gas is gone from the eye.

Predictably, postoperative positioning is much more difficult in children. We often position children face down the first night after surgery. They can be held face down on a parent's lap. On the second postoperative day, we have the child remain elevated in an infant seat for all activities for 2 weeks unless otherwise indicated to prevent the child from bumping his or her head, hitting his or her eye, or burrowing into the mattress or pillow. Children also can badly injure the eye with a flailing arm or fist after vitreous surgery. For this reason, we use elbow restraints and a Fox shield to protect the eye postoperatively. We also are concerned about amblyopia that has been encouraged by patching and postoperative medications. In unilateral cases, we use atropine drops in both eyes for 5 days to try and reduce the chance of amblyopia by atropinizing just the postoperative eye.

REFERENCES

1. Hairston RJ, Maguire AM, Vitale S, et al. Morphometric analysis of pars plan development in humans. *Retina* 1997;17:135–138.
2. Verstraeten TC, Chapman C, Hartzer M, et al. Pharmacologic induction of posterior vitreous detachment in the rabbit. *Arch Ophthalmol* 1993;111:849–854.
3. Margherio AR, Margherio RR, Hartzer M, et al. Plasmin enzyme-assisted vitrectomy in traumatic pediatric macular holes. *Ophthalmology* 1998;105:1617–1620.
4. Ferrone PJ, Trese MT, Williams GA, et al. Good visual acuity in an adult population with marker posterior segment changes secondary to retinopathy of prematurity. *Retina* 1998;18:335–338.
5. Chang S, Lincoff H, Coleman DJ, et al. Perfluorocarbon gases in vitreous surgery. *Ophthalmology* 1985;92:651–656.

PREOPERATIVE MANAGEMENT OF THE INFANT AND CHILD

SCOTT M. STEIDL

OBTAINING THE PREOPERATIVE HISTORY

Prior to surgery, a history is needed for preoperative planning. Important information to obtain include a history of prematurity with date of birth, medical conditions, patient's age and sex, age at the time of the condition's diagnosis, family history, known trauma, type or stage of the condition if applicable, and any previous visual acuity information. If surgical procedures were performed, the dates, intraoperative and postoperative complications, type of surgery, location and number of sclerotomy sites, postoperative course, visual rehabilitation with type used, amount of amblyopic patching, final visual acuity, and length of follow-up can be helpful.

General anesthesia is used for operations on infants, children, and most young adults undergoing retinal surgery. The anesthetists should be experienced with general anesthesia for small infants and children. Because malignant hyperthermia is a possible complication of general anesthesia in children, a history should inquire into any previous anesthetic problem with the patient or close relatives. Susceptible patients can be given anesthesia and only develop malignant hyperthermia with a second general anesthesia operation. Therefore, patients with a history suggestive of malignant hyperthermia should be treated appropriately (1). Fortunately, if the problem is recognized in time, treatment is available (2).

Preoperative Discussion

Preoperative evaluation includes a presentation of the risks and benefits to the parents. Most parents are willing to follow a surgeon's suggestions, even if the chances of improvement are small. In some cases, this plays into parental concern about doing what's best for the child, a topic that tugs at every parent's heart. Many parents are willing to do anything to help a dismal prognosis, even if there is little chance for functional improvement. Therefore, the surgeon must

guide parents toward an understanding of realistic and likely outcomes and discuss whether observation alone, rather than surgical intervention, is a reasonable option.

CONSIDERATIONS WITH GENERAL ANESTHESIA IN CHILDREN AND INFANTS

Infants younger than 1 year with a history of prematurity are at risk for developing apnea following general anesthesia. Risk factors include young postconceptual age, early gestational age, and anemia (hematocrit <30%). Apnea may manifest many hours after surgery. Even short periods of apnea, <60 seconds in duration, have been associated with bradycardia and decreased hemoglobin oxygen saturation. Therefore, former premature babies may require admission to the hospital for postoperative monitoring. Patients using topical echothiophate (phospholine iodide) or isoflurophate [diisopropyl fluorophosphate (DFP)] for accommodative esotropia may develop prolonged paralysis with depolarizing muscle relaxants, such as succinylcholine due to systemic absorption of these cholinesterase inhibitors. These relaxants should not be used for patients taking echothiophate or DFP.

Postoperative Observation

Some infants will require monitoring even after uncomplicated eye surgery. Protocols vary among institutions, but typically, younger infants, and infants with a history of lung disease, anemia, or apnea will require overnight observation. A protocol used at the University of Maryland suggests that postoperative cardiac and respiratory monitoring for 18 hours is required for (i) preterm infants who manifest apnea of >15 seconds' duration or symptomatic apnea in the recovery room, (ii) preterm infants with anemia (hematocrit <30% within 2 weeks of surgery), (iii) preterm infants with gestational age 35 to 36 weeks with postconceptual age 54 weeks or less, (iv) preterm infants with gestational age 32 to

34 weeks with postconceptual age 56 weeks or less, (v) preterm infants with gestational age 28 to 31 weeks with postconceptual age 60 weeks or less, (vi) preterm infants with gestational age 25 to 27 weeks with postconceptual age 64 weeks or less, (vii) preterm infants with ongoing manifestations of apnea or bradycardia at home, and (viii) preterm infants who exhibit a complicated postoperative course who cannot safely be cared for in an outpatient setting.

Oculocardiac Reflex

The oculocardiac reflex may be induced during scleral buckle operations by pulling on extraocular muscles. This autonomic response is mediated by stretch receptors within the extraocular muscles and leads to reflexive bradycardia, possible atrioventricular block, and even asystole. The oculocardiac reflex typically does not cause significant cardiac problems and may be blocked by retrobulbar and local anesthetics, although not by general anesthesia. Systemic atropine or glycopyrrolate prevents the reflex if cardiac dysrhythmia is observed and can be used prophylactically (3).

CONDITIONS LEADING TO RETINAL SURGERY IN INFANTS

A discussion of vitreous surgery in infants is largely a discussion of retinopathy of prematurity (ROP) surgery and is covered elsewhere in the text (see Chapters 26 and 27). However, other less common conditions that cause retinal detachment in infants include familial exudative vitreoretinopathy (see Chapter 28), which can present within the first few months of life (4), persistent fetal vasculature (see Chapter 30), which usually presents as leukocoria in infancy (5), and incontinentia pigmenti, an X-linked dominant condition associated with whorl-like skin pigmentation, dental anomalies, optic atrophy, cataracts, and nystagmus. Hemorrhage caused by birth trauma or shaken baby syndrome can be observed in infants as well. Little can be done to determine visual potential once macular dragging, macular folding, or retinal detachment has begun. However, if any occurs within the first few months of life, the prognosis is generally poor. Irreversible damage is likely a combination of developmental and amblyopic effects on the retina and visual system.

Retinopathy of Prematurity

In the late stages of ROP, vitreoretinal traction on the retina, from fibrovascular tissue originating from the retinal ridge, can cause complex retinal detachments. The severity

of retinal detachment depends on the clock-hour extent of the fibrous tissue formation. Once retinal detachment occurs, it can progress rapidly, although this is not always observed. In the worst scenarios, peripheral detachments posterior to the ridge can proceed to total retinal detachment within 1 day, and total detachments can become closed funnels within 1 week. Scleral buckling has been used to treat milder forms of traction retinal detachment in acute ROP (6,7). Its effectiveness and indications remain controversial. Surgery for early stage 4 disease also can be managed by lens-sparing vitrectomy, where instruments are placed 0.5 mm posterior to the limbus and a vitrectomy is done without removal of the lens (8). There are two major approaches to vitrectomy for advanced stage 5 ROP with closed funnel detachments. These techniques are transcorneal "closed" vitrectomy, where the cornea remains intact, and the "open sky" technique, where the cornea is removed for surgical access and sutured in place at the end of the case (9,10) (see Chapter 27). Anatomic success rates vary from 13% (11) to 76% (12). Functional success is generally poor, but in some cases ambulatory vision may be achieved.

Incontinentia Pigmenti

Incontinentia pigmenti or Bloch-Sulzberger syndrome is an X-linked dominant condition. It is characterized by skin pigmentation in lines and whorls, alopecia, dental anomalies, optic atrophy, cataracts, nystagmus, chorioretinal and conjunctival pigmentation, and peripheral retinal avascularity. The ocular presentation can be extremely variable and can resemble ROP. In early stages, peripheral avascular zones can be present with extraretinal neovascularization at the junction of vascularized and avascular retina. At this stage, laser to the avascular area may prevent later fibrovascular proliferation, retinal folds, and retinal detachment. Surgery for selected cases is appropriate because successful reattachment of the retina has been accomplished in some advanced cases.

Nonaccidental Trauma (Shaken Baby Syndrome)

When children are injured from abuse, multiple retinal hemorrhages are commonly seen. The pathogenesis of retinal hemorrhage is thought to involve shearing forces due to acceleration and deceleration, and possible associated increase in intraocular venous pressure (13). Vision loss in shaken baby syndrome may be due to retinal damage, optic atrophy, cortical damage, and amblyopia caused by visual deprivation due to blood in the vitreous. Vitrectomy to remove vitreous blood may be indicated in an effort to prevent amblyopia. However, brain injuries can limit visual potential (14).

CONDITIONS LEADING TO RETINAL SURGERY IN CHILDREN

Retinal Detachment

Pediatric retinal surgery usually is done for repair of retinal detachment. Retinal detachment may be "tractional," due to pulling of the retina from membranous growth on the retinal surface or in the vitreous cavity, or "rhegmatogenous," caused by retinal tears. Retinal detachments also may be caused by fluid exudation in the face of ocular inflammation. For example, exudative retinal detachment occasionally occurs after intense scatter laser treatment for threshold ROP.

Retinal tears and holes can be caused by vitreous traction on the retinal surface. This tractional force may lead to "horseshoe tears," macular holes, giant tears, or retinal dialysis. Traction-induced retinal tears and holes are commonly the result of trauma in pediatric patients. The superonasal and inferotemporal quadrants are the most commonly involved sites (15,16). "Tobacco dust" can be seen in the vitreous when a tear has occurred, and it is virtually pathognomonic of a retinal break. It represents intravitreous retinal pigment epithelial cells, which migrate through the break and can be seen by biomicroscopy as fine particulate, darkly colored particles in the anterior vitreous cavity.

Peripheral horseshoe tears are not as common in children because they usually are the result of posterior vitreous detachment occurring later in life. Autopsy studies have found that the incidence of posterior vitreous detachment was 63% by the eighth decade of life (17). A giant retinal tear is larger than a horseshoe tear, although both are typically formed by vitreous tractional forces. Giant tears extend over an area of 90 degrees or more (18) and often occur at the vitreous base rather than at the ora serrata. Giant tears may arise spontaneously, but approximately 25% occur in association with ocular trauma (19,20). This percentage is likely higher in children due to their higher rate of trauma-induced injuries. Traumatic macular holes are caused by traumatic separation of the retina from the vitreous (21), usually the result of blunt injury. Traumatic dialysis results when the retina tears from its attachment at the ora serrata. The inferotemporal quadrant is involved in about 75% of cases of traumatic dialysis after trauma (22).

In the pediatric age group, improvement of vision is possible if retinal detachments are repaired. Improvement is less likely if retinal detachment or occlusion of the optical media has been present for an extended period of time because of occlusion amblyopia. The duration of time when this complication can occur is shorter, the younger the infant or child. This time may decrease to a matter of months in the very young child. If the child is younger than 6 years, there is an extremely high chance of amblyopia, which decreases the functional success of vitreous surgery.

Persistent Fetal Vasculature

Persistent fetal vasculature usually is a unilateral condition associated with a smaller eye (23). Eye size usually is measured by corneal diameter, which can be obtained with the patient under anesthesia. Presentation at time of surgery ranged from 1 month to 7 years in one study and includes leukocoria, strabismus, nystagmus, and, in older children, decreased vision (5). Procedures that have been done for complications of persistent fetal vasculature include scleral buckle surgery, vitrectomy, anterior or pars plana cataract removal, and glaucoma filtration surgery with or without valve placement (24).

Toxocara Canis

Toxocariasis in humans is caused predominantly by *Toxocara canis* and presents clinically as either visceral larva migrans or ocular larva migrans. *Toxocara canis* is found worldwide in dogs (25). Infection of humans may occur by ingestion of eggs from the soil, contaminated hands, or less frequently by ingestion of the larval stage from undercooked meat. Seroprevalence rates in children (aged 1–11 years) in the United States range between 4.6% and 7.3% (26). Enzyme-linked immunosorbent assay (ELISA) titers of 1:32 are indicative of visceral larva migrans (78% sensitivity, 92% specificity) (27). A lack of calcifications on computed tomography helps to rule out retinoblastoma as a differential diagnosis when mass lesions occur (28). Upon biopsy, granulomatous reactions with neutrophil and eosinophil infiltrates are seen, occasionally with the larvae located in the center of the reaction (29). Steroids are frequently used to decrease inflammation. Various other treatments, including photocoagulation, cryopexy, and vitrectomy, have been used to manage the other manifestations of this condition. Occasionally, vitrectomy may be done to acquire vitreous for ELISA testing when the diagnosis is in question or to manage tractional detachment or endophthalmitis.

Penetrating Injuries

In children, ocular contusions are the primary cause of retinal detachment (30). They typically occur in males, and the majority of traumatic detachments are the result of blunt trauma (31–33).

Seventy-five percent of the retinal breaks found after blunt trauma are retinal dialyses. Retinal dialyses are present in up to 85% of traumatic retinal detachment cases (34–36). Detachments after penetrating injuries commonly involve development of intravitreal proliferative membranes (see also Chapter 32).

Marfan Syndrome

Marfan syndrome is an autosomal dominant abnormality of collagen. Patients with Marfan syndrome appear to have one of several point mutations in chromosome 15, band 21, the site of the fibrillin gene (37). The findings can include increased height, long extremities, increased lower body to upper body ratio, and an arm span exceeding the patient's height. The ocular features of Marfan syndrome include myopia, ectopia lentis, and retinal detachment. Of 12 eyes examined in one series, 10 had up to 16 diopters of myopia (38). Retinal detachment has been reported to occur in 9% of phakic eyes and 19% of aphakic eyes (39). The greater extent of vitreous loss during cataract surgery may be a factor contributing to increased risk for the development of retinal detachment (40). Based on an analysis of a group of 160 patients with Marfan syndrome, Maumenee (41) found that rhegmatogenous retinal detachment did not occur in eyes with normal axial length.

Stickler Syndrome

Stickler syndrome is an autosomal dominant trait closely linked to the structural gene for type II collagen (42). Systemic findings include degeneration of joints, joint laxity, hyperextensibility of the ankles, cleft of the secondary palate, sunken nasal bridge, and mandibular hypoplasia. Hearing loss may occur. Cataracts develop in 50% of patients. Characteristic fundus findings include transvitreous strands and vitreous liquefaction. Lattice degeneration and complicated retinal detachments may develop. Retinal detachments usually occur in the second decade, but they may occur earlier and may be complicated by development of giant retinal tears (43).

AMBLYOPIA AND PEDIATRIC RETINAL SURGERY

Surgical Timing

Amblyopia is certain to occur after stage 5 ROP has developed (44). All efforts should be directed to preventing stage 5 ROP. However, if it occurs, surgery should be performed early, as soon as vascular activity is reduced. Correlation between timing of surgery, postsurgical complications, and final visual acuity is limited. In general, authors advocate timely surgical intervention for stage 4 ROP. Based on long-term visual results, one study showed vision as good as 20/63 after surgery for stage 4B ROP (45). Good results were attributed to timely intervention. Stage 5 eyes in this study did poorly. In a different series, vision of 20/100 to 20/800 measured as grating acuity was achieved in 58.2% of cases with stage 5 ROP eyes using open sky vitrectomy (46). These authors found the best results were achieved in children between 6 and 12 months of age. Most agreed that eyes without active disease should be operated on as quickly as possible. Active proliferative disease conferred a risk of intraoperative hemorrhage and postoperative complications. Dilated iris and retinal vessels may indicate increased disease

activity and are considered in the decision to proceed with surgery. Surgery might best be postponed if retinal convexity, which is suggestive of exudative retinal detachment, is observed (47). Poor outcome with postoperative retinal proliferation is more likely with active proliferative ROP. In general, waiting increases the likelihood of surgical success for stage 5 ROP and decreases anesthesia risk, but it increases the likelihood of diminished retinal function and profound amblyopia.

Incorporating the Possibility of Deprivational Amblyopia into Surgical Planning

In children younger than 6 years, there is a high rate of amblyopia with surgery. This reduced likelihood of good postoperative vision must be taken into account when planning surgery with unilateral disease (44). The most critical period for amblyopia is in the first few months of life. The most critical period for stereopsis is the first 2 years of life. Media opacity can lead to both anisometropia (induced myopia) initially and deprivational amblyopia later.

The four main types of amblyopia are refractive, deprivational, strabismic, and organic. Deprivational amblyopia is by far the worst. Complete occlusion of an eye in kittens in the first 3 months of life results in the stimulation of the striate cortex only by the normal eye (48). Critical periods in the development of visual acuity include birth to 5 years when visual acuity is developing, about 2 months to 8 years when deprivation is effective in causing amblyopia, and about 7 years to the teenage years and beyond when recovery from amblyopia can be obtained (49). In general, the first few months are critical for development of deprivation amblyopia, but sensitivity persists until much later. In the macaque monkey, monocular deprivation affects absolute sensitivity to light, sensitivity to contrast, sensitivity to wavelength, and binocular summation (50). Correction of visual deprivation before age 4 months in humans appears to produce less visual loss, but we generally have difficulty specifying the level of functional correction within this period. If the eye is deprived between 6 and 30 months of age, finger counting is typically the best visual acuity achieved (51). With stereopsis, the critical period appears to be the first 2 years of life. In general, surgeons recommend surgery to remove media opacities without delay, after diagnosis has been made.

Postoperative Management of Amblyopia

Once surgery is undertaken, rehabilitation requires intensive amblyopia therapy for young age groups, especially those in the first few months of life. Treatment focuses on three main principles: first, maintaining a clear visual axis; second, focusing the retinal image; and third, forced use of the eye. Children are generally out of risk for development of amblyopia beyond age 6 years (52).

Scleral buckling procedures typically cause myopia, and some of this may be relieved by removal of the buckle. This may in part be due to refractive amblyopia. Single eye surgery can cause unilateral myopia. If the myopia is significant, these children rarely do well. Most postoperative cases should be seen for evaluation and possible refraction and lens fitting within 1 week of surgery. Occlusion therapy may be needed. In the first 6 months of life, a reduced occlusion schedule may be used to allow for development of binocularity. The common recommendation is for close follow-up at intervals of no more than 1 week per year of age during periods of aggressive patching (53).

Amblyopia that is deprivational or organic in nature is difficult to treat. Organic amblyopia is associated with structural damage to the retina. Therapy for macular structural anomalies, including macular scars and myopia, can achieve moderate success after full-time occlusion therapy in unilateral cases (54). Duration of amblyopia treatment is proportional to the child's age. Maintenance therapy usually is needed until visual maturation around age 7 to 10 years.

DIAGNOSTIC ECHOGRAPHY IN INFANTS

Retinoblastoma

In infants, the most common use of echography (see Chapter 5) is in the evaluation of leukokoria and conditions that may lead to leukokoria (Table 20-1). Retinoblastoma is the condition that must always be kept in mind when dealing with infantile and early childhood ocular abnormalities. Its

manifestations are variable and include decreased vision, strabismus, a white pupil (leukokoria), and uveitis. Echography has been shown to be useful in the diagnosis and evaluation of retinoblastoma (55). Retinoblastomas may be unilateral or bilateral, unifocal or multifocal, or endophytic (on the inner retinal surface) or exophytic (on the outer retinal surface). They also may be diffuse without nodularity presenting with uveitis in the slightly older child. This is called diffuse infiltrative retinoblastoma (56,57). Retinoblastomas are typically dome shaped. Internal reflectivity usually is seen to different degrees, based on the amount of calcification within the lesion. Calcium can be dense or diffuse. Baseline tumor measurements are needed so that size can be monitored during treatment. The differential diagnosis of retinoblastoma includes ROP, persistent fetal vasculature, Coats disease, toxocariasis, cysticercosis, and endophthalmitis. Although these other conditions rarely contain calcium, it has been reported in Coats disease, and there are overlaps in findings among all of them. A comprehensive evaluation including other forms of diagnostic imaging may be required.

Retinopathy of Prematurity

ROP usually is a bilateral condition, commonly associated with very low birth weight or premature babies, often after a history of oxygen use. Echography typically is used in stage 4 eyes to evaluate the extent and height of a retinal detachment and to determine whether it has a convex (in exudative stage 4 ROP) or concave configuration (in traction stage 4 ROP). In stage 5 eyes, echography can be used to determine the

TABLE 20-1. CONDITIONS ASSOCIATED WITH LEUKOKORIA[a]

Condition	Main Echographic Finding	Axial Eye Length	Unilateral/Bilateral
Retinoblastoma	Calcified mass	Normal	Unilateral/bilateral
Retinopathy of prematurity (stage 5)	Total retinal detachment with retinal loops	Short	Bilateral
Persistent hyperplastic primary vitreous	Vitreous band from lens to optic nerve	Short	Unilateral
Coats disease	Exudative retinal detachment	Normal	Unilateral
Toxocara canis	Peripheral granuloma, retinal folds and posterior traction, retinal detachment	Normal	Unilateral
Endophthalmitis	Vitreous opacities	Normal	Unilateral
Cysticercosis	Cyst with scolex	Normal	Unilateral
Medulloepithelioma (diktyoma)	Ciliary body mass with cystic cavities	Normal	Unilateral

[a] The main echographic findings for the most common conditions associated with leukokoria are listed.
From Byrne FB, Green RL. Ultrasound of the eye and orbit. St. Louis: Mosby Year Book, 1992:202, with permission.

TABLE 20-2. CONDITIONS ASSOCIATED WITH TRAUMA IN THE PEDIATRIC POPULATION

Blunt trauma
   Anterior segment
      Hyphema
      Cataract
      (Sub)luxated lens
      Ruptured lens capsule
   Posterior segment
      Vitreous hemorrhage
      Retinal tear
      Retinal dialysis
      Retinal detachment
      Edema of retinochoroid layer
      Posterior scleral rupture

Penetrating trauma
   Anterior segment
      Hyphema
      Shallow anterior chamber
      Ruptured lens capsule
   Posterior segment
      Vitreous hemorrhage (posterior vitreous detachment)
      Hemorrhagic track through the vitreous
      Posterior scleral rupture
      Retinal detachment
      Hemorrhagic choroidal detachment
      Scleral fold

Foreign bodies
   Intraocular foreign bodies
      Metallic
      Spherical
      Glass and organic material
      Air bubbles
   Orbital foreign bodies

From Byrne FB, Green RL. Ultrasound of the eye and orbit. St. Louis: Mosby Year Book, 1992:96, with permission.

retinal detachment configuration. Stage 5 ROP may present with a funnel detachment either tightly closed posteriorly or both posteriorly and anteriorly. With anterior detachment, the retina is pulled toward the posterior lens surface creating peripheral loops or retinal troughs. Hemorrhage with cholesterol crystals can be seen under the retina (58).

Persistent Fetal Vasculature

In the affected eye, the globe typically is smaller and the lens may be thinner. A band may be seen extending from the posterior lens to the optic nerve, representing persistence of the fetal vasculature. The band that develops may cause traction retinal detachment and, in rare cases, total retinal detachment.

Coats Disease

Coats disease usually is a unilateral disease that may lead to severe exudative retinal detachments. In less severe cases, partial retinal detachment or retinal thickening may be detected.

DIAGNOSTIC ECHOGRAPHY IN CHILDREN

In older children, echography is most commonly required to evaluate ocular injuries. These issues are more prevalent in the pediatric population, but the principles are the same as with adult diagnostic evaluation of ocular injury.

Trauma

Trauma is a common cause of severe vision loss in children. Echography is of great benefit when the eye structures are opacified, the patient is in great pain, or the patient is unwilling to open lids (Table 20-2). A "nonpressure" technique can be used in the face of a possible ruptured globe, with the ultrasound probe placed over the lids using methylcellulose or ultrasound gel.

Vitreous Hemorrhage

When vitreous hemorrhage occurs after trauma, the possibility of a retinal tear, retinal detachment, or choroidal detachment must be considered (Table 20-3). Dots and lines representing intravitreous blood are seen on B scan. The greater the density of the hemorrhage, the more highly reflective are the dots. Blood may drift downward in the eye with gravity. In some cases of older children and young adults, a posterior vitreous detachment may occur, and

TABLE 20-3. CONDITIONS ASSOCIATED WITH VITREOUS HEMORRHAGE IN THE PEDIATRIC POPULATION

Infant
   Retinopathy of prematurity
   Coats disease
   Norrie disease
   Persistent fetal vasculature
   Trauma/shaken baby syndrome
   Postsurgical

Child
   Trauma
   Congenital retinoschisis
   Persistent fetal vasculature
   Spontaneous retinal tears
   Sickle cell retinopathy
   Dysproteinemias
   Diabetic retinopathy
   Systemic lupus erythematosus
   Postsurgical
   Acute retinal necrosis
   Candidiasis
   Cytomegalovirus retinitis
   Toxoplasmosis
   Leukemia
   Retinal vein occlusion

blood may create the appearance of a pseudomembrane on the posterior vitreous face. However, in most children, the vitreous remains formed and attached to the retina. Blood can layer within the vitreous and become sequestered within the formed gel. These layers of blood may create highly reflective membranes noted on ultrasonography similar to that seen in retinal detachment. Other clues are then used to exclude the possibility of retinal detachment, including the absence of attachment of the membrane to the optic nerve, reduced reflectance when gain is reduced, discontinuous appearance of the membrane, and occasional appearance of swirling of the membrane when the patient is asked to turn the eye. However, blood within formed vitreous in a child may not move with eye movement and can be misdiagnosed as retinal detachment.

Tractional Vitreous Detachment

In children with vascular diseases such as persistent fetal vasculature, incontinentia pigmenti, familial exudative vitreoretinopathy, ROP, or inflammatory detachments associated with *Toxocara canis,* toxoplasmosis, or peripheral uveitis, traction on the retinal surface can cause a focal retinal detachment. Traction detachments show minimal movement on dynamic ultrasonography and often are concave in configuration.

Rhegmatogenous Retinal Detachments

Retinal detachments generally occur from retinal breaks, such as horseshoe tears, giant tears, or a dialysis, or traction. A dialysis of the peripheral retina may be detected by observing disinsertion of the retina from the ora serrata. Spontaneous dialysis of the retina typically occurs in the inferior temporal retinal periphery. Inferotemporal dialysis also is common after trauma. The retina may only be shallowly detached, but the vision can be significantly impaired. A very peripheral disinsertion of the retina and a shallow retinal detachment are often the echographic findings with a retinal dialysis. Frequent echographic studies are suggested after trauma if media opacity obscures the view. This is especially true if a ruptured globe is present due to the increased risk of retinal detachment.

Hemorrhagic Choroidal Detachments

Hemorrhagic choroidal detachments may develop after penetrating or perforating trauma. They are dome shaped and do not shift with eye movement. They can extend anterior to the ora serrata and often remain attached at the vortex vein ampullae. The location of the detachments may determine the approach to surgical repair. Scleral folds in a soft eye may be mistaken for small choroidal detachments as well as foreign bodies and scleral buckles (59).

Foreign Bodies

A foreign body is more precisely detected by echography than computed tomographic scanning, especially if it is located next to the scleral wall (60). Metallic foreign bodies are highly reflective and often irregular in shape. They vary in size and may cause shadowing of orbital structures. Anterior foreign bodies may be more difficult to image. An immersion technique can be useful in visualizing anteriorly located foreign bodies, but often computed tomographic scanning is more useful in these cases. Both BBs and gas bubbles may form a highly echogenic pattern on echography. An air bubble in front of a foreign body can produce a signal that is not easily differentiated from the foreign body itself (61).

Dislocated Lens

Blunt trauma usually is the cause of lens dislocation in children. Lens subluxation is possible in other conditions such as Marfan syndrome and homocystinuria. When a lens is dislocated into the posterior segment, it must be distinguished from tumors. Usually it is mobile and associated with vitreous membranes. Internal reflectivity will vary based on lens clarity.

VISUAL EVOKED POTENTIALS

The infant visual system continues to mature after birth up to age 6 months to 1 year. Peak latencies of the flash and pattern visual evoked potential (VEP) decrease as the pathways myelinate (62). The pattern VEP has been shown to be a valid estimate of visual acuity in preverbal children when the retina is attached (63). It also has been shown to be a good indicator of amblyopia (64). The sweep VEP was designed to be a rapid objective estimate of amblyopia, and it has provided important information on diagnosis of amblyopia. In eyes in which the retina is attached, VEP function may provide information regarding the integrity of the retina. The VEP also may be used to assess postoperative retinal function. A study of 25 diabetic eyes found flicker VEP results to reliably predict the functional visual outcome 6 months after surgery (65).

In the setting of a poor retinal view from media opacities, optic nerve function can be assessed by obtaining a flash VEP if the retina is attached. In a state of retinal detachment, bright flash VEP may identify eyes with visual function (66). With partial retinal attachment, a flash VEP gives a gross indication of optic nerve function if at least part of the macula is functional. When retinal detachment involves the entire retina, there is no evidence that the VEP is of predictive value regarding postoperative visual potential (67). Some surgeons obtain a VEP in the setting of total retinal detachment. In this case, a recordable VEP waveform would indicate the presence of light perception. However, the absence of a VEP signal in the setting of retinal detachment does not rule out the possibility of light perception. For this reason, the VEP has limited value as an aid for surgical planning.

SUMMARY

It is presently within our grasp to manage many infantile presentations of advanced ROP with surgical treatments. In older children, retinal surgical techniques used in adults are often effective in managing trauma, as well as conditions prone to retinal detachment such as Stickler and Marfan syndromes. Despite these successes, a discrepancy often exists between anatomic and functional outcome. For this reason, care must be taken to explain this distinction to parents and give realistic expectations for ultimate function and visual acuity. Amblyopia is a significant concern for children younger than 6 years. The most critical period for amblyopia development is in the first months of life; therefore, severe infantile retina disease nearly always will result in some degree of amblyopia. Still, media opacity from vitreous hemorrhage that is cleared early can afford an opportunity for visual development. Echography may be helpful in a great number of situations when evaluating the child with retinal disease in whom fundus evaluation is limited due to media opacities. Echography also may be helpful when a diagnosis is uncertain, and characteristic echographic findings will support a diagnosis. VEP evaluation of the retina may offer preoperative information, such as macular and optic nerve function when the macula is attached. However, its value in predicting future retinal function is limited in the case of total retinal detachment.

REFERENCES

1. American Academy of Pediatrics Section on Anesthesiology: evaluation and preparation of pediatric patients undergoing anesthesia. *Pediatrics* 1996;98:502.
2. Strazis KP, Fox AW. Malignant hyperthermia: a review of published cases. *Anesth Analg* 1993;77:297.
3. Mirakhur RK, Jones CJ, Dundee JW. Atropine or glycopyrrolate for the prevention of OCR in children undergoing squint surgery. *Br J Anaesthesiol* 1982;71:66.
4. Pendergast SD, Trese MT. Familial exudative vitreoretinopathy results of surgical management. *Ophthalmology* 1998;105:1015–1023.
5. Dass AB, Trese MT. Surgical results of persistent hyperplastic primary vitreous. *Ophthalmology* 1999;106:280–284.
6. Trese MT. Scleral buckling for retinopathy of prematurity. *Ophthalmology* 1994;101:23–26.
7. Ricci B, Santo A, Ricci F, et al. Scleral buckling surgery in stage 4 retinopathy of prematurity. *Graefes Arch Clin Exp Ophthalmol* 1996;234:S38–S41.
8. Capone A, Trese MT. Lens sparing vitreous surgery for tractional stage 4a retinopathy of prematurity retinal detachments. *Ophthalmology* 2001;108:2068–2070.
9. Hirose T, Katsumi O, Mehta MC, et al. Vision in stage 5 retinopathy of prematurity after retinal reattachment by open-sky vitrectomy. *Arch Ophthalmol* 1993;111:345–349.
10. deJuan E, Machemer R. Retinopathy of prematurity. Surgical technique. *Retina* 1987;7:63–69.
11. McPherson AR, Hittner HM, Moura RA, et al. Treatment of retrolental fibroplasia with open-sky vitrectomy. In: McPherson AR, Hittner HM, Kretzer FL, eds. *Retinopathy of prematurity: current concepts and controversies.* Toronto: BC Decker, 1986:225–234.
12. Mintz-Hittner HA, O'Malley RE, Kretzer FL. Long-term form identification vision after early, closed, lensectomy-vitrectomy for stage 5 retinopathy of prematurity. *Ophthalmology* 1997;104:454–459.
13. Greenwald M. The shaken baby syndrome. *Semin Ophthalmol* 1990;5:202.
14. Matthews GP, Das A. Dense vitreous hemorrhages predict poor visual and neurological prognosis in infants with shaken baby syndrome. *J Pediatr Ophthalmol Strabismus* 1996;33:260.
15. Cox MS, Schepens CL, Freeman HM, et al. Retinal detachment due to ocular contusion. *Arch Ophthalmol* 1966;76:678.
16. Runyan TE. *Concussive and penetrating injuries of the globe and optic nerve.* St. Louis: CV Mosby, 1975.
17. Foos RY. Posterior vitreous detachment. *Trans Am Acad Ophthalmol Otolaryngol* 1974;76:480.
18. Leaver PK, Lean JS. Management of giant retinal tears using vitrectomy and silicone oil fluid exchange. A preliminary report. *Trans Ophthalmol Soc UK* 1981;101:189.
19. Freeman HM. Treatment of giant retinal tears. In: McPherson A, ed. *New and controversial aspects of retinal detachment.* New York: Harper & Row, 1968:391–399.
20. Aylward GW, Cooling RJ, Leaver PK. Trauma-induced retinal detachment associated with giant retinal tears. *Retina* 1993;13:136.
21. Margherio RR, Schepens CL. Macular breaks: diagnosis, etiology and observations. *Am J Ophthalmol* 1972;74:219.
22. Kennedy CJ, Parker CE, McAllister IL. Retinal detachment caused by retinal dialysis. *Aust N Z J Ophthalmol* 1997;25:25–30.
23. Charles S, Katz A, Wood B. *Vitreous microsurgery, 3rd ed.* Philadelphia: Lippincott Williams & Wilkins, 2002:231.
24. Mittra RA, Huynh LT, Ruttman MS, et al. Visual outcomes following lensectomy and vitrectomy for combined anterior and posterior persistent hyperplastic primary vitreous. *Arch Ophthalmol* 1998;116:1990–1994.
25. Glickman LT, Schantz PM. Epidemiology and pathogenesis of zoonotic toxocariasis. *Epidemiol Rev* 1981;3:230.
26. Herrmann N, Glickman LT, Schantz PM. Seroprevalence of zoonotic toxocariasis in the United States: 1971–1973. *Am J Epidemiol* 1985;122:890.
27. Glickman LT, Schantz P, Dombrsoke R. Evaluation of serodiagnostic tests for visceral larva migrans. *Am J Trop Med Hyg* 1978;27:492.
28. Wan WL, Cano MR, Pince KJ. Echographic characteristics of ocular toxocariasis. *Ophthalmology* 1991;98:28.
29. Dent JH, Nichols RL, Beaver PC. Visceral larva migrans: with a case report. *Am J Pathol* 1956;32:777.
30. Cox MS, Schepens CL, Freeman HM. Retinal detachment due to ocular contusion. *Arch Ophthalmol* 1966;76:678.
31. Malbran E, Dodds R, Hulsbris R. Traumatic retinal detachment. *Mod Probl Ophthalmol* 1972;10:479.
32. Dumas JJ. Retinal detachment following contusion of the eye. *Int Ophthalmol Clin* 1967;7:19.
33. Goffstein R, Burton TC. Differentiating traumatic from nontraumatic retinal detachment. *Ophthalmology* 1982;89:361.
34. Tasman W. Peripheral retinal changes following blunt trauma. *Trans Am Ophthalmol Soc* 1972;70:190.

35. Sellors PJ, Mooney D. Fundus changes after traumatic hyphaema. *Br J Ophthalmol* 1973;57:600.

36. Eagling EM. Ocular damage after blunt trauma to the eye. Its relationship to the nature of the injury. *Br J Ophthalmol* 1974;58:126.

37. Dietz H, Cutting GR, Pyeritz RE, et al. Marfan syndrome caused by a recurrent de novo missense mutation in the fibrillin gene. *Nature* 1991;352:337.

38. Allen RA, Straatsma BR, Apt L, et al. Ocular manifestations of the Marfan syndrome. *Trans Am Acad Ophthalmol Otol* 1967;71:18.

39. Cross HE, Jensen AD. Ocular manifestations in the Marfan syndrome and homocystinuria. *Am J Ophthalmol* 1973;75:405.

40. Jarrett WH II. Dislocation of the lens: a study of 166 hospitalized cases. *Arch Ophthalmol* 1967;78:289.

41. Maumenee IH. The eye in the Marfan syndrome. *Trans Am Ophthalmol Soc* 1981;79:684.

42. Francomano CA, Liberfarb RM, Hirose T, et al. The Stickler syndrome: evidence for close linkage to the structural gene for type II collagen. *Genomics* 1987;1:293.

43. Billington BM, Leaver PK, McLeod D. Management of retinal detachment in the Wagner-Stickler syndrome. *Trans Ophthalmol Soc UK* 1985;104:875.

44. Charles S, Katz A, Wood B. *Vitreous microsurgery, 3rd ed.* Philadelphia: Lippincott Williams & Wilkins, 2002:231.

45. Trese MT, Droste PJ. Long term postoperative results of a consecutive series of stages 4 and 5 retinopathy of prematurity. *Ophthalmology* 1998;105:992–997.

46. Hirose T, Katsumi O, Mehta MC, et al. Vision in stage 5 retinopathy of prematurity after retinal reattachment by open-sky vitrectomy. *Arch Ophthalmol* 1993;111:345–349.

47. Charles S. *Vitreous microsurgery, 2nd ed.* Baltimore: Williams & Wilkins, 1987:160.

48. Wiesel T. Postnatal development of the visual cortex and the influence of environment. *Nature* 1982;299:583–591.

49. Daw NW. Critical periods and amblyopia. *Arch Ophthalmol* 1998;116:502–505.

50. Harwerth RS, Smith EL, Duncan GC, et al. Multiple sensitive periods in the development of the primate visual system. *Science* 1986;232:235–238.

51. Vaegan TD. Critical period for deprivation amblyopia in children. *Trans Ophthalmol Soc UK* 1979;99:432–439.

52. Keech RV, Kutschke PJ. Upper age limit for the development of amblyopia. *J Pediatr Ophthalmol Strabismus* 1995;32:89–93.

53. Simon JW, Parks MM, Price EC. Severe visual loss resulting from occlusion therapy for amblyopia. *J Pediatr Ophthalmol* Strabismus 1987;24:244–246.

54. Bradford GM, Kutschke PJ, Scott WE. Results of amblyopia therapy in eyes with unilateral structural abnormalities. *Ophthalmology* 1992;99:1616–1621.

55. Byrne FB, Green RL. *Ultrasound of the eye and orbit.* St. Louis: Mosby Year Book,1992:196.

56. Steidl S, Hirose T, Sang D, et al. Difficulty in excluding the diagnosis of retinoblastoma in cases of advanced Coats' disease: a clinicopathologic report. *Ophthalmologica* 1996;210:336–340.

57. Byrne FB, Green RL. *Ultrasound of the eye and orbit.* St. Louis: Mosby Year Book, 1992:196.

58. Steidl SM, Hirose T. Subretinal organization in stage 5 retinopathy of prematurity. *Graefes Arch Clin Exp Ophthalmol* 2003;241:263–268.

59. Byrne FB, Green RL. *Ultrasound of the eye and orbit, 2nd ed.* Philadelphia: Mosby, 2002:99.

60. Byrne FB, Green RL. *Ultrasound of the eye and orbit.* St. Louis: Mosby Year Book,1992:107.

61. Guthoff R. *Ultrasound in ophthalmologic diagnosis.* New York: Thieme,1991:58–59.

62. Barnet AB, Friedman SL, Weiss IP, et al. VEP development in infancy and early childhood: a longitudinal study. *Electroencephalogr Clin Electrophysiol* 1980;49:476–489.

63. McCulloch DL, Taylor LJ, Whyte HE. Visual evoked potentials and visual prognosis following perinatal asphyxia. *Arch Ophthalmol* 1991;109:229–233.

64. Sokol S, Bloom B. Visual evoked cortical responses of amblyopes to a special altering stimulus. *Invest Ophthalmol* 1973;12:936–939.

65. Schonfeld CL, Schneider T, Korner U, et al. Prognostic factors in vitreous surgery for proliferative diabetic retinopathy. *Ger J Ophthalmol* 1994;3:137–143.

66. Clarkson JG, Jacobson SG, Frazier-Byrne S, et al. Evaluation of eyes with stage-5 retinopathy of prematurity. *Graefes Arch Clin Exp Ophthalmol* 1986;227:332–334.

67. Charles S, Katz A, Wood B. *Vitreous microsurgery, 3rd ed.* Philadelphia: Lippincott Williams & Wilkins, 2002:220.

GENERAL ANESTHESIA
IN PREMATURE INFANTS

P. ANTHONY MEZA

The premature or very low birth weight infant (VLBW) afflicted with retinopathy of prematurity (ROP) is extremely delicate and requires great consideration and attention when undergoing general anesthesia. An experienced practitioner in pediatric anesthesiology best meets these requirements. This chapter is no replacement for a textbook of pediatric anesthesiology, but it does provide a description of our anesthetic techniques and the reasons we use these techniques when caring for the infant with ROP.

The following is an overview of the anesthetic implications of neonatal anatomy and physiology based on general anesthesia concerns and organized by systems: (i) The central nervous system has lower anesthetic requirements in neonates, an immature blood brain barrier, and an immature central respiratory drive with the potential for apnea; (ii) Within the cardiovascular system, cardiac output is rate-dependent, and bradycardia must be treated aggressively. There must be patency of the ductus arteriosus and foramen ovale; thus, air bubbles must be avoided; (iii) In the respiratory system, one must consider the anatomic features of difficult intubation (relatively large head and short neck in relation to rest of the body) and short trachea, with risk of endobronchial intubation increased. The possibility of damaged lungs may be present, resulting from respiratory distress of the newborn, leaving the VLBW infant with bronchopulmonary dysplasia (BPD); (iv) Metabolic concerns include relatively high oxygen consumption and rapid desaturation with apnea.; (v) Hematologic issues that will need to be monitored include larger blood volume per kilogram in relation to other age groups and increased amounts of fetal hemoglobin, requiring higher hematocrit for adequate oxygen delivery; (vi) Pharmacologic points to remember include the possibility of immature drug metabolism and elimination (narcotics are metabolized more slowly) and immature hepatic enzyme function; (vii) The renal system is unable to concentrate or dilute urine; therefore, excessive sodium or water infusions should be avoided; (viii) Temperature regulation requires adequate body warming. This is due to a high neonatal body surface area to volume ratio,

which leads to rapid heat loss. An inability to shiver contributes to this problem; (ix) Endocrine system management necessitates glucose supplementation. This typically is given as glucose infusion at 4 mL/kg/hour D10W (6–7/kg/min).

A preoperative hemoglobin level should be near 10 g/dL. Some premature neonates at about age 2 months will reach their physiologic nadir of hemoglobin around 8 g/dL. Many of these infants with significant airway disease may be on diuretic therapy. If a blood specimen for electrolytes is obtained by heel stick or other peripheral means, it may hemolyze and give a falsely elevated potassium level. If a blood sample for potassium level is essential, then a venous sample should be obtained.

First and foremost for the anesthetist is concern about the amount of respiratory compromise experienced by the VLBW infant. The degree of respiratory compromise may be mild, in which case the child requires no supplemental oxygen. In this scenario, the anesthetist must be aware of the VLBW infant's decreased functional residual capacity and increased compliance of the neonatal chest wall. In addition, there is decreased oxygen carrying capacity due to residual fetal hemoglobin. Physiologic anemia is generally encountered at about age 2 months in the VLBW infant, when the hemoglobin level may be as low as 8 g/dL. Regardless of the fitness of the VLBW infant presenting for general anesthesia, the anesthetist must always be concerned about the possibility of postanesthetic apnea. In a recent study, postanesthetic apnea occurred at an incidence of 26% for infants younger than 44 weeks' postconceptual age (PCA) and 3% for infants older than 44 weeks' PCA. All VLBW infants younger than 60 weeks should be observed with apnea monitoring for at least 12 hours after general anesthesia. All infants older than 60 weeks' PCA with a history of prematurity who are still on apnea monitors at home will require apnea monitoring after general anesthesia.

The VLBW premature infant can present with severe respiratory compromise, as with moderate-to-severe BPD. In BPD, there is a loss of the small airways and alveoli and an increase in airway and pulmonary arterial smooth muscle.

These factors make reactive bronchoconstriction and pulmonary arterial vasoconstriction more likely to occur. Pulmonary ventilation perfusion mismatch, leading to hypoxemia, can occur with any stress, especially those brought on by general anesthesia. The lungs of the infant with BPD will also have a variable amount of destructive fibrosis affecting both the airways and the pulmonary vasculature. The VLBW infant may have lung disease that ranges between mild BPD to BPD so severe that continuous mechanical ventilation is required.

Because the VLBW infant usually will require endotracheal intubation and mechanical ventilation early in life, the incidence of subglottic stenosis is increased. Care must used in placing appropriately sized endotracheal tubes so that subglottic stenosis is not exacerbated and subglottic edema is avoided.

RAE oral endotracheal tubes (endotracheal tubes with a premolded curvature at the standard lip level) are best not used in premature VLBW infants because the molded curves usually place the tip of endotracheal tube below the carina, resulting in endobronchial intubation and one-lung ventilation.

Mechanical ventilation with anesthesia ventilators can be difficult for VLBW infants. The best anesthesia ventilators have settings for a minimum weight of 3 kg. These infants, who may weigh less than this, are best ventilated in the pressure control mode. If the anesthesia ventilator has only a volume ventilation mode available, it may be impossible to use for the VLBW neonate. Care must used in setting the peak inspiratory pressure (PIP). The PIP must be set high enough to ensure adequate ventilation but low enough to prevent barotrauma and the catastrophic complication of pneumothorax, which can easily lead to death in the VLBW infant. When mechanical ventilation is not easily accomplished, even if pressure control ventilation is available, manual ventilation by hand with close attention to PIP is recommended.

The neonate should be transported from the neonatal intensive care unit to the operating room in an isolette so that adequate body temperature can be easily maintained. Supplementary oxygen delivery is used as needed when transporting the VLBW infant. Monitoring by pulse oximetry and electrocardiography also should be available for transport of the neonate to the operating room.

Some neonates will arrive in the operating room breathing room air; others will arrive intubated, requiring complete ventilatory assistance.

The operating room temperature should be warmed to 27°C (80°F) prior to arrival of the neonate. Warm air blankets are used on the operating room table on which the neonate will be placed. Maintaining normothermia for the neonate is essential.

After routine monitoring of the electrocardiogram, noninvasive blood pressure cuff, pulse oximetry, and temperature probe and placement of a neonatal-sized precordial

stethoscope, induction of general anesthesia may begin. We have found carefully performed general anesthesia to be safe for the infant with ROP. A 1997 British study found that infants with ROP undergoing cryosurgery had fewer and less severe complications receiving general anesthesia compared to those who received only topical anesthesia for cryosurgery.

When no intravenous (IV) access is available prior to anesthetic induction, we prefer an anesthetic face mask inhalation induction with sevoflurane, oxygen, and air mixture.

Sevoflurane has the advantages, such as rapid uptake and less noxious odor, over the currently available inhalational anesthetic agents. Nitrous oxide, if used at all, must be administered with extreme caution. Nitrous oxide increases the pulmonary artery pressure in adults and older children, may increase the risk of hypoxemia, and must be discontinued 15 minutes prior to the injection of air into the eye. Prior to placing the anesthetic face mask on the neonate, a roll of surgical towels is placed under the shoulders of the neonate to extend the neck slightly. This maneuver helps maintain a patent airway by aligning the oral, pharyngeal, and laryngeal axes and facilitates orotracheal intubation. An appropriately sized oral airway may be placed at this time to help maintain the airway. After general inhalational anesthesia has been established, IV access is sought. The level of inhalational agent (usually sevoflurane) will be decreased to avoid hypotension during the search for a suitable vein for establishing IV access. For infants weighing 3 kg or less who must have their airway secured quickly, an awake intubation may be performed with or without IV access.

Establishing IV access can be difficult, even for the most experienced practitioner. Recommendations for success in establishing an IV in these neonates are basic. The anesthetist managing the airway cannot be the person obtaining IV access. Attention to the airway of the neonate requires the full attention of that anesthetist. Adequate lighting must be available. Appropriately sized equipment, such as a small tourniquet, and small IV catheters (24 and 22 gauge) are necessary. After a target vein is identified and the tourniquet placed, the skin surrounding the target vein is held slightly taut. This will help prevent movement of the target vein when the skin is pierced by the tip of the IV cannula. The skin should be pierced 1 to 2 mm away from the desired point of entry of the target vein to avoid having the IV cannula pass through the target vein when the skin is pierced. Once the skin is pierced, the target vein should be entered with a deliberate 1- to 2-mm thrust of the IV cannula tip so that the target vein will not pushed aside with the movement of the IV cannula. When it is estimated that 1 to 2 mm of the IV cannula is in the lumen of the target vein, the plastic IV cannula can be advanced. It is helpful to have a T-piece with Luer-Lok connected to the hub of the IV cannula to allow injection of medications without large IV fluid boluses. If medications are administered through the injection

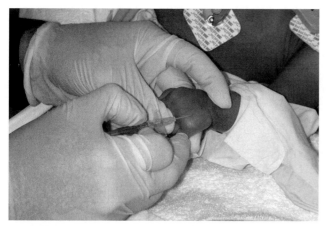

FIGURE 21-1. Skin of the area of the target vein is held taut as the tip of the intravenous cannula enters the skin 1 to 2 mm away from the target vein.

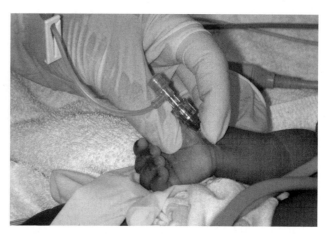

FIGURE 21-3. Intravenous catheter is connected to the intravenous tubing with a Luer-Lok T-piece.

ports along the IV tubing, they may not reach the neonate for a long period of time due to the low flow rate of the IV fluid required by the neonate. When IV access must be established quickly to administer emergency medication, it is recommended that a 25- or 23-gauge butterfly be placed in a scalp vein or other easily visualized vein. A plastic IV cannula then can be placed after the clinical situation is stabilized. As soon as IV access is established, we recommend the administration of IV atropine 0.02 mg/kg to prevent bradycardia from laryngoscopy and other causes. If laryngospasm occurs, succinylcholine can be administered intravenously quickly without the concern of bradycardia from administered succinylcholine (Figs. 21-1 through 21-4).

Only preservative-free saline can be used as a flush solution for these neonates, because flush solutions containing benzyl alcohol can precipitate acidosis in small babies.

For short procedures that allow easy access to the neonate's airway, the laryngeal mask airway (LMA) is ideal. The LMA has been shown to provide a satisfactory airway in infants with BPD during minor surgical procedures and re-

sults in fewer respiratory problems compared to an endotracheal tube. Procedures such as extended eye examination under anesthesia and laser surgery, allow for easy placement of an LMA and rapid reinsertion of the LMA, should it become dislodged. We do not recommend the use of the LMA for open eye procedures where the patient's entire head and neck are covered by surgical drapes and easy access to the LMA would not be available. We have had one extreme situation of a neonate with severe reactive airway disease accompanying BPD. In this situation, the bronchospasm was precipitated by intubation. An LMA was used successfully for an open eye procedure, but great care was taken by the surgical and anesthesia teams to secure and not dislodge the LMA during the procedure. Use of the LMA for an open eye procedure is the rare exception and is not recommended unless the infant does not tolerate intubation well.

When we are certain we have adequate ventilation via mask airway, have established IV access, and plan to proceed with oral endotracheal intubation, we administer rocuronium 1 mg/kg IV for muscle relaxation.

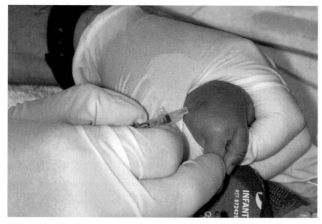

FIGURE 21-2. Target vein is entered with a deliberate 1- to 2-mm thrust of the intravenous cannula into the vein.

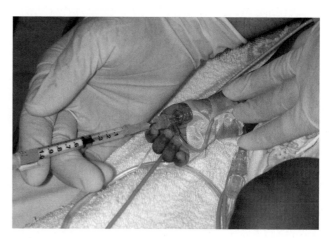

FIGURE 21-4. Medications are administered directly at the site of the T-piece.

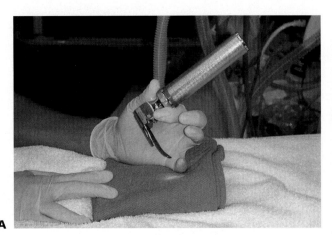
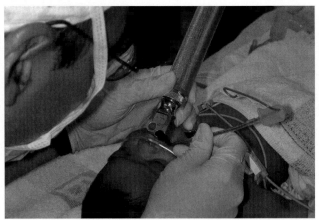

A   B

FIGURE 21-5. Laryngoscope is held close to the laryngoscope blade.

Prior to commencing anesthetic induction, the three sizes of uncuffed endotracheal tubes (2.5-, 3.0-, and 3.5-mm internal diameter) used in neonates should be available, with stylets in place. For most neonates, a laryngoscope fitted with a Miller 0 laryngoscope blade is the instrument of choice for intubation. The anesthetist should hold the laryngoscope handle close to the laryngoscope blade to allow use of his or her fifth finger to apply external pressure over neonate's cricoid cartilage. This pressure pushes the glottis into view when the tip of the laryngoscope blade is pulling up on the neonate's epiglottis. During laryngoscopy, this maneuver will maximize the chances of good visualization of the glottis of the neonate for successful intubation (Figs. 21-5 and 21-6).

For maintenance of general anesthesia, we generally change over from sevoflurane to isoflurane because isoflurane is less toxic when given for a long period of time. We rarely administer any narcotic to these neonates for ROP surgery because of their decreased ability to metabolize narcotics and our desire to establish a normal respiratory pattern as soon as possible after anesthesia to facilitate extuba-

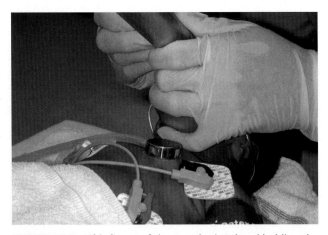

FIGURE 21-6. Fifth finger of the anesthetist's hand holding the laryngoscope is used to place pressure over the infant's cricoid cartilage.

tion. For neonates who will remain intubated for a long period after surgery with general anesthesia, we titrate small amounts of fentanyl IV.

We have encountered a few neonates who have severe reactive airway disease and do not tolerate more than moderate-to-low inspired concentrations of sevoflurane or isoflurane. In these cases, we have used low concentrations of sevoflurane or isoflurane augmented with propofol infusion. We begin the propofol infusion at 100 µg/kg/min and titrate up or down as the clinical situation requires. We use rocuronium for muscle relaxation as needed.

CRISIS AND TREATMENT OF BRONCHOSPASM

One of the most difficult anesthetic complications to deal with when anesthetizing the VLBW infant for ROP surgery is bronchospasm. Although rare, bronchospasm occurs in the VLBW infant with moderate-to-severe BPD, at about 1 to 3 months after birth. The bronchospasm, which probably is a combination of airway smooth muscle and arterial smooth muscle contraction, can be of sudden onset and lead to rapid oxygen desaturation. Bronchospasm can be very difficult to treat. If it does not abate with positive pressure via face mask or endotracheal tube, we administer epinephrine IV in 1-µg boluses until the bronchospasm improves or the heart rate is >215 beats/min. Sometimes increasing the sevoflurane concentration helps relieve the bronchospasm; at other times, the sevoflurane must be discontinued to stop the bronchospasm. It is important to emphasize that this type of sudden severe bronchospasm is rare.

Because of limited respiratory reserve, the VLBW infant with BPD should not receive elective general anesthesia when the infant has an upper respiratory infection (URI). Infants and children with a URI are more likely to have respiratory complications. These patients already have significant respiratory compromise and should not be placed at greater risk than necessary when receiving general anesthesia for ROP surgery.

TABLE 21-1. WILLIAM BEAUMONT HOSPITAL BASIC PEDIATRIC ANESTHESIA DRUGS

Drug	Dose	Drug	Dose
Atracurium	0.5 mg/kg	Naloxone	0.1 mg/kg
Atropine	0.01–0.02 mg/kg	Furosemide	0.2–1 mg/kg
STP (IV)	4–6 mg/kg	Pentobarbital (IM)	4–6 mg/kg
STP (PR)	25–30 mg/kg	Ketamine (IV)	1–2 mg/kg
Fentanyl	1–2 μg/kg	Ketamine (IM)	5–10 mg/kg
Glycopyrrolate	5–10 μg/kg	Tylenol	10–15 mg/kg
Succinylcholine	1–1.5 mg/kg	Versed (IV)	0.07–0.08 mg/kg
Succinylcholine (IM)	3–5 mg/kg	Versed (PO)	0.5–1.0 mg/kg
Neostigmine	0.05 mg/kg	Versed (nasal)	0.3 mg/kg
Vecuronium	0.1 mg/kg	Meperidine (IV)	1–1.5 mg/kg
Chloral hydrate	50–100 mg/kg	Meperidine (IM)	1 mg/kg
Diazepam (IV)	0.1 mg/kg	Zemuron	0.6–1.6 mg/kg
Methohexital (IV)	1–2 mg/kg	Pavulon	0.05–0.1 mg/kg
Droperidol	0.01–0.05 mg/kg	Propofol	4–6 mg/kg
Morphine	0.05–0.1 mg/kg	Ondansetron	0.1 mg/kg
Ephedrine	0.1 mg/kg		

STP, sodium pentothal.

These infants may require a full 6 weeks to recover from a URI to be suitable for elective general anesthesia.

EXTUBATION IN OPERATING ROOM VERSUS TRANSPORT TO NEONATAL INTENSIVE CARE UNIT WITH SLOW EXTUBATION

Most VLBW infants aged 4 months or older with mild-to-moderate lung disease will tolerate extubation in the operating room after the ROP eye surgery is completed. Some of the VLBW infants in this age group with severe lung disease will require postoperative ventilatory support. Most of the VLBW infants will require postoperative apnea monitoring, and many of these infants are on continuous apnea monitoring at home.

CONCLUSION

Anesthetic care of the VLBW infant for ROP surgery requires a trained pediatric anesthetist. These patients require extra time and consideration because of the fragility of their physical condition caused by the multiple medical problems of extreme prematurity.

Tables 21-1 through 21-8 list the medication, endotracheal, and LMA guidelines we use at William Beaumont Hospital, Royal Oak, Michigan.

TABLE 21-2. ENDOTRACHEAL TUBE SIZE AND LENGTH BY WEIGHT AND AGE

Weight or Age	Internal Diameter (mm)	Length to Lips (cm)
Weight		
<1500 g	2.5 uncuffed	Wt in kg + 6.0 cm
1,500–5,000 g	3.0 uncuffed	Wt in kg + 6.0 cm
75 kg, 6 mo	3.5 uncuffed	12–13
Age		
6–18 mo	3.5–4.0 uncuffed	13–14
18 mo to 3 yr	4.0–4.5 uncuffed	13.0–14.0
3–5 yr	4.5	13.5–14.5
5–6 yr	5.0	15.5–17.0
6–8 yr	5.5–6.0	17.0–19.0
8–10 yr	5.5–6.0	19.0–20.0
10–12 yr	6.0–6.5	20.0–20.5
12–14 yr	6.5–7.0	21.0–22.0
14–16 yr	7.0–7.5	22.0–23.0

Depth of insertion for the neonate + wt in kg + 6.0 cm. This gives length from distal tip to corner of mouth. External diameter of the endotracheal tube approximates the size of the patient's little finger. Cuffed endotracheal tubes are recommended after age 6 years. Tube tip should be halfway between thorax inlet and carina. All tubes are checked for placement by auscultation and if necessary by x-ray film. When ventilating for life support at usual pressures, the uncuffed endotracheal tube should leak at 20 cm H_2O inspiratory pressure. The general tube size rules used after age 1 year:

$$\text{Tube size} = \left[\frac{16 + age}{4}\right] \text{ or } \left[\frac{age \text{ of patient in yr}}{4}\right] + 4 \text{ or}$$

$$\left[\frac{\text{height of patient in cm}}{20}\right] = \text{Size internal diameter (mm) of}$$

endotracheal tube.

TABLE 21-3. LMA PATIENT SELECTION GUIDELINES

LMA Mask Size	Patient Size	Maximum Cuff Volume (Air)
1	Neonates/infants up to 5 kg	Up to 4 mL
1.5	Infants 5–10 kg	Up to 7 mL
2	Infants/children 10–20 kg	Up to 10 mL
2.5	Children 20–30 kg	Up to 14 mL
3	Children 30–50 kg	Up to 20 mL
4	Adults 50–70 kg	Up to 30 mL
5	Adults 70–100 kg	Up to 40 mL
6	Adults >100 kg	Up to 50 mL

LMA, laryngeal mask airway.

TABLE 21-4. MAC CONCENTRATIONS OF COMMON ANESTHETIC AGENTS IN CHILDREN

Agent	Neonates	1–6 months	6–12 months	12–24 months	Children
Desflurane	9.16%	9.42%	9.92%	8.72%	7.89%
Enflurane				−1.69%	
Halothane	0.87%	1.2%	1.98%	0.97%	0.87%
Isoflurane	**1.6%**	**1.87%**	**1.8%**	**1.6%**	**1.6%**
N_2O (predicted)					109%
Sevoflurane	3.2%	3.2%	2.5%	2.5%	2.49%

MAC, minimum alveolar concentration.

TABLE 21-5. PHARMACOLOGIC THERAPY FOR ACUTE INTRAOPERATIVE BRONCHOSPASM

The following treatments should be initiated after eliminating other causes of intraoperative wheezing or airway obstruction:

1. Deepen anesthesia with inhalational agents or opioids

2. P-agonist bronchodilators (albuterol, metaproterenol) using metered dose inhalers through the endotracheal tube

    b. Epinephrine infusion 0.01–0.1 μg/kg/min

4. Methylxanthines: aminophylline 5–7 mg/kg IV load over 30 min; infusion 0.6–1 mg/kg/h (therapeutic level: 10–20 μg/mL)

5. Corticosteroids
    a. Hydrocortisone 5 mg/kg IV q6h
    b. Methylprednisolone 1 mg/kg IV load, then 0.8 mg/kg q4–6h

TABLE 21-6. TREATMENT OF PAIN IN THE POSTANESTHESIA CARE UNIT

Mild to moderate
  Ketorolac 0.75–1.0 mg/kg IV
  Ibuprofen 10 mg/kg PO
  Acetaminophen 10–15 mg/kg PO/PR

Moderate to severe [usually begin with 1/2l (one half) dose and titrate effect]
  Morphine 0.1 mg/kg
  Demerol 1.0 mg/kg
  Fentanyl 1.0 μg/kg IV
  Codeine 1.0 mg/kg PO

TABLE 21-7. PEDIATRIC RESUSCITATION MEDICATIONS

Epinephrine[a]	First dose: IV/IO: 0.01 mg/kg (1:10,000)
	ET: 0.1 mg/kg (1:1,000)
	Subsequent doses
	IV/IO/ET: 0.1 mg/kg (1:1,000)
	Doses up to 0.2 mg/kg of 1:1,000 may be effective
	Repeat every 3–5 min
Atropine[a]	0.02 mg/kg/dose IV; using a minimum of 0.1 mg
	Dose may be repeated to a maximum of 1 mg for children or 2 mg for adolescents.
Adenosine	0.1 mg/kg fast IVP (double and repeat if necessary)
Sodium bicarbonate	1 mEq/kg/dose IV
25% Dextrose	1–2 cc/kg/dose IV
Calcium chloride	20 mg/kg/dose IV
Lidocaine[a]	1 mg/kg/dose IV
Bretylium	5 mg/kg/dose IV; subsequent dose may be doubled
Naloxone (Narcan)[a]	0.1 mg/kg/dose IV
Defibrillation	2 J/kg (double and repeat if unsuccessful)
	Internal paddles dosage is considerably less
	10 J/kg is used to defibrillate an adult heart
Cardioversion	0.5 J/kg (double and repeat if unsuccessful)

[a]*May also give endotracheally.*

TABLE 21-8. CARDIOVASCULAR DRIPS

Drug	Concentration	Dose
Epinephrine	1:1,000 (1 mg/mL), 1-mL ampule	[a]0.6 mg/kg diluted with D5W to total 100 mL[a]
		Start at 0.1 μg/kg/min
Isoproterenol	1:5,000 (1 mg/mL), 0.5-mL ampule	[a]0.6 mg/kg diluted with D5W to total 100 mL[a]
		Start at 0.1 μg/kg/min
Norepinephrine	1:1,000 (1 mg/mL), 4-mL ampule	[a]0.6 mg/kg diluted with D5W to total 100 mL[a]
		Start at 0.1 μg/kg/min
Dopamine	40 mg/mL, 5-mL vial	6.0 mg/kg diluted with D5W to total 100 mL[b]
		Start at 5 μg/kg/min.
Dobutamine	250-mg powdered vial	6.0 mg/kg diluted with D5W to total 100 mL[b]
		Start at 5 μg/kg/min
Nitroprusside	10 mg/mL, 5-mL vial	Start at 0.25–0.50 μg/kg/min
		Titrate to needed effect or maximum of 6.0 μg/kg/min
Neonatal use	Dilute 5-mL vial with 5-mL D₅W	0.3 mL/kg diluted with D5W to total 100 mL
		Start at 0.5 μg/kg/min, which will be 1.0 mL/h
Lidocaine	40 mg/mL (4%), 5-ml vial	Load: 1 mg/kg maximum
		75 mg maintenance drip: 20–50 μg/kg/min

[a]For isoproterenol, norepinephrine, and epinephrine, 1.0 mL/h provides 0.1 μg/kg/min.
[b]Each *l* mL/h infused will provide the same number of μg/kg/min of dopamine or dobutamine (or 1.0 mL/h provides 1.0 μg/kg/min).

SUGGESTED READING

1. Gregory GA, ed. *Pediatric anesthesia, 3rd ed.* New York: Churchill Livingstone, 1994.
2. Cook DR, Marcy JH, eds. *Neonatal anesthesia.* Pasadena: Appleton Davies, Inc. 1988.
3. Haigh P, Chiswick M, O'Donoghue E. Retinopathy of prematurity: systemic complications associated with different anaesthetic techniques at treatment. *Br J Ophthalmol* 1997;81: 283–287.
4. Ferrari L, Goudsouzian N. The use of the laryngeal mask airway in children with pulmonary dysplasia. *Anesth Analg* 1995;81: 310–313.
5. Seefelder C. Challenges in neonatal anesthesia. Presented at Practical Aspects of Pediatric Anesthesia, Harvard Medical School, The Children's Hospital, Massachusetts General Hospital, May 22–24, 2002.

SURGICAL APPROACHES TO INFANT AND CHILDHOOD RETINAL DISEASES: NONINVASIVE METHODS

MICHAEL T. TRESE
ANTONIO CAPONE, JR.

ANESTHETIC CONSIDERATIONS RELATIVE TO EXAMINATION

Several considerations must be weighed when deciding what an infant, child, or family can withstand relative to examination with or without anesthesia.

The clearest goal is an examination that provides accurate information and effective treatment whether or not anesthesia is needed. Some children will allow effective examination and treatment without anesthesia whereas others will not. Sometimes it is necessary to attempt examination without anesthesia; if it is not tolerated by the child or the family, then anesthesia can be used. The appropriate risks of anesthesia are outlined elsewhere in this text. Although a lid speculum and scleral depression are often used, with experience, the necessary information can be obtained using the doll's-eyes phenomenon and a 28-diopter lens with indirect ophthalmoscopy. By turning the infant's head, the eyes will stay directed in the original field of gaze, making it easier to examine the peripheral retina in that field.

NEODYMIUM:YTTRIUM-ALUMINUM-GARNET TREATMENT

Indications

Although uncommon, the need to open secondary membranes after cataract surgery occurs in children and can be performed using the neodymium:yttrium-aluminum-garnet (Nd-YAG) laser.

Equipment

The 1064-nm Nd-YAG laser in a slitlamp delivery system is used. We do not use a contact lens and usually have the parent in the treatment room with the child. When general anesthesia is necessary, some surgeons use ceiling-mounted YAG lasers or other adaptations for the operating room.

Anesthesia

We have found that some children as young as 3 years can cooperate for YAG treatment with the slitlamp delivery system using topical anesthesia. For those unable to be treated awake, general anesthesia is used.

Procedure

We use the conventional slitlamp delivery system, often without a contact lens. We usually set up the laser parameters prior to bringing the child into the laser room. The child's attention span is customarily short, and the procedure requires some patience. The child is seated (on the parent's lap if necessary), and the child's attention is directed to the physician.

Postoperative Care

The intraocular pressure is checked 1 hour after the procedure and the following day, if possible.

Complications

Damage to the intraocular lens (IOL) is possible.

Outcomes

In our experience, successful capsular opening is achieved approximately 80% of the time without the need for general anesthesia.

DIODE OR ARGON LASER PHOTOCOAGULATION

Indications

Probably the most common pediatric retinal laser procedure is peripheral ablation for stage 3 retinopathy of prematurity (ROP) (see Chapter 27) (1–4). Peripheral ablation is also used for familial exudative vitreoretinopathy and incontinentia pigmenti or other retinal vascular diseases. Additional information regarding management of tumors or Coats disease is discussed elsewhere in the text (see Chapters 14, 15, and 29). Laser is also used for retinal breaks, tears, and dialyses.

Equipment

Photocoagulation can be performed with a number of different lasers. For ROP, ablation of the avascular zone is performed with indirect delivery using one of several laser wavelengths: (i) argon green (visible) wavelength, (ii) 810 nm (infrared), or (iii) 532 nm (visible). In contrast to the argon green lasers, the 810- and 532-nm lasers are small and portable, and they can be plugged into a standard wall socket. The lasers can be diode systems alone (810 nm) or in combination with a frequency-doubled YAG (532 nm). The benefit of the 810 nm diode laser is that it is less likely to cause lens damage because the wavelength is not absorbed by hemoglobin of persistent tunica vasculosa lentis.

In older children undergoing laser for a retinal break or for ablation of vascular abnormalities in Coats disease, slit-lamp delivery of laser is accomplished with a contact lens, such as a quadrispheric lens or Goldmann three-mirror lens. For children with peripheral lesions, the indirect delivery system is used.

Anesthesia

Anesthesia varies depending on the age and cooperation of the child. For premature infants, consultation with the neonatologist or anesthesiologist at the hospital is essential. The agents selected for sedation and the decision of whether intubation is to be used are determined by the neonatologist.

For young children requiring laser for peripheral breaks, general anesthesia may be necessary. However, with a cooperative child, laser can be performed in the office setting and often is easier for the child if the indirect delivery system is used. However, those accustomed to contact lenses often tolerate laser using contact lens delivery

Procedure

For treatment of ROP, we prefer the 810-nm diode indirect laser, although others have used green lasers. The theoretical advantage of the diode is less absorption of laser energy by hemoglobin within persistent tunica vasculosa lentis. The

spot size is determined by the condensing lens and the distance from the eye, and is an approximation at best. The power, direction, and interval between spots can be determined. Settings are adjusted based on the pigmentation of the fundus and the appearance of the spot size on the retina. We prefer slightly whitened retina and not chalk-white lesions. Often settings can be started at 200 ms and 100 to 200 mW. Once an adequate burn is achieved, we use the repeat mode to deliver spots. We try not to exceed a power of 500 mW and 500 ms to achieve retinal lesions. We believe that excessive power might contribute to the complication of anterior segment ischemia. The laser records a number of spots delivered that can be vastly different from the number of lesions that appear at the retinal surface. However, it is important to maintain focus at the retinal surface when treating to avoid unwanted laser energy to other ocular structures.

We prefer to treat infants with threshold ROP in the neonatal intensive care unit (NICU) under the supervision of a neonatologist. However, the choice often depends upon the hospital, anesthesia department, operating room, and NICU. Sometimes, the better approach is to treat the infant in the operating room. It is helpful to work out a plan that is suitable for all involved in the care of the premature infant. Some physicians believe that an intubated child is stressed less by the lid speculum and scleral depression. We believe a wire lid speculum makes it easier to treat the superior and inferior retina, but whatever the treating physician is comfortable with is acceptable. Postoperatively, antiinflammatory drops may be considered because cells can be seen in some eyes after treatment; however, topical antiinflammatory drops are not necessary. There is no absolute number of laser spots that is necessary, but the goal of treatment should be to treat all avascular retina with a nearly confluent pattern. We define nearly confluent as spots placed one half a spot size apart. In the horizontal meridian, we place spots a full spot size apart to reduce possible damage to the long posterior ciliary nerves.

Children who have been discharged from the NICU prior to needing treatment usually are treated in the operating room with mask or laryngeal mask general anesthesia upon readmission to the hospital.

For treatment of Coats vascular lesions, we often use longer duration spots to safely ablate the lesion and reduce the risk of hemorrhage. This is possible in older, more cooperative patients with Coats disease. In younger children, we prefer cryotherapy to laser for the treatment of Coats lesions, particularly if the retina is detached. Indocyanine green (ICG) can be infused prior to treatment with the 810-nm diode laser. The laser energy is preferentially absorbed by ICG within the Coats lesions. Thus, less energy is needed to cause thrombosis. This "photodynamic therapy" reduces the damage to surrounding retina.

For treatment of peripheral breaks or lattice degeneration, we often use the following parameters: (i) for contact lens delivery: 100- to 200-μm spot size, 100- to 200-ms duration, 100-mW power adjusted, depending on whether a Goldmann or quadrispheric lens is used; (ii) for indirect delivery: 28- or 20-diopter indirect lens (spot size varies depending on lens and position of physician treating), 100- to 200-ms duration, and 100-mW (green laser) or 200-mW (810-nm diode) power.

Postoperative Care

Customarily, postoperative drops are not needed. However, for extensive cryotherapy, a subconjunctival steroid injection is often administered.

Complications

In order to apply appropriate peripheral ablation, the complications of treatment should be appreciated. Although complications of peripheral ablation are few, two are of note and should be explained to the patient's family. Cataract has been described as a complication of laser photocoagulation for ROP. The cataract itself probably has two potential etiologies. One is the presence of the tunica vasculosa lentis remnant. If an argon green laser is used, the light is absorbed by the blood in the vessels of the persistent tunica vasculosa lentis, the lens capsule ruptures, and the lens can swell resulting in a cataract (5,6). This mechanism can be minimized by using an 810-nm diode laser. However, cataract has also been reported with the 810-nm diode laser and even after cryotherapy treatment for ROP. These treatments might potentially cause cataract by another mechanism involving partial anterior segment ischemia. We believe this is due to overtreatment in the horizontal meridian by ablative therapy and that less treatment reduces the risk (7). The horizontal meridian is the easiest area to treat, and perhaps scleral depression reduces circulation of the large posterior ciliary vessels. An even more severe complication of peripheral ablation is full-blown anterior segment ischemia with cataract iris atrophy and hypotony that can lead to phthisis bulbi. In these eyes, the retina usually does not detach as in the usual progression of ROP. Effusive detachment can appear rarely after laser and is more often observed after cryotherapy.

Outcomes

Specific outcomes for ROP are presented in the tables in Chapter 26. See Chapter 29 for outcomes of Coats disease.

Fluorescein Angiography

Fluorescein angiography (see Chapter 5) is now available for young children and can be done in the operating room. Dosing or dye is available in the package insert by weight. We use a contact wide-angle camera for angiography.

CRYOTHERAPY

Indications

Prior to the availability of indirect laser, cryotherapy had been popular for peripheral ablation for ROP and other retinal diseases. With the development of the indirect laser, cryotherapy is used less often to treat ROP because it causes swelling of the ocular tissues, more globe manipulation, inflammation, reduced blood–retinal barrier (8), and, in some cases, effusive retinal detachment. Cryotherapy is used when laser cannot be delivered to the eye because of vitreous hemorrhage, extensive tunica vasculosa lentis, or poorly dilating pupil preventing adequate treatment of the periphery. Occasionally, it is necessary to perform a small conjunctival incision in order to treat very posterior retina. When this is needed, the procedure is performed in the operating room.

Equipment

Equipment includes cryotherapy unit, probe (preferably curved), and lid speculum.

Anesthesia

Anesthesia used depends on the age of the child. Topical tetracaine or subconjunctival lidocaine can be used in older children, whereas general anesthesia is used in infants.

Procedure

The eye is widely dilated. The child lies down on a table and an anesthetic is given. If the conjunctiva is opened, the eye is prepped in sterile fashion and the patient is draped. A drop of 10% povidone-iodine in placed into the conjunctival cul-de-sac. The cryotherapy probe (we prefer a curved probe) is placed onto the conjunctiva and, while indirect ophthalmoscopy is performed, a cryotherapy freeze is placed where desired (in avascular retina, on a vascular lesion in Coats disease, or around an open break). When the retina begins to whiten, the freezing is stopped so as to avoid overtreatment.

Postoperative Care

In eyes with conjunctival incisions, postoperative antibiotic drops are used for about 5 days. In eyes with moderately extensive cryotherapy, a subconjunctival steroid injection is used.

Complications

Complications of cryotherapy include bleeding from the choroid, damage to the sclera, and even perforation of the globe, but fortunately these complications are extremely rare. The choroidal effusion caused by cryotherapy can reabsorb over time, but there may be irreversible damage to the retinal pigment epithelium (RPE) and photoreceptors when cryoablative therapy is used.

Cryotherapy is commonly used to treat retinal tears and is very effective. Cryotherapy had been believed to contribute to proliferative vitreoretinopathy (PVR) development by releasing RPE cells from the subretinal space through the retinal break into the vitreous. However, the risk seems small clinically if care is taken to avoid treating the area of bare RPE cells. Laser and cryoablative treatment for retinoblastoma is found in the retinoblastoma chapter.

Outcomes

Outcomes for ROP are given in Chapter 26 and for Coats lesions in Chapter 29.

PHOTODYNAMIC THERAPY

Indications

In older children, photodynamic therapy has been used with some success for retinal and choroidal vascular lesions, such as choroidal hemangiomas (9) and choroidal neovascularization (10).

Equipment

Equipment used includes laser that emits 689- to 692-nm light, verteporfin (Visudyne), contact lens, scale, and infusion.

Anesthesia

The child must be old enough to cooperate with local topical anesthesia, such as proparacaine.

Order of Procedure

The use of photodynamic therapy in children is still being studied. Variations in the method have been reported, depending on the nature of the lesion (8–12). The child is weighed to determine the amount of drug to be infused (6 mg/m^2). The dye is mixed per standard recommendations, and the appropriate amount is infused over 10 minutes. At 15 minutes, laser is delivered over the lesion with a spot size equal to 1000 microns + the greatest linear diameter. Methods have varied, but in several cases of choroidal hemangioma, energy of 50 to 100 J/cm^2 at an intensity of 600 mW/cm^2 has been delivered over 83 seconds (13,14). In cases of large choroidal hemangiomas, large nonoverlapping (8) or overlapping (15) consecutive spots can be delivered to treat the extent of the lesion.

Postoperative Care

Topical drops are not routinely used. Patients are seen back in the clinic within 3 to 4 months.

Complications

From our experience, the risk is small and the literature is scant. Anticipated complications would be similar to those in adults, including the possibility of posttreatment-related bleeding in approximately 4% of eyes. Serous retinal detachment can occur with tumor treatment, similar to that seen with thermal laser treatment.

Outcomes

Initial results in adults with choroidal hemangioma are encouraging, with flattening of serous retinal detachments, improvement in visual acuity, and little or no recurrence given limited follow-up.

REFERENCES

1. Cryotherapy for Retinopathy of Prematurity Cooperative Group. Multicenter trial of cryotherapy for retinopathy of prematurity: preliminary results. *Arch Ophthalmol* 1988;106:471–479.
2. Goggin M, O'Keefe M. Diode laser for retinopathy of prematurity: early outcome. *Br J Ophthalmol* 1993;77:559–562.
3. Capone A, Diaz-Rohena R, Sternberg P, et al. Diode laser photocoagulation for zone 1 threshold retinopathy of prematurity. *Am J Ophthalmol* 1993;116:444–450.
4. Ling CS, Fleck BW, Wright E, et al. Diode laser treatment for retinopathy of prematurity: structural and functional outcome. *Br J Ophthalmol* 1995;79:637–641.
5. Capone A, Drack AV. Transient lens changes after diode laser retinal photoablation for retinopathy of prematurity. [Letter] *Am J Ophthalmol* 1994;118:533–535.
6. Palmer EA. The continuing threat of retinopathy of prematurity. [Editorial] *Am J Ophthalmol* 1996;122:420–423.
7. Banach MJ, Ferrone PJ, Trese MT. A comparison of dense versus less dense diode laser photocoagulation patterns for threshold retinopathy of prematurity. *Ophthalmology* 2000;107:324–328.
8. Jaccoma EH, Conway BP, Campochiaro PA. Cryotherapy causes extensive breakdown of the blood-retinal barrier: a comparison with argon laser photocoagulation. *Arch Ophthalmol* 1985;103:1728–1730.
9. Anand R. Photodynamic therapy for diffuse choroidal hemangioma associated with Sturge Weber syndrome. *Am J Ophthalmol* 2003;136:758–760.
10. Mimouni KF, Bressler SB, Bressler NM. Photodynamic therapy with verteporfin for subfoveal choroidal neovascularization in children. *Am J Ophthalmol* 2003;135:900–902.
11. Anand R. Photodynamic therapy for diffuse choroidal hemangioma associated with Sturge Weber syndrome. *Am J Ophthalmol* 2003;136:758–760.
12. Mimouni KF, Bressler SB, Bressler NM. Photodynamic therapy with verteporfin for subfoveal choroidal neovascularization in children. *Am J Ophthalmol* 2003;135:900–902.
13. Robertson DM. Photodynamic therapy for choroidal hemangioma associated with serous retinal detachment. *Arch Ophthalmol* 2002;120:1155–1161.
14. Barbazetto I, Schmidt-Erfurth U. Photodynamic therapy of choroidal hemangioma: two case reports. *Graefes Arch Clin Exp Ophthalmol* 2000;238:214–221.
15. Schmidt-Erfurth UM, Michels S, Kusserow C, et al. Photodynamic therapy for symptomatic choroidal hemangioma: visual and anatomic results. *Ophthalmology* 2002;109:2284–2294.

SURGICAL APPROACHES TO INFANT AND CHILDHOOD RETINAL DISEASES: INVASIVE METHODS

MICHAEL T. TRESE
ANTONIO CAPONE, JR.

There are many common issues relative to invasive approaches in children. This chapter outlines these issues irrespective of the disease for which these techniques are used. The pertinent features of the invasive techniques are explained in each section relative to a specific disease.

SCLERAL BUCKLE

Performing a scleral buckling procedure in the face of the growing child's eye presents a few issues not present in the adult eye. Scleral buckling should always be presented to the family as a procedure, particularly in an infant, who may require a second operation to divide the buckle in order to not inhibit eye growth or induce persistent anisometropic amblyopia (1). It has been shown in retinopathy of prematurity (ROP) that up to 12 diopters of anisometropic amblyopia can be induced by scleral buckling (2). Scleral buckles used in acute retinopathy of prematurity are used primarily in the face of combined effusive and tractional retinal detachment, but over the last several years they have been used increasingly less, having been replaced by lens-sparing vitrectomy techniques. Scleral buckle for rhegmatogenous retinal detachments in children remains an important therapeutic tool. Vitreous surgery is difficult, and all epiretinal proliferation in children cannot be removed because the vitreous is firmly adherent to the inner retinal surface. Scleral buckling can be used in conjunction with vitreoretinal surgical techniques or alone for rhegmatogenous retinal detachments even when there is minimal proliferative vitreoretinopathy. The child presenting with a rhegmatogenous retinal detachment should be evaluated for both trauma or another congenital predisposing condition, such as Stickler syndrome.

The scleral buckle we use in children is a tire and an encircling element. We use a 2.5-mm solid silicone band (such as a 240-style) to encircle the eye, a large (e.g., 2.5-mm) sponge (such as a 5025-style) for the buckling elements, and nylon sutures for scleral fixation of the sponge and silicone band (Fig. 23-1). Others have advocated using solid silicone buckles, with the size determined by the localization on the sclera of the areas of pathology and the size of the eye. In children, we use a proportionally larger buckle than we might use in the adult eye because of the aggressive nature of the proliferative vitreoretinopathy seen in children following rhegmatogenous detachments. Treatment around the dialysis or retinal break(s) is often performed with cryotherapy. Breaks are localized on the sclera, and the buckle is chosen to support the breaks adequately (approximately 2 mm beyond the anterior and posterior extents of the break localized on sclera). Intrascleral mattress sutures are placed approximately 2 mm farther apart than the width of the buckling element. If drainage of subretinal fluid is considered, we prefer a scleral cutdown and use diathermy to cause the sclera fibers to retract and expose the choroid. Diathermy is placed onto the choroid once it is exposed and prior to release of subretinal fluid. Transillumination may be performed to locate so as to avoid perforating large choroidal vessels. A preplaced mattress suture of 7-0 silk is placed into the lips of the scleral cutdown. Tension on the rectus muscle sutures is lessened. Then, subretinal fluid is released with a cold thin perforating electrode. In cases with thick subretinal fluid that is difficult to drain, a 5-0 Vicryl needle (S-14) can be used to create a small opening in the choroid. When perforating, care is taken not to stick the needle into the eye but rather to pierce and lift up on the knuckle of choroid protruding from the scleral cutdown site.

It often is difficult to ascertain symptoms in the younger, especially preverbal, child. Therefore, the child often already has some proliferative vitreoretinopathy on the presenting examination. We believe larger buckles can be helpful in overcoming the tractional forces caused by the proliferative vitreoretinopathy. Customarily, the child is evaluated approximately 3 months after scleral buckling to determine if division of the buckle is possible. We usually do not remove the buckling element *in toto* but leave the large buckling el-

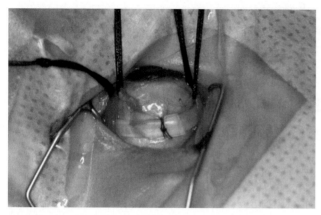

FIGURE 23-1. Image of scleral buckle in place. Position of the encircling element, a 2.5-mm solid silicone band, is shown. Sponge elements are often used to create a large indentation to overcome lesser amounts of proliferative vitreoretinopathy (PVR).

ement in place and divide the encircling band in an area where the retina is flat without any clinical evidence of traction. In children, capsular tissue can form rapidly around the scleral buckle, even after a relatively short period of time. This is noted on attempted division of the encircling band. The band can be located by tapping gently in the area where it is suspected with a closed pair of forceps. Once the band's location is determined, a hockey stick–like blade can be used to make a 2- to 3-mm incision through the capsule in the direction along the length of the band. The band then can often be lifted from the sclera and divided with scissors. After longer periods of time, even 6 to 12 months, the band might rarely erode into or through the sclera. In that situation, it is important to avoid any deep tissue dissection. Sometimes division of the band over the larger buckling element can be performed. In the author's experience, it is extremely rare that redetachment results after division of the encircling elements, particularly in eyes where buckling has been performed for a predominantly nonrhegmatogenous retinal detachment.

Drainage of subretinal fluid is always an important consideration. Drainage should be considered in all eyes where all traction is relieved and the areas of the retina and retinal pigment epithelium are similar (see earlier). If the retina is stretched and all traction is not removed, drainage of subretinal fluid can be dangerous and lead to retinal breaks. Therefore, drainage is rarely performed in ROP and familial exudative vitreoretinopathy (FEVR). Drainage might be considered in these cases if there is a total retinal detachment with extensive amounts of subretinal fluid; then, often only partial drainage is performed to reduce the risk of iatrogenic retinal tears. In addition, unless there is an existing retinal break, which makes intraretinal drainage possible in vitreous surgery, external drainage is more desirable. This is true because it is unlikely that the posterior hyaloid can be mechanically removed in a child during vitreous surgery.

VITREOUS SURGERY

Vitreous surgery over the last 15 years has become increasingly useful in pediatric retinal diseases. As better understanding of the pathophysiology of these retinal diseases evolves, the role of vitreous surgery in altering the mechanical scaffolding of the vitreous or the biochemical interactions present in the vitreous cavity expands. From an instrumentation standpoint, three-port and two-port vitrectomy, and open sky vitrectomy, can be used for pediatric indications. The authors most commonly use two-port vitrectomy with a variety of instruments that allow two-hand dissection (Table 23-1). These are the wide-angle high-flow light pipe, the infusion spatula, the infusion forceps, and retractable lighted pick (Fig. 23-2). These, in addition to the vitreous cutter and membrane peeler cutter (MPC) scissors, make up the instrumentation customarily used by the authors for vitreous surgery in infants and children. The viewing system used is an operating microscope with adjustable horizontal and vertical movement (X-Y) and the BIOM wide-angle viewing system. At this time, there does not appear to be a significant advantage to using smaller than 20-gauge instruments. In fact, some stiffer proliferative tissue may be difficult to deform and draw into the smaller port. Smaller instruments may become useful with the future development of enzymatic manipulation of vitreous collagen. They may have the advantage of being more safely and freely moved behind the lens and across the phakic eye.

TABLE 23-1. PEDIATRIC VITREOUS SURGERY INSTRUMENT LIST

Wide-field, high-flow end irrigator: 5614 Synergetics

Irrigating spatula: 28.30 Synergetics

Directional dull illuminated pick: 5617 Synergetics (retractable lighted pick)

Irrigating forceps: 11.10 Synergetics

EZ butterfly set: 367297 Becton-Dickinson

Knife illuminated (20 gauze): TR 980661 Escalon Medical

Three-way infusion tubing: 16579 Synergetics

Light fiber illuminated: 5605 Synergetics

Infusion cannula 20 gauge × 6 mm: 3032 Synergetics

Gas C3F8: TR9089 Escalon-Trek Medical

Solution BSS irrigating 500 mL: 65079550 Alcon

Drape: Ophthy w/ pouch: 8065103020 Alcon

Suture: Ethicon

Nylon 5-0: 7731G S-24 Spatula OR 749G RD-1 Spatula

Vicryl 7-0: J546G

C_3F_8, perfluoro octane; BSS, balanced salt solution.

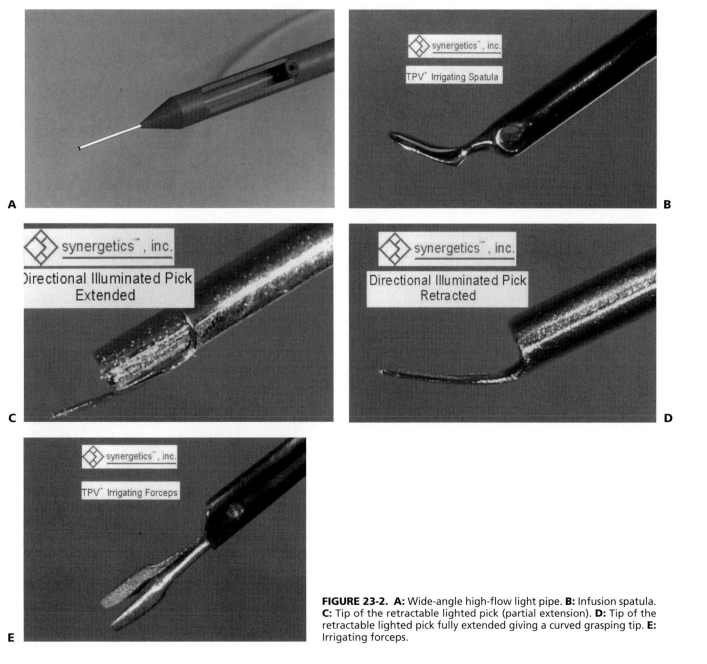

FIGURE 23-2. A: Wide-angle high-flow light pipe. **B:** Infusion spatula. **C:** Tip of the retractable lighted pick (partial extension). **D:** Tip of the retractable lighted pick fully extended giving a curved grasping tip. **E:** Irrigating forceps.

The location of the sclerotomies often is determined by the anatomy of the pathology and the age of the child. The premature eye does not have a pars plana; therefore, entry into the vitreous cavity should be performed through the pars plicata approximately 0.5 mm posterior to the limbus. A developed pars plana is not present until 8 to 9 months post-term (3). In retinal detachments, with vitreoretinal membranes that contact the posterior lens capsule, a lensectomy-vitrectomy often is required to relieve the vitreous traction and permit the retina to reattach. We often use a 23-gauge butterfly needle (Fig. 23-3), bent so as to allow infusion into the anterior chamber without contacting the corneal endothelium, while the vitreous cutter is used to remove the lens within the capsule. The entry for the lensectomy-vitrectomy in the premature eye is located immediately posterior to the limbus through the iris root directed into the lens anterior to the equator of the lens. This avoids the possibility of injuring the retina pulled anteriorly into the posterior chamber. When the lens is aspirated, the capsule is removed using a broad flat Sutherland forceps. The Sutherland forceps grasps the capsule approximately one third of the distance from the equator to the posterior pole of the lens; in that fashion, frequently all of the capsule can be removed at once. Complete removal of the capsule is essential to remove all of the cells that can lead to subsequent retinal iridal adhesions postoperatively.

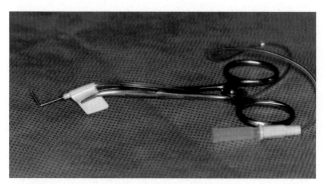

FIGURE 23-3. A 23-gauge butterfly needle mounted on a hemostat to be used as infusion with a sharp tip.

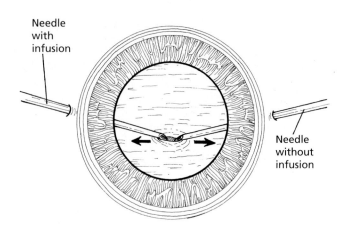

FIGURE 23-4. Artist's drawing of two needles being used to open retrolenticular tissue by cutting through a small central opening with very little posterior pressure and then separating the tips to avoid traction on the periphery.

Retrolental, preretinal tissue in many pediatric eyes with ROP is in contact with retinal tissue. It is important to open this retrolenticular tissue without affecting the retina beneath or peripheral to it. This opening is created with the sharp point of the 23-gauge infusion butterfly needle or a disposable 26-gauge needle on a TB syringe. The retrolenticular tissue in stage 5 ROP, when an anteriorly closed funnel detachment is present, is approached in a cross-action fashion, trying to dissect an opening without creating traction on the peripheral retina (Fig. 23-4). Traction on the peripheral retina can cause a retinal dialysis, almost uniformly a procedure failure. The retrolenticular tissue then can be dissected using two-hand dissection with the infusion spatula and forceps, either Grieshaber-Sutherland forceps or other positive action forceps that can grasp tissue using one hand and allow tissue to be spread or cut using the other hand. We call this *lamellar dissection* (Fig. 23-5). Particularly in ROP, FEVR, and other vitreoretinal dystrophies where the vitreous is formed in solid and liquid sheets, it is possible to perform lamellar dissection, peeling off one layer of preretinal membrane or vitreous at a time. This allows the surgeon to approach the retina safely, taking advantage of the collapsed layers of vitreous collagen. The MPC scissors also can be used to divide, in a sharp fashion, this tissue from the retinal surface.

Another technique involves using the retractable lighted pick with the pick extended in one hand and the infusion spatula beneath tissue adherent to, but not part of, the retina in the other hand. The instruments are pulled away from each other, thus avoiding inducing traction on the peripheral or other areas of the retina (Fig. 23-6). This frequently permits large areas of tissue to be stripped from the retinal surface, which can exert both circumferential and radial traction on the retina.

The goals of vitreous surgery in the pediatric eye must be considered differently from those in adult eyes. It is not necessary, and is dangerous, to try to remove all vitreous or preretinal membranous tissue from the inner retinal surface. Particularly in diseases such as ROP, much of the preretinal tissue is attached and sometimes is anatomically part of the

retinal surface. Often preretinal membranes can be segmented and left in place after the main vectors of vitreoretinal traction have been relieved. This technique minimizes the risk of damage to the extremely thin peripheral retina.

Also, unlike adult vitreoretinal surgery in which iatrogenic breaks can be managed by removal of preretinal membranes, retinotomies, and endophotocoagulation, iatrogenic retinal breaks in most pediatric retinal diseases usually result

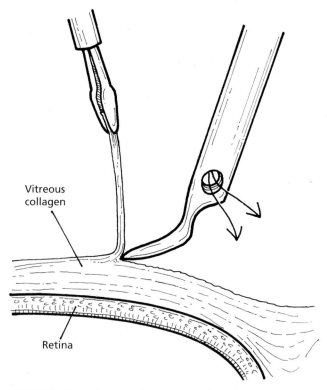

FIGURE 23-5. Artist's drawing showing the infusion spatula dissecting a vitreous collagen lamella that is held by forceps. This technique is called *two-hand lamellar dissection.*

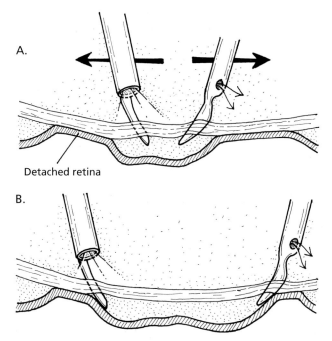

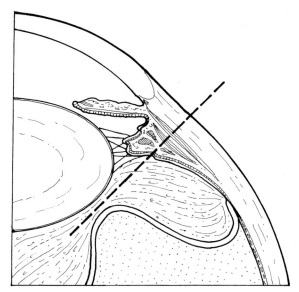

FIGURE 23-7. Artist's drawing showing the entry site into the sheet of tissue that extends between the lens and circumferential ridge of retina. The *dotted line* shows the *ab interno* sweeping of the MVR blade.

FIGURE 23-6. Artist's drawing showing the use of the retractable lighted pick and irrigating spatula to strip tissue from the retina. The two instruments are gently separated, thus dissecting the epiretinal tissue from the retina.

in inoperable retinal detachments, even with the use of laser, perfluorocarbon, and silicone oil, because of the inability to completely dissect the vitreous from the inner retinal surface. The guiding tenant of pediatric vitreous surgery should be to use extreme caution to not create a retinal break. This is often difficult because of the convoluted nature of the retinal anatomy and the fact that the retina can be stretched into an appearance unfamiliar to most surgeons. This is particularly true in ROP, FEVR, congenital retinoschisis, and persistent fetal vasculature syndrome.

Modification of the lens-sparing vitrectomy may be required in some cases. The entry must be made where there is adequate space between the lens and the neurosensory retina. As the surgeon becomes more familiar with this technique, a larger number of eyes can be operated upon by adapting to anatomic differences in this way. Very often there are spaces between circumferential or radial folds of retina and the posterior lens capsule. The surgeon can create entry wounds at sites other than the customary 9 and 3 o'clock positions. It may be necessary to enter through the sclera with a microvitreoretinal (MVR) blade and make an incision between the retinal fold and posterior lens by what we have described as an *ab interna* incision. This *ab interna* incision is made by placing the MVR blade through the sheet of tissue between the circumferential retinal fold and the posterior lens capsule and drawing back, extending the internal incision by cutting parallel to the lens capsule. The opening between the preretinal tissue or retinal fold and the posterior lens capsule can be extended from 90 to 120 degrees of arc (Fig. 23-7). En-

try into these eyes also requires care to avoid the lens equator. This is accomplished by pointing the MVR blade posteriorly, parallel to the visual axis. As the point of the blade comes into view, the blade is angled toward the center of the eye, avoiding contact with the clear lens material. The same angle of entry is used with all other surgical instruments such as the MPC scissors, intraocular forceps, and light pipe (Fig. 23-8).

The dissections within the eye are dictated based on the anatomy of each disease and are discussed in greater detail in individual chapters. Intraocularly, several vitreous substitutes may be used.

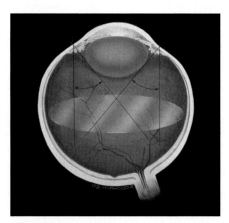

FIGURE 23-8. Artist's drawing showing the path of instrument entry for lens-sparing vitrectomy, first straight back paralleling the visual axis and then toward the center of the eye. This allows access to all areas posterior to the equator of the eye.

Vitreous Infusion

The infusion fluids used for vitreous surgery are balanced salt solution (BSS) Plus and lactated Ringer solution. We customarily use BSS Plus in our main infusion, which is delivered through the wide-angle high-flow infusion light pipe. However, a manifold system with three tubes split from a single one extending from a hung bottle of lactated Ringer solution, permits infusion to the infusion spatula, infusion forceps, and 23-gauge butterfly needle at the initial part of the surgery. The butterfly can then be easily replaced with an infusion contact lens for higher-magnification dissection customarily required in the posterior pole. This manifold requires only one bottle of lactated Ringer solution and one bottle of BSS Plus for the course of our vitrectomy. Other tamponades commonly used in adult vitreoretinal surgery include sodium hyaluronate (Healon), perfluorocarbon liquids, long-acting gases, and silicone oil. In pediatric two-port vitrectomies, we use air at the end of the case to facilitate closure of the sclerotomy wounds (4). If submacular blood is present, we place the child face down overnight using an air bubble to displace the blood. We tend not to use expanding gases in young children because of the inability to get reliable postoperative intraocular pressure measurements without an examination under anesthesia and the inability to obtain adequate postoperative positioning. If it is necessary to use a long-acting gas bubble, we use 10% C3F8. Families are cautioned that until the air/gas is gone from the eye, nitrous oxide anesthesia, air travel, and high altitudes should be avoided to prevent expansion and contraction of the bubble and, thus, dangerously high or low intraocular pressures. We place a bracelet on the child to caution against using N_2O anesthesia while air or other gases are in the vitreous cavity.

In addition, we use viscoelastic substances, such as Healon, to separate tight retinal folds and facilitate dissection of proliferative tissue. Care must be taken not to inject the Healon under such force that either a peripheral dialysis or posterior retinal break is created. To control the force, a foot-activated pump can be used with a special adaptor for viscodissection. In addition, the use of perfluorocarbon liquids must be performed cautiously, as the weight of perfluorocarbon can tear the very thin retinal periphery. Perfluorocarbons are used when all traction has been relieved and mainly to displace subretinal blood. The use of silicone oil, both by itself and in conjunction with perfluorocarbon liquids, has helped us to displace blood from the posterior pole (5). In some circumstances, perfluorocarbon and silicone oil used together and left in the eye temporarily, can result in retinal reattachment. The child must remain on his or her back for up to 1 week. The perfluorocarbon liquid is then removed and the silicone oil replaced. This technique has been most helpful in FEVR and will be explained in greater depth in Chapter 28 (5). In addition, we have found silicone oil to be a great help in eyes with long-standing hypotony from ciliary body destruction or detachment.

Pharmacologic Adjuncts

The use of intraocular agents, such as autologous plasmin enzyme, to assist vitreous surgery has been reported only in pilot studies to date and will demand the rigors of a randomized prospective controlled clinical trial to determine its ultimate usefulness (6,7). However, at this time, the authors use autologous plasmin when the vitreous needs to be completely removed from the retinal surface. In addition, antimetabolites, such as 5-fluorouracil, occasionally are used to suppress intraocular proliferation, particularly in traumatized eyes with epithelial downgrowth or fibrous ingrowth. The 5-fluorouracil, has both antiproliferation and antiinflammatory inhibitors. These agents require human subjects approval if they are to be used for research data collection.

Occasionally, *n*-butyl or *n*-octyl cyanoacrylate can be used to seal a retinal break created during vitreous surgery and permit successful retinal reattachment (8). This procedure requires a relatively dry retinal surface and is performed after fluid–air exchange. It is most easily accomplished with open sky vitrectomy because the instruments used to inject glue often get fluid in their tips when placed into the vitreous cavity. The fluid interacts with the cyanoacrylate, causing it to solidify before the glue can be placed onto the retinal break. In an open sky technique, the corneal is removed, permitting direct access to the retina. A carefully placed drop of cyanoacrylate onto the retinal break can result in an instantaneous seal. This technique is less frequently used. Future development of other retinal glues and enzymatic vitreolysis will facilitate pediatric retinal surgery.

REFERENCES

1. Trese MT. Scleral buckling for retinopathy of prematurity. *Ophthalmology* 1994;101:23–26.
2. Maguire AM, Trese MT. Lens-sparing vitreoretinal surgery in infants. *Arch Ophthalmol* 1992;110:284–286.
3. Hairston RJ, Maguire AM, Vitale S, et al. Morphometric analysis of pars plana development in humans. *Invest Ophthalmol Vis Sci* 1992;33:1197.
4. Stirpe M, Michels RG. *Sodium hyaluronate in anterior and posterior segment surgery*. Padova, Italy: Fidia Spa, Abano Terme Publishers, 1989.
5. Shaikh S, Trese M. Retinal reattachment facilitated by short term perfluorocarbon liquid tamponade in a case of FEVR and rhegmatogenous retinal detachment. *Retina* 2002;22: 674–676.
6. Trese MT, Williams GA, Hartzer MK. A new approach to stage 3 macular holes. *Ophthalmology* 2000;107:1607–1611.
7. Verstraeten TC, Chapman C, Hartzer M, et al. Pharmacologic induction of posterior vitreous detachment in the rabbit. *Arch Ophthalmol* 1993;111:849–854.
8. Hartnett ME, Hirose T. Cyanoacrylate glue in the repair of retinal detachment associated with posterior retinal breaks in infants and children. *Retina* 1998;18:125–129.

PEDIATRIC RHEGMATOGENOUS RETINAL DETACHMENT

ANTONIO CAPONE, JR.
MICHAEL T. TRESE

OVERVIEW

Epidemiology

There are few reported series of rhegmatogenous retinal detachment (RRD) in children most likely due to the low incidence. However, in affected patients, the rate of vision-threatening pathology in the companion eye can be as high as 90% (1). Although RRD has an incidence of approximately 12.4 cases per 100,000 population (2), RRD occurring in the pediatric age group (birth to 18 years) accounts for only 3.2% to 5.6% of the total number of RRD in the population (approximately 0.38–0.69 per 100,000 population).

Etiology

When considered across all age groups, RRD occurs following trauma in approximately 11% of cases (3,4). Approximately 40% of pediatric RRD occurs secondary to ocular trauma (1,5). Pediatric retinal detachments unrelated to globe-disrupting trauma in children or acute retinopathy of prematurity (ROP) in infants are seen most often in association with myopia, both isolated ocular or syndrome associated, or following intraocular surgery (2,3). This chapter discusses RRD secondary to myopia or previous ocular surgery.

Public Health Considerations

Although the incidence of RRD in children is low, there is a high incidence of bilateral retinal detachment or other disorders limiting vision in children (1). In our series, 75% of eyes with pediatric RRD and nearly half of the companion eyes presented with vision worse than 20/800 (1).

Considerable financial and emotional investment is incurred when the decision is made to attempt repair. However, pediatric RRDs are generally repaired successfully with contemporary vitreoretinal surgical techniques. Multiple surgical procedures often are necessary, partly due to the tendency for children to present late to the physician and have already with advanced pathology. The tendency toward bilateral ocular disease and the finding that nearly 40% of the repaired eyes have better or equal visual acuity compared to the companion eye at final follow-up make a compelling case for proceeding with surgical repair. Often, it will not be "just a spare eye."

CLINICAL PRESENTATION

Poor visual acuity is generally the presenting symptom. Retinal detachment usually is detected on an otherwise routine examination, on routine follow-up to a surgical procedure, or as a consequence of parental awareness of leukocoria.

For those patients who are able to determine the duration of time that vision loss was present in the affected eye, the mean duration is several weeks, ranging from immediate awareness to many months (1). In studies including all age groups, the mean time to presentation usually is much less than 30 days (3). Children who developed RRD often have bilateral ocular abnormalities predisposing them to poor vision in both eyes (Fig. 24-1). Consequently, it is difficult for them to compare vision in both eyes or to appreciate a difference in vision, analogous to the scenario of an adult developing RRD after penetrating keratoplasty (6). Thus, it often is difficult to discern a definite time when vision loss from RRD started.

The tendency for late diagnosis at presentation is an important feature of pediatric retinal detachment, with predictable consequences. Pediatric RRD typically presents as macula-off (80%) (1,5,7). In contrast, macula-off RRD occurs less frequently in adults. In 342 eyes with RRD from patients with mean age of 52.8 years, the macula was detached in only 56.5% of the eyes (8). Proliferative vitreoretinopathy (PVR) was present at initial diagnostic examination in approximately half of all eyes (Fig. 24-2) (1), which is in line with reports by Sternberg et al. (6) and Wa-

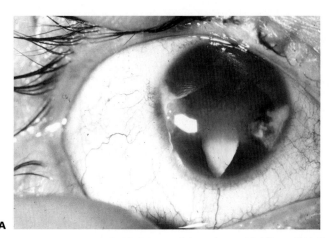

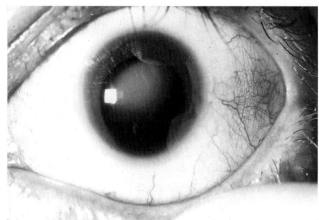

FIGURE 24-1. Adult patient with bilateral iris **(A, B)** and optic nerve coloboma. The right eye has band keratopathy and chronic retinal detachment.

terhouse et al. (9) of RRD after previous ocular surgery in which PVR was observed at initial presentation in 39% and 41% of adult patients, respectively.

A single retinal break or horseshoe retinal tear is commonly the cause of RRD. Giant retinal tears (Fig. 24-3) are generally seen in association with syndromes such as Stickler syndrome type 1. Conversely, retinal dialyses are seen most often following intraocular surgical procedures (1).

ETIOLOGIES

Pathologic Myopia-Associated Rhegmatogenous Retinal Detachment

Nonsyndromic Pathologic Myopia in Otherwise Healthy Infants and Children

Myopia is a significant public health problem associated with an increased risk of visual loss. Significant morbidity in

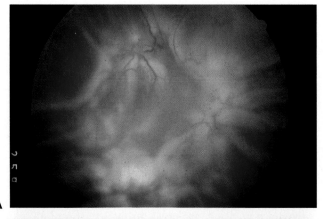

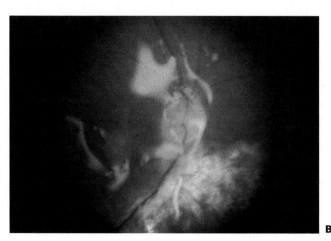

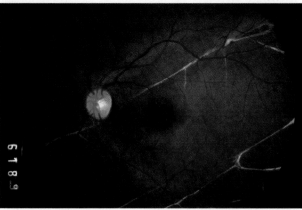

FIGURE 24-2. A: Total retinal detachment with associated proliferative vitreoretinopathy. **B:** Posterior pole image of the same eye shown in panel **A** following vitreoretinal surgery, completely attached under silicone oil. **C:** Strands of subretinal proliferative vitreoretinopathy, without retinal detachment.

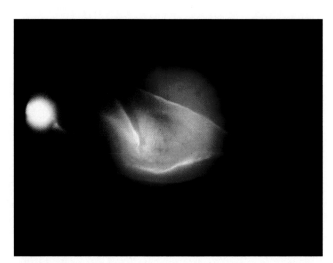

FIGURE 24-3. Retina folded over itself with bare retinal pigment epithelium in an eye with a giant retinal tear.

adults occurs as a result of high myopia (more than −4.00 diopters), most notably retinal detachment, myopic degeneration (both atrophic and neovascular), and glaucoma. Following trauma, juvenile retinal detachment is most commonly associated with myopia. Although the prevalence of myopia is low in otherwise healthy children, juvenile-onset myopia is of clinical interest for two reasons: (i) because of the opportunity for prevention of high myopia later in life, and (ii) because of its association with many systemic and ocular diseases that may require therapeutic intervention.

Epidemiology of Myopia

Myopia typically begins after age 6 years and progresses most rapidly through age 16 years. Nearly 6% of childhood blindness in the United States is attributable to myopia (10). It affects approximately 25% of all individuals in the United States overall (11). Juvenile-onset myopia is considerably more common in Asia (12), with the highest incidence in the world said to be among Singapore Chinese children (13). The incidence worldwide is thought to be increasing (14).

One explanation for the increase in juvenile myopia is that younger generations may be more likely to be exposed to myopigenic factors (discussed later) than their elders. Alternatively, among populations with a low incidence of "simple high myopia," myopia may be more strongly associated with systemic and ocular problems (15).

Pathogenesis

The "nature versus nurture" debate regarding the development of myopia is longstanding. Evidence to date suggests that heredity and environment both likely play a role in juvenile-onset myopia (4). Evidence supporting the role of heredity in myopia include the following: (i) myopia is more common in several ethnic groups; (ii) both syndromic and autosomal dominant pedigrees have been described; and (iii) an increasing number of genetic loci are being implicated.

There is controversy, however, regarding the difficulty in distinguishing shared genes from shared environment. Both influences are addressed here.

Environmental Factors. *Near activity.* Studies in humans and animals strongly suggest that retinal defocus interferes with emmetropization and results in myopia (16–18). Presumably, image blur occurs in the setting of tasks requiring near vision and results in axial elongation. These data serve as the basis for refractive therapies for juvenile-onset myopia in otherwise healthy school-aged children, as described later.

Light exposure. Daily illumination patterns are thought to influence ocular development, evidenced by the observation that postnatal ocular elongation occurs primarily during the day (19). Several reports implicated light exposure in the development of myopia, particularly with increased nighttime ambient light exposure during sleep in children younger than 2 years (20) and in adult law students (21). This is an area of considerable controversy, however, because other investigators have noted no impact of light exposure on the development of myopia (22,23).

Education. Although advanced educational level often is associated with myopia, it is universally considered to be an associative phenomenon, related to near activity, light exposure, or some other environmental factor.

Nonsyndromic Pathologic Myopia Associated with Nonhereditary Ocular Disease

Prematurity

The pathogenesis of myopia in patients with more severe ROP is a topic of considerable debate, currently without consensus. The pattern of refractive development also differs from that of both full-term infants and premature infants without severe ROP. The degree of myopia is related to the depth of the anterior chamber, the thickness of the lens, and the change in axial length. Myopia is not related to keratometric value.

Ocular as well as systemic factors, including duration of oxygen exposure and central nervous system microenvironment, may play a role. Prior reports have noted increased severity of ROP is associated with an increased prevalence of myopia. Cryotherapy has been implicated as well. A recent publication by the Cryotherapy for Retinopathy of Prematurity Cooperative Group suggests that cryotherapy does not change refractive status in eyes with severe ROP. The authors contend that cryotherapy prevents retinal detachment and allows refractive error assessment in some eyes in which high myopia is likely to be manifest. A recent randomized study reported a lower incidence of high myopia in eyes with severe ROP treated with laser photocoagulation (24), in addition to superior structural outcome and visual function (25).

Retinal detachment occurs infrequently later in childhood. There are no good published data on this topic. It is the authors' experience that RRD in older children who had ROP fell into two demographic groups. Between the ages of 4 and 8 years, traction-rhegmatogenous detachments seemed to occur primarily in boys. There often was a history of trauma, with tears or round holes occurring as a consequence of localized vitreous detachment and retinal traction. In the second group, RRD in early adolescence seemed more common in young females.

Stimulus Deprivation Myopia

Unilateral progressive myopia has been described following a variety of conditions that result in stimulus deprivation, including congenital ptosis (26), corneal opacification (27), cataract (Fig. 24-4A to C) (28), and vitreous hemorrhage (29).

Syndromic Pathologic Myopia

Ocular

Twin studies suggest a high degree of heritability, approximately 85% (30) of the spherical equivalent myopia, supporting the impact of parental refractive error. Several investigators have described genetic loci associated with nonsyndromic high myopia. Both X-linked (MYP1) (31) and autosomal loci (18p11.31 designated MYP2, 12q23.1-24 designated MYP3, and 7q36 for AD high myopia) (32–34) have been reported.

Systemic

Genetic loci have been identified for a variety of systemic syndromes with myopia as a component. The most common of these are the Stickler syndromes and Marfan syndrome.

Autosomal Dominant Vitreoretinopathies.

These vitreoretinopathies include the Stickler syndromes, erosive vitreoretinopathy, and Wagner disease. They are characterized by abnormal vitreous gel structure ("optically empty vitreous") and associated retinal changes, most commonly myopia. Although the latter two are commonly mentioned along with the Stickler syndromes, each is a distinct clinical entity. With the exception of cataract, noted in Stickler syndromes and Wagner disease, anterior segment abnormalities are uncommon. Associated systemic stigmata are seen only in Stickler syndrome. Only Stickler syndrome and erosive vitreoretinopathy are associated with a high incidence of retinal detachment. At the genetic level, the Stickler syndromes occur as a consequence of a defect mapping to chromosome 12q13.11. The other two entities both have been localized to chromosome 5q13–14, as have other vitreoretinopathies (35).

Stickler Syndromes.

The Stickler syndromes (hereditary or progressive oculoarthropathy) types 1 and 2 are the most common causes of retinal detachment in children, occurring as a consequence of collagen mutation. Myopia, an "optically empty vitreous," and retinal detachment are frequent ocular features. The most common form is associated with the 54 exon-containing gene located on chromosome 12q13.11–p13.2, which codes for type II collagen (type 1 Stickler, collagen 2A1) (36) and demonstrates a "membranous" vitreous. The less commonly encountered form of Stickler syndrome (type 2) is due to a defect in the collagen 11A1 gene involved in type XI collagen production (37) and maps to chromosomal locus 1p21. Such patients have fibrillar or "beaded" vitreous. Mutation in the collagen 11A2 gene results in a systemic Stickler phenotype without ocular

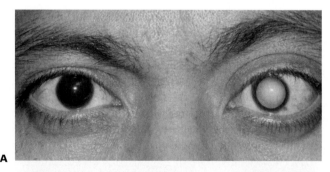

A

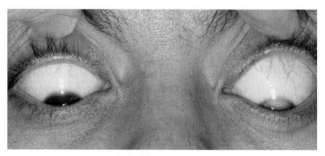

B

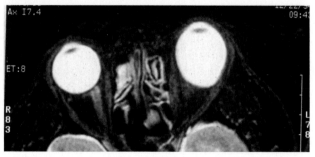

C

FIGURE 24-4. A: External image of an adult male with a dense traumatic cataract since early childhood resulting in leukocoria, stimulus deprivation, and related increase in axial length of the left eye. **B:** Note the marked curvature of the lower eyelid during downward gaze due to asymmetry in axial length, mimicking the Munson sign typically seen in patients with keratoconus. **C:** T2-weighted magnetic resonance image demonstrating marked asymmetry in axial length, with an appreciably larger left eye.

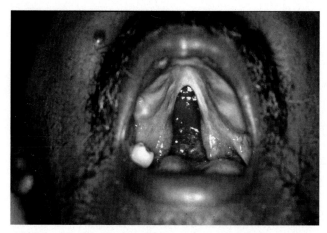

FIGURE 24-5. Cleft palate in a patient with Stickler syndrome who presented with a retinal detachment due to giant retinal tear.

findings (type III) (38) mapping to chromosomal locus 6p21.3. Direct DNA testing is available for all three loci to confirm the diagnosis or for prenatal testing.

Deafness, orofacial features (Fig. 24-5), and arthritis are associated components of type 1 Stickler syndrome (39). More than 17 mutations have been described for the highly penetrant type 1 gene (40) with considerable phenotypic variability. Some patients present without associated systemic features and a fundus appearance characterized by a radial perivascular retinal degeneration. The vitreoretinal degeneration of type 1 Stickler syndrome may be visible in the first decade with retinal holes and tears occurring within the lesion and at its margins (41,42).

Individuals with type 1 Stickler syndrome (collagen 2A1 mutation) have a high risk of RRD in childhood, approximately 50% (43,44). The RRDs in Stickler syndrome are unusual, perhaps because the typical posterior vitreous separation is lacking as a mechanism. As is true of Marfan syndrome, multiple retinal breaks and giant retinal tears are common.

Erosive Vitreoretinopathy. Brown et al. (45) described this clinical entity in 1994. In 1995, they reported that this condition may be allelic to Wagner disease and mapped to chromosome 5q13–14 (46). Similar to Wagner disease, retinal pigment epithelial changes, poor night vision, visual field defects, and abnormal electroretinographic findings are characteristic. Such features are not noted in Stickler syndrome patients. In contrast to Wagner disease, RRDs occur in approximately 50% of patients, similar in incidence to that of retinal detachment in Stickler syndrome. In 1999, the locus was refined to the 5q14.3 region (47).

Wagner Disease. Wagner disease (48) also is inherited as an autosomal dominant condition. Retinal detachment was not noted in the original description, and osteoarthropathy

is not a feature of Wagner disease. Wagner disease has not been demonstrated to exist beyond a single pedigree (49), in which the genetic abnormality has been localized to chromosome 5q13–14 (50). Subsequent examination of 60 members of Wagner's original pedigree reported a low incidence of RRDs in childhood and a high incidence of retinal detachment (50%) after age 45 years, with a high prevalence of peripheral traction retinal detachments and chorioretinal atrophy and cataract in older affected individuals (51). Thus, Wagner disease is often incorrectly categorized with Stickler disease, but there are differences. Wagner disease rarely presents with RD in childhood, whereas Stickler syndromes do. When retinal detachments do occur in Wagner disease, they usually do so later in life—after age 45 years and often are tractional as opposed to rhegmatogenous.

Marfan Syndrome. Marfan syndrome is due to a mutation in the fibrillin 1 gene (FBN1, locus 15q21.1) (52–54). Skeletal, cardiovascular, and ocular findings are characteristic of the autosomal dominant syndrome. Ectopia lentis with superotemporal displacement, lens coloboma (Fig. 24-6), and axial high myopia with scleral thinning are common ocular findings.

Retinal detachment occurs in 5% to 11% of patients, increasing to 8% to 38% in association with ectopia lentis or following lens surgery (55–57). Retinal detachment typically occurs in the third decade but can occur in childhood. There is a high relative prevalence of giant retinal tear, bilateral retinal detachment, total retinal detachment, macula-off retinal detachment, and PVR on initial presentation (58).

Other Myopia-Associated Syndromes. Myopia-associated systemic syndromes include Knobloch syndrome (collagen 18A1, associated with neuronal migratory defects and mapped to 21q22.3) (59,60), osteogenesis imperfecta type 1 (collagen 1A2) (61), and others (62–64).

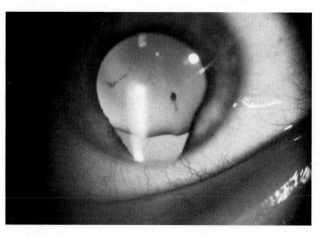

FIGURE 24-6. Lens coloboma in a child with Marfan syndrome.

Other Conditions

Colobomatous Rhegmatogenous Retinal Detachment

Colobomata can occur in the iris, lens, ciliary body, retina, choroid, and optic nerve. They are described as "typical" when they occur in inferonasal locations. Additional ocular findings can include microphthalmia, microcornea, cataract, and retinal detachment. The high incidence of associated systemic defects (approximately 40%) underscores the importance of pediatric referral (65).

Optic nerve coloboma (Fig. 24-7) occurs as a consequence of incomplete closure of the optic stalk in weeks 5 to 7 of embryogenesis. Optic nerve coloboma may occur sporadically or in association with multisystem abnormalities (66–70). In general, the visual potential in an eye with an optic nerve coloboma correlates with the foveal anatomy (71). Discerning foveal anatomy may pose a challenge because of the alteration of foveal detail (72). Chorioretinal colobomas are known to predispose to retinal detachment [4%–43%, depending on the series (73–76), with the "true" incidence likely on the order of 8% (74)]. The retina overlying the choroidal defect is thin and prone to breaks within or along the margin of the coloboma.

Retinal detachments associated with coloboma can occur in infancy but most typically are seen in childhood. Rarely, they may resolve spontaneously (77,78A). Visual acuity typically is poor, even with successful repair.

Juvenile Dialysis

Retinal dialysis is defined as a break at the junction of the retina and the pars plana, typically along the course of the ora serrata. The vast majority of retinal dialyses occur as a consequence of trauma. Dialyses, in general and following trauma, are more common in the inferotemporal quadrant. However, most dialyses detected in the superonasal quadrant are associated with a history of preceding trauma

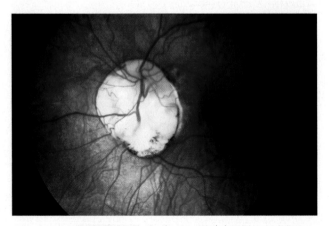

FIGURE 24-7. Optic nerve coloboma.

(78B,79). Idiopathic retinal dialyses accounted for approximately 2% of retinal detachments in one series, typically occurring in the inferotemporal quadrant of young adult eyes.

Retinal detachment associated with retinal dialysis often is subclinical. Associated findings include demarcation lines, retinal cysts, peripheral microcystoid degeneration, and yellow-white vitreous opacities (80). PVR is seen rarely, perhaps due to the overlying vitreous base impeding access of cells to the central vitreous cavity.

Retinal detachments from idiopathic retinal dialyses have been a subject of debate (81), considered by some to represent a distinct clinical entity. Reports of bilateral involvement (82,83) have been cited in support of this contention. Bilateral nontraumatic retinal dialysis is an indication for examination of family members.

Atopic Dermatitis

Atopic dermatitis, a chronic pruritic skin condition, is an allergic form of eczema primarily affecting infants, children, and young adults. Onset usually is in infancy, often with a positive family history of atopic disease. Prevalence is on the order of 10% in the United States and up to 20% in Japan. The incidence of atopic dermatitis is thought to be rising (84,85), with retinal detachments in such patients representing approximately 3% of RRDs seen in Japan. RRD typically occurs in early adulthood but may be seen in late adolescence (86).

Eyelid dermatitis, blepharitis, conjunctivitis, cataract, and keratoconus are recognized anterior segment associations. Retinal detachment has been reported in 6% to 10% of Japanese patients (87,88). The peripheral fundus is characterized by a "fluffy" appearance, with signs of vitreous base contraction (wrinkling of the pars plana epithelium and oral dialyses) (89). Retinal breaks often are multiple and located at the ora serrata or in the nonpigmented ciliary body epithelium. Retinal detachments are generally low lying and asymptomatic, although giant retinal tears occur as well (90). Intense pruritus prompts frequent eye rubbing and face slapping, thought to play a role in causing retinal or ciliary body breaks. Scleral buckle with thorough peripheral retinopexy is advocated for this reason. Maruyama et al. (91) suggest that moderate-to-dense anterior chamber angle pigmentation in patients with atopic dermatitis is a sign of breaks of the peripheral retina or ciliary body epithelium and should be an indication of meticulous peripheral retinal examination.

Postsurgical

Eyes that have undergone ophthalmic surgical procedures (for cataract, strabismus, corneal transplantation, or glaucoma tube shunt) often fare considerably worse than previously unoperated eyes. In our published series, the postoperative subgroup included all eyes with RRD and known antecedent intraocular surgery (1). This group included eyes with juvenile glaucoma, congenital cataracts, Peter anomaly, juvenile retinoschisis, and the sequelae of these disorders and accounted for 34% (10/29) of eyes in this series. We qualified them by the procedure performed immediately prior to the development of RRD. None of the eyes developed a recognized retinal detachment intraoperatively. Of these 10 eyes, 6 were aphakic, 5 had undergone pars plana vitrectomy, 2 had Molteno tube placement, 1 had trabeculectomy, 1 had suprachoroidal drainage, and 1 had penetrating keratoplasty. The risk for RRD after Molteno glaucoma implant surgery was reported as 5.0% with a median patient age of 9 years (92). Retinal detachment following other ophthalmic surgeries is not well documented, except for extracapsular cataract extraction for which the incidence of retinal detachment is estimated to be 0.02% to 3.6% (93).

MANAGEMENT

Prevention of Myopia in Otherwise Healthy Infants and Children

The main approaches to prevent or slow myopic progression in otherwise normal children are either pharmacologic, including muscarinic antagonists such as atropine or pirenzepine (94), or refractive, including bifocals in place of single-vision lenses (95) or rigid contact lenses (96,97). A topical formulation of pirenzepine is under evaluation in a clinical trial (The Myopia Control Study). In general, however, neither the pharmacologic nor the refractive strategy has met with clinically significant success.

Prevention of Nonhereditary Myopia in Infants and Children

Prematurity

A significant opportunity is available to minimize myopia in association with ROP requiring peripheral retinal ablation. The available body of clinical data, taken together, indicates that laser photocoagulation is the preferred method of treatment.

Stimulus Deprivation Myopia

Conditions likely to result in stimulus deprivation should be corrected promptly. Infantile vitreous hemorrhage may occur in several clinical scenarios: most commonly in normal infants as a result of birth trauma, spontaneous bleeding from a persistent hyaloid vessel, or secondary to thrombocytopenia or ROP. Although the data are limited, significant stimulus deprivation in a newborn from dense vitreous hemorrhage has produced axial myopia on the order of −11 diopters and amblyopia within a matter of 4

weeks (98). Waiting for spontaneous clearance of hemorrhage from the formed infant vitreous is not a practical clinical option because waiting can result in anisometropia or amblyopia. Lens-sparing vitreous surgery is indicated soon after diagnosis, within 7 to 10 days in the newborn infant.

Surgical Considerations

The management of pediatric RRD varies with the clinical circumstances. General recommendations are given in the following.

Some general principles bear mention. RRD with PVR often requires combined scleral buckle and vitrectomy. Silicone oil tamponade can be used for many pediatric RRDs repaired by vitrectomy and is used in initial as well as repeat vitrectomy, whether or not in combination with scleral buckle. Giant retinal tears are repaired with vitrectomy, endolaser, and silicone oil in most instances, and the lens often is sacrificed to facilitate meticulous vitreous removal. Autologous plasmin enzyme, still not clinically available, is used to assist vitrectomy in colobomatous detachments and schisis-rhegmatogenous detachment.

Complications of silicone oil in children are similar to those seen in adults: secondary intraocular pressure elevation, band keratopathy, oil emulsification (Fig. 24-8), and cataract.

Syndromic Myopia

Several of the syndromic conditions associated with myopia in infants and children have unique vitreoretinal features, described earlier. Accurate diagnosis is important to discuss visual prognosis and guide genetic counseling.

The high rate of bilaterality of retinal detachment in Stickler and Marfan syndromes, particularly from giant retinal tears, justifies consideration of prophylactic retinopexy

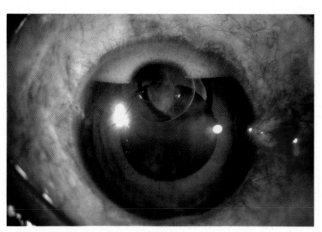

FIGURE 24-8. Emulsified silicone oil accumulated in the superior anterior chamber angle ("inverse hypopyon") in a child.

of the fellow eye in these patients (99). Treatment should be circumferential, not focal, because normal-appearing retina is vulnerable to retinal detachment from circumferential vitreous traction (99).

Although posterior vitreous separation may not always be present as a precipitating factor in RRD in children, removal of the hyaloid appears important to minimize the probability of retinal redetachment. Enzymatic vitreolysis of the hyaloideoretinal junction presently is experimental but appears to be useful. It seems to eliminate the need for scleral buckle because the risk of anterior PVR is minimized. In addition, hyaloidal vitreolysis theoretically eliminates the preretinal scaffold on which cells migrate and proliferate to cause PVR. Circumferential laser and silicone tamponade are commonly used. Perisilicone proliferation (Fig. 24-9) may occur despite use of enzymatic vitreolysis. Indications for removal of silicone oil are similar to those in adults, and, in our experience, the complications that occur (cataract, glaucoma) are also similar.

Colobomatous Retinal Detachment

Retinal detachments can be caused by retinal breaks within normal retina outside the coloboma or from a retinal break within a coloboma. Retinal detachment caused by the latter can be uniquely challenging to repair. When this is the mechanism of retinal detachment, the posterior hyaloid typically is attached, particularly firmly at the edge of the coloboma.

Repair of the retinal detachment usually is accomplished by vitrectomy with either gas or temporary silicone oil tamponade. Autologous plasmin enzyme is useful in facilitating posterior hyaloidal detachment. If the break within the coloboma is not closed primarily with cyanoacrylate, laser retinopexy is performed around the circumference of the coloboma to achieve chorioretinal adhesion (100). If the break is not closed directly, there is significant probability that silicone oil will track into the subretinal space via the

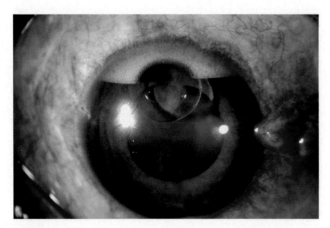

FIGURE 24-9. Peripapillary perisilicone proliferation and associated shallow tractional posterior retinal detachment.

open break within the coloboma, which likely is the same path that accounts for the RRD (101). The source of the subretinal fluid causing retinal detachment in other diseases with optic nerve anomalies has been proposed to be cerebrospinal fluid, although this is believed to be the less likely cause (102).

Juvenile Dialysis

Asymptomatic retinal detachment from retinal dialysis can be repaired with scleral buckle or stabilized with retinopexy. Repair of symptomatic retinal dialysis typically is accomplished by a scleral buckling procedure (see Chapter 23). Light cryopexy is applied along the dialysis edge. Subretinal fluid drainage usually is not necessary for recent-onset dialyses and is reserved for chronic dialyses with viscous subretinal fluid. Overall, anatomic and visual outcome for detachments from retinal dialysis, both traumatic and idiopathic, is typically quite good.

Surgery for Other Pediatric Rhegmatogenous Retinal Detachments

Detachment of the fovea, particularly repeated retinal detachment, has a devastating effect on visual acuity in children. Primary retinal detachment due to a single retinal break or idiopathic retinal dialysis with no PVR or low-grade PVR is managed with a scleral buckle. Predictably, such eyes have the best prognosis, with repair rates reported at 80% or more (5).

Eyes that have undergone prior surgical intervention with penetrating keratoplasty or glaucoma tube shunt often fare considerably worse than eyes with no history of antecedent surgery. In our series (1), anatomic reattachment after one or more procedures was achieved in 80% of myopic eyes with primary RRD, but only 44% of eyes that had undergone prior intraocular surgery. Taken as a group, most repairable eyes will require more than one surgical procedure to effect retinal reattachment, with a mean of approximately two surgeries (range 1–5 per eye).

Although anatomic reattachment is its necessary precedent, functional outcome is the ultimate measure of success. In our series of pediatric RRD, repaired eyes had a substantial improvement in visual acuity. Among children for whom final visual acuity was available for both eyes (n = 21), 8 (38%) of these 21 patients had equal or better final visual acuity in the affected eye after surgical repair as in the companion eye (1).

CONCLUSIONS

- The incidence of childhood retinal detachment is low and is seen most often in association with myopia.
- There is often a high rate of vision-threatening pathology in the companion eye.

- Heredity and environment both likely play a role in myopia.
- Modification of presumed causative factors for myopia has done little to mitigate the progression of juvenile-onset myopia in otherwise healthy children.
- Pediatric RRDs generally are repaired successfully with contemporary vitreoretinal surgical techniques.
- Multiple surgical procedures often are necessary to repair pediatric RRDs, partly because of the high incidence of PVR at the initial presentation.
- Syndromic retinal detachment in children should be managed aggressively, with serious consideration of prophylactic retinopexy of the fellow eye.
- Laser retinopexy should be used in infants with threshold or acute severe ROP requiring peripheral retinal ablation, instead of cryopexy, in order to minimize associated myopia.
- Stimulus deprivation due to dense cataract or vitreous hemorrhage should be managed by prompt lensectomy or vitrectomy, respectively, to reduce the possibility of anisometropia or amblyopia. Consultation with a pediatric ophthalmologist is essential.

REFERENCES

1. Fivgas GD, Capone A Jr. Pediatric rhegmatogenous retinal detachment. *Retina* 2001;21:101–106.
2. Haimann MH, Burton TC, Brown CK. Epidemiology of retinal detachment. *Arch Ophthalmol* 1982;100:289–292.
3. Haimann MH, Burton TC, Brown CK. Epidemiology of retinal detachment. *Arch Ophthalmol* 1982;100:289–292.
4. Laatikainen L, Tolppanen EM. Characteristics of rhegmatogenous retinal detachment. *Acta Ophthalmol* 1985;63:146–154.
5. Winslow RL, Tasman W. Juvenile rhegmatogenous retinal detachment. *Ophthalmology* 1978;85:607–618.
6. Sternberg P, Meredith TA, Stewart MA, et al. Retinal detachment in penetrating keratoplasty patients *Am J Ophthalmol* 1990;109:148–152.
7. Hilton GF, Norton EW. Juvenile retinal detachment. *Mod Probl Ophthalmol* 1969;8:325–341.
8. Laatikainen L, Tolppanen EM. Characteristics of rhegmatogenous retinal detachment. *Acta Ophthalmol* 1985;63:146–154.
9. Waterhouse WJ, Lloyd ME, Dugel PU, et al. Rhegmatogenous retinal detachment after Molteno glaucoma implant surgery. *Ophthalmology* 1994;101:665–671.
10. National Advisory Eye Council. Strabismus, Amblyopia and Visual Processing Panel (1999–2003) Vision Research: A National Plan. NIH Publication 98-4120. Washington, DC: National Institutes of Health, 1998.
11. Wang Q, Klein B, Klein R, et al. Refractive status in the Beaver Dam Eye Study. *Invest Ophthalmol Vis Sci* 1994;35:4344–4347.
12. Lin LL, Shih YF, Tsai CB, et al. Epidemiologic study of ocular refraction among schoolchildren in Taiwan in 1995. *Optom Vis Sci* 1999;76:275–281.
13. Saw SM, Carkeet A, Chia KS, et al. Component dependent risk factors for ocular parameters in Singapore Chinese children. *Ophthalmology* 2002;109:2065–2071.
14. Saw SM, Katz J, Schein OD, et al. Epidemiology of myopia. *Epidemiol Rev* 1996;18:175–187.
15. Marr JE, Halliwell-Ewen J, Fisher B, et al. Associations of high myopia in childhood. *Eye* 2001;15:70–74.
16. Norton T. Animal models of myopia: learning how vision controls the size of the eye. *Inst Lab Anim Res* J 1999;40:59–77.
17. Wildsoet CF. Active emmetropization: evidence for its existence and ramifications for clinical practice. *Ophthalmic Physiol Opt* 1997;17:279–290.
18. Gwiazda J, Thorn F, Bauer J, et al. Myopic children show insufficient accommodative response to blur. *Invest Ophthalmol Vis Sci* 1993;34:690–694.
19. Stone RA. Neural mechanisms and eye growth control. In: Tokoro T, ed. *Myopia updates: Proceedings of the 6th International Conference on Myopia.* New York: Springer-Verlag, 1997:241–254.
20. Quinn GE, Shin CH, Maguire MG, et al. Myopia and ambient lighting at night. *Nature* 1999;399:113–114.
21. Loman J, Quinn GE, Kamoun L, et al. Darkness and near work: myopia and its progression in third-year law students. *Ophthalmology* 2002;109:1032–1038.
22. Gwiazda J, Ong E, Held R, et al. Myopia and ambient night-light lighting. *Nature* 2002;404:144.
23. Zadnik K, Jones LA, Irvin BC, et al. Myopia and ambient night-light lighting. *Nature* 2000;404:143–144.
24. Connolly BP, Ng EY, McNamara JA, et al. A comparison of laser photocoagulation with cryotherapy for threshold retinopathy of prematurity at 10 years: part 2. Refractive outcome. *Ophthalmology* 2002;109:936–941.
25. Ng EY, Connolly BP, McNamara JA, et al. A comparison of laser photocoagulation with cryotherapy for threshold retinopathy of prematurity at 10 years: part 1. Visual function and structural outcome. *Ophthalmology* 2002;109:928–934.
26. Gusek-Schneider GC, Martus P. Stimulus deprivation myopia in human congenital ptosis: a study of 95 patients. *J Pediatr Ophthalmol Strabismus* 2001;38:340–348.
27. Twomey JM, Gilvarry A, Restori M, et al. Ocular enlargement following infantile corneal opacification. *Eye* 1990;4:497–503.
28. Zhang Z, Li S. The visual deprivation and increase in axial length in patients with cataracts. *Yan Ke Xue Bao* 1996;12:135–137.
29. Mohney BG. Axial myopia associated with dense vitreous hemorrhage of the neonate. *J AAPOS* 2002;6:348–353.
30. Hammond CJ, Snieder H, Gilbert CE, et al. Genes and environment in refractive error: the twin eye study. *Invest Ophthalmol Vis Sci* 2001;42:1232–1236.
31. Schwartz M, Haim M, Skarsholm D. X-linked myopia: Bornholm eye disease-linkage to DNA markers on the distal part of Xq. *Clin Genet* 1990;38:281–286.
32. Young TL, Ronan SM, Drahozal LA, et al. Evidence that a locus for familial high myopia maps to chromosome 18p. *Am J Hum Genet* 1998;63:109–119.
33. Young TL, Ronan SM, Alvear A, et al. A second locus for familial high myopia maps to chromosome 12q. *Am J Hum Genet* 1998;63:1419–1424.
34. Naiglin L, Gazagne C, Dallongeville F, et al. A genome wide scan for familial high myopia suggests a novel locus on chromosome 7q36. *J Med Genet* 2002;39:118–124.
35. Black GC, Perveen R, Wiszniewski W, et al. A novel hereditary developmental vitreoretinopathy with multiple ocular abnormalities localizing to a 5-cM region of chromosome 5q13–q14. *Ophthalmology* 1999;106:2074–2081.
36. Knowlton RG, Weaver EJ, Struyk AF, et al. Genetic linkage analysis of hereditary arthro-ophthalmopathy (Stickler syndrome) and the type II procollagen gene *Am J Hum Genet* 1989;45:681–688.
37. Richards AJ, Yates JRW, Williams R, et al. A family with Stickler syndrome type 2 has a mutation in the COL11A1 gene re-

sulting in the substitution of glycine 97 by valine in alpha-1 (XI) collagen. *Hum Mol Genet* 1996;5:1339–1343.

38. Vikkula M, Mariman ECM, Lui VCH, et al. Autosomal dominant and recessive osteochondrodysplasias associated with the COL11A2 locus. *Cell* 1995;80:431–437.

39. Snead MP, Yates JR. Clinical and molecular genetics of Stickler syndrome. *J Med Genet* 1999;36:353–359.

40. Donoso LA, Edwards AO, Frost AT, et al. Clinical variability of Stickler syndrome: role of exon 2 of the collagen COL2A1 gene. *Surv Ophthalmol* 2003;48:191–203.

41. Donoso LA, Edwards AP, Frost AT, et al. Identification of a stop codon mutation in exon 2 of the collagen 2A1 gene in a large Stickler syndrome family. *Am J Ophthalmol* 2002;134: 720–727.

42. Parma ES, Korkko J, Hagler WS, et al. Radial perivascular retinal degeneration: a key to the clinical diagnosis of an ocular variant of Stickler syndrome with minimal or no systemic manifestations. *Am J Ophthalmol* 2002;134:728–734.

43. Richards AJ, Martin S, Yates JR, et al. COL2A1 exon 2 mutations: relevance to the Stickler and Wagner syndromes. *Br J Ophthalmol* 2000;84:364–371.

44. Donoso LA, Edwards AO, Frost AT, et al. Identification of a stop codon mutation in exon 2 of the collagen 2A1 gene in a large Stickler syndrome family. *Am J Ophthalmol* 2002;134: 720–727.

45. Brown DM, Graemiger RA, Hergersberg M, et al. Genetic linkage of Wagner disease and erosive vitreoretinopathy to chromosome 5q13–14. *Ophthalmology* 1995;113:671–675.

46. Brown DM, Graemiger RA, Hergersberg M, et al. Genetic linkage of Wagner disease and erosive vitreoretinopathy to chromosome 5q13–14. *Arch Ophthalmol* 1995;113:671–675.

47. Perveen R, Hart-Holden N, Dixon MJ, et al. Refined genetic and physical localization of the Wagner disease (WGN1) locus and the genes CRTL1 and CSPG2 to a 2- to 2.5-cM region of chromosome 5q14.3. *Genomics* 1999;57:219–226.

48. Wagner H. Ein bisher unbekanntes Erbleiden des Auges (Degeneratio hyaloideo-retinalis hereditaria) beobachtet im Kanton Zurich. *Klin Monatsbl Augenheilkd* 1938;100:840.

49. Parke DW II. Stickler syndrome: clinical care and molecular genetics. *AJO* 2002;134:746–748.

50. Brown DM, Graemiger RA, Hergersberg M, et al. Genetic linkage of Wagner disease and erosive vitreoretinopathy to chromosome 5q13–14. *Ophthalmology* 1995;113:671–675.

51. Graemiger RA, Niemeyer G, Schneeberger SA, et al. Wagner vitreoretinal degeneration: follow-up of the original pedigree. *Ophthalmology* 1995;102:1830–1839.

52. Milewicz DM, Pyeritz RE, Crawford ES, et al. Marfan syndrome: defective synthesis, secretion, and extracellular matrix formation of fibrillin by cultured dermal fibroblasts. *J Clin Invest* 1992;89:79–86.

53. Magenis RE, Maslen CL, Smith L, et al. Localization of the fibrillin (FBN) gene to chromosome 15, band q21.1. *Genomics* 1991;11:346–351.

54. Nijbroek G, Sood S, McIntosh I, et al. Fifteen novel FBN1 mutations causing Marfan syndrome detected by heteroduplex analysis of genomic amplicons. *Am J Hum Genet* 1995;57:8–21.

55. Maumenee IH. The eye in the Marfan syndrome. *Trans Am Ophthalmol Soc* 1981;79:684–733.

56. Cross HE, Jensen AD. Ocular manifestations in the Marfan syndrome and homocystinuria. *Am J Ophthalmol* 1973;75:405–420.

57. Jarret WH Jr. Dislocation of the lens: a study of 166 hospitalized cases. *Arch Ophthalmol* 1967;78:289–296.

58. Sharma T, Gopal L, Shanmugam MP, et al. Retinal detachment in Marfan syndrome: clinical characteristics and surgical outcome. *Retina* 2002;22:423–428.

59. Kliemann SE, Waetge RT, Suzuki OT, et al. Evidence of neu-

ronal migration disorders in Knobloch syndrome: clinical and molecular analysis of two novel families. *Am J Med Genet* 2003;119:15–19.

60. Sertie AL, Sossi V, Camargo AA, et al. Collagen XVIII, containing an endogenous inhibitor of angiogenesis and tumor growth, plays a critical role in the maintenance of retinal structure and in neural tube closure (Knobloch syndrome). *Hum Mol Genet* 2002;9:2051–2058.

61. Superti-Furga A, Pistone F, Romano C, et al. Clinical variability of osteogenesis imperfecta linked to COL1A2 and associated with a structural defect in the type I collagen molecule. *J Med Genet* 1989;26:358–362.

62. Weaver RG Jr, Martin T, Zanolli MD. The ocular changes of incontinentia pigmenti achromians (hypomelanosis of Ito). *J Pediatr Ophthalmol Strabismus* 1991;28:160–163.

63. Yang CI, Chen SN, Yang ML. Excessive myopia and anisometropia associated with familial exudative vitreoretinopathy. *Chang Gung Med J* 2002;25:388–392.

64. Brody JA, Hussels I, Brink E, et al. Hereditary blindness among the Pingelapese people of Eastern Caroline Islands. *Lancet* 1970;13:1253–1257.

65. Postel EA, Pulido JS, McNamara JA, et al. The etiology and treatment of macular detachment associated with optic nerve pits and related anomalies. *Trans Am Ophthalmol Soc* 1998;96: 73–88; discussion 88–93.

66. Russell-Eggitt IM, Blake KD, Taylor DSI, et al. The eye in the CHARGE association. *Br J Ophthalmol* 1990;74:421–426.

67. Dureau P, Attie-Bitach T, Salomon R, et al. Renal coloboma syndrome. *Ophthalmology* 2001;108:1912–1916.

68. Temple IK, MacDowall P, Baraitser M, et al. Focal dermal hypoplasia (Goltz syndrome). *J Med Genet* 1990;27:180–187.

69. Temple IK, Brunner H, Jones B, et al. Midline facial defects with ocular colobomata. *Am J Med Genet* 1990;37:23–27.

70. Warburg M. Classification of microphthalmos and coloboma. *J Med Genet* 1993;30:664–669.

71. Olsen TW, Summers CG, Knobloch WH. Predicting visual acuity in children with colobomas involving the optic nerve. *J Pediatr Ophthalmol Strabismus* 1996;33:47–51.

72. Olsen TW. Visual acuity in children with colobomatous defects. *Curr Opin Ophthalmol* 1997;8:63–67.

73. Morrison DA, Fleck B. Prevalence of retinal detachments in children with chorioretinal colobomas. [Letter] *Ophthalmology* 1999;106:645–646.

74. Jesberg DO, Schepens CL. Retinal detachment associated with coloboma of the choroid. *Arch Ophthalmol* 1961;65:163–173.

75. Patnaik B, Kalsi R. Retinal detachment with coloboma of the choroid. *Ind J Ophthalmol* 1981;29:345–349.

76. Gopal L, Badrinath SS, Kumar KS, et al. Optic disc in fundus coloboma. *Ophthalmology* 1996;103:2120–2126.

77. Shami M, McCartney D, Benedict W, et al. Spontaneous retinal reattachment in a patient with persistent hyperplastic primary vitreous and an optic nerve coloboma. *Am J Ophthalmol* 1992;114:769–771.

78A. Bochow TW, Olk RJ, Knupp JA, et al. Spontaneous reattachment of a total retinal detachment in an infant with microphthalmos and an optic nerve coloboma. *Am J Ophthalmol* 1991;112:347–348.

78B. Cox MS, Schepens CL, Freeman HM. Retinal detachment due to ocular contusion. *Arch Ophthalmol* 1966;76:678; Tasman W. Peripheral retinal changes following blunt trauma. *Trans Am Ophthalmol Soc* 1972;70:190; Johnson PB. Traumatic retinal detachments. *Br J Ophthalmol* 1974;58:126.

79. Zion VM, Burton TC. Retinal dialysis: pathology and pathogenesis. *Retina* 1982;2:94–116.

80. Kinyoun JL, Knobloch WH. Idiopathic retinal dialysis. *Retina* 1984;4:9–14.

81. Ross WH. Retinal dialysis: lack of evidence for a genetic cause. *Can J Ophthalmol* 1991;26:309–312.

82. Smiddy WE, Green WR. Idiopathic retinal dialysis. *Retina* 1984;4:9–14.

83. Brown GC, Tasman WS. Familial retinal dialysis. *Can J Ophthalmol* 1980;15:193–195.

84. Larsen FS, Hanifin JM. Epidemiology of atopic dermatitis. *Immunol Allergy Clin NA* 2002;22:1–25.

85. Hida T, Tano Y, Okinami S, et al. Multicenter retrospective study of retinal detachment associated with atopic dermatitis. *Jpn J Ophthalmol* 2000;44:407–418.

86. Katsushima H, Miyazaki I, Sekine N, et al. Incidence of cataract and retinal detachment associated with atopic dermatitis. *Nippon Ganka Gakkai Zasshi* 1994;98:495–500.

87. Nakano E, Iwasaki T, Osanai T, et al. Ocular complications of atopic dermatitis. *Nippon Ganka Gakkai Zasshi* 1997;101: 64–68.

88. Taniguchi H, Ohki O, Yokozeki H, et al. Cataract and retinal detachment in patients with severe atopic dermatitis who were withdrawn from the use of topical corticosteroid. *J Dermatol* 1999;26:658–665.

89. Matsuo T, Shiraga F, Matsuo N. Intraoperative observation of the vitreous base in patients with atopic dermatitis and retinal detachment. *Retina* 1995;15:286–290.

90. Azuma N, Hida T, Katsura H, et al. Retrospective survey of surgical outcomes on rhegmatogenous retinal detachments associated with atopic dermatitis. *Arch Ophthalmol* 1996;114:281–285.

91. Maruyama I, Katsushima H, Suzuki J, et al. Pigmentation on anterior chamber angle in eyes of patients with atopic dermatitis. *Jpn J Ophthalmol* 1999;43:535–538.i

92. Waterhouse WJ, Lloyd ME, Dugel PU, et al. Rhegmatogenous retinal detachment after Molteno glaucoma implant surgery. *Ophthalmology* 1994;101:665–671.

93. Scheie HG, Morse PH, Aminlari A. Incidence of retinal detachment following cataract extraction. *Arch Ophthalmol* 1973;89: 293–295.

94. Luft WA, Ming Y, Stell WK. Variable effects of previously untested muscarinic receptor antagonists on experimental myopia. *Invest Ophthalmol Vis Sci* 2003;44:1330–1338.

95. Gwiazda J, Hyman L, Hussein M, et al., and the COMET Group. A randomized clinical trial of progressive addition lenses versus single vision lenses on the progression of myopia in children. *Invest Ophthalmol Vis Sci* 2003;44:1492–1500.

96. Walline JJ, Mutti DO, Jones LA, et al. The contact lens and myopia progression (CLAMP) study: design and baseline data. *Optom Vis Sci* 2001;78:223–233.

97. Katz J, Schein OD, Levy B, et al. A randomized trial of rigid gas permeable contact lenses to reduce progression of children's myopia. *Am J Ophthalmol* 2003;136:82–90.

98. Mohney BG. Axial myopia associated with dense vitreous hemorrhage of the neonate. *J AAPOS* 2002;6:348–353.

99. Freeman HM. Fellow eyes of giant retinal breaks. *Trans Am Ophthalmol Soc* 1978;76:343–382.

100. McDonald HR, Lewis H, Brown G, et al. Vitreous surgery for retinal detachment associated with choroidal coloboma. *Arch Ophthalmol* 1991;109:1399–1402.

101. Bartz-Schmidt KU, Heimann K. Pathogenesis of retinal detachment associated with morning glory disc. *Int Ophthalmol* 1995;19:35–38.

102. Haik BG, Greenstein SH, Smith ME, et al. Retinal detachment in the morning glory anomaly. *Ophthalmology* 1984;91:1638–1647.

CONGENITAL X-LINKED RETINOSCHISIS

PAUL A. SIEVING
IAN M. MACDONALD
MICHAEL T. TRESE

HISTORY AND PREVALENCE

The first description of a retinopathy similar to what we now call *congenital X-linked retinoschisis* (CXLRS) was given to two brothers by Haas (1) in 1898. The term *retinoschisis* (RS) was introduced by Wilczek (2) in 1935, and the condition was recognized as an X-linked recessive trait that affects essentially only males by Mann and MacRae (3) in 1938. The prevalence of congenital juvenile RS is approximately 1:5,000 to 1:25,000, depending upon which population is studied. Affected males typically have characteristic foveal schisis and an electroretinogram (ERG) that shows selective reduction of the amplitude of the b-wave. The peripheral retina also may be involved, with splitting of the layers internal to the retina or, in severe cases, full-thickness retinal detachment. The trait is passed genetically to these affected males by their mothers. These female carriers usually cannot be identified clinically because they show no retinal findings and have normal ERG responses. They are identified clinically only through pedigree analysis. In rare cases, female carriers have been reported to have white flecks or areas of schisis involving the peripheral retina (4). Subsequent to identification of the RS gene in 1997 (5), molecular deoxyribonucleic acid (DNA) diagnostic testing is being offered and may prove helpful for women at risk of carrying the trait for RS.

CLINICAL SYMPTOMS AND SIGNS

The range of clinical findings in CXLRS is broad, and many diagnoses may be mistaken before a definite diagnosis is established (Table 25-1). Although CXLRS is relatively uncommon, like all of the monogenic retinal and macular dystrophies, it competes with Stargardt macular dystrophy as the most common form of juvenile macular degeneration affecting males. Less flagrant cases of CXLRS can be overlooked on cursory fundus examination. Not infrequently, one finds CXLRS masquerading behind a misdiagnosis of "amblyopia," and it should be high in the differential disease list if family history indicates an X-linked inheritance of visual abnormality.

Affected males have poor central vision, which typically comes to parental attention during early childhood and nearly always by the first vision screening examination in school. Reduced acuity typically is found, usually in the range from 20/60 to 20/120. Fundus examination reveals bilateral foveal schisis in virtually all patients at some point in their history and can be the only physical finding. The foveal schisis appears as a spokewheel pattern with areas of retinal folds surrounding the microcysts (Fig. 25-1). The human fovea is incompletely developed at birth and does not reach adult conformation until age 15 months (6). Hence, one can anticipate that the "spokewheel" intraretinal parafoveolar cysts of CXLRS may not be fully clinically apparent at birth.

The maculopathy may progress later in life, with macular atrophy developing in patients in their 50s and 60s. Peripheral RS occurs in the inferotemporal quadrant in approximately half of patients (7). The schisis may progress toward the central retina. Peripheral chorioretinal scars may mimic a healed chorioretinitis; macular scars also can occur. These scars can be circumferential and located posterior to peripheral schisis cavities (Fig. 25-1C).

A pseudopapillitis may occasionally be seen with optic nerve pallor. The nerve head may show a dragged disc appearance. A single case report by Pearson and Jagger (8) described a patient with a vitreous hemorrhage who was identified with optic disc neovascularization and peripheral retinal vessel tortuosity. Laser panretinal photocoagulation resulted in regression of the disc neovascularization (8). Tortuous fine vessels at the optic disc also have been noted by other authors (9).

"Veils" consisting of partial thickness retinal layers occur in the vitreous, along with overlying retinal vessels, in <50% of cases and can result in vitreous hemorrhage. Full-thickness retinal detachment occurs occasionally, and repair usually is not successful. The frequency of retinal detachment is ≤10% in our clinical practices. In patients who have adapted to darkness, the onset of light may create an unusual whitish appearance of the normal retinal reflex, a condition termed the *Mizuo phenomenon* (10). This condition is believed to result from abnormal potassium processing in the retina. In pa-

TABLE 25–1. DIFFERENTIAL DIAGNOSIS OF RETINOSCHISIS

Diagnosis	Differentiating Features
Amblyopia	Absence of macular cysts on clinical examination Absence of shallow schisis (best identified by OCT testing) ERG b-wave is not selectively reduced (i.e., not electronegative)
Chorioretinitis	Associated inflammatory signs No family history of maculopathy
Cystoid macular edema	Signs of diabetic retinopathy or previous ocular surgery No family history of maculopathy
Degenerative retinoschisis (45)	Associated with aging in an older population No family history of other affected males Occurs in females as well as males
Goldmann-Favre (26)	Autosomal recessive inheritance (i.e., women also affected) Central coarse microcysts and peripheral schisis with no vitreous veils ERG a-wave and b-wave both are reduced moderately to severely
Retinitis pigmentosa	Various modes of inheritance (also can be X-linked) Optic nerve pallor, vessel narrowing, pigment dispersion not just at the demarcation of areas of schisis ERG a-wave and b-wave both are reduced moderately to severely
Rod-cone dystrophy with retinoschisis (46)	ERG a-wave and b-wave both are reduced moderately to severely
Stargardt macular dystrophy (47)	Autosomal recessive disorder, usually with fundus flecks and significant macular atrophy.
Wagner disease (27)	Autosomal dominant inheritance Pigmentary changes, normal macula, myopia ERG b-wave is not selectively reduced (i.e., not electronegative)

ERG, electroretinogram; OCT, optical coherence tomography.

tients with RS who have undergone a vitrectomy, this phenomenon disappears, presumably as a result of removing the interface between the retina and the vitreous (11).

DIAGNOSTIC STUDIES

Young patients with CXLRS usually have a normal retinal fluorescein angiogram, but older patients may show macular window defects in areas of retinal pigment epithelial changes. Peripheral vascular changes can be noted with angiography, with areas of peripheral retinal nonperfusion and leakage of dye from abnormal retinal capillaries (12) and leakage into vitreous veils (9). Obligate carriers of CXLRS have a normal angiogram (9).

Although many visual function tests may be performed during the investigation of patients with presumed CXLRS, the ERG is one of the most clinically instructive tests. The dark-adapted ERG in patients with CXLRS shows reduction in the amplitude of the b-wave, whereas the a-wave remains normal (13). This configuration is termed an *electronegative response* because of the suppression, or loss of amplitude, of the positive-going b-wave, which normally rises above baseline from the negative-going a-wave (Fig. 25-2).

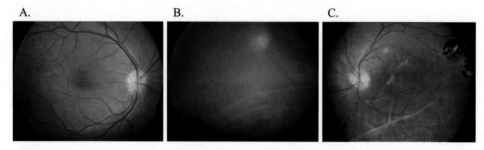

FIGURE 25-1. Fundus photographs showing variability in congenital X-linked retinoschisis. **A:** Affected male (QC) with spokewheel pattern of foveal cysts. **B:** Affected male (UL) with "vitreous veils" of the inferonasal quadrant. **C:** Affected male (TF) with chorioretinal scars posterior to peripheral schisis cavities and molecular diagnosis of 208 G→A mutation (gly70ser) in exon 4 of the *RS1* gene.

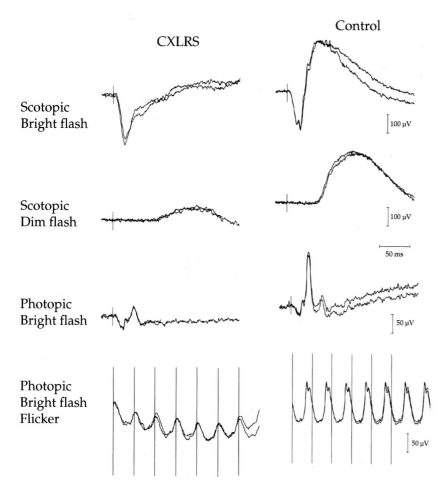

Scotopic
Bright flash

Scotopic
Dim flash

Photopic
Bright flash

Photopic
Bright flash
Flicker

CXLRS

Control

100 μV

100 μV

50 ms

50 μV

50 μV

FIGURE 25-2. "Electronegative" full-field ERG in congenital X-linked retinoschisis (CXLRS). CXLRS-affected male shows typical electroretinogram with b-wave reduction but a-wave preservation in dark-adapted recordings, compared with a normal individual (control).

The "electronegative waveform" is the most frequent presentation of full-field ERG change in CXLRS. Although an electronegative ERG response is not pathognomonic exclusively of CXLRS, only a few other retinal dystrophies result in this waveform configuration, and finding this ERG type in a suspect male is clinically confirmatory of CXLRS. Alternatively, observing an electronegative ERG response should heighten clinical suspicions for CXLRS. A normal ERG does not, however, rule out the possibility of CXLRS, because a patient with a confirmed mutation in the *RS1* gene (arg213trp) and a normal ERG was reported by Sieving et al. (14).

Unfortunately, female carriers of CXLRS cannot be identified through electrophysiologic analysis, because the a- and b-waves of the ERG are normal. One study proposed that the scotopic threshold response (a specialized form of ERG response) might be a method of identifying carriers; however, no abnormality was noted in obligate female carriers (15). Final thresholds of the dark-adaptation curve and the phases of cone and rod adaptation occur at the appropriate time. The Arden ratio of the electrooculogram is normal (13).

The b-wave was thought to result from depolarization of the Müller cell after potassium release and depolarization of the bipolar cells (16). Observation of selective reduction in the amplitude of the b-wave and the structural role of the

Müller cell in spanning cross sections of the retina suggested that the primary defect of CXLRS was in the Müller cell. This hypothesis has since been challenged by immunohistochemical studies of CXLRS gene expression.

The a-wave in CXLRS is of normal amplitude and latency. Studies on 15 males with CXLRS showed no significant effect on the dynamics of phototransduction as measured by the responses of the a-wave to intense light flashes in the dark-adapted state (17). The photopic flicker ERG responses in patients with CXLRS will show a reduction in amplitude and a delay in the phase. These findings are consistent with abnormal signaling in the ON and OFF pathways beyond the photoreceptors (18).

Multifocal ERG (mfERG) is a technique to assess macular responses. Alterations in the shapes of the mfERG have been associated with RS in the mouse model and in males affected with RS (19,20). Although the relative sensitivity is unknown compared to the full-field ERG, mfERG may be useful for studying the severity of macular involvement. However, mfERG may not be able to differentiate the degree of functional loss associated with foveal schisis, as witnessed in a study of twin males aged 22 years affected by CXLRS (Fig. 25-3). Although one twin had vision at the level of legal blindness, the other twin had vision of 20/40.

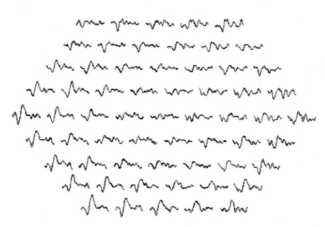

FIGURE 25-3. Multifocal electroretinogram (mfERG) waveforms from congenital X-linked retinoschisis–affected male (right eye of a 22-year-old) shows significant amplitude reduction of all responses. Fixation gives minimal response, whereas the perimacular responses at 20 degrees from fixation show recognizable waveforms. Recorded with Dawson, Trick, Litzkow (DTL) electrodes and dilated pupils.

Their fundus examinations were similar, and the waveforms of the mfERG were similar.

Optical coherence tomography (OCT) testing has expanded our knowledge of congenital RS (21). OCT has revealed schisis lesions that frequently lie deeper in the retina than previously thought, often in the midretinal layers. In addition, areas thought clinically to be intact can show large areas of shallow schisis across the macula by OCT. We have called this observation *flat* or *lamellar schisis,* and it is found in the macular area between the arcades (Fig. 25-4). This lamellar schisis may be associated with an abnormal ERG, but as mentioned previously, CXLRS can occur with a normal ERG.

OCT monitoring can be informative in both presurgical and postsurgical situations. Azzolini et al. (21) were among the first to investigate the fundus using OCT. They observed cleavage planes in the macula in both nerve fiber and outer retinal layers, which goes beyond the traditional clinical conceptions of retinal delamination occurring only at the retinal surface. OCT findings may also correlate with surgical outcomes. In one case in which surgical intervention was performed bi-

laterally, one eye that had good recovery of visual function showed disappearance of the macular schisis by OCT, whereas the fellow eye with similar surgery but no resolution of the macular schisis on OCT failed to recover visual function.

We are now using OCT combined with the clinical appearance to classify CXLRS into four types based on the presence of foveal cysts only (type 1), foveal cysts by clinical examination and a lamellar macular schisis detected by OCT (type 2), findings of type 2 CXLRS with peripheral schisis (type 3), or foveal cysts and peripheral schisis (type 4) (Table 25-2) (unpublished data). At this time, it is not known if one type progresses to another during the course of a person's lifetime. Currently, OCT examination has only been possible in children who are old enough to sit in position for the testing equipment; however, a system to be used in the operating room is under development that will allow evaluation of infants with congenital RS during an examination under anesthesia. This classification system will allow better testing of therapeutic interventions, genetic or other, as they become available.

MANAGEMENT

Surgical Treatment of Retinal Detachment with Congenital Retinoschisis

Rhegmatogenous retinal detachment in CXLRS can be challenging. Usually, the rhegmatogenous component involves an outer- and inner-wall hole in an area of peripheral schisis. The inner-wall holes are often easy to find and can be very large. By themselves, these inner wall holes do not lead to full thickness retinal detachment and do not require treatment. The search for outer-wall holes can be more difficult, and these holes must be closed to successfully repair the retinal detachment. When the outer-wall hole is not obvious, the most common site is at the posterior border of the peripheral schisis cavity and normal retina. These eyes are often repaired with a scleral buckle encompassing the outer- and often inner-wall holes. The advantage of a scleral buckle is that it is less invasive than vitrectomy. In addition, a disadvantage of vitrectomy in infant eyes with CXLRS is that the hyaloid

A

B

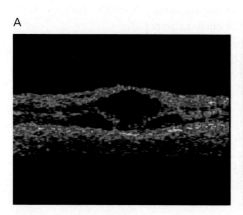

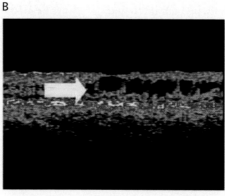

FIGURE 25-4. Ocular coherence tomographic findings of eyes with congenital retinoschisis. **A:** Foveal schisis. **B:** Lamellar schisis in area of clinically normal-appearing parafoveal macular retina *(white arrow).*

TABLE 25–2. CLASSIFICATION SYSTEM FOR CONGENITAL X-LINKED RETINOSCHISIS

CXLRS Type	Foveal Cystic Schisis (Clinical Examination)	Lamellar Macular Schisis (OCT Testing)	Peripheral Schisis
Type 1 foveal	+	−	−
Type 2 foveolamellar	+	+	−
Type 3 complex	+	+	+
Type 4 foveoperipheral	+	−	+

CXLRS, congenital X-linked retinoschisis; OCT, optical coherence tomography.

cannot be easily peeled from the retina. It seems that peeling of the posterior vitreous may be damaging, particularly in type 2 and 3 eyes, which have shallow, flat macular schisis that may not be clinically apparent. It is the authors' experience that type 2 and 3 CXLRS are clinically more complex and difficult to handle. Enzymatic degradation of the vitreoretinal junction may give a less traumatic separation and allow more complete relief of vitreoretinal traction. If buckling fails, we perform a vitrectomy because it allows us to treat the outer-wall break with laser after internal drainage and flattening the retina. Vitrectomy often involves removal of the inner wall of the schisis cavity, which may move freely in the vitreous cavity with eye movement. This movement of the inner leaflet may contribute to shearing forces that contribute to progression of the schisis cavity. At this time, we have no way to reconnect the anterior to the posterior leaflet of retina after they split. The technique of inner-wall retinectomy is best performed in eyes with type 4 congenital RS, in which macular flat schisis is not seen on OCT.

Tractional retinal detachment is a second form of retinal detachment that can occur in CXLRS, in which the retinal detachment occurs posterior to the peripheral schisis cavity and involves the fovea with a shallow macular detachment. This can be difficult to determine clinically, but it may be detectable by OCT testing. The visual acuity in these eyes can improve after vitrectomy in which the hyaloid is removed from the macular area. In one report, visual acuity improved from 20/200 to 20/50 (21). These eyes are best operated in type 4 CXLRS, but if the child has type 2 or 3 CXLRS and requires vitrectomy, no inner-wall retinectomy is performed.

In eyes with type 2 or 3 CXLRS that do undergo retinectomy, proliferation can form along the anterior surface of the anterior leaflet of the schisis. As this tissue contracts, the anterior schisis leaflet can scroll up, further splitting the retina. Although both gas and silicone oil have been used as a postoperative tamponade, we tend to use silicone oil in younger children who cannot position or those suspected to be type 2 or 3 CXLRS.

Other therapeutic options for CXLRS, which conceivably may be possible in the future, include (i) gene therapy, (ii) reattachment of the inner and outer leaflet with a combination of mechanical techniques and biologic interventions, and (iii) enzymatic vitreolysis to eliminate foveal traction (22). This may prevent progression in CXLRS.

DIFFERENTIAL DIAGNOSIS

Isolated cases of CXLRS offer no opportunity to examine other family members and not infrequently are mislabeled as some other disorder (Table 25-1). Amblyopia, retinal dialysis, congenital infection, and retinitis pigmentosa (RP) as the initial referring diagnoses later diagnosed as CXLRS in a cohort of 56 males in 16 British families (23). An isolated case of a male CXLRS does not imply a new mutation, because the female carrier mother essentially never exhibits clinical signs of the trait and has normal vision. New mutations have been reported for CXLRS (24), but such instances are exceedingly uncommon.

The maculopathy in cases of rod–cone dystrophy or Stargardt disease may mimic RS, particularly because the dark choroid sign is not always present in Stargardt disease, particularly in the autosomal dominant form from *ELOVL4* gene mutations (25). An X-linked pattern of inheritance should differentiate CXLRS from these conditions. In general, Stargardt disease and rod–cone dystrophy do not exhibit an ERG with selective reduction in the amplitude of the b-wave.

Goldmann-Favre syndrome is an autosomal recessive vitreoretinopathy that causes poor vision in early infancy. Affected individuals have coarse macular cysts and peripheral lattice degeneration that could be confused with RS. There are no vitreous veils as seen in CXLRS. Unlike CXLRS, Goldmann-Favre patients complain of night blindness and have a markedly reduced ERG (26).

Wagner disease is an autosomal dominant disorder characterized by myopia and vitreous syneresis (27). Retinal detachment is a frequent complication and might be confused with RS. The macula usually is normal but may show pigmentary changes. Although the ERG may be abnormal in patients with Wagner disease, selective b-wave reduction is not seen.

ENVIRONMENTAL FACTORS

Clinical impression indicates that trauma can exacerbate vision loss in CXLRS. As the cellular pathology is known to result from molecular alteration of the retinoschisin molecule, which normally has biologic adhesive properties conveyed by its discoidin domain (5), CXLRS disease may leave the retina vulnerable to mechanical shock and injury. Prudent medical advice at this time warrants advising CXLRS affected males to avoid boxing and other excessive body contact sports. Environmental factors otherwise are not suspected as contributing to the etiology or progression of the condition. The authors' clinical experience thus far suggests that eyes with type 2 or 3 CXLRS are seemingly more likely to have severe injury from mild, direct ocular trauma; therefore, these patients should be advised to use eye protection.

HUMAN HISTOLOGIC STUDIES

Condon et al. (28) reported on the eye pathology of two patients with CXLRS from one family. The older patient, aged 55 years, died from metastatic cancer. Both eyes were available for study. Apart from the areas of schisis, the photoreceptor and outer nuclear layers were well preserved. In the retina adjacent to areas of schisis, there were rosettes of cells around the lumen, and some cells had processes resembling those of photoreceptors. The macular photoreceptors were either degenerate or absent and were replaced by uncharacterized amorphous material with fibrils. The younger patient, a nephew of the older patient, developed neovascular glaucoma in one eye, which was enucleated at age 33 years and therefore available for study. A similar amorphous material was found in the areas of schisis in the eye. We speculate that this material was retinoschisin and that the anomalous protein interfered with normal cell–cell interactions. The rosettes and anomalous cell processes may reflect the role that normal retinoschisin is proposed to play in the maintenance of the photoreceptor synapse. Unfortunately, there have not been any recent studies using immunohistochemistry and modern microscopy to further define the pathology of human eyes affected by CXLRS.

GENE STRUCTURE

The gene for CXLRS, *RS1,* was mapped by conventional strategies and then cloned from the region of interest by Sauer et al. (5). The gene is composed of six exons that encode a 224-amino-acid protein called retinoschisin. In certain populations, founder mutations may be found in the *RS1* gene, which represent most cases of CXLRS. Of CXLRS patients with Finnish ancestry, 95% have one of three mutations in the *RS1* gene: E72K (214 G→A), G74V (221 G→T), and G109R (325 G→C) (29).

PROTEIN STRUCTURE AND FUNCTION

The protein product of the *RS1* gene is called retinoschisin. Recent evidence from many sources suggests that the photoreceptor is an abundant and possibly primary site of synthesis of the protein. Grayson et al. (30) showed by ribonucleic acid (RNA) expression studies that retinoschisin is present in the photoreceptor layer. Further, retinoschisin was localized not only in the photoreceptors but also in the inner retina, which suggests that the protein is secreted or transported to sites beyond the photoreceptors. To support this hypothesis, they demonstrated that retinoschisin was secreted by differentiated retinoblastoma (Weri-Rb1) cells, implying that retinoschisin is normally produced by the photoreceptor and then secreted. Similarly, Molday et al. (31) demonstrated that antibody to retinoschisin bound to photoreceptors and bipolar cells and not Müller cells and ganglion cells—finally challenging the accepted hypothesis that retinoschisin was a Müller cell defect. In addition, we recently observed that retinoschisin is expressed by nearly all retinal neurons during development and in the adult retina (31A) (Fig. 25-5).

The retinoschisin protein has a single discoidin domain that is thought to function in maintaining cell adhesion to extracellular matrix proteins and other cells (5). This function may be particularly important in maintaining the photoreceptor synapse with the bipolar cell (32). The fact that the predominant mutations are missense and occur in the discoidin domain supports this concept of structure and function of retinoschisin (33).

MOUSE MODEL

A mouse model of CXLRS has been generated by homologous DNA insertion across the endogenous retinoschisin *RS1* gene (32). The ERG of the male *RS1h-/Y* mice is similar to CXLRS patients in showing a selective b-wave reduction. However, this mouse model shows an additional and severe

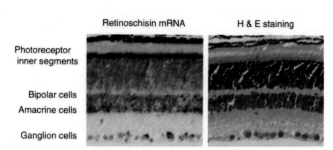

FIGURE 25-5. Gene expression of retinoschisin in the normal adult mouse retina. **Left:** *In situ* hybridization of retinoschisin mRNA, particularly of the photoreceptor inner segments, and of bipolar cells, amacrine cells, and ganglion cells. **Right:** Hematoxylin and eosin staining of normal adult mouse retina. (Courtesy of Dr. Yuichiro Takada.)

effect on the cone ERG. The retina of the *RS1h-/Y* mouse has a significant loss of its normal architecture, including areas of schisis in between cells in the inner nuclear layer (32). This finding supports the hypothesis of a functional role of retinoschisin in maintaining cell–cell adhesion.

GENETIC PHENOTYPIC VARIANTS

Mutations in the CXLRS gene are thought to be highly penetrant and to result in clinical disease. Mutations cluster in two regions of the gene. Missense mutations predominate overwhelmingly in exons 4, 5, and 6, whereas exons 1, 2, and 3 are susceptible to major deletions, splice site mutations, and introduction of a stop codon, all of which would cause loss of normal protein function. The severity and clinical characteristics of the disease associated with missense mutations present with relatively similar and clinically familiar severity (7,34,35). One report indicates that *RS1* mutations that cause truncation or nonexpression of the protein may have greater clinical severity due to the absence of the RS protein (34).

CXLRS disease severity may vary among family members. One example is of identical twin boys with CXLRS identified in early infancy with nystagmus and similar fundus findings of foveal RS. Neither twin has since experienced any complications from CXLRS. The refraction of one twin at age 2 years 3 months was +5.00 +2.50 ×105 (OD) and +6.00 +2.25 ×90 (OS). His vision remained stable throughout his early childhood and remained at 20/200 when last tested at age 22 years. The intervention of low-vision specialists and appropriate support for learning were instrumental in his successful primary education and allowed him to obtain a college degree. His identical twin brother was never as hyperopic as his sibling, +3.75 OU, and never demonstrated the same degree of nystagmus in early infancy. His mother thought his vision was normal. He never required intervention by low-vision aids and has maintained approximately 20/40 vision in both eyes. He completed a degree in science at the same university as his brother (see also Chapter 33).

There may be considerable variability in the effect of mutations of *RS1* on retinal phenotype. For example, a mutation in *RS1* (cys223arg or C223R) was identified in a small Chinese family. At age 22 months, the proband had typical features of CXLRS with foveal and peripheral RS. His mother had no phenotype, but his grandfather had a phenotype consistent with Bietti crystalline retinopathy (36). Bietti crystalline dystrophy is not known to follow an X-linked pattern of inheritance. An autosomal recessive form of Bietti crystalline dystrophy has been mapped to 4q35, but the gene has yet to be identified (37).

Sporadic cases of bilateral symmetrical maculopathy, without known family history of other affected males, can be particularly challenging to the clinician who is trying to establish a diagnosis and prognosis for the patient and family. Electrophysiologic testing and supplemental molecular genetic analysis are key diagnostic aids. Mutation analysis can identify mutations in the *RS1* gene in approximately 90% of males (34). The usefulness of supplementation molecular genetic analysis is exemplified by the report by Nakamura et al. (38) of a patient with the referring diagnosis of bull's-eye maculopathy and selective reduction in the b-wave of the ERG. The possibility of CXLRS was raised by this clinical finding, and the patient was subsequently shown to have a novel mutation (ala100pro) in the *RS1* gene (38).

Retinal findings in CXLRS may include schisis and white retinal flecks simulating fundus albipunctatus (39). All of the patients with CXLRS and white flecks presented by Hotta et al. (40) had foveal schisis. Therefore, the flecks were not seen without other classic features of CXLRS. Similarly, the CXLRS patients described by van Schooneveld and Miyake (39) with white retinal flecks had a maculopathy consistent with juvenile RS.

MANAGEMENT OF AMBLYOPIA AND STRABISMUS IN CONGENITAL X-LINKED RETINOSCHISIS

The ophthalmic care of a child with RS should carefully evaluate and treat refractive errors, strabismus, and amblyopia. Roesch et al. (41) reported that almost 20% of children with CXLRS had significant vision loss in childhood, and that half of this vision loss in childhood was due to complications of the disorder: retinal detachment, vitreous hemorrhage, and neovascular glaucoma. Fifty-seven eyes of patients with RS younger than age 9 years had a mean visual acuity of 20/64. Cataract was found in 11 eyes of the children and adolescents, representing 6% of the entire cohort, and was associated with severe retinopathy.

George et al. (23) noted a bimodal age of presentation of CXLRS in childhood. One group presented early with strabismus and nystagmus at a mean age of 1.88 years, and the second group presented at a mean age of 6.7 years with only poor vision. Of their cohort of 56 males, 30% had strabismus, and corrective strabismus surgery had universally been performed before the diagnosis of CXLRS was uncovered. The proportion of cases associated with strabismus (30%) is identical to that reported by Roesch et al. (41). The number of cases with esotropia and exotropia in their study was almost identical; however, the likelihood of poor vision (<20/200) and severe schisis was highest in the group with exotropia. The fact that amblyopia and strabismus coexist with CXLRS should increase our surveillance of these patients throughout childhood.

In the British cohort, 50% of patients had hyperopia >2 diopters (D). The proportion in the age range susceptible to amblyopia was not defined. Eleven percent had anisometropia >1.5 D, and in 5 of 6 patients, the eye that was more ametropic developed amblyopia. The more extensive Canadian cohort of Roesch et al. (41) reported on refractive errors in 183 eyes. Half the eyes were hyperopic, and most of these had <2 D of hyperopia. Again, the refractive errors of the pediatric group were not defined. In study of Japanese patients, the mean refractive error of 12 eyes of patients younger than age 13 years was 1.33 D (SD = 2.73) (42). Correction of refractive errors and early intervention with amblyopia therapy are prudent throughout the period of visual development in children.

VISION REHABILITATION AND LOW-VISION AIDS

RS-affected males will benefit from visual aids. Acuity typically is between 20/60 and 20/120 during teenage and middle-aged years. Such levels of vision are amenable to help with low-vision aids, including hand-held spectacle magnifiers and telescopes. These can be provided by low-vision specialists. The primary visual deficit occurs in central vision, although peripheral vision fields can be impaired to some degree but often to a far less extent than progressive retinal dystrophies, such as retinitis pigmentosa. Changes in dark adaptation normally are minor in RS and do not cause significant night blindness.

GENETICS COUNSELING AND ETHICAL CONSIDERATIONS

Genetic counseling is advised for families in which CXLRS is found to affect males. In keeping with the nature of an X-linked recessive trait, this condition affects only the males. Female carriers suffer no visual sequelae of the carrier state, either on visual function or in retinal structure. Targeted counseling is advised for females who have a brother with CXLRS, because these women have a 50% chance of inheriting the *RS1* gene carrier state. Carriers subsequently could have affected male offspring. With the identification of the *RS1* gene, molecular genetic diagnosis is available to determine whether or not these women are carriers. Ethical questions are raised by molecular diagnostic testing of females at risk for the carrier state prior to their age of consent, because this is useful solely for family planning and would not otherwise affect their need for medical intervention.

Each request for carrier testing should be considered on its own merits. In some instances, carrier testing of young girls could contribute to counseling of other family members. If the result affects the child's reproductive choice, then it is recommended that testing be deferred until the child is at an age of consent and is able to understand the issues (43).

FUTURE TREATMENTS BASED ON RESEARCH

The retinoschisin protein acts biologically as a cell adhesion factor through properties of the discoidin domain. In the absence of this protein, or from a functional deficit due to misfolding of the protein, or from defective secretion to the extracellular matrix (44), retinal structural integrity will be impaired and subject to lamellar separation or retinal detachment. Therapeutic intervention may be theoretically possible by restoring the function or providing a substitute, normally functioning, wild-type protein to structurally stabilize the retina. To this end, gene therapy studies recently have shown that delivery of *RS-1* to adult *RS1h* knockout mice restores the ERG b-wave, demonstrating a rescue of physiological function (unpublished data). In the future, gene delivery may afford an opportunity to use protein replacement as a treatment strategy to stabilize the retina of affected males with CXLRS.

REFERENCES

1. Haas J. Über das Zusammenvorkommen von Veränderungen der Retina und Choroidea. *Arch Augenheilkd* 1898;37:343–348.
2. Wilczek M. Ein der netzhautspaltung (retinoschisis) mit einer offnung. *Zeit Augenhlkd* 1935;85:108–116.
3. Mann I, MacRae A. Congenital vascular veils in the vitreous. *Br J Ophthalmol* 1938;22:1–10.
4. Kaplan J, Pelet A, Hentati H, et al. Contribution to carrier detection and genetic counselling in X linked retinoschisis. *J Med Genet* 1991;28:383–388.
5. Sauer CG, Gehrig A. Positional cloning of the gene associated with X-linked juvenile retinoschisis. *Nat Genet* 1997;17:164–170.
6. Hendrickson AE, Yuodelis C. The morphological development of the human fovea. *Ophthalmology* 1984;91:603–612.
7. Eksandh LC, Ponjavic V, Ayyagari R, et al. Phenotypic expression of juvenile X-linked retinoschisis in Swedish families with different mutations in the XLRS1 gene. *Arch Ophthalmol* 2000; 118:1098–1104.
8. Pearson R, Jagger J. Sex linked juvenile retinoschisis with optic disc and peripheral retinal neovascularisation. *Br J Ophthalmol* 1989;73:311–313.
9. Ewing CC, Cullen AP. Fluorescein angiography in X-chromosomal maculopathy with retinoschisis (juvenile hereditary retinoschisis). *Can J Ophthalmol* 1972;7:19–28.
10. de Jong PT, Zrenner E, van Meel GJ, et al. Mizuo phenomenon in X-linked retinoschisis. Pathogenesis of the Mizuo phenomenon. *Arch Ophthalmol* 1991;109:1104–1108.
11. Miyake Y, Terasaki H. Golden tapetal-like fundus reflex and posterior hyaloid in a patient with x-linked juvenile retinoschisis. *Retina* 1999;19:84–86.
12. Keunen JE, Hoppenbrouwers RW. A case of sex-linked juvenile retinoschisis with peripheral vascular anomalies. *Ophthalmologica* 1985;191:146–149.
13. Peachey NS, Fishman GA, Derlacki DJ, et al. Psychophysical and electroretinographic findings in X-linked juvenile retinoschisis. *Arch Ophthalmol* 1987;105:513–516.
14. Sieving PA, Bingham EL, Kemp J, et al. Juvenile X-linked retinoschisis from XLRS1 Arg213Trp mutation with preservation of the electroretinogram scotopic b-wave. *Am J Ophthalmol* 1999;128:179–184.

15. Murayama K, Kuo C, Sieving PA. Abnormal threshold ERG response in X-linked juvenile retinoschisis, evidence for a proximal retinal origin of the human STR. *Clin Vis Sci* 1991;6:317–322.

16. Karowski CJ, Proenza LM. Relationship between Muller cell responses, a local transretinal potential, and potassium flux. *J Neurophysiol* 1977;40:244–259.

17. Khan NW, Jamison JA, Kemp JA, et al. Analysis of photoreceptor function and inner retinal activity in juvenile X-linked retinoschisis. *Vision Res* 2001;41:3931–3942.

18. Kondo M, Sieving PA. Primate photopic sine-wave flicker ERG: vector modeling analysis of component origins using glutamate analogs. *Invest Ophthalmol Vis Sci* 2001;42:305–312.

19. Seeliger MW, Weber BH, Besch D, et al. MfERG waveform characteristics in the RS1h mouse model featuring a "negative" ERG. *Doc Ophthalmol* 2003;107:37–44.

20. Huang S, Wu D, Jiang F, et al. The multifocal electroretinogram in X-linked juvenile retinoschisis. *Doc Ophthalmol* 2003;106:251–255.

21. Azzolini C, Pierro L, Codenotti M, et al. OCT images and surgery of juvenile macular retinoschisis. *Eur J Ophthalmol* 1997;7:196–200.

22. Verstraeten TC, Chapman C, Hartzer M, et al. Pharmacologic induction of posterior vitreous detachment in the rabbit. *Arch Ophthalmol* 1993;111:849–854.

23. George ND, Yates JR, Moore AT. Clinical features in affected males with X-linked retinoschisis. *Arch Ophthalmol* 1996;114:274–280.

24. Gehrig A, Weber BH, Lorenz B, et al. First molecular evidence for a de novo mutation in RS1 (XLRS1) associated with X linked juvenile retinoschisis. *J Med Genet* 1999;36:932–934.

25. Griesinger IB, Sieving PA, Ayyagari R. Autosomal dominant macular atrophy at 6q14 excludes CORD7 and MCDR1/PBCRA loci. *Invest Ophthalmol Vis Sci* 2000;41:248–255.

26. Fishman GA, Jampol LM, Goldberg MF. Diagnostic features of the Favre-Goldmann syndrome. *Br J Ophthalmol* 1976;60:345–353.

27. Brown DM, Graemiger RA, Hergersberg M, et al. Genetic linkage of Wagner disease and erosive vitreoretinopathy to chromosome 5q13–14. *Arch Ophthalmol* 1995;113:671–675.

28. Condon GP, Brownstein S, Wang NS, et al. Congenital hereditary (juvenile X-linked) retinoschisis. Histopathologic and ultrastructural findings in three eyes. *Arch Ophthalmol* 1986;104:576–583.

29. Huopaniemi L, Rantala A, Forsius H, et al. Three widespread founder mutations contribute to high incidence of X-linked juvenile retinoschisis in Finland. *Eur J Hum Genet* 1999;7:368–376.

30. Grayson C, Reid SN, Ellis JA, et al. Retinoschisin, the X-linked retinoschisis protein, is a secreted photoreceptor protein, and is expressed and released by Weri-Rb1 cells. *Hum Mol Genet* 2000;9:1873–1879.

31. Molday LL, Hicks D, Sauer CG, et al. Expression of X-linked retinoschisis protein RS1 in photoreceptor and bipolar cells. *Invest Ophthalmol Vis Sci* 2001;42:816–825.

31a. Takada Y, Fariss RN, Tanikawa A, et al. A retinal neuronal developmental wave of retinoschisin expression begins in ganglion cells during layer formation. *Invest Ophthalmol Vis Sci* 45;2004 (in press).

32. Weber BH, Schrewe H, Molday LL, et al. Inactivation of the murine X-linked juvenile retinoschisis gene, Rs1h, suggests a role of retinoschisin in retinal cell layer organization and synaptic structure. *Proc Natl Acad Sci U S A* 2002;99:6222–6227.

33. Retinoschisis Consortium. Functional implications of the spectrum of mutations found in 234 cases with X-linked juvenile retinoschisis. *Hum Mol Genet* 1998;7:1185–1192.

34. Sieving PA, Yashar BM, Ayyagari R. Juvenile retinoschisis: a model for molecular diagnostic testing of X-linked ophthalmic disease. *Trans Am Ophthalmol Soc* 1999;97:451–464; discussion 464–469.

35. Inoue Y, Yamamoto S, Okada M, et al. X-linked retinoschisis with point mutations in the XLRS1 gene. *Arch Ophthalmol* 2000; 118:93–96.

36. Weinberg DV, Sieving PA, Bingham EL, et al. Bietti crystalline retinopathy and juvenile retinoschisis in a family with a novel RS1 mutation. *Arch Ophthalmol* 2001;119:1719–1721.

37. Jiao X, Munier FL, Iwata F, et al. Genetic linkage of Bietti crystallin corneoretinal dystrophy to chromosome 4q35. *Am J Hum Genet* 2000;67:1309–1313.

38. Nakamura M, Ito S, Terasaki H, et al. Japanese X-linked juvenile retinoschisis: conflict of phenotype and genotype with novel mutations in the XLRS1 gene. *Arch Ophthalmol* 2001;119:1553–1554.

39. van Schooneveld MJ, Miyake Y. Fundus albipunctatus-like lesions in juvenile retinoschisis. *Br J Ophthalmol* 1994;78:659–661.

40. Hotta Y, Nakamura M, Okamoto Y, et al. Different mutation of the XLRS1 gene causes juvenile retinoschisis with retinal white flecks. *Br J Ophthalmol* 2001;85:238–239.

41. Roesch MT, Ewing CC, Gibson AE, et al. The natural history of X-linked retinoschisis. *Can J Ophthalmol* 1998;33:149–158.

42. Kato K, Miyake Y, Kachi S, et al. Axial length and refractive error in X-linked retinoschisis. *Am J Ophthalmol* 2001;131:812–814.

43. Clarke A. The genetic testing of children. Working Party of the Clinical Genetics Society (UK). [Comment] *J Med Genet* 1994; 31:785–797.

44. Wu WW, Molday RS. Defective discoidin domain structure, subunit assembly, and endoplasmic reticulum processing of retinoschisin are primary mechanisms responsible for X-linked retinoschisis. *J Biol Chem* 2003;278:28139–28146.

45. Lewis H. Peripheral retinal degenerations and the risk of retinal detachment. *Am J Ophthalmol* 2003;136:155–160.

46. Noble KG, Carr RE, Siegel IM. Familial foveal retinoschisis associated with a rod-cone dystrophy. *Am J Ophthalmol* 1978;85:551–557.

47. Peralta S, Santori M. Degenerazione maculare centrale tipo Stargardt associata ad alterazione vitreali congenite. *Ann Ottal* 1967; 93:237–242.

26

RETINOPATHY OF PREMATURITY: CURRENT UNDERSTANDING BASED ON CLINICAL TRIALS AND ANIMAL MODELS

JANET R. McCOLM
MARY ELIZABETH HARTNETT

CLINICAL RETINOPATHY OF PREMATURITY, RISKS, AND ENVIRONMENTAL FACTORS

Prevalence

Of the 14,000 to 16,000 premature infants weighing <1,250 g born each year in the United States, 9,000 to 10,500 will develop retinopathy of prematurity (ROP), 1,100 to 1,500 will require treatment, and 400 to 600 will become legally blind (1). These estimates are similar to those reported in the late 1970s (2), even though advancements in ROP management have led to better visual outcomes. This is due in part to progress in neonatal care and greater survival of infants at the highest risk for ROP, namely, those born weighing <1,000 g (3). Thus, ROP continues to be a serious health concern. The costs of acute neonatal and chronic long-term care, as well as the cost to society for life-long blindness and visual impairment (4), justify ongoing research and means to achieve effective treatment (5).

History: From Retrolental Fibroplasia to Retinopathy of Prematurity

Retrolental fibroplasia (RLF) (Fig. 26-1) was first recognized in the 1940s (6) as the cicatricial form of the most severe stage of ROP, stage 5 ROP. The white pupil found in the eyes of a premature infant, approximately 32 weeks' gestational age (6), represented a retrolental fibrovascular membrane behind which existed a total retinal detachment. Once high and uncontrolled oxygen delivery was recognized as a cause of RLF (7), efforts to regulate oxygen were initiated, and, as a result, RLF was nearly completely obliterated. However, ROP reappeared with increased survival of young gestational age and very low birth weight premature infants and with emerging neonatal care throughout the world. We now recognize that multiple factors are involved in the development of ROP, and the role of supplemental oxygen ap-

pears more complex (see section on Environmental Factors). In addition, the recognition of earlier stages of ROP has both facilitated investigation into the causes of ROP (see section on Animal Models) and led to treatment (see section on Screening and Management and Chapter 22) to reduce the risk of retinal detachment.

International Classification of Retinopathy of Prematurity Characterizes Progression of Retinopathy of Prematurity

The International Classification of Retinopathy of Prematurity (ICROP) was developed to describe the early levels of severity of ROP based on several parameters: zone, stage, extent of stage, and presence of plus disease (8). The zone of ROP refers to 1 of 3 areas that best describes the retinal area that has apparent intraretinal vascularization (Fig. 26-2). Normally, in development, vascularization of the retina starts posteriorly with early vascularization around the optic nerve disputed to be a result of angioblast growth or vasculogenesis. From these early vessels, further proliferation and migration extends vascularization toward the ora serrata. Zone I is the retinal area encompassed by a circle centered around the optic nerve with a radius equivalent to two times the distance from the optic nerve to the fovea. Zone II is the area outside zone I but within a circular area centered on the optic nerve with a radius equivalent to the distance from the optic nerve to the nasal horizontal ora serrata. Zone III is the remaining crescent. Where there is no retinal vascularization, an avascular area is clinically apparent peripheral to vascularized retina. The stage of ROP defines the clinical appearance of the retina at the junction of vascularized retina and the avascular area. There are five stages. In stage 1, a line is apparent (Fig. 26-3). In stage 2, there is a ridge having obvious

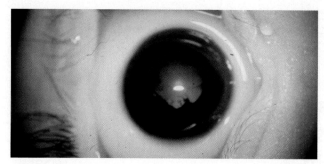

FIGURE 26-1. Eye of infant with retrolental fibrovascular membrane from stage 5 ROP. Total retinal detachment, determined by ultrasonogram, exists posterior to the white retrolental membrane.

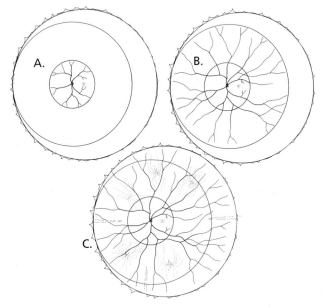

FIGURE 26-2. Circular zones I (A), II (B), and III (C) drawn onto schematic of fundus. Zone 1 is the least mature and encompasses the smallest area of retina with developed retinal vasculature.

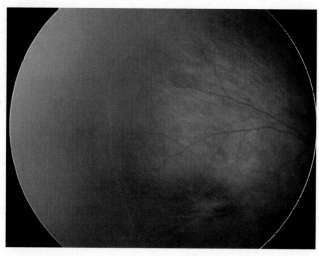

FIGURE 26-4. Stage 2 retinopathy of prematurity with islands of neovascular tissue extending from the ridge.

volume (Fig. 26-4). In stage 3 ROP, there is neovascularization growing onto the vitreous at the ridge (Fig. 26-5). Stage 4 ROP is partial retinal detachment (Fig. 26-6, Fig. 27-1D), 4A without macular involvement and 4B with macular involvement. Stage 5 ROP is total retinal detachment and is described as closed where the retina is adherent to itself or open where it is not (see Figure 27-25). In some cases of stage 5 ROP, there is a peripheral area of attached avascular retina causing a peripheral retinal trough. The extent of ROP refers to the number of clock hours of the highest stage. Plus disease refers to dilatation and tortuosity of the retinal arterioles and veins in the posterior pole (Fig. 26-7; see also Fig. 27-2) and is based on a standard photograph

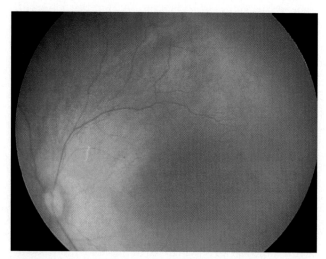

FIGURE 26-3. Stage 1 retinopathy of prematurity seen as a discontinuous white, tortuous line between vascularized (posterior) and avascular (peripheral) retina temporally.

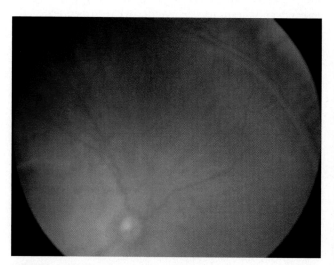

FIGURE 26-5. Image of eye treated with laser to avascular retina (upper right of field). Note stage 3 neovascularization extending into vitreous. Some blood is seen within the neovascular tissue.

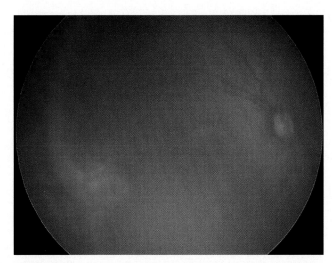

FIGURE 26-6. Early stage 4A retinopathy of prematurity with exudation posterior to the ridge. The elevated retina extending superiorly and inferiorly from area of exudation at 9 o'clock appears out of focus.

published in the Multicenter Trial of Cryotherapy for Retinopathy of Prematurity (CRYO-ROP) (9). In later clinical trials, the definition of plus disease was changed to include less severe degrees of vascular tortuosity and dilatation (Table 26-1, STOP-ROP, HOPE-ROP) (10,11).

Age of Onset

Most infants that develop some form of ROP do so at about 32 weeks' postmenstrual age (PMA). PMA equals gestational age plus age after birth in weeks (12,13). Threshold disease, at which the risk of a poor outcome approached

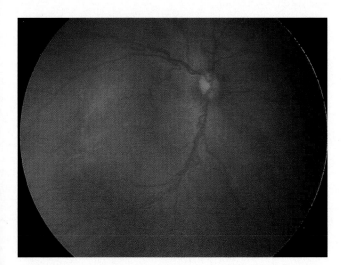

FIGURE 26-7. Moderate plus disease present posteriorly as dilated, tortuous vessels around the optic nerve.

50% (see later), peaks at approximately 37 weeks' PMA (10,14), and type 1 prethreshold ROP (see section on Prethreshold and Threshold Retinopathy of Prematurity), where risk of a poor outcome is ≥15%, at approximately 35 weeks (15). Eyes that rapidly progress to prethreshold ROP have a greater risk of developing threshold ROP (14,16) and will develop threshold disease at an earlier PMA. When infants achieve 45 weeks' PMA without developing prethreshold ROP, they have a low risk of developing threshold ROP or of having a poor outcome (Table 26-2) (13).

Course of Retinopathy of Prematurity

Most ROP regresses; >90% of stages 1 and 2 do not develop threshold ROP (12). However, typically, ROP progresses before it regresses. In about 6% of infants born weighing <1,251 g, threshold ROP develops. Without treatment, this results in an unfavorable outcome in about 50% of eyes (17). Even after treatment for threshold ROP, 20% to 30% of eyes will experience an unfavorable outcome (18). However, based on outcome data from the Early Treatment for Retinopathy of Prematurity (ETROP) trial (Table 26-1), treatment at a less severe level of ROP, i.e., for type 1 prethreshold ROP (Table 26-2), reduces poor visual and functional outcomes at 9-month follow-up compared to waiting until threshold ROP develops (15,19).

Prethreshold and Threshold Retinopathy of Prematurity

Based on the CRYO-ROP Study, threshold ROP is defined as the level of severity of ROP at which the risk of an unfavorable anatomic outcome (Table 26-3) approached 50% (9,17) and was diagnosed by the presence of five contiguous or eight total clock hours of stage 3 ROP in zones I or II with plus disease (Fig. 26-8). Because a high frequency (87%) of zone I eyes had an unfavorable outcome in the CRYO-ROP study, later studies such as Supplemental Therapeutic Oxygen to Prevent Prethreshold Retinopathy of Prematurity (STOP-ROP) (10) and High-Oxygen-Percentage Retinopathy of Prematurity (HOPE-ROP) (11) defined threshold ROP less stringently for zone I eyes (Table 26-4). Prethreshold ROP defined eyes at high risk of developing threshold ROP and that should be monitored closely. In the ETROP trial, prethreshold ROP was further subdivided based on the risk of an unfavorable outcome. Eyes with high risk were defined as having ≥15% risk, whereas eyes at low risk had <15% risk of an unfavorable outcome. An unfavorable outcome was primarily based on 1 of 4 categories of visual function as tested with Teller acuity cards (15). Secondary outcomes were based on structure where poor outcomes were a retinal fold or detachment involving the macula, or a retrolental opacity blocking the visual axis. Type 1 prethreshold ROP was defined as zone I, any stage ROP with plus disease, zone I,

TABLE 26–1. MAJOR CLINICAL TRIALS IN RETINOPATHY OF PREMATURITY

Trial (Enrollment)	Criteria	Number Enrolled	Endpoint (Follow-up)
CRYO-ROP (1/1/86 – 1/22/88)	<1251 g BW; survived 28 days of life; no major systemic or ocular anomalies	4099 (291 with threshold ROP randomized to cryo or observation[a], 247 analyzed at 10 yr)	Reports at 3 mo, 1 through 10 yrs. (9, 17, 18, 20–22)
CRYO-ROP Natural History Study[a] (1/1/86 – 1/22/88)	See above	1208 survived 1 yr and followed (69 had threshold ROP randomized to cryo or observation)	App 3 mo, 5.5 yr
CRYO-ROP (1/1/86 – 1/22/88)	See above	See above	See above
LIGHT-ROP (7/95-3/97)	<1251 g BW and GA <31 weeks; NICU admission within 24 hr of birth	409 (205 wore goggles and 204 did not)	Through regression of ROP; 6 mo follow up
STOP-ROP (2/94-3/99)	prethreshold in one eye; <94% SaO_2 in RA, no lethal anomalies or ocular congenital anomalies	649 (325 given O_2 to achieve 89-94% SaO_2 (Con), 324 given O_2 to achieve 96-99% SaO_2 (S))	3 mos after 40 weeks PMA
HOPE-ROP (1/96-3/99 concurrent with STOP-ROP)	prethreshold in one eye and median SaO_2 >94%	136 HOPE-ROP compared to 229 STOP-ROP infants enrolled from 15 hospitals	Through development of threshold ROP or regression of ROP
Laser compared to cryotherapy for threshold ROP (1990-1991)	threshold ROP; bilateral randomized to laser in one eye and cryo in other	66 patients treated (39 with bilateral disease); at 10 yrs, 25 patients analyzed (19 bilateral)	10 years
Vitamin E meta-analysis of 6 controlled clinical trials (1978-1981)	≤ 1500 g BW	536/704 infants received vitamin E prophylaxis and 551/714 were control; all completed trials	varied
ETROP (10/99 – 10/02)	<1251 g BW; prethreshold	828 infants (730 studied); 401 type 1 prethreshold (high risk or ≥ 15% risk of unfavorable outcome), 329 low risk (< 15% risk)	9 mos PMA

[a] 240 had bilateral disease and were treated with cryotherapy (cryo) in one eye and observed in the fellow eye. In 51 asymmetric eyes, treatment was randomly assigned to either cryo or observation.
[b] For the 1-year and 3½-year studies, Teller acuity vision was determined. For the 5½- and 10-year outcome studies, testing using the ETDRS visual acuity chart was also performed.

TABLE 26–1. *Continued*

Rationale (Hypothesis)	Outcome Measures	Results
Treatment of avascular zone in threshold ROP reduces poor visual and structural outcomes	Visual function[b]; structural findings; (Table 26.3)	At 10 years; 44.4% cryo vs. 62.6% observation had <20/200 and 27.2% vs. 47.9% had unfavorable structural outcomes; p<0.001 (18). (Table 26. 2)
A. Factors associated with development of threshold ROP or unfavorable macular outcome	Systemic factors; ocular factors	A. young GA, multiple births, out-of-nursery birth, low BW (14); white race (14, 30); zone I ROP, plus disease, stage 3 (14); > 6 clock hours stage 3 (31); iris vessel dilatation (64). (Table 26. 2)
B. Factors associated with increased risk of prethreshold progressing to threshold ROP	See above	B. Lower PMA at ROP diagnosis; zone I at 1st exam; rapid progression to prethreshold; plus disease at 1st prethreshold exam; white race (14, 16). (Table 26. 2)
Light reduction and reducing ultraviolet light reduces ROP	Primary – any ROP; secondary – prethreshold or threshold (CRYO-ROP definitions; [Table 26.4])	54% goggles vs 58% no goggles developed ROP; 15% goggles vs 14% no goggles developed either prethreshold or threshold ROP; p=NS (84). No difference in myopia at 6 mos.
Oxygen supplementation relieves the hypoxic stimulus (for stage 3 ROP) caused through normal retinal differentiation and oxygen consumption	Threshold ROP or worse; 3 mo follow up for structural outcome	Threshold ROP in at least one eye in 48% Con vs. 41% S; prethreshold without plus disease 46% Con vs. 32% S developed threshold ROP (10). (Table 26.7; See also HOPE-ROP below)
Fewer HOPE-ROP infants would progress to threshold ROP than STOP-ROP infants	Threshold ROP (adverse) or regressed ROP (positive)	HOPE-ROP infants progressed less frequently (25%) to threshold ROP than STOP-ROP (46%), but when race, GA, PMA at prethreshold, zone I disease, plus disease at prethreshold were controlled, p=0.0623 (11).
Laser to the avascular zone of threshold ROP reduces untoward outcomes to the same degree as cryotherapy	Structural outcome by indirect ophthalmoscopy and review of fundus images; BCVA by ETDRS testing; refractive status	Mean visual acuity 20/66 for laser vs. 20/182 for cryotherapy eyes: p=0.0152 (34,38); (Table 26. 6); Cost of treatment of ROP with cryotherapy ($1801) and laser ($678); treatment cost-effective (5).
Antioxidant vitamin E reduces oxidative damage to particularly vulnerable polyunsaturated fatty acids of retina	Any ROP; stage 3+ ROP	39.8% of vitamin E compared to 43.5% control had any ROP; 2.4% of vitamin E vs 5.3% control developed stage 3+ ROP; p<0.02 (97). Unable to assess adverse effects of vitamin E from meta-analysis.
Early treatment with ≥15% risk of unfavorable outcome will reduce blindness (based on model of risk factors to assign risk of blindness without treatment)	BCVA at 9 mos corrected age (Teller Acuity Cards); secondary outcomes retinal structure, myopia, amblyopia, strabismus	Reduced unfavorable visual outcome (19.5% to 14.5%, p=.01); reduced unfavorable structural outcome (15.6% to 9.1%; p<.001) (15).

BCVA, best-corrected visual acuity; BW, birthweight; Con, conventional oxygen; ETDRS, Early Treatment Diabetic Retinopathy Study visual acuit; GA, gestational age; MO, month; NICU, neonatal intensive care unit; PMA, postmenstrual age; PUFA, polyunsaturated fatty acids; RA, room air; ROP, retinopathy of prematurity; S, supplemental oxygen.

TABLE 26–2. LATER STUDIES PERFORMED ON ORIGINAL CRYO-ROP COHORT

31.1% treated vs. 51.4% control in 273/279 had unfavorable structural outcome at 3 mo (17)

44.4% treated vs. 62.6% control ($p < 0.001$) ≤20/200; 27.2% treated vs. 47.9% control had either partial retinal detachment with foveal involvement, total RD or other unfavorable outcome at 10 years (18)

Zone I ROP (16 eyes) at 10 years had unfavorable VA ≤20/200 (18); unfavorable structural outcome in 88% treated and 94% control [8.24 odds ratio that zone I eyes have an unfavorable macular outcome compared to zone II (14)]

At 5.5 yr in eyes with attached retinas, 13.4% cryotherapy-treated vs. 20% control had ≥20/40 (due to sample size) (22)

Contrast sensitivity followed visual acuity results; in eyes with favorable outcomes, there was no difference in contrast sensitivity between treated and untreated eyes at 10 yr (23)

In natural history cohort (n = 1,208), strabismus surgery was performed in 6% and amblyopia therapy in 7%, whereas in those that developed threshold ROP (n = 257), strabismus surgery was performed in 10% and amblyopia therapy in 20% (24)

Myopia was increased in premature infants and was directly related in degree to the severity of ROP (25)

For 247 tested of original 291 children enrolled, rates of retinal detachment increased in control group between 5.5 yr (38.6%) and 10 y (41.4%) whereas treated eyes remained stable (22%) (18)

Visual fields somewhat smaller in threshold ROP vs. no ROP groups; in infants with bilateral threshold ROP and measurable visual acuity OU, treated eyes had 6–7 degrees smaller fields than untreated eyes (26)

Acute ROP involutes naturally on average at 38.6 wks PMA, with 90% involuting before 44 wks PMA (27)

ROP level of severity associated with functional disability at age 5.5 yr (28)

Increased (200 × adult prevalence) blue-yellow color defects in preterm infants, not related to ROP severity, birth weight, gestational age, or treatment with cryotherapy (29)—tested at 5.5 yr

Retinal conditions indicating a risk of poor outcome were not observed before 31 wks PMA or 4 wks chronologic age in 99% of combined CRYO-ROP and LIGHT-ROP. Infants that attained 45 wks PMA and did not develop prethreshold ROP had minimal risk (13)

In natural history cohort of 4,099 infants, 51 (3.2%) of 1,584 black infants and 160 (7.4%) of 2,158 white infants developed threshold ROP. Race was significant in logistic regression analysis, accounting for gestational age, birth weight, multiple births, sex, and transport status ($p < 0.001$) (30)

Unfavorable structural and nearly all unfavorable visual acuity outcomes occurred in eyes with stage 3 ROP of ≥6 clock hours in zone I or II with plus disease (31)

Based on known nonocular and ocular risk factors (14) at birth, onset of ROP and prethreshold ROP, and rate of progression of ROP, individual estimates of risk of threshold ROP and of an unfavorable 3-mo outcome after treatment or observation are computed and become basis for ETROP trial (16,32)

PMA, postmenstrual age (gestational age plus chronological age in weeks); RD, retinal detachment; ROP, retinopathy of prematurity; OU, both eyes.

TABLE 26–3. UNFAVORABLE RETINAL OUTCOMES

Favorable
    Essentially normal posterior pole (near periphery and zone I), including angle of vessels
    Abnormal angle of major temporal vascular arcade in the posterior pole
    Macular ectopia
    Stage 4A partial retinal detachment, retinoschisis, or fold in the posterior pole (fovea spared)

Unfavorable
    Stage 4B partial retinal detachment retinoschisis, or fold—all with foveal involvement
    View of macula (and presumably patient's central vision) blocked by partial cataract, retrolental membrane, or corneal opacity due to ROP
    Stage 5 retinal detachment, total retinoschisis, or retrolental membrane
    Entire view of posterior pole and near periphery is blocked by total cataract or total corneal opacity from ROP
    Enucleation for any reason

Unable to grade
    Unable to determine (e.g., view impossible because of corneal opacity unrelated to ROP or because of miotic pupil)
    None of the above (e.g., extreme vascular attenuation, optic atrophy)

ROP, retinopathy of prematurity.

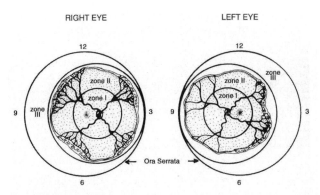

RIGHT EYE   LEFT EYE

FIGURE 26-8. Artist rendition of threshold disease defined in the Multicenter Trial of Cryotherapy for Retinopathy of Prematurity (CRYO-ROP) study as five contiguous or eight total clock hours of stage 3+ in zone I or II.

stage 3 ROP without plus disease, and zone II, stage 2 or 3 with at least two quadrants of plus disease based on the standard photograph from the CRYO-ROP study (9). Treatment of the peripheral retina with laser for type 1 prethreshold ROP is recommended (Table 26-1) (15). These definitions provide guidelines for managing infants with acute ROP.

TABLE 26–4. DEFINITIONS OF PRETHRESHOLD AND THRESHOLD ROP

Prethreshold ROP

Zone I, any stage
Zone II, stage 2 with plus[a] disease
Zone II, stage 3 less than threshold
Prethreshold classification used for Early Treatment for Retinopathy of Prematurity Trial
  Type 1 (high-risk prethreshold where risk of unfavorable outcome is ≥15%) (15)
    Zone I, any stage with plus[b] disease
    Zone I, stage 3 without plus[b] disease
    Zone II, stage 2 or 3 with plus[b] disease
  Type 2 (low-risk prethreshold ROP where risk of unfavorable outcome is <15%) (15)
    Zone I, stage 1 or 2 without plus[b] disease
    Zone II, stage 3 without plus[b] disease

Threshold ROP

Zone I[a] or II, stage 3 (five contiguous or eight total clock hours with plus disease)
[a]The definition of threshold ROP was different for the CRYO-ROP and STOP-ROP studies: (i) for STOP-ROP, plus disease was defined as two quadrants of posterior pole dilation/tortuosity, whereas in CRYO-ROP it was defined as about four quadrants of posterior pole dilation/tortuosity, and (ii) for STOP-ROP, a less stringent definition of threshold disease was given for zone I eyes that included any ROP with plus disease or any stage 3 with or without plus disease.
[b]Based on standard photograph used in CRYO-ROP studies; requires two quadrants of plus disease (similar to criteria used in STOP-ROP study)

ROP, retinopathy of prematurity.

Diagnosis

An accurate diagnosis of ROP is essential to detect eyes that require urgent treatment for threshold ROP and, in eyes at low or moderate risk of threshold ROP, to determine when the follow-up examination should be performed. To obtain an accurate diagnosis, a complete retinal examination must be performed in a well-dilated infant using an indirect ophthalmoscope and, often, scleral depression. Once the infant's eyes are fully dilated and the infant is swaddled, a drop of topical anesthetic is instilled into one eye and a lid speculum is inserted. Initially no scleral depression is performed so as to reduce possible blanching of plus disease. The retinal vessels are assessed for vascular dilatation and tortuosity in each of the four quadrants first, in the vascular arcades around the optic nerve (Fig. 26-7), and second in the periphery (Fig. 26-9). Scleral depression can be useful to determine the zone of intraretinal vascularization. Determination of zone I is made either by estimating the circle surrounding the optic nerve having a radius of twice the distance from the optic nerve to the fovea or by viewing the image of the fundus through a 28-diopter lens with the optic nerve in the center. If the retinal vasculature does not extend beyond the image size of the 28-diopter lens, then vessels are likely within zone I. Zone II is retinal vascularization beyond zone I but not within one disc diameter of the nasal two clock-hours of the ora serrata, e.g., 8 to 10 o'clock OS or 2 to 4 o'clock OD (10). Zone III is the remaining avascular temporal area of retina (Fig. 26-2).

There can be difficulties examining the lightly pigmented, blonde fundus, or deeply pigmented fundus. In the blonde fundus (Fig. 26-10), the choroidal vessels are apparent, and the examiner may mistake these for retinal vessels.

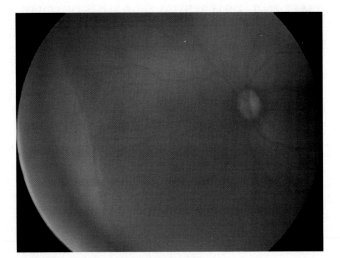

FIGURE 26-9. Peripheral plus disease noted by dilated and tortuous retinal arterioles and veins in the peripheral retina extending into the ridge.

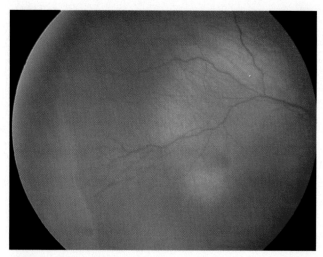

FIGURE 26-10. Blonde fundus permits visualization of deeper choroidal vessels that can be mistaken for retinal blood vessels.

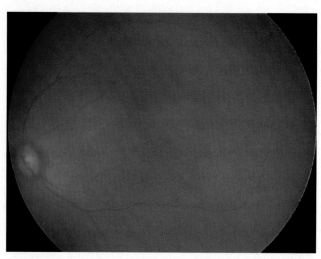

FIGURE 26-11. Deeply pigmented fundus reduces the contrast between melanin of retinal pigment epithelium and choroid and hemoglobin of retinal vessels, making it difficult to visualize retinal vessels.

In the deeply pigmented fundus (Fig. 26-11), it can be difficult to visualize the retinal vessels against the dark, pigmented background. In both of these cases, the 20-diopter lens can improve diagnostic ability.

Classically, at the junction of vascularized and avascular retina, the examiner determines the stage of ROP and the clock-hour extent of each stage. The clock-hour extent of the highest stage, the zone, and the presence or absence of plus disease are recorded. The clock-hour extent may be less important in determining eyes at risk of an unfavorable outcome that should have laser treatment (15,19) but still is important in determining eyes at risk of progressive stage 4 ROP after laser treatment (33).

The same procedure is performed in the fellow eye.

Differential Diagnosis

The differential diagnosis of ROP includes familial exudative vitreoretinopathy (FEVR) (see Chapter 28), Norrie disease, incontinentia pigmenti, congenital retinal fold, *Toxocara canis* infection (see Chapter 16), and causes of leukocoria (Table 26-5). A white pupil, referred to as *leuko-*

TABLE 26–5. DIFFERENTIAL DIAGNOSIS OF LEUKOCORIA

Cornea	Mesodermal dysgenesis including mutations of the PAX gene family; mucopolysaccharidoses, mucolipidoses, fucosidosis, mannosidosis, Farber and other storage diseases; congenital glaucoma; aniridia (sporadic); infectious causes, e.g., syphilis, interstitial keratitis, rubella, CMV; birth trauma; dermoid; fetal alcohol syndrome; late stage 5 ROP; and others
Lens	Lenticonus; congenital cataract; infectious (rubella, viral, toxocariasis, toxoplasmosis); inflammatory (juvenile rheumatoid arthritis, sarcoidosis); metabolic (hypocalcemia, hypoglycemia, diabetes mellitus, mannosidosis, galactosemia, galactokinase deficiency, Lowe aminoaciduria, homocystinuria); traumatic (amniocentesis or other trauma); Alport syndrome (also with fleck retinopathy and corneal dystrophy); aniridia; persistent fetal vasculature (PFV); Stickler; late stage 5 ROP; and others
Vitreous	Hemorrhage (nonaccidental and accidental trauma, retinoblastoma, persistent hyaloid artery bleed, PFV, ROP, protein C deficiency, Terson syndrome, disseminated intravascular coagulation disorder); inflammation/uveitis (*Toxocara canis*, toxoplasmosis, peripheral uveitis, CMV retinitis, endophthalmitis, sarcoidosis); tumor seeding or hemorrhage from retinoblastoma; and others
Retinal/choroidal	PFV; ROP; congenital retinal fold; Norrie disease; incontinentia pigmenti; optic nerve abnormalities (coloboma, peripapillary staphyloma, morning glory syndrome); tumor (retinoblastoma, medulloepithelioma, medulloblastoma); Coats disease; trauma (accidental, nonaccidental, amniocentesis injury); X-linked retinoschisis; retinal detachment; and others

CMV, cytomegalovirus; ROP, retinopathy of prematurity; PFV, persistent fetal vasculature.

coria, can occur from media opacities at any level from the cornea to the retina. The history of prematurity and low birth weight are the most helpful historical data in the differential diagnosis of ROP.

Clinical Symptoms and Signs

There are no symptoms of acute ROP, nor can a specific visual behavior in the preterm newborn herald a concern for ROP. Therefore, effective screening is essential.

Screening and Management

The screening protocol at each neonatal intensive care unit (NICU) should be based on published recommendations and preferences of the screening ophthalmologists, neonatologists, and NICU nurses. All at-risk infants should be identified and receive adequate dilated retinal evaluations at appropriate times. The Joint Statement of the American Academy of *Pediatrics* (approved March 1997), the American Association for Pediatric Ophthalmology and Strabismus (approved October 1996), and the American Academy of Ophthalmology (approved November 1996) provided the following guidelines for infants who should be screened for ROP: (i) all infants born weighing ≤1,500 g or ≤28 weeks' gestational age and (ii) infants born weighing >1,500 g but who experience an unstable course. The first examination should be performed prior to hospital discharge, at 4 to 6 weeks after birth, or between 31 and 33 weeks' PMA. An analysis of the combined data from the CRYO-ROP and Light Reduction in ROP (Light-ROP) studies was performed to determine the lowest PMA when retinal features were present that indicated a risk of an

unfavorable outcome. From this analysis, recommendations were made that the first screening examination be conducted prior to 31 weeks' PMA or 4 weeks' chronologic age, whichever was later (Table 26-2) (13).

Examinations should be repeated periodically, e.g., every 2 weeks if there is no ROP, weekly with any ROP, and more frequently with prethreshold ROP. If intraretinal vascularization proceeds toward the ora serrata, examinations are performed less frequently. Signs indicating that the risk of visual loss from ROP is minimal include PMA of 45 weeks, intraretinal vascularization into zone III without previous zone II ROP, and complete intraretinal vascularization determined on two consecutive examinations (13). When any of these signs is present, screening can be discontinued and the focus of care changed to that of visual rehabilitation.

If threshold disease develops, treatment with laser, preferable to cryotherapy (Table 26-6) (34), should be performed within 72 hours (see Chapter 22 for guidelines). Treated eyes are followed closely, often weekly or more frequently, for signs of regression, need for further laser, or possible vitreoretinal surgery if progressive stage 4 ROP develops (see Chapter 27).

Prevention

ROP is a disease of premature infants. Therefore, reducing the number of premature births, such as through good prenatal care (35), reduction in teenage pregnancies (36), and avoidance of illegal drug use (37), would reduce the number of infants at risk for ROP.

To reduce the incidence of ROP, in the 1960s, NICUs began to monitor oxygen delivery to the preterm newborn, particularly in the perinatal period so as to avoid high oxy-

TABLE 26–6. LASER COMPARED TO CRYOTHERAPY FOR TREATMENT OF THRESHOLD ROP

	Laser-Treated	Cryotherapy-Treated	*p* Value
Mean ETDRS VA (all cases)	20/66	20/182	0.0152
Mean ETDRS VA (bilateral cases)	20/66	20/152	0.033
Unfavorable outcome	2 eyes (10%)	4 eyes (19%)	Too few eyes for meaningful statistics
Macular dragging (bilateral; *n* = 13)	Score = 0.39	Score = 1.15	0.018
Myopia (diopters)	−4.48	−7.65	0.019
Axial length (mm)	22.9	21.7	0.024
Lens thickness (mm)	3.95	4.33	<0.001

Laser-treated eyes 5.2 times more likely to have 20/50 visual acuity (VA). Linear regression analysis revealed poor correlation ($r = 0.36$, $p = 0.14$, $n = 18$) in best-corrected visual acuity (BCVA) between eyes of the same infant with bilateral disease and had one eye treated with laser and the fellow eye with cryotherapy. For laser-treated eyes that lacked retinal dragging, BCVA was predicted to be 20/32, but for cryotherapy-treated eyes (34), BCVA was predicted to be 20/50.
The thickness of the lens was most strongly correlated to refractive outcomes in both laser-treated ($r = 0.885$, $p < 0.001$) and cryotherapy-treated eyes ($r = 0.591$, $p = 0.026$) (38).
ETDRS, Early Treatment Diabetic Retinopathy Study visual acuity testing standards.

gen levels, such as those used when RLF was first recognized (6). NICUs now have the technology to maintain oxygen within predetermined "safe" limits, defined by the Fetus and Newborn Committee of the American Academy of Pediatrics and American College of Obstetricians and Gynecologists (39). However, several studies provide evidence that not only the concentration but also the variability of oxygen are factors in the development and severity of ROP (40,41) (see section on Effects of Environmental Factors, Oxygen).

To prevent blindness from ROP in the preterm infant, screening is important to detect threshold ROP. The CRYO-ROP study (17), the STOP-ROP study (10), and other studies (34) have shown that laser treatment or cryotherapy delivered to the avascular zones of eyes with threshold ROP within 72 hours reduced unfavorable outcomes and vision loss (Table 26-3). The ETROP trial refined the definition of eyes at risk of threshold ROP and an unwanted outcome: all zone I eyes with any ROP and plus disease, zone I eyes with stage 3 ROP without plus disease, zone II eyes with stages 2 or 3 ROP and plus disease (Table 26-1) (15,19). If treatment for threshold ROP is adequate but ROP progresses to stage 4 ROP with certain retinal features (33) or in eyes with stage 5 ROP, vitreoretinal surgery is considered. Finally, visual rehabilitation is important to treat amblyopia and myopia that occur more commonly in prematurely born children and even more often in those who had ROP, compared to infants born full term (Table 26-2) (24,25). Later segmentation of encircling elements used to treat stage 4 ROP or rhegmatogenous retinal detachment (42) reduces optical irregularities, permits growth of the globe (43), and may improve visual outcomes.

Vision Rehabilitation

Vision rehabilitation is important in all premature infants with or without ROP. Premature infants are more likely to require strabismus surgery, to be treated for amblyopia, and to be myopic than full-term infants (Table 26-2) (24,25,44). These conditions are even more common in premature infants who had more severe levels of ROP and threshold disease (24,25,38,44) than those with milder ROP. Infants with macular heterotopia may have potential for visual acuity (45); therefore, correction of refractive errors and treatment of amblyopia are indicated. For the aphakic infant who had retinal detachment repair, visual rehabilitation with special adjustments for low vision is recommended (see Chapter 33). Even when grating acuity cannot be measured, low vision can be stratified into levels characterized by the presence of light perception in different fields of gaze (46) and may be important to infant and child development. Treatment of aphakic amblyopia and aphakia is controversial, particularly in the infant after successful retinal reattachment of stage 5 ROP. Macular vi-

sion is not likely to develop, but aphakic spectacles are believed by vision teachers to improve the peripheral vision of the child (Perkins School of the Blind, Watertown, MA). In the child with macular acuity in one eye and aphakic amblyopia in the fellow eye, spectacle wear also provides protection against ocular trauma. We recommend that infants be managed by a pediatric ophthalmologist for visual rehabilitation starting at an earlier age than that recommended for full-term infants and that children be enrolled in an early intervention program that enhances the use of all of the senses.

Role of Other Physicians and Health Care Providers

A team approach and effective communication are important in the care of the premature infant. During the time that the infant is in the NICU, the core caregivers include the neonatologist, the screening ophthalmologist, and the nursing staff. Often a nurse manager or ophthalmic technician can facilitate communication between the ophthalmologist and the NICU to assure that eye drops are given at the appropriate time, consultation reports are available for the examining ophthalmologist to fill out, and the individual infant's nurse is available to assist and monitor for apnea and bradycardia during the examination. We prefer to have a nurse, fellow physician, or trained technician assist by securely holding the swaddled infant during the examination. It is important to provide a written consultation for all infants and to communicate with the neonatologist, especially about infants with progressing ROP. Ongoing communication with the parents helps to avoid any possible surprise if treatment is urgently needed.

Once the infant is discharged from the NICU, follow-up examinations for the retina and later for visual rehabilitation are important. Often, a written information booklet is given to parents or guardians with emphasis placed on the importance of the timing of appointments. A system is required to reschedule infants as soon as possible if appointments are missed and requires training of the office staff to assure infants needing urgent appointments are examined. When repeated appointments are missed, we send a certified letter to the parents or guardians. Once the risk of ROP is reduced, follow-up with a pediatric ophthalmologist and in an early intervention program is important for visual rehabilitation.

Ethical Considerations

Ethical questions arise when working in neonatal intensive care. Each question is taken on an individual basis, accounting for the infant's general condition and fellow eye, and is addressed by a team that may include the neonatologist, parents, and ophthalmologists. For example, it is universally agreed that stage 5 ROP should be prevented, and efforts are made to accomplish this. Careful monitoring of eyes after treatment for threshold ROP is essential to diagnose progressive stage 4 ROP that might be repaired with a lens-sparing vitrectomy (47,48). However, cases of stage 5 ROP can occur when an infant is too sick to undergo treatment for threshold ROP, when treatment for threshold ROP does not prevent retinal detachment, or when infants are lost to follow-up despite efforts to prevent this. The question may arise as to whether heroic surgery should be performed to reattach the retina in an eye with stage 5 ROP in a preterm infant with multiple medical conditions. Evidence exists that low vision can be stratified in infants with repaired retinal detachments from stage 5 ROP (46) and can be useful in children when at a level believed to have little value in adults (49). Still, long-term benefits of low vision on child development and quality of life are difficult to study and remain largely unknown.

Worldwide Impact on Child Blindness, Including Public Health Issues

ROP is a growing cause of blindness, especially in middle-income developing countries where neonatal care is now emerging, and is discussed in detail in Chapter 18.

Risk Factors

Severe Retinopathy of Prematurity

The greatest single risk factor for developing ROP is being born prematurely (40,50–63). However, we now know much more about the risks of progression of the disease. The CRYO-ROP study provided data from the natural history cohort (Table 26-1) on ocular and systemic characteristics associated with increased risk of ROP, progression to threshold ROP, and development of an unfavorable macular outcome (Table 26-3) (14). An important ocular risk factor was zone I. If, at 32 weeks' PMA, incomplete vascularization in zone I was present, 32.8% of eyes developed threshold ROP, compared to 9.3% with incomplete vascularization in zone II. Eyes with zone I ROP also were at high risk of developing threshold ROP. Other ocular risk factors for developing threshold ROP included plus disease, stage 3 ROP (14), ≥6 clock-hours stage 3 (31), and iris vessel dilatation (64). Nonocular risk factors associated with the development of threshold ROP included young gestational age, multiple births, out-of-nursery birth, low birth weight (14), and Caucasian race (Table 26-1) (14,30). Once prethreshold ROP developed, the risk of developing threshold ROP was about the same given these factors. For each 100-g increase in birth weight, there was a 27% decrease in the percentage of infants who developed threshold ROP. Black race was associated with a 65% lower chance of developing threshold ROP compared to Caucasian race if any ROP was present and a 51% decreased chance of develop-

ing threshold if prethreshold ROP developed. Once threshold ROP developed, the risk of an unfavorable anatomic outcome (Table 26-3) was about the same in Blacks as for Caucasians (14). Factors associated with increased risk of prethreshold progressing to threshold ROP included lower PMA at the diagnosis of any ROP, ROP in zone I at the first screening examination, rapid progression of ROP to prethreshold characteristics, plus disease at the first prethreshold examination, and white race (14,16).

There have been few other studies of race and risk of ROP in premature infants. However, an earlier study performed in the United Kingdom demonstrated that Asians had a greater risk of developing ROP than Caucasians and that this perceived risk was related to an increased survival of Asians (53). Another small study reported that native Alaskans were more susceptible to ROP compared to nonnative Alaskans (65). Although race cannot be addressed using animal models, different strains of rats were shown to develop different degrees of severity of retinopathy under the same conditions (66).

Unfavorable Macular Outcome

In the initial natural history report, ocular characteristics associated with an unfavorable macular outcome included zone I ROP, plus disease, and stage 3 ROP (Table 26-1) (14). Eyes with zone I ROP had an odds risk of 8.24 toward developing an unfavorable outcome compared to zone II ROP (14). For each clock hour of stage 3 ROP greater than 5 clock hours, there was a 26% increased risk of an unfavorable macular outcome (14). Stage 3 ROP with plus disease in zone II was associated with a 62% risk of an unfavorable result compared to stage 3 ROP without plus disease in zone II in which the risk was 3%. In the 5.5-year report from the natural history cohort of CRYO-ROP (31), an unfavorable anatomic outcome occurred in 62.5% of zone I eyes compared to 44.2% of zone II eyes. All unfavorable anatomic outcomes in this cohort from CRYO-ROP occurred in eyes with 6 or more clock hours of stage 3 ROP with plus disease in zones I or II (31).

Predicting Progressive Stage 4 Retinopathy of Prematurity Requiring Surgery

Few studies have provided information regarding risk factors associated with progressive stage 4 ROP requiring surgical intervention. Clinical trials have not been funded to pursue this question. To address this question, we studied features of 72 eyes of 36 infants who had been treated with laser for threshold ROP. Features were abstracted from examinations made 1 week prior to the development of stage 4 ROP that was found to progress over time or 2 weeks after laser in eyes that had regression of threshold ROP. Eyes were stratified into two groups based on whether progressive stage 4 ROP or regressed stage 3 ROP occurred. A generalized estimating equation model was used to account for within-subject variability and determine predictive features of progressive stage 4 ROP. Features assessed included clock hours of ridge elevation, quadrants of plus disease, quadrants of neovascularization, and vitreous state. Ridge elevation was defined as white thickened tissue at the junction of vascularized and avascular retina. Absence of ridge meant that no or only a line denoted the junction. Plus disease was defined as dilated and tortuous retinal arterioles and veins. The presence of only dilated veins in a quadrant was counted as a half quadrant. The vitreous state was defined as hazy, with hemorrhage, or vitreous condensation permitting visualization of the regressed primary vitreous structures. The following features predicted progressive stage 4 ROP: ≥6 clock hours of ridge elevation ($p = 0.0248$), ≥2 quadrants of plus disease ($p = 0.0490$), and vitreous haze ($p = 0.0039$) (33). Neovascularization did not predict progressive stage 4 ROP; however, in a separate analysis, it was associated with a poor surgical outcome (67).

Effects of Environmental Factors and Nonocular Treatments on Retinopathy of Prematurity

Oxygen

The relationship of oxygen to the development of ROP is complex and incompletely understood. Metabolic and oxygen needs increase during the development of the retinal vasculature and the maturation of the neural retina and photoreceptors (68). Early retinal vessels are also sensitive to fluctuations in outside oxygen delivery. A number of factors also affect oxygen delivery to the retinal vasculature and neural retina in the premature infant, including poor blood oxygenation secondary to immature lungs and respiratory disease, anemia of prematurity, and changes in the ratio of fetal to adult hemoglobin affecting oxygen affinity to hemoglobin.

During the 1950s when ROP was initially described, high, unregulated oxygen at the time of birth was found to

TABLE 26–7. RESULTS FROM STOP-ROP STUDY

	Conventional Oxygen (89%–94% SaO$_2$)	Supplemental Oxygen (96%–99% of SaO$_2$)	p Value
Threshold ROP	48%	41%	0.032, NS[a]
Prethreshold without plus	46%	32%	0.004 post-hoc analysis
Prethreshold with plus	52%	57%	0.484 post-hoc analysis
3-mo unfavorable retinal structure (excluding ectopia)	4.4%	4.1%	NS
Macular ectopia at 3 mo	3.9%	3.9%	NS
3- to 6-mo unfavorable retinal structure (excluding ectopia) after treatment for threshold ROP	9.2%	13.2%	NS
Macular ectopia at 3–6 mo	6.3%	7.7%	NS
Pneumonia and/or chronic lung disease exacerbations	8.5%	13.2%	0.066
Infants with baseline lung disease	10.6%	18.7%	0.051
Infants without baseline lung disease	6.5%	6.8%	0.93
Hospitalized at 50 wks PMA	6.8%	12.7%	0.012[b]
On oxygen at 50 wks PMA	37%	46.8%	0.02[b]
On diuretics at 50 wks PMA	24.4%	35.8%	0.002[b]

[a] The target alpha value was 0.025, deliberately conservative to allow for preplanned sequential testing. To balance the benefits and risks of supplemental oxygen, a number-needed-to-treat analysis was performed. This analysis compares the number of infants with prethreshold retinopathy of prematurity (ROP) who would have to be treated with supplemental oxygen to spare an infant from retinal surgery to the number of infants treated with supplemental oxygen to be expected to cause one episode of pulmonary exacerbation. The number requiring supplemental oxygen to prevent an adverse retinal event was 13.2 and to cause a pulmonary exacerbation was 13.7. Pulmonary events were not lethal, although they did prolong hospitalizations (10,82).

[b] The proportion of infants who experienced any one or more of these adverse pulmonary events by 3 months' corrected age was 57% (supplemental) vs. 46% (conventional), $p = 0.005$, and was unaffected after adjusting for baseline covariates of race, ROP severity, gestational age, and pulmonary status.

PMA, postmenstural age (gestational age plus chronologic age in weeks); NS, not significant.

be a significant factor that led to severe ROP (69). Efforts then to reduce oxygen concentration led to reduced blindness but also increased pulmonary and cerebral morbidity. Although today's NICUs provide oxygen in a controlled fashion at lower inspired O_2 than when ROP was first recognized, ROP continues to cause blindness. However, high oxygen, proposed as an important risk factor for ROP in the past (7,69,70), now is no longer an independent risk factor for ROP (71) because oxygen levels are lower and better controlled.

Because of ethical considerations—inability to obtain retinal tissue and to adequately experiment in the human infant—animal models have been created by varying oxygen concentrations to induce retinal avascularity followed by intravitreous neovascularization (see section on Animal Models). Early models of oxygen-induced retinopathy (OIR) and some of the current models exposed animals to constant high oxygen followed by room air to create avascular areas of retina first, and to a variable degree, subsequent intravitreous neovascularization (72–74). These models showed that high concentrations of oxygen led first to large areas of avascular retina, with subsequent development of intravitreous neovascularization, when animals were placed into room air (72). These models were useful in understanding the events of acute ROP in the 1950s but do not describe the oxygen delivery currently used in neonatal care. Later studies showed that retinopathy could be reduced in animals exposed to the conditions described if the animals were rescued with oxygen supplementation (75–77). Based on these findings, a large multicenter clinical trial, STOP-ROP (10), was designed to test supplemental oxygen as a strategy to prevent threshold ROP (Table 26-7). In a *post hoc* analysis, the study showed reduced progression to threshold ROP in a subgroup of infants treated with supplemental oxygen (to achieve SaO_2 of 96%–99%) who had prethreshold ROP without plus disease.

More recently, in current neonatal medical practice, with the aid of transcutaneous oxygen monitoring, studies have found that oxygen variability, even within clinically predetermined acceptable ranges [PaO_2 of 45–75 mmHg (39)], was associated with ROP (40,78). Animals rescued in variable supplemental oxygen (21%–28% O_2) developed more severe intravitreous neovascularization than those rescued in constant supplemental oxygen therapy (79). A recent study reported a lower incidence of threshold ROP in premature infants nursed in slightly lower oxygen saturation levels than that recommended in current guidelines (41). This study also trained the nursing staff to maintain fewer fluctuations in inspired O_2 but did not report on possible associated adverse pulmonary and cerebral events. We speculate that these infants might not have developed as large peripheral avascular areas and therefore were at lower risk of threshold ROP (80). This is based on our recent animal data that oxygen fluctuations around a lower than normal mean oxygen were associated with a reduced peripheral avascular area (81).

These studies demonstrate that the effect of oxygen on the development and progression of ROP is not as straightforward as whether high or low oxygen is delivered to premature infants who develop ROP. Ongoing investigation is necessary to understand the relationships among oxygen concentration, variability and timing of oxygen delivery, and other medical conditions.

Light

Light was proposed as a causative factor in ROP because light leads to a release of free radicals that can cause oxidative damage, death of endothelial cells, and release of angiogenic compounds. Expression of tumor necrosis factor-α and vascular endothelial growth factor (VEGF) during retinal neovascularization can be initiated by lipid hydroperoxides (83). However, the retina is most metabolically active in the dark; thus, the release of oxidative compounds conceivably might be greater than that released when the retina is illuminated. The Light-ROP study (84) (Table 26-1) was designed to test the effect of reduced light to the preterm infant's retinas on the development of ROP. Infants were randomized to either a group in which infants wore goggles that reduced ultraviolet light exposure within 24 hours of birth or a group in which infants did not. There was no evidence that reduced light exposure had an effect on the incidence of ROP or the severity of ROP when it developed (84).

Steroids

Prenatal steroids administered to women in preterm labor have resulted in reduced infant mortality and morbidity, primarily through improved lung function. There is evidence from several small studies that prenatal steroids are protective for the development of ROP (62,85,86). Later administration of steroids, for example, when treating lung disease, has been reported to have an adverse effect (87,88) or no effect (89–91) on the incidence of ROP. Adverse effects appear to be more likely when steroids are given more than 3 weeks postnatally (88) and less likely when used within 2 weeks of birth (89,90).

In a rat model of OIR (see section on Animal Models), an angiostatic steroid, anecortave acetate, believed to prevent endothelial cell migration, greatly reduced intravitreous neovascularization (92) with little to no effect on normal retinal vascular development. Dexamethasone inhibited both normal retinal growth and pathologic intravitreous neovascularization in rabbits (93). Further investigation into possible effects of steroids on ROP is warranted.

Vitamin E

Oxidative stress has been linked to ROP through a number of mechanisms related to oxygen delivery to retinal tissue in the premature infant. The retina is susceptible to oxidative damage because of (i) its abundance of polyunsaturated fatty acids, the double bonds of which are vulnerable to peroxidation reactions (94); (ii) its high metabolic rate and rapid rate of oxygen consumption (95); and (iii) through its vulnerability to light toxicity. In addition, the premature infant has an inability to induce oxidative scavenging mechanisms during times of oxygen stress (96).

A number of early studies tested the use of antioxidants, such as vitamin E, to reduce ROP in infants. A meta-analysis of six of these studies (97) found a 52% overall reduction in the incidence of intravitreous neovascularization in ROP when infants were given vitamin E (Table 26-1). Sepsis or late-onset necrotizing enterocolitis reported in earlier vitamin E studies did not occur in a later study performed by the same group and was attributed to improved immunologic function with ongoing development of the preterm infant (98). Vitamin E therapy has also been reported in association with a greater incidence of intraventricular hemorrhage in the premature infant (99).

Surfactant

Surfactant therapy that has increased survival in very low birth weight premature infants initially appeared to be beneficial in reducing the incidence of ROP (100). However, follow-up studies have failed to confirm this (57,58,101,102). The most recent studies found a reduced incidence of severe ROP in preterm infants treated with surfactant therapy (103); however, these studies used historic controls (104). In a meta-analysis, inositol, an essential nutrient and important in maturation of surfactant, was shown to significantly reduce the incidence of ROP (105).

Carbon Dioxide

Clinical studies that analyzed intermittent blood gas samples found that both hypocarbia (51) and hypercarbia (51,106,107) were associated with the development of ROP. The only study that analyzed continuous transcutaneously monitored CO_2 showed no association between absolute blood CO_2 level or variability and the subsequent development of ROP (108).

The evidence from animal models, however, is unequivocal. Hypercarbia alone (109) and metabolic acidosis (110) have induced retinopathy in rats. When hypercarbia is combined with variable oxygen (109), the severity of disease is increased.

CO_2 affects the retinal vasculature by causing dilatation of vessels in part through relaxation of retinal pericytes (111). With vessel dilatation, oxygenation (112) and blood flow (113) are increased to the retina. The damaging effect of CO_2 in animal models has been speculated to be through increased delivery of oxygen to the retina, followed by a reduced stimulus for the release of hypoxia-induced angiogenic factors, such as VEGF and, in turn, delay retinal vascular development.

A recent small trial in ventilated preterm infants that allowed the level of carbon dioxide to passively rise to between 45 and 55 mmHg $PaCO_2$ showed no difference in the incidence of ROP (114) compared to infants who were ventilated to maintain $PaCO_2$ levels of 35 to 45 mmHg.

Other Risk Factors and Treatments

Other small studies have described additional risk factors for ROP, including intraventricular hemorrhage (115), respiratory distress syndrome, bronchopulmonary dysplasia, and patent ductus arteriosus (62). Bilirubin, through its antioxidant qualities, was proposed as a protective compound against ROP; however, elevated bilirubin was not found to be protective against ROP (116) and was speculated to be a risk factor in one study (117). D-Penicillamine, used to treat hyperbilirubinemia, was found to be associated with reduced ROP. A review of two clinical trials showed a reduced risk of ROP in preterm infants who were treated with D-penicillamine (118). Iron, a known oxidant, has been implicated indirectly through studies of blood transfusions, anemia, and erythropoietin use. Blood transfusions have been associated with increased risk of ROP development (59,119), as has the use of erythropoietin (120). However, anemia has been found to be both slightly protective in one study (121) and associated with ROP in another study (122).

There was no association between mean arterial blood pressure measurement and ROP reported in an observational study that measured minute intraarterial blood pressure in newborn preterms over the first week of life (123).

Several studies have compared the incidence in ROP between twins and singletons and have found no difference in risk once birth weight was taken into account (124,125).

DEVELOPMENT OF RETINAL VASCULATURE INFORMED BY MODELS OF OXYGEN-INDUCED RETINOPATHY

From human examination came the ICROP classification and the observation that the larger the retinal avascular zone in ROP, the greater are the risks of intravitreous neovascularization (8) and its consequences, retinal detachment, and blindness (80). The specific mechanisms leading to ROP in humans remain unknown and are difficult to study in human infants. Investigations into the mechanisms of disease are facilitated through the use of models of OIR (see section on Animal Models).

Normal Retinal Vascular Development

Studies of retinal vascular development have demonstrated that spindle-shaped mesenchymal precursor cells appear around the optic disc region at postnatal day 5 in the cat

(126) and before 15 weeks' gestation in the human (127). These spindle cells migrate toward the ora serrata and cover much of the retina in early development. Astrocytes appear after the spindle cells and by 25 weeks' gestation cover much of the human retina, at which time the spindle cells are virtually nonexistent (127). The spindle cells are reported to aggregate into formations that ultimately define the retinal vasculature. Controversy exists as to whether these spindle cells are (i) precursors to endothelial cells (126,127) or angioblasts; (ii) precursors to astrocytes (128) and, that once differentiated, play an important role in intraretinal endothelial cell migration and angiogenesis; or (iii) an entirely separate population of cells. There also are likely differences among species that must be considered when interpreting the data.

Once early vessels surround the optic nerve, it is agreed that some new vessels sprout from existing vessels through a process of angiogenesis. A proposed theory is that VEGF, an angiogenic factor up-regulated in response to hypoxia (129–132), is necessary for physiologic angiogenesis during retinal vascular development (131) and acts as a survival factor for newly formed vessels (133). Astrocytes sense the physiologic hypoxia (126) in the avascular retinal area [devoid of retinal vasculature and, therefore, hypoxic (134)] and, in response, release VEGF (135), which causes endothelial cell proliferation, migration, and angiogenesis (135). As endothelial cells migrate from existing vessels and develop into intraretinal vessels, the stimulus for continued VEGF up-regulation from hypoxia is relieved locally (135). This angiogenesis is important for continued vascular growth of the inner retinal vascular plexus to the peripheral-most extent of the retina and for the subsequent development of the outer retinal plexus. The reduced hypoxic stimulus to express VEGF in the vascularized retina is also believed to be important in the subsequent remodeling of newly formed vessels through programmed cell death, or apoptosis, of endothelial cells (133). In addition, fluctuations in oxygen have been shown to increase the expression of specific isoforms that may play a role in pathologic intravitreous neovascularization (136). Thus, changes in local tissue oxygen level are believed to be important to normal retinal vascular development through the effect on growth factor expression.

Vascular Endothelial Growth Factor and Intravitreous Neovascularization

In models of OIR, VEGF was also associated with pathologic intravitreous neovascularization (129,137–139). Other growth factors that are angiogenic stimulators also may play a role in ROP. Some of these include hepatocyte growth factor (140), basic fibroblast growth factor (141), and insulin-like growth factor-1 (IGF-1) (142). However, VEGF is recognized as one of the most important factors causing pathologic intravitreous neovascularization in many retinovascular diseases, including ROP, and models of them

(143–145). VEGF is up-regulated by hypoxia (131,132) and reactive oxygen intermediates (146), both of which occur in retinovascular disease (83,145,147). In experimental models, when the action of VEGF was blocked, intravitreous neovascularization was significantly reduced (138,139,148). VEGF mRNA was also expressed in the avascular zone of a human infant eye that had had threshold ROP (149). However, blockade of the actions of VEGF is not likely to be the most effective treatment for ROP. Blocking the effect of VEGF in animal models of ROP led to reduced intravitreous neovascularization and increased areas of avascular retina (138). Thus, although intravitreous neovascularization was prevented, the stimulus to further neovascularization remained. The specific mechanisms of physiologic and pathologic neovascularization require further investigation.

Astrocytes in Retinal Vascular Development and Intravitreous Neovascularization

In feline retina, astrocytes release VEGF and are important for endothelial cell migration within the retina rather than into the vitreous (150). In felines exposed to extreme hyperoxia (70%–80% O_2) for 4 days, astrocyte degeneration occurred upon return to room air and was postulated to result from relative hypoxia (126). In rats raised in 24-hour cycles alternating between hyperoxia (75% O_2) and room air (21% O_2), astrocyte apoptosis occurred in the avascular retina upon return to room air. Some migration of endothelial cells into the vitreous occurred adjacent to areas of degenerated, apoptotic astrocytes (150). Thus, it appeared that intact astrocytes were necessary to contain newly formed retinal vessels within the retina. This has not been proven in human ROP, however. Other cells, including smooth muscle cells and pericytes, also are important in retinal vessel development and maturation.

Animal Models

Animal models permit investigation into retinal vascular development and the proposed causes of ROP because the full-term newborn of many species is born with incompletely vascularized retinas. The most common strategy used to produce a neovascular response (stage 3 ROP) in OIR models is, first, to expose the newborn animal to high constant oxygen for several days and, second, to expose the animal to room air (Table 26-8). Areas of avascular retina develop following hyperoxia and are postulated to be a result of both delayed development and loss of newly developed vessels, sometimes termed *vasoobliteration*. This experimental approach mimicked the conditions of neonatal care in the 1950s when preterm newborns were ventilated in high oxygen immediately upon birth and then weaned back to room air over time. Oxygen conditions used in most models of OIR do not mimic those used in neonatal care today, where

TABLE 26–8. ANIMAL MODELS OF RETINOPATHY OF PREMATURITY (OXYGEN-INDUCED RETINOPATHY)

Species	Insult	Room Air	Neovascularization	Avascularity	Ridge Elevation	Retinal Detachment	Comments	Plus Disease	Regress	Reference No.
Mouse	P7–12 75% O_2	P12–44	Yes in 100% of pups Max at P21	Central	No	No	P7 when hyaloid regressed	No (dilated tortuous vessels at P14	Yes	74
Mouse	P0–P5 90%–95% O_2	Up to P20	Yes in 30%–65% of pups Max at P13–17	Peripheral	No	No	Also hyaloidal proliferation	No	Yes	171
Rat	P0–14 Cycled O_2 50%–10% every 24 h	P14–18	Yes in 100% of pups Max at P18	Peripheral	No	No		No	Yes	152
Rat	P0–11 Cycled O_2 80% for 21 then 21% for 30 min	P11–18	Yes in 94% of pups Max at P18	Peripheral	No	No	Addition of 10% CO_2 to this model results in increased severity of disease (173)	No	Yes	172
Rat	P0–14 80% O_2	Up to P25	No	Some central, but mostly peripheral	No	No		No	Yes	173
Rat	P0–14 Min-by-min fluctuations in O_2 (range 9%–42%	No	No	Peripheral	No	No	Oxygen profile exactly as experienced by a preterm infant that developed severe ROP	No	Yes	151

Rat	P0–7 10% CO_2	Up to P12	Yes in 19% of pups	Peripheral	No	No	Addition of variable oxygen to this model results in increased severity of disease (174)	No	Not reported	109
Rat	P2–7 Twice daily gavage with NH_4Cl	Up to P12	Yes in 36% of pups	Peripheral	No	No	Litter size artificially enlarged to 25 pups	No	Not reported	175
Rat	P2–7 Twice daily gavage with acetazolamide	Up to P12	Yes in 29% of pups	Peripheral	No	No	Litter size artificially enlarged to 25 pups	No	Not reported	110
Cat	P0–4 70%–80% O_2	Up to P88	Yes % of kittens not reported Earliest at P11 Max at P18	Peripheral	No	No	Neovascular vessels were leaky	No	Yes	72, 176
Dog	P0–4 95%–100% O_2	Up to P45	Yes in 100% of pups Earliest was P22	Peripheral	"Ridge" includes astrocytes but is not defined as in humans	Folds	Ongoing neovascular response	Yes	Not at 40 days post-insult	154, 177

oxygen is strictly regulated and infants rarely experience a prolonged period of hyperoxia followed by hypoxia. A rat model of OIR that uses fluctuating oxygen mimicking the extremes and frequency of fluctuations of that of a human preterm infant reported peripheral retinal avascularity and retinal vascular irregularities, although not neovascularization, compared to control (151). When the same extremes in oxygen were used, but the duration of each was extended to alternating cycles of 24-hour hyperoxia followed by hypoxia, the resulting disease was similar to that of human stage 3 ROP (152).

In rodent and cat models of ROP, spontaneous regression of the neovascular response occurs and the retinal vessels assume, at least morphologically, a normal vasculature, although evidence exists that this vasculature does not respond normally to oxygenation (153). No model of OIR has yet produced stage 5 ROP or total retinal detachment, the most severe form in human infants. The closest has been achieved in the beagle puppy, in which there is a prolonged neovascular response compared to other animal models and retinal folds have been reported at age 45 days (154).

GENETICS

The similarities between Norrie disease, X-linked FEVR (see Chapter 28), and the retinal vascular changes seen in ROP led to an investigation of the Norrie disease gene mutations in infants with severe ROP (155). The Norrie gene product (156) is believed to be important in providing recognition signals for neuronal and retinal connections and angiogenesis during retinal development (155). Transgenic mice failing to produce the protein, normally found in the inner retina, cerebellum, and olfactory epithelium (157), undergo abnormal retinal development from focal disorganization in only one layer of the retina to a complete loss of cells in all layers. In addition, there are abnormalities in the retinal vasculature with persistence of the hyaloid artery (158), suggesting that this gene may be necessary for the regulation of retinal vascular development. Finally, the animals have an attenuated b-wave (157), suggesting a defect in the inner retinal layers. In a study of 12 infants (including monozygotic twins), 4 had mutations in the translated region of the third exon of the Norrie gene. Another large study reported that the prevalence of Norrie disease gene defects in children with severe ROP was 3%, compared to zero in controls (159). However, a further study of 118 individuals [87 preterm infants of whom 57 had severe ROP (15 prethreshold, 33 threshold, 1 stage 4B, and 3 stage 5 ROP) and 31 parents] failed to show polymorphisms in the translated part of the Norrie disease gene. Five polymorphisms were reported in the nontranslated portion of the gene. This study did not support the association between the Norrie disease gene and severe ROP (160). More work clearly is needed to define the role of genetic mutations.

FUTURE TREATMENTS BASED ON RESEARCH

Two small studies that measured levels of circulating IGF-1 in preterm infants found that infants with low IGF-1 had delayed physical growth (161) and were more likely to develop ROP (162,163). IGF-1 also has been shown to be important in the development of the normal retinal vasculature (164) and acts synergistically with VEGF to increase VEGF signaling (165). Therefore, low IGF-1 may result in arrested retinal vessel development in preterm infants. Because the size of the avascular area of the retina is directly related to the development of ROP (80), there has been interest in supplementing infants who have low endogenous IGF-1 with IGF-1 in order to reduce ROP. However, there is concern that supplementation with IGF-1, a growth factor that enhances the signaling capabilities of VEGF, might also increase the neovascular pathology associated with VEGF (145). Therefore, the timing and administration of such a treatment needs to be investigated carefully.

The administration of anti-VEGF or anti-VEGF receptor therapies is unlikely to be risk-free. Animal studies in which these treatments were used to treat OIR (139,166) have reported varying degrees of success (138). However, VEGF is critical for normal retinal vascularization (168) and endothelial cell survival (133), findings suggesting that blocking VEGF without understanding its properties and time of action during development is unlikely to be without side effects.

Placental growth factor-1, which only binds VEGF receptor 1 (VEGFR1), decreased hyperoxia induced retinal vasoobliteration and resulted in less intravitreous neovascularization in a mouse model of OIR (169). This suggests that preferential stimulation of specific receptors of VEGF may provide a means to target unwanted intravitreous neovascularization and still promote normal retinal vascular development.

Retrospective studies have supported managing of infants in lower levels of oxygen (170) or with reduced variability in oxygen (40). Both of these parameters were tested in a small clinical trial with excellent results (41) and low pulmonary or neurologic sequelae, supporting plans to develop a multicenter trial. However, although these studies may reduce the incidence of ROP, long-term follow-up is essential to determine possible future morbidity from pulmonary and neurologic problems associated with managing infants in lower oxygen. Future studies will test low oxygen saturations from shortly after birth up to 32 weeks' PMA and its effect on the development of prethreshold ROP.

Surgery for stage 4 ROP has led to improved visual (46) and anatomic (67) outcomes. Several technical advances have made it possible to intervene early in the small eye of the premature infant and include: (i) two-port vitrectomy using illuminated infusing cannulas and instruments, (ii) small incision surgery using 25-gauge instruments, and (iii) future development of enzymatic vitreolysis to relieve vitreous traction especially at the vitreoretinal interface. Although advancements in surgery are essential for certain stages of ROP, future hope rests in a better understanding of the molecular mechanisms of ROP that would lead to prevention.

REFERENCES

1. NEI Press Statement. National Eye Institute, 2-7-2000. May 21, 2003.
2. Phelps DL. Retinopathy of prematurity: an estimate of vision loss in the United States—1979. *Pediatrics* 1981;67:924–925.
3. Allen MB, Donohue PK, Dusman AE. The limit of viability—neonatal outcome of infants born at 22 to 25 weeks' gestation. *N Engl J Med* 1993;329:1597–1601.
4. Javitt JJ, Dei, Cas R, et al. Cost-effectiveness of screening and cryotherapy for threshold retinopathy of prematurity. *Pediatrics* 1993;91:859–866.
5. Brown GC, Brown MM, Sharma S, et al. Cost-effectiveness of treatment of threshold retinopathy of prematurity. *Pediatrics* 1999;104:e47.
6. Terry TL. Extreme prematurity and fibroblastic overgrowth of persistent vascular sheath behind each crystalline lens: (1) preliminary report. *Am J Ophthalmol* 1942;25:203–204.
7. Campbell K. Intensive oxygen therapy as a possible cause of retrolental fibroplasia. A clinical approach. *Med J Aust* 1951;2:48.
8. The Committee for the Classification of Retinopathy of Prematurity. An international classification of retinopathy of prematurity. *Arch Ophthalmol* 1984;102:1130–1134.
9. Cryotherapy for Retinopathy of Prematurity Cooperative Group. Multicentre trial of cryotherapy for retinopathy of prematurity. Preliminary results. *Arch Ophthalmol* 1988;106:471–479.
10. The STOP-ROP Multicenter Study Group. Supplemental Therapeutic Oxygen for Prethreshold Retinopathy of Prematurity (STOP-ROP), a randomized, controlled trial. I: primary outcomes. *Pediatrics* 2000;105:295–310.
11. McGregor ML, Bremer DL, Cole C, et al. Retinopathy of prematurity outcome in infants with prethreshold retinopathy of prematurity and oxygen saturation >94% in room air: the High Oxygen Percentage in Retinopathy of Prematurity Study. *Pediatrics* 2002;110:540–544.
12. Palmer EA, Flynn JT, Hardy RJ, et al. Incidence and early course of retinopathy of prematurity. *Ophthalmology* 1991;98:1628–1640.
13. Reynolds JD, Dobson V, Quinn GE, et al. CRYO-ROP and LIGHT-ROP Cooperative Study Groups. Evidence-based screening criteria for retinopathy of prematurity: natural history data from the CRYO-ROP and LIGHT-ROP Studies. *Arch Ophthalmol* 2002;120:1470–1476.
14. Schaffer DB, Palmer EA, Plotsky DF, et al. Prognostic factors in the natural course of retinopathy of prematurity. *Ophthalmology* 1993;100:230–237.
15. Early Treatment for Retinopathy of Prematurity Cooperative Group. Revised indications for the treatment of retinopathy of prematurity: results of the Early Treatment for Retinopathy of Prematurity Randomized Trial. *Arch Ophthalmol* 2003;121:1684–1694.
16. Hardy RJ, Palmer EA, Schaffer DB, et al. Outcome-based management of retinopathy of prematurity. Multicenter Trial of Cryotherapy for Retinopathy of Prematurity Cooperative Group. *JAAPOS* 1997;1:46–54.
17. Cryotherapy for Retinopathy of Prematurity Cooperative Group.
18. Cryotherapy for Retinopathy of Prematurity Cooperative Group. Multicenter Trial of Cryotherapy for Retinopathy of Prematurity ophthalmological outcomes at 10 years. *Arch Ophthalmol* 2001;119:1110–1118.
19. Fielder AR. Preliminary results of treatment of eyes with high-risk prethreshold retinopathy of prematurity in the Early Treatment for Retinopathy of Prematurity Randomized Trial. *Arch Ophthalmol* 2003;121:1769–1771.
20. Cryotherapy for Retinopathy of Prematurity Cooperative Group. Multicenter Trial of Cryotherapy for Retinopathy of Prematurity: one-year outcome - structure and function. *Arch Ophthalmol* 1990;108:1408–1416.
21. Cryotherapy for Retinopathy of Prematurity Cooperative Group. Multicenter Trial of Cryotherapy for Retinopathy of Prematurity: three and a half year outcome-structure and function. *Arch Ophthalmol* 1993;111:339–344.
22. Cryotherapy for Retinopathy of Prematurity Cooperative Group. Multicenter Trial of Cryotherapy for Retinopathy of Prematurity: Snellen visual acuity and structural outcome at 51/2 years after randomization. *Arch Ophthalmol* 1996;114: 417–424.
23. Cryotherapy for Retinopathy of Prematurity Cooperative Group. Contrast sensitivity at age 10 years in children who had threshold retinopathy of prematurity. *Arch Ophthalmol* 2001;119:1129–1133.
24. Repka MX, Summers CG, Palmer EA, et al. The incidence of ophthalmologic interventions in children with birth weights less than 1251 grams. Results through 5 1/2 years. Cryotherapy for Retinopathy of Prematurity Cooperative Group. *Ophthalmology* 1998;105:1621–1627.
25. Quinn GE, Dobson V, Kivlin J, et al. Prevalence of myopia between 3 months and 5 1/2 years in preterm infants with and without retinopathy of prematurity. *Ophthalmology* 1998;105:1292–1300.
26. Quinn GE, Dobson V, Hardy RJ, et al. Visual fields measured with double-arc perimetry in eyes with threshold retinopathy of prematurity from the Cryotherapy for Retinopathy of Prematurity Trial. *Ophthalmology* 1996;103:1432–1437.
27. Repka MX, Palmer EA, Tung B. Involution of retinopathy of prematurity. *Arch Ophthalmol* 2000;118:645–649.
28. Msall ME, Phelps DL, GiGaudio KM, et al. Severity of neonatal retinopathy of prematurity is predictive of neurodevelopmental functional outcome at age 5.5 years. *Pediatrics* 2000;106:998–1005.
29. Dobson V, Quinn GE, Abramov I, et al. Color vision measured with pseudoisochromatic plates at five-and-a-half years in eyes of children from the CRYO-ROP study. *Invest Ophthalmol Vis Sci* 1996;37:2467–2474.
30. Saunders RA, Donahue ML, Christmann LM, et al. Racial variation in retinopathy of prematurity. The Cryotherapy for Retinopathy of Prematurity Cooperative Group. *Arch Ophthalmol* 1997;115:604–608.
31. Cryotherapy for Retinopathy of Prematurity Cooperative Group. Multicenter Trial of Cryotherapy for Retinopathy of Prematurity: natural history ROP: ocular outcome at 5(1/2) years in premature infants with birth weights less than 1251g. *Arch Ophthalmol* 2002;120:595–599.
32. Hardy RJ, Palmer EA, Dobson V, et al. Risk analysis of prethreshold retinopathy of prematurity. *Arch Ophthalmol* 2003;121:1697–1701.
33. Hartnett ME, McColm JR. Retinal features predictive of progression to stage 4 ROP. *Retina* 2004;24:237–241.
34. Ng EY, Connolly BP, McNamara JA, et al. A comparison of laser photocoagulation with cryotherapy for threshold retinopathy of

prematurity at 10 years: part 1. Visual function and structural outcome. *Ophthalmology* 2002;109:928–934.

35. Vintzileos AM, Ananth CV, Smulian JC, et al. The impact of pre-natal care in the United States on preterm births in the presence and absence of antenatal high-risk conditions. *Am J Obstet Gynecol* 2002;187:1254–1257.

36. Akinbami LJ, Schoendorf KC, Kiely JL. Risk of preterm birth in multiparous teenagers. *Arch Pediatr Adolesc Med* 2000; 154:1101–1107.

37. Datta-Bhutada S, Johnson HL, Rosen TS. Intrauterine cocaine and crack exposure: neonatal outcome. *J Perinatol* 1998;18: 183–188.

38. Connolly BP, Ng EY, McNamara JA, et al. A comparison of laser photocoagulation with cryotherapy for threshold retinopathy of prematurity at 10 years: part 2. Refractive outcome. *Ophthalmology* 2002;109:936–941.

39. Fetus and Newborn Committee of the AAP. Clinical considerations in the use of oxygen. In: Freeman RK, Poland RL, Hauth JC, et al., eds. *Guidelines for perinatal care.* Elk Grove Village, IL: American Academy of Pediatrics and American College of Obstetricians and Gynecologists, 2002: Chapter 8.

40. Cunningham S, Fleck BW, Elton RA et al. Transcutaneous oxygen levels in retinopathy of prematurity. *Lancet* 1995;346: 1464–1465.

41. Chow LC, Wright KW, Sola A. Can changes in clinical practice decrease the incidence of severe retinopathy of prematurity in very low birth weight infants? *Pediatrics* 2003;111:339–345.

42. Greven CM, Tasman W. Rhegmatogenous retinal detachment following cryotherapy in retinopathy of prematurity. *Arch Ophthalmol* 1989;107:1017–1018.

43. Chow DR, Ferrone PJ, Trese MT. Refractive changes associated with scleral buckling and division in retinopathy of prematurity. *Arch Ophthalmol* 1998;116:1446–1448.

44. Choi MY, Park IK, Yu YS. Long term refractive outcome in eyes of preterm infants with and without retinopathy of prematurity: comparison of keratometric value, axial length, anterior chamber depth, and lens thickness. *Br J Ophthalmol* 2000;84:138–143.

45. Reynolds J, Dobson V, Quinn GE, et al. Prediction of visual function in eyes with mild to moderate posterior pole residua of retinopathy of prematurity. *Arch Ophthalmol* 1993;111:1050–1056.

46. Hartnett ME, Rodier DW, McColm JR, et al Long-term vision results measured with teller acuity cards and a new light perception projection scale after management of late stages of retinopathy of prematurity. *Arch Ophthalmol* 2003;121:991–996.

47. Capone A, Trese MT. Lens-sparing vitreous surgery for tractional stage 4A retinopathy of prematurity retinal detachments. *Ophthalmology* 2001;108:2068–2070.

48. Maguire AM, Trese MT. Visual results of lens-sparing vitreoretinal surgery in infants. *J Pediatr Ophthalmol Strabismus* 1993; 30:28–32.

49. Seaber JH, Machemer R, Eliott D, et al. Long-term visual results of children after initially successful vitrectomy for stage V retinopathy of prematurity. *Ophthalmology* 1995;102:199–204.

50. Campbell PB, Bull MJ, Ellis FD, et al. Incidence of retinopathy of prematurity in a tertiary newborn intensive care unit. *Arch Ophthalmol* 1983;101:1686–1688.

51. Shohat M, Reisner SH, Krikler R, et al. Retinopathy of prematurity: incidence and risk factors. *Pediatrics* 1983;72:159–163.

52. Hammer ME, Mullen PW, Ferguson JG, et al. Logistic analysis of risk factors in acute retinopathy of prematurity. *Am J Ophthalmol* 1986;102:1–6.

53. Ng YK, Fielder AR, Shaw DE, et al. Epidemiology of retinopathy of prematurity. *Lancet* 1988;1235–1238.

54. Prendiville A, Schulenburg WE. Clinical factors associated with retinopathy of prematurity. *Arch Dis Child* 1988;63:522–527.

55. Batton DG, Roberts C, Trese M, et al. Severe retinopathy of prematurity and steroid exposure. *Pediatrics* 1992;90:534–536.

56. Flynn JT, Bancalari E, Snyder ES, et al. A cohort study of transcutaneous oxygen tension and the incidence and severity of retinopathy of prematurity. *N Engl J Med* 1992;326:1050–1054.

57. Rankin SJ, Tubman TRJ, Halliday HL, et al. Retinopathy of prematurity in surfactant treated infants. *Br J Ophthalmol* 1992;76:202–204.

58. Repka MX, Hardy RJ, Phelps DL, et al. Surfactant prophylaxis and retinopathy of prematurity. *Arch Ophthalmol* 1993;111:618–620.

59. Cooke RWI, Clark D, Hickey-Dwyer M, et al. The apparent role of blood transfusions in the development of retinopathy of prematurity. *Eur J Pediatr* 1993;152:833–836.

60. Fleck BW, Wright E, Dhillon B, et al. An audit of the 1995 Royal College of Ophthalmologists guidelines for screening for retinopathy of prematurity applied retrospectively in one regional neonatal intensive care unit. *Eye* 1995;9[6 Suppl]:31–35.

61. Hesse L, Eberl W, Schlaud M, et al. Blood transfusion. Iron load and retinopathy of prematurity. *Eur J Pediatr* 1997;156:465–470.

62. Higgins RD, Mendelsohn AL, DeFeo MJ, et al. Antenatal dexamethasone and decreased severity of retinopathy of prematurity. *Arch Ophthalmol* 1998;116:601–605.

63. Costeloe KL, Hennessy E, Gibson AT, et al. The EPICure study: outcomes to discharge from hospital for infants born at the threshold of viability. *Pediatrics* 2000;106:659–671.

64. Kivlin JD, Biglan AW, Gordon RA, et al. Early retinal vessel development and iris vessel dilatation as factors in retinopathy of prematurity. *Arch Ophthalmol* 1996;114:150–154.

65. Arnold RW, Kesler K, Avila E. Susceptibility to retinopathy of prematurity in Alaskan Natives. *J Pediatr Ophthalmol Strabismus* 1994;31:192–194.

66. Gao G, Li Y, Fant J, et al. Difference in ischemic regulation of vascular endothelial growth factor and pigment epithelium-derived factor in Brown Norway and Sprague Dawley rats contributing to different susceptibilities to retinal neovascularization. *Diabetes* 2002;51:1218–1226.

67. Hartnett ME. Features associated with surgical outcome in patients with stages 4 and 5 retinopathy of prematurity. *Retina* 2003;23:322–329.

68. Weiter JJ, Zuckerman R, Schepens CL. A model for the pathogenesis of retrolental fibroplasias based on the metabolic control of blood vessel development. *Ophthalmic Surg* 1981;13: 1013–1017.

69. Kinsey VE. Cooperative study of retrolental fibroplasia and the use of oxygen. *Arch Ophthalmol* 1956;56:481–543.

70. Patz A. The role of oxygen in retrolental fibroplasia. *Am J Ophthalmol* 1982;94:715–743.

71. Gallo JE, Jacobsen L, Broberger U. Perinatal factors associated with retinopathy of prematurity. *Acta Paediatr* 1993;82: 829–834.

72. Ashton N, Ward B, Serpell G. Effect of oxygen on developing retinal vessels with particular reference to the problem of retrolental fibroplasia. *Br J Ophthalmol* 1954;38:397–430.

73. Patz A, Eastham A, Higginbotham DH, et al. Oxygen studies in retrolental fibroplasia. *Am J Ophthalmol* 1953;36:1511–1522.

74. Smith LEH, Wesolowski E, McLellan A, et al. Oxygen induced retinopathy in the mouse. *Invest Ophthalmol Vis Sci* 1994;35: 101–111.

75. Phelps DL, Rosenbaum AL. Effects of marginal hypoxemia on recovery from oxygen induced retinopathy in the kitten model. *Pediatrics* 1984;73:731–736.

76. Phelps DL. Reduced severity of oxygen-induced retinopathy in kittens recovered in 28% oxygen. *Pediatr Res* 1988;24:106–109.

77. Chan-Ling T, Gock B, Stone J. Supplemental oxygen therapy: basis for noninvasive treatment of retinopathy of prematurity. *Invest Ophthalmol Vis Sci* 1995;36:1215–1230.

78. Saito Y, Omoto T, Cho Y, et al. The progression of retinopathy of prematurity and fluctuation in blood gas tension. *Graefes Arch Clin Exp Ophthalmol* 1993;231:151–156.

79. Berkowitz BA, Berlin ES, Zhang W. Variable supplemental oxygen during recovery does not reduce retinal neovascular severity in experimental ROP. *Curr Eye Re*s 2001;22:401–404.

80. Flynn JT. Retinopathy of prematurity. *Pediatr Clin North Am* 1987;34:1487–1516.

81. McColm JR, Cunningham S, Wade J, et al. Hypoxic oxygen fluctuations produce less severe retinopathy than hyperoxic fluctuations in a rat model of retinopathy of prematurity. *Pediatr Res* 2004;55:1-7–113.

82. Hay WW, Bell EF. Oxygen therapy, oxygen toxicity and the STOP-ROP trial. *Pediatrics* 2000;105:424–425.

83. Armstrong D, Ueda T, Ueda T, et al. Expression of TNF-alpha and VEGF during retinal neovascularization is initiated by lipid hydroperoxide. *Angiogenesi*s 1997;2:174–184.

84. Reynolds JD, Hardy RJ, Kennedy KA, et al. Lack of efficacy of light reduction in preventing retinopathy of prematurity. *N Engl J Med* 1998;338:1572–1576.

85. Console V, Gagliardi L, De Giorgi A, et al. Retinopathy of prematurity and antenatal corticosteroids. The Italian ROP Study Group. *Acta Bio-Med Ateneo Parmense* 1997;68[Suppl 1]: 75–79.

86. Rowlands E, Ionides ACW, Chinn S, et al. Reduced incidence of retinopathy of prematurity. *Br J Ophthalmol* 2001;85:933–935.

87. Haroon PM, Dhanireddy R. Association of postnatal dexamethasone use and fungal sepsis in the development of severe retinopathy of prematurity and progression to laser therapy in extremely low-birth-weight infants. *J Perinatol* 2001;21: 242–247.

88. Halliday HL, Ehrenkranz RA. Delayed (>3 weeks) postnatal corticosteroids for chronic lung disease in preterm infants (Cochrane Review). *Cochrane Database Syst Rev* 2003;2:CD001145.

89. Halliday HL, Ehrenkranz RA. Early postnatal (<96 hours) corticosteroids for preventing chronic lung disease in preterm infants (Cochrane Review). *Cochrane Database Syst Rev* 2003;1: CD001146.

90. Halliday HL, Ehrenkranz RA. Moderately early (7–14 days) postnatal corticosteroids for preventing chronic lung disease in preterm infants (Cochrane Review). *Cochrane Database Syst Rev* 2001;1:CD001144.

91. Cuculich PS, DeLozier KA, Mellen BG, et al. Postnatal dexamethasone treatment and retinopathy of prematurity in very-low-birth-weight neonates. *Biol Neonate* 2001;79:9–14.

92. Penn JS, Rajaratnam VS, Collier RJ, et al. The effect of an angiostatic steroid on neovascularization in a rat model of retinopathy of prematurity. *Invest Ophthalmol Vis Sci* 2001;42:283–290.

93. Lawas-Alejo PA, Slivka S, Hernandez H, et al. Hyperoxia and glucocorticoid modify retinal vessel growth and interleukin-1 receptor antagonist in newborn rabbits. *Pediatr Res* 1999;45: 313–317.

94. Daemen FJM. Vertebrate rod outer segment membranes. *Biochim Biophys Acta* 1973;300:255.

95. Rodieck W. Structure of the retinal epithelium and receptor inner segments. In: Rodieck W, ed. *The vertebrate retina: Principles of structure and function.* WH Freeman and Company, San Francisco: 1973:159.

96. Askikainen TM, Heikkilä P, Kaarteenaho-Wiik R, et al. Cell-specific expression of manganese superoxide dismutase protein in the lungs of patients with respiratory distress syndrome, chronic lung disease, or persistent pulmonary hypertension. *Pediatr Pulmonol* 2001;32:193–200.

97. Raju TNK, Langenberg P, Bhutani V, et al. Vitamin E prophylaxis to reduce retinopathy of prematurity: a reappraisal of published trials. *J Pediatr* 1997;131:844–850.

98. Johnson L, Quinn GE, Abbasi S, et al. Severe retinopathy of prematurity in infants with birth weights less than 1250 grams: incidence and outcome of treatment with pharmacologic serum levels of vitamin E in addition to cryotherapy from 1985 to 1991. *J Pediatr* 1995;127:632–639.

99. Phelps DL, Rosenbaum AL, Isenberg SJ, et al. Tocopherol efficacy and safety for preventing retinopathy of prematurity: a randomized, controlled, double-masked trial. *Pediatrics* 1987;79: 489–500.

100. Repka MX, Hudak ML, Parsa CF, et al. Calf lung surfactant extract prophylaxis and retinopathy of prematurity. *Ophthalmology* 1992;99:531–536.

101. Holmes JM, Cronin CM, Squires P, et al. Randomized clinical trial of surfactant prophylaxis in retinopathy of prematurity. *J Pediatr Ophthalmol Strabismus* 1994;31:189–191.

102. Pennefather PM, Tin W, Clarke MP, et al. Retinopathy of prematurity in a controlled trial of prophylactic surfactant treatment. *Br J Ophthalmol* 1996;80:420–424.

103. Termote J, Schalij-Delfos NE, Cats BP, et al. Less severe retinopathy of prematurity induced by surfactant replacement therapy. *Acta Paediatr* 1996;85:1491–1496.

104. Termote J, Schalij-Delfos NE, Brouwers HAA, et al. New developments in neonatology: less severe retinopathy of prematurity? *J Pediatr Ophthalmol Strabismus* 2000;37:142–148.

105. Howlett A, Ohlsson A. Inositol for respiratory distress syndrome in preterm infants. *Cochrane Database Syst Rev* 2000;4: CD000366.

106. Tsuchiya S, Tsuyama K. Retinopathy of prematurity birth weight, gestational age and maximum PaCO$_2$. *Tokai J Exp Clin Med* 1987;12:39–42.

107. Brown DR, Milley JR, Ripepi UJ, et al. Retinopathy of prematurity. Risk factors in a five-year cohort of critically ill premature neonates. *Am J Dis Child* 1987;141:154–160.

108. Gellen B, McIntosh N, McColm JR, et al. Is the partial pressure of carbon dioxide in the blood related to the development of retinopathy of prematurity? *Br J Ophthalmol* 2001;85: 1044–1045.

109. Holmes JM, Zhang S, Leske DA, et al. Carbon-dioxide induced retinopathy in the neonatal rat. *Curr Eye Res* 1998;17:608–616.

110. Zhang S, Leske DA, Lanier WL, et al. Preretinal neovascularization associated with acetazolamide-induced systemic acidosis in the neonatal rat. *Invest Ophthalmol Vis Sci* 2001;42:1066–1071.

111. Chen Q, Anderson DR. Effect of CO$_2$ on intracellular pH and contraction of retinal capillary pericytes. *Invest Ophthalmol Vis Sci* 1997;38:643–645.

112. Berkowitz BA. Adult and newborn rat inner retinal oxygenation during carbogen and 100% oxygen breathing. *Invest Ophthalmol Vis Sc*i 1996;37:2089–2098.

113. Stiris T, Odden J-P, Hansen TWR, et al. The effect of arterial PCO$_2$—variations on ocular and cerebral blood flow in the newborn piglet. *Pediatr Res* 1989;25:205–208.

114. Mariani G, Cifuentes J, Carlo WA. Randomised trial of permissive hypercapnia in preterm infants. *Pediatrics* 1999;104: 1082–1088.

115. Brown DR, Biglan AW. Retinopathy of prematurity: the relationship with intraventricular hemorrhage and bronchopulmonary dysplasia. *J Pediatr Ophthalmol Strabismus* 1990;27:268–271.

116. DeJonge MH, Khuntia A, Maisels MJ, et al. Bilirubin levels and severe retinopathy of prematurity in infants with estimated gestational ages of 23 to 26 weeks. *J Pediatr* 1999;135:102–104.

117. Milner JD, Aly HZ, Ward LB, et al. Does elevated peak bilirubin protect from retinopathy of prematurity in very low birth-weight infants. *J Perinatol* 2003;23:208–211.

118. Phelps DL, Lakatos L, Watts JL. D-Penicillamine for preventing retinopathy of prematurity in preterm infants (Cochrane Review). *Cochrane Database Syst Rev* 2001;1:CD001073.

119. Dani C, Reali MF, Bertini G, et al. The role of blood transfusions and iron intake on retinopathy of prematurity. *Early Hum Dev* 2001;62:57–63.

120. Romagnoli C, Zecca E, Gallini F, et al. Do recombinant human erythropoietin and iron supplementation increase the risk of retinopathy of prematurity? *Eur J Pediatr* 2000;159:627–628.

121. Englert JA, Saunders RA, Purohit DM, et al. The effect of anemia on retinopathy of prematurity in extremely low birth weight infants. *J Perinatol* 2001;21:21–26.

122. Rekha S, Battu RR. Retinopathy of prematurity: incidence and risk factors. *Ind Pediatr* 1996;33:999–1003.

123. Cunningham S, Symon AG, Elton RA, et al. Intra-arterial blood pressure reference ranges, death and morbidity in very low birth-weight infants during the first seven days of life. *Early Hum Dev* 1999;56:151–165.

124. Friling R, Rosen SD, Monos T, et al. Retinopathy of prematurity in multiple-gestation, very low birth weight infants. *J Pediatr Ophthalmol Strabismus* 1997;34:96–100.

125. Brown BA, Thack AB, Song JC, et al. Retinopathy of prematurity: evaluation of risk factors. *Int Ophthalmol* 1998;22:279–283.

126. Chan-Ling T, Gock B, Stone J. The effect of oxygen on vasoformative cell division: Evidence that 'physiological hypoxia' is the stimulus for normal retinal vasculogenesis. *Invest Ophthalmol Vis Sci* 1995;36:1201–1214.

127. Hughes S, Yang H, Chan-Ling T. Vascularisation of the human fetal retina: roles of vasculogenesis and angiogenesis. *Invest Ophthalmol Vis Sci* 2000;41:1217–1228.

128. Fruttiger M. Development of the mouse retinal vasculature: angiogenesis versus vasculogenesis. *Invest Ophthalmol Vis Sci* 2002;43:522–527.

129. Pierce EA, Avery RL, Foley ED, et al. Vascular endothelial growth factor/vascular permeability factor expression in a mouse model of retinal neovascularization. *Proc Natl Acad Sci U S A* 1995;92:905–909.

130. Shweiki D, Itin A, Soffer D, et al. Vascular endothelial growth factor induced by hypoxia may mediate hypoxia-initiated angiogenesis. *Nature* 1992;359:843–845.

131. Klagsbrun M, D'Amore PA. Regulators of angiogenesis. *Annu Rev Physiol* 1991;53:217–239.

132. Forsythe JA, Jiang BH, Iyer NV, et al. Activation of vascular endothelial growth factor gene transcription by hypoxia-inducible factor 1. *Mol Cell Biol* 1996;16:4604–4613.

133. Alon T, Hemo I, Itin A, et al. Vascular endothelial growth factor acts as a survival factor for newly formed retinal vessels and has implications for retinopathy of prematurity. *Nat Med* 1995;1:1024–1028.

134. Ernest JT, Goldstick TK. Retinal oxygen tension and oxygen reactivity in retinopathy of prematurity in kittens. *Invest Ophthalmol Vis Sci* 1984;25:1129–1134.

135. Stone J, Itin A, Alon T, et al. Development of retinal vasculature is mediated by hypoxia-induced vascular endothelial growth factor (VEGF) expression by neuroglia. *J Neurosci* 1995;15:4738–4747.

136. McColm JR, Geisen P, Hartnett ME. VEGF isoforms and their expression after a single episode of hypoxia or repeated fluctuations between hyperoxia and hypoxia: relevance to clinical ROP. *Mol Vis* 2004;10:512–520.

137. Dorey CK, Aouididi S, Reynaud X, et al. Correlation of vascular permeability factor/vascular endothelial growth factor with extraretinal neovascularization in the rat. *Arch Ophthalmol* 1996;114:1210–1217.

138. McLeod DS, Taomoto M, Cao J, et al. Localization of VEGF receptor-2 (KDR/Flk-1) and effects of blocking it in oxygen-induced retinopathy. *Invest Ophthalmol Vis Sci* 2002;43:474–482.

139. Robinson GS, Pierce EA, Rook SL, et al. Oligodeoxynucleotides inhibit retinal neovascularization in a murine model of proliferative retinopathy. *Proc Natl Acad Sci U S A* 1996;93:4851–4856.

140. Gille J, Khalik M, König V, et al. Hepatocyte growth factor/scatter factor (HGF/SF) induces vascular permeability factor (VPF/VEGF) expression by cultured keratinocytes. *J Invest Dermatol* 1998;111:1160–1165.

141. Seghezzi G, Patel S, Ren CJ, et al. Fibroblast growth factor-2 (FGF-2) induces vascular endothelial growth factor (VEGF) expression in the endothelial cells of forming capillaries: an autocrine mechanism contributing to angiogenesis. *J Cell Biol* 1998;141:1659–1673.

142. Smith LEH, Kopchick JJ, Chen W, et al. Essential role of growth hormone in ischemia-induced retinal neovascularization. *Science* 1997;276:1706–1709.

143. Miller JW, Adamis AP, Shima DT, et al. Vascular endothelial growth factor/vascular permeability factor is temporally and spatially correlated with ocular angiogenesis in a primate model. *Am J Pathol* 1994;145:574–584.

144. Tolentino MJ, Miller JW, Gragoudas ES, et al. Intravitreous injections of vascular endothelial growth factor produce retinal ischemia and microangiopathy in an adult primate. *Ophthalmology* 1996;103:1820–1828.

145. Aiello LP, Avery RL, Arrigg PG, et al. Vascular endothelial growth factor in ocular fluid of patients with diabetic retinopathy and other retinal disorders. *N Engl J Med* 1994;331:1480–1487.

146. Kuroki M, Voest E, Amano S, et al. Reactive oxygen intermediates increase vascular endothelial growth factor expression *in vitro* and *in vivo*. *J Clin Invest* 1996;98:1667–1675.

147. Penn JS. Oxygen-induced retinopathy in the rat: possible contribution of peroxidation reactions. *Doc Ophthalmol* 1990;74:179–186.

148. Bainbridge JWB, Mistry A, De Alwis M, et al. Inhibition of retinal neovascularization by gene transfer of soluble VEGF receptor sFLT-1. *Gene Ther* 2002;9:320–326.

149. Young TL, Anthony DC, Pierce E, et al. Histopathology and vascular endothelial growth factor in untreated and diode laser-treated retinopathy of prematurity. *JAAPOS* 1997;1:105–110.

150. Zhang Y, Stone J. Role of astrocytes in the control of developing retinal vessels. *Invest Ophthalmol Vis Sci* 1997;38:1653–1666.

151. Cunningham S, McColm JR, Wade J, et al. A novel model of retinopathy of prematurity simulating preterm oxygen variability in the rat. *Invest Ophthalmol Vis Sci* 2000;41:4275–4280.

152. Penn JS, Henry MM, Wall PT, et al. The range of PaO2 variation determines the severity of oxygen induced retinopathy in newborn rats. *Invest Ophthalmol Vis Sci* 1995;36:2063–2070.

153. Berkowitz BA, Penn JS. Abnormal panretinal response pattern to carbogen inhalation in experimental retinopathy of prematurity. *Invest Ophthalmol Vis Sci* 1998;39:840–845.

154. McLeod DS, D'Anna SA, Lutty GA. Clinical and histopathologic features of canine oxygen-induced proliferative retinopathy. *Invest Ophthalmol Vis Sci* 1998;39:1918–1932.

155. Shastry BS, Pendergast SD, Hartzer MK, et al. Identification of missense mutations in the Norrie disease gene associated with advanced retinopathy of prematurity. *Arch Ophthalmol* 1997;115:651–655.

156. Meindl A, Berger W, Meitinger T, et al. Norrie disease is caused by mutations in an extracellular protein resembling C-terminal globular domain of mucins. *Nat Genet* 1992;2:139–143.

157. Berger W. Molecular dissection of Norrie disease. *Acta Anat* 1998;162:95–100.

158. Richter M, Gottanka J, May CA. Retinal vasculature changes

in Norrie Disease mice. *Invest Ophthalmol Vis Sci* 2003;39: 2450–2457.

159. Hiraoka M, Berinstein DM, Trese MT, et al. Insertion and deletion mutations in the dinucleotide repeat region of the Norrie disease gene in patients with advanced retinopathy of prematurity. *J Hum Genet* 2001;46:179–181.

160. Young, T, Hutcheson KA, Quinn GE, et al. Screening of Norrie disease gene mutations in retinopathy of prematurity. Presented at the third international meeting on ROP, Anaheim, California, November 13, 2003.

161. Hikino S, Ihara K, Yamamoto J, et al. Physical growth and retinopathy of prematurity in preterm infants: involvement of IGF-1 and GH. *Pediatr Res* 2001;50:732–736.

162. Hellstrom A, Peruzzu C, Ju M, et al. Low IGF-1 suppresses VEGF-survival signalling in retinal endothelial cells: direct correlation with clinical retinopathy of prematurity. *Proc Natl Acad Sci U S A* 2001;98:5804–5808.

163. Hellstrom A, Engstrom E, Hard A-L, et al. Postnatal serum insulin-like growth factor 1 deficiency is associated with retinopathy of prematurity and other complications of premature birth. *Pediatrics* 2003;112:1016–1020.

164. Hellstrom A, Carlsson B, Niklasson A, et al. IGF-1 is critical for normal vascularization of the human retina. *J Clin Endocrinol Metab* 2002;87:3413–3416.

165. Smith LEH, Shen W, Peruzzu C, et al. Regulation of vascular endothelial growth factor-dependent retinal neovascularization by insulin-like growth factor-1 receptor. *Nat Med* 1999;5: 1390–1395.

166. Aiello LP, Pierce EA, Foley ED, et al. Suppression of retinal neovascularization *in vivo* by inhibition of vascular endothelial growth factor (VEGF) using soluble VEGF-receptor chimeric proteins. *Proc Natl Acad Sci U S A* 1995;92:10457–10461.

167. Duh EJ, Yang HS, Suzuma I, et al. Pigment epithelium-derived factor suppresses ischemia-induced retinal neovascularization and VEGF-induced migration and growth. *Invest Ophthalmol Vis Sci* 2002;43:821–829.

168. Ozaki H, Seo M-S, Ozaki K, et al. Blockade of vascular endothelial cell growth factor receptor signalling is sufficient to completely prevent retinal neovascularisation. *Am J Pathol* 2000;156:697–707.

169. Shih SC, Ju M, Liu N, et al. Selective stimulation of VEGFR-1 prevents oxygen-induced retinal vascular degeneration in retinopathy of prematurity. *J Clin Invest* 2003;112:50.

170. Tin W, Milligan DWA, Pennefather PM, et al. Pulse oximetry, severe retinopathy, and outcome at one year in babies of less than 28 weeks gestation. *Arch Dis Child (Fetal Neonat Ed)* 2001;84:106–110.

171. Browning J, Wylie CK, Gole G. Quantification of oxygen-induced retinopathy in the mouse. *Invest Ophthalmol Vis Sci* 1997;38:1168–1174.

172. Reynaud X, Dorey KC. Extraretinal neovascularisation induced by hypoxic episodes in the neonatal rat. *Invest Ophthalmol Vis Sci* 1994;35:3169–3177.

173. Ashton N, Blach R. Studies on developing retinal vessels: effect of oxygen on the retinal vessels of the ratling. *Br J Ophthalmol* 1961;45:321–340.

174. Holmes JM, Zhang S, Leske DA, et al. The effect of carbon dioxide on oxygen-induced retinopathy in the neonatal rat. *Curr Eye Res* 1997;16:725–732.

175. Holmes JM, Zhang S, Leske DA, et al. Metabolic acidosis-induced retinopathy in the neonatal rat. *Invest Ophthalmol Vis Sci* 1999;40:804–809.

176. Chan-Ling T, Tout S, Hollander H, et al. Vascular changes and their mechanisms in the feline model of retinopathy of prematurity. *Invest Ophthalmol Vis Sci* 1992;33:2128–2147.

177. McLeod DS, Crone SN, Lutty GA. Vasoproliferation in the neonatal dog model of oxygen-induced retinopathy. *Invest Ophthalmol Vis Sci* 1996;37:1322–1333.

RETINOPATHY OF PREMATURITY: EVOLUTION OF STAGES 4 AND 5 ROP AND MANAGEMENT

A. EVOLUTION TO RETINAL DETACHMENT AND PHYSIOLOGICALLY BASED MANAGEMENT

MICHAEL T. TRESE
ANTONIO CAPONE, JR.

Retinopathy of prematurity (ROP) is a retinal vascular disease that affects premature infants during the neonatal period and can progress to retinal detachment and blindness. Over the last half century, much interest has been shown in the disease, and many contributions have been made through clinical series, retrospective comparative studies, and randomized, prospective trials. The evidence addressing the pathophysiology of the acute stages of ROP (1) (Figs. 27-1 and 27-2) and the knowledge obtained from clinical trials that has helped to develop the current medical management are discussed in Chapter 26. This chapter addresses the management of ROP and a theory of the pathophysiology of stage 4 ROP to provide a means of current clinical management (2).

STAGE 3 RETINOPATHY OF PREMATURITY IN POSTERIOR RETINOPATHY OF PREMATURITY

Neovascularization in ROP can have two appearances. In typical stage 3 ROP, neovascularization immediately posterior to the ridge extends up and grows onto the vitreous scaffold (Fig. 27-1C). In the second less common type, flat neovascularization lies on the retinal surface. This second type is often present in zone I or posterior zone II and has a lacy appearance without ridge tissue. Occasionally, as a confusing feature to the ophthalmologist, there is a hint of a small white line at the anterior aspect of the flat neovascularization.

Although most screening today is carried out by individual ophthalmologists using indirect ophthalmoscopy, photographic screening is gaining popularity, particularly for documenting features such as posterior flat neovascularization and plus disease. It offers advantages over drawings for both clinical management and clinical trials. For example, pilot studies showed the correlation between clinical examination and photographic assessment of plus disease to be very high, approaching 100% (3). This study supports the benefit of photographic assessment in clinical management. However, there can be limitations in documenting more peripheral plus disease, retinal detachment, and neovascularization even using wide-angle imaging. Also, the cost for most units is high. It is hoped that advancements in technology will provide better resolution in wide-angle imaging and reduced cost so that the benefits of imaging, such as improved documentation of ROP and fundus development, can be achieved.

PATHOGENESIS OF LATE STAGES OF RETINOPATHY OF PREMATURITY

Studies of the pathogenesis of the late stages of ROP associated with retinal detachment are difficult because of the inability to obtain tissue during the acute development of stage 4 and 5 ROP. This in part accounts for the sparse literature on the pathogenesis of retinal detachment in ROP. We speculate on possible mechanisms for the two most commonly seen configurations of retinal detachment in ROP. Evidence of this is based on histologic, biochemical, and clinical observations of eyes affected with advanced ROP (stages 3, 4, and 5) and with the morphologically similar retinal detachment of familial exudative vitreoretinopathy (FEVR) (4,5). We base the management of ROP on these observations.

Retinal vascular assembly is carried out intrauterinely in a relatively hypoxic setting (6,7). The hyaloid vasculature or primary vitreous fills the developing vitreous cavity with blood vessels, which initially have many attachments to the developing retina. During development, these attachments

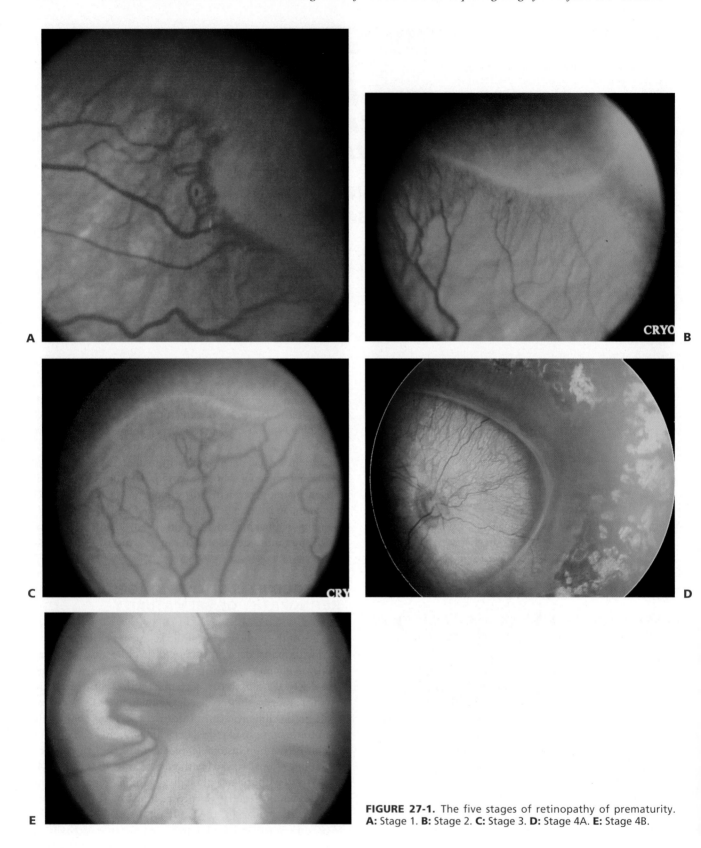

FIGURE 27-1. The five stages of retinopathy of prematurity.
A: Stage 1. **B:** Stage 2. **C:** Stage 3. **D:** Stage 4A. **E:** Stage 4B.

undergo involution. The last of these vascular structures to regress is the hyaloid artery. Involution of the hyaloid vasculature and tunica vasculosa lentis occurs through apoptosis and is generally complete by 40 weeks' postmenstrual age. However, the primary vitreous can persist, with a wide spectrum of clinical features previously referred to as *persistent hyperplastic primary vitreous* and more recently referred to as *persistent fetal vasculature syndrome* (8,9).

In the full-term infant, secondary vitreous consists of a dense collagen gel that replaces the primary vitreous, except in the areas of the vitreous canals where the former primary vitreous attachments to the retina and optic nerve existed. The most well known of these is the Cloquet canal. There is evidence that the retinal vascular assembly and involution of the hyaloid system and tunica vasculosa lentis by apoptosis are partly affected by vascular endothelial growth factor (VEGF) (Figs. 27-3 and 27-4) (6,10,11). The production and assembly of collagen gel might be a result of several cells, including hyalocytes, influenced by growth factor signals and extracellular matrix mediators (12).

VEGF has been shown to be important in normal retinal vascular development, survival of newly formed vessels, and pathologic neovascularization (see Chapter 26). It also causes microvascular permeability.

In the fetus, wound healing responses and scar formation differ depending on the time *in utero*. For example, fetal regenerative wounds heal without scar formation in the second and early third trimesters (13). Transforming growth factor-β_1 (TGF-β_1) has been widely studied regarding its effects on wound healing and in the eye. It leads to excessive scar formation in fetal wounds and contributes to hyaluronic acid synthesis (14). It differentially affects adult and fetal fibro-blast migration and hyaluro-

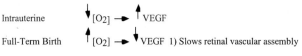

FIGURE 27-3. Effect of vascular endothelial growth factor in normal vascular development.

nan synthesis (15). In addition, it down-regulates VEGF in cell culture (12). Although direct evidence is lacking, TGF-β is present in fetal development and conceivably could affect collagen structure, vascularity, and wound healing in the eye. These processes could participate in the development of retinal detachment seen in stage 4 (Fig. 27-1D) and 5 ROP (Fig. 27-1E).

CLINICAL FEATURES OF RETINAL DETACHMENT IN RETINOPATHY OF PREMATURITY

The International Classification of Retinopathy of Prematurity (ICROP) describes retinal detachments as stage 4A, 4B, and 5 (1,2). Others have also used the term *predominantly effusive* and *predominantly tractional* to further classify these detachments (16,17). The predominantly effusive retinal detachment has a characteristic shape. The retina is convex toward the examiner and smooth with fluid extending primarily posterior to the ridge detaching the ridge and macula. This detachment begins at the ridge and is believed to be a result of leakage from vascular structures into the subretinal space creating subretinal fluid that might vary from relatively clear to turbid or bright red. Some of the components of this subretinal fluid are blood products (17). This detachment is much less common now that cryotherapy is used less frequently than laser (Figs. 27-4 to 27-6).

The second type is the stage 4B predominantly tractional detachment (Fig. 27-7). This detachment has peaked retinal folds pulled toward the center of the eye and tortuous vessels. The retinal ridge may circumferentially contract and pull the retina toward the center of the eye. Frequently, prior to detachment, a central stalk and scaffolding of spokes extending to the retina becomes increasingly visible and is appreciated with endoillumination during vitreous surgery. The network can be predominantly posterior when associated with regression of posterior hyaloid structures, predominantly anterior when associated with regressed structures of the tunica vasculosa lentis, or both. This tractional form of retinal detachment is common if detachment occurs after laser treatment has reduced the vascularity, producing a "quiet" eye with less effusion into the subretinal space.

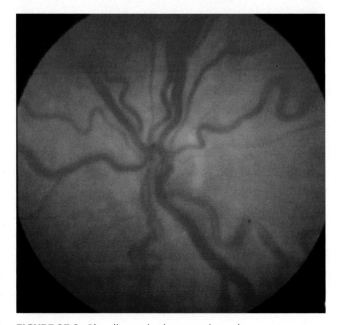

FIGURE 27-2. Plus disease in the posterior pole.

Pre-Term Birth   ↑[O2] ⟶ ↓VEGF

Phase 1: Causes temporary cessation of normal retinal vascular development

and

1) ↑ Apoptosis of hyaloid, vasculature, and tunica vasculosa lentis

2) Arrest of the developing retinal vasculature leaves a variable area
    of avascular retina

3) Creates area of relative retinal ischemia (dose dependent)

Phase 2: Ischemia ⟶ ↑VEGF

A. Causes retinal vessels to progress ⟶ regression

or

B. Extraretinal (pre and/or subretinal) neovascularization ⟶ ROP

Stages 3 and 4 effusive RD

and

↓ Apoptosis of the hyaloid and tunica vasculosa lentis

Clinical Correlate

1) Visible hyaloid structure

2) Rubeosis iridis

FIGURE 27-4. Retinopathy of prematurity (ROP) vascular phases and effusive retinal detachment phase biochemically.

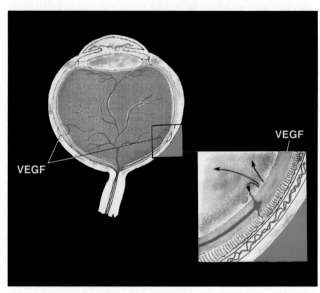

FIGURE 27-5. Schematic drawing showing the area of highest vascular endothelial growth factor concentration anterior to the advancing retinal vascular ridge. The **inset** shows the relationship of developing intraretinal and extraretinal vascularization contributing to the formation of subretinal blood (effusive retinal detachment) and the areas of cellular elements (primary vitreous and tunica vasculosa lentis) contributing to predominantly tractional retinal detachment.

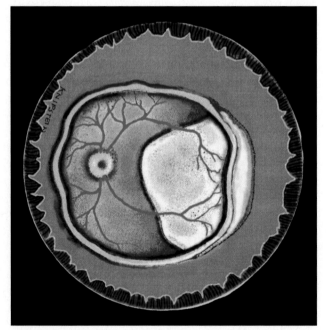

FIGURE 27-6. Artist's drawing showing the predominantely effusive 4B retinal detachment of retinopathy of prematurity extending from the ridge to include the center of the fovea. Subretinal fluid may be clear to turbid.

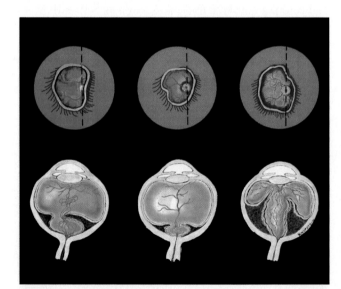

FIGURE 27-7. Artist's drawing of a predominantly tractional 4B retinal detachment of retinopathy of prematurity with asymmetrical traction by posterior cellular elements (hyaloid vasculature), the symmetrical traction by predominantly posterior cellular elements, and the configuration resulting by traction of predominantly anterior cellular elements (tunica vasculosa lentis). Upper row shows appearance with indirect ophthalmoscope. Lower row depicts cross-section of condition in upper row.

MECHANISM OF PREDOMINANTLY EFFUSIVE 4B RETINAL DETACHMENT

The mechanism for predominantly effusive 4B retinal detachment is an extension of the mechanism of the neovascular process described earlier. It has been known for years that the primary content of subretinal fluid in ROP was blood (17). Sang et al. (18) observed vessels in the subretinal space of humans in a histologic study; however, the pathogenesis of the subretinal neovascularization is enigmatic. Okamoto et al. (19) developed a transgenic mouse model in which VEGF expression was linked to the rhodopsin promoter and observed intraretinal and subretinal neovascularization as a result of increased expression of VEGF in the outer retina. Although direct clinical evidence is lacking, this model supports the notion that VEGF expressed in the retina can lead to subretinal neovascularization, leakage of fluid into the subretinal space, and thus retinal detachment, characteristics clinically noted in the predominantly effusive form of stage 4B retinal detachment (Fig. 27-6)

MECHANISM OF PREDOMINANTLY TRACTIONAL 4B RETINAL DETACHMENT

The predominantly tractional retinal detachment of stage 4B ROP involves one of the most interesting features of retinal detachment evolution in the premature child's eye. The often ignored involuting hyaloid system and tunica vasculosa lentis play an important role in tractional retinal detachment in ROP. Eyes with predominantly tractional 4B develop sharply peaked retinal folds. These folds can be seen to be attached to spokes connecting to the central stalk. This stalk often is not visible until endoillumination is used at surgery. The stalk always extends to the disc and can have other direct isolated strands connecting to the retina at or posterior to the ROP ridge. The anterior aspect of the stalk often connects to the posterior lens surface.

The traction generally has a dominant direction first toward the center of eye and then posterior toward the optic nerve or anteriorly toward the lens (Fig. 27-7). With progression from preterm through birth and thereafter, the vitreous organizes and the circumferential folds are often drawn centrally. Clear to turbid subretinal fluid can be present.

A possible scenario is outlined. An infant is examined a few weeks after premature birth during the period of slowed retinal vascular development and active apoptosis of the hyaloid system and tunica vasculosa lentis. At that time, only the hyaloid vessel or a few persistent vessels at the lens may be visible. The continued retinal ischemia from avascular retina drives an increase in angiogenic activity, such as through increased VEGF action, with a

reduction in apoptosis of the hyaloid endothelium resulting in clinically visible hyaloid vasculature and rubeosis iridis. In addition, an increase in proteolytic enzymes might release or activate growth factors within extracellular matrix that result in fibrosis. One possible candidate is TGF-β_1, which aggravates the scarring process in fetal tissue and allows formation of hyaluronic acid. Increased concentration of hyaluronic acid in the secondary vitreous then would promote liquefied vitreous noted in eyes with late stages of ROP. This liquefied vitreous would provide less internal tamponade and allow the retina to be pushed (effusive) or pulled (tractional) toward the center of the eye. The increased scar tissue may account for the cicatricial phase seen in the classic "retrolental fibroplasia" of late stage 5 ROP (Fig. 27-8). Surgical specimens of infant eyes operated for ROP provide evidence for regressing vascular elements within the stalk likely from the hyaloid vasculature (Fig. 27-9 to 27-11).

It has been our clinical observation that eyes that show more prominent clinical evidence of the regressed hyaloid structure following laser often develop retinal detachment shortly after this observation is made. In a study of late ROP, vitreous haze and the appearance of the vitreous organization in front of the lens in eyes treated for threshold ROP predicted progression of stage 4A ROP (20). We speculate this is the clinical correlate of reduced apoptosis and activated TGF-β_1 supporting hypocellular gel contraction. In addition, prominent or persistent iris vessels at 34 to 35 weeks' postmenstrual age were associated with increased risk of threshold ROP and a higher risk of retinal detachment (21). We speculate this increase in iris vessel activity reflects a resurgence of the VEGF activity.

Phase 3   ↑VEGF → Vascular Effects (↑Vessel Growth, ↓apoptosis)

and

→ Activates Plasminogen Activators (PA)

PA activates plasminogen to plasmin enzyme

which manipulates extracellular matrix and

activates TGFB1

TGFB1 - down regulates VEGF

and

Promotes excessive scarring in fetal tissue

(Stage 4-5 Tractional ROP)

Phase 4   Cycles of fetal wound healing contributing to predominantly

tractional retinal detachment

FIGURE 27-8. Retinopathy of prematurity (ROP) tractional retinal detachment phases. Shown is the biochemical cycle leading to the cicatricial stage of ROP (4–5) predominantly tractional retinal detachment (phases 1 and 2 are shown in Fig. 27-4).

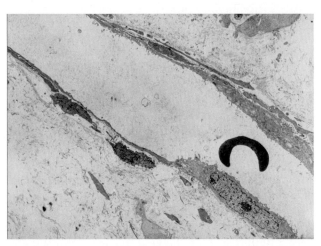

FIGURE 27-9. Transmission electron micrograph of the stalk material with vascular elements consistent with hyaloid vascular structures (magnification ×4,000).

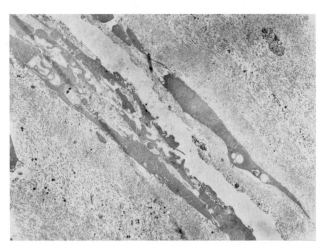

FIGURE 27-10. Transmission electron micrograph showing oriented dense collagen around the regressing vascular structure of the central stalk (hyaloid vasculature) (magnification ×5280).

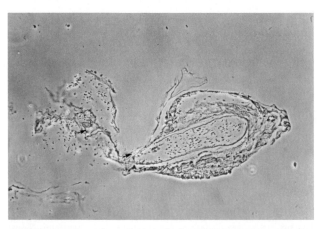

FIGURE 27-11. Light micrograph showing apoptotic cells *(arrows)* in a vitreous stalk removed from a patient undergoing surgery for retinopathy of prematurity. Cells were stained using an Apoptag (Oncor Inc.) kit, which labels the 3'-OH DNA ends generated by DNA fragmentation during apoptosis (×220).

REFERENCES

1. The Committee for the Classification of ROP: an international classification of ROP. *Arch Ophthalmol* 1984;102:1130–1134.
2. The Committee for the Classification of ROP: an international classification of ROP. *Int Ophthalmol* 1985;8:3–10.
3. Schwartz SD, Harrison SA, Ferrone PJ, et al. Telemedical evaluation and management of retinopathy of prematurity using a fiberoptic digital fundus camera. *Ophthalmology* 2000;107:25–28.
4. Shastry BS, Trese MT. Familial exudative vitreoretinopathy: further evidence for genetic heterogeneity. [Letter] *Am J Med Genet* 1997;69:217–218.
5. Shastry BS, Pendergast SC, Hartzer MK, et al. Identification of missense mutations in the Norrie disease gene associated with advanced retinopathy of prematurity. *Arch Ophthalmol* 1997; 115:651–655.
6. Pierce EA, Foley ED, Smith LE. Regulation of vascular endothelial growth factor by oxygen in a model of retinopathy of prematurity. *Arch Ophthalmol* 1996;114:1219–1228.
7. Aiello LP, Avery RL, Arrigg PG, et al. Vascular endothelial growth factor in ocular fluid of patients with diabetic retinopathy and other retinal disorders. *N Engl J Med* 1994;331:1480–1487.
8. Goldberg MF. Persistent vasculature (PFV): an integrated interpretation of signs and symptoms associated with persistent hyperplastic primary vitreous (PHPV). LIV Edward Jackson Memorial Lecture. *Am J Ophthalmol* 1997;124:587–626.
9. Dass AB, Trese MT. Persistent hyperplastic primary vitreous. In: Yanoff M, Duker J, eds. *Ophthalmology.* London: Times Mirror International, 1998.
10. Smith LEH. Oxygen-induced retinopathy in the mouse. *Invest Ophthalmol Vis Sci* 1994;35:101–111.
11. Penn JS. Variable oxygen exposure causes preretinal neovascularization in the newborn rat. *Invest Ophthalmol Vis Sci* 1993; 34: 576–585.
12. Mandriota SJ, Menoud PA, Pepper MS. Transforming growth factor B$_1$ down-regulates vascular endothelial growth factor receptor 2/flk-1 expression in vascular endothelial cells. *J Biol Chem* 1996;271:11500–11505.
13. Longaker MT, Whitby DJ, Adzich NS, et al. Studies in fetal wound healing. VI. Second and early third trimester fetal wound demonstrate rapid collagen deposition without scar formation. *J Pediatr Surg* 1990;25:63–69.
14. Krummel TM, Michna BA, Thomas BL, et al. Transforming growth factor beta (TGF-beta) induces fibrosis in a fetal wound model. *J Pediatr Surg* 1988;23:647–652.
15. Ellis IR, Schor SL. Differential effects of TGF-β1 on hyaluronan synthesis by fetal and adult skin fibroblasts: implications for cell migration and wound healing. *Exp Cell Res* 1996; 228: 326–333.
16. Trese MT. Retinopathy of prematurity. In: *Retina,* 2nd ed. St. Louis: Mosby-Year Book, 1994:2449–2462.
17. Trese MT. Surgical results of stage V retrolental fibroplasia and timing of surgery. *Ophthalmology* 1984;91:461–466.
18. Sang DN, Hirose T, Soque J. Histopathology and immunopathology of retinal detachment in retinopathy of prematurity. In: Shapiro MJ, Biglan AW, Miller MM, eds. *Retinopathy of prematurity.* Chicago: 1993:219–222.
19. Okamoto N, Tobe T, Hackett SF, et al. Animal model. Transgenic mice with increased expression of vascular endothelial growth factor in the retina. A new model of intraretinal and subretinal neovascularization. *Am J Pathol* 1997;151:281–291.
20. Hartnett ME, McColm JR. Retinal features predictive of progression to stage 4 ROP. *Retina* 2004;24:237–241.
21. Kivlin JD, Biglan AW, Gordon RA, et al. Early retinal vessel development and iris vessel dilatation as factors in retinopathy of prematurity. *Arch Ophthalmol* 1996;114:150–154.

B. TREATMENT OF RETINOPATHY OF PREMATURITY: PERIPHERAL RETINAL ABLATION AND VITREORETINAL SURGERY

ANTONIO CAPONE, JR.
MARY ELIZABETH HARTNETT
MICHAEL T. TRESE

The indications for photocoagulation for ROP have been changed based on the Early Treatment for Retinopathy of Prematurity (ETROP) trial to include eyes with severe ROP (see Chapter 26). Essential is the diagnosis of plus disease, requiring two quadrants of vessels with a certain level of tortuosity and dilation (Fig. 27-2). Photocoagulation is delivered through a dilated pupil using a 20-diopter (D) or 28-D condensing lens. Initial laser settings vary depending on the laser wavelength and fundus pigmentation. Settings of 200 mW for power and 100 ms for duration are used initially and titrated until a laser burn with a gray or gray-white appearance is visible. For flat neovascularization, laser is applied to avascular retina beneath the neovascularization (Figs. 27-12 and 27-13). The endpoint is near-confluent ablation, with burns spaced one-half burn width apart (Fig. 27-14), from the ora serrata up to, but not including, the ridge for 360 degrees (1). At the conclusion of the treatment session, the retina is inspected for "skip areas" to ensure peripheral retinal ablation has been complete.

Some physicians treat with topical steroids and cycloplegics one to two times per day. The eyes are reexamined within 1 week. Persistent plus disease or fibrovascular proliferation may indicate inadequate treatment, in which case additional treatment is indicated in the areas where skip areas are present.

COMPLICATIONS OF PERIPHERAL LASER RETINOPEXY FOR RETINOPATHY OF PREMATURITY

Complications from peripheral retinal ablation for ROP are relatively uncommon. Acute anterior segment complications include burns of the cornea, iris, or tunica vasculosa lentis (2,3). Laser burns too high in power may result in rupture of the Bruch's membrane and acute focal choroidal hemorrhage, or delayed exudative choroidal detachment. Clinically significant anterior segment hemorrhage is rarely encountered (4). Mild anterior segment inflammation following treatment is common and may result in formation of posterior synechiae. Vitreous hemorrhage may occur if laser is applied to the ridge of extraretinal fibrovascular proliferation. Cataract is the most common visually significant late complication (5,6), anticipated to occur in approximately 1% of eyes (7). Anterior segment ischemia (Fig. 27-15) resulting in iris atrophy, cataracts, hypotony (8), and occasionally phthisis (9) is fortunately among the least common complications of peripheral retinal ablation for ROP.

VITREORETINAL SURGERY FOR RETINOPATHY OF PREMATURITY

Although retinal ablation is effective in a majority of cases of threshold ROP, a substantial number progress to retinal detachment. Detachment is often seen associated with areas of incomplete peripheral ablation ("skip areas") or in eyes with inexorably progressive disease, usually in posterior zones II or I. The risk of lifelong visual impairment is substantially greater once retinal detachment develops.

SURGICAL ANATOMY OF RETINOPATHY OF PREMATURITY-RELATED RETINAL DETACHMENT

Fibrous proliferation and contraction of neovascularization along the ridge and onto the overlying vitreous precede traction retinal detachment. Condensation of vitreous into sheets and strands acts as a scaffold for further extension of the fibrovascular tissue. Traction along the retinal surface and contraction of the posterior hyaloid face contribute to distortion of the posterior pole architecture. The configuration of the retinal detachment in ROP depends primarily on

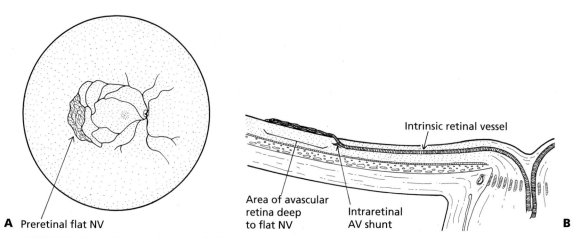

FIGURE 27-12. Artist's drawing of **A. (left):** avascular retina beneath the flat neovascularization and **B. (right):** cross-section near optic nerve.

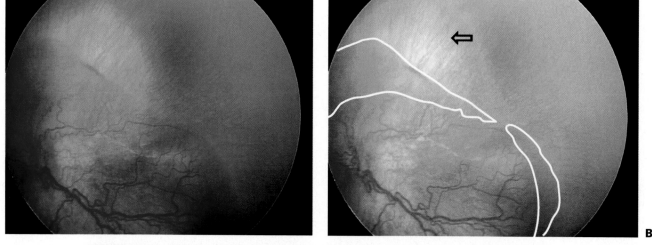

FIGURE 27-13. A: Wide-angle fundus image of stage 3 retinopathy of prematurity (ROP) in zone I. **B:** Note prominent choroidal vasculature visible through pale premature retinal pigment epithelium *(black arrow)* and flat arcuate syncytium of stage 3 ROP *(white-dotted outline).* The posterior aspect of the neovascular lobule is bordered by shunt vessels coursing circumferentially. [Images courtesy of Christine A. Gonzales, M.D., and the ROP Photographic Screening Trial (Photo-ROP) Study Group.]

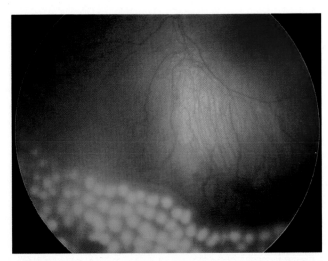

FIGURE 27-14. Near-confluent laser ablation with burns spaced one-half burn width apart, up to—but not including—the ridge.

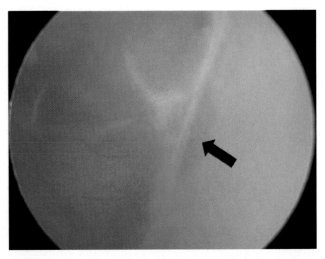

FIGURE 27-16. Contraction of proliferation intrinsic to the circumferential ridge, resulting in a radial fold. Resolved nasal stage 4A retinopathy of prematurity-related tractional retinal detachment following lens-sparing vitreous surgery.

the location of the ridge and the orientation of vectors of vitreoretinal traction. Tractional forces are exerted in the following ways:

1. *Intrinsic to retina* (Fig. 27-16). These forces consist of proliferation intrinsic to the ridge itself causing a tractional vector that cannot be removed surgically. Contraction of this circumferential vector results in a radial fold. It can be addressed by scleral buckle alone when it is the sole tractional vector located near or anterior to the equator.
2. *Ridge-to-lens* (Fig. 27-17). The most common and easily conceptualized traction vector, and the most important

to interrupt surgically, often extends circumferentially from the ridge toward the midperipheral lens.

3. *Ridge-to-ridge* (Fig. 27-18). This vector extends as a sheet across the "mouth" of the developing funnel-shaped retinal detachment.
4. *Ridge-to-ciliary body* (Fig. 27-19). This vector extends from the ridge anteriorly toward the ciliary body.
5. *Ridge-to-retina*. This traction extends from the elevated ridge back toward the portion of the retina just anterior to the original location of the ridge.
6. *Disc stalk*. There are three variants of the proliferative tissue extending from the optic disc: (a) a typically very ad-

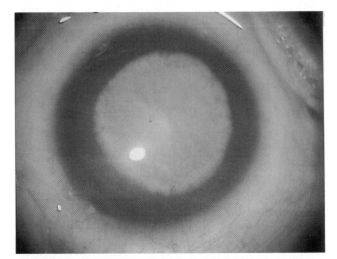

FIGURE 27-15. Right eye of a patient with zone II threshold retinopathy of prematurity (ROP) treated 4 weeks earlier using a diode laser (1,400 spots, 240 mW, 200 ms). There is a dense cataract with pigment on the anterior lens surface. Also present, although not apparent in this photograph, were posterior synechiae, a shallow anterior chamber with iridocorneal touch nasally, and mild corneal edema.

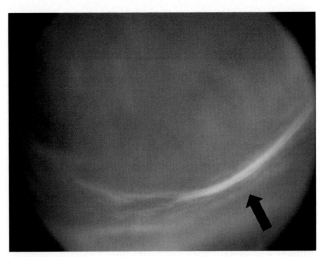

FIGURE 27-17. Proliferation extending anteriorly from the ridge toward the lens. Tractional stage 5 retinopathy of prematurity-related retinal detachment in an anteriorly open—posteriorly open funnel configuration. Traction originates at the ridge in a circumferential, pursestring pattern that draws the retina anteriorly and centrally.

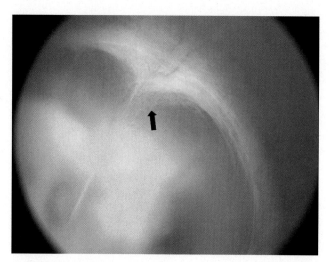

FIGURE 27-18. Sheet of proliferation originating from the ridge and extending across the "mouth" of the funnel-shaped retinal detachment toward the contralateral ridge. Stage 4B retinopathy of prematurity (ROP)-related tractional retinal detachment resulting in retrolental fibroplasia mimicking stage 5 ROP.

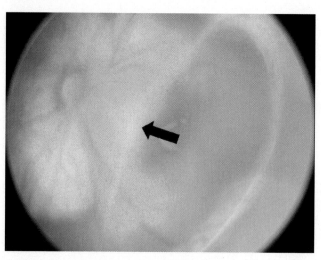

FIGURE 27-20. Central "T-shaped" stalk extending transvitreally from the optic disk (out of focus) anteriorly to join with the ridge-to-ridge sheet. Contraction of proliferation intrinsic to the circumferential ridge, resulting in a radial fold.

herent epiretinal sheet extending along the retinal surface to the ridge often seen in eyes in which the ridge is located posterior to the equator; (b) a transvitreal stalk extending to the ridge usually seen in eyes with an equatorial ridge; and (c) a transvitreal sheet extending from ridge-to-ridge sheet usually seen in eyes with a ridge located anterior to the equator (Fig. 27-20).

Some or all of these components are present in ROP-related retinal detachments. The configuration of the detachment is determined by the overall tractional contribution of the relative force vectors.

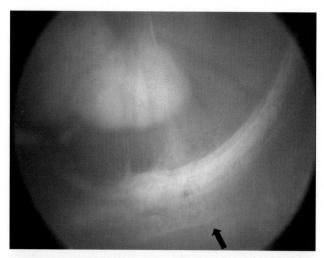

FIGURE 27-19. Sheet of proliferation originating from the ridge extends anteriorly toward the ciliary processes in the inferior portion of the image. Stage 4B retinopathy of prematurity-related tractional retinal detachment 1 week following vitreous surgery. Haze is a result of mild postoperative vitreous hemorrhage. Note reattachment of temporal retina, peripheral temporal laser scars, faint visibility of optic nerve head in the center of the image, and arcuate residual nasal peripheral proliferation.

Surgical Goals

The advanced stages of ROP (stages 4A, 4B, and 5) are poorly understood. Common misconceptions are that macula-sparing (stage 4A) partial retinal detachments are benign and that surgery should be deferred until the macula is detached. Rather, once a stage 4A detachment is progressive, we believe that surgery should be performed to prevent macular detachment. However, if stage 4B or 5 ROP occurs, surgical reattachment of the retina can still provide some level of vision that is of greater use for the developing infant than the same level of vision is for the adult (10). Lens-sparing vitrectomy is the preferred treatment for posterior disease and most forms of tractional progressive stage 4 ROP, whereas scleral buckle may be useful for rhegmatogenous detachments, some effusive detachments, and those where the main tractional component is the sole tractional vector located near or anterior to the equator (Fig. 27-16). The specific tasks of surgical intervention for ROP-related retinal detachments vary depending on the tractional components causing retinal detachment.

The goal for extramacular retinal detachment (stage 4A ROP) is an undistorted or minimally distorted posterior pole, total retinal reattachment, and preservation of the lens and central fixation vision (Figs. 27-21 and 27-22). Scleral buckle (11,12) and vitrectomy (13) have been used to manage stage 4A ROP. Disadvantages of scleral buckle for stage 4A ROP are the dramatic anisometropic myopia (14) and the second intervention required for transection or removal so that the eye can continue to grow. More importantly, however, not all tractional forces can be alleviated with scleral buckling alone. Vitreous surgery can interrupt progression of ROP from stage 4A to stages 4B or 5 by

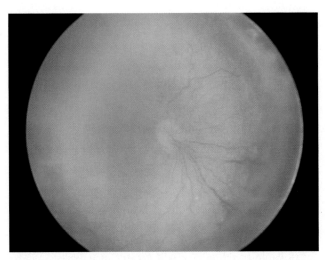

FIGURE 27-21. Nasal stage 4A retinopathy of prematurity-related tractional retinal detachment located in zone I in a 38-week-old infant 1 month following laser.

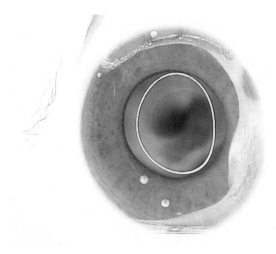

FIGURE 27-23. Stage 4B retinopathy of prematurity (ROP)-related tractional retinal detachment resulting in retrolental fibroplasia mimicking stage 5 ROP.

directly addressing transvitreous traction resulting from fibrous proliferation. In experienced hands, lens-sparing vitrectomy allows primary retinal reattachment in 90% of eyes with stage 4A ROP. Early visual outcomes appear encouraging as well. In a cohort of 11 consecutive eyes of children able to cooperate with Teller visual acuity testing (mean age 2.5 years), Snellen equivalent was 20/80 or better in eight eyes (73%) (15). In a retrospective comparison of stage 4 ROP treated with scleral buckle or lens-sparing vitrectomy, progressive stage 4 ROP was prevented after one procedure in 7 of 11 eyes treated with lens-sparing vitrectomy com-

pared to only 5 of 16 eyes treated with scleral buckle ($p = 0.03$; exact Chi-square) (16).

Surgery for tractional retinal detachments involving the macula is performed to minimize retinal distortion and prevent total retinal detachment (stage 5). The practical surgical goal is to reattach as much of the retina as is possible. Partial residual retinal detachment in such eyes is common (Figs. 27-23 and 27-24). The functional goal for stage 4B eyes is ambulatory vision.

The surgical goal for stage 5 ROP is to reattach as much of the retina as possible. As with stage 4B detachments, par-

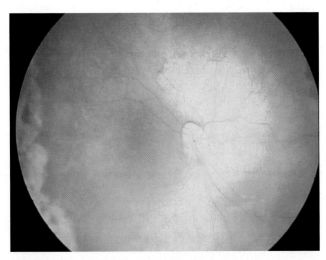

FIGURE 27-22. Resolved nasal stage 4A retinopathy of prematurity-related tractional retinal detachment following lens-sparing vitreous surgery. Straightening of the vessels inferonasal to the optic disc is the only residuum of the tractional detachment following vitrectomy.

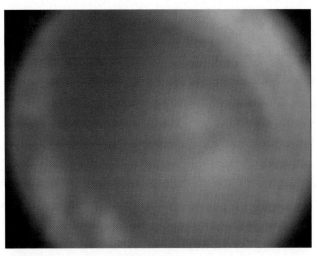

FIGURE 27-24. Stage 4B retinopathy of prematurity-related tractional retinal detachment 1 week following vitreous surgery. Haze is a result of mild postoperative vitreous hemorrhage. Note reattachment of temporal retina, peripheral temporal laser scars, faint visibility of optic nerve head in the center of the image, and arcuate residual nasal peripheral proliferation.

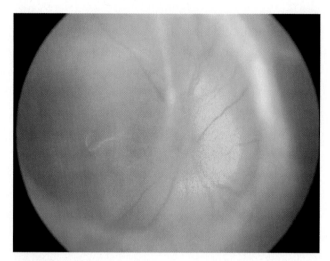

FIGURE 27-25. Tractional stage 5 retinopathy of prematurity-related retinal detachment in an anteriorly open–posteriorly open funnel configuration. Traction originates at the ridge in a circumferential, pursestring pattern that draws the retina anteriorly and centrally.

tial residual retinal detachment is common. Form vision can be preserved following vitrectomy for stage 5 ROP (Fig. 27-25) (17,18). Lower levels of vision can be measured by detecting the perception of light in different fields of vision as determined in different levels of illumination (19). This measurement permits one to stratify low levels of vision and then follow low vision in infants treated for stage 5 ROP. Maximal recovery of vision following the insult of macula-off retinal detachment and interruption of visual development in infants may take years.

Timing of Surgery

ROP-related detachments may appear stable in the first few weeks or months after peripheral retinal ablation. Yet neither the stability of the partial detachment (6) nor visual acuity is predictable from the retinal appearance in infants with ROP. This is particularly true for untreated eyes (3) or those with incomplete peripheral retinal ablation. Visual outcome of eyes with even partial ROP-related retinal detachment is generally poor by age 4.5 years. In the cohort of 61 eyes from the Multicenter Trial of Cryotherapy for Retinopathy of Prematurity (CRYO-ROP) study with partial retinal detachment 3 months after threshold, only six eyes had vision of 20/200 or better at age 4.5 years (20,21). The difficulty exists in determining whether an eye with residual or recurrent features of threshold ROP will develop progressive stage 4 ROP or show regression after laser treatment. One retrospective study of retinal features in eyes treated with laser for threshold ROP determined that ≥6 clock hours of ridge elevation, ≥2 quadrants of plus disease, and vitreous haze were predictive of progressive stage 4 ROP and that these features should indicate to the ophthalmologist that this patient likely will require surgery to

prevent stage 4B ROP. The study was retrospective and did account for the correlation between eyes in the same infant by using a generalized estimating equation model (22).

When ROP-related retinal detachments occur, they can progress—often very gradually—for years. In general, the earlier the surgical intervention the better, as the prognosis for vision is best when the detachment is least extensive. In eyes with stage 4 detachments and thorough peripheral retinal ablation, surgery typically is done between 38 and 42 weeks postconceptional age (23).

An exception to this rule is the eye with active vascularity. In the setting of stage 4 ROP in an actively vascular eye with marked plus disease that lacked prior peripheral retinal laser ablation, it often is better to treat the avascular peripheral retina first and wait to perform surgery. The risk of uncontrollable bleeding is much greater in actively vascular eyes. If the eye has a stage 5 retinal detachment with significant vascular activity, one may need to wait several weeks for the vascular activity to quiet.

Surgical Approach

Scleral Buckle

We rarely perform scleral buckle for ROP-related retinal detachment. A scleral buckle also can be tried first in eyes that have peripheral detachments or eyes in which there is a likelihood that the lens will need to be removed to address the surgical goals. The element of choice for scleral buckle in infants is a no. 40 or 240 silicone band. If possible, the band is placed to support the ridge as one would support a retinal tear, with the encircling element supporting the ridge along the anterior portion of the element. The buckle is placed along the greater curvature of the eye in order to minimize migration of the band, which occurs commonly in infants. Sutures are imbricated to provide height. The anterior chamber is tapped with a 30-gauge needle to normalize intraocular pressure. In eyes with substantial subretinal fluid, drainage through an external sclerotomy, using a scleral cutdown, diathermy, and release of subretinal fluid, can be carried out to permit tightening of the band, intraocular pressure (IOP) reduction, and reattachment of the retina.

Lens-Sparing Vitrectomy

If vitreoretinal pathology is accessible because the lens and retrolenticular vitreous are not involved, the lens can be spared. A lens-sparing vitrectomy is our preferred approach for stage 4A and many stage 4B detachments. Lens-sparing vitreoretinal surgery is uniquely suited to the management of stage 4 ROP. Maguire and Trese (24) reported the technique initially for eyes with subtotal posterior retinal detachment involving the macula.

An infusing light pipe or pic, vitreous cutter, and MPC scissors are used in the procedure. The eye is entered through the pars plicata at a clock hour advantageous to approaching the existing traction. A core vitrectomy is performed addressing the organized vitreous in four planes: transvitreous ridge-to-ridge, ridge-to-periphery, ridge-to-lens, and tentacles from the central stalk of organized vitreous extending from the optic nerve head to the ridge. When this dissection is complete, a fluid–air exchange is performed. During the fluid–air exchange, the retina is not forced to reattach; rather, only a bubble is placed into the eye. The sclerotomies are closed and the child positioned such that the air bubble encourages the retina to reattach and displace subretinal blood from the posterior pole. However, much subretinal fluid is reabsorbed over weeks in the postoperative period after the bubble has disappeared.

Lensectomy and Vitrectomy

There are cases of advanced ROP in which scleral buckle is not likely to work or has failed to prevent progression, and lensectomy clearly is required in order to address the surgical goals. In these cases, the lens and retrolenticular vitreous are involved. This is the case for some stage 4B and most stage 5 ROP-related retinal detachments.

The surgical goals can be achieved in two ways. The usual approach is a closed technique. However, with a very tight closed—closed funnel stage 5 detachment, the open-sky approach may be considered because it provides better access for dissection of the preretinal membrane than the closed approach. For this type of stage 5 ROP, it also is safer because there is less risk that the posteriorly infusing balanced salt solution would cause a peripheral dialysis.

In the closed technique, either infusing instruments, such as an irrigating light pipe, light pic, or spatula, may be used, or an infusion is placed through the limbus inferiorly. Sometimes the infusion is a bent 25-gauge butterfly needle inserted through the limbus and taped onto the drape or lid to maintain it in position. A portion of the iris often is sacrificed for visualization and to minimize reproliferation along the posterior iris. Bimanual dissection techniques are used to free the retina from traction as much is possible.

In the open-sky technique, the cornea is trephined and placed into either tissue culture media or Optisol. Bimanual dissection is used to circumcise the retrolental preretinal membrane under direct visualization through the operating room microscope. Continued dissection of membranes within the funnel of the retinal detachment is then completed. To facilitate dissection of preretinal membranes from detached retina within the funnel, a viscoelastic substance is used to spread tissue planes. To optimize visualization, a flat glass contact lens is used. The viscoelastic can be used to push the retina posteriorly away from the iris and anterior structures. Drainage of subretinal fluid can be performed to allow the retina to settle back, but care is taken not to forcefully attempt to reattach

the retina so as to avoid iatrogenic breaks. Much of the retina is permitted to reattach over weeks or months in the postoperative period.

ENZYMATIC VITREOLYSIS

Several studies have shown the benefit of enzymes to create a posterior vitreous detachment. Use of plasmin and chondroitinase have been used successfully in humans, although long-term results have not been reported (25).

ADULT RETINOPATHY OF PREMATURITY

As infants afflicted with ROP have matured, the ophthalmic community has gained experience with "adult ROP." Early nuclear sclerotic cataract, glaucoma (26), exudative retinopathy (27), and rhegmatogenous retinal detachment (28) are a few of the sequelae of ROP prompting the need for lifelong ophthalmic monitoring of formerly premature infants. Rhegmatogenous retinal detachment in adults with ROP is challenging to repair because of irregular tears, atrophied peripheral retina, and abnormalities of the vitreoretinal interface, especially in areas of formerly avascular retina. Scleral buckling with large elements supporting the vitreous base, which often is posteriorly displaced, or a combination of vitrectomy with scleral buckling may improve initial success.

CONCLUSION

The body of information germane to caring for ROP—from infancy to adulthood—continues to grow. It is hoped that greater knowledge of the pathophysiology of ROP at the cellular level will afford novel and more effective therapeutic strategies. Pharmacologic stabilization of aberrant angiogenesis may be one approach. Surgical intervention offers the potential for preservation of vision for eyes with ROP-related retinal detachment, particularly if it is addressed prior to macular distortion or detachment.

REFERENCES

1. Banach MJ, Ferrone PJ, Trese MT. A comparison of dense versus less dense diode laser photocoagulation patterns for threshold retinopathy of prematurity. *Ophthalmology* 2000;107:324–328.
2. Lambert SR, Capone A Jr, Cingle KA, et al. Cataract and phthisis bulbi after laser photoablation for threshold retinopathy of prematurity. *Am J Ophthalmol* 2000;129:585–91.
3. Kaiser RS, Trese MT. Iris atrophy, cataracts, and hypotony following peripheral ablation for threshold retinopathy of prematurity. *Arch Ophthalmol* 2001;119:615–617.
4. Simons BD, Wilson MC, Hertle RW, et al. Bilateral hyphemas and cataracts after diode laser retinal photoablation for retinopathy of prematurity. *J Pediatr Ophthalmol Strabismus* 1998;35:185–187.

5. Capone A Jr, Drack AV. Transient lens changes after diode laser retinal photoablation for retinopathy of prematurity. *Am J Ophthalmol* 1994;118:533–535.

6. Christiansen SP, Bradford JD. Cataract in infants treated with argon laser photocoagulation for threshold retinopathy of prematurity. *Am J Ophthalmol* 1995;119:175–180.

7. O'Neil JW, Hutchinson AK, Saunders RA, et al. Acquired cataracts after argon laser photocoagulation for retinopathy of prematurity. *JAAPOS* 1998;2:48–51.

8. Ferrone PJ, Banach MJ, Trese MT. Cataract and phthisis bulbi after laser photocoagulation for threshold retinopathy of prematurity. *Am J Ophthalmol* 2001;132:948–949.

9. Lambert SR, Capone A Jr, Cingle KA, et al. Cataract and phthisis bulbi after laser photoablation for threshold retinopathy of prematurity. *Am J Ophthalmol* 2000;129:585–591.

10. Seaber JH, Machemer R, Elliott D, et al. Long-term visual results of children after initially successful vitrectomy for stage V retinopathy of prematurity. *Ophthalmology* 1995;102:199–204.

11. Trese MT. Scleral buckling for retinopathy of prematurity. *Ophthalmology* 1994;101:23–26.

12. Greven C, Tasman W. Scleral buckling in stages 4B and 5 retinopathy of prematurity. *Ophthalmology* 1990;97:817–820.

13. Capone A Jr, Trese MT. Lens-sparing vitreous surgery for tractional stage 4A retinopathy of prematurity retinal detachments. *Ophthalmology* 2001;108:2068–2070.

14. Chow DR, Ferrone PJ, Trese MT. Refractive changes associated with scleral buckling and division in retinopathy of prematurity. *Arch Ophthalmol* 1998;116:1446–1448.

15. Prenner JL, Capone Jr A, Trese MT. Visual outcomes in patients with stage 4A retinal detachments from retinopathy of prematurity. Presented at the Association for Research in Vision and Ophthalmology Annual Meeting, Fort Lauderdale, Florida, May 2003.

16. Hartnett ME, Maguluri S, McColm J, et al. Comparison of retinal outcomes after scleral buckle or lens-sparing vitrectomy for Stage 4 retinopathy of prematurity. *Retina* (in press).

17. Trese MT, Droste PJ. Long-term postoperative results of a consecutive series of stages 4 and 5 retinopathy of prematurity. *Ophthalmology* 1998;105:992–997.

18. Mintz-Hittner HA, O'Malley RE, Kretzer FL. Long-term form identification vision after early, closed, lensectomy-vitrectomy for stage 5 retinopathy of prematurity. *Ophthalmology* 1997;104:454–459.

19. Hartnett ME, Rodier DW, McColm JR, et al. Long-term vision results measured with Teller Acuity Cards and a New Light Perception Projection Scale after management of late stages of retinopathy of prematurity. *Arch Ophthalmol* 2003;121:991–996.

20. Gilbert WS, Quinn GE, Dobson V, et al. Partial retinal detachment at 3 months after threshold retinopathy of prematurity. Long-term structural and functional outcome. *Arch Ophthalmol* 1996;114:1085–1091.

21. Palmer EA, Flynn JT, Hardy RJ, et al. Incidence and early course of retinopathy of prematurity. *Ophthalmology* 1991;98:1628–1640.

22. Hartnett ME, McColm JR. Retinal features predictive of progression to stage 4 ROP. *Retina* 2004;24:237–241.

23. Capone A Jr, Trese MT. Lens-sparing vitreous surgery for tractional stage 4A retinopathy of prematurity retinal detachments. *Ophthalmology* 2001;108:2068–2070.

24. Maguire AM, Trese MT. Lens-sparing vitreoretinal surgery in infants. *Arch Ophthalmol* 1992;110:284–286.

25. Trese MT. Enzymatic vitreous surgery. *Semin Ophthalmol.* 2000;15:116–121.

26. Gallo JE, Holmstrom G, Kugelberg U, et al. Regressed retinopathy of prematurity and its sequelae in children aged 5–10 years. *Br J Ophthalmol* 1991;75:527–531.

27. Brown MM, Brown GC, Duker JS, et al. Exudative retinopathy of adults: a late sequela of retinopathy of prematurity. *Int Ophthalmol* 1994–95;18:281–285.

28. Kaiser RS, Trese MT, Williams GA, et al. Adult retinopathy of prematurity. Outcomes of rhegmatogenous retinal detachments and retinal tears. *Ophthalmology* 2001;108:1647–1653.

FAMILIAL EXUDATIVE VITREORETINOPATHY

MICHAEL T. TRESE
ANTONIO CAPONE, JR.

HISTORY AND OVERVIEW

Familial exudative vitreoretinopathy (FEVR) was first described by Criswick and Schepens (1) in 1969. Because this condition was reported after the description of retinopathy of prematurity (ROP) and the ocular findings resembled those in ROP but were observed in full-term babies, it often had been referred to as ROP in full-term infants. Several reports in the literature have suggested that ROP can occur in infants with birth weight >1,800 g (2). We believe that this is unlikely and that these eyes were really cases of FEVR. The differential diagnoses are discussed later in this chapter.

FEVR is a retinal vascular disease in which the peripheral retinal vessels fail to grow into the far peripheral retina, leaving areas of avascular retina. In its more severe form, FEVR is a lifelong active retinal vascular disease with variable periods of quiescence. At the juncture of avascular and vascularized retina there often is a line of vascular buds that are distinct from the typical neovascularization of ROP and the telangiectatic vessels of Coats disease. FEVR has great variability in presentation, course, and inheritance pattern. Benson (3) investigated the natural history of FEVR. Benson observed, and we agree, that people who present with FEVR prior to age 3 years have a worse prognosis and that there can be very long quiet periods, a decade or more, in this retinovascular process (4).

Other than the obvious difference in birth weight associated with ROP, the most significant difference is that FEVR can be a lifelong vascularly active process.

GENETICS

The most common pattern of inheritance for FEVR is autosomal dominant, although families with X-linked and autosomal recessive forms have been reported. The loci for two autosomal dominant forms (EVR1 and EVR3) and an X-linked form (EVR2) of FEVR have been mapped (5–8). EVR1 and EVR3 are both on chromosome 11 and have been localized to 11q13–q23 (9) and 11p13–p12 (10), respec-

tively. Robitaille et al. (11) demonstrated that mutations in the frizzled-4 gene *(FZD4)* cause EVR1 and suggested that *FZD4* plays a role in retinal angiogenesis. EVR2 is associated with missense mutations in the Norrie disease gene (6,12,13), and it has been suggested that the protein encoded by the Norrie disease gene may be required for normal expression of transforming growth factor-β (TGF-β). Thus, when the encoded protein is abnormal or missing, the eyes do not produce appropriate levels of endogenous TGF-β; therefore, the vascular endothelial growth factor (VEGF) cycle is unchecked by TGF-β down-regulation (14). This has been supported by animal work by Zhao and Overbeek (15). They developed a mouse model that does not express TGF-β in the eye, has an avascular peripheral retina, and develops retinal detachment (Fig. 28-1). These results suggest that pharmacologic agents that down-regulate VEGF or up-regulate TGF-β might be helpful in this retinal vascular disease.

Although genetic diagnostic tests to detect mutations are not yet feasible for most cases of FEVR, referral of patients to a clinical geneticist for counseling is recommended. After obtaining a thorough family and medical history, the clinical geneticist may be able to provide information about research laboratories that would be helpful to the patient.

CLINICAL DIAGNOSIS

The clinical diagnosis often is made by the examiner saying, "This looks like ROP, but the child was full term." The features of FEVR include areas of avascular peripheral retina and findings of vascular buds at the junction of the avascular and vascularized retina, as well as dragged vessels (Fig. 28-2) in the posterior pole and retinal folds (Fig. 28-3), which can be in contact with the lens. Large amounts of subretinal exudate can be present, and total retinal detachment due to exudative and proliferative forces can be seen (Fig. 28-4). Histologically, inflammatory elements are found that may support the proliferative process (16). A positive family history also may be helpful in making a diagnosis. However, the lack of a diagnosis of

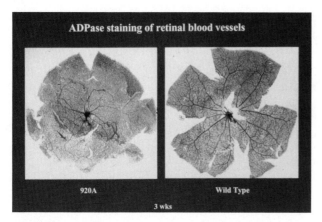

FIGURE 28-1. Flat mount mouse retina (wild-type) shows vascularization to the periphery. The retina of the mouse, which does not express transforming growth factor-β in the eye, shows an avascular peripheral retina similar to familial exudative vitreoretinopathy. If left alone, the eyes will progress to develop retinal detachment.

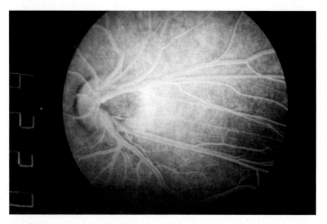

FIGURE 28-2. Fluorescein angiographic image showing the dragged vessels of the posterior pole. This is often seen in familial exudative vitreoretinopathy but also presents in other pediatric retinal diseases. Note the temporal dragging of the nasal vessels before they course nasally.

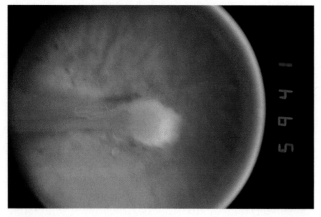

FIGURE 28-3. Now tightly dragged retina fold. Note the retinal vessels are drawn into the fold, and there are large areas of attached avascular retina. What appears to be optic nerve tissue, is actually the retina being dragged across the nerve.

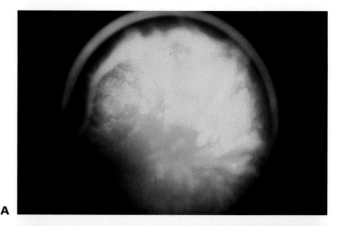

A

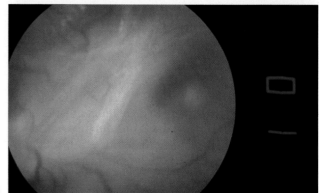

B

FIGURE 28-4. A: Wide-angle photograph of an eye affected by severe familial exudative vitreoretinopathy with avascular peripheral neovascular buds, subretinal exudate, and shallow total retinal detachment. This eye shows a predominantly exudative retinal detachment. **B:** Eye with organized vitreous causing a predominantly tractional retinal detachment in this area, with a resultant retinal fold.

FEVR in family members does not rule out a diagnosis of FEVR; for example, in one study no family history was found in 55% of cases (14). In addition, FEVR shows variable expression (e.g., mild avascular peripheral retina without significant exudate or detachment) and incomplete penetrance (mutation present but asymptomatic). Therefore, if the diagnosis of FEVR is suspected, a thorough peripheral retinal examination should be recommended for family members.

As mentioned earlier, the presentation of FEVR can be variable, and a classification system that somewhat parallels the International Classification of Retinopathy of Prematurity (ICROP) has been proposed. The FEVR classification system has five stages (Table 28-1). The classification system ranges from avascular periphery alone to total retinal detachment with and without active exudation.

The bilateral and unilateral features of FEVR have been used and can be helpful for diagnosis. In one series, 85% of eyes were bilaterally involved and 15% were unilaterally involved (14). Bilaterally involved patients need not be symmetrical (both eyes with the same stage). One eye can be severely involved with great exudation whereas the other eye

TABLE 28-1. CLINICAL CLASSIFICATION OF FAMILIAL EXUDATIVE VITREORETINOPATHY

Stage	Clinical Feature
1	Avascular retinal periphery without extraretinal vascularization
2	Avascular retinal periphery with extraretinal vascularization Without exudate With exudate
3	Retinal detachment—subtotal, not involving fovea Primarily exudative Primarily tractional
4	Retinal detachment—subtotal, involving fovea Primarily exudative Primarily tractional
5	Retinal detachment—total Open funnel Closed funnel

can be at a more minor FEVR stage. The diagnosis often is made by examining the less involved eye because the features for diagnosis may not be recognizable in the more involved end-stage eye. In addition, careful examination of newborns can be helpful in identifying involved eyes at earlier stages. As in most pediatric retinal diseases where severe retinal detachment can occur, if both eyes are involved, the more involved eye is often smaller than the less involved eye. Fluorescein angiography has been performed in FEVR but is not needed to make the diagnosis (17).

CLINICAL COURSE

FEVR eyes that present in the first year of life have a much worse prognosis. Benson (3) noted that children who presented in the first 3 years of life had a worse prognosis. However, in our opinion, presentation in the first year of life is even worse. Children often present because of reduced visual attention, strabismus, or leukocoria.

We believe that FEVR likely is underdiagnosed, with earlier milder stages of FEVR diagnosed as congenital retinal folds and more severely involved eyes diagnosed as congenital retinal detachments. This misdiagnosis seems to be less common as ophthalmologists become more aware of FEVR.

DIFFERENTIAL DIAGNOSIS

The differential diagnosis for FEVR includes ROP (easily ruled out by birth weight) and Norrie disease (genetic testing is available, but the result of genetic testing is negative in 20% of children with Norrie disease). Retinoblastoma must

be ruled out. Most of the time this can be done easily by clinical examination alone, but occasionally computed tomographic scanning is necessary when leukocoria is the presenting sign. Other more rare diseases, such as persistent fetal vasculature syndrome in the end stage, can look similar to FEVR. Persistent fetal vasculature syndrome (PFV) is more commonly unilateral and FEVR more commonly bilateral. Incontinentia pigmenti also can have findings similar to FEVR but often can be ruled out by the lack of skin or dental involvement.

TREATMENT

Like many treatments for pediatric retinal diseases, early intervention often results in better visual results. Screening is particularly important in preverbal children. FEVR often has a progressive long-term course, with periods of waxing and waning, and requires lifelong screening, particularly with new symptoms such as reduced vision or floaters. Because the stimulus for neovascularization in the avascular retina is similar to that in ROP, we recommend treating the avascular peripheral retina with laser if any vascular irregularity is present at the juncture of the avascular and vascularized retina. We also recommend treating any avascular retina in children younger than 3 years with FEVR of stage 2 or greater (Table 28-1). In our experience, these eyes have a generally poor prognosis. We treat these eyes with laser ablation using a pattern similar to the retinal ablation for ROP, adding near-confluent spots, one-half spot size from one another. We do not recommend monitoring these eyes until they develop exudates. We recommend treatment to prevent exudation before it occurs because laser or cryotherapy becomes less effective once subretinal fluid and exudation develop. Drainage of subretinal fluid followed by laser or cryotherapy often is disappointing because the fluid is so thick and difficult to drain.

At this time, we reserve scleral buckling for eyes with a rhegmatogenous component to their retinal detachment (14). Vitrectomy has a considerable role in the management of eyes with severe FEVR and vitreous hemorrhage, exudation, and tractional retinal detachment (14,18–20). We advocate separating the vitreous from the retina both mechanically and with enzymatic vitreolysis, such as with autologous plasmin (21). We believe that the vitreous plays a major role in the pathogenesis of FEVR. This vitreous is composed of liquid and solid sheets, with the posterior hyaloid firmly attached to the retina, and often is attached by cellular pegs leading to retinal folds and tractional retinal detachment. We use a two-port vitrectomy technique with an infusing instrument and another lighted instrument to perform two-hand dissection of the posterior hyaloid as much as possible. For the initial vitrectomy, high frequency (1,000–1,800 cuts/min) cutting is used. Aspiration is varied, but for thick membranes involving the lens, suction can be increased to 300 mmHg and cutting reduced to about 300 cuts/min. For work close to the retina, the suction is reduced and the cutting rate increased. It usually is possible to get sheets of vitreous off the retina, but a clean retinal surface is impossible to achieve through mechanical dissection only. The posterior hyaloid that remains on the retinal surface can lead to progressive retinal traction and contribute to continued vascular exudation. We believe that the use of enzymatic vitreolysis using a compound such as plasmin can remove vitreous from the retinal surface. Silicone oil then helps to stabilize the eye, perhaps by providing long-term tamponade to maintain retinal attachment and reduce the stimulus for vascular leakage. Others report success with lensectomy and vitrectomy (19,22).

OUTCOMES

It has been reported that the mechanical stripping of vitreous yields a success rate for retinal reattachment of 63% to 86% and visual improvement in 35% to 71% (14,18–20).

One feature of FEVR that makes analysis of surgical success difficult is the long periods of inactivity and later worsening in the nonvitrectomized eye. We have seen inactivity for 20 years before resumption of the process. We believe that silicone oil may reduce the number of episodes of reactivation and should be considered in eyes that have been undergone previous vitreous surgery and have signs of ongoing activity. The oil usually is not removed. We recommend silicone oil that is less likely to emulsify, i.e., is a pure form or has higher centistokes (5,000 cs).

Like ROP, FEVR requires early screening of possibly affected individuals; laser ablation when vascular irregularities are noted, particularly in affected children younger than 3 years; and vitreoretinal surgery, often with silicone oil when retinal detachment persists. In the future, pharmacologic therapy may be the best way to approach FEVR to offset the effects of growth factors, such as VEGF, as we learn more about their mechanisms of actions.

As the genetics of FEVR are further explored, the disease may become a candidate for gene therapy. It appears as though FEVR will continue to be a threat to children's vision, but through better awareness of its diagnosis, screening, and earlier treatment, the number of children blinded from FEVR hopefully will be reduced.

REFERENCES

1. Criswick VG, Schepens CL. Familial exudative vitreoretinopathy. *Am J Ophthalmol* 1969;68:578–594.

2. Schulman J, Jampol LM, Schwartz H. Peripheral proliferative vitreoretinopathy in a full-term infant. *Am J Ophthalmol* 1980; 90:509–514.

3. Benson WE. Familial exudative vitreoretinopathy. *Trans Am Ophthalmol Soc* 1995;93:473–521.

4. Smith L. Pathogenesis of retinopathy of prematurity. *Acta Paediatr* 2002;91(Suppl):26–28.

5. Fuchs S, Kellner U, Wedemann H, et al. Missense mutation in the Norrie disease gene associated with X-linked exudative vitreoretinopathy. *Hum Mutat* 1995;6:257–259.

6. Shastry BS, Hejtmancik JF, Plager DA, et al. Linkage and candidate gene analysis of X-linked familial exudative vitreoretinopathy. *Genomics* 1995;27:341–344.

7. Shastry BS, Pedergast SD, Hartzer MK, et al. Identification of missense mutations in the Norrie disease gene associated with advanced retinopathy of prematurity. *Arch Ophthalmol* 1997; 115:651–655.

8. Plager DA, Orgel IK, Ellis FD, et al. X-linked recessive familial exudative vitreoretinopathy. *Am J Ophthalmol* 1992;114:145–148.

9. Muller D, Orth U, Van Nouhuys CE, et al. Mapping of the autosomal dominant exudative vitreoretinopathy locus (EVRI) by multipoint linkage analysis in four families. *Genomics* 1994;20: 317–319.

10. Downey LM, Keen TJ, Roberts E, et al. A new locus for autosomal dominant familial exudative vitreoretinopathy maps to chromosome 11p12–13. *Am J Hum Genet* 2001;68:778–781.

11. Robitaille J, MacDonald MLE, Kaykas A, et al. Mutant frizzled-4 disrupts retinal angiogenesis in familial exudative vitreoretinopathy. *Nat Genet* 2002;32:326–330.

12. Shastry BS, Trese Mt. Familial exudative vitreoretinopathy: further evidence of genetic heterogeneity. *Am J Med Genet* 1997; 69:217–218.

13. Shastry BS, Hejtmancik JF, Trese MT. Identification of novel missense mutations in the Norrie disease gene associated with one X-linked and four sporadic cases of familial exudative vitreoretinopathy. *Hum Mutat* 1997;9:396–401.

14. Pendergast SD, Trese MT. Familial exudative vitreoretinopathy. Results of surgical management. *Ophthalmology* 1998;105: 1015–1023.

15. Zhao S, Overbeek PA. Elevated TGF beta signaling inhibited ocular vascular development. *Dev Biol* 2001;237:45–53.

16. Boldrey EE, Egbert P, Gass JD, et al. The histopathology of familial exudative vitreoretinopathy. A report of two cases. *Arch Ophthalmol* 1985;103:238–241.

17. Canny CL, Oliver GL. Fluorescein angiographic findings in familial exudative vitreoretinopathy. *Arch Ophthalmol* 1976; 94:1114–1120.

18. Tasman W, Augsburger JJ, Shields JA, et al. Familial exudative vitreoretinopathy. *Trans Am Ophthalmol Soc* 1981;79:211–226.

19. Ikeda T, Tano Y, Tsujikawa K, et al. Vitrectomy fro rhegmatogenous or tractional retinal detachment with familial exudative vitreoretinopathy. *Ophthalmology* 1999;106:1081–1085.

20. Glazer LC, Maguire A, Blumenkranz MS, et al. Improved surgical treatment of familial exudative vitreoretinopathy in children. *Am J Ophthalmol* 1995;120:471–479.

21. Margherio AR, Margherio RR, Hartzer M, et al. Plasmin enzyme-assisted vitrectomy in traumatic pediatric macular holes. *Ophthalmology* 1998;105:1617–1620.

22. Williams JG, Trese MT, Williams GA, et al. Autologous plasmin enzyme in the surgical management of diabetic retinopathy. *Ophthalmology* 2001;108:1902–1905.

COATS' DISEASE

FRANCO M. RECCHIA
ANTONIO CAPONE, JR.
MICHAEL T. TRESE

In 1908, George Coats, curator of the Royal London Ophthalmic Hospital, described the clinical and histologic features of an ophthalmic disorder "characterized by the presence in some part of the fundus of an extensive mass of exudation" and sometimes accompanied by "very peculiar forms of vascular disease" (1). Coats observed that the disorder had a slow, insidious onset and occurred most frequently in one eye of otherwise healthy boys. The prominent findings were raised patches of flocculent, yellow-white exudates, usually in the posterior pole, and always beneath retinal vessels. Vascular anomalies, retinal hemorrhage, cystic retinal degeneration, and subretinal accumulations of fibrous tissue were evident microscopically. The disorder was seldom quiescent and progressed slowly to retinal detachment, cataract, glaucoma, and phthisis bulbi (1).

More than 90 years after Coats seminal article, the cause, pathogenesis, and classification of Coats' and related diseases remain controversial. From the natural history of the disease and technologic and therapeutic advances, preservation of good visual function has been possible with prompt intervention and careful follow-up.

HISTORICAL CONTEXT AND CLASSIFICATIONS

Coats originally classified his cases of exudative retinopathy into three groups: (i) those without marked vascular disease, (ii) those with marked vascular disease, and (iii) those with "large arteriovenous communications" (1). He observed that groups 1 and 2 were similar and believed that they likely shared a common pathophysiology (1). In 1912, Coats combined groups 1 and 2 and termed them *exudative retinitis.* He eliminated the third group, which later became known as *von Hippel angiomatosis retinae* (2) (see Chapter 15). Coincidentally, in 1912, Leber (3) described a nonexudative retinal degeneration characterized by "multiple miliary aneurysms." He concluded, and most authorities today agree, that his findings represented a milder or earlier stage of Coats' disease (4–7).

The typing of Coats' disease has engendered much controversy. Some authors distinguish between a congenital or juvenile form (Coats' disease) and an adult form (Coats reaction or Coats' syndrome) that occurs in patients older than 30 years. Others insist that the Coats' name should be applied only to cases originating in childhood (8,9). It is agreed, however, that the clinical, pathologic, and angiographic findings can be identical in juvenile and adult patients (10–14). The focus of this chapter is the entity that occurs before age 16 years and is characterized by microvascular anomalies and retinal exudation.

Various classifications of Coats' disease have been proposed by different authors, although none is formally or universally agreed upon (15–17). Gomez Morales (15) studied 51 patients between the ages of 1 and 34 years and classified the disease into five grades based on clinical appearance and progression: (i) isolated focal exudates; (ii) massive elevated exudation; (iii) partial retinal detachment; (iv) total retinal detachment; and (v) secondary complications such as uveitis, glaucoma, or cataract. In a modification of this scheme, Sigelman (16) designated retinal telangiectasis as the initial stage. Recently, Shields et al. (17) proposed a similar classification that may have useful application to clinical prognosis. In their system, Coats' disease is classified as follows: (i) telangiectasias only; (ii) telangiectasias and exudation; (iii) exudative retinal detachment; (iv) total detachment with secondary glaucoma; and (v) advanced end-stage disease.

EPIDEMIOLOGY (PREVALENCE, ENVIRONMENTAL FACTORS)

The epidemiologic and clinical features described in recent clinical series correspond with that originally reported by Coats. Cases can present as early as the first month and as late as the eighth decade of life, but approximately two thirds present before age 10 years (14,15,18,19). Younger patients appear to be afflicted more rapidly and with more severe progression. In a series of 75 patients with advanced disease reported by Haik (20), 30 (40%) presented before age 2 years. At all ages, the disease usually is unilateral (90%); if bilateral, it shows asynchronous progression (10,21–23). From 70% to 90% of affected children are boys. No racial or ethnic predilection has been shown. The precise incidence and prevalence of Coats' disease are unknown.

No environmental factors have been shown to cause or influence the severity of Coats' disease.

GENETIC ASSOCIATIONS

A genetic cause for Coats' disease has been proposed based on several observations: (i) the association of retinal telangiectasias with muscular dystrophy and deafness in one family (24); (ii) occurrence of exudative retinopathy in a few members of families with retinitis pigmentosa (25–27); and (iii) the case of a mother purported to have unilateral retinal telangiectasias and a son with Norrie disease (28). Cytogenetic studies of isolated cases have demonstrated pericentric inversion of chromosome 3 in one child and a partial deletion of chromosome 13 in another (29,30). However, the overwhelmingly sporadic occurrence of Coats' disease precludes any substantive genetic linkage studies.

Black et al. (28) investigated a mother with "a unilateral variant of Coats' disease" and her son afflicted with Norrie disease. Both carried a missense mutation in the Norrie disease (NDP) gene, which has been implicated in retinal vasculogenesis (31). Archived tissue from nine eyes enucleated for Coats' disease then was analyzed, and a mutation in the NDP gene was found in retinal tissue from one eye. The authors postulated that Coats' telangiectasias arise from somatic mutation in the NDP gene (28). The possibility that the mutation represented a naturally occurring polymorphism was not conclusively eliminated, however. DNA analysis of a child with coexisting Coats' disease and congenital retinoschisis failed to reveal mutations in either the NDP gene or the retinoschisin (RS) gene (33).

In a study of five families with a specific form of retinitis pigmentosa (designated RP12), 5 of 8 patients with an associated Coats'-like exudative vasculopathy demonstrated mutations in the CRB1 (crumbs homolog 1) gene. Mutations in the CRB1 gene also are seen in patients with RP12 and a small percentage of patients with Leber congenital amaurosis (33). It remains unclear, however, whether the exudative changes seen in such cases are truly an independent genetic event or merely are secondary to vascular endothelial decompensation associated with the retinal degeneration.

WORLDWIDE IMPACT

Coats' disease is a rare disorder and does not impact many children throughout the world; however, the disease can have a negative impact on the quality of life of those who are affected. Coats' disease is included on the National Organization of Rare Disorders Web site *(http://www.rarediseases.org/search/rdbdetail_abstract.html?disname=Coats'%20Disease)*.

PATHOLOGY AND PATHOPHYSIOLOGY

The source of Coats' disease remains unclear. Reese (5) observed periodic acid–Schiff staining of basement membrane under the endothelium of retinal veins and theorized that deposition of polysaccharide led to atresia and occlusion of vessel lumina, "thereby occasioning vascular ectasia and the formation of collateral channels." Wise (34) speculated that local retinal hypoxia awakened "a dormant vasoproliferative factor," stimulating growth of new vessels from veins and capillaries. Imre (35) postulated an endocrine source based on increased urinary excretion of 17-ketosteroids and 11-oxysteroids.

Histologic and ultrastructural studies support Coats original speculation "that some of the vascular changes are primary" and lead to the classic histopathologic findings of vessel thickening and hyalinization, interspersed with thinning and loss of endothelial elements (1,22,36,37). It is believed that breakdown of the blood–retinal barrier, at the level of the endothelium, causes plasma leakage into vessel walls, which become necrotic and disorganized and form dilatations and telangiectasias. Further leakage into adjacent retinal tissue produces the recognizable intraretinal and subretinal cholesterol exudates, hemorrhage, cysts, edema, lymphocytic infiltration, and deposition of lipid and fibrin (38,39). These changes lead to degeneration of the neural retina and to infiltration by phagocytic, lipid-laden "ghost" cells, which appear to be transformed retinal pigment epithelial cells (40). Clinically, these microscopic changes manifest as irregular, raised patches of yellow-white or yellow-green material, often with superficial hemorrhage. Partial serous retinal detachment may ensue and worsen with increasing vasculopathy and exudation. The exudation can be so abundant that it drains into the orbit and stimulates an inflammatory reaction (41).

CLINICAL FEATURES, SYMPTOMS, AND SIGNS

The most common signs of disease are strabismus, leukocoria, and visual impairment detected on routine vision screening. One child presented with turbid yellow fluid filling the anterior chamber (42). Up to 25% of patients can be asymptomatic, with diagnosis occurring during routine ophthalmic examination (43). The hallmark funduscopic findings in Coats' disease are vascular telangiectasias and massive subretinal and intraretinal exudates (Fig. 29-1). Affected vessels display an irregular caliber, focal telangiectasias, aneurysmal dilatations ("light bulbs") and sheathing by yellow cholesterol deposits. Microaneurysms can occur in all parts of the vascular bed but most commonly arise from capillaries (6). In the series of Henkind and Morgan (44), vascular abnormalities, although not always apparent clinically, were found histologically in all cases.

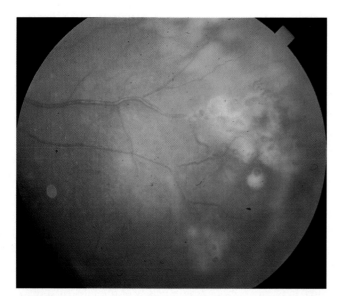

FIGURE 29-1. Peripheral fundus photograph of a 4-year-old boy with Coats' disease. Characteristic vascular abnormalities with extensive intraretinal and subretinal exudation are seen.

The earliest changes involve the equatorial and peripheral retina, with the temporal quadrants and the sector temporal to the fovea most commonly involved (19,45). The posterior pole is involved less frequently than the periphery (6,19,20,46). In a series of 112 eyes, Spitznas et al. (6) found lipid deposits in the central retina in fewer than 50%, with concomitant vascular changes in 17%. Shields et al. (18) observed retinal telangiectasias restricted to the macula in 1%.

The macula can become involved directly, by exudation from macular telangiectasias or indirectly by accumulation of exudate from peripheral retinal telangiectasias (Figs. 29-2 and 29-3A) (4,47). The macular exudate is yellow and occurs in continuous broad sheets that can form subretinal

mounds (10,16). Macular edema, exudative macular detachment, and organization into a disciform mass in the macula can ensue, resulting in significant visual decline (4).

The optic disc can appear hyperemic (10). The vitreous remains clear until advanced stages. Then, vitreous condensation and contraction of vitreoretinal connections lead to retinal detachment and vitreous hemorrhage. Intraretinal macrocysts can develop, likely as a result of longstanding retinal detachment (18,46,48).

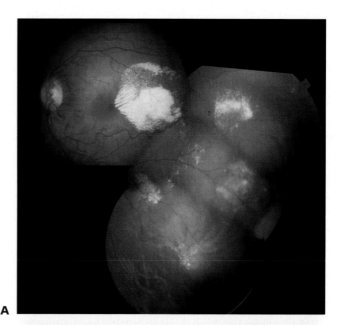

A

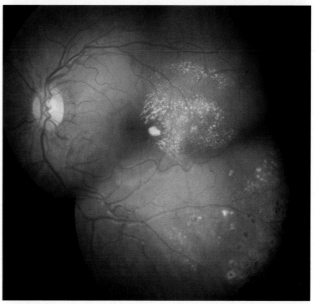

B

FIGURE 29-3. Montage of the left eye of a 10-year-old girl with Coats' disease before and after treatment. **A:** There are peripheral vascular changes (most notably inferotemporally) with associated intraretinal hemorrhage and intraretinal lipid. Visual acuity at this time had declined to 20/40, most likely as a result of macular exudation. **B:** Eight months following peripheral scatter laser photocoagulation to the areas of vascular change inferotemporally, the macular exudate has begun to resolve. Visual acuity improved to 20/25.

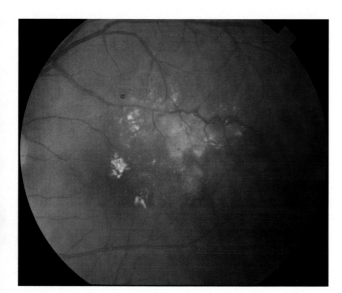

FIGURE 29-2. Fundus photograph showing massive accumulation of lipid exudates and subretinal fluid in the macula.

In the early stage of Coats' disease, ocular abnormalities outside the fundus are rare. Isolated associated findings include congenital retinoschisis, uveal coloboma, choroidal angioma, morning glory disc, and microphthalmos (13,20,32,43,49). There is one report of bilateral Coats' disease associated with infantile cataracts, congenital glaucoma, and later ketotic hypoglycemia (33). A fundus appearance resembling Coats' disease is seen in up to 4% of patients with retinitis pigmentosa (51).

SYSTEMIC ASSOCIATIONS

The overwhelming majority of children with Coats' disease are otherwise healthy. Previous toxoplasmosis has been reported in a few cases and epilepsy in one case (13,14,43). Reese (5) noted the rare occurrence of telangiectasias elsewhere in the body and suggested an association with Osler-Weber-Rendu disease.

Retinal changes typical of incipient Coats' disease are seen commonly in patients with the familial syndrome of facioscapulohumeral muscular dystrophy (24,52). In a cohort of 64 patients with this disorder, retinal telangiectasias were documented angiographically in 48 (75%) (53). There are isolated reports of Coats' disease in patients with trisomy 8 mosaic (20), Turner syndrome (54), frontoparietal circumscribed scleroderma (55), mandibulofacial dysostosis (Hallermann-Streiff syndrome) (56), familial renal-retinal dystrophy (Senior-Loken syndrome) (57), Cornelia de Lange syndrome (58), ichthyosis hystrix (epidermal nevus syndrome) (59), bone marrow hypoplasia (60), and vascular anomalies of the central nervous system (61).

DIAGNOSTIC STUDIES

Intravenous fluorescein angiography is helpful in children with Coats' disease, for both diagnosis and identification of treatable areas. Retinal telangiectasias produce the characteristic "light bulb" appearance and fluoresce dramatically. Capillaries can appear dilated but more often are occluded and are replaced by large arteriovenous shunts within areas of nonperfused retina (6,19). In the late phases of the angiogram, fluorescein dye can leak from aneurysmal vessels to produce a pattern of cystoid macular edema or subretinal pooling (13).

Ultrasonography provides safe and effective evaluation of leukocoria in which the diagnosis of Coats' disease is uncertain. Findings supporting the diagnosis of Coats' disease include poorly mobile retinal detachment; convolution and looping of the peripheral retina; dispersed subretinal cholesterol opacities exhibiting constant slow convection movements; and absence of a mass lesion or calcification (62). However, there can be overlap of findings for different diagnoses depending on the diseases and their stages.

Computed tomography (CT) facilitates the differentiation of Coats' disease from retinoblastoma. Intraocular calcifications are much more common in retinoblastoma and are readily seen radiographically. Partially calcified nodules can occur in Coats' disease but almost exclusively in phthisical eyes (28,46,63). More typical CT findings in Coats' disease are homogeneous opacification of the vitreous cavity, homogeneous subretinal densities, distinct retinal detachment, and lack of subretinal enhancement following administration of iodinated contrast dye (20,64).

Use of magnetic resonance imaging (MRI) provides greater tissue delineation, thus allowing differentiation between solid intraocular tumors, i.e., noncalcific or minimally calcified exophytic retinoblastoma, and nonneoplastic conditions causing retinal detachment. In Coats' disease, there is hyperintensity of the subretinal space on T1-weighted images, hyperintensity or hypointensity of the subretinal space on T2-weighted images, and linear enhancement of retinal detachment following infusion of gadolinium contrast dye (65). The variation in MRI findings likely relates to the variability of the composition of subretinal exudate and the extent of retinal detachment (66).

Analysis of subretinal fluid obtained intraoperatively by fine-needle aspiration can confirm the diagnosis of Coats' disease and permit safe and more thorough drainage. Colorless plates of cholesterol crystals, large pigment-laden cells, and fat-laden macrophages are present in Coats' disease and not in retinoblastoma (67,68). Fine-needle aspiration is not recommended as part of routine evaluation, however, because of the risk of seeding the orbit with malignant cells in cases of retinoblastoma. The measurement of lactate dehydrogenase in the aqueous humor has been studied, but this practice is not recommended because of the wide and nonspecific range of results (20,69–71).

DIFFERENTIAL DIAGNOSIS

Accurate diagnosis of Coats' disease, especially in advanced stages, can be difficult. In a series of 62 histologically confirmed cases, Coats' disease was the primary clinical diagnosis in only 13 (21%) (46). It must be distinguished from other conditions, some of them life threatening, that cause leukocoria, strabismus, or intraocular mass lesions. The differential diagnosis of Coats' disease is given in Table 29-1.

The most serious of these lesions is retinoblastoma (see Chapter 14), the most common primary intraocular malignancy in children. In cases of retinoblastoma, the age at diagnosis (average 18 months) is younger than in Coats' disease. Retinoblastoma has no gender predilection, bilaterality occurs in roughly one third of cases (72) from a germline mutation, and even in unilateral cases up to 19% have an

TABLE 29-1. DIFFERENTIAL DIAGNOSIS OF JUVENILE COATS' DISEASE

Retinoblastoma	Ocular toxocariasis
Von Hippel angiomatosis retinae	Incontinentia pigmenti
Retinopathy of prematurity	Pars planitis
Familial exudative vitreoretinopathy	Choroidal hemangioma
Persistent fetal vasculature	

underlying germline mutation. Ophthalmoscopically, the retinoblastoma lesion is pink, highly vascular, and often contains calcifications. Difficulty in differentiating retinoblastoma from Coats' disease arises most often in cases of exophytic retinoblastoma, in which the tumor grows into the subretinal space and causes a large exudative retinal detachment. In such instances, typical radiographic findings (usually from CT or MRI) can help confirm the diagnosis (20,65). Differentiating diffuse infiltrating retinoblastoma from Coats' disease can be difficult (73) because this form of retinoblastoma occurs at a later age and does not always demonstrate calcification (74).

Von Hippel angiomatosis retinae (see Chapter 15) is associated with renal cell carcinoma, pheochromocytoma, and vascular tumors of the central nervous system and viscera. Typically, this phakomatous lesion appears as a yellow or reddish balloonlike mass with a feeding arteriole and a draining venule. It is bilateral in 30% to 50% of cases, becomes symptomatic in early adulthood, and can be inherited in an autosomal dominant fashion. Genetic testing currently is available.

Familial exudative vitreoretinopathy (FEVR) and retinopathy of prematurity (ROP) can cause peripheral retinal vascular abnormalities. However, the vascular changes seen in FEVR and retinopathy of prematurity usually are bilateral and located at the vitreoretinal interface, not within the retina, as in Coats' disease. Additional diagnostic clues include a family history of FEVR or blindness or a history of premature birth. Persistent fetal vasculature syndrome (formerly known as *persistent hyperplastic primary vitreous*) occurs congenitally in an often microphthalmic eye. Ocular toxocariasis is suspected by a history of contact with puppies and is confirmed by serologic testing.

MANAGEMENT

Natural History

If untreated, Coats' disease most often deteriorates progressively at a variable rate. According to Gomez Morales (15), of 22 untreated patients followed for an average of 5 years, 14 (64%) developed total retinal detachment and 7 (32%) developed secondary glaucoma. Of the five patients in whom the disease appeared stable, the youngest was 7 years old. All four patients younger than 4 years

progressed rapidly to retinal detachment. Ridley et al. (75) confirmed that the rapidity of decline appears to correlate directly with the severity of disease and a younger age at presentation (15). In the series of advanced disease (exudative retinal detachment with subretinal mass) reported by Haik (20), 20 (80%) of 25 untreated eyes developed glaucoma or phthisis within 5 years, and 14 required enucleation. Factors that portend clinical and visual decline include extensive telangiectasias (involving three or more quadrants), diffuse exudation, presence of retinal macrocysts, and macular involvement (13,17,23,76,77).

Spontaneous regression of telangiectasias with resorption of subretinal fluid has been reported in rare instances (10,78). However, given the natural clinical course of the vast majority of children with Coats' disease, observation of actively leaking retinal telangiectasias is not recommended.

Treatment and Outcomes

Given the discouraging natural history of Coats' disease, early treatment, preferably at the time of diagnosis, is advised. All abnormal vasculature and areas of nonperfusion are treated to prevent progression of disease and, ultimately, to preserve vision.

Initial therapy of Coats' disease with antibiotics, corticosteroids, vitamins, and x-ray irradiation proved unsuccessful (79). In 1943, Guyton and McGovern (80) reported successful resolution of exudate with the application of diathermy coagulation to abnormal vascular proliferation. In the 1960s, direct photocoagulation, with xenon arc or argon laser, was used with encouraging results (15).

In many cases of early Coats' disease, elimination of telangiectasias and aneurysms will inhibit further exudation, induce resorption of already-formed exudate, and lead to resolution of serous detachments (12,19,76). Photocoagulation of peripheral vascular lesions can lead to resolution of macular exudates (Fig. 29-3A and B) (7,23,38). Favorable results are more likely to be obtained in early stages of disease (involvement of only one or two retinal quadrants) and in cases where treatment can be applied over areas of vascular, rather than exudative, changes (7). Multiple ablative treatments often are required to contain the vascular activity completely, and recurrences may be seen over a decade following successful treatment (17–19). In anticipation of recurrence, patients with Coats' disease should be examined every 6 months.

In their experience with 124 eyes with Coats' disease, Shields et al. (17) observed anatomic stabilization or improvement, defined as diminution of telangiectasias or resorption of exudate or subretinal fluid, in three fourths of cases. Only one fifth, however, achieved vision of better than 20/200. Sixteen percent required enucleation, most commonly for neovascular glaucoma. Older children and those presenting with retinal telangiectasias only (Shields stage 1) or minimal extrafoveal exudation (Shields stage 2A) are most likely to achieve vision of 20/200 or better. Visual outcomes of less than 20/200 are most often attributable to persistent retinal detachment, macular exudates, and subfoveal fibrosis and are more likely in eyes with extensive disease (17).

Cryotherapy, either alone or in combination with laser photocoagulation, is effective, especially in advanced cases with significant exudation (19). Complications of cryotherapy include posterior subcapsular cataract, proliferative vitreoretinopathy, and total retinal detachment (4,13). Because of the risk of retinal detachment, no more than two quadrants are treated with cryotherapy at one session.

In cases of partial retinal detachment, initial reapposition of the retina to the retinal pigment epithelium may be accomplished by drainage of subretinal fluid, with or without scleral buckling (19,81). Ablation of abnormal vessels is thus facilitated and is more likely to be effective.

Surgical treatment of children with advanced Coats' disease is directed more toward preservation of ocular comfort and cosmesis. Macular damage often is significant by the late stages of the disease, and visual potential is severely limited. Silodor et al. (82) used intraocular infusion, drainage of subretinal fluid, and cryotherapy in seven blind eyes and avoided enucleation in all seven. Six comparable eyes, left untreated, all eventually were enucleated (82). Advanced vitreoretinal surgical techniques have been used to salvage eyes with exudative and tractional retinal detachments and can maintain low levels of vision (81,83).

LONG-TERM MANAGEMENT AND VISUAL REHABILITATION

Parents of a child diagnosed with Coats' disease must be prepared for the sometimes inexorable course of the disease and the need for frequent monitoring and repeated treatment usually requiring general anesthesia. Most children with Coats' disease are otherwise healthy and live normal, productive lives. Visual rehabilitation with pediatric ophthalmologists and low-vision specialists is important in most cases of Coats' disease, particularly in the 10% of children with bilateral ocular involvement. With bilateral disease, there is the risk of total blindness. In these cases, the children and their siblings should be encouraged to learn the Braille alphabet.

ROLE OF OTHER PHYSICIANS AND PROFESSIONALS

Children can develop painful, neovascular glaucoma. Consultation with pediatric glaucoma specialists may be useful in some cases to reduce intraocular pressure, preserve the eye, and reduce pain. There are social and psychological considerations associated with a child growing up with a disfigured or phthisical eye. If enucleation is considered, the physician should consider the emotional trauma of the procedure and strive for an aesthetically acceptable surgical result. Consultation with an oculoplastic surgeon and an ocular prosthetic specialist can be helpful. Psychological support and occupational rehabilitation also can be helpful in certain cases. The importance of eye protection is stressed to all children with Coats' disease to reduce the risk of eye trauma while promoting normal daily activities and exercise. Children and families are counseled as to the importance of lifelong eye examinations.

FUTURE TREATMENT

Improvements in therapy and prognosis for children with Coats' disease are predicated foremost on a better understanding of its pathogenesis. In the absence of an identifiable genetic defect, preparation of an animal model is challenging. It is hoped that knowledge gained from the study of other vascular retinopathies, such as retinal angiomatosis or diabetic retinopathy, can be applied to Coats' disease. Pharmacologic modulation of vascular permeability, vasculogenesis, and lipid metabolism can hold promise as therapies for this debilitating disease.

REFERENCES

1. Coats G. Forms of retinal disease with massive exudation. *R Lond Ophthalmic Hosp Rep* 1908;17:440–525.
2. Coats G. Über Retinitis exsudativa (Retinitis haeorrhagica externa). *Graefes Arch Ophthalmol* 1912;81:275–327.
3. Leber TH. Über eine durch Vorkommen multipler Miliaraneurysmen characterisierte Form von Retinaldegeneration. *Graefes Arch Ophthalmol* 1912;81:1–14.
4. Gass JDM. *Stereoscopic atlas of macular diseases: diagnosis and treatment,* 3rd ed. St. Louis: Mosby, 1987.
5. Reese AB. Telangiectasis of the retina and Coats' disease. *Am J Ophthalmol* 1956;42:1–8.
6. Spitznas M, Joussen F, Wessing A, et al. Coats' disease. *Graefes Albrecht Graefes Arch Klin Exp Ophthalmol* 1975;195:241–250.
7. Theodossiadis GP, Bairaktaris-Kouris E, Kouris T. Evolution of Leber's military aneurysms: a clinicopathological study. *J Pediatr Ophthalmol Strabismus* 1979;16:364–370.
8. Duke-Elder S, Dobree JH. Coats' syndrome. In: Duke-Elder S, ed. *System of ophthalmology.* London: Kimpton, 1967:164–178.
9. Manschot WA, DeBruijn.WC. Coats' disease: definition and pathogenesis. *Br J Ophthalmol* 1967;51:145–157.
10. Campbell FP. Coats' disease and congenital vascular retinopathy. *Trans Am Ophthalmol Soc* 1976;74:365–424.
11. Green WR. Coats' disease. In: Spencer WH, ed. *Ophthalmic pathology.* Philadelphia: WB Saunders, 1996:700–708.
12. Spitznas M, Joussen F, Wessing A. Treatment of Coats' disease with photocoagulation. *Albrecht Von Graefes Arch Klin Exp Ophthalmol* 1976;199:31–37.
13. Tarkkanen A, Laatikainen L. Coats' disease: clinical, angiographic, histopathological findings and clinical management. *Br J Ophthalmol* 1983;67:766–776.

14. Woods AC, Duke JR. Coats' disease I. Review of the literature, diagnostic criteria, clinical findings, and plasma lipid studies. *Br J Ophthalmol* 1963;47:385–412.

15. Gomez Morales A. Coats' disease. Natural history and results of treatment. *Am J Ophthalmol* 1965;60:855–864.

16. Sigelman J. *Retinal diseases: pathogenesis, laser therapy, and surgery.* Boston: Little, Brown and Company, 1984.

17. Shields JA, Shields CL, Honavar SG, et al. Classification and management of Coats' disease: The 2000 Proctor lecture. *Am J Ophthalmol* 2001;131:572–583.

18. Shields JA, Shields CL, Honavar SG, et al. Clinical variations and complications of Coats' disease in 150 cases: the 2000 Sanford Gifford memorial lecture. *Am J Ophthalmol* 2001;131: 561–571.

19. Egerer I, Tasman W, Tomer T. Coats' disease. *Arch Ophthalmol* 1974;92:109–112.

20. Haik BG. Advanced Coats' disease. *Trans Am Ophthalmol Soc* 1991;89:371–476.

21. Imre G. Coats' disease. *Am J Ophthalmol* 1962;54:175–191.

22. McGettrick PM, Loeffler KU. Bilateral Coats' disease in an infant (a clinical, angiographic, light and electron microscopic study). *Eye* 1987;1:136–145.

23. Theodossiadis GP. Some clinical, fluorescein-angiographic, and therapeutic aspects of Coats' disease. *J Pediatr Ophthalmol Strabismus* 16:257–262.

24. Small RG. Coats' disease and muscular dystrophy. *Trans Am Acad Ophthalmol Otolaryngol* 1968;72:225–231.

25. Spallone A, Carlevaro G, Ridling P. Autosomal dominant retinitis pigmentosa and Coats'-like disease. *Int Ophthalmol* 1985;8: 147–151.

26. Lanier JD, McCrary JA III, Justice J. Autosomal recessive retinitis pigmentosa and Coats' disease. A presumed familial incidence. *Arch Ophthalmol* 1976;94:1737–1742.

27. Khan JA, Ide CH, Strckland MP. Coats'-type retinitis pigmentosa. *Surv Ophthalmol* 32:317–332.

28. Black GC, Perveen R, Bonshek R, et al. Coats' disease of the retina (unilateral retinal telangiectasis) caused by somatic mutation in the NDP gene: a role for norrin in retinal angiogenesis. *Hum Mol Genet* 1999;2031–2035.

29. Skuta GL, France TD, Stevens TS, et al. Apparent Coats' disease and pericentric inversion of chromosome 3. *Am J Ophthalmol* 1987;104:84–86.

30. Genkova P, Toncheva D, Tzoneva M, et al. Deletion of 13q12.1 in a child with Coats' disease. *Acta Paediatr Hung* 1986;27: 141–143.

31. Richter M, Gottanka J, May CA, et al. Retinal vasculature changes in Norrie disease mice. *Invest Ophthalmol Vis Sci* 1998;39:2450–2457.

32. Berinstein DM, Hiraoka M, Trese MT, et al. Coats' disease and congenital retinoschisis in a single eye: a case report and DNA analysis. *Ophthalmologica* 2001;215:132–135.

33. den Hollander AI, Heckenlively JR, van den Born LI, et al. Leber congenital amaurosis and retinitis pigmentosa with Coats'-like exudative vasculopathy are associated with mutations in the crumbs homologue 1 (CRB1) gene. *Am J Hum Genet* 2001;69: 198–203.

34. Wise GN. Coats' disease. *AMA Arch Ophthalmol* 1957;58: 735–746.

35. Imre G. Coats' disease and hyperlipemic retinitis. *Am J Ophthalmol* 64:726–728.

36. Egbert PR, Chan C, Winter FC. Flat preparations of the retinal vessels in Coats' disease. *J Pediatr Ophthalmol* 1976;13: 336–339.

37. Tripathi R, Ashton N. Electron microscopical study of Coats' disease. *Br J Ophthalmol* 1972;55:289–301.

38. Farkas TG, Potts AM, Boone C. Some pathologic and biochemical aspects of Coats' disease. *Am J Ophthalmol* 1973;75:289–301.

39. Green WR. Bilateral Coats' disease. Massive gliosis of the retina. *Arch Ophthalmol* 1967;77:378–383.

40. Takel Y. Origin of ghost cell in Coats' disease. *Invest Ophthalmol* 1976;15:677–681.

41. Judisch JF, Apple DJ. Orbital cellulites in an infant secondary to Coats' disease. *Arch Ophthalmol* 1980;98:2004–2006.

42. Patel HK, Augsburger JJ, Eagle RC Jr. Unusual presentation of advanced Coats' disease. *J Pediatr Ophthalmol Strabismus* 1995;32:120–122.

43. Chisholm IA, Foulds WS, Christison D. Investigation and therapy of Coats' disease. *Ophthalmol Soc U K* 1974;94:355–341.

44. Henkind P, Morgan G. Peripheral retinal angioma with exudative retinopathy in adults (Coats' lesion). *Br J Ophthalmol* 1966;50:2–11.

45. Fox KR. Coats' disease. *Metab Pediatr Ophthalmol* 1980;4: 121–124.

46. Chang M, McLean IW, Merritt JC. Coats' disease: a study of 62 histologically confirmed cases. *J Pediatr Ophthalmol Strabismus* 1984;21:163–168.

47. Lee ST, Friedman SM, Rubin ML. Cystoid macular edema secondary to justafoveolar telangiectasias in Coats' disease. *Ophthalmic Surg* 1991;22:218–221.

48. Goel S, Augsburger JJ. Hemorrhagic retinal macrocysts in advanced Coats' disease. *Retina* 1991;11:437–440.

49. Kremer I, Cohen S, Izhak RB, et al. An unusual case of congenital unilateral Coats's disease associated with morning glory optic disc anomaly. *Br J Ophthalmol* 1985;69:32–37.

50. Wilensky JT, Goldberg MF, Ziyai F, et al. Infantile cataracts, Coats' disease, and ketotic hyperglycemia. *J Pediatr Ophthalmol* 1976;13:75–79.

51. Pruett RC. Retinitis pigmentosa: clinical observations and correlations. *Trans Am Ophthalmol Soc* 1983;81:693–735.

52. Gurwin EB, Fitzsimons RB, Sehmi KS, et al. Retinal telangiectasias in facioscapulohumeral muscular dystrophy with deafness. *Arch Ophthalmol* 1985;103:1695–1700.

53. Fitzsimons RB, Gurwin EB, Bird AC. Retinal vascular abnormalities in facioscapulohumeral muscular dystrophy. *Brain* 1987;110:631–648.

54. Cameron JD, Yanoff M, Frayer WC. Coats' disease and Turner's syndrome. *Am J Ophthalmol* 1974;78:852–854.

55. Neki AS, Sharma A. Ipsilateral Coat's reaction in the eye of a child with en coup de saber morphoea: a case report. *Ind J Ophthalmol* 1992;40:115–116.

56. Newell SW, Hall BD, Anderson CW, et al. Hallermann-Streiff syndrome with Coats' disease. *J Pediatr Ophthalmol Strabismus* 1994;31:123–125.

57. Schuman JS, Lieberman KV, Friedman AH, et al. Senior-Loken syndrome (familial renal-retinal dystrophy) and Coats' disease. *Am J Ophthalmol* 1985;100:822–827.

58. Folk JC, Genovese FN, Biglan AW. Coats' disease in a patient with Cornelia de Lange syndrome. *Am J Ophthalmol* 1981;91: 607–610.

59. Burch JV, Leveille AS, Morse PH. Ichthyosis hystrix (epidermal nevus syndrome) and Coats' disease. *Am J Ophthalmol* 1980;89:25–30.

60. Kajtar P, Mehes K. Bilateral Coats' retinopathy associated with aplastic anemia and mild dyskeratotic signs. *Am J Med Genet* 1994;49:374–377.

61. Robitaille JM, Monsein L, Traboulsi EI. Coats' disease and central nervous system venous malformation. *Ophthalmic Genet* 1996;17:215–218.

62. Atta HR, Watson NJ. Echographic diagnosis of advanced Coats' disease. *Eye* 1992;6:80–85.

63. Senft SH, Hidayat AA, Cavender JC. Atypical presentation of Coats' disease. *Retina* 1994;14:36–38.

64. Katz NNK, Margo CE, Dorwart RH. Computed tomography with histopathologic correlation in children with leukocoria. *J Pediatr Ophthalmol Strabismus* 1984;21:50–56.

65. De Potter P, Shields CL, Shields JA. The role of magnetic resonance imaging in children with intraocular tumors and simulating lesions. *Ophthalmology* 1996;103:1774–1783.

66. Lai WW, Edward DP, Weiss RA, et al. Magnetic resonance imaging findings in a case of advanced Coats' disease. *Ophthalmic Surg Lasers* 1996;27:234–238.

67. Haik BG, Koizumi J, Smith ME, et al. Fresh preparation of subretinal fluid aspirations in Coats' disease. *Am J Ophthalmol* 1985;100:327–328.

68. Kremer I, Nissenkorn I, Ben-Sira I. Cytologic and biochemical examination of the subretinal fluid in diagnosis of Coats' disease. *Acta Ophthalmol* 1989;67:342–346.

69. Das A, Roy IS, Maitra TK. Lactate dehydrogenase level and protein pattern in the aqueous humour of patients with retinoblastoma. *Can J Ophthalmol* 19983;18337–18339.

70. Jakobiec FA, Abramson D, Scher R. Increased aqueous lactate dehydrogenase in Coats' disease. *Am J Ophthalmol* 1978;85:686–689.

71. Lifshitz T, Tessler Z, Maor E, et al. Increased aqueous lactic dehydrogenase in Coat's disease. *Ann Ophthalmol* 1987;19:116–119.

72. Shields JA, Parsons HM, Shields CL, et al. Lesions simulating retinoblastoma. *J Pediatr Ophthalmol Strabismus* 1991;26:338–340.

73. Steidl SM, Hirose T, Sang D, et al. Difficulties in excluding the diagnosis of retinoblastoma in cases of advanced Coats' disease: a clinicopathologic report. *Ophthalmologica* 1996;210:336–340.

74. Shields CL, Honavar S, Shields JA, et al. Vitrectomy in eyes with unsuspected retinoblastoma. *Ophthalmology* 2000;107:2250–2255.

75. Ridley ME, Shields JA, Brown GC, et al. Coats' disease. Evaluation of management. *Ophthalmology* 1982;89:1381–1387.

76. Harris GS. Coats' disease, diagnosis and treatment. *Can J Ophthalmol* 1970;5:311–320.

77. Budning AS, Heon E, Gallie BL. Visual prognosis of Coats' disease. *J AAPOS* 1998;2:356–359.

78. Deutsch TA, Rabb MF, Jampol LM. Spontaneous regression of retinal lesions in Coats' disease. *Can J Ophthalmol* 1982;17:169–172.

79. McGrand JC. Photocoagulation in Coats' disease. *Trans Ophthalmol Soc U K* 1970;90:47–56.

80. Guyton JS, McGovern FH. Diathermy coagulation in the treatment of angiomatosis retinae and of juvenile Coats' disease: report of two cases. *Am J Ophthalmol* 1943;26:675–684.

81. Schmidt-Erfurth U, Lucke K. Vitreoretinal surgery in advanced Coats' disease. *Ger J Ophthalmol* 1995;4:32–36.

82. Silodor SW, Augsburger JJ, Shields JA, et al. Natural history and management of advanced Coats' disease. *Ophthalmic Surg* 1988;19:89–93.

83. Yoshizumi MO, Kreiger AE, Lewis H, et al. Vitrectomy techniques in late-stage Coats'-like exudative retinal detachment. *Doc Ophthalmol* 1995;90:387–394.

30

PERSISTENT FETAL VASCULATURE SYNDROME (PERSISTENT HYPERPLASTIC PRIMARY VITREOUS)

MICHAEL T. TRESE
ANTONIO CAPONE, JR.

Persistent hyperplastic primary vitreous (PHPV) is an ocular assembly disorder in which fetal vasculature does not regress. It is unilateral approximately 90% of the time. The process does not tend to be progressive during the course of the child's life, but tractional intraocular changes can occur later, most likely due to eye growth. Recently, the term *persistent fetal vasculature* (PFV) *syndrome* has been introduced (1) and is a better name because it addresses the fact that persistent hyaloid vessels and tunica vascular lentis can persist and lead to a spectrum of structural changes within the eye. Other chapters in this textbook deal with the embryologic development of the vitreous and retina. However, in order to appreciate the process of PFV syndrome, we must recall that the hyaloid system, also referred to as the *primary vitreous,* is more than just the hyaloid vessel that extends from the optic nerve to the back of the lens. The hyaloid vasculature actually fills the vitreous cavity and has many attachments to the retinal surface. The hyaloid system usually is regressed by 28 to 30 weeks' gestational age, and the remnant of the hyaloid vessels can exist within the Cloquet canal after birth (2). The tunica vasculosa lentis includes anterior and posterior divisions encircling the human lens. Anteriorly, the tunica vasculosa lentis includes the lens and has attachments that extend to the pupillary frill of the iris and onto the anterior lens surface (Fig. 30-1). Posterior to the lens, the tunica vasculosa lentis covers the lens and interdigitates with the hyaloid system. It also is attached to the ciliary process (Fig. 30-2). When the tunica vasculosa lentis persists, the lens does not form properly. The tunica vasculosa lentis usually persists more prominently at the posterior lens surface and can create a lens opacity. In typical anterior PFV syndrome, no lens capsule is present posteriorly, making peeling tissue from the posterior lens impossible (3).

PFV syndrome has a spectrum of presentations depending on the degree of involution of the hyaloid and tunica vasculosa lentis. PFV syndrome can be associated with varying amounts of retinal dysplasia, which frequently is the rate-limiting step for postoperative vision beyond that from anisometropic aphakic amblyopia following lens removal in this predominantly unilateral process.

PFV syndrome can present with predominant features of the tunica vasculosa lentis without much or any posterior hyaloid component (Fig. 30-3) (4). Alternatively, the hyaloid vasculature can persist with little in the way of regressed tunica vasculosa lentis (Figure 30-4). Eyes with predominantly hyaloid changes often are referred to as *posterior PFV syndrome* and those with predominantly tunica vasculosa changes as *anterior PFV syndrome.*

Although PFV syndrome (PHPV) has been recognized for many years, a single gene for PFV syndrome has not been identified. Certainly, the PFV syndrome process, which involves an interrupted genetically programmed involution of embryonic vessels and the assembly of the lens and retinal tissue, is considered likely to have a genetic etiology. A six-generation consanguineous Pakistani family showing linkage to chromosome 10q11–q21 has been reported (5). The abnormal gene in this family has not yet been found, and whether or not it will explain other PFV syndrome cases remains to be determined. Additionally, mutations in the *PAX6* gene were detected recently in patients with optic nerve malformations that included PFV syndrome (6).

When bilateral PFV syndrome is present, Norrie disease must be ruled out (6a). Although Norrie disease is commonly thought to mimic persistent fetal vascular syndrome, it often has a more severe hemorrhagic and dysplastic retinal detachment. In some circumstances (<27%), hearing or central nervous system abnormalities are present (7,8). Other systemic associations have been reported with PFV syndrome, most often in association with central nervous system problems (9). However, many of these reports do not rule out mutations in the Norrie disease gene. Associations have also been reported with oculo-palatal-cerebral syndrome (10), intrauterine herpes simplex virus infection (11), intrauterine exposure to clomiphene, oral-facial-digital syndrome, anterior and posterior colobomas or even cystic globes (12,13), and tuberous sclerosis (14).

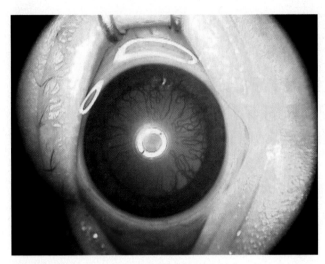

FIGURE 30-1. Persistent anterior tunica vasculosa lentis vessels. These vessels are persistent, are not neovascularization, and are best referred to as *rubeosis iridis.*

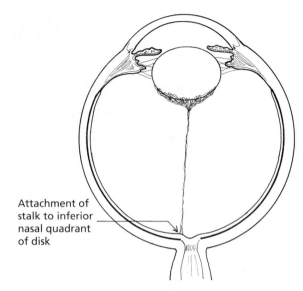

FIGURE 30-3. Illustration of the opaque posterior lens tissue, elongated ciliary processes, and fine stalk extending to the disc. This is predominantly anterior persistent fetal vasculature syndrome.

Attachment of stalk to inferior nasal quadrant of disk

CLINICAL PICTURE

PFV syndrome is customarily described as the involved eye being a smaller eye with a posterior lens opacity, elongated ciliary processes, and, if visible, a stalk that extends from the lens posterior to the optic disc (Fig. 30-5). There is variability in clinical presentation. In our experience, the severity of anterior segment appearance, globe size, severity of lens involvement, or vascular appearance does *not* predict the amount of retinal dysplasia, which in turn often determines the eye's visual result.

Ultrasound, computed tomographic scanning, magnetic resonance imaging, and visual evoked potential testing have not been reliable in predicting retinal dysplasia. However, of these modalities, visual evoked potential testing is perhaps the most helpful (15). If a response is present, then it can be helpful in the decision whether to recommend surgery for a retinal detachment. This is most helpful when the other eye is uninvolved, and the waveforms can be compared.

The problem of PFV syndrome can be divided into two components that affect vision: the media opacity and retinal changes (both dysplasia and traction). The stalk also can cause traction on the posterior lens capsule leading to poste-

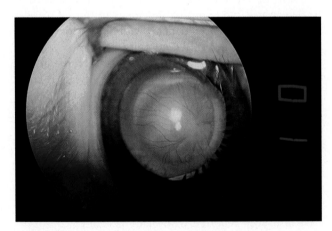

FIGURE 30-2. Vessels extending from the lens surface to the ciliary processes. These vessels can be divided with little bleeding after the central vessel is treated with diathermy.

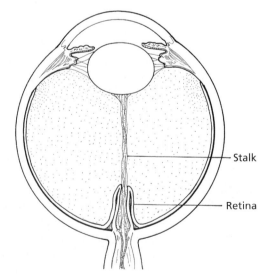

FIGURE 30-4. Illustration of the stalk attachment to the lens, obstructing the visual axis. Retina is draped around the stalk or hyaloid tissue. Bending the stalk can pinch retinal vessels.

Stalk

Retina

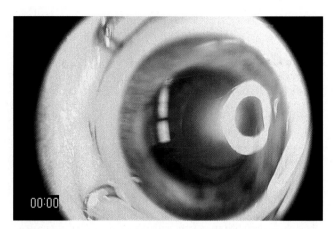

FIGURE 30-5. Typical persistent fetal vasculature syndrome with a smaller eye, elongated ciliary processes, and media opacity.

rior lenticonus (Fig. 30-6). In addition, traction on the ciliary body can lead to hypotony.

Media opacities are addressed similarly to congenital cataract and, for the most part, are handled by lens removal, refraction, and amblyopia therapy (16). The tractional effects and retinal dysplastic features are not as well understood. The stalk itself can be a simple columnlike structure that extends from the lens to the optic nerve or posterior retina or can be an inverted Y shape with a second or even third arm that attaches to the disc and elsewhere on the retinal surface. The stalk can exert traction on the retina, leading to areas of tractional retinal detachment. The stalk can insert anteriorly on the lens either centrally, involving the visual axis, or eccentrically, sparing the visual axis of the lens. If the stalk is eccentric, no change in visual acuity is noticed

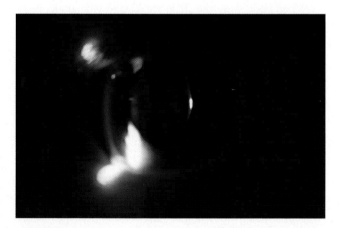

FIGURE 30-6. Slitlamp photograph showing the bowing of the posterior lens surface in the child with an eccentric stalk who did not have surgery as an infant and developed posterior lenticonus.

in the very young child, but strabismus can result. If there is a visual axis opacity, the problem usually is discovered at the newborn screening. The child with a stalk eccentric to the visual axis often presents with strabismus later in life, at age 9 to 10 months (17).

The tractional component on the lens is perhaps even less well known. The eccentric stalk that leaves the visual axis clear does not always need surgical intervention. Tractional effects on the lens or retina determine whether surgical intervention with division of the stalk is necessary. Retinoscopy, giving a scissorslike reflex, can help to identify progressive posterior lenticonus as a result of the traction of the fixed stalk on the posterior lens surface during eye growth.

The traction on the ciliary body is primarily a function of the tunica vasculosa lentis and must be relieved in order to avoid one of the complications of the long-term PFV syndrome, hypotony, which we believe is due to prolonged ciliary body traction resulting in either ciliary process damage or ciliary body detachment.

Retinal dysplasia has a wide range of clinical presentations and can involve the retinal circulation and the cellular retina. We divide retinal dysplasia into macroscopic and microscopic types. *Macroscopic dysplasia* is defined as changes easily visible with the operating microscope or indirect ophthalmoscope. *Microscopic dysplasia* occurs at the cellular or vascular level. Although at present we have no way to determine cell dysplasia, vascular dysplasia can be assessed by fluorescein angiography. An example of vascular dysplasia is the lack of a capillary-free zone. This finding can be missed without angiography and might account for some of the poor vision after successful surgery. It is not unusual for a surgeon to anticipate good vision after surgery for PFVS based on the clinical appearance of the retina. After a reasonable course of amblyopia therapy, the doctor might find that vision better than 20/100 is not possible. The converse also can be true: that eyes with unusual appearing posterior poles can sometimes achieve better vision. Recently, we found that alterations in the foveal circulation detected by fluorescein angiography predicted foveal hypoplasia and poor central visual acuity. However, such changes may not always be detectable. We use fluorescein angiography and a full examination under anesthesia to determine if the foveal structure is good enough to merit continued amblyopia therapy. If the child is older, optical coherence tomographic testing can be performed to further define foveal architecture.

The surgeon should be aware that intrinsic retinal vessels can be pulled onto the stalk tissue and occasionally can be dragged one to two thirds the length of the stalk toward the lens. In addition, retinal tissue can cloak the stalk, giving it more substance. This requires great care to divide only stalk tissue, not retina or intrinsic retinal vessels. This could lead to a retinal hole or bleeding, followed by a retinal ischemic event (Fig. 30-7).

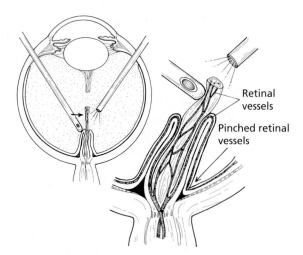

Retinal vessels

Pinched retinal vessels

FIGURE 30-7. Illustration of moving the stalk tissue to determine if intrinsic retinal circulation is in the stalk tissue. If moving the stalk changes the retinal vascular flow, then the surgical goal is to only minimally dissect the stalk.

DIFFERENTIAL DIAGNOSIS

The differential diagnosis depends on the ocular appearance. For leukocoria, the most important differential diagnosis is retinoblastoma. Retinoblastoma must be ruled out. It is uncommon to see retinoblastoma in a smaller eye. PFV syndrome often is unilateral and involves the smaller eye. Without a good view into the eye, retinoblastoma must be ruled out prior to any intraocular surgery. Computed tomographic scanning to detect intraocular calcifications in retinoblastoma is helpful. Further discussion is found in Chapter 14. The other differential diagnostic considerations are congenital cataract, Norrie disease, Walker-Warburg syndrome, and trisomy (18). Familial exudative vitreoretinopathy, incontinentia pigmenti, and retinopathy of prematurity are included in the differential diagnosis when eyes have total retinal detachments and retrolental fibrous tissues (19).

TREATMENT

Many series reported in the literature describe surgical management of PFV syndrome or PHPV (15,20,21). These series present anatomic and visual results and complication rates. These studies are very hard to compare, particularly when assessing the visual outcomes because visual outcomes are dependent on retinal dysplasia, the timing of surgery, and postoperative amblyopic therapy (21,22).

We describe here the techniques we use in the management of three distinctly different presentations of PFV syndrome: (i) the typical form with significant media opacity and hyaloid stalk remnant, (ii) the eccentric stalk with variable changes in the posterior pole, and (iii) the less common combination of posterior coloboma, PFV syndrome, and

microphthalmia. In eyes with significant media opacity from congenital cataract, rapid intervention is advised.

Typical Persistent Fetal Vasculature Syndrome

The eye presents with leukocoria in a child usually shortly after birth, within 1 to 2 weeks. No obvious systemic changes are present, retinoblastoma is ruled out, and the involved eye usually is somewhat smaller than the fellow eye. The lens itself is clear anteriorly with an opaque posterior surface. You may or may not be able to see around the opacity in the lens. You may see some elongated ciliary processes, depending on the degree of pupillary dilatation. The pupil may be difficult to dilate because of the anterior tunica vasculosa lentis (TVL). The surgical approach we prefer is a two-port technique. We first use a 23-gauge butterfly fashioned for infusion and vitreous cutter to remove the lens material. We prefer entry made through the iris root and dissection posterior to the iris. When the opaque tissue is removed, diathermy is used to treat the central vessel. The opaque tissue and lens zonules are divided from the ciliary processes. The lens and opaque tissue is removed, usually using the vitreous cutter with care to circumcise the stalk tissue. The eye with PFV syndrome can harbor choristomatous tissue in this opaque lens tissue, such as cartilage that is not removable with the vitreous cutter. This dense cartilage tissue sometimes can be divided with scissors and removed in small pieces, or it may need to be moved to the anterior chamber and removed through the limbus as a foreign body (23).

Once the position and size of the stalk are determined, the surgeon can manage the stalk tissue. It is helpful to remember that the average hyaloid remnant often is inserted slightly nasal to the visual axis on the posterior aspect of the lens and often inserts into the inferior nasal quadrant of the disc.

When addressing the stalk, we used a wide-angle, high-flow light pipe (Synergetics) and MPC scissors (Alcon). The stalk is inspected for areas of hyaloid tissue that are not covered by retinal tissue or retinal vessels. The stalk is pushed from side to side before dividing it to see if pushing the vessels in the stalk alters the retinal circulation (Fig. 30-7). If it does, then we are likely to leave the stalk longer. It is not necessary to remove the entire stalk. Often one does not see the disc tissue well during its dissection. Stalk tissue can continue to regress after surgery and, rarely, completely disappears over many months. There often are fine areas of organized vitreous that support the stalk posteriorly. These can be hyaloid remnants and should be divided in a fashion that keeps the stalk from falling toward the center of the macula.

At the end of dissection, a fluid–air exchange is performed, and the child is positioned face down for the first night. Postoperative drops include a cycloplegic, steroid, and antibiotic. A metal shield and elbow restraints are used to protect the eye from ocular trauma. The eye is examined 1 day following surgery.

Persistent Fetal Vasculature Syndrome with Eccentric Stalk

The child generally presents to the ophthalmologist or pediatrician with strabismus at age 9 to 10 months. The stalk of tissue is attached eccentric to the visual axis and extends posteriorly creating traction on the posterior lens surface and posterior lenticonus, as well as traction on the retina in the posterior pole of the eye (Fig. 30-8) (17). These eyes can have a pigmented demarcation line from the effect of retinal traction. If traction is not exerted on the lens capsule or retina, or perhaps if the stalk is lax, then the eye may not require surgical intervention.

If surgery is determined to be necessary, the technique is much different than that of typical PFV syndrome. Although retinal dysplasia perhaps has the primary effect on visual outcome, amblyopia and anisometropia amblyopia also are factors. It has been shown that lensectomy, even at age 10 months, can result in good vision (16). In eyes with PFV syndrome and an eccentric stalk, the stalk and its traction can be addressed using a lens-sparing vitrectomy. The main differences in the techniques are that (i) entry is through the pars plicata avoiding the lens, and (ii) the first step is to divide the stalk without vitrectomy first or diathermy of the stalk (17). Any manipulation of the stalk can result in damage to the posterior lens capsule around the area of attachment of the stalk to the lens (exaggerated Mittendorf dot). After the stalk is divided, the anterior remnant is not manipulated. This anterior stalk tissue can also partially involute over time. After being divided, the posterior stalk tissue often immediately retracts several millimeters during surgery, demonstrating the force exerted by the stalk tissue. After entry into the eye and division of the stalk, the vitrectomy techniques are the same as those described for typical PFV syndrome. In one series managed in this fash-

ion, the majority of children showed improvement of function and resolution of strabismus without muscle surgery following vitreous surgery (17).

Persistent Fetal Vasculature Syndrome with Posterior Coloboma

PFV syndrome with posterior coloboma can present with both typical opaque media and eccentric stalks. In these eyes, the considerations of PFV syndrome are similar to those described earlier. In addition, the coloboma may involve the center of the macula (Fig. 30-9). We have found that fluorescein angiography can be helpful in defining the presence of a capillary-free zone, which can predict the development of the fovea in a child less than 3 months post term (Fig. 30-10). We have also examined a child who had an eccentric stalk in one eye that allowed visualization of the posterior pole and a much smaller fellow eye with opaque media. The eye with a view of the posterior pole had a large posterior coloboma. On fluorescein angiography, the capillary-free zone had alterations predictive of a poorer foveal development. The second eye with no view of the posterior pole and a 7-mm cornea was operated by lensectomy-vitrectomy and removal of the stalk. The eye also had a coloboma but, on clinical examination, a potentially better foveal anatomy. Despite being much smaller than the fellow eye, this eye achieved 20/60 vision with 3-year follow-up, whereas the larger fellow eye had 20/400 vision. The visual evoked potential had predicted some retinal function in the smaller eye with opaque media.

PFV syndrome and coloboma may be a continuum of optic pit coloboma and morning glory disc (24,25).

All of these surgical approaches must be followed by careful and continuing visual rehabilitation emphasizing refractive testing and amblyopia techniques. The importance of this must be made clear with the parents, because the surgical technique itself will not result in full visual potential without postoperative visual rehabilitation.

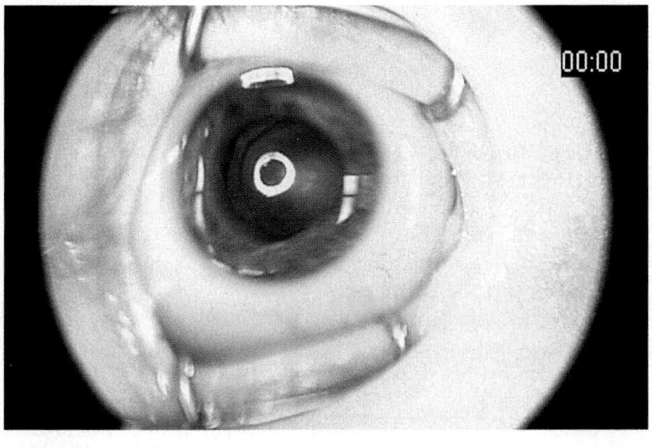

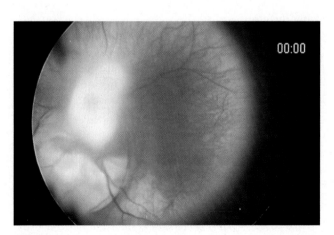

FIGURE 30-8. Location of the eccentric stalk attaching to the posterior lens surface.

FIGURE 30-9. Persistent fetal vasculature syndrome stalk extending from the coloboma.

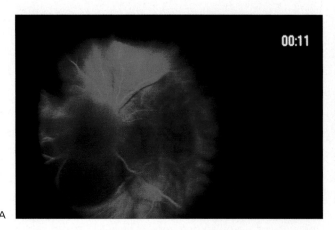
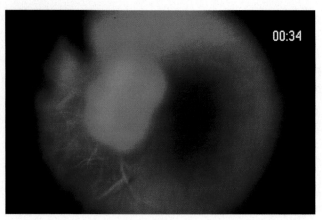

FIGURE 30-10. A: Fluorescein angiogram demonstrating altered macular architecture. **B:** Stalk tissue fluorescence in the late phase of the angiogram.

Surgical complications are similar to those of any vitreoretinal surgery. However, PFV syndrome surgery appears to have a higher risk for postoperative glaucoma, reported in 32% of eyes in one study (26). In the author's experience, hypotony can be a lasting problem for eyes with PFV syndrome. We believe this is due to ciliary process damage or detachment of the ciliary body.

The visual results following surgical therapy for PFVS range from 20/20 to no light perception (NLP), depending on surgical complications, the extent of retinal dysplasia, and amblyopia therapy.

Often parents are concerned about the cosmetic issues of a child with one eye that is much smaller than the other. In these children, the first consideration should be visual, but if that is resolved and vision is not possible for that eye, then cosmetic consideration is appropriate. There are differing opinions on the effect of a smaller globe and orbital development. Some believe that a small globe will not permit normal growth of the orbit and will result in a smaller orbit. Others believe that any globe will stimulate orbital growth. We have used conformers and prosthetics to stretch the lids and a safety spectacle to protect the other eye and detract from the prosthetic eye. Enucleation is rarely needed.

PFV syndrome has a variety of presentations and possible anatomic and visual results. Although no distinct genetic mutation has been found for unilateral typical PFV syndrome, the genetic changes of Norrie disease give us hope that such a mutation may be found and that gene therapy may be possible for these children.

REFERENCES

1. Goldberg MF. Persistent fetal vasculature (PFV): an integrated interpretation of signs and symptoms associated with persistent hyperplastic primary vitreous (PHPV). LIV Edward Jackson Memorial Lecture. *Am J Ophthalmol* 1997;124:587–626.
2. Barishak YR. *Embryology of the eye and its adnexa,* 2nd rev ed. Basel, Switzerland: S. Karger, 2001:80.
3. Spencer WH. *Ophthalmic pathology: an atlas and textbook,* 3rd ed, vol. 1. Philadelphia: WB Saunders, 1985:439.
4. deJuan E Jr, Farr A, Noorily S. Retinal detachment in infants. In: Ryan SJ, Wilkinson CP, eds. *Retina,* 3rd ed., vol. 3, Surgical retina. St. Louis: Mosby, 2001:2506.
5. Khaliq S, Hameed A, Ismail M, et al. Locus for autosomal recessive nonsyndromic persistent hyperplastic primary vitreous. *Invest Ophthalmol Vis Sci* 2001;42:2225–228.
6. Azuma N, Yamaguchi Y, Handa H, et al. Mutations of the PAX6 gene detected in patients with a variety of optic-nerve malformations. *Am J Hum Genet* 2003;72:1565–1570.
6a. deJuan E Jr, Farr A, Noorily S. Retinal detachment in infants. In: Ryan SJ, Wilkinson CP, eds. *Retina,* 3rd ed., vol. 3, Surgical retina. St. Louis: Mosby, 2001:2501.
7. Enyedi LB, deJuan E. Ultrastructural study of Norrie's disease. *Am J Ophthalmol* 1991;111:439–445.
8. Esakowitz L, Clark C: A genetic linkage study of a family with Norrie's disease. *Eye* 1988;2:443–447.
9. Marshman WE, Jan JE, Lyons CJ. Neurologic abnormalities associated with persistent hyperplastic primary vitreous. *Can J Ophthalmol* 1999;34:17–22.
10. Pellegrino JE, Engel JM, Chavez D. Oculo-palatal-cerebral syndrome: a second case (review). *Am J Med Genet* 2001;99: 200–203.
11. Corey RP, Flynn JT. Maternal intrauterine herpes simplex virus infection leading to persistent fetal vasculature. *Arch Ophthalmol* 2000;118:837–840.
12. Tsai PS, O'Brien JM. Retinal hamartoma in oral-facial-digital syndrome. *Arch Ophthalmol* 1999;117:963–965.
13. Pasquale LR, Romayananda N, Kubacki J, et al. Congenital cystic eye with multiple ocular and intracranial anomalies. *Arch Ophthalmol* 1991;109:985–987.
14. Milot J, Michaud J, Lemieux N, et al. Persistent hyperplastic primary vitreous with retinal tumor in tuberous sclerosis: report of a case including tumoral immunohistochemistry and cytogenetic analyses. *Ophthalmology* 1999;106:630–634.
15. Dass AB, Trese MT. Surgical results of persistent hyperplastic primary vitreous. *Ophthalmology* 1999;106:280–284.
16. Hosal BM, Biglan AW, Elhan AH. High levels of binocular function are achievable after removal of monocular cataracts in children before 8 years of age. *Ophthalmology* 2000;107: 1647–1655.
17. Shaikh S, Trese MT. Lens-sparing vitrectomy in predominantly posterior persistent fetal vasculature syndrome in eyes with non-axial lens opacification. *Retina* 2003;23:330–334.

18. Heggie P, Grossniklaus HE, Roessmann U, et al. Cerebro-ocular dysplasia-muscular dystrophy syndrome. Report of two cases. *Arch Ophthalmol* 1987;105:520–524.

19. Chang-Godinich A, Paysse EA, Coats DK, et al. Familial exudative vitreoretinopathy mimicking persistent hyperplastic primary vitreous. *Am J Ophthalmol* 1999;127:469–471.

20. Mittra RA, Huynh LT, Ruttum MS, et al. Visual outcomes following lensectomy and vitrectomy for combined anterior and posterior persistent hyperplastic primary vitreous. *Arch Ophthalmol* 1998;116:1190–1194.

21. Karr DJ, Scott WE. Visual acuity results following treatment of persistent hyperplastic primary vitreous. *Arch Ophthalmol* 1986;104:662–667.

22. Alexandrakis G, Scott IU, Flynn HW Jr, et al. Visual acuity outcomes with and without surgery in patients with persistent fetal vasculature. *Ophthalmology* 2000;107:1068–1072.

23. Shiraki K, Moriwaki M, Kohno T. Incising the thick retrolental fibrovascular tissue with a hooked sclerotome in persistent hyperplastic primary vitreous. *Ophthalmic Surg Lasers* 1999;30:758–761.

24. Apple DJ. New aspects of colobomas and optic nerve anomalies. *Int Ophthalmol Clin* 1984;24:109.

25. Daufenbach DR, Ruttum MS, Pulido JS, et al. Chorioretinal colombas in a pediatric population. *Ophthalmology* 1998;105:1455–1458.

26. Johnson CP, Keech RV. Prevalence of glaucoma after surgery for PHPV and infantile cataracts. *J Pediatr Ophthalmol Strabismus* 1996;33:14–17.

SURGICAL APPROACHES TO UVEITIS

MELANIE H. ERB
BARUCH D. KUPPERMANN

Childhood uveitis is generally considered a medical subspecialty within the field of ophthalmology, and the mainstay of therapy is aggressive control of ocular inflammation with corticosteroids. Occasionally, surgical intervention is necessary in the pediatric uveitic patient. Diagnostic surgery may be needed in the pursuit of the underlying diagnosis. Therapeutic surgery may be needed to treat the multitude of complications that occur in an eye that has been chronically and recurrently inflamed. In the past, surgery often was attempted hesitantly because of a high incidence of complications, including uncontrolled postoperative inflammation, hypotony, and phthisis. Two advances have contributed to safer surgical intervention in uveitic eyes. The first advance is more aggressive control of chronic and recurrent inflammation by ophthalmologists using corticosteroids or immunosuppressants. The second advance is improved microsurgical instruments and techniques in anterior segment and vitreoretinal surgery (1,2).

Corticosteroids comprise the cornerstone of therapy for uveitis. Vigilant control of intraocular inflammation prevents or curtails the complications of uveitis that cause irreversible ocular structural damage. Aggressive treatment is crucial at the time of diagnosis, with frequent topical corticosteroid dosing. Periocular or systemic corticosteroids may be needed to gain adequate control of the inflammation. Steroid tapering schedules should continually be reevaluated and readjusted to abolish the recurrence of a low-grade inflammation. Even low-grade inflammation will continue to wreak damage to ocular structures. Patients who receive long-term steroid therapy may develop unacceptable side effects at the dosages needed to control the inflammation. In these patients, immunosuppressant medications may need to be added as steroid-sparing agents.

The decision to proceed with therapeutic surgery on a child for the complications of uveitis is a difficult one and must be considered carefully (Table 31-1). Operating on an eye that has been repeatedly or chronically inflamed is very different from operating on an eye that has not been inflamed (1). Surgery in pediatric uveitic eyes is daunting to even the most accomplished cataract surgeon because of the unknown risks faced intraoperatively and the uncertainty of the postoperative course (3,4). Surgery is frequently technically challenging because of corneal opacification, posterior synechiae, iris vasculature delicacy, excessive bleeding, pupillary membranes, and miotic pupil (5). The combination of the pediatric heightened immune response and a uveitic eye often results in a fierce postoperative inflammatory response following the most exquisite, gentle operation. Eyes may become hypotonous or phthisical. Thus, the decision to operate must not be taken lightly.

On the other hand, delayed surgical intervention in these children may lead to permanent structural damage to the eye, causing irreversible macular pathology and optic nerve pathology that will limit any future postsurgical ability of achieving a good visual outcome. Delayed intervention also may result in visual loss from amblyopia and strabismus in this patient population. There is a point in the course of the disease where the benefits of surgery outweigh the risks.

The essential element for a successful surgery is careful control of inflammation. Details on control of inflammation during and after surgery are given under specific surgical sections that follow. It is important to work closely with a pediatric ophthalmologist to manage and reduce possible amblyopia. The age of the child at the time of surgery, the presence or absence of amblyopia, and the presence of irreversible retinal or optic nerve pathology are the primary factors influencing the outcome of surgery in the pediatric uveitic patient.

This chapter first discusses diagnostic surgical procedures that may be indicated in the pursuit of the diagnosis of uveitis. The chapter then discusses some of the many therapeutic surgical procedures that are used to treat the complications of uveitis that occur in a recurrent or chronically inflamed eye. The chapter finishes with specific surgical approaches to a few of the more common pediatric uveitides, such as ocular toxocariasis, sarcoidosis, intermediate uveitis, and juvenile rheumatoid arthritis (JRA)-associated uveitis.

DIAGNOSTIC SURGERY

Diagnostic surgery may be necessary to arrive at the underlying diagnosis of uveitis. Pursuing a diagnosis is help-

TABLE 31-1. SURGICAL CONSIDERATIONS IN PEDIATRIC UVEITIS

1. The prevention of the complications of uveitis and associated ocular structural damage is preferable to surgery. Bouts of inflammation must be completely controlled; thus the secondary complications of cataract, glaucoma, and maculopathy development may be curtailed. Often the limiting factor to postsurgical visual acuity is the presence of irreversible macular pathology, optic nerve pathology, and amblyopia.

2. Operating on an eye that has been repeatedly or chronically inflamed is very different from operating on an eye that has not been inflamed. The alterations in ocular tissue after recurrent inflammation make ophthalmic surgery challenging to even the most accomplished ophthalmic surgeon. The pediatric uveitic eye may respond with explosive postoperative inflammation following the most exquisite, gentle operation.

3. Surgery for the complications of uveitis is best undertaken after inflammation has been quiescent for as long as possible. Aggressive control of perioperative and postoperative inflammation is essential for all surgery and laser procedures. Adjunctive steroid therapy should be generously used preoperatively, intraoperatively, and postoperatively.

4. When uveitis affects the visual acuity in a child, it should be stressed that a successful surgery is only part of the visual rehabilitation in a child. Vigilant postoperative amblyopia therapy is equally important with proper postoperative spectacles or contact lens, orthoptic evaluation, and occlusion therapy.

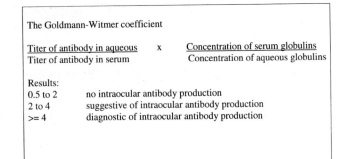

FIGURE 31-1. Goldmann-Witmer coefficient.

ful in understanding the natural history of the disease and potential complications of the disease. A surgical procedure for diagnosis is reasonable if (i) noninvasive studies have been performed and have failed to disclose the underlying cause of the patient's uveitis; (ii) the patient is unresponsive to medical therapy and alternative diagnoses are being considered; (iii) the patient develops significant ocular or systemic complications during therapy and more diagnostic information is needed to guide therapy; or (iv) malignancy is suspected.

Anterior Chamber Paracentesis

Indications

Anterior chamber paracentesis is an easily performed technique that provides a small amount of aqueous humor for analysis. In the inflamed eye, the breakdown of the blood–eye barrier results in antibody titers and immunoglobulin concentrations in the aqueous humor that may be higher than normal. Thus, samples of both aqueous humor and serum must be obtained on the same day for simultaneous measurement of immunoglobulin and antibody to control for the increased aqueous humor values from diffusion from breakdown of blood–eye barriers. The Goldmann-Witmer coefficient is used to help us reasonably conclude whether there is a localized antibody production in the eye (Fig. 31-1) (6).

Procedure

The anterior chamber is entered at the limbus with a 30-gauge needle on a tuberculin syringe and about 0.2 mL of aqueous humor can usually be obtained. This small amount of fluid must be handled carefully. The aqueous humor usually should be used for cell studies and antibody measurement. However, if an infection is suspected, the aqueous humor can be cultured instead. Use of aqueous humor for cultures will reduce the volume available for cell studies and antibody measurement. If a larger amount of aqueous humor is required to complete the necessary studies, reaspiration of the anterior chamber typically can be performed safely within several minutes of the initial tap, once the anterior chamber has been reformed by production of more aqueous humor. Importantly, if an infectious organism is suspected, the vitreous provides both a higher yield of positive cultures and more material for culture, allowing more types of cultures to be performed.

Vitrectomy

Indications

Diagnostic vitrectomy should be considered when noninvasive methods have failed to establish a diagnosis in severe, sight-threatening uveitis. The goal of diagnostic vitrectomy is to attempt to determine the cause of inflammation, thus modifying and directing medical treatments.

Vitreous specimens may be obtained by either vitrectomy or direct vitreous aspiration. A diagnostic vitrectomy is preferable to a vitreous aspiration. With a three-port vitrectomy, a larger volume of vitreous sample can be obtained under direct visualization. Additionally, there is more control over the amount of vitreous traction produced during the procedure, and the intraocular pressure (IOP) can be controlled during the procedure.

Procedure

A diagnostic vitrectomy is performed using a standard three-port vitrectomy procedure. A longer infusion tip

(4–6 mm) often is required in an eye with uveitis to accommodate scleral thickening, choroidal edema, or retinal separation that is frequently encountered (6). Direct visualization to confirm proper location of the infusion cannula within the vitreous cavity is essential before turning on the infusion in these patients.

The initial specimen in a diagnostic vitrectomy should be obtained undiluted, before the infusion port is turned on. A small amount of vitreous, 0.5 to 1 mL, should be obtained by using the vitrectomy instrument on low suction with the infusion line turned off. The sample is aspirated directly into a syringe through a three-way stopcock attached to the suction tubing. Next, the infusion line is opened and 10 mL of vitreous washings is aspirated into a separate syringe through the three-way stopcock. A therapeutic vitrectomy may then be performed in standard fashion, if necessary.

Both the undiluted vitreous aspirate and the vitreous washings should be immediately sent for microbiologic and cytologic analysis. Millipore filtration should be performed on vitreous washings to concentrate any microorganisms and cellular elements (2). The filter can be cut up and sent for culture or cytology. The washings can be processed for immunohistochemical staining, and cellular specimens can be sorted for monoclonality and cell subtyping. Polymerase chain reaction and cDNA probes may be used to detect DNA from many infectious agents, such as the herpetic viruses and *Toxoplasma gondii*.

Retinal or Chorioretinal Biopsy

Indications

Occasionally, neither aqueous nor vitreous specimens will provide a useful answer. In certain infectious conditions, the inflammatory process is localized primarily to the retina or choroid. The vitreous may contain few or none of the responsible microorganisms; thus, a diagnostic vitrectomy would provide little information. A retinal biopsy may be indicated when there is a macula-threatening lesion unresponsive to therapy or suspicion of malignancy, and this may be undertaken at the time of retinal detachment repair. Chorioretinal biopsy may be considered in patients with severe, sight-threatening, medically unresponsive inflammation and is an alternative to diagnostic enucleation.

Procedure

The retinal biopsy site should be carefully selected to maximize diagnostic yield and to minimize intraoperative and postoperative complications. If possible, a location in the superior retina will allow for postoperative gas tamponade of the retinal biopsy site. A location posterior to the equator allows easier surgical access. The biopsy site should be at the border of normal retinal and active retinal disease; a biopsy of quiescent retinal disease or atrophic retina will have poor yield for diagnostic information.

A vitrectomy is performed, and the site for retinal biopsy is identified. If the retina was previously detached with a large tear, intraocular scissors can be used to obtain a sample of the tissue. If the retina is not detached, the endolaser is used to surround the identified site with a triple row of laser photocoagulation. A retinotomy is made, and saline is injected under the retina to create a bleb. Intraocular scissors are used to complete the retinectomy. Forceps are used to grasp the specimen and remove it from the eye (6). Care should be taken to not lose the retinal biopsy sample as the forceps leave the eye at the sclerotomy site. The retina is then reattached with pneumatic air–fluid exchange. The retina is inspected, and any retinal breaks are treated with endolaser. The sclerotomies are closed, and gas is exchanged with air.

The chorioretinal biopsy site should be carefully selected with location criteria similar to those used for a retinal biopsy site. However, a location anterior to the equator allows surgical access to the site from the eye wall. A standard three-port pars plana vitrectomy is performed, and the biopsy site is carefully identified with indirect ophthalmoscopy. The area is localized on the surface of the eye with scleral depression and marked with a pen. A triple row of photocoagulation is placed surrounding the biopsy site with the laser indirect ophthalmoscope to reduce bleeding and the risk of retinal detachment (6). The eye is filled with air. A scleral flap, 6 mm × 6 mm, with hinge at posterior aspect, is made as thick as possible. The inner bed is surrounded by diathermy. An inner rectangle of remaining sclera, choroid, and retina, 4 mm × 3 mm, is incised with a needle knife and then is removed with retinal scissors. The specimen is carefully grasped at the corner and removed. The scleral flap is sutured closed. The eye is then filled with gas.

The retinal or chorioretinal biopsy specimen should be carefully subdivided into three sections. The first section is sent for light and electron microscopy; the second section is sent for viral or fungal culture or polymerase chain reaction analysis; and the third section is sent for immunohistochemical studies to determine the type of predominant immune response (2).

THERAPEUTIC SURGERY

Despite optimal medical therapy to control ocular inflammation, therapeutic surgery may be needed to treat the complications and sequelae of chronic inflammation. The following are therapeutic surgical procedures that may be indicated in the treatment of the complications of uveitis. It must be remembered that operating on an eye that has been repeatedly or chronically inflamed is very different from operating on an eye that has not been inflamed. The alterations in ocular tissue after recurrent inflammation make ophthalmic surgery challenging to even the most accomplished ophthalmic surgeon. The pediatric uveitic eye may respond with explosive postoperative inflammation following the most gentle operation. Maximum control of inflammation preoperatively, intraoperatively, and postoperatively allows the greatest chance of a successful surgery.

Band Keratopathy

Indications

Calcium hydroxyapatite may accumulate in the epithelial basement membrane, basal epithelium, and Bowman membrane in children with chronic uveitis such as JRA, sarcoidosis, or chronic intermediate uveitis (7). These deposits can become densely white with a rough surface that elevates the epithelium and results in pain, foreign body sensation, recurrent corneal erosions, and decreased vision. Indications for surgery are for vision rehabilitation, ocular surface improvement with decreased corneal erosions, or enhancement of the ophthalmologist's view to perform adequate ocular examinations.

Band keratopathy may be removed by disodium ethylenediaminetetraacetic acid (EDTA) chelation and superficial keratectomy. An alternative method of removal of band keratopathy is with excimer laser phototherapeutic keratectomy (PTK); however, this often leaves a highly irregular base due to the nonuniformity of the calcium density in the band across the cornea (8). PTK effectively treats the ocular surface symptoms, but the improvement in visual acuity is variable. Stewart and Morrell (9) reported that of the patients with band keratopathy who underwent PTK for visual rehabilitation, 55% had an improvement or no change in visual acuity, whereas 45% had a decrease in visual acuity. Of the patients who underwent PTK for ocular surface improvement, 83% had an improvement in symptoms. Chelation with EDTA remains the mainstay of surgical therapy for band keratopathy and should be attempted prior to PTK. In chronically inflamed eyes, such as in children with JRA-associated uveitis, multiple recurrences of band keratopathy usually occur, which may require multiple future treatments.

Procedure

Although chelation can be performed with local anesthesia, general anesthesia usually is necessary for these pediatric patients. Foster has described his technique for EDTA chelation and superficial keratectomy (1). The epithelium overlying the calcium deposition is removed with a no. 15 Bard-Parker blade by wiping off the epithelium, ensuring that no cuts are made in the Bowman membrane. After the epithelium is removed, a well, which can be made from a cut back-end of a 3-mL plastic syringe, is positioned over the affected area, cut side up. Solution of 0.35% EDTA is placed in the watertight well and held in position for 5 minutes, to chelate calcium in the affected area while protecting the limbal stem cells. The well is removed, and the cornea is irrigated with balanced salt solution. The no. 15 blade is used

to scrape the loosened flakes of calcium. The procedure is repeated as many times as necessary to remove the calcium from the central cornea. Care must be taken to avoid scarring of the Bowman membrane in the visual axis. Cycloplegic and antibiotic medications are instilled, a continuous-wear bandage soft contact lens is placed, and the eye is patched. Topical antibiotic and steroid are used postoperatively. Bandage contact lens, cycloplegia, and oral analgesics help with pain control. The epithelium generally has covered the corneal surface within 1 week following surgery, and the bandage soft contact lens can be removed.

Glaucoma

Mechanisms of Glaucoma in the Uveitis Setting

Glaucoma may occur in the uveitic patient as a consequence of severe anterior segment inflammation. The mechanism of intraocular pressure (IOP) elevation in the uveitic eye is complex, and a combination of mechanisms may coexist in the eye with uveitis. The five major causes of secondary glaucoma in patients with uveitis are secondary angle closure from posterior synechiae causing pupillary block and iris bombe, secondary angle closure by peripheral anterior synechiae, blockage of the trabecular meshwork by inflammatory debris, active trabeculitis, or steroid-induced IOP rise. Additionally, active inflammation may suppress ciliary body function with a decrease in IOP. Thus, IOP in the actively inflamed eye may be higher or lower than in the uninflamed eye. Topical steroid administration may relieve trabeculitis and reduce IOP. Topical corticosteroids may increase IOP from either reactivated ciliary body function or a steroid-induced IOP rise. Increased IOP with the addition of corticosteroid may complicate the management of the pediatric uveitic patient who needs the corticosteroid for treatment of inflammation and for prevention of ocular damage from chronic inflammation.

Angle Closure Glaucoma

Indications

Patients with uveitis may develop posterior synechiae sufficient to produce relative pupillary block, iris bombé, and secondary angle closure. Ordinarily in a patient with nonuveitic pupillary block glaucoma, laser peripheral iridotomy is the therapeutic procedure of choice. However, in the inflamed eye of a pediatric uveitic patient, the laser peripheral iridotomy commonly closes. Moreover, the young age of the pediatric patient makes laser procedures difficult. A large surgical iridectomy under general anesthesia is the procedure of choice in the pediatric uveitic patient with pupillary block and secondary angle closure.

Procedure

Surgical iridectomy consists of five steps: (i) incision, (ii) exteriorization of the iris, (iii) excision of the iris, (iv) repositioning of the iris, and (v) closure of the incision. The incision may be made in the sclera under a conjunctival flap or through clear cornea. Although it is more difficult to prolapse the iris tissue through a clear corneal incision, the conjunctiva will be spared for future glaucoma surgery.

A partial thickness incision is made perpendicularly into clear cornea. Preplaced sutures are then placed on either side of the corneal incision to facilitate spreading of the corneal wound. The corneal incision is then continued perpendicularly until the anterior chamber is entered. Gentle pressure on the posterior lip of the wound usually will prolapse the iris into the wound. The prolapsed "knuckle" of iris is then excised. If the iris does not prolapse, then the anterior chamber must be entered with fine nontoothed forceps to grasp the iris. After iridectomy, the iris usually will spontaneously return into the anterior chamber. If the iris remains prolapsed, radial massage from wound to central cornea with a smooth instrument will result in spontaneous repositioning of iris back into the anterior chamber. The wound is closed with 10-0 nylon suture. Corticosteroid is injected subconjunctivally.

Uveitic Glaucoma

Raised IOP in patients with uveitis may lead to visual loss. Patients with chronic uveitis, who develop intractable glaucoma, are notoriously difficult to treat (10). Medical therapy often proves inadequate in controlling IOP, necessitating surgical intervention. Conventional filtering procedures, such as trabeculectomy, are known to fail more frequently in inflamed eyes than in noninflamed eyes. Although some studies report fairly successful 1- and 2-year results of trabeculectomy, with or without antimetabolites, the long-term success rate of trabeculectomy in patients with uveitic glaucoma is quite poor (11–14). Glaucoma drainage implants have been reported by some studies to have fairly successful 1- and 2-year results, with continued, moderate long-term success at 5 and 10 years (12,15–18).

After trabeculectomy, the extensive inflammatory response of the pediatric eye and the recurrent or chronic nature of inflammation result in fibrous tissue growth and subsequent closure of the filtering bleb over time. Although adjunctive antimetabolites may keep the filtering bleb open in the initial few weeks or months after surgery, recurrent inflammation may later close the filtering bleb. Thus, the long-term success rate of filtering surgery has a decreasing chance of success in these pediatric uveitic patients over time. One- and two-year success rates after trabeculectomy without antimetabolite therapy ranges from 67% to 92% (11–14). Hoskins et al. (11) reported a 67% success rate at 1 year; Hill et al. (12) reported 81% and 73% success rates at 1 and 2 years; and Stavrou et al. (13) reported 92% and 83% success rates at 1 and 2 years . However, at 5 years, the success rates decrease dramatically. Towler et al. (14) reported that the success rate fell from an 80% at 2 years to 30% at 5 years. With the addition of antimetabolites to trabeculectomy,

Towler et al. (14) reported an improvement to 50% of patients still controlled at 5 years.

Some studies report reasonable success rates using glaucoma drainage devices for control of uveitic glaucoma. More importantly, the long-term success rates remain fairly good. Choroidal effusions, hypotony, and cystoid macular edema comprise the most common postoperative complications. The 1- and 2-year success rates after glaucoma drainage devices range from 92% to 94% (12,15–18). A 91.7% success rate at both 1 and 2 years with IOPs of 5 to 21 mmHg was reported in 24 eyes treated with Baerveldt glaucoma drainage implant (15). A 94% success rate at 1 year with IOP ≤21 mmHg was reported in 21 eyes treated with Ahmed valve implantation (16), whereas a 79% success rate at both 1 and 2 years with IOP of 6 to 21 mmHg with Molteno device implantation (12). A 95% success at 27 months and a 90% success at 52 months with IOP ≤22 mmHg with Molteno device implantation was reported in 27 eyes with secondary glaucoma caused by JRA (17). In a prospective case series of 40 eyes, the probability of the Molteno implant to control IOP ≤21 mmHg was calculated to be 87% at 5 years and 77% at 10 years after surgery (18).

In the child with uveitis, surgery is best undertaken after the inflammation is maximally controlled with corticosteroid or immunosuppressant medications for as long as possible preoperatively in patients undergoing nonurgent glaucoma surgery. A glaucoma drainage device may be implanted in standard fashion between Tenon fascia and sclera and secured in place. The silicone tube is tied off if the Baerveldt implant is used. The tube is placed through either the limbus or the pars plana in vitrectomized eyes. The tube and its insertion site are covered with a patch of preserved donor sclera. Topical corticosteroids are used postoperatively. Maximum control of inflammation preoperatively, intraoperatively, and postoperatively allows the greatest chance of a successful surgery.

In the pediatric aphakic uveitic patient, postoperative amblyopia therapy is vital with proper spectacles or aphakic contact lens. If a glaucoma drainage implant is placed in a vitrectomized, aphakic, pediatric patient, a pars plana tube placement will better allow contract lens fitting following surgery (1).

Cataract

Cataract is one of the most common complications of uveitis, with a prevalence of up to 50% and can be attributed to chronic inflammation and corticosteroid use (19,20). Cataract surgery in pediatric uveitic eyes is daunting to even the most accomplished cataract surgeon because of the unknown risks faced intraoperatively and the uncertainty of the postoperative course (3,4). The uveitic cataract frequently is technically challenging with posterior synechiae, iris vasculature delicacy, pupillary membranes, miotic pupil, and corneal opacification (5). There may be permanent damage to ocular structures before the cataract surgery such as maculopathy, chronic macular edema, epiretinal membrane, glaucomatous optic neuropathy, or cyclitic membrane with associated hypotony and progressive phthisis, which may limit a good visual outcome after surgery. The combination of the pediatric heightened immune response and a uveitic eye often results in a fierce postoperative inflammatory response following the most careful operation.

Indications

Indications for cataract surgery in the child with uveitic cataract include visual rehabilitation, prevention or treatment of amblyopia, and enhancement of the ophthalmologist's view of the posterior segment for ongoing assessment of the optic nerve and retina.

Cataract extraction with intraocular lens (IOL) implantation has become increasingly successful over the past 20 years as a result of improved microsurgical techniques and viscoelastics, as well as more rigorous control of recurrent inflammation and chronic low-grade inflammation (1,2). Currently, cataract extraction with endocapsular posterior chamber IOL is an accepted practice in the management of many adults with uveitic cataract, provided the inflammation has been quiescent for a sustained period before surgery (21). However, the decision whether to implant an IOL in a pediatric patient with uveitis remains controversial.

Procedure

The surgical technique for cataract extraction in a child with uveitis should include removal of the cataract, including the posterior capsule, all retrolenticular and cyclitic membranes, and most of the vitreous. Historically, pars plana lensectomy with pars plana vitrectomy was the procedure of choice (22). For the pars plana approach, the lens and posterior and anterior capsules are cut and aspirated with an ocutome probe. This is followed by a near-total vitrectomy. Removal of the lens capsule and anterior hyaloid must be performed in an attempt to eliminate the "scaffold" along which secondary membranes may subsequently form (19). This reduces the likelihood of subsequent posterior synechiae and cyclitic membrane formation and decreases the need for postoperative neodymium:yttrium-aluminum garnet (Nd:YAG) laser capsulotomy, which may be difficult in small children and which may often incite further inflammation (22–25). A surgical peripheral iridectomy should be made if recurrent or chronic inflammation is anticipated.

Cataract extraction may be accomplished by a combined limbal approach with phacoemulsification and pars plana vitrectomy. During the limbal approach, synechiolysis, pupillary stretching, and iris hooks are used as needed for adequate exposure. Then a capsulorrhexis, hydrodissection, and phacoemulsification are performed in standard fashion,

and the incision is closed. This is followed by a pars plana approach for complete posterior capsule excision, followed by a near-total vitrectomy.

The decision whether to implant an IOL in a pediatric patient with uveitis remains controversial. The decision must be carefully considered and must be tailored to both the patient and the risk of recurrent inflammation. If the disease course predicts recurrent inflammation or chronic inflammation, the child is at extremely high risk of developing thick perilenticular membranes, severe postoperative inflammation, and iris capture. The IOL itself may provide a stimulus for intraocular inflammation and structural support for inflammatory membranes, which can result in ciliary body dysfunction, ocular hypotony, and chronic macular edema. Treatment of these membranes with Nd:YAG capsulotomy can incite further inflammation and reformation of membranes. Even with surgical posterior capsulectomy, retrolental membranectomy, and total vitrectomy, significant perilenticular membranes may persist or recur. In addition, chronic inflammation refractory to therapy or cyclitic membranes can result in hypotony and, ultimately, IOL removal is required (21). Patients at highest risk of required IOL explantations are young patients with JRA, as periodic flareups of uveitis were still occurring, and in patients with chronic low-grade peripheral uveitis (21). IOL implantation is contraindicated in children with JRA-associated uveitic cataract (1,2,19,26).

The choice of IOL may affect postoperative inflammation and formation of perilenticular membranes. Acrylic lenses may be the least inflammogenic (27,28). Report (27) of a randomized, double-masked trial of 36 adult uveitic eyes that had implantation with one of four IOLs: silicone, polymethylmethacrylate (PMMA), heparin-coated PMMA, or acrylic lenses, acrylic lenses appeared to provide the best overall result when evaluated for postoperative inflammation, posterior capsular opacification (PCO) rates, cystoid macular edema, and final visual acuity. Of 140 adult uveitic eyes that had implantation with silicone, PMMA, heparin-coated PMMA, or acrylic lens, the acrylic lens resulted in a lower PCO rate (28). The choice of IOL in the pediatric uveitic eye remains to be studied. The use of heparin in the infusion solution for pediatric uveitic cataract surgery is controversial (29,30).

Management of Inflammation

The essential element for successful cataract surgery is vigilant control of inflammation preoperatively, perioperatively, and postoperatively. Cataract surgery has an increased chance for a successful outcome if it is performed after the inflammation has been quiescent for as long as possible, ideally more than 3 months. Surgery in the presence of active inflammation carries a much higher potential for complications. The optimal time to operate is after the active inflammatory phase of the uveitis has burned out (31).

This is particularly true in case of intermediate uveitis in which the inflammation may remit without recurring. If this is not practical, the next best time to operate is after the uveitis has been inactive for several months with corticosteroid treatment. This is true in cases of acute intermittent inflammation. In some patients with chronic inflammation, it is impossible to completely quiet the eye. Although attempts should be made to maximally quiet the eye, surgery should not be delayed to the point of leading to irreversible ocular damage. If the level of inflammation cannot be assessed, the eye should be prophylactically treated for a few days as though active inflammation were present (2).

Systemic immunosuppressive therapy in the form of low-dose methotrexate may be needed for adequate preoperative control of inflammation in children with JRA-associated uveitis. In 2003, a favorable outcome was reported in five children (six eyes) younger than 13 years with JRA-associated uveitis who underwent standard phacoemulsification cataract extraction without a posterior capsulectomy and with posterior chamber IOL implantation (32). Postoperative visual acuity was 20/40 or better in all six eyes. Median follow-up was 44 months. Preoperatively, four children (five eyes) were on low-dose methotrexate immunosuppressive therapy for a median length of 1.25 years before surgery. Preoperatively, two children (three eyes) were on additional immunosuppressants or systemic corticosteroids. All eyes received frequent topical corticosteroid therapy for a median of 2 weeks preoperatively and 8.5 weeks postoperatively. Five eyes required Nd:YAG capsulotomy. One eye needed a subsequent surgical posterior capsulectomy and pars plana vitrectomy. The authors concluded that children with JRA-associated uveitis might have favorable surgical outcomes after cataract surgery with posterior chamber IOL implantation provided they had adequate long-term preoperative and postoperative control of intraocular inflammation with systemic immunosuppressive therapy and intensive perioperative topical corticosteroid therapy.

Perioperative control of inflammation is vital, as the pediatric uveitic eye often has an intense postoperative inflammatory reaction. The goal of perioperative medications is to control and reduce the anticipated severe postoperative inflammation. Although specific medications and dosing schedules vary, the concepts are similar. In general, patients should be given oral and topical corticosteroids and nonsteroidal antiinflammatory drugs (NSAIDs) for 1 to 3 days preoperatively, even if there is no evidence of active inflammatory disease. Intraoperatively, patients should receive a periocular steroid injection and may receive an intravenous bolus of steroid. Periocular injections may be delivered to the retroseptal space or the subtenon space. In small children, 20 mg of triamcinolone acetonide is effective (33). Postoperatively, patients should receive aggressive topical steroids and NSAIDs, along with oral steroids and NSAIDs. Perioperative steroid remains superior to perioperative cyclosporine in preventing severe postoperative inflammation (2).

Postoperatively, the eye may appear quiet at first but then may respond with a violent inflammatory reaction with significant dense fibrin and an outpouring of protein within the eye. This inflammatory response peaks about 48 hours after surgery and lasts for 5 to 6 days after the surgery, even in the presence of high doses of systemic corticosteroids. Pediatric uveitis patients should be examined every day for the first 5 to 7 days postoperatively (2). Occasionally, a severe dense fibrin that is refractory to steroids and NSAIDs may occur in the anterior chamber within 6 days after surgery. Recombinant tissue plasminogen activator (rt-PA) can be used to clear severe dense fibrin in the anterior chamber. A report on 11 pediatric eyes, three with uveitis, who developed dense fibrin clots after cataract surgery that was refractory to intensive prednisolone acetate and cycloplegic agents showed a benefit of rt-PA (34). Injection of rt-PA, 100 μL of 10 μg/100 μL, into the anterior chamber thought a limbal paracentesis resulted in complete resolution of fibrin formation in all eyes except for two eyes in a JRA patient, usually within 24 hours.

Visual Rehabilitation

It is imperative to remember that a successful operation is only part of the visual rehabilitation in a child. Postoperative amblyopia therapy in conjunction with a pediatric ophthalmologist is equally important with proper postoperative spectacles or contact lenses, orthoptic evaluation, and occlusion therapy. Parents must be constantly educated about amblyopia therapy. Despite excellent anatomic outcomes, visual rehabilitation for aphakic eyes may be suboptimal, because many patients of this age are unable or refuse to wear aphakic contact lens or aphakic spectacles (35). Among children, contract lens intolerance is reported to range from 17% to 38% (26,36). The frequent concomitant occurrence of band keratopathy makes contact lens fitting difficult. Multiple lost contact lenses carry a substantial expense. Children often are intolerant of aphakic spectacles because of the weight and aniseikonia. The age of the child at the time of surgery, the presence or absence of amblyopia, and the presence of irreversible retinal or optic nerve pathology are the primary factors influencing the outcome of cataract surgery in the pediatric uveitic patient.

Vitreoretinal Surgery

Pars plana vitrectomy may be performed for the many vitreoretinal complications secondary to chronic uveitis. Vitreous removal may have a curative or moderating effect on the clinical course in patients with intermediate uveitis, JRA-associated uveitis, and sarcoidosis. Indications for pars plana vitrectomy include persistent vitreous opacification, medically unresponsive vitritis, traction retinal detachment, impending retinal detachment, epiretinal membrane creating significant distortion or heterotropia, cyclitic membrane, prevention or treatment of amblyopia, and enhancement of the ophthalmologist's view of the posterior segment for ongoing assessment of the optic nerve and retina. These patients frequently have cataract, posterior synechiae, and vitreous opacification that must be addressed either prior to or at the time of vitreoretinal surgery. Final visual prognosis often is limited by the presence of macular or optic nerve pathology.

Indications

There are four objectives in pars plana vitrectomy in patients with chronic uveitis. The first is to remove opacities in the visual axis. The second is to remove vitreomacular membranes producing retinal traction or epiretinal membranes causing macular pucker. The third is to remove cyclitic membranes or thickened anterior cortical hyaloid causing hypotony. The fourth is to alter the course of vitreous inflammation refractory to medical therapy or persistent cystoid macular edema.

Remove Opacities in the Visual Axis
In cases of vitreous inflammation refractory to medical therapy, a pars plana vitrectomy is performed to clear the visual axis by removal of media opacities and vitreous debris.

Alter the Course of Vitreous Inflammation Refractory to Medical Therapy
Vitrectomy may alter the course of inflammation and result in stabilization of the disease by removing immunocompetent cells and inflammatory mediators from the vitreous cavity (23,24,37). Vitrectomy may potentially reduce cystoid macular edema either by eliminating the contact between an inflamed vitreous body and the macula or by allowing better penetration or distribution of corticosteroids (22,24,38). However, others have noted that although vitrectomy removes vitreous debris and appears to allow for easier intraocular penetration of corticosteroid, no change in the inflammation process was observed (2).

Remove Vitreomacular Membranes
Membranectomy may be performed after pars plana vitrectomy to remove inflammatory membranes from the retina and ciliary body. Anteroposterior vitreomacular traction from an inflamed vitreous body may result in chronic cystoid macular edema or may create a shallow traction retinal detachment. Tangential traction caused by epiretinal membranes cause decreased vision and secondary cystoid macular edema. These membranes can be removed successfully at the time of vitrectomy by delamination or *en bloc* techniques. Traction also may lead to retinal breaks in atrophic retina, creating a combined traction-rhegmatogenous detachment, which may be repaired during pars plana vitrectomy.

Remove Cyclitic Membranes or Thickened Anterior Cortical Hyaloid
A cyclitic membrane may occur and may result in hypotony. Chronic traction of the ciliary body from a cyclitic membrane or a thickened anterior cortical hyaloid will result in ciliary body detachment and reduced aqueous humor formation. Pars plana vitrectomy and cyclitic membrane removal can be performed to reattach the ciliary body. A skilled assistant is required to assist in scleral depression in the region of the ciliary body so that the surgeon can dissect and remove the inflammatory membrane or surgically segment it to reduce traction.

Procedure

Vitreoretinal surgery is performed using a standard three-port vitrectomy procedure. A longer infusion tip (4—6 mm) is often required in uveitis patients to accommodate scleral thickening, choroidal edema, or retinal separation that is frequently encountered in an eye with uveitis (1). Direct visualization to confirm proper location of the infusion cannula within the vitreous cavity is important before turning on the infusion in these patients.

The infusion is turned on, and the endoillumination probe and vitrectomy cutter are introduced. A complete vitrectomy is performed. Preretinal membranes are dissected or stripped from the retinal surface using a combination of scissors, membrane picks, and forceps. If there is vitreous base exudation or neovascularization, it may be treated with laser scatter photocoagulation or cryopexy. Indirect ophthalmoscopy is used at the completion of the vitrectomy to search for any other retinal pathologies, such as retinal tears. If present, they are treated with retinal laser or cryopexy. Long-acting gas or silicone oil tamponade may be needed. Unless contraindicated, corticosteroids are injected in the vitreous space and periocularly. The corticosteroids greatly assist in controlling excessive postoperative inflammation and fibrin formation. Regional and intraocular corticosteroids are contraindicated in a patient with a possible infectious etiology.

Management of Inflammation

Surgery has an increased chance for a successful outcome if it is performed after the inflammation has been quiescent for as long as possible, ideally more than 3 months. Occasionally, this cannot be obtained, and surgery must be performed while the eye is still inflamed, such as in surgery for medically unresponsive uveitis. Surgery in the presence of active inflammation carries a much higher potential for surgical complications.

Perioperative control of inflammation is vital, as the pediatric uveitic eye often has an intense postoperative inflammatory reaction. Postoperative fibrin and inflammation may promote cyclitic membrane formation and/or proliferative vitreoretinopathy. Final visual acuity will be influenced by the presence of macular scarring, cystoid macular edema, macular ischemia, or retinal necrosis. Patients have better visual prognoses if they presented with a macula-on retinal detachment.

Lasers

In the nonuveitic eye, lasers often are used to perform peripheral iridotomy and posterior capsulotomy, to cut pupillary membranes, and to treat retinal or subretinal neovascularization. Any laser procedure may incite an extensive inflammatory response in a uveitic eye. Periprocedural control of inflammation is important, with frequent topical corticosteroid dosing and consideration of periocular or systemic corticosteroids.

Surgical Iridectomy Preferable to Peripheral Iridectomy

Patients with uveitis may develop posterior synechiae sufficient to produce relative pupillary block subsequent iris bombe configuration, narrow angles, and possibly angle closure glaucoma. Ordinarily, laser peripheral iridotomy is the therapeutic procedure of choice. In the pediatric uveitic patient, the positioning of a child at the Nd:YAG laser is difficult. Additionally, chronic or recurrent inflammation often will result in subsequent closure of the laser peripheral iridotomy. A surgical iridectomy performed with the patient under general anesthesia is preferable to laser peripheral iridotomy in the pediatric uveitic patient.

Posterior Capsulotomy versus Surgical Posterior Capsulotomy

Cataract formation is a frequent complication of uveitis. After phacoemulsification cataract extraction with posterior chamber IOL implantation, thick perilenticular membranes often form in the pediatric population, particularly in patients with chronic or recurrent uveitis. These perilenticular membranes may result in ciliary body dysfunction, ocular hypotony, and chronic macular edema. The thick inflammatory membranes often require multiple sessions of Nd:YAG capsulotomy, which often may incite further inflammation, and they may subsequently reaccumulate. Eventually, surgical posterior capsulectomy, retrolental membranectomy, and total vitrectomy may be necessary. If IOL implantation is attempted in a pediatric uveitic patient, especially a patient with JRA, a posterior capsulectomy with removal of the anterior hyaloid face and a thorough near-total vitrectomy should be considered in attempts to eliminate the "scaffold" along which secondary membranes may subsequently form (19). This reduces the likelihood of subsequent posterior synechiae and cyclitic membrane formation and decreases the need for postoperative Nd:YAG laser capsulotomy, which may be difficult in small children (22–25,39).

Panretinal or Segmental Photocoagulation for Retinal Neovascularization (Sarcoidosis)

Patients with sarcoidosis may develop large areas of retinal capillary nonperfusion and secondary retinal or disc neovascularization. Both retinal and disc neovascularization may regress in patients with sarcoidosis in up to 50% of patients treated by systemic medical therapy alone (40,41). When persistent or progressive peripheral retinal neovascularization causes recurrent vitreous hemorrhage, laser photocoagulation may be required to eliminate the neovascularization. Local grid treatment or cryopexy is applied to the areas of ischemia adjacent to retinal neovascularization. Fluorescein angiography can define the areas of ischemia and help direct photocoagulation. Laser photocoagulation usually is followed by a significant increase in cystoid macular edema (40). Steroid therapy should be used in combination with laser treatment to blunt the inflammatory response. When disc neovascularization causes recurrent vitreous hemorrhage, panretinal photocoagulation may be required to eliminate the disc vessels.

Peripheral Neovascularization (Intermediate Uveitis)

Patients with intermediate uveitis may develop peripheral retinal neovascularization. These patients have thick ropy neovascularization in the far periphery extending over the ora serrata, which often is obscured from visualization by pars plan exudation and vitreitis. In patients with unremitting chronic pars planitis that is recalcitrant to steroid or NSAID therapy, cryotherapy and scatter laser photocoagulation of the peripheral retina have been reported to be effective in causing regression of peripheral neovascularization and reduction of inflammatory activity. This treatment can reduce the frequency of vitreous hemorrhage and may reduce the severity of the intermediate uveitis and cystoid macular edema. Cryotherapy is thought to reduce inflammation by eliminating the inflammation stimulus in the peripheral retinal tissue (42,43). Reduction in neovascularization may be caused by direct vessel ablation or by destruction of ischemic retinal tissue (43,44).

In children, cryotherapy is performed with general anesthesia. Retrobulbar anesthesia is given for intraoperative and postoperative pain control. Cryotherapy is applied directly to the areas of exudation at the pars plana using a double freeze-thaw technique (25,42). The ice ball should be seen to cover the exudative area and neovascularization. Uninvolved pars plana and retina are treated one cryotip width beyond the involved area. In areas where the visualization of the ice ball is precluded, freezing should be continued for a time interval similar to that required in adjacent areas with adequate visualization. Periocular steroids are administered following the procedure. The procedure may be repeated in 3 to 4 months if there is residual disease. Cryotherapy was first advocated in 1973 (42) and was later reported to eliminate inflammation in 78% of 27 eyes (45). Visual acuity improved or remained unchanged in 89% of eyes and eliminated the need for corticosteroids therapy in 90% of eyes.

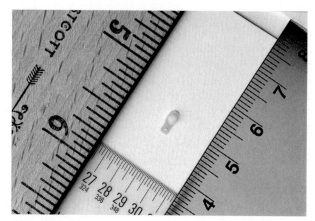

FIGURE 31-2. Fluocinolone acetonide reservoir device (Retisert, Bausch & Lomb, Rochester, NY) alongside rulers.

Panretinal scatter photocoagulation has been shown to be effective in the treatment of peripheral neovascularization associated with intermediate uveitis. Regression of neovascularization, improvement of cystoid macular edema, and stabilization of inflammation were reported in 10 eyes with scatter diode or argon photocoagulation treatment, either alone or in combination with pars plana vitrectomy (38).

Three rows of photocoagulation are delivered to the inferior retinal periphery, just posterior to the area of exudation or neovascularization. Treatment may be carried out with either argon endophotocoagulation or an indirect ophthalmoscopic delivery system using argon or diode photocoagulation. Laser photocoagulation appears to be a safe and effective alternative to cryotherapy and is a useful adjunct during a therapeutic pars plana vitrectomy.

SLOW-RELEASE STEROID TREATMENT FOR UVEITIS

Two sustained-release, steroid-based drug delivery devices currently are under development. Although neither has yet been approved for marketing by the United States Food and Drug Administration (FDA), both are in phase III clinical trial testing as of this date. One device is a reservoir-based, surgically implanted device containing 0.5 mg of fluocinolone acetonide; it is designed to release the drug over a 3-year period. The device initially was developed by Control Delivery Systems (Watertown, MA) and now is licensed by Bausch & Lomb (Rochester, NY) (Fig. 31-2). The device has been shown to be extremely effective for the treatment of uveitis, even in patients who have had poor control of their disease with aggressive systemic therapy (Figs. 31-3 and 31-4) (46). A large phase III clinical trial evaluating the use of the fluocinolone implant in patients with refractory uveitis is underway, and children between the ages of 13 and 18 years are allowed in the trial, although most of the patients in the trial are adults.

Fluocinolone Implantation Procedure

The procedure for surgical implantation of the fluocinolone implant is similar to that of the ganciclovir implant, which was developed by the same two companies. A limbal-based conjunctival peritomy is performed in the inferotemporal quadrant using Westcott scissors and 0.3 forceps. The inferotemporal quadrant is not used if there is significant pathology of the vitreous base in that location; an alternate site is chosen, with a preference for an inferior-based location. All episcleral vessels are cauterized using eraser-type cautery.

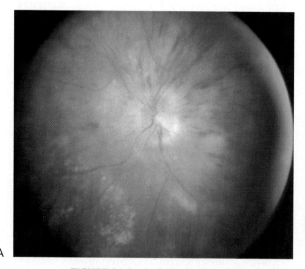
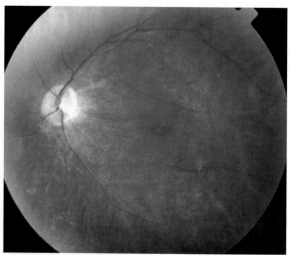

FIGURE 31-3. A: Color fundus photograph 1 year before fluocinolone acetonide implant. Optic nerve swelling and peripapillary necrotizing retinitis with intraretinal hemorrhage are seen. Image taken with a 30-degree fundus camera. **B:** Six months after fluocinolone acetonide implant. Healed retinitis. Image taken with a 50-degree fundus camera.

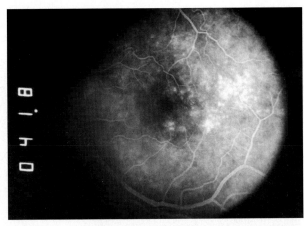 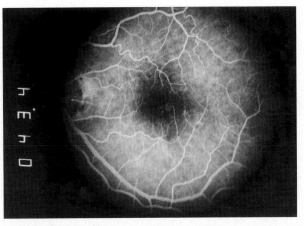

FIGURE 31-4. Fluorescein angiogram taken just before **(A)** and 4 months after **(B)** fluocinolone acetonide device implantation. Mid arteriovenous phase **(A)** and late phase **(B)** are shown. (Courtesy of Glenn Jaffee, MD.)

A 3.5-mm circumferential incision is performed 4 mm from the limbus using a 15-degree blade or the equivalent. The wound is inspected to assure that the uvea has been adequately incised. The fluocinolone implant, which has a double-armed 9-0 prolene suture with TG-175 needles passed through the eyelet at the base of the strut, is grasped with nontoothed forceps and thrust through the incision into the vitreous cavity. All prolapsed vitreous is excised with a vitrector. The implant is sutured into place by grasping the needle of the anterior arm of the suture and performing a radial full scleral thickness bite through the wound emerging through the scleral 2 mm anterior to the wound. The process is repeated using the needle attached to the posterior arm of the suture, going full thickness though the wound emerging 2 mm posterior to the wound. The elevated aspect of the implant housing the drug should face the center of the eye. The implant is tied firmly into place using a 3-1-1 knot, with the ends of the suture left long after the needles have been cut off. The rest of the wound is closed with two radial sutures of 9-0 prolene (one on either side of the central anchoring suture) tied with a 2-1-1 knot, with the suture ends cut short and the knots rotated into the sclera. The long ends of the central anchoring suture are tucked under the radial sutures on either side. The conjunctiva is closed using either plain gut or vicryl suture. The implant is inspected with indirect ophthalmoscopy to assure that it is appropriately placed in the vitreous cavity. Standard subconjunctival injections of antibiotic and steroid are given at the end of the procedure.

Dexamethasone Implantation Procedure

The other sustained-release, steroid-based drug delivery technology that is under development is a dexamethasone bioerodible device designed to release drug over a 4- to 6-week period (Oculex Pharmaceuticals, Sunnyvale, CA)

(Fig. 31-5). A phase III trial using an office-based, 23-gauge injectable device is in the final planning stages. Previously, a 20-gauge surgically implantable device was shown to be effective in five boys with chronic cystoid edema associated with intermediate uveitis (Fig. 31-6). The device that is entering phase III testing will not require surgical cutdown and will be injected using a 23-gauge needle through the pars plana inferotemporally. Patients in the trial will have persistent macular edema caused by diabetic retinopathy, central retinal vein occlusion, branch retinal vein occlusion, uveitis, or postcataract removal Irvine-Gass syndrome refractory to medical management or laser.

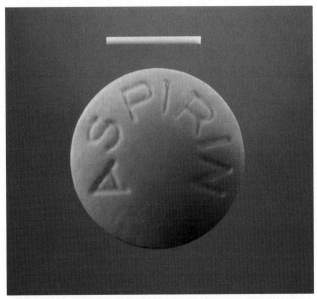

FIGURE 31-5. Dexamethasone bioerodible device (Posurdex, Oculex Pharmaceuticals, Sunnyvale, CA) alongside an aspirin. (Courtesy of Oculex Pharmaceuticals.)

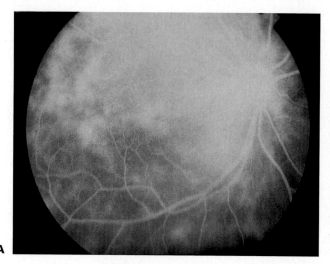
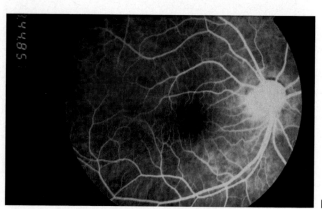

FIGURE 31-6. Fluorescein angiogram of a 12-year-old boy with intermediate uveitis with chronic cystoid macular edema just before **(A)** and 2.5 months after **(B)** dexamethasone bioerodible device implantation.

SURGICAL APPROACH TO UVEITIS BY DISEASE

This chapter finishes with specific surgical approaches to a few of the more common pediatric uveitides: ocular toxocariasis, sarcoidosis, intermediate uveitis, and JRA-associated uveitis. The focus of this section of the chapter is on the specific surgical approaches for the complications and sequelae of these uveitides. For a detailed discussion on the epidemiology, histopathology, ocular and systemic signs and symptoms, diagnostic tests, and medical treatments of ocular toxocariasis, sarcoidosis, intermediate uveitis, and JRA-associated uveitis, please refer to Chapters 16 and 17.

Ocular Toxocariasis

Ocular toxocariasis is a monocular disease that affects children.

Pathogenesis

Toxocariasis is an infectious disease caused by the invasion of tissue by larvae of *Toxocara canis*. *Toxocara canis* is a roundworm of dogs. It is a ubiquitous worldwide parasite. The incidence of infected puppies has been estimated to vary from 33% to 100% worldwide (47). Human infection occurs when a child ingests soil containing ova. The ova hatch in the small intestine, and the larvae pass through intestinal wall. The larvae migrate to various tissues, including the eye, where they may wander about aimlessly for weeks or months, or the larvae may become encysted by a focal granulomatous reaction, where they can remain alive for months or years (48). The adult worms do not develop in humans; thus, *Toxocara* eggs will not be found in the stool of an infected person.

Ocular toxocariasis typically affects children at an average age of 7.5 years (range 2–31 years); 80% of the cases occur in children younger than age 16 years (49). Intermediate uveitis from *Toxocara* is almost always unilateral, whereas idiopathic intermediate uveitis is bilateral in 70% to 90% of cases (50); thus, ocular toxocariasis must be suspected in all cases of unilateral intermediate uveitis, particularly in children.

Clinical Signs

Ocular toxocariasis presents in a variety of clinical patterns. A variable amount of vitreous inflammation is present. The main ocular findings include peripheral retinochoroiditis, posterior retinochoroiditis, also called a *posterior pole granuloma,* and vitreitis. Fibrous traction bands may result in epiretinal membrane formation, traction retinal detachment, and combined traction-rhegmatogenous retinal detachment. Vitreoretinal surgery has been shown to be effective in clearing inflammatory debris from the vitreous cavity and reattaching the macula in some eyes with retinal detachment (51).

The posterior pole granuloma is a white, elevated, intraretinal or subretinal mass from 0.5 to 4 disc diameters in size, with traction bands from mass to the macula or to the optic disc (Fig. 31-7). The granuloma is the larva of *Toxocara* surrounded by an eosinophilic abscess with a granulomatous inflammatory reaction (52). In the periphery, hazy white inflammatory masses may be seen at the pars plana (Fig. 31-8) and often are associated with retinal folds extending posteriorly toward the optic disc. Traction bands from these inflammatory masses to the optic disc may result in a retinal fold through the macula, macular traction, or macular dragging. *Toxocara* endophthalmitis usually presents with a white eye and little pain but with marked vitreous inflammation,

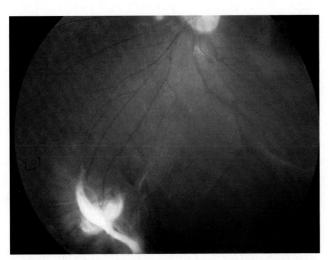

FIGURE 31-7. Posterior pole of an 8-year-old boy with inflammatory granuloma caused by *Toxocara canis*. Note traction on the surrounding retina. Vitreitis has been controlled with systemic prednisone.

granulomatous keratic precipitates, and anterior chamber inflammation. A white retrolental mass, which represents an organization of the inflammatory process into a cyclitic membrane between a detached retina and lens, may occur and must be differentiated from retinoblastoma. Amblyopia also may occur as a complication of toxocariasis.

Diagnosis

The diagnosis of ocular toxocariasis usually is presumptive based on the clinical findings and correlation with serum antibodies to *T. canis* measured by serologic enzyme-linked immunoabsorbent assay. A 1:8 dilution is considered positive in the presence of the appropriate clinical findings (48). In cases where the diagnosis is uncertain, enzyme-linked

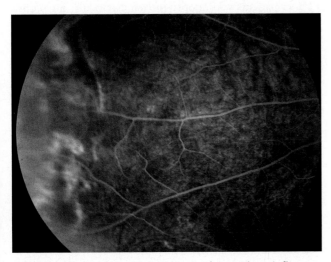

FIGURE 31-8. Fluorescein angiogram of pars plana inflammatory exudation in an 8-year-old boy with ocular toxocariasis.

immunoabsorbent assay on aqueous or vitreous biopsy specimens may facilitate the diagnosis. The presence of eosinophils in aqueous or vitreous biopsy specimens also suggests the diagnosis of toxocariasis.

Medical Management

Ocular toxocariasis is treated medically. Therapy is directed at the inflammatory response to prevent inflammation-induced tissue injury and secondary membrane formation. The inflammation is treated with corticosteroids, either topically or periocularly. Systemic prednisone administered at a rate of 0.5 to 1 mg/kg/day may be added, if needed. If the inflammation is refractory to steroid treatment, therapy with anthelmintics directed at the larvae itself may be attempted. Thiabendazole 50 mg/kg/day for 7 days has been proposed if steroid therapy failed (53). There have been reports of clinical improvement of ocular toxocariasis treated with thiabendazole (25 mg/kg twice a day for 5 days), albendazole (800 mg twice a day for 6 days), and mebendazole (100 to 200 mg twice a day for 5 days) (54).

Indications for Surgery

Intraocular inflammation may lead to macular detachment through either direct vitreomacular traction or epiretinal membrane formation creating macular pucker. Traction also may lead to retinal breaks in atrophic retina, creating a combined traction-rhegmatogenous detachment. A pars plana vitrectomy may be beneficial for patients who have not had a satisfactory response to medical treatment or for those who have marked vitreous fibrosis and tractional complications. Indications for surgery are traction retinal detachment, epiretinal membrane creating significant distortion or heterotropia, impending retinal detachment, or cyclitic membrane. When a retinal detachment appears inevitable, early vitrectomy to eliminate the vitreous traction band from the granuloma has been successful, providing the preoperative visual acuity was good (55).

Surgical Management

For traction macular detachment, pars plana vitrectomy and membrane peeling may be performed in a manner similar to that for other types of epiretinal membrane (55). The fibrous membranes located between the peripheral granuloma and the optic disc usually have extensions into the underlying retina and need to be carefully lifted off from the retinal surface before they can be severed. These membranes usually remain tightly adherent to the optic disc and peripheral granuloma; therefore, they often need to be circumcised rather than delaminated or peeled. Because the granulomas appear to be an intimal part of the retina, attempts to extirpate the retinal granuloma usually are unsuccessful and may cause undesirable complications. Therefore, the granulomas usually are left in place. In most cases, macular traction can be released without removal of the granuloma, although scleral buckling is necessary in some cases.

Outcomes

The use of pars plana vitrectomy for traction retinal detachment and/or impending macular detachment has been reported. Anatomic success for reattachment ranges from 66% to 83% (55–57). However, the rate of redetachment is fairly high, ranging from 24% to 48%. Vitreous surgery to treat macular traction due to *T. canis* was reported in 1977 (58). Later, 12 (71%) of 17 eyes attained retinal reattachment after vitreoretinal surgery for retinal detachment associated with complications of toxocariasis (56). Fifteen eyes (88%) had stabilization or improvement in visual acuity. Redetachment occurred in 4 (24%) of 17 eyes. In a series in which 10 (83%) of 12 eyes attained retinal reattachment after vitrectomy for traction macular disorders associated with toxocariasis, nine eyes (75%) had stabilization or improvement in visual acuity (55). Redetachment occurred in 5 (42%) of 12 eyes and was associated with epiretinal membrane proliferation. The presence of a preoperative tractional fold through the macula was associated with a poor final visual outcome. In 12 eyes with toxocariasis-associated complications, although only 9 had traction-related macular problems (57). The other eyes had vitreous opacification alone. Of those with traction detachment, 6 (66%) of 9 eyes were reattached, and these cases improved or were stabilized visually. Redetachment occurred in three eyes (33%). Recovery of the intraocular larvae usually is not possible, except in rare cases, because of the small size of the organism (approximately 18–21 μm) or because of destruction of the organism by inflammatory cells. The unintentional extraction of toxocariasis larvae during vitreoretinal surgery was reported (59).

Postoperative Care

It is essential to remember that a successful operation is only part of the visual rehabilitation in a child. Postoperative amblyopia therapy in conjunction with a pediatric ophthalmologist is necessary. The primary factors influencing the outcome of surgery for the complications of ocular toxocariasis are factors such as the age of the patient, disease duration before diagnosis, preexisting amblyopia, and compromise of the macula. The prognosis for improved visual acuity and normal binocular vision is better when the onset of the disease occurs in older patients and the disease is detected early in its course.

Sarcoidosis

Sarcoidosis is an idiopathic, noncaseating granulomatous inflammatory disease that may affect any part of the body, most commonly the lungs, but may include the eye and orbit, lymphatics, heart, kidneys, musculoskeletal system, and skin (60). The incidence of sarcoidosis is 6 to 10 in 100,000 (61). It is 10 times more frequent among African Americans than among Caucasians (62). Although 75% of affected patients are between 20 and 50 years old, sarcoidosis may occur in children (63).

Children aged 5 years or younger may develop a childhood sarcoid arthritis (64). The classic triad of symptoms consists of skin, eye, and joint lesions; initial pulmonary involvement is rare. It can be easily misdiagnosed as JRA, which also presents with joint and eye findings (65,66). However children with JRA-associated uveitis usually suffer from pauciarticular arthritis, are antinuclear antibody (ANA) positive, and rarely develop skin lesions, whereas children with sarcoidosis usually develop polyarthritis, are ANA negative, often exhibit skin lesions in the form of erythema nodosum, and have elevated serum angiotensin-converting enzyme (ACE) (67).

Diagnosis

Initial systemic workup consists of a chest radiograph, and serum ACE, lysozyme, serum and urine calcium, and liver enzymes (67). If the results of these studies are negative, chest computed tomography, gallium scan, and pulmonary function test should be performed. Gallium scanning shows uptake in lacrimal and parotid glands, also known as a *panda sign*. Sarcoidosis may first present with uveitis only, with a negative workup, and with extraocular manifestations evolving slowly over several years (68). Thus, laboratory and radiologic tests should be repeated periodically in "sarcoid suspects" (67).

The definitive diagnosis of sarcoidosis is a histopathologic one and has been made by biopsy of the parotid gland, lung, conjunctiva, skin, or lacrimal gland (67). Conjunctival biopsy is a simple procedure to perform on easily accessible tissue with a low complication rate. Random conjunctival biopsies have been reported to be positive in 55% to 71% of patients with biopsy-proven extraocular sarcoidosis (69,70) and in 28% of patients with suspected sarcoidosis (69). True sarcoid granulomas may be too small to be seen with slitlamp examination, and prominent nodules often turn out to be large follicles, an ectopic lacrimal gland, or foreign body fibrosis rather than noncaseating granulomas (71). Because true sarcoid granulomas are often too small to be seen with slitlamp examination, random conjunctival biopsy may be reasonable.

Conjunctival Biopsy

The lower fornix is the preferred site for conjunctival biopsy. The lower lid is retracted and a strip of stretched conjunctiva is excised with Westcott scissors. The optimal size of biopsy specimen is approximately 1 cm long × 3 mm wide. A topical antibiotic is instilled and pressure is applied for 5 to 10 minutes to prevent hemorrhage and soft tissue edema. No suturing is needed. There have been no reports of infection or symblepharon formation after conjunctival biopsy. Multiple sectioning is recommended because the noncaseating granulomas may be sporadic throughout the conjunctival tissue (70).

Clinical Signs

The ocular manifestations of sarcoidosis in children are similar to those seen in adults and include granulomatous anterior uveitis, posterior uveitis, pars planitis, periphlebitis, macular edema, epiretinal membrane, branch retinal vein occlusion, retinal neovascularization, traction retinal detachment, conjunctival and iris granulomas, and keratoconjunctivitis sicca. Severe visual loss worse than 20/200 has been reported in 6% to 24% of patients with ocular sarcoidosis and is more common in patients with chronic posterior uveitis (68,72).

Medical Management

Sarcoidosis is primarily treated medically. Treatment should be directed toward absolute control of the inflammation to minimize any potential ocular complications and structural damage. Mild anterior uveitis is treated with topical corticosteroids and cycloplegics. Systemic steroids are indicated in refractory anterior uveitis and in patients with posterior uveitis, retinal neovascularization, or optic nerve compromise. If inflammation persists with systemic steroids, the addition of oral NSAIDs may be useful. Immunosuppressive medications such as azathioprine, cyclosporine, methotrexate, or cyclophosphamide may be required for refractory disease or as part of a steroid-sparing strategy (72–74).

Surgical Indications

Vitreoretinal surgery occasionally may be needed to remove nonclearing vitreous hemorrhages, peel epiretinal membranes, repair traction or rhegmatogenous retinal detachment, or remove inflammatory debris from the vitreous cavity. Additionally, the complications of chronic uveitis, such as band keratopathy, glaucoma, and cataract, may need to be treated surgically.

The major cause of poor visual outcome in these patients is macular pathology such as cystoid macular edema and epiretinal membrane. Vitreous hemorrhage secondary to retinal neovascularization may cause decreased visual acuity. Secondary glaucoma may occur as a consequence of severe anterior segment inflammation. Band keratopathy or cataract may develop as a consequence of chronic uveitis.

Surgical Management

Iris Nodules

Surgical excision of iris nodules may help in the diagnosis and control of sarcoid uveitis refractory to medical manage-

ment. The surgical excision of iris nodules for histopathologic confirmation of the diagnosis of sarcoidosis in two 10-year-old boys in whom anterior uveitis was refractory to medical management was reported (75) and resulted in control of inflammation. The authors hypothesize that the iris granuloma may become a focus of continued cytokine production and ocular inflammation, and they suggested that total surgical excision of the iris masses may help in the diagnosis and control of sarcoid uveitis refractory to medical management.

Cataracts

Cataracts may form as a result of recurrent inflammation from ocular sarcoidosis. Cataract extraction may be achieved through limbal approach with phacoemulsification or through a pars plana approach with lensectomy in combination with a pars plana vitrectomy. Placement of an IOL in young patients who will experience future flareups of inflammation or have an anticipated chronic course of inflammation places them at high risk for developing thick retrolental membranes, severe postoperative inflammation, iris capture, chronic cystoid macular edema, or hypotony. In a retrospective analysis of 102 patients with sarcoidosis-associated uveitis (73), the successful implantation of a posterior chamber lens during cataract surgery was reported in 19 (90.5%) of 21 adult eyes; however, the success rate is likely to be much lower in the pediatric eye with sarcoidosis-associated uveitis. After cataract extraction and IOL implantation, young patients and patients with sarcoidosis were reported to have a marked postoperative flareup of inflammation accompanied by significant fibrin and protein within the eye that peaked 48 hours after surgery and persisted for 5 to 6 days postoperatively (2). The consideration of placing an IOL is similar to the earlier discussion for other uveitic conditions. Removal of the vitreous scaffold intraoperatively (19), careful control of inflammation with high-dose steroids during the first postoperative week, and follow-up within 5 to 7 days after surgery are important (2). Tissue plasminogen activator can be used to clear severe dense fibrin in the anterior chamber.

Glaucoma

Secondary glaucoma with sarcoid uveitis appears to be a particularly poor prognostic sign and is associated with severe vision loss (76). Glaucoma associated with uveitis usually is notoriously difficult to treat. Conventional filtering surgery has a lower chance of success in these patients with ongoing uveitis because recurrent inflammation promotes fibrous tissue growth and subsequent closure of the filtering bleb. Some studies report reasonable success rates using glaucoma drainage devices, i.e., success rates of 77% to 94% with follow-up from 1 to 10 years, with choroidal effusions, hypotony, and cystoid macular edema being the most common postoperative complications (12,15–18).

Vitreoretinal Complications

Retinal complications of ocular sarcoidosis include retinal vasculitis, peripheral retinal and disc neovascularization, choroidal nodules or granulomas with overlying sensory retinal detachment, subretinal neovascularization, epiretinal membrane proliferation, and traction retinal detachment. Patients with sarcoidosis may develop large areas of retinal capillary nonperfusion and secondary retinal or disc neovascularization. Both retinal and disc neovascularization may regress in patients with sarcoidosis in up to 50% of patients treated by systemic medical therapy alone (40,41). When persistent or progressive peripheral retinal neovascularization causes recurrent vitreous hemorrhage, laser grid photocoagulation or cryopexy may be applied to areas of ischemia as defined by fluorescein angiography. Laser photocoagulation usually is followed by a significant increase in cystoid macular edema (40). Steroid therapy should be used in combination with laser treatment to blunt the anticipated inflammatory response. When disc neovascularization causes recurrent vitreous hemorrhage, panretinal photocoagulation may be required to cause regression of the disc vessels. Vitrectomy has a role in removing nonclearing vitreous hemorrhages that result from peripheral retinal or disc neovascularization. Active neovascularization at the time of surgery may be treated with endophotocoagulation or peripheral cryopexy. Vitrectomy may be needed for epiretinal membrane peeling or for repair of traction or rhegmatogenous retinal detachment.

Pars plana vitrectomy clears the visual axis by removing media opacities and vitreous debris in patients with vitreous inflammation refractory to medical therapy. Vitrectomy may alter the course of inflammation and result in stabilization of the disease by removing immunocompetent cells and inflammatory mediators from the vitreous cavity (23,24,37). Vitrectomy may potentially reduce cystoid macular edema either by eliminating the contact between an inflamed vitreous body and the macula or by allowing better penetration or distribution of corticosteroids (22,24,38).

In the pediatric sarcoid-associated uveitis patient, surgery is best undertaken after the eye has been quiescent for as long as possible. Perioperative inflammation must be rigorously controlled with aggressive topical, periocular, and possibly systemic corticosteroid use. Maximum control of inflammation preoperatively, intraoperatively, and postoperatively allows the greatest chance of a successful surgery.

Intermediate Uveitis

Intermediate uveitis is a relatively common bilateral disease that affects otherwise healthy children and young adults. The course is variable, ranging from a mild self-limiting disease to a chronic disease with exacerbations and remissions. The main ocular finding is a marked exudative response in the peripheral retina and inflammation in the anterior vitreous. Vision loss is most commonly due to vitreous debris, cystoid macular edema, epiretinal membrane, and cataract. Vitreoretinal surgery may be needed for clearing of vitreous debris as well as attenuation of inflammation and the exudative response. Cryotherapy or panretinal scatter photocoagulation may be used for peripheral neovascularization. Uveitic cataract may be treated with surgerical intervention.

Intermediate uveitis is an idiopathic intraocular inflammatory syndrome of the peripheral retina and pars plana, which is known by many names, most commonly pars planitis and peripheral uveitis. Intermediate uveitis has been reported in 16% to 33% of all uveitis cases presenting among children (77). The age of onset ranges from 5 to 65 years, with the mean occurrence in the third decade of life (25). Severe cases tend to present at an earlier age, whereas older patients have a milder form of the disease. From 70% to 90% of cases are bilateral, although the majority of cases are asymmetric (78).

Symptoms and Signs

Patients with intermediate uveitis often present with minimal symptoms, which may include floaters or blurred vision but no pain, photophobia, or redness of the eye. A mild anterior chamber inflammation may be present or absent. Posterior subcapsular cataracts are the most common anterior segment complication, ranging from 15% to 60% (79,80). The incidence of glaucoma is quite low, reported to be 8% in one large series (80). Vitreous cells are the most characteristic sign for intermediate uveitis, ranging from mild to severe. Large gray-white or yellow exudative aggregates, also called *snowbanks,* may be present during active pars planitis. White collagen bands at the pars plana may be seen chronically in some patients, even during periods of quiescence. Vitreous yellow-white aggregates, also called *snowballs,* may be seen inferiorly. Vitreous inflammation tends to be mild early in the course of disease, but the vitreous can later become organized and opacified (22,25). Peripheral retinal neovascularization may occur, resulting in vitreous hemorrhage. Cystoid macular edema is the most common cause of permanent visual loss, and it may occur in 30% to 60% of patients (25,79) Serous, traction, rhegmatogenous, and combined retinal detachments occur in 5% of eyes. Optic disc edema is not uncommon.

The clinical course of intermediate uveitis may range from a mild course with complete remission to a relentlessly progressive course with severe exudation, neovascularization, and resistance to therapy, which is seen more often in children (78,81). Brockhurst and Schepens (81) described four different groups as defined by their clinical course. A mild course with complete remission was seen in 31% of patients, a mild chronic course in 49%, a severe chronic course in 15%, and a relentlessly progressive course in 5%. Others (80) found 19% to have mild inflammation, 42% moderate inflammation, and 39% severe inflammation in their group of patients with intermediate uveitis who were followed 10 years later.

Diagnosis

The differential diagnosis of intermediate uveitis includes many causes of vitreous inflammation. It is imperative to exclude infectious causes, because antimicrobial therapy may be curative. Infectious entities in the differential diagnosis include Lyme disease, toxocariasis, Whipple disease, tuberculosis, syphilis, human T-cell leukemia virus type 1, Epstein-Barr virus, and catscratch disease. Equally important is the exclusion of intermediate uveitis associated with underlying systemic disease such as sarcoidosis, Behcet disease, multiple scleroses, or intraocular lymphoma. Initial laboratory studies include a complete blood count with differential (myeloproliferative and infectious disease), ACE (sarcoidosis), chest X-ray film (sarcoidosis and tuberculosis), tuberculin skin test (purified protein derivative [PPD]) with anergy panel, microhemagglutinin *Treponema pallidum* (MHATP) or fluorescent treponemal antibody absorption test (FTA-ABS) (syphilis), and antinuclear antibody (systemic lupus erythematosis [SLE] and other connective tissue diseases), with consideration of Lyme or *Toxocara* antibody testing (25).

Management

Having excluded treatable infections and noninfectious entities, treatment of intermediate uveitis may begin. Intermediate uveitis is treated medically and is directed toward the complications and sequelae of intraocular inflammation such as cystoid macular edema, cataract, vitreous opacity, peripheral neovascularization, or retinal detachment. A five-step regimen has been proposed (50) that is a modified approach based on a four-step regimen initially described in 1984 (39): (i) topical corticosteroid for anterior segment inflammation with periocular corticosteroid injections; (ii) oral NSAIDs should inflammation recur following the third injection, with topical NSAIDs in the presence of cystoid macular edema; (iii) systemic corticosteroids should inflammation persist or recur despite the previous interventions; (iv) peripheral retinal cryopexy or indirect laser photocoagulation should pars planitis recur following the sixth regional steroid injection; and (v) pars plana vitrectomy versus immunosuppressive chemotherapy, such as cyclosporin A at a dosage of 2 to 5 mg/kg/day should inflammation be recalcitrant to the preceding modalities. Many antimetabolites and immunosuppressive drugs have been tried, including cyclosporine, methotrexate, azathioprine, 6-mercaptopurine, cyclophosphamide, and chlorambucil (49).

Peripheral Laser or Cryotherapy

In patients with unremitting chronic pars planitis that is recalcitrant to steroid or NSAID therapy, cryotherapy and scatter laser photocoagulation of the peripheral retina have been reported effective in causing regression of peripheral neovascularization and reduction of inflammatory activity (42,43) and vitreous hemorrhage (43,44). For discussion, see earlier section: "Lasers-Peripheral Neovascularization (Intermediate Uveitis)."

Vitrectomy

In patients with vitreous opacities impairing vision, causing amblyopia, or obscuring the ophthalmologist's view of the periphery, pars plana vitrectomy is an effective treatment for visual rehabilitation as well as attenuation of inflammation. Pars plana vitrectomy with or without pars plana lensectomy is used to treat certain complications of intermediate uveitis, such as vitreous opacification, traction retinal detachment, vitreous hemorrhage, and epiretinal membrane formation. In cases of vitreous inflammation refractory to medical therapy, pars plana vitrectomy clears the visual axis by removal of media opacities and vitreous debris. Vitrectomy also may alter the course of inflammation and result in stabilization of the disease by removing immunocompetent cells and inflammatory mediators from the vitreous cavity (23,24,37). Vitrectomy may potentially reduce cystoid macular edema either by eliminating the contact between an inflamed vitreous body and the macula or by allowing better penetration or distribution of corticosteroids (22,24,38). General guidelines for vitrectomy for medically refractory intermediate uveitis include (i) removal of the posterior hyaloid; (ii) removal of as much anterior vitreous as possible; (iii) careful inspection of the periphery, looking for neovascularization and occult retinal breaks that can be treated with endolaser photocoagulation; and (iv) maximal perioperative control of inflammation with intravitreous, periocular, and possibly systemic corticosteroid use.

Cataract Surgery

Cataract formation is another complication of intermediate uveitis. Cataract extraction may be achieved through limbal approach with phacoemulsification or through a pars plana approach with lensectomy in combination with a pars plana vitrectomy. If a concurrent vitreous opacity exists, combined pars plana lensectomy and core vitrectomy is classically the procedure of choice. A combined limbal cataract extraction and pars plana vitrectomy approach also can be used.

Implantation of a posterior chamber IOL is dependent on the risk of future or chronic inflammation. A peripheral iridectomy should be made if recurrent or chronic inflammation is anticipated.

In the child with intermediate uveitis, surgery is best undertaken after the eye has been quiet for as long as possible. Perioperative inflammation must be rigorously controlled with aggressive topical, periocular, and possibly systemic corticosteroid use. Maximum control of inflammation preoperatively, intraoperatively, and postoperatively allows the greatest chance for a successful surgery.

Juvenile Rheumatoid Arthritis

JRA is a chronic arthritis of at least 3 months' duration that affects children younger than 16 years (82–84). The estimated prevalence is 113 per 100,000, with an annual incidence of 14 cases per 100,000 in the United States (5). The course of JRA-associated uveitis is predominantly chronic, lasting a mean of 19.7 years (85), with a relapsing and remitting course in 60% of patients and an unremitting course in 20% of patients. Only 20% of patients have a single episode of intraocular inflammation (86).

Symptoms and Signs

JRA-associated uveitis is a binocular disease that affects children. The clinical course is predominantly chronic. The main ocular finding is a chronic iridocyclitis with associated complications of uveitis, such as band keratopathy, cataract, and secondary glaucoma, amblyopia, and strabismus. Surgical treatment of refractory glaucoma or cataract may be necessary. These children are at increased risk for intraoperative complications due to permanent structural changes from chronic inflammation and are at increased risk for postoperative complications from an excessive postoperative inflammatory response and recurrent inflammation, which is the norm.

JRA-associated uveitis is the most common cause of anterior uveitis in childhood and is associated with significant ocular morbidity (87). The degree of final visual loss was correlated with the degree of visual loss at onset and that the risk of ocular complications were correlated with the severity of inflammation observed at the initial examination as defined by the presence of posterior synechiae (88). Other factors that correlated with poor visual prognosis were pauciarticular arthritis (four or fewer joints affected), young age at onset, female gender, ANA positivity, and rheumatoid factor negativity. Associated band keratopathy occurs in 6% to 66%, associated cataract in 18% to 71%, and associated glaucoma in 11% to 38% (20). Blindness, with a visual acuity worse than 20/200, ranged from 0% to 41% (20). Chronic or recurrent uveitis eventually caused the complications of cataract, glaucoma, hypotony, vitreous organization, optic neuropathy, or macular edema.

Medical Management

JRA-associated uveitis is primarily treated medically. Treatment should be directed toward absolute control of the inflammation with medications, which must be administered over the numerous years of this chronic disease. Although topical and periocular corticosteroid injections remain the first-line therapy for anterior uveitis, up to 61% of patients with JRA-associated uveitis either do not respond to corticosteroid treatment or require prolonged therapy, with its attendant side effects (88). If inflamma-

tion persists with frequent topical steroid dosing or continues to recur every time corticosteroids are tapered and withdrawn, the addition of chronic oral NSAIDs may be useful (89). Refractory inflammation should be treated with once-a-week low-dose methotrexate therapy, i.e., 0.5 mg/kg once per week. In one large study, virtually no toxicity was found in 127 patients in whom low-dose methotrexate was given for the management of JRA-associated joint disease (26,90). Other immunomodulatory agents such as cyclosporine, azathioprine, or chlorambucil may be considered if continued inflammation with loss of vision occurs despite these measures (5).

Surgical Indications

Children with JRA-associated uveitis may require surgical treatment for refractory glaucoma, cataract, or band keratopathy. These patients are at increased risk for intraoperative and postoperative complications due to chronic inflammation. Even if the eye appears clinically quiet preoperatively, it often responds to surgery with excessive bleeding, postoperative inflammation, and unexpected postoperative IOP responses such as ocular hypertension or hypotony. General anesthesia with endotracheal intubation may be complicated by the presence of cervical arthritis or spondylitis, temporomandibular joint inflammation with restriction of movement, or micrognathia. The decision to proceed with surgery for the complications of JRA-associated uveitis in a child is difficult and must be considered carefully.

Cataract Surgery
Cataracts occur in 18% to 71% of patients with JRA-associated uveitis and can be attributed to chronic inflammation and corticosteroid use (19,20). Cataract surgery in JRA-associated uveitic eyes is daunting to even the most accomplished cataract surgeon because of the unknown risks that can occur intraoperatively and the uncertainty of the postoperative course (3,4). Surgery is frequently technically challenging because of posterior synechiae, iris vasculature delicacy, pupillary membranes, miotic pupils, and corneal opacification (5). The combination of the heightened pediatric immune response and a uveitic eye often results in a violent postoperative inflammatory response. Loss of vitreous or retention of cortical material may exacerbate intraocular inflammation. Indications for cataract surgery include visual rehabilitation, prevention or treatment of amblyopia, and enhancement of the ophthalmologist's view of the posterior segment for ongoing assessment of the optic nerve and retina. Given the risk of surgery, the unexpected postoperative course, and likely aphakia, prevention of cataract in patients with JRA is preferable (1). Chronic steroid therapy that results in cataract development should be eschewed, and chronic NSAID therapy or low-dose methotrexate therapy should be considered.

The surgical technique for cataract extraction in the child with JRA should include removal of the cataract, including the posterior capsule, all retrolenticular and cyclitic membranes, and most of the vitreous. Historically, pars plana lensectomy with pars plana vitrectomy was the procedure of choice (22). For the pars plana approach, the lens and posterior and anterior capsules are cut and aspirated with an ocutome probe. This is followed by a near-total vitrectomy and removal of the lens capsule, anterior hyaloid, and vitreous scaffold to reduce secondary membrane formation (19). A surgical peripheral iridectomy should be performed if recurrent or chronic inflammation is anticipated.

An alternative approach to cataract extraction may be accomplished by a combined limbal approach with phacoemulsification and pars plana vitrectomy. During the limbal approach, synechiolysis, pupillary stretching, and iris hooks are used as needed for adequate exposure. Capsulorrhexis, hydrodissection, and phacoemulsification are performed in standard fashion, and the incision is closed. This is followed by a pars plana approach for complete posterior capsule excision, followed by a near-total vitrectomy.

IOL implantation has not been recommended in patients with JRA-associated uveitis (1,2,19,26). The IOL may provide a stimulus for intraocular inflammation and structural support for inflammatory membranes, which may induce irreversible ocular pathology. Thus, patients with JRA usually have been left aphakic after cataract surgery, necessitating the use of aphakic spectacles or contact lenses. Despite excellent anatomic outcomes, visual rehabilitation for aphakic eyes may be suboptimal because many patients of this age are unable or refuse to wear aphakic contact lens or aphakic spectacles (7). Among children, contract lens intolerance is reported to be 17% to 38% (26,36). The frequent concomitant occurrence of band keratopathy makes contact lens fitting difficult. Multiple lost contact lenses carry a substantial expense. Children often are intolerant of aphakic spectacles because of the weight and aniseikonia.

Cataract Surgery Outcomes

The results of cataract extraction with or without IOL implantation in patients with JRA-associated uveitis historically have been abysmal. In a report of 162 eyes with extracapsular cataract extraction, only 30% of patients had visual acuity of 20/40 or better, and 48% of patients had a visual acuity of hand motion or worse (91). With the advent of improved microsurgical instruments and techniques, seven of eight eyes of adults and children with JRA-associated uveitis that had standard phacoemulsification cataract extraction, without a posterior capsulectomy, and posterior chamber IOL implantation achieved a final visual acuity better than 20/40 (92). However, all three patients aged 13 years or younger had postoperative results inferior to those of adult patients at a median follow-up of 14 months. The children's eyes developed persistent postoperative inflammation, posterior synechiae, and pupillary membranes. The authors

concluded that in selected adults with cataracts caused by JRA-associated uveitis, standard phacoemulsification cataract extraction with IOL implantation may have excellent results. They cautioned that IOL implantation in children with JRA merits further investigation.

In another report (93), the results of five eyes of children aged 4 to 8 years who had JRA-associated uveitis after phacoemulsification cataract extraction, posterior capsulectomy, anterior vitrectomy, and IOL placement and four eyes of children aged 3 to 8 years after pars plana lensectomy and vitrectomy without IOL placement were examined. The patients were followed for 5 years. Visual acuity with IOL was 6/6, 6/60, 6/240, light perception (LP), and hand motion (HM) whereas visual acuity with aphakia was 6/9, LP in 2 patients, and no light perception (NLP) in 1 patient. Four of five patients with IOL implantation required a subsequent surgical retrolental membranectomy and total vitrectomy. Preoperative topical or systemic corticosteroids or immunosuppressive treatment were not reported in any children. After surgery, each child received a retroorbital injection of methylprednisolone and an intravenous bolus of hydrocortisone. Postoperatively, each child received hourly topical corticosteroids for 1 week that was tapered on an individual basis. Although the outcomes were poor, the patients were mildly better with IOL implantation.

In 2003, favorable outcomes with IOL implantation with cataract surgery were reported in children with JRA-associated uveitis (32). Five children (six eyes) younger than 13 years with JRA-associated uveitis underwent standard phacoemulsification cataract extraction without posterior capsulectomy and posterior chamber IOL implantation. Postoperative visual acuity was 20/40 or better in all six eyes. Median follow-up was 44 months. Preoperatively, four children (five eyes) were on low-dose methotrexate immunosuppressive therapy for a median length of 1.25 years before surgery. Preoperatively, two children (three eyes) were on additional immunosuppressants or systemic corticosteroids. All eyes received frequent topical corticosteroids for a median of 2 weeks preoperatively and 8.5 weeks postoperatively. Five eyes required Nd:YAG capsulotomy. One eye needed a subsequent surgical posterior capsulectomy and pars plana vitrectomy. The authors concluded that with adequate long-term preoperative and postoperative control of intraocular inflammation with systemic immunosuppressive therapy and intensive topical perioperative corticosteroid therapy, children with JRA-associated uveitis may have favorable surgical outcomes after cataract surgery with posterior chamber IOL implantation.

Management of Inflammation

It is critical that cataract surgery with or without IOL implantation be attempted after absolute and sustained control of uveitis for a minimum of 3 months in patients with JRA. Long-term preoperative systemic immunosuppressive therapy and aggressive perioperative topical corticosteroids may vastly improve the outcome of cataract extraction in children with JRA and may allow for IOL implantation for improved visual rehabilitation. For aphakic children, vigilant postoperative amblyopia therapy is critical, and patients should be followed in conjunction with a pediatric ophthalmologist with proper aphakic contact lens or spectacles, orthoptic evaluation, and occlusion therapy.

Glaucoma Surgery

Elevated IOP frequently accompanies uveitis in patients with JRA. The incidence of glaucoma in patients with JRA varies between 11% and 38% (20). The prognosis for patients who develop glaucoma with JRA is poor. One group (91) reported a 35% incidence of NLP vision in children with uveitis and glaucoma. Medical therapy often proves inadequate for controlling IOP, necessitating surgical intervention.

Glaucoma Surgery Outcomes

Trabeculectomy in children with chronic intraocular inflammation often is unsuccessful. The increased failure rate of filtration procedures in children has been postulated to be secondary to decreased scleral rigidity and accelerated healing of the Tenon capsule in the younger population (2). In addition, the extensive inflammatory response of the pediatric eye, as well as possible recurrent or chronic inflammation, results in fibrous tissue growth and subsequent closure of the filtering bleb over time. Although adjunctive 5-fluorouracil may keep the filtering bleb open in the initial few weeks or months after surgery, recurrent inflammation may later close the bleb (2). Thus, the long-term success rate of filtering surgery has a decreasing chance of success in these patients over time.

The success rate with glaucoma drainage devices is slightly more encouraging. Twenty-seven eyes with secondary glaucoma due to JRA had Molteno implant and were followed for 40 months (17). A successful outcome with IOP >5 mmHg and ≤23 mmHg was achieved in 89% of patients. Life-table analysis success rates were 95% after 27 months and 90% after 52 months. Postoperative complications included flat anterior chamber, tube blockage by iris or vitreous, cataract, cornea-tube touch, choroidal detachment, corneal edema, and corneal abrasion.

The inflammation should be maximally controlled with corticosteroid or immunosuppressant medications for as long as possible preoperatively in patients undergoing nonurgent glaucoma surgery. The glaucoma drainage device can be implanted in standard fashion between tenon fascia and sclera and secured in place. The tube is placed through either the limbus or the pars plana in vitrectomized eyes. The tube and its insertion site are covered with a patch of preserved donor sclera. Topical corticosteroids are used postoperatively. If a glaucoma drainage implant is placed in a vitrectomized, aphakic, pediatric patient, a pars plana tube placement will better allow contract lens fitting following surgery (1).

Band Keratopathy

Band keratopathy is observed in 6% to 66% of patients with advanced JRA-associated uveitis (20) and can be removed by EDTA chelation and superficial keratectomy. For discussion see "Therapeutic Surgery: Band Keratopathy Section of this Chapter."

Management of Inflammation

In the child with JRA-associated uveitis, surgery is best undertaken after the eye has been quiescent for as long as possible. Systemic immunosuppressive therapy with low-dose methotrexate prevents the complications of both chronic inflammation and chronic corticosteroid use. It also allows an improved chance of successful surgery with adequate control of inflammation. Perioperative inflammation must be rigorously controlled with aggressive topical, periocular, and possibly systemic corticosteroid use. Maximum control of inflammation preoperatively, intraoperatively, and postoperatively allows the greatest chance of a successful surgery.

REFERENCES

1. Foster CS, Opremcak EM. Therapeutic surgery: cornea, iris, cataract, glaucoma, vitreous, retinal. In: Foster CS, Vitale AT, eds. *Diagnosis and treatment of uveitis.* Philadelphia: WB Saunders, 2002:222–235.
2. Nussenblatt RB, Whitcup SM, Palestine AG. Role of surgery in the patient with uveitis. In: Nussenblatt RB, Whitcup SM, Palestine AG, eds. *Uveitis: fundamentals and clinical practice,* 2nd ed. St. Louis: Mosby, 1996:135–152.
3. Okhravi N, Lightman SL, Towler HMA. Assessment of visual outcome after cataract surgery in patients with uveitis. *Ophthalmology* 1999;106:710–722.
4. Alió JL, Chipont E. Phacoemulsification in patients with uveitis. In: Lu LW, Fine IH, eds. *Phacoemulsification in difficult and challenging cases.* New York: Thieme, 1999:65–74.
5. Foster CS, O'Brien JM. Childhood arthritis and anterior uveitis. In: Albert DM, Jakobiec FA, eds. *Principles and practice of ophthalmology,* 2nd ed. Philadelphia: WB Saunders, 2000:4542–4554.
6. Opremcak EM, Foster CS. Diagnostic surgery. In: Foster CS, Vitale AT, eds. *Diagnosis and treatment of uveitis.* Philadelphia: WB Saunders, 2002:215–221.
7. O'Connor GR. Calcific band keratopathy. *Trans Am Ophthalmol Soc* 1972;70:58–85.
8. Campos M, Nielson S, Szerenyi K, et al. Clinical follow-up of phototherapeutic keratectomy for the treatment of corneal opacities. *Am J Ophthalmol* 1993;115:433–440.
9. Stewart OG, Morrell AJ. Management of band keratopathy with excimer phototherapeutic keratectomy: visual, refractive, and symptomatic outcome. *Eye* 2003;17:233–237.
10. Panek WC, Holland GN, Lee DA, et al. Glaucoma in patients with uveitis. *Br J Ophthalmol* 1990;74:223–227.
11. Hoskins HD Jr, Hetherington J Jr, Shaffer RN. Surgical management of the inflammatory glaucomas. *Perspect Ophthalmol* 1977;1:173–181.
12. Hill RA, Nguyen QH, Baerveldt G, et al. Trabeculectomy and Molteno implantation of glaucomas associated with uveitis. *Ophthalmology* 1993;100:903–908.
13. Stavrou P, Mission GP, Rowson JJ, et al. Trabeculectomy in uveitis. *Ocul Immunol Inflamm* 1995;3:209–215.

14. Towler HMA, Bates AK, Broadway DC. Primary trabeculectomy with 5-fluorouracil for glaucoma secondary to uveitis. *Ocul Immunol Inflamm* 1995;3:163–170.

15. Ceballos EM, Parrish RK, Schiffman JC. Outcome of Baerveldt glaucoma drainage implants for the treatment of uveitic glaucoma. *Ophthalmology* 2002;109:2256–2260.

16. Da Mata A, Burk SE, Netland PA, et al. Management of uveitic glaucoma with Ahmed glaucoma valve implantation. *Ophthalmology* 1999;106:2168–2172.

17. Valimaki J, Airaksinen JA, Tuulonen A. Molteno implantation for secondary glaucoma in juvenile rheumatoid arthritis. *Arch Ophthalmol* 1997;115:1253–1256.

18. Molteno ACB, Sayawat N, Herbison P. Otago glaucoma surgery outcome study: long-term results of uveitis with secondary glaucoma drained by Molteno implants. *Ophthalmology* 2001;108:605–613.

19. Kanski JJ. Juvenile arthritis and uveitis. *Surv Ophthalmol* 1990;34:253–267.

20. Edelsten C, Lee V, Bentley CR, et al. An evaluation of baseline risk factors predicting severity in juvenile idiopathic arthritis associated uveitis and other chronic anterior uveitis in early childhood. *Br J Ophthalmol* 2002;86:51–56.

21. Foster CS, Stavrou P, Zafirakis P, et al. Intraocular lens removal patients with uveitis. *Am J Ophthalmol* 1999;128:31–37.

22. Mieler WF, Will BR, Lewis H, et al. Vitrectomy in the management of peripheral uveitis. *Ophthalmology* 1988;95:859–864.

23. Algvere P, Alanko H, Dickhoff K, et al. Pars plana vitrectomy in the management of intraocular inflammation. *Acta Ophthalmol* 1981;59:727–736.

24. Diamond JG, Kaplan HF. Uveitic effect of vitrectomy combined with lensectomy. *Ophthalmology* 1979;86:1320–1329.

25. Saperstein DA, Capone A Jr, Aaberg TM. Intermediate uveitis. In: Albert DM, Jakobiec FA, eds. *Principles and practice of ophthalmology,* 2nd ed. Philadelphia: WB Saunders, 2000:1225–1235.

26. Foster CS, Barrett R. Cataract development and cataract surgery in patients with juvenile rheumatoid arthritis-associated iridocyclitis. *Ophthalmology* 1993;100:809–817.

27. Papaliodis GN, Nguyen QD, Samson CM, et al. Intraocular lens tolerance in surgery for cataracta complicata: assessment of four implant materials. *Semin Ophthalmol* 2002;17:120–123.

28. Alio JR, Chipont E, BenEzra D, et al. International ocular inflammation society, study group of uveitis cataract surgery. *J Cataract Refract Surg* 2002;28:2096–2108.

29. Bayramlar H, Keskin UC. Heparin in the irrigation solution during cataract surgery. *J Cataract Refract Surg* 2002;28:2070–2071.

30. Kruger A, Amon M, Abela-Formanek C, et al. Effect of heparin in the irrigation solution on postoperative inflammation and cellular reaction on the intraocular lens surface. *J Cataract Refract Surg* 2002;28:87–92.

31. Michelson JB, Nozik RA, eds. *Surgical treatment of ocular inflammatory disease.* Philadelphia: JB Lippincott, 1988.

32. Lam LA, Lowder CY, Baerveldt G, et al. Surgical management o cataract in children with juvenile rheumatoid arthritis-associated uveitis. *Am J Ophthalmol* 2003;125:772–778.

33. Helm CJ, Holland GN. The effects of posterior subtenon injection of triamcinolone acetonide in patients with intermediate uveitis. *Am J Ophthalmol* 1995;120:55–64.

34. Klais CM, Hattenbach LO, Steinkamp GWK, et al. Intraocular recombinant tissue-plasminogen activator fibrinolysis of fibrin formation after cataract surgery in children. *J Cataract Refract Surg* 1999;25:357–362.

35. Koenig SB, Mieler WF, Han DP, et al. Combined phacoemulsification, pars plana vitrectomy, and posterior chamber intraocular lens insertions. *Arch Ophthalmol* 1992;110:1101–1104.

36. Hiles DA. Visual acuities of monocular IOL and non-IOL aphakic children. *Ophthalmology* 1980;87:1296–1300.

37. Bacskulin A, Eckardt C. Result of pars plana vitrectomy in chronic uveitis in children. *Ophthalmologie* 1993;90:434–439.

38. Park SE, Mieler WF, Pulido JS. Peripheral scatter photocoagulation for neovascularization associated with par planitis. *Arch Ophthalmol* 1995;113:1277–1280.

39. Kaplan HJ. Intermediate uveitis (pars planitis, chronic cyclitis)—a four step approach to treatment. In Saari KM, ed. *Uveitis update.* Amsterdam: Excerpta Medica, 1984:169–172.

40. Graham EM, Stanford MR, Shilling JS, et al. Neovascularization associated with posterior uveitis. *Br J Ophthalmol* 1987;71:826–833.

41. Duker JS, Brown GC, McNamara JA. Proliferative sarcoid retinopathy. *Ophthalmology* 1988;95:1680–1686.

42. Aaberg TM, Cesarz TJ, Flickinger RR. Treatment of peripheral uveoretinitis by cryotherapy. *Am J Ophthalmol* 1973;75:685–688.

43. Josephberg RG, Kanter ED, Jaffee RM. A fluorescein angiographic study of patients with pars planitis and peripheral exudation (snowbanking) before and after cryopexy. *Ophthalmology* 1994;101:1262–1266.

44. Phillips WB II, Bergren RL, McNamara JA. Pars planitis presenting with vitreous hemorrhage. *Ophthalmic Surg* 1993;24:630–631.

45. Devenyi RG, Mieler WF, Lambrou FH, et al. Cryopexy of the vitreous base in the management of peripheral uveitis. *Am J Ophthalmol* 1988;106:135–138.

46. Jaffe GJ, Ben-Nun J, Guo H, et al. Fluocinolone acetonide sustained drug delivery device to treat severe uveitis. *Ophthalmology* 2000;107;2024–2033.

47. Mok CH. Visceral larva migrans. *Clin Pediatr* 1968;7:565–573.

48. Shields JA. Ocular toxocariasis. A review. *Surv Ophthalmol* 1984;28:361–380.

49. Brown DH. Ocular Toxocara canis. II. Clinical review. *J Pediatr Ophthalmol* 1970;7:182–191.

50. Vitale AT, Zierhut M, Foster CS. Intermediate uveitis. In: Foster CS, Vitale AT, eds. *Diagnosis and treatment of uveitis.* Philadelphia: WB Saunders, 2002:844–857.

51. Amin HI, McDonald RF, Han DP, et al. Vitrectomy update for macular traction in ocular toxocariasis. *Retina* 2000;20:80–85.

52. Dent JH, Nichols RL, Beaver PC, et al. Visceral larva migrans. *Am J Pathol* 1956;32:777–803.

53. Dinning WJ, Gillespie SH, Cooling RJ, et al. Toxocariasis: a practical approach to management of ocular disease. *Eye* 1988;2:580–582.

54. Dietrich A, Auer H, Titti M, et al. Ocular toxocariasis in Austria. *Dtsch Med Wochenschr* 1998;123:626–630.

55. Small KW, McCuen BW, deJuan E Jr, et al. Surgical management of retinal traction caused by Toxocariasis. *Am J Ophthalmol* 1989;108:10–14.

56. Hagler WS, Pollard ZF, Jarrett WH, et al. Results of surgery for ocular Toxocara canis. *Ophthalmology* 1981;88:1081–1086.

57. Rodriguez A. Early pars plana vitrectomy in chronic endophthalmitis of toxocariasis. *Graefes Arch Clin Exp Ophthalmol* 1986;224:218–220.

58. Triester G, Machemer R. Results of vitrectomy for rare proliferative and hemorrhagic diseases. *Am J Ophthalmol* 1977;84:394–412.

59. Maguire AM, Green WR, Michels RG, et al. Recover of intraocular Toxocara canis by pars plana vitrectomy. *Ophthalmology* 1990;97:675–680.

60. Smith JA, Foster CS. Sarcoidosis and its ocular manifestations. *Int Ophthalmol Clin* 1996;36:109–125.

61. Chan CC, Wetzig RP, Palestine AG, et al. Immunohistopathology of ocular sarcoidosis. Report of a case and discussion of immunopathogenesis. *Arch Ophthalmol* 198;105:1398–1402.

62. Hunter DG, Foster CS. Systemic manifestations of sarcoidosis. In: Albert DM, Jakobiec FA, eds. *Principles and practice of*

ophthalmology, 2nd ed. Philadelphia: WB Saunders, 2000: 4606–4615.

63. Mayers M. Ocular sarcoidosis. *Int Ophthalmol Clin* 1990;30:257–263.

64. Hoover DL, Khan JA, Giangiacomo J. Pediatric ocular sarcoidosis. *Surv Ophthalmol* 1986;30:215–228.

65. Cancrini C, Angelini F, Colavita M, et al. Erythema nodosum: a presenting sign of early onset sarcoidosis. *Clin Exp Rheumatol* 1998;16:337–339.

66. Sahn EE, Hampton MT, Garen PD, et al. Preschool sarcoidosis masquerading as juvenile rheumatoid arthritis: two case reports and a review of the literature. *Pediatr Dermatol* 1990;7:208–213.

67. Stavrou P, Foster CS. Sarcoidosis. In: Albert DM, Jakobiec FA, eds. *Principles and practice of ophthalmology,* 2nd ed. Philadelphia: WB Saunders, 2000:710–725.

68. Rothova A, Alberts C, Glasius E, et al. Risk factors for ocular sarcoidosis. *Doc Ophthalmol* 1989;72:287–296.

69. Karcioglu AZ, Brear R. Conjunctival biopsy in sarcoidosis. *Am J Ophthalmol* 1985;99:68–73.

70. Nicholls CW, Eagle RC, Yanoff M, et al. Conjunctival biopsy as an aid in the evaluation of the patients with suspected sarcoidosis. *Ophthalmology* 1980;87:287–291.

71. Spaide FR, Ward DL. Conjunctival biopsy in the diagnosis of sarcoidosis. *Br J Ophthalmol* 1990;74:469–471.

72. Karma A, Huhti E, Poukkula A. Course and outcome of ocular sarcoidosis. *Am J Ophthalmol* 1988;106:467–472.

73. Akova YA, Foster CS. Cataract surgery in patients with sarcoidosis-associate uveitis. *Ophthalmology* 1994;101:473–479.

74. Dana M-R, Merayo-Lloves J, Schaumberg DA, et al. Prognosticators for visual outcome in sarcoid uveitis. *Ophthalmology* 1996;103:1846–1853.

75. Ocampo VVD, Foster CS, Baltatzis S. Surgical excision of iris nodules in the management of sarcoid uveitis. *Ophthalmology* 2001;108:1296–1299.

76. Jabs DA, Johns CJ. Ocular involvement in chronic sarcoidosis. *Am J Ophthalmol* 1986;102:297–301.

77. Hogan JU, Kimura SJ, O'Connor GR. Peripheral retinitis and chronic cyclitic in children. *Trans Ophthalmol Soc UK* 1965;85:39–52.

78. Aaberg TM, Cesarz TJ, Flinckinger RR. Treatment of pars planitis. I. Cryotherapy. *Surv Ophthalmol* 1977;22:120–125.

79. Malinowski SM, Folk JC, Pulido JS. Pars planitis. *Curr Opin Ophthalmol* 1994;5:72–82.

80. Smith RE, Godfrey WA, Kimura. SJ. Chronic cyclitis. I. Course and visual prognosis. *Trans Am Acad Ophthalmol Otolaryngol* 1973;77:760–768.

81. Brockhurst RJ, Schepens CL. Uveitis. IV. Peripheral uveitis: the complication of retinal detachment. *Arch Ophthalmol* 1968;80:747–753.

82. Cassidy JT, Levinson JE, Bass JC, et al. A study of classification criteria for a diagnosis of juvenile rheumatoid arthritis. *Arthritis Rheum* 1986;29:274–281.

83. Brewer EJ Jr, Bass JC, Cassidy JT, et al. Criteria for the classification of juvenile rheumatoid arthritis. *Bull Rheum Dis* 1972; 23:712–719.

84. Brewer EJ, Bass J, Baum J, et al. Current proposed revision of JRA criteria. *Arthritis Rheum* 1977;20:195–199.

85. David J, Cooper C, Hickey L, et al. The functional and psychological outcome of juvenile chronic arthritis in young adulthood. *Br J Rheumatol* 1994;33:876–881.

86. Rosenberg AM. Uveitis associated with juvenile rheumatoid arthritis. *Semin Arthritis Rheum* 1987;16:158–173.

87. Kanski JJ. Care of children with anterior uveitis. *Trans Ophthalmol Soc UK* 1981;101:387–390.

88. Wolf MD, Lichter PR, Ragsdale CG. Prognostic factors in the uveitis of juvenile rheumatoid arthritis. *Ophthalmology* 1987;94: 1242–1248.

89. Olson NY, Lindsley CB, Godfrey WA. Nonsteroidal anti-inflammatory drug therapy in chronic childhood iridocyclitis. *Am J Dis Child* 1988;142:1289–1292.

90. Giannini EH, Brewer EJ, Kuzmina N, et al. Methotrexate in resistant juvenile rheumatoid arthritis. Results of the USA-USSR double-blind, placebo-controlled trial. *N Engl J Med* 1992;326: 1043–1049.

91. Kanski JJ, Shun-Shin GA. Systemic uveitis syndromes in childhood: an analysis of 340 cases. *Ophthalmology* 1984;91: 1247–1252.

92. Probst LE, Holland EJ. Intraocular lens implantation in patient with juvenile rheumatoid arthritis. *Am J Ophthalmol* 1996;122: 161–170.

93. BenEzra D, Cohen E. Cataract surgery in children with chronic uveitis. *Ophthalmology* 2000;107:1255–1260.

32

TRAUMA

FERENC KUHN
ROBERT MORRIS
VIKTÓRIA MESTER

Injury is dramatic because it is sudden and almost always unexpected. The victim recognizes that trauma occurs but assumes it occurs to someone else. Ocular trauma is particularly serious because people fear blindness.

Eye injury carries even more pronounced psychological implications when a child is involved. Adults perceive children as vulnerable, innocent, and special. In many societies, children care for their aging parents. Consequently, ophthalmologists who treat injured children must be prepared to properly deal with overwhelming emotional reactions (1).

There are additional factors that make dealing with the injured child difficult. First, certain unavoidable injuries may have occurred when the child was in the womb or was being born. Taking a truthful history may be impossible because of the child's age or desire to hide the facts for fear of being caught in partaking in certain activities. A perpetrator would want to conceal his or her involvement in a child victim's injury to avoid criminal prosecution. The child's visual system is still developing and vulnerable to amblyopia due to deprivation or media opacities. The child can resist cooperation with the examination. The eye grows to 85% of its axial length by age 2 years and continues growth by 1% annually (2), so interventions, such as scleral buckles, may interfere with this growth. In addition, the orbital tissues continue to grow and rely on the normal volume of the eye to expand appropriately. The tissues of the injured eye or orbit may respond differently and be prone to intraocular scarring (3,4) more in a child than in an adult. The orbital floor is immature before puberty and overlies a small maxillary sinus, making the bones easy to bend and fracture rather than shatter so that muscle entrapment commonly results (5).

Finally, the term *child* presents a unique problem to the ophthalmologist because it encompasses those just born (age 0 years) to older individuals, but the upper age limit varies greatly in the trauma literature, from 9 to 20 years (6–13). A further potential source for misinterpretation is how this upper age level is described. When "children aged 0 to 12 years" is used, this is unambiguous, implying that children within this age range were studied. However, when "under 12" years is used, it is unclear as to whether those aged 12 years were included in the study. Furthermore, an unambiguous description such as "under 17" (14) can become ambiguous if improperly cited: "0 to 17" (15). Such inaccuracies present no problems in adults in whom an error of 1 year or even a decade is without significance, but they may lead to biased conclusions in children.

In this chapter, we define children as those aged 0 to 18 years ("under 19"). As much as possible, we also try to standardize the referenced literature (see later) so that data can be compared. Because of the differences in epidemiology, management, and prognosis, we tried to present data broken down for different age groups.

STANDARDIZED LANGUAGE OF OCULAR INJURIES: BIRMINGHAM EYE TRAUMA TERMINOLOGY

Without a system that unambiguously defines the type of mechanical trauma an eye has sustained, it is impossible for ophthalmologists to (i) properly describe the injured globe's condition to a colleague, (ii) present and interpret the result of research in journals and at scientific meetings, or (iii) conduct accurate and unbiased *Medline* searches. If no systematic source exists to define ocular trauma terms, ophthalmologists must rely on terms determined by subjective factors such as one's own institution of training, place of practice, personal experience, or peer pressure. This varied background historically led to terms such as *nonpenetrating laceration* (16) and *anterior globe nonperforating injury* (17), which are difficult to interpret.

An ideal system provides unambiguous definitions for all possible types of mechanical eye injury. The Birmingham Eye Trauma Terminology (BETT) was designed with these goals in mind.

This comprehensive system (18), now adopted worldwide, has an unambiguous definition for each of its terms so that a 1:1 relationship exists between term and injury. No term describes more than a single clinical condition; conversely, no clinical condition is described by more than a single term. Regardless of injury type, the tissue of reference is always the entire globe. Thus, there is no need to specify the tissue involved. For example, in a corneal penetrating injury, corneal defines the location of the wound, not the type of trauma (Fig. 32-1).

The *wall of the eye* is defined as the sclera and/or cornea, regardless of whether there is choroidal or retinal involvement, which may be difficult or impossible to verify. There are two major injury categories, depending on whether a full-thickness wound of the eye wall is present: *open globe injury* or *closed globe injury.*

In the closed globe category, a lamellar (partial-thickness) laceration is distinguished from a contusion. A lamellar laceration does not violate the entire width of the tissue (Fig. 32-1A), whereas a contusion is caused by a blunt object that transfers its kinetic energy without creation of a full-thickness wound. Contusions were described historically in the literature as blunt trauma (19).

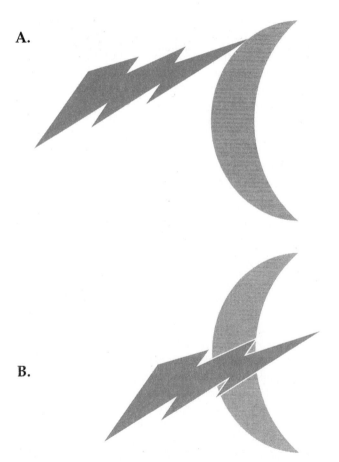

A.

B.

FIGURE 32-1. The tissue of reference, not just the term used, determines the injury type. **A:** The tissue of reference is the *cornea.* This is a penetration *into* the cornea but not into the inside of the eye; therefore, it is a *closed globe* injury. **B:** The tissue of reference is the *globe.* This is a penetration *through* the cornea, into the inside of the eye; therefore, it is an *open globe* injury.

In the open globe category, ruptures and lacerations are differentiated. The underlying cause of a *rupture* is elevated intraocular pressure (IOP), which is the result of energy transfer from a blunt object. Consequently, the wound occurs by internal pressure pushing out against the eye wall, and frequently there is loss of the globe's contents with tissue prolapse or extrusion. The wound is not necessarily at the impact site but usually at the site of least resistance. An example is an eye that was operated on remotely in time for cataract and then sustained an impact with a blunt object several years later. The wound most likely will form at the cataract surgical incision rather than at the point of impact. Ruptures have the worst prognosis of all injury types, in part because injury is not localized to the point of impact (20). It is important prognostically not to describe all open globe injury types as rupture (15,21).

A *laceration* is caused by a sharp object. The wound always occurs at the impact site and always by energy transmitted from outside the eye to the inside of the globe. An exception is the exit wound in perforating trauma. The object entering the eye can exit by the same route, be retained, or exit at a site distant from the entry wound.

When a single wound is present, it is termed *penetrating* injury, in which the object exits through the entry wound. If the agent exits via a different wound, a *perforating* injury is encountered ("through and through injury"). An *intraocular foreign body* (IOFB) injury is similar to a penetrating injury but is distinguished because of its special management and prognostic implications due to the presence of foreign material inside the eye. The confusion caused by two different terms (penetrating, perforating) to describe the same type of injury (22) now is prevented with the BETT (Table 32-1, Fig. 32-2).

EPIDEMIOLOGY

To identify areas where prevention can be effective, valid epidemiologic data are helpful. Epidemiologic studies of ocular trauma have been published (5,7–12,14–17,21–57), although comparative analysis is difficult because there are differences in target population; definition of pediatric, country, or region surveyed; type of study (whether hospital or population based); and method and length of surveillance. Relevant clinical information as discussed in the following includes injury types, circumstances of injury, tissue involvement, and functional outcomes.

Literature Review

Children suffer a disproportionate number of eye injuries (58,59), sustaining 27% to 52% of all ocular trauma (28,42,60). Injury was the leading cause of monocular blindness in children (61). Among children 0 to 14 years, 27% presented with trauma (44). Of open globe trauma, 26% occurred in children in a US study (21). In a population-based

TABLE 32-1. DEFINITIONS IN THE BIRMINGHAM EYE TRAUMA TERMINOLOGY[a]

Term	Definition	Comments
Eye wall	Sclera and cornea	Although technically the wall of the eye has not one but three tunics (coats) posterior to the limbus, for clinical purposes it is best to restrict the term *eye wall* to the rigid structures of the sclera and cornea.
Closed globe injury	Eye wall does not have a full-thickness wound	Rarely, a contusion and a lammellar laceration may coexist.[a]
Lamellar laceration	Eye wall has a partial-thickness wound	
Contusion	No wound	Energy transfer from object to globe causes damage inside the eye wall.
Open globe injury	Eye wall has a full-thickness wound	Cornea and/or sclera sustained a through-and-through injury. Depending on the inciting object's characteristics and the injury's circumstances, ruptures and lacerations are distinguished. The choroid and the retina may be intact, prolapsed, or damaged.
Rupture	Full-thickness wound of the eye wall caused by a blunt object. Impact results in momentary increase of the IOP and an inside-out injury mechanism	Eye is a ball filled with incompressible liquid. Blunt object with sufficient momentum creates energy transfer over a large surface area, greatly increasing IOP. Eye wall gives way at its weakest point, which may or may not be at the impact site. Actual wound is produced by an inside-out force; consequently, tissue herniation is very frequent and can be substantial.
Laceration	Full-thickness wound of the eye wall, usually caused by a sharp object. Wound occurs at the impact site by an outside-in mechanism	Further classification is based on whether an exit wound or IOFB also is present. Occasionally, an object may create a posterior (exit) wound while remaining, at least partially, intraocular (IOFB).[a]
Penetrating injury	Single laceration of the eyewall, usually caused by a sharp object	No exit wound has occurred. If more than one *entrance* wound is present, each must have been caused by a different agent.
Intraocular foreign body injury	Retained foreign object/s causing entrance laceration(s)	An IOFB is technically a penetrating injury but is grouped separately because of different clinical implications (treatment modality, timing, endophthalmitis rate, etc.).
Perforating injury	Two full-thickness lacerations (entrance exit) of the eye wall, usually caused by a sharp object or missile	The two wounds must have been caused by the same agent.

[a] Rarely, the injury is so atypical that characterization is very difficult. The clinician should use his or her best judgment, based on the information provided here.
IOFB, intraocular foreign body; IOP, intraocular pressure.

report from Maryland, it was estimated that the incidence rate was 15.2 per 100,00 population-years for those aged 0 to 15 years (53). Children constituted 16% to 35% of those hospitalized for trauma (58,62–64) and 21% of trauma-related emergency room visits by those under 15 years (65). In a study from Scotland, 22% of hospitalized cases were under 15 years (66). Of assault-related injuries, 17% targeted children 0 to 18 years in a survey solely on open globe trauma (67). In a report from Oman on almost 700 children aged 6 to 12 years examined, the prevalence of traumatic monocular visual damage was 0.19% (36).

Children from poor socioeconomic populations have a greater risk (26) with an inverse relationship between injury risk and family income and education level (41). Those under 5 years may be most at risk (41). In a study from Scotland (8), the relative risk of an eye injury was 2.16 among those aged 0 to 14 years. The risk to bystanders also was significant, with a victim rate of up to 44% in a study from Brazil (41).

Young children are disproportionally represented among those within the pediatric group with eye injuries. Among children 0 to 19 years, the mean was age 7 years in a study in Scotland (38). In the age group from 0 to 14 years, 88% of injuries occurred in those aged 5 years or older (48). The proportion of eye injuries involving those under 15 years is approximately one third to one half (14,41,43).

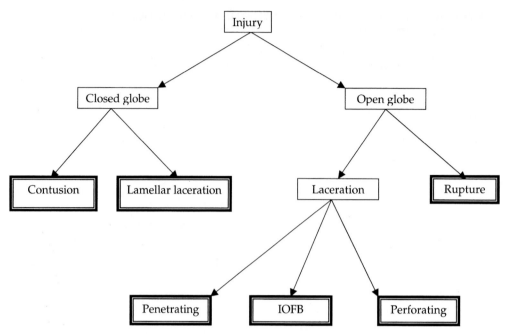

FIGURE 32-2. *Double-framed boxes* show the diagnoses used in clinical practice.

Male preponderance is less in children than in adults. This is speculated to be the result of different time exposure to risk factors (8). Still, males are more likely to be affected than females by a ratio of 4:1 (61). The ratio increases with increasing age (53). In several studies, 65% to 82% of patients were male (10,22,48,56), even when only open globe injuries were analyzed (47,52).

The home is the most common place where ocular trauma occurred, reported in 37% (10) to 51% (38) of cases. Higher rates of domestic trauma were reported when only open globe injuries were surveyed: 34% (37) to 75% (47,55).

Local factors influence the cause of the injury. Most reports identified sports as the most common activity resulting in eye injury. However, a Nigerian survey identified that 30% of injuries occurred during domestic activities, such as fetching firewood, gardening, and collecting seeds, and that 24% occurred during play and sports (56). Most (59%) injuries were found to be agent related in India (57), bows and arrows were the most common cause (15%), and household appliances were second (14%) (48). In one US study, 32% of injuries was shown to be agent related or caused directly by toys (16). In a separate US study, accidental blows and falls were responsible for 37% of injuries (53).

Sports and play are the most common activities that lead to eye injuries. Forty-one percent of all sports-related trauma occurred in children under 15 years of age, and more than 70% were sustained by those under 25 years (31) (Table 32-2).

Air guns are a serious, preventable source of eye injuries. In one study from Kansas and Seattle (12), the average vic-

tim was 11 years old and 51% were shot by a friend or sibling. A total of 71% of the shootings was unintentional, and 3% of the victims died. The consequences of air-gun related eye injury are severe: 32% lost an eye and 53% lost light perception (49). In the greater Ottawa area from 1974 to 1993, 60% of enucleations were performed for trauma among those under 18 years; of these, 25% were caused by air guns (39).

War games and paint ball injuries constitute a new source of ocular trauma, especially if these sports are played in a nonorganized or unofficial capacity. In a review of the 101 reported cases, only 12% of patients wore eye protection, and even this may have been inadequate, i.e., goggles instead of face guards. The trauma often was severe. Only 43% of eyes had final visual acuity of 20/40 or greater (40).

Fireworks are another easily preventable source of pediatric eye injury (Fig. 32-3). In Sweden, 75% (54) and in Austria 49% (11) of fireworks-related injuries affected those under 18 years (54). Eye involvement occurred in 29% to 38% of all fireworks injuries (54). Although two thirds of fireworks-related injuries were caused by legal devices (50), bottle rockets were the main culprit for eye trauma. They caused 80% of the 185 injuries in the Eye Injury Registry of Alabama (35) and also affected bystanders in 67% of the cases (35). The average charge for treatment of fireworks-related injuries was reported as $1,385 in 1966 (50).

Motor vehicle crashes cause eye injury rates of 11% (53) to 12% (17), but these injuries are less common mainly due to enforcement of seat belt and child seat laws.

Serious assaults are an uncommon source of eye trauma in children, although a review of hospitalized trauma in

TABLE 32-2. SPORT AS A CAUSE OF PEDIATRIC EYE INJURIES: LITERATURE REVIEW

Proportion of Sports-Related Injuries Among Total	Study Origin	Reference No.
74% (play included)	Jordan	10
27% among those under 15 years	United States	53
16%	Scotland	38
27%	Sweden	54
15% (32% baseball, 10% basketball)	United States	17
10% (31% baseball, 15% basketball)	United States	42
15% among open globe injuries (71% caused by darts)	England	37
Soccer increasingly important source	United States	31
Sports responsible for most orbital fractures	United States	5
Sports responsible for 16% of enucleations	United States	31

Scotland (38) found a 14% rate. Before being banned in 1989, lawn darts were responsible for several cases of serious eye injury (51).

Among open globe injuries, mostly sharp objects (55) are the culprit: 67% in one study (47). In another report, the breakdown was darts 16%, glass 15%, and knives 14% (45). In a large city, guns were responsible for open globe injuries in 22%, sticks and tree branches 11%, and missiles 9% (15). Projectiles (22%), sticks (10%), and falls (10%) are common sources (22) of eye trauma; however, reports of less common causes include magpies (32), tarantula's hairs, and bites by other spiders (68–70). Education regarding sharp toys (34) and the danger of explosion from glass bottles and caps is important (71–76).

Having an adult present usually is believed to reduce the injury risk. In one study, most injuries occurred during unsupervised play (52).

Most reports found no difference in the laterality of eye involvement in ocular trauma. However, among those injured by exploding glass bottles, the left eye was more likely to be involved (77,78). However, champagne cork injuries often caused right eye trauma (79). Among children with self-inflicted injuries, the right eye was involved in 83% (55).

Children sustain the entire spectrum of ocular trauma seen in adult patients. In one study, 28% of injuries involved the adnexa and 72% the globe (42). Burns are not a common cause of serious eye injury; the cornea is involved in only 1% of injuries. The outcome in most survivors was good, with rare permanent complications (25). In one study in which 54% of the cases were open and 42% were closed globe trauma, 4% were chemical injuries (22). Open globe trauma constituted 9% to 56% (22,28,42,48,57) and as high as 84% (7) of all cases among children. In a survey of open globe injuries, 34% of those injured were children under 15 years (45). Penetrating trauma was more common than rupture in open globe injuries (79% vs 13%) (61). In a study on those hospitalized for trauma in Scotland (38), 65% were contusion, 28% were open globe, and 4% had IOFBs. Trauma was responsible for 62% of retinal detachments in those 19 years and under (46).

Data from the United States Eye Injury Registry

The United States Eye Injury Registry (USEIR), the surveillance arm of the American Society of Ocular Trauma (ASOT), is the world's largest database on serious eye injuries and is a model for affiliate registries operating under identical guidelines in more than 30 countries. The USEIR collects and publishes information on all types of "ocular

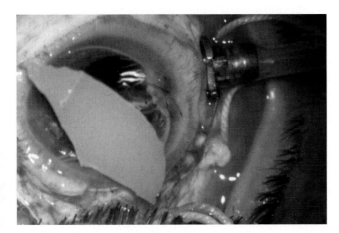

FIGURE 32-3. Large piece of plastic removed from an eye with a fireworks injury.

TABLE 32-3. PLACE OF INJURY IN A UNITED STATES EYE INJURY REGISTRY STUDY OF SERIOUS EYE INJURIES

	Group AD (Aged ≥ 19 Years)	Group CH (Aged 0–18 Years)	Group A (Aged 0–4 Years)	Group B (Aged 5–14 Years)	Group C (Aged 15–18 Years)
Total no. of cases	7,605	3,941	535	2,282	1,124
Home	34%	59%	84%	85%	33%
Industrial premises	28%	0.2%	0.7%	0.6%	6.8%
Street and highway	19%	11%	5%	6%	23%
Sports and recreation	11%	17%	5.6%	18%	20%
Farm	3%	1.6%	1.7%	1.2%	02.3%
School	1.6%	7%	0.06%	7%	11%

Courtesy of LoRetta Mann.

trauma that threaten permanent and significant structural or functional change to the eye/adnexa" (35,80–83). The USEIR encourages all ophthalmologists to report on the epidemiology and clinical characteristics of serious eye injuries via the Internet (*useironline.org* in the United States and *weironline.org* internationally).

The pediatric patients were divided into three age groups: 0 to 4 years [group A, n = 560 (13%)]; 5 to 14 years [group B; n = 2,485 (57%)]; and 15 to 18 years [group C, n= 1,288 (30%)]. This represents the largest dataset of pediatric injuries available, the epidemiologic and clinical details of which we analyzed for the purpose of this chapter. In addition to presenting information on the pediatric age group, we also provide data on the adult patients (aged 19 and above, group AD) for comparison.

The male-to-female ratio in group AD was 4.5:1 and in group CH was 3.4:1, with the following breakdown: group A: 1.9:1; group B: 3.6:1; and group C: 4.1:1. These ratios confirm the trend reported in many publications that the male-to-female ratio increases with age.

In group AD, information on eyewear at the time of the incident was known in 6,076 of cases; of these, none was worn in 90%, prescription or sunglasses in 3%, and safety glasses in 3%. In group CH, information on eyewear at the time of the incident was known in 3,175 of cases; of these, none was worn in 98%, prescription or sunglasses in 1%, and safety glasses in less than 1%. Children were less likely to wear eye protection than adults.

Injuries to bystanders often are not reported in the literature, although bystanders are commonly the victims. Fifteen percent of the 6,283 known cases in group AD and 37% of the 3,090 known cases in group CH were bystanders. The risk of sustaining a bystander injury was twice as high in children than in adults.

The place of injury varied with age (Table 32-3). In developed countries, the home was the most common place of injury. The younger the child, the greater was the risk of sustaining trauma in the home. The risk of sports-related injuries increased with the child's age.

The older the child, the more similar were the causes of the injury to those seen in adults (Table 32-4).

There was a consistent, although unexplained, shift with age from right eye to left eye preponderance.

The posterior segment was involved in group AD in 44% and in group CH in 43%. Retinal detachment was found in 10% in group AD, 8% in group CH, 4.6% in group A, 7.8% in group B, and 10% in group C. Almost half of serious eye injuries involved the posterior segment, which is the primary factor in determining the final outcome. The rate of retinal detachment increased with age. We found no difference in the number of surgeries performed on children versus adults (Table 32-5).

The initial visual acuities are given in Table 32-6. *Final visual acuity,* defined as at least 1 month postoperatively for this study, was available for 3,562 eyes in group AD and 1,750 eyes in group CH. The results are given in Table 32-7.

EVALUATION

General Ophthalmologic Examination

History taking is always an art, and it is an especially difficult one when a child is injured (61). Children who are too young commonly are not able to recall the events accurately because they may not have the capability to recall important details or differentiate between what is significant and what is not, are overwhelmed by fright or pain, are in denial, or

TABLE 32-4. SOURCE OF INJURY IN A UNITED STATES EYE INJURY REGISTRY STUDY OF SERIOUS EYE INJURIES

	Group AD (Aged ≥ 19 Years)	Group CH (Aged 0–18 Years)	Group A (Aged 0–4 Years)	Group B (Aged 5–14 Years)	Group C (Aged 15–18 Years)
Total no. of cases	8,544	4,241	539	2,445	1,257
Hammering on metal	6.3%	1.2%	0.2%	11%	2.2%
Various sharp objects	23%	22%	40%	23%	12%
Various blunt objects	33%	29%	14%	31%	34%
Fall	5.3%	2.7%	9.5%	2.3%	0.8%
Gunshot/air gun	6%/0.8%	3.2%/14%	0.07%/6.9%	1.6%/18%	7.5%/8.5%
Motor vehicle crash	11%	6.9%	4%	3.6%	15%
Fireworks	2.3%	10%	3.1%	11%	11%
Burn	2.8%	1.1%	2%	0.6%	1.8%
Explosion	2.8%	1.6%	0.6%	1.8%	1.8%
Lawn equipment	2.3%	1.2%	0.9%	1.4%	0.8%

Courtesy of LoRetta Mann.

TABLE 32-5. NUMBER OR SURGICAL PROCEDURES PERFORMED IN A UNITED STATES EYE INJURY STUDY OF SERIOUS EYE INJURIES

	Group AD (Ages ≥ 19 Years)	Group CH (Ages 0–18 Years)
Total no. of cases	7,625	4,412
No surgery	8.7%	8.9%
One surgery	68%	75%
Two surgeries	17%	13%
Three surgeries	4.6%	3.9%
Four or more surgeries	1.5%	1.4%

Coutesy of LoRetta Mann.

TABLE 32-6. AGE-RELATED INITIAL VISUAL ACUITY IN A UNITED STATES EYE INJURY REGISTRY STUDY OF SERIOUS EYE INJURIES

Visual Acuity Category[a]	Group AD (Aged ≥19 Years)	Group CH (Aged 0–18 Years)	Group A (Aged 0–4 Years)	Group B (Aged 5–14 Years)	Group C (Aged 15–18 Years)
NLP	684 (10)	195 (6)	12 (6)	100 (5)	78 (8)
LP to HM	1,954 (29)	865 (28)	56 (29)	550 (28)	259 (26)
1/200 to 19/200	825 (12)	385 (12)	17 (9)	232 (12)	136 (13)
20/200 to 20/50	1329 (19)	648 (21)	27 (14)	433 (22)	188 (19)
20/40 or greater	2015 (30)	1053 (33)	80 (42)	634 (33)	339 (34)
Total	6,807 (100)	3,146 (100)	192 (100)	1,949 (100)	1,000 (100)

Values are given as number (percent). Percentages do not add up to 100 because of rounding.
[a] The visual acuity categories are identical to those used in the development of the Ocular Trauma Score (20).
HM, hand motion; LP, light perception; NLP, no light perception. Courtesy of LoRetta Mann.

TABLE 32-7. AGE-RELATED VISUAL OUTCOMES IN A UNITED STATES EYE INJURY REGISTRY STUDY OF SERIOUS EYE INJURIES

Visual Acuity Category[a]	Group AD (Aged ≥ 19 Years)	Group CH (Aged 0–18 Years)	Group A (Aged 0–4 Years)	Group B (Aged 5–14 Years)	Group C (Aged 15–18 Years)
NLP	479 (14)	154 (9)	15 (10)	82 (8)	57 (11)
LP to HM	399 (11)	132 (8)	15 (10)	80 (8)	37 (7)
1/200 to 19/200	328 (9)	137 (8)	17 (12)	82 (8)	38 (7)
20/200 to 20/50	598 (17)	344 (20)	16 (11)	213 (20)	115 (22)
20/40 or greater	1754 (49)	983 (56)	81 (56)	624 (58)	278 (53)
Total	3,562 (100)	1,750 (100)	144 (100)	1018 (100)	525 (100)

Values are given as number (percent). Percentages do not add up to 100 because of rounding.
[a] The visual acuity categories are identical to those used in the development of the Ocular Trauma Score (20).
HM, hand motion; LP, light perception; NLP, no light perception. Courtesy of LoRetta Mann.

fear punishment with disclosure of facts. Fabrication (Munchausen syndrome) is not uncommon with children (44); therefore, it is important to find an adult eyewitness, although this usually is not possible. If a caregiver was present at the time of the injury, a word of caution is in order: he or she also may be interested in giving false information (see shaken baby syndrome later in this chapter). Table 32-8 lists the most important questions to which the ophthalmologist should obtain answers. As a general rule, the ophthalmologist should trust the observations from examination and be skeptical if the findings and the child's description of events are in conflict.

It may be advisable for the ophthalmologist not to wear a white laboratory coat when dealing with smaller children, who commonly associate a white coat with something bad, such as pain.

Bilateral injury occurs in less than 3% of injuries in children. The unaffected eye offers an excellent control to which the injured eye can be compared if there is any doubt regarding the diagnosis.

The evaluation starts with an external inspection. The ophthalmologist must look for any injury-related tissue damage or foreign material on the lids and bones, the position of the globes whether exophthalmic or enophthalmic, and any asymmetry in the appearance of the eyes or orbits. A recent picture can provide a basis for comparison. If possible, the child is asked to move the eyes in all directions to see if motility is retained. Motility restriction presents early with blowout fractures if it is the trap door type (84). Small lid wounds may hide thin, long, and potentially life-threatening intraorbital foreign bodies that can protrude intracranially. When a penetrating orbital injury and systemic symptoms are present, always suspect brain injury (85). The history often is negative with organic intraorbital foreign

bodies. Therefore, the skin and conjunctiva are carefully examined (86).

Dog bites to skin and lacrimal system can cause severe infections, even death (87).

The globe is first examined with a penlight. Before any examination, the ophthalmologist can reassure the child that all of the procedures will not be painful and then can carefully examine the child so as not to create pain. The penlight examination will help detect large foreign bodies (Fig. 32-4), significant prolapse of intraocular tissues, and large subcutaneous and subconjunctival hemorrhages. The penlight examination permits examination of the pupils and their reaction to light.

Examining very young or uncooperative small children may require physical restraining. For this, at least one assistant may be necessary. Help provided by the parent or somebody known to the child is valuable and also involves the parent as a supportive participant in the overall management of the injured child. If no parent is available, a second assistant may be necessary. The child should be placed on a flat surface, preferably onto a sheet that can be rolled around to immobilize all four of the child's extremities. The parent sits at the child's legs and holds both legs and the arms while the assistant, sitting at the child's head, holds the head.

Once the inspection is over, the ophthalmologist may perform a careful physical examination. Careful palpation is not always recommended because although it may aid in finding bone dislocation, subcutaneous foreign bodies, and crepitus, it also may cause pain and prove to be counterproductive. It is, however, important to always examine the orbit, because orbital fractures are rather common in children, and orbital imaging may be more appropriate (88).

If the lids are swollen, the child continues to squeeze them, or the need for surgical intervention is obvious, then

TABLE 32-8. THE MOST IMPORTANT QUESTIONS TO ASK WHEN A CHILD IS INJURED[a]

Question	Comment
What happened?	General circumstances.
What was the object that caused the injury?	If the consequences of the injury are in obvious conflict with the answer, for e.g., a small wound with iris prolapse is found and the child says he was injured when a soccer ball hit him, the ophthalmologist must carefully rephrase the question.
Where can the object that caused the injury be found?	Being able to examine the object can yield a wealth of important information.
Is there a person who played a key role in the injury?	Another child or adult who caused the injury.
When did the event occur?	67% of children present after the critical first 24 hours (7).
Where did the injury take place?	Is it possible that the agent was soil contaminated?
What were the symptoms that occurred instantly and how have they changed since?	Most important is vision. Ask for as many details as possible.
	When asking about pain, remember that the answer may be unreliable and that there is an inverse relationship between pain and the severity of the condition: a corneal abrasion may cause severe pain and marked symptoms whereas a rupture with extensive tissue prolapse may involve minimal or no pain.
What treatment has been administered?	Ask for local (washout, foreign body removal, bandage) as well as general (pills, etc.).
When did the child last eat or drink, what and how much?	Anesthesiologists rarely undertake putting the child to sleep if the last meal was within 6 hours.
Is there an eyewitness?	
Was the eye normal before the injury?	Ask for previous surgery, injury, amblyopia.
Did the child wear prescription (protective/sun) glasses at the time the injury occurred?	Nonsafety glasses may be protective in some cases but also may cause injury by shattering.
Does the child have any systemic disease/condition?	If yes, what medications does he take and when were they taken last?
Is the child allergic to any known substance?	
How is the child's tetanus immunization status?	When and what type of tetanus shot was administered?

[a] These are some of the most basic questions: According to the injury's specific circumstances, the line of questions has to be modified in each individual case. The order must be changed accordingly, and, in some cases, e.g., chemical injury, questions should be asked *after* emergency care has been delivered.

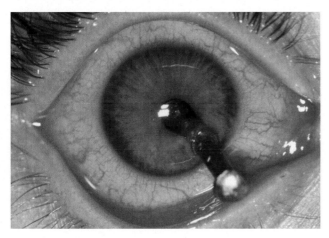

FIGURE 32-4. Intraocular but protruding foreign body raises a dilemma if the child is referred: should it be removed first? Although the decision must be made on a case-by-case basis, the general rule is *not* to remove it (see text for further details).

no effort should be made to forcibly open the lids. The risk of causing further tissue prolapse in an open globe injury is too great. It is preferred to have a thorough examination under sedation or mask anesthesia in the operating room (Fig. 32-5). Oral medication should be avoided so that general anesthesia remains an option. Consent for possible surgery is obtained with the examination under anesthesia (EUA) consent so that repair, if necessary, is performed under one anesthetic.

If possible, visual acuity should be determined in both eyes. If the child is willing to cooperate but cannot read, then illiterate charts, Allen cards, or the "E" sign can be used.

In older children and in younger children willing to cooperate, a slitlamp examination should be performed. A full evaluation should be attempted, from the skin to the anterior vitreous. On the conjunctiva, areas of hemorrhage are examined. Smaller and thin hemorrhages usually are without significance, but large and thick hemorrhages may hide scleral wounds. If a conjunctival laceration is found, it is important to remember that a scleral wound also may be present, and its location can be remote to the area beneath the conjunctival laceration. Especially thick and widespread hemorrhagic chemosis raises the possibility of orbital fracture, foreign body, or hemorrhage. Bilateral periorbital hemorrhage should alert the ophthalmologist to the possibility of cranial fracture. If it is not possible to exclude with certainty that there is no scleral wound under the subconjunctival hemorrhage, exploratory surgery is recommended.

When examining the cornea, the examiner must look for epithelial abrasions and ulcerations, stromal opacities, and wounds. Rose bengal stain can show damaged epithelial cells and fluorescein can show epithelial loss. Signs and symptoms are not consistent in determining the severity or even the presence of corneal abrasions (89). For certain stromal injuries, such as those associated with foreign bodies, indirect, retroillumination, or sclerotic scatter can be useful. If a piece of glass is embedded deep in the cornea, it may be preferable to use the slitlamp to remove it because it can become invisible under the direct illumination of the operating microscope. If a laceration is found, it must be determined whether the wound is full thickness. After instilling a drop of 2% fluorescein and viewing under light emitted through a blue filter, a green stream is visible if aqueous is leaking from the anterior chamber (Seidel sign). Sometimes slight pressure on the eye is necessary to observe the phenomenon. Not all full-thickness wounds require suturing, whereas some partial-thickness wounds may require suturing, for example, if the flap is displaced.

The anterior chamber must be evaluated for the presence of foreign bodies, flare, inflammatory cells, fibrin, pus, blood, and vitreous. A shallow anterior chamber may indicate aqueous loss, an anteriorly displaced lens, or a hemorrhagic or serous choroidal detachment, whereas a deep chamber may signal a lens that has been extruded or is posteriorly dislocated, or an open globe injury.

The iris is examined under both direct illumination and retroillumination for full-thickness or stromal defects and sphincter tears. However, an iridodialysis or iridodonesis also may be present. To detect iridodonesis, eye movement is necessary.

The pupils are evaluated to determine their shape, size, and location, whether they are of equal size, and if they are equally reactive to direct and consensual light. If no pupillary light reaction is detected, the presence or absence of an afferent pupillary defect (APD) is determined. The focused light from a penlight or ophthalmoscope is swung away from the intact to the injured eye. Normally, both pupils constrict to light after a brief period of relative darkness. However, if there is inadequate light perception or transmission from the injured eye, the pupil in the intact eye will dilate, not constrict. Although both pupils should dilate if an APD in the injured eye is present, the advantage of inspecting the uninjured eye is that the pupils may not react in the directly traumatized eye for reasons other than an APD, such as an iris sphincter tear. The presence of an APD has a poor prognostic significance (20). If leukocoria is found, the ophthalmologist should always ask if trauma has occurred to the eye (90).

Intraocular pressure (IOP) is rarely measured. It may be assessed digitally unless an open wound is present. A low IOP is not always present with an occult wound.

The lens is examined for its presence, whether the anterior (and, more importantly, the posterior) lens capsule has been violated, clarity, position (dislocation or luxation), stability (phacodonesis), zonular rupture (often with vitreous prolapse), and presence of an intralenticular foreign body. All of these lens pathologies can occur in eyes with open globe injury and, with the exception of intralenticular for-

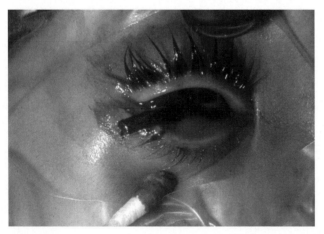

FIGURE 32-5. Child with an injury that obviously required surgical intervention. Further evaluation was not performed; the eye is examined only under general anesthesia and careful draping.

eign body, with closed globe injuries. For instance, contusion commonly causes anterior capsular rupture and cataract (91) and, less commonly, isolated posterior capsular lesions. Of eyes undergoing surgery for traumatic cataract, one third (92) to one half (93) were found to have posterior capsular ruptures.

The anterior vitreous is examined for the presence of foreign bodies and white, pigmented, or blood cells. A retinal detachment also can be visible.

Indirect ophthalmoscopy should be performed on the injured child's eyes. Ideally, the pupils are dilated with sterile, short-acting, topical medications. Mydriatics should not be used in the presence of an obvious open wound, and their use should always be documented. The retinal periphery usually is difficult to examine (28). Although retinal detachment is occasionally found, children usually present late with retinal detachment (94).

Most of the pathologies described can occur in closed or open globe injuries. Table 32-9 presents a differential diagnosis.

Finally, it is of crucial importance that the child receives care as necessary from other specialists. Certain relationships between ocular and systemic symptoms should be remembered. For example, bradycardia and somnolence are common with hyphema (95). The oculocardiac reflex, which consists of nausea, bradycardia, and hypotension, is common in children with orbital fractures and muscle entrapment (5).

Imaging Studies

In the hands of an experienced clinician, ultrasonography is helpful for detecting foreign bodies, posterior full-thickness wounds, lens luxation, vitreous hemorrhage, posterior vitreous detachment, and retinal detachment in children (96). It also provides a simple method to follow intraocular events longitudinally. It typically should not be used in eyes with open globe trauma, although small wounds with minimal risk of tissue extrusion are suitable for ultrasonography in cooperative children.

Of the radiologic studies, computed tomography is the most valuable. It avoids physical contact with the eye, and it can detect very small IOFBs and intraocular and intraorbital pathologies, including vitreous hemorrhage, retinal detachment, and orbital fractures. Magnetic resonance imaging provides visualization of even finer details of soft tissue lesions. Plain x-ray films are used less often today because of the relatively high rate of false-positive and especially false-negative results.

No radiologic method is 100% accurate. Computed tomography and magnetic resonance imaging are positive in about 50% of cases with organic intraorbital foreign bodies (65).

An extensive overview of the advantages and disadvantages of various imaging studies in patients with ocular trauma is given in reference 97.

TABLE 32-9. PROBABILITY OF SELECTED TRAUMA-RELATED PATHOLOGIES IN DIFFERENT TYPES OF GLOBE INJURY

Pathology	Contusion	Penetrating Injury	Rupture
Subconjunctival hemorrhage	+	+	+
Corneal wound	−	+	∓
Limbal wound	−	±	+
Posterior wound	−	−	±
Tissue prolapse in wound	−	+	+
Hyphema	+	+	+
Vitreous prolapse into anterior chamber	+	∓	+
Lens lost	−	−	±
Lens dislocated	−	∓	±
Cataract	+	+	+
Vitreous hemorrhage	+	+	+
Commotio retinae	+	−	∓
Peripheral retinal tear	±	±	±
Macular hole	±	−	∓
Retinal detachment	+	+	+
Choroidal rupture	±	−	∓

−, no or very rare; ∓, rare; ±, relatively common; +, common.

COUNSELING

Empathy is as important a part of the true physician's armamentarium, as are knowledge, expertise, and experience. An ophthalmologist who wants to offer the best possible care must understand that he or she is not treating a tissue or an organ but a *person.* This person underwent an experience that was traumatic not only to the eye but also to the soul and mind. The child and family must be offered physical care and mental support—not just drugs and a surgical repair—as well as information, comfort, hope, understanding, compassion, and even affection.

Once the evaluation is completed and the ophthalmologist has a reasonably comprehensive understanding of the eye's condition, what treatment options are available, and what each option can offer, they must be discussed with the persons involved.

In adults, the "target" of counseling is primarily the patient, although it is recommended that the immediate family, usually the spouse, also be included (98). In the case of an injured child, the task is much more complex because the primary decision-maker is not the child but the parent. How much detail should be shared with the child is a decision that must be made on a case-by-case basis. Often the parent decides whether and how much should be disclosed to the child.

From personal experience, we believe the best alternative is to be honest with the parents. There is no advantage to hiding the severity of the condition, even if it may appear to lessen the shock experienced by many parents. It is important to build trust and establish a relationship that will last throughout the entire treatment period, which may take years. The parents should believe that although the doctor–patient relationship was started by chance, not choice, they can have total confidence that the best possible care is provided for their child. Conversely, if the ophthalmologist believes that a colleague can offer better treatment, he or she should initiate the referral.

Honest, straightforward, and compassionate ophthalmologists not only will enjoy the rewards of a good personal relationship with the parents and the child but also may lessen their risk of being targeted in legal action. For this, the ophthalmologist must provide adequate information to the parents so that they together choose the treatment option to pursue. Prognostic information should be as specific as possible. It is better to err slightly on the pessimistic side.

MANAGEMENT AND DECISION MAKING

Before the ophthalmologist decides to treat the consequences of the injury, he or she must answer the three *"E"* questions: Does the team have the *E*xpertise, *E*xperience, and *E*quipment to do an optimal job? If the answer to any of these fundamental questions is "no," the child should be referred to a colleague.

During the evaluation and as the treatment plan is finalized, the ophthalmologist must focus on the *child* and on the *eyeball,* not on individual tissue injuries. The goal is to restore as much of the globe's function as possible or at least to preserve a comfortable eye; enucleation is a last resort that should be avoided if possible.

The ophthalmologist should recognize that general ocular trauma guidelines are somewhat different in children. Almost all open globe injuries in a child require suturing to avoid reopening. In adults, waiting for 24 to even 72 hours does not increase the risk of endophthalmitis (99). Although this also is true in children, the risk of inadvertent tissue extrusion by putting pressure on the eye is greater in children, especially in younger ones. Therefore, it is recommended that the wound be closed as soon as possible. If the child is transferred, the eye must be covered with a firm, resistant shield, and the child must be refrained from touching the eyes, even if it requires immobilization of the hands. It is not necessary to start antibiotic therapy, but tetanus prophylaxis is appropriate. Personal communication between institutions and physicians is important, as is complete documentation, actual copies of imaging studies performed (not only readings), and a list of medications administered. If the child presents with an intraocular but protruding foreign body (Fig. 32-4), it usually is better not to remove it before referral. It is important to prevent the child from removing the foreign body during transit.

Whether the surgeon chooses a staged approach (for instance, wound cleansing and closure initially, followed by cataract removal and intraocular lens (IOL) implantation later) or a comprehensive reconstruction in a single setting depends upon the eye's condition and the surgeon's expertise. The advantage of one procedure to achieve globe restoration and function can be outweighed by several disadvantages. First, it can be difficult to appreciate the extent of damage to all of the involved tissues and anticipate the outcome of a long, complicated surgical case. Second, the risk of intraoperative complications, such as major hemorrhage, is greater. Third, visibility through an inflamed or injured cornea may be compromised. Finally, wound leakage is more likely to occur in inflamed, injured tissues. For these reasons, it usually is advisable to perform reconstruction in stages in eyes with posterior segment injury.

It is important to emphasize repeatedly to parents, siblings, and the child that protective eye wear and protection against additional eye trauma are necessary during the postoperative period and for the remainder of life.

Following are important points to remember when surgically managing ocular trauma in the pediatric patient. It often is helpful to work in teams with other experts; however, because this is not always possible, information on the surgical repair of tissue other than the posterior segment is provided.

Lids and Orbit

- Full-thickness wounds of the eyelid, however small, may hide injuries that can involve the globe, the deep orbital structures, the sinuses, and even the brain.
- Repairing eyelid wounds is rarely urgent. The initial 6-0 silk suture is placed at the lid margin to align the gray line. Deep sutures using 5-0 Dexon then are used to reapproximate the tarsus edges, avoiding iatrogenic corneal injury. The orbicularis muscle may have to be approximated, again with 5-0 Dexon sutures. Finally, the lid is sutured using 6-0 silk; avoid eyelash imbrications.
- Orbital fractures commonly require surgery in children (88). For blowout or internal fractures, early surgical intervention is recommended (84).
- Intraorbital foreign bodies can be left if they are inert, such as metal or glass, but they should be removed if they are organic or contaminated (86). If a ferrous object needs to be extracted, a powerful permanent intraocular magnet may be valuable (100).

Lacrimal System

- Although some claim that it is unnecessary to reconstruct both canaliculi (101), most authors disagree (102), stating that both the upper and the lower canaliculi should be repaired.
- To prevent irregular wound healing leading to a "pigtail" configuration, it is important to identify the proximal end of the severed canaliculus during repair. Thus, adequate exposure, magnification under bright illumination, and irrigation may be necessary.
- Starting with the damaged canaliculus, silicone tubing is placed in both the upper and lower canaliculi. The nasal end is tied loosely and the knots allowed to retract into the nose.
- Simple reapproximation of the lacerated overlying soft tissue combined with bicanalicular silicone intubation proved highly successful in managing canalicular lacerations (103).
- It is recommended to wait for at least 2 months before removing the silicone tubing.

Conjunctiva

- For thick subconjunctival hemorrhages, determine whether an occult scleral wound is present.
- Foreign bodies usually can be removed easily from the bulbar conjunctiva with a cotton-tipped applicator, under topical anesthesia. Objects that are on the tarsal conjunctiva cause much more pain because they scratch the cornea with each blink, and they are more difficult to remove. For removal, the upper lid must be everted, which is impossible if the child does not cooperate and continues to squeeze the eyelids shut. Calming words and re-

peated explanations work; force does not. If the object is in the upper fornix, double eversion using a Desmarres retractor is necessary.
- Small lacerations do not need to be sutured. For large lacerations, absorbable sutures such as Vicryl should be used. The significance of a conjunctival wound is primarily (i) whether a scleral wound lies beneath and (ii) that a hidden scleral wound may be located at some distance from the conjunctival wound.

Cornea

- Abrasions usually are treated with antibiotics and cycloplegics. Topical anesthetics must not be used for pain relief because of adverse effects on wound healing, and bandage contact lenses are rarely needed. Both anatomically and functionally, not patching is at least as effective (104), if not more so (105), as patching. Foregoing patching is preferred by most children.
- For recurrent erosions, topical hyperosmotic agents such as 5% sodium chloride, an extended-wear bandage contact lens, surgical debridement, stromal micropunctures, and even excimer laser may be tried.
- Superficial foreign bodies usually can be removed with a cotton-tipped applicator, following adequate topical anesthesia and careful explanation. For deep foreign bodies, a careful decision as to whether removal is necessary must be made. Inert materials that cause no interference with vision may be left in place. If removal is advisable, extreme care must be taken to avoid pushing the object intraocularly. In most cases, the operating microscope should be used, and light anesthesia may be needed (glass is easy to find under the slit lamp, but difficult to find under the operating microscope).
- Although small and firmly self-sealing wounds can be left alone or treated with a topical hyperosmotic agent or tissue glue, most open wounds require closure with sutures. All tissues and any external substance (iris, vitreous, foreign bodies, etc.) must be removed from the wound first and the edges thoroughly cleaned with forceps, cellulose sponge, or irrigation. Some basic principles in suturing corneal wounds include the following:

1. The goal is to create a wound that is watertight, minimizes astigmatism, maintains as regular a surface as possible, minimizes scarring that would later interfere with vision, and minimizes flattening of the corneal dome shape.
2. It is important to identify anterior and posterior edges of the wound so as to properly align them.
3. Unless the wound is circumferential and in the periphery, interrupted—rather than running—sutures are recommended (Fig. 32-6). The most ideal suture material is nylon, 9-0 or 10-0.
4. The sutures should be full thickness to achieve proper alignment of the corneal layers and to eliminate poste-

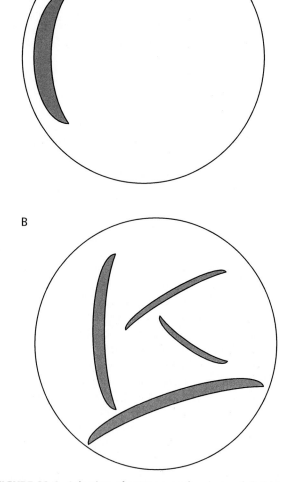

FIGURE 32-6. Selection of suture type for closing full-thickness corneal wounds. **A:** Circumferential wound can be closed with running suture because it will actually enhance the dome shape of the cornea. **B:** Any other wound is best closed using interrupted sutures to minimize the flattening effect.

rior gaping. All sutures should be at a 90-degree angle to the wound edge.

5. Suturing is begun at the limbus, at the bend of the wound's angle, or at other landmarks, such as a pigmentation line. If the wound is corneoscleral, start at the limbus, then suture the corneal, and finally the scleral wound.

6. If the wound is long, start with long and tight bites at the periphery and continue toward the center with gradually shorter and looser suture bites. Avoid sutures in the visual axis as much as possible.

7. If the compression zones of the already introduced sutures do not meet, use longer bites or put sutures in-between the existing ones. If corneal tissue is truly missing, it is first determined whether the corneal edge is rolled inward. If not, a more compressive suture or tissue glue, such as *n*-butyl or *n*-octyl cyanoacrylate, may be used. A bandage contact lens or penetrating keratoplasty is rarely necessary, although the latter can be successful (106). If loose corneal fragments are present, it is better to try to suture them back rather than remove them.

8. Once the corneal wound is repaired, reflection from the corneal surface of a Flieringa ring can determine if any suture is too tight. It is then removed and replaced, as necessary, to minimize astigmatism.

9. All sutures knots are buried to minimize irritation and promote healing.

10. The avascular cornea may take a few months to heal. Removal of sutures depends on the wound's length, its appearance, and other considerations, such as the child's possible exposure to ongoing trauma.

Sclera

- If the wound is anterior, make sure it is visible in its entirety; expose the area at the wound edges sufficiently to ensure that no part of the wound remains hidden.
- If the wound is posterior, it is important *not* to expose the wound in its entirety. The anterior aspect is closed before the posterior peritomy and wound closure are performed (Fig. 32-7).
- If the wound is under an extraocular muscle, a traction suture or muscle hook may be sufficient to provide exposure. However, because the sclera is the thinnest under the muscle, sometimes it is necessary to disinsert the muscle to avoid putting pressure on the globe.
- Attempted surgical closure is not recommended for wounds that extend posterior to the equator in which suture introduction would increase the risk of tissue extrusion. As with all open wounds, tissue, especially retina and uvea, should be cleared from between the wound lips. The retina must be carefully reposited. A viscoelastic substance can be used to prevent reextrusion during suture introduction. Vitreous should be removed as completely as possible. However, it can be difficult to excise completely.
- For most wounds, 6-0 or 8-0 Vicryl is adequate to allow permanent closure. For long wounds, some prefer nonabsorbable materials, such as nylon or silk.
- Prophylactic cryopexy over the scleral wound is not recommended. Treatment is performed only around visible retinal breaks or areas suspicious for harboring a retinal defect. Laser is preferred to cryopexy.

Anterior Chamber

- The incidence of hyphema is 17 per 100,000 population-years (107).

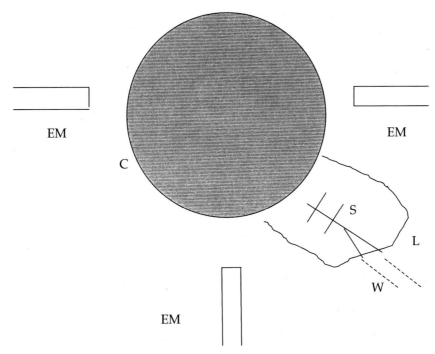

FIGURE 32-7. "Close-as-you-go" technique to suture a scleral wound that extends posteriorly. C, cornea; EM, extraocular muscle; L, line showing sclera already exposed; S, sutures; W, wound.

- In eyes with closed globe trauma, topical corticosteroids and oral aminocaproic acid are considered. Surgical blood or fibrin removal rarely is necessary, but if the IOP is elevated and cannot be medically controlled, surgical evacuation is recommended. Liquefied blood can be washed out using repeated irrigations through a single paracentesis or with a bimanual technique combining irrigation of the anterior chamber with one syringe and evacuation with the other. For a clotted hyphema, a larger incision is necessary, and forceps or the vitrectomy probe can be used. For the latter, considerable experience and a simultaneous infusion are necessary. In considering evacuation of a hyphema in a patient with sickle cell disease or sickle cell trait, the threshold for IOP is lower than that for patients without these conditions. It is important to maintain hydration and perioperative oxygenation and avoid extraocular muscle removal, excessive cryopexy, and diuretic agents that reduce IOP, such as carbonic anhydrase inhibitors or mannitol.
- In eyes with open globe injury, the goal is to leave the anterior chamber cleared of blood or fibrin. New incisions are preferred to using the original wound, because fibrin can reform within minutes.
- If an intracameral foreign body is found, a viscoelastic substance may facilitate removal. Should the object be lodged in the angle, the extraction incision should be at least 90 degrees away from the IOFB to allow adequate room for manipulating instruments.
- The more peripheral the paracentesis, the more likely is the iris to prolapse through it and anterior synechiae to

subsequently form. The use of a viscoelastic substance between the iris and wound can reduce this risk. However, a viscoelastic substance can raise the IOP postoperatively. We prefer air for this reason. Air also is useful to determine whether vitreous is present in the anterior chamber.
- Although age is not a risk factor for rebleeding in hyphema (107), sickle cell trait (108), black race (109), high IOP, and initial visual acuity 20/200 or less (110) are. Aminocaproic acid treatment is especially important in these high-risk children (109).
- Secondary bleeding occurs in 7.6% to 12% (111) and is a risk factor for poor outcome. In one report, 91% of eyes with one episode of rebleeding as opposed to 77% with more than one rebleed achieved 20/30 final vision (107).
- Outpatient management has been found acceptable, but careful counseling is crucial (111).

Iris and Pupil

- The iris is much more important than its cosmetic significance would suggest: it provides a barrier between the anterior and posterior compartments of the eye, and it regulates the amount of incoming light to the retina. Therefore, restoration of the iris diaphragm is very important. However, it is also important to maintain enough of a pupillary opening to permit adequate examination of the retina (see below).
- Iris prolapse commonly occurs with anteriorly located full-thickness wounds. In most cases, even if the injury is

older than 24 hours, the iris remains viable. Viable iris can be cleaned of contaminating debris and reposited. It is less traumatic and more effective to pull the iris with a small hook introduced through a paracentesis opposite the wound than to push it back through the wound.

- Simple lacerations are sutured using the McCannel method (112). A similar suture can be used to manage an iridodialysis. In both cases, the knot should be buried or internalized.

- If the pupil is permanently dilated, a single or pursestring suture allows adequate constriction. It is important to avoid making the pupil too small so that the retina can be examined adequately thereafter.

- Transpupillary membranes may have to be removed if they cause pupillary block, angle closure, and secondary glaucoma, or if they interfere with the child's vision. They may contain blood vessels or have such firm connections to surrounding structures that their forced removal can lead to complications more severe than those that initially indicated surgery. Therefore, manipulations should be careful and kept to a minimum.

- In the case of aniridia, an iris print contact lens, corneal tattooing, or implantation of an open type iris diaphragm (113) are the most viable alternatives.

Lens

- Traumatic cataract (i) reduces vision in the child and, in the young child, increases the risk of amblyopia, (ii) reduces the ability of the ophthalmologist to examine the retina, and (iii) signals a more severe intraocular injury. Both the vitreous hemorrhage and retinal detachment rates are significantly higher in the presence of a cataract (93).

- In children, it may take only a few hours for a lens to become cataractous and swollen. Cataract removal and even IOL implantation have been reported with penetrating keratoplasty (114).

- Injury to the lens capsule, even the presence of an intralenticular foreign body, does not necessarily mean that cataract formation is inevitable (115).

- Because of the strong connections between the posterior lens capsule and the anterior vitreous, intracapsular lens removal should not be attempted in children.

- Because the lens is soft in children, simple aspiration is technically adequate. However, because the posterior lens capsule often is violated, vitrectomy instrumentation often is used (lensectomy), rather than a simple irrigation/aspiration cannula to reduce placement of additional traction on the peripheral retina (116).

- Either a limbal or pars plana approach is used to perform a posterior capsulectomy and anterior vitrectomy (117). Because posterior capsular opacification occurs in up to 100% (118) of cases, capsulectomy and anterior vitrectomy are recommended primarily by most (119), although not all (120), surgeons.

- In children, antiamblyopia therapy is especially important in visual rehabilitation. There are several methods proposed (119): contact lens, epikeratophakia (121), and IOL. Today most agree that the IOL is the most reliable method (118), preferably after early lensectomy (122). The decision to insert the IOL during the primary surgery or as a secondary procedure (123) is determined by the injury, but, with proper case selection, either can yield excellent results.

- Following cataract removal, the surgeon should perform indirect ophthalmoscopy to determine the extent of the posterior segment injury. If extensive posterior segment injury is present, concurrent IOL implantation should not be performed.

- In eyes with primary IOL implantation and no posterior segment involvement, acute pigment dispersion and inflammation remain the most important immediate complications, but they rarely cause significant problems (123). The most common early complication is severe fibrinous anterior uveitis (51%), which is especially prominent in patients with dark irides (92).

- In eyes undergoing secondary IOL implantation, the IOL often is placed onto the capsule because the remaining capsules will have scarred together. In primary IOL implantation, some authors claim to have fewer complications with in-the-sulcus implantation (118), whereas others claim success with in-the-bag IOL placement (124), but the final outcome is equally good (119).

- After implanting an IOL with a power calculated in the standard fashion, there will be an overcorrection subsequently if the child is under 8 years because of the myopic shift from the eye's normal growth. Undercorrection, gradually decreasing from +6 D at age 1 to plano at age 7, has been suggested as a controversial solution (125). Some advocate providing contact lenses to address continued ocular growth. Often these thinner lenses are better tolerated than are thick aphakic contact lenses. Patients must undergo appropriate contact lens fitting and antiamblyopia therapy until emmetropia develops. Eye growth, with the consequent myopic shift, after cataract removal and IOL implantation is believed to be a normal process and not due to the procedure (126).

- If the lens is subluxed but no other serious complications are present and vision is good, there is no need for removal. Should surgery be necessary, vitrectomy instrumentation is preferred because there is a high chance of encountering vitreous.

- If the lens is dislocated anteriorly, urgent removal is necessary to prevent corneal damage and IOP elevation. If the lens is in the vitreous cavity, a complete vitrectomy must be performed before the lens is extracted. Because the lens is soft in children, a lensectomy is most conveniently performed in the vitreous using vitreous instrumentation.

Vitreous

- The most common vitreous pathology is hemorrhage. Vitreous hemorrhage reduces a child's vision, increases the risk of amblyopia, and prevents visualization of the retina by the ophthalmologist. It is associated with an increased risk of intraocular proliferation, particularly in the setting of open globe injuries (127). In closed globe injuries without retinal detachment, ultrasonography is performed at regular intervals to determine whether a retinal or choroidal detachment is present. Surgical intervention is indicated when the hemorrhage starts to organize or a retinal detachment develops. If a vitreous hemorrhage is found in an eye with an open globe injury, a vitrectomy should be performed, preferably 7 to 14 days post injury. In children, mechanical removal of the posterior cortical vitreous often is impossible. Therefore, enzymatic vitreolysis, such as with 0.4 IU autologous plasmin (128), may be of help in the future when it becomes available. If the vitreous does not readily detach, careful shaving of the vitreous and release of obvious traction are performed.
- For anterior wounds in the region of the vitreous base, vitreous base dissection is performed to remove hemorrhage and the scaffold onto which proliferating cells migrate in the proliferative vitreoretinopathy (PVR) process. High-speed vitreous instruments (1,000–1,800 cuts/min) and peristaltic pumps facilitate safe shaving of the vitreous base. Because vitreous can be difficult to remove in young children, care is taken to avoid additional trauma in releasing vitreous traction.
- For an IOFB, surgery is indicated (see following).

Retina

Injuries in children often are more complex than in adults because of problems related to postoperative inflammation, tractional retinal detachment, and PVR (61,129–131). Subretinal membrane formation and preretinal PVR are common in open globe injuries. PVR may be more pronounced in children, particularly in open globe injuries (3,132). In one series of open globe injuries, primary vitrectomy and/or lensectomy were necessary in 22%, and 24% of these needed a third or more surgeries (61). Vitrectomy performed within 2 weeks was believed to prevent PVR development and improve the prognosis (61). Risk factors include trauma (especially with long and posterior wounds, perforating injury, and lens loss), vitreous hemorrhage, retinal detachment, and persistent inflammation. In the USEIR, we found no significant difference in the PVR rates between groups AD and CH. However, the risk was more than twice as high in group A than in group C.

Peripheral breaks developed in 9% to 12% of contusions (19). Contusion-related defects are more likely to be located near the ora, not at the equator as in nontraumatic cases. Dialysis is the most common type of retinal break and the

inferotemporal quadrant the most common location. Dialyses can be managed with scleral buckle alone when there is little or no vitreous organization in contusions, whereas in open globe injuries, vitreous surgery often is required with or without scleral buckle. Choroidal rupture can lead to severe vision loss if the macula is involved. Subretinal fibrosis commonly occurs (Fig. 32-8).

Up to 16% of the breaks may be giant tears, which have the highest risk of PVR development. A giant tear differs from a dialysis in that the giant tear's pathogenesis is secondary to vitreous base contraction, whereas a dialysis is believed to be a disinsertion at the ora serrata. Therefore, the giant tear is observed at the margin of the vitreous base and usually the posterior margin. The dialysis is observed at the ora serrata. A giant tear, whether associated with open or closed globe trauma, should be treated to prevent retinal detachment formation with prompt vitrectomy, careful vitreous traction release, and vitreous base shaving. According to some authors, a scleral buckle often is considered in pediatric traumatic giant tears. A buckle, however, can distort the globe and increase the risk of posterior slippage of the giant tear. For this reason, a broad, only moderately high buckle is recommended for giant tears less than 360 degrees in extent (a buckle is unnecessary for 360-degree giant tears). Laser is preferred to cryotherapy because it is believed less likely to incite PVR development. However, it may be necessary to treat the extents of the giant tear with cryotherapy so as to assure adequate treatment up to the ora serrata and prevent extension of the giant tear, a task often difficult with laser alone. Finally, silicone oil is considered in pediatric cases, especially if compliance with adequate postoperative positioning is in question (129). Leaving heavy perfluorocarbon liquid in the eye for a few days is a controversial approach. The authors of this chapter rarely if ever use scleral buckling or cryopexy for giant tears.

In eyes with perforating injury, careful early vitrectomy to remove the scaffold connecting the entry and exit wounds and a prophylactic retinectomy around the exit wound may help reduce the high PVR rate (author's unpublished data).

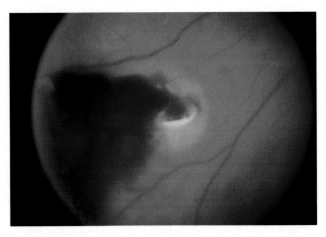

FIGURE 32-8. Choroidal rupture and subretinal fibrosis following contusion injury.

Silicone oil use has been found satisfactory in children (129). PVR can recur postoperatively and can include subretinal band and/or preretinal membrane formation.

- Macular holes should be operated on as soon as possible. Removal of the internal limiting membrane measurably increases the success rate but may be difficult in the pediatric patient (133).
- Retinal detachment may be slow to develop even after open globe trauma. In one study, 30% did not present until 2 years postinjury (134). After closed globe injury, only 12% of patients with retinal detachment presented acutely, 30% within 1 month, 50% within 8 months, and 20% after 2 years (135). Myopia is a risk factor for retinal detachment development after trauma, but lattice degeneration is not. Traumatic retinal detachment has a rather poor outcome in children: in one series, only 56% of eyes had long-term reattachment because of PVR (136). The anatomic success ranged from 25% to 48% (129,131,137). Vision of finger counting or better occurred in 20% to 33% (129,131,137).
- Management of eyes with IOFBs differs in several aspects from that of eyes without them (Fig. 32-9). Because of the higher incidence of endophthalmitis, earlier, even immediate, surgery may be indicated. The intraocular magnet is the optimal tool to remove ferrous IOFBs (100), but often IOFBs are not metallic and require removal with intraocular forceps. The treatment of additional pathology is similar to that in eyes without IOFB.

Issues Related to the Entire Globe

- Fewer than 3% of trauma-related cases of endophthalmitis occurs in children, and the microbiologic spectrum also is different. *Streptococcus* species are more common (138). In addition to using intravitreous antibiotics, vitrectomy should be performed early.

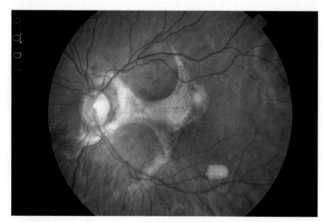

FIGURE 32-9. Retinal and vitreous hemorrhage with an intraretinal foreign body.

- Amblyopia must be managed to preserve and restore as much vision in the injured eye as possible. Trauma is the greatest risk factor for trauma to the fellow nonamblyopic eye, occurring in 63% of all cases (139).
- In a study of open globe injuries in a pediatric population, 7% of eyes had to be enucleated (47). If enucleation must be performed, an implant that is 2 mm smaller in diameter than the axial length of the removed eye is recommended (140).

PROGNOSIS

- Although visual outcome is worse if the corneal center, rather than the corneal periphery, is involved or if significant astigmatism is present (141), the final visual acuity is primarily determined by the extent of involvement of the posterior segment (56,106).
- In a large study, a major factor influencing the outcome was whether PVR developed. PVR was most common following perforating injury (186× higher risk compared to contusion) and was second most common following rupture (23×) (142). Eyes with PVR had a 12× increased risk for poor final visual acuity. PVR presented earliest after perforating injury (1.3 months), somewhat later after rupture (2.1 months), and latest after IOFB injuries (3.1 months). Young age was not a risk factor for PVR development, but vitreous hemorrhage, retinal detachment, expelled lens, vitreous prolapse, poor postinjury vision, and a posterior wound were risk factors. PVR appeared to be more common (94) and aggressive (130) in children. Other studies found no differences (143).
- In several studies, rupture, missile injury, retinal detachment, and age under 4 years were found to be poor prognostic factors (30,119). Another report found that age 9 years or under had a poor prognosis (61). Open globe trauma had a much worse outcome than did contusion (41,144). The outcome in open globe injuries (145) and in fireworks trauma (11) is worse in children than in adults. Surgery for retinal detachment and PVR also has a poorer prognosis in children than adults (61). In one study, 92% of eyes with closed globe injuries, as opposed to 15% with open globe trauma, achieved final visual acuity of 20/40 (48). Among open globe injuries, the more posterior the trauma, the worse the outcome (45).
- Most authors found initial visual acuity to be a crucial prognostic indicator (30), whereas others found no such relationship (61). Wound length, but not wound location, was found to have predictive value (30).
- Eyes requiring only one procedure to treat an open globe injury have better outcomes then those undergoing multiple surgeries (47). Only 25% of contused eyes had visual impairment, [whereas 70% of eyes with open globe trauma did] (16). Overall, the prognosis in children is guarded and depends on several factors: the extent of injury, when treat-

ment is sought, the postoperative inflammatory response and PVR, and amblyopia therapy. In one study, 29% of eyes became blind (22) and 32% to 81% had visual impairment (9,47,38,52,55). Monocular blindness occurred in up to 33% of patients (9).

SPECIAL CASES

Intrauterine and Perinatal Injuries

It is extremely rare that amniocentesis causes ocular trauma, although this cause of trauma has been described if amniocentesis is performed in the second or third trimester (14). During delivery, globe and adnexal injuries occur in 12%; the retinal hemorrhage rate is 11% (146). Forceps delivery can cause retinal hemorrhages in up to 47% of infants; the complications range from corneal leukoma to tractional retinal detachment, and even choroidal rupture (147). The injuries occur as a result of compression of the globe between the orbital roof and the forceps blade (148). Among neonates nursed under radiant warmers, no permanent eye damage attributable to near- or far-wavelength infrared radiation was found (149).

Nonaccidental Trauma (Child Abuse)

Nonaccidental trauma typically occurs in a male child younger than 6 months and is three times more common among African Americans than Caucasians. Injuries from shaken baby syndrome (SBS) are responsible for more than 1,200 deaths per year in the United States, with a death rate of 29% (150,151). Fewer than 20% of victims have a good outcome (150). A single shaking may be responsible, although it may be combined with direct trauma (shaken impact injury). Of the perpetrators, 90% were males. The key to diagnosis is a significant disparity between the alleged mechanism and the observed injuries. A retinal hemorrhage in a 6-week-old child probably is SBS, not birth trauma. The typical hemorrhage is flame shaped and central (150). Indirect ophthalmoscopy must be performed on the entire fundus. An intraocular hemorrhage was present in 83% of cases (93% of eyes) of SBS, and 85% of these were bilateral (151).

Other common findings include subdural hematoma in 70%, seizure in 67%, and bruise and long bone fracture in 13%, but common presenting signs include diarrhea, bradycardia, hypothermia, irritability, and seizures (151,152). Even in patients with cerebral edema, optic disc edema is rare. Retinal hemorrhage rarely occurs after accidental trauma or cardiopulmonary resuscitation (27).

The following are associated with a poor outcome or high mortality rate: nonreactive pupil and midline shift of brain structures, ventilatory requirement (152), lack of visual response, poor pupillary response, perimacular folds (151), and submembranous hemorrhagic macular cysts (153), reported to have an associated 50% death rate (151).

Poor visual outcome was correlated with cerebral injury (151). The most severe trauma was associated with vitreous and choroidal hemorrhages, followed by retinal detachment, subhyaloid, intraretinal, or perineural hemorrhages, and finally subdural hemorrhages (154).

Sports Injuries

Protective eyewear is critical to prevent sports-related eye trauma (13). Examples include the following: baseball (155), paint ball (40,156,157), soccer (31), and ice hockey (158). An excellent overview of sports-related injuries and their prevention has been put together by Paul Vinger, M.D., for the Protective Eyewear Certification Council, 2003 (available at *www.protecteyes.org*) (see also the section on Epidemiology).

Animal-Related Trauma

Dog bites pose danger not only because they can cause severe lid and lacrimal system lacerations, but also because the canine oral flora contains pathogens that can cause severe infections and even death (87). Injury also may result from spider bites (70) and tarantula hairs (68).

Self-Inflicted Injuries

The right eye is involved 83% of the time, most commonly with open globe trauma from a sharp tool poked into the eye. The prognosis usually is very poor. Self-enucleation also can occur (55).

Laser Pointers

Laser pointers pose little danger (159). Legal devices made in the United States are five times as powerful as those allowed by European standards and may be of more concern.

Globe Penetration During Strabismus Surgery

Needles causing full-thickness scleral wounds occur in 3 (160) to 4 (161) per 1,000 operations and are more common in myopic eyes. Complications such as endophthalmitis and retinal detachment are extremely rare. No treatment may be necessary. If a visible retinal lesion is present, laser retinopexy may be performed. Occasionally, a scleral patch graft is required (160).

PREVENTION

- As a general rule, a ban (whether it relates to boxing by children, air gun use, darts, or private use of fireworks) is much more effective than adult supervision (12,29,35,45,50,51,53,162–166).

- Appropriate protective eyewear has a very high success rate of preventing sports-related injuries. Even if the injured eye is lost, the ophthalmologist should prescribe protective eyewear for the fellow eye to avoid being accused of negligence (13).
- Seat belts are highly effective in older children (38). It is advised that children be in the back seats (167). Small children should be seated in specially designed child seats. With the use of child seats, the death rate of children under 10 years decreased 23.9% in Alabama (AAA, 2003). Booster seats are recommended for older children. Do not place a rear-facing seat in front of the air bag.
- Serious penetrating injuries with endophthalmitis can result from hypodermic needles (33). Other penetrating trauma has been reported with toothpicks (168).
- Elastic (bungee) cords cause severe trauma and should be avoided or redesigned (169).

REFERENCES

1. Steiner GC PL. Severe emotional response to eye trauma in a child: awareness and intervention. *Arch Ophthalmol* 1992;110: 753–754.
2. Weiss H, Koussett B, Ross E, et al. Simple microphthalmos. *Arch Ophthalmol* 1989;107:1625–1630.
3. Guillaume J, Godde-Jolly D, Haut J. Surgical treatment of traumatic retinal detachment in children under 15 years of age. *J Fr Ophthalmol* 1991;14:311–319.
4. Han D, Abrams G, Aaberg T. Surgical excision of the attached posterior hyaloid. *Arch Ophthalmol* 1988;106:988–1000.
5. Egbert J, May K, Kersten R, et al. Pediatric orbital floor fracture: direct extraocular muscle involvement. *Ophthalmology* 2000; 107:1875–1879.
6. Maltzman B, Pruzon H, Mund M. A survey of ocular trauma. *Surv Ophthalmol* 1976;21:285–290.
7. Ariturk N, Sahin M, Oge I, et al. The evaluation of ocular trauma in children between ages 0–12. *Turkish J Pediatr* 1999; 41:43–52.
8. Desai P, MacEwen C, Baines P, et al. Epidemiology and implications of ocular trauma admitted to hospital in Scotland. *J Epidemiol Community Health* 1996;50:436–441.
9. Chan T, O'Keefe M, Bowell R, et al. Childhood penetrating eye injuries. *Irish Med J* 1995;88:168–170.
10. Al-Bdour M, Azab M. Childhood eye injuries in North Jordan. *Int Ophthalmol* 1998;22:269–273.
11. Sacu S, Segur-Eltz N, Stenng K, et al. Ocular firework injuries at New Year's eve. *Ophthalmologica* 2002;216:55–59.
12. Bratton S, Dowd M, Brogan T, et al. Serious and fatal air gun injuries: more than meets the eye. *Pediatrics* 1997;100: 609–612.
13. Drack A, Kutschke P, Stair S, et al. Compliance with safety glasses wear in monocular children. *J Pediatr Ophthalmol Strabismus* 1993;30:249–252.
14. Rapoport I, Romem M, Kinek M, et al. Eye injuries in children in Israel. A nationwide collaborative study. *Arch Ophthalmol* 1990;108:376–379.
15. Rudd J, Jaeger E, Freitag S, et al. Traumatically ruptured globes in children. *J Pediatr Ophthalmol Strabismus* 1994;31:307–311.
16. LaRoche G, McIntyre L, Schertzer R. Epidemiology of severe eye injuries in childhood. *Ophthalmology* 1988;95:1603–1607.
17. Cascairo M, Mazow M, Prager T. Pediatric ocular trauma: a retrospective survey. *J Pediatr Ophthalmol Strabismus* 1994;31: 312–317.
18. Kuhn F, Morris R, Witherspoon CD, et al. A standardized classification of ocular trauma terminology. *Ophthalmology* 1996; 103:240–243.
19. Eagling E. Ocular damage after blunt trauma to the eye. Its relationship to the nature of the injury. *Br J Ophthalmol* 1974;58:126–140.
20. Kuhn F, Maisiak R, Mann L, et al. The Ocular Trauma Score (OTS): prognosticating the final vision of the seriously injured eye. In: Kuhn F, Pieramici D, eds. *Ocular trauma: principles and practice.* New York: Thieme, 2002:14–22.
21. Dunn E, Jaeger E, Jeffers J, et al. The epidemiology of ruptured globes. *Ann Ophthalmol* 1992;24:405–410.
22. Takvam J, Midelfart A. Survey of eye injuries in Norwegian children. *Acta Ophthalmol Scand* 1993;71:500–505.
23. Adeoye A. Eye injuries in the young in Ile-Ife, Nigeria. *Nigerian J Med* 2002;11:26–29.
24. Al Salem M, Ismail L. Eye injuries among children in Kuwait: pattern and outcome. *Ann Trop Paediatr* 1987;7:274–277.
25. Boone K, Boone D, Lewis RN, et al. A retrospective study of the incidence and prevalence of thermal corneal injury in patients with burns. *J Burn Care Rehabil* 1998;19:216–218.
26. Dandona L, Dandona R, Srinivas M, et al. Ocular trauma in an urban population in southern India: the Andhra Pradesh Eye Disease Study. *Clin Exp Ophthalmol* 2000;28:350–356.
27. Drack A, Petronio J, Capone A. Unilateral retinal hemorrhages in documented cases of child abuse. *Am J Ophthalmol* 1999;128: 340–344.
28. Elder M. Penetrating eye injuries in children of the West Bank and Gaza strip. *Eye* 1993;7:429–432.
29. Enger C, Schein O, Tielsch J. Risk factors for ocular injuries caused by air guns. *Arch Ophthalmol* 1996;114:469–474.
30. Farr A, Hairston R, Humayun M, et al. Open globe injuries in children: a retrospective analysis. *J Pediatr Ophthalmol Strabismus* 2001;38:72–77.
31. Horn E, McDonald H, Johnson R, et al. Soccer ball-related retinal injuries: a report of 13 cases. *Retina* 2000;20:604–609.
32. Horsburgh B, Stark D, Harrison J. Ocular injuries caused by magpies. *Med J Austral* 1992;157:756–759.
33. Jalali S, Das T, Majji A. Hypodermic needles: a new source of penetrating ocular trauma in Indian children. *Retina* 1999;19: 213–217.
34. Jeng B, Steinemann T, Henry P, et al. Severe penetrating ocular injury from ninja stars in two children. *Ophthalmic Surg Lasers* 2001;32:336–337.
35. Kuhn F, Morris R, Witherspoon CD, et al. Serious fireworks-related eye injuries. *Ophthalmic Epidemiol* 2000;7:139–148.
36. Lithander J, Al Kindi H, Tonjum A. Loss of visual acuity due to eye injuries among 6292 school children in the Sultanate of Oman. *Acta Ophthalmol Scand* 1999;77:697–699.
37. Luff A, Hodgkins P, Baxter R, et al. Aetiology of perforating eye injury. *Arch Dis Child* 1993;68:682–683.
38. MacEwen C, Baines P, Desai P. Eye injuries in children: the current picture. *Br J Ophthalmol* 1999;83:933–936.
39. Marshall D, Brownstein S, Addison D, et al. Air guns: the main cause of enucleation secondary to trauma in children and young adults in the greater Ottawa area in 1974–93. *Can J Ophthalmol* 1995;30:187–192.
40. Mason JR, Feist R, White MJ. Ocular trauma from paintball-pellet war games. *South Med J* 2002;95:218–222.
41. Moreira CJ, Debert-Ribeiro M, Belfort RJ. Epidemiological study of eye injuries in Brazilian children. *Arch Ophthalmol* 1988;106:781–784.

42. Nelson L, Wilson T, Jeffers J. Eye injuries in childhood: demography, etiology, and prevention. *Pediatrics* 1989;84: 438–441.
43. Niiranen M, Raivio I. Eye injuries in children. *Br J Ophthalmol* 1981;65:436–438.
44. Olver J, Hague S. Children presenting to an ophthalmic casualty department. *Eye* 1989;3:415–419.
45. Patel B. Penetrating eye injuries. *Arch Dis Child* 1989;64: 317–320.
46. Rosner M, Treister G, Belkin M. Epidemiology of retinal detachment in childhood and adolescence. *J Pediatr Ophthalmol Strabismus* 1987;24:42–44.
47. Rostomian K, Thach A, Isfahani A, et al. Open globe injuries in children. *J AAPOS* 1998;2:234–238.
48. Saxena R, Sinha R, Purohit A, et al. Pattern of pediatric ocular trauma in India. *Indian J Pediatr* 2002;69:863–867.
49. Shuttleworth G, Galloway P. Ocular air-gun injury: 19 cases. *J R Soc Med* 2001;94:396–369.
50. Smith G, Knapp J, Barnett T, et al. The rockets' red glare, the bombs bursting in air: fireworks-related injuries to children. *Pediatrics* 1996;98:1–9.
51. Sotiropoulos S, Jackson M, Tremblay G, et al. Childhood lawn dart injuries. Summary of 75 patients and patient report. *Am J Dis Child* 1990;144:980–982.
52. Soylu M, Demircan N, Yalaz M, et al. Etiology of pediatric perforating eye injuries in southern Turkey. *Ophthalmic Epidemiol* 1998;5:7–12.
53. Strahlman E, Elman M, Daub E, et al. Causes of pediatric eye injuries. A population-based study. *Arch Ophthalmol* 1990;108: 603–606.
54. Sundelin K, Norrsell K. Eye injuries from fireworks in Western Sweden. *Acta Ophthalmol Scand* 2000;78:61–64.
55. Thompson C, Kumar N, Billson F, et al. The aetiology of perforating ocular injuries in children. *Br J Ophthalmol* 2002;86: 920–922.
56. Umeh R, Umeh O. Causes and visual outcome of childhood eye injuries in Nigeria. *Eye* 1997;11:489–495.
57. Vasnaik A, Vasu U, Battu R, et al. Mechanical eye (globe) injuries in children. *J Pediatr Ophthalmol Strabismus* 2002;39: 5–10.
58. Schein O, Hibberd P, Shingleton B. The spectrum and burden of ocular injury. *Ophthalmology* 1988;95:300–395.
59. Monestam E, Bjornstig U. Eye injuries in northern Sweden. *Acta Ophthalmol* 1991;69:1–5.
60. Hemo Y, Ben Ezra D. Traumatic cataracts in young children; correction of aphakia by intraocular lens implantation. *Ophthalmic Paediatr Genet* 1987;8:203–207.
61. Jandeck C, Kellner U, Bornfeld N, et al. Open globe injuries in children. *Graefes Arch Ophthalmol* 2000;238:420–426.
62. Zagelbaum B, Tostanoski J, Kerner D, et al. Urban eye trauma. A one-year prospective study. *Ophthalmology* 1993;100: 851–856.
63. Grin T, Nelson L, Jeffers J. Eye injuries in childhood. Pediatrics 1987;80:13–17.
64. Klopfer J, Tielsch J, Vitale S, et al. Ocular trauma in the United States: eye injuries resulting in hospitalization, 1984 through 1987. *Arch Ophthalmol* 1992;110:838–842.
65. Nash E, Margo C. Patterns of emergency department visits for disorders of the eye and ocular adnexa. *Arch Ophthalmol* 1998; 116:1222–1226.
66. Desai P, MacEwen C, Baines P, et al. Incidence of cases of ocular trauma admitted to hospital and incidence of blinding outcome. *Br J Ophthalmol* 1996;80:592–596.
67. Dannenberg A, Parver L, Fowler C. Penetrating eye injuries related to assault. *Arch Ophthalmol* 1992;110:849–852.
68. Chang P, Soong H, Barnett J. Corneal penetrations by tarantula hairs. *Br J Ophthalmol* 1991;75:253–254.
69. Teske S, Hirst L, Gibson B, et al. Caterpillar-induced keratitis. *Cornea* 1991;10:317–321.
70. Jarvis R, Neufeld M, Westfall C. Brown recluse spider bite to the eyelid. *Ophthalmology* 2000;107:1492–1496.
71. Al Salem M, Sheriff SM. Ocular injuries from carbonated soft drink bottle explosions. *Br J Ophthalmol* 1984;68:281–283.
72. Grinbaum A, Ashkenazi I, Treister G, et al. Exploding bottles: eye injury due to yeast fermentation of an uncarbonated soft drink. *Br J Ophthalmol* 1994;78:883.
73. Gupta AK, Nadiger M, Moraes O. Ocular injury from a carbonated beverage bottle. *J Pediatr Ophthalmol Strabismus* 1980; 17:394–395.
74. Savir H. Ocular injuries from exploding beverage bottles. *Arch Ophthalmol* 1979;97:1544.
75. Sellar PW, Johnston PB. Ocular injuries due to exploding bottles of carbonated drinks. *BMJ* 1991;303:176–177.
76. Viestenz A, Kuchle M. Eye contusions caused by a bottle cap. A retrospective study based on the Erlangen Ocular Contusion Register. *Ophthalmologe* 2002;99:105–108.
77. Sloan SH. Champagne cork injury to the eye. *Trans Am Acad Ophthalmol Otolaryngol* 1975;79:OP889–OP892.
78. Archer D, Galloway N. Champagne-cork injury to the eye. Lancet 1967;2:487–489.
79. Kuhn F, Mester V, Morris R, et al. Serious eye injuries caused by bottles containing carbonated drinks. *Br J Ophthalmol* 2004;88:69–71.
80. Kuhn F, Collins P, Morris R. Epidemiology of motor vehicle crash-related serious eye injuries. *Accident Analysis Prevention* 1994;26:385–390.
81. Kuhn F, Mester V, Witherspoon CD, et al. Epidemiology and socioeconomic impact of eye injuries. In: Alfaro V, Liggett P, eds. *Vitrectomy in the management of the injured globe.* Philadelphia: Lippincott Raven, 1998:17–24.
82. Kuhn F, Mester V, Berta A, Morris R. Epidemiology of serious ocular trauma: the United States Eye Injury Registry (USEIR) and the Hungarian Eye Injury Registry (HEIR). *Ophthalmologe* 1998;95:332–343.
83. May D, Kuhn F, Morris R, et al. The epidemiology of serious eye injuries from the United States Eye Injury Registry. *Graefes Arch Clin Exp Ophthalmol* 2000;238:153–157.
84. Bansagi Z, Meyer D. Internal orbital fractures in the pediatric age group: characterization and management. *Ophthalmology* 2000;107:829–836.
85. Paucic-Kirincic E, Prpic I, Gazdik M, et al. Transorbital penetrating brain injury caused by a toy arrow: a case report. *Pediatr Rehabil* 1997;1:191–193.
86. Nasr A, Haik B, Fleming J, et al. Penetrating orbital injury with organic foreign bodies. *Ophthalmology* 1999;106:523–532.
87. Slonim C. Dog bite-induced canalicular lacerations: a review of 17 cases. *Ophthal Plast Reconstr Surg* 1996;12:218–222.
88. Hatton M, Watkins L, Rubin P. Orbital fractures in children. *Ophthal Plast Reconstr Surg* 2001;17:174–179.
89. Rittichier K, Roback M, Bassett K. Are signs and symptoms associated with persistent corneal abrasions in children? *Arch Pediatr Adolesc Med* 2000;154:370–374.
90. Guemes A, Wright K, Humayun M, et al. Leukocoria caused by occult penetrating trauma in a child. *Am J Ophthalmol* 1997;124:117–119.
91. Zabriskie N, Hwang I, Ramsey J, et al. Anterior lens capsule rupture caused by air bag trauma. *Am J Ophthalmol* 1997;123:832–833.
92. Gradin D, Yorston D. Intraocular lens implantation for traumatic cataract in children in East Africa. *J Cat Refract Surg* 2001;27:2017–2025.
93. Mester V, Kuhn F. Lens. In: Kuhn F, Pieramici D, eds. *Ocular trauma: principles and practice.* New York: Thieme, 2002: 180–196.

94. Sadeh A, Dotan G, Bracha R, et al. Characteristics and outcomes of paediatric rhegmatogenous retinal detachment treated by segmental scleral buckling plus an encircling element. *Eye* 2001;15:31–33.

95. Cohn J, Scagliotti D, Deutsch T. Bradycardia with traumatic hyphema in children. *J Pediatr Ophthalmol Strabismus* 1987;24: 315–317.

96. Ramji F, Slovis T, Baker J. Orbital sonography in children. *Pediatr Radiol* 1996;26:245–258.

97. Harlan J Jr, Ng E, Pieramici D, eds. *Evaluation.* New York: Thieme, 2002.

98. Morris R, Witherspoon C, Kuhn F, eds. *Counseling the patient and the family.* New York: Thieme, 2002.

99. Barr C. Prognostic factors in corneoscleral lacerations. *Arch Ophthalmol* 1983;101:919–924.

100. Kuhn F, Heimann K. Ein neuer Dauermagnet zur Entfernung intraokularer ferromagnetischer Fremdkoerper. *Klin Monatsbl Augenheilkd* 1991;198:301–303.

101. Smit T, Mourits M. Monocanalicular lesions: to reconstruct or not. *Ophthalmology* 2000;107:1310–1312.

102. Jordan D. To reconstruct or not. *Ophthalmology* 2000;107: 1022–1023.

103. Kersten R, Kulwin D. "One-stitch" canalicular repair. A simplified approach for repair of canalicular laceration. *Ophthalmology* 1996;103:785–789.

104. Michael J, Hug D, Dowd M. Management of corneal abrasion in children: a randomized clinical trial. *Ann Emerg Med* 2002; 40:67–72.

105. Campanile T, St. Clair D, Benaim M. The evaluation of eye patching in the treatment of traumatic corneal epithelial defects. *J Emerg Med* 1997;15:769–774.

106. Dana M, Schaumberg D, Moyes A, et al. Outcome of penetrating keratoplasty after ocular trauma in children. *Arch Ophthalmol* 1995;113:1503–1507.

107. Agapitos P, Noel L, Clarke W. Traumatic hyphema in children. *Ophthalmology* 1987;94:1238–1241.

108. Nasrullah A, Kerr N. Sickle cell trait as a risk factor for secondary hemorrhage in children with traumatic hyphema. *Am J Ophthalmol* 1997;123:783–790.

109. Lai J, Fekrat S, Barron Y, et al. Traumatic hyphema in children: risk factors for complications. *Arch Ophthalmol* 2001;119: 64–70.

110. Rahmani B, Jahadi H, Rajaeefard A. An analysis of risk for secondary hemorrhage in traumatic hyphema. *Ophthalmology* 1999;106:380–385.

111. Coats D, Viestenz A, Paysse E, et al. Outpatient management of traumatic hyphemas in children. *Binocul Vis Strabismus Q* 2000;15:169–174.

112. McCannel M. A retrievable suture idea for anterior uveal problems. *Ophthalmic Surg Lasers* 1976;7:8–103.

113. Heimann K, Konen W. Künstliches Irisdiphragma für die Silikonölchirurgie. *Fortschr Ophthalmol* 1990;87:329–330.

114. Zaidman G, Ramirez T, Kaufman A, et al. Successful surgical rehabilitation of children with traumatic corneal laceration and cataract. *Ophthalmology* 2001;108:338–342.

115. Pieramici D, Capone AJ, Rubsamen P, et al. Lens preservation after intraocular foreign body injuries. *Ophthalmology* 1996; 103:1563–1567.

116. Malukiewicz-Wisniewska G, Kaluzny J, Lesiewska-Junk H, et al. Intraocular lens implantation in children and youth. *J Pediatr Ophthalmol Strabismus* 1999;36:129–133.

117. Ahmadieh H, Javadi M, Ahmady M, et al. Primary capsulectomy, anterior vitrectomy, lensectomy, and posterior chamber lens implantation in children: limbal versus pars plana. *J Cataract Refract Surg* 1999;25:768–775.

118. BenEzra D, Cohen E, Rose L. Traumatic cataract in children: correction of aphakia by contact lens or intraocular lens. *Am J Ophthalmol* 1997;123:773–782.

119. Zwaan J, Mullaney P, Awad A, et al. Pediatric intraocular lens implantation. Surgical results and complications in more than 300 patients. *Ophthalmology* 1998;105:112–118.

120. Crouch EJ, Pressman S, Crouch E. Posterior chamber intraocular lenses: long-term results in pediatric cataract patients. *J Pediatr Ophthalmol Strabismus* 1995;32:210–218.

121. Morgan K, Marvelli T, Ellis GJ, et al. Epikeratophakia in children with traumatic cataracts. *J Pediatr Ophthalmol Strabismus* 1986;23:108–114.

122. Churchill A, Noble B, Etchells D, et al. Factors affecting visual outcome in children following uniocular traumatic cataract. *Eye* 1995;9:285–291.

123. DeVaro J, Buckley E, Awner S, et al. Secondary posterior chamber intraocular lens implantation in pediatric patients. *Am J Ophthalmol* 1997;123:24–30.

124. Pandey S, Ram J, Werner L, et al. Visual results and postoperative complications of capsular bag and ciliary sulcus fixation of posterior chamber intraocular lenses in children with traumatic cataracts. *J Cataract Refract Surg* 1999;25:1576–1584.

125. Enyedi L, Peterseim M, Freedman S, et al. Refractive changes after pediatric intraocular lens implantation. *Am J Ophthalmol* 1998;126:772–781.

126. Kora Y, Shimizu K, Inatomi M, et al. Eye growth after cataract extraction and intraocular lens implantation in children. *Ophthalmic Surg Lasers* 1993;24:467–475.

127. Cleary P, Ryan S. Histology of wound, vitreous, and retina in experimental posterior penetrating eye injury in the rhesus monkey. *Am J Ophthalmol* 1979;882:221–231.

128. Margherio A, Margherio R, Hartzer M, et al. Plasmin enzyme-assisted vitrectomy in traumatic pediatric macular holes. *Ophthalmology* 1998;105:1617–1620.

129. Scott I, Flynn HJ, Azen S, et al. Silicone oil in the repair of pediatric complex retinal detachments: a prospective, observational, multicenter study. *Ophthalmology* 1999;106:1399–1407.

130. Moisseiev J, Vidne O, Treister G. Vitrectomy and silicone oil injection in pediatric patients. *Retina* 1998;18:221–227.

131. Ferrore P, McCuen IB, de Juan EJ, et al. The efficacy of silicone oil for complicated retinal detachments in the pediatric population. *Arch Ophthalmol* 1994;112:773–777.

132. Glaser B, Michels R, Kupperman B. *Medical and surgical retina.* St. Louis: CV Mosby, 1991.

133. Kuhn F, Morris R, Mester V, et al. Internal limiting membrane removal for traumatic macular holes. *Ophthalmic Surg Lasers* 2000;31:308–315.

134. Cox M, Freeman H. Retinal detachment due to ocular penetration. I. Clinical characteristics and surgical results. *Arch Ophthalmol* 1978;96:1354–1361.

135. Cox M, Schepens C, Freeman H. Retinal detachment due to ocular contusion. *Arch Ophthalmol* 1966;76:678–685.

136. Cekic O, Batman C, Totan Y, et al. Management of traumatic retinal detachment with vitreon in children. *Int Ophthalmol* 1999;23:145–148.

137. Guillaume J, Godde-Jolly D, Haut J, et al. Surgical treatment of traumatic retinal detachment in children under 15 years of age. *J Fr Ophthalmol* 1991;14:311–319.

138. Alfaro D, Roth D, Laughlin R, et al. Paediatric post-traumatic endophthalmitis. *Br J Ophthalmol* 1995;79:888–891.

139. Rahi J, Logan S, Timms C, et al. Risk, causes, and outcomes of visual impairment after loss of vision in the non-amblyopic eye: a population-based study. *Lancet* 2002;360:597–602.

140. Kaltreider S, Peake L, Carter B. Pediatric enucleation: analysis of volume replacement. *Arch Ophthalmol* 2001;119:379–384.

141. Baxter R, Hodgkins P, Calder I, et al. Visual outcome of childhood anterior perforating eye injuries: prognostic indicators. *Eye* 1994;8:349–352.

142. Cardillo J, Stout J, LaBree L, et al. Post-traumatic proliferative vitreoretinopathy. The epidemiologic profile, onset, risk factors, and visual outcome. *Ophthalmology* 1997;104:1166–1173.

143. Sternberg PJ, de Juan EJ, Michels R. Penetrating ocular injuries in young patients. Initial injuries and visual results. *Retina* 1984;4:5–8.

144. Jaouni Z, O'Shea J. Surgical management of ophthalmic trauma due to the Palestinian Intifada. *Eye* 1997;11:392–397.

145. Apt L, Sarin L. Causes for enucleation of the eye in infants and children. *JAMA* 1962;181:948–953.

146. Jain I, Singh Y, Gupta A. Ocular hazards during birth. *J Pediatr Ophthalmol Strabismus* 1980;17:14–16.

147. Estafanous M, Seeley M, Traboulsi E. Choroidal rupture associated with forceps delivery. *Am J Ophthalmol* 2000;129:819–820.

148. Honig M, Barraquer J, Perry H, et al. Forceps and vacuum injuries to the cornea: histopathologic features of twelve cases and review of the literature. *Cornea* 1996;15:463–472.

149. Baumgart S, Knauth A, Casey F, et al. Infrared eye injury not due to radiant warmer use in premature neonates. *Am J Dis Child* 1993;147:565–569.

150. Lancon J, Haines D, Parent A. Anatomy of the shaken baby syndrome. *Anat Rec* 1998;253:13–18.

151. Kivlin J. A 12-year ophthalmologic experience with the shaken baby syndrome at a regional children's hospital. *Trans Am Ophthalmol Soc* 1999;97:545–581.

152. McCabe C, Donahue S. Prognostic indicators for vision and mortality in shaken baby syndrome. *Arch Ophthalmol* 2000;118:373–377.

153. Kuhn F, Morris R, Mester V, et al. Terson's syndrome. Results of vitrectomy and the significance of vitreous hemorrhage in patients with subarachnoid hemorrhage. *Ophthalmology* 1998;105:472–477.

154. Green M, Lieberman G, Milro C, et al. Ocular and cerebral trauma in non-accidental injury in infancy: underlying mechanisms and implications for paediatric practice. *Br J Ophthalmol* 1996;80:282–287.

155. Danis R, Hu K, Bell M. Acceptability of baseball face guards and reduction of oculofacial injury in receptive youth league players. *Injury Prevent* 2000;6:232–234.

156. Hargrave S, Weakley D, Wilson C. Complications of ocular paintball injuries in children. *J Pediatr Ophthalmol Strabismus* 2000;37:338–343.

157. Thach A, Ward T, Hollifield R, et al. Ocular injuries from paintball pellets. *Ophthalmology* 1999;106:533–537.

158. Pashby T. Eye injuries in Canadian amateur hockey. *Can J Ophthalmol* 1985;20:2–4.

159. Sethi C, Grey R, Hart C. Laser pointers revisited: a survey of 14 patients attending casualty at the Bristol Eye Hospital. *Br J Ophthalmol* 1999;83:1164–1167.

160. Awad A, Mullaney P, Al-Hazmi A, et al. Recognized globe perforation during strabismus surgery: incidence, risk factors, and sequelae. *JAAPOS* 2000;4:150–153.

161. Noel L, Bloom J, Clarke W, et al. Retinal perforation in strabismus surgery. *J Pediatr Ophthalmol Strabismus* 1997;34:115–117.

162. Participation in boxing by children, adolescents, and young adults. American Academy of Pediatrics Committee on Sports Medicine and Fitness. *Pediatrics* 1997;99:134–135.

163. Fireworks-related injuries to children. American Academy of Pediatrics: Committee on Injury and Poison Prevention. *Pediatrics* 2001;108:190–191.

164. Levitz L, Miller J, Uwe M, et al. Ocular injuries caused by fireworks. *JAAPOS* 1999;3:317–318.

165. Colby D. Serious childhood injuries caused by air guns. *CMAJ* 1991;145:1200–1202.

166. Shanon A, Feldman W. Serious childhood injuries caused by air guns. *CMAJ* 1991;144:723–725.

167. Lueder G. Air bag-associated ocular trauma in children. *Ophthalmology* 2001;107:1472–1475.

168. Budnick L. Toothpick-related injuries in the United States, 1979 through 1982. *JAMA* 1984;252:796–797.

169. Da Pozzo S, Pensiero S, Perissutti P. Ocular injuries by elastic cords in children. *Pediatrics* 2000;106:E65.

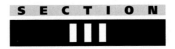

SECTION

III

VISUAL REHABILITATION OF INFANTS AND CHILDREN WITH LOW VISION

VISUAL REHABILITATION OF THE INFANT AND CHILD

LEA HYVÄRINEN

Rehabilitation of visually impaired infants and children is a necessary part of early intervention and requires close collaborative work with therapists, special teachers, and educators to support these children's development and learning. More than half of the children with vision impairment have one or more other impairments (1). Therefore, early intervention and special education must be coordinated with the requirements of several therapies and educational approaches. Because many children have neurologic deficits, therapies and day care have to be planned together with the child's neurologist and therapists. Neurologists and neuropsychologists are often an important part of the low-vision team.

Impaired vision affects all areas of development. Early intervention should consider all developmental areas in each case and find an answer to the basic question, "How much vision is there for the present use in different functions and for the development of each particular function?" The most important areas of functioning where vision plays a central role are as follows:

- Interaction and communication
- Motor functions
- Balance
- Visual spatial concepts
- Auditory spatial concepts
- Object permanence
- Language
- Incidental learning
- Social skills

An infant with multiple impairments may have other areas of development where impaired vision causes problems. Therefore, it is wise to write for each infant a list of functions that need to be addressed during each assessment and those at certain ages.

In pediatric surgical services, active rehabilitation starts before and continues immediately after surgical intervention. Growth and developmental issues are central in the care. Loss of vision, even of a moderate degree, frightens and worries families. Loss of vision in both eyes often is felt to be the most severe loss of a multiply impaired infant. Therefore, immediate early intervention is important in ophthalmology. Anticipated functional vision should be discussed with the family before surgery, especially whether surgery is likely to prevent further vision loss, improve vision, or just save the globe. This discussion should be put in the context of the child's developmental stage, if possible. At an early developmental stage, both eyes may appear to have the same level of visual function; however, as the child matures, the impaired eye's visual function may not keep up with the fellow eye and thus be seen by parents as a worsening in vision. If the parents have false hopes of the infant becoming sighted by surgery alone and do not understand the importance of visual rehabilitation, they may not be active in stimulating the infant before surgery. Disappointment after the surgery may prevent the parents' participation by months and may cause severe depression in the whole family. Early intervention should not be seen as something happening after all surgical interventions are over but as an integral part of the interventions.

In planning rehabilitation of older children, the same functions are important as were important during the first years; however, development of social skills, communication strategies, special learning techniques, and orientation and mobility become the content of special education.

In all pediatric rehabilitation, not only is the infant or child considered but also the whole family, including parents, siblings, grandparents, and even neighbors. Numerous administrative decisions are based on the ophthalmologist's report. Therefore, the reports should describe the child's vision and vision-related functions in an understandable way, supporting the development of the child (2).

The nature of visual impairment in children was officially discussed preceding the International Council for the Education of the Visually Handicapped (ICEVH) Conference in Bangkok in 1992 (3). The World Health Organization (WHO) and the ICEVH called an expert group to a meeting to discuss pediatric low vision. That meeting resulted in a statement with two important details that make the definition of pediatric low vision different from the WHO classification of visual impairment in adult persons:

1. Pediatric low vision includes visual functions other than visual acuity and visual field

2. "This working definition of pediatric low vision is solely designed for reporting purposes and SHOULD NOT be used for eligibility for services."

The Bangkok Working Definition is related to reporting to the WHO and concurs with the International Classification of Diseases. The other visual functions that should be included in the definition of pediatric low vision are low contrast sensitivity, loss of dark adaptation, and other equally disabling functions. This recommendation is not known in most surgical services; therefore, children are assessed as if they were small adults, even if they are infants.

The International Classification of Functioning, Disabilities and Health for adults contains a list of activities considered in the assessment of disability (4):

- Learning and applying knowledge
- General tasks and demands
- Communication
- Mobility
- Self-care
- Domestic life
- Interpersonal interactions and relationships
- Major life areas
- Community
- Social life
- Civic life

These functional areas are present in the life of young children in a simpler framework. Activity areas to be assessed can be restricted to four (2):

- Communication and interaction
- Orientation and mobility
- Activities of daily life
- Sustained near-vision tasks

However, a child may have specific problems related to other impairments that need to be considered as well.

To someone who has worked with visually impaired children, it is rather obvious if a child uses techniques typical of

blind children or of those with low vision to perform a certain task or whether the child uses techniques typical of normally sighted children. The prerequisite is that the evaluator knows the differences and can detect the change in technique when the child switches from one to another. Visually impaired children use different techniques for different tasks, depending on the type of vision loss.

Children with central scotomas and low visual acuity may need high magnification, even a closed-circuit television to read, or they may prefer Braille and talking books when longer texts need to be read. They may have no problems in orientation and movement in known places where they use techniques typical of normally sighted children but still may have problems in unknown places. Thus, there is variation in techniques used by blind persons or those severely visually impaired for sustained near-vision tasks compared to those techniques used by normally sighted individuals for orientation in known environments.

If we assess the use of the techniques in each of the four main functional areas—communication, orientation and mobility, daily living skills, and sustained near-vision tasks such as reading and writing—we obtain useful information for planning special education (Table 33-1). Variation may be caused by changes in visual acuity, contrast sensitivity, visual field, or visual adaptation to changes in luminance level.

If we describe the findings in a diagram, we can fine tune the description by using lines to depict variation in the use of the different techniques, for example, as a function of luminance if the child has poor night vision.

Although we can describe the techniques used and thus the needs of intervention and special education, numbers are sometimes needed when classifying the level of visual impairment. We can depict the functional situation with one number by giving points to the three different techniques. If we give 3 points to blind techniques, 2 to low-vision techniques, and 1 point to techniques typical to the normally sighted, the variation is between 12 and 4 points:

12 points: functional blindness
11–10 points: severe low vision
9–8 points: moderate low vision
7–6 points: mild low vision
5 points: near-normal
4 points: normal sighted functions

TABLE 33-1. ASSESSMENT OF TECHNIQUES USED IN THE FOUR MAIN FUNCTIONAL AREAS

	This Child Uses		
	Blind Techniques	Low-vision Techniques	Sighted Techniques
In Communication		X ——————————— X	
In O&M	X ——————————— X		
In ADL	X ——————————— X		
In SNVT		X ——————————— X	

ADL, activities of daily life; O&M, orientation and mobility; SNVT, sustained near-vision tasks.

By combining this numeric classification and the description of variation of functioning as a table, we are able to give clear information about the degree of impairment and the type and degree of disability. This aids in clarifying the need for services for the child.

Children with retinitis pigmentosa (RP) are a large group of children with good visual acuity. Another large and growing group is children with vision loss due to brain damage. Like children with RP, children with cerebral visual impairment often have normal or near-normal visual acuity but may have difficulties in the following areas:

- Recognizing people's faces
- Recognizing facial expressions
- Perception of motion
- Perception of objects standing still
- Perception of object-background
- Perception and comprehension of pictures
- Eye–hand coordination
- Orientation in egocentric space at near and orientation in environment
- Creating a whole of its components

Assessment and classification of young visually impaired infants need to include all areas of early development so that proper techniques are taught to infants. Severely visually impaired infants develop their communication and interaction, motor skills, spatial concepts, object permanence, language, and social skills in different ways from sighted children because their experiences of the environment and other people are different from those of normally sighted infants. These developmental areas and the possibility of incidental learning need to be considered separately. When this is done, the need of special therapies can be defined.

Assessment of the child is not the only area of concern in planning early intervention. Children are part of a family that needs support and special teaching to cope with the deviations from usual interaction and learning strategies of the child. The family doctor should be involved in early intervention so that the needs of the parents and siblings are known and taken care of. Often contact with other families with similar experiences helps to decrease worries related to the future of a disabled child.

The pediatric International Classification of Functioning, Disability and Health should be completed in 2004 and will give us a much-needed foundation for work in early intervention and special education.

DEVELOPMENT OF VISION AND VISION-RELATED FUNCTIONS IN VISUALLY IMPAIRED INFANTS AND CHILDREN

Although development of visual functions may be well known by the parents, therapists, and teachers, it is good to have a list of milestones of normal vision development (5) at hand when discussing the child's development with the par-ents and caretakers. When they see how many questions there are in the normal development, it makes explanations of the many deviating functional areas easier to comprehend and accept. It helps the parents to understand in which areas their child's environment needs to be modified so that it is stimulating and gives opportunity to optimal learning. Rehabilitation of children with low vision and of blind children should be rewarding for the practitioner, the child, and the family (12) (Table 33-2).

Development of Vision-Related Functions in Visually Impaired Children

Oculomotor functions and abnormal interaction often are the cause of worries that bring an infant to a pediatrician when an infant is otherwise healthy. When normal eye movements do not develop, the eyes have slow roving movements or nystagmus. Sometimes nystagmus is a benign inherited motor nystagmus that may be related to mild-to-moderate vision impairment. If vision impairment is due to damage of the posterior pathways, the infant may have normal-looking eyes with no nystagmus or rotatory nystagmus that may not be diagnosed.

Oculomotor functions, fixation, tracking, convergence, saccades, and accommodation are routine observations that do not require much time. When observing accommodative efforts during dynamic retinoscopy, refractive error without cycloplegia is simultaneously measured. Later when the eye is examined under cycloplegia, basic refraction is assessed. Accommodation and refraction are the two cornerstones of information that the other members of the early intervention team cannot measure and thus must receive from the ophthalmologist.

TABLE 33-2. NORMAL DEVELOPMENTAL MILESTONES OF VISION

Age (Months)	Behavior
0–1	Turns eyes and head to look at light sources; horizontal tracking near midline; eye contact at 6–8 weeks
2–3	Intense eye contact and interaction; vertical and circular tracking; interested in mobiles
3–6	Watches own hands; trains hand movements, reaches toward and later grasps hanging objects; observes toys falling and rolling away, shifts fixation across midline; visual sphere of attention widens gradually
7–10	Notices small bread crumbs, first touches them, then develops pincer grasp; interested in pictures; recognizes partially hidden objects
11–12	Visual orientation at home; looks through window and recognizes people; recognizes pictures; plays hide-and-seek

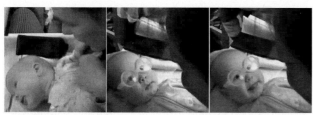

FIGURE 33-1. This healthy infant had not developed eye contact at the age of 4 months. Instead, she turned her head away when somebody wanted to communicate with her. She had been diagnosed as having infantile autism because she seemed to "avoid eye contact." Her accommodation did not function at all, and she was 1 diopter hyperopic. When +4.0 lenses were put in front of her eyes, she immediately looked surprised and after a few seconds developed a normal social smile and good eye contact with her mother. Like many other infants who have difficulties in developing smooth accommodation, she developed esotropia after a few weeks at a time when she started to accommodate. (From L. Hyvärinen's homepage, www.lea-test.fi, Assessment of Vision: Vision in Early Development.)

Accommodation often develops late and remains insufficient in infants with poor vision and/or with brain damage-related visual impairment. Accommodation can be roughly assessed both by using dynamic retinoscopy and by testing the effect of near correction on the interaction of the infant (Fig. 33-1). The effect of near-correction lenses is so often beneficial that they should be assessed in the care of every infant with low vision.

Fixation of normally developing infants may be stable at birth and is expected to be functioning well at the age of 6 weeks. To elicit fixation, tracking, and saccades in a young visually impaired infant, a large brightly colored object with good contrast is used. Often high-contrast black-and-white objects are used as fixation targets. The target does not need to be black and white, because high luminance contrast can be achieved by using light and dark shades of any color.

Fixation difficulties may persist even if central vision develops. Among children with CVI, there is a group whose most impairing visual disorder is inability to fixate. Their gaze glides past the target so that they may be able to see it as a "snapshot" image. If they are asked to look at a target, their eyes may turn upwards and there is simultaneous head thrust backwards. These children's therapists and teachers need to be taught that commands to fixate must not be used. Visual information that a child should look at needs to be placed near him or her and its presence mentioned with a brief description of what the content of the object or picture is and what the child may use it for. Video recording is helpful in explaining the child's difficulties in fixation if it can be taken through a transparent text held on a glass surface (Fig. 33-2).

When a child who is starting to read has cerebral palsy or another motor problem that affects fixation, accommodation, saccadic function, and reading, these need to be assessed in detail. The child is allowed to choose first the text

size, then the spacing on the computer screen. Usually the size can be slightly reduced when the optimal spacing is found. If the child still needs to use a finger to fixate the letters, reading is so time consuming and requires so much of the child's brain capacity that it cannot be used as the main learning medium and auditory materials should be considered. Because of the poor motor functions of the hands and often concomitant hypersensitive or hyposensitive skin, these children usually cannot use Braille. Assessment of auditory memory and auditory orientation in space is important as a part of functional assessment of all visually impaired children.

A teaching situation that simultaneously uses techniques typical to blind persons, i.e., the auditory mode, and techniques typical of the normally sighted, i.e., pictures (if the child has good picture perception and picture comprehension), often is experienced to be difficult by the kindergarten teacher, the classroom teachers, and their aides. Visual and auditory functions need to be discussed in detail with the teacher and the teacher's aide, and an itinerary teacher should visit the child regularly to help teach them how to use auditory materials. It is not generally understood that converting written materials to auditory materials is a special education skill, especially in mathematics and whenever formulas, tables, or footnotes are in the text. Children with cerebral palsy may use text and auditory material simultane-

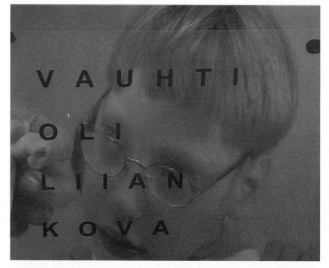

FIGURE 33-2. This boy with severe motor problems had visual acuity of 0.6 (20/30) with single symbols and therefore had not been considered visually impaired. He preferred using 48-point text with 38-point spacing on the computer screen. Even then he could read letters only when he pointed at each letter. Because his hand movements were slow and inaccurate and he needed help in getting the finger to the correct letter, reading was very slow. In such a situation, auditory learning materials and assessment of auditory memory are important. (From L. Hyvärinen's homepage, www.lea-test.fi, Assessment of Vision: Lectures at San Francisco State, November 15, 2003, Slide 41.)

ously and thus get support from the layout of the page in memorizing the content.

Tracking and saccades of tiny infants may be a combination of head and eye movements until the age of 3 to 5 months of corrected age. At age 3 months, a normally developing infant fixates and follows a high-contrast picture of a smiling face of 5-cm diameter moving at a distance of 30 cm. If a prematurely born infant has brain damage, differentiation of eye movements from head movements may not occur if the infant is not specially trained. In some cases, brain damage prevents the development of normal eye movements even if there is useful vision and training of oculomotor functions is practiced as a part of physiotherapy early on.

Congenital strabismus should always lead to the following question: Does this infant have signs of more generalized brain damage than the involvement of one or two oculomotor functions? If there is brain damage, it changes our approach to treatment of the infant. The infant may have impaired vision of the strabismic eye, not so much because of deprivation but because of anatomic changes in the optic pathways of both eyes. Therefore, patching requires careful observations and may not improve the function of the strabismic eye.

Covering of an amblyopic eye of an infant with brain damage initially needs to be for only a few seconds when the infant is exploring something with his or her hands and vision. Because the tactile, haptic, and kinesthetic information remains when the leading eye is briefly covered, the infant has better possibility of coping with abnormal visual information. By repeating the short covering several times a day during a few days, it becomes obvious how well the infant tolerates patching. If patching makes the infant immobile, upset, or sleepy, it disturbs the child too much and does not improve vision in the amblyopic eye.

A visually impaired infant and child with only one functioning eye should have protective glasses so that accidental loss of sight in the only eye would be prevented.

Development of macular vision varies widely in normal infants and young children, and the range of visual acuity remains great even in older children with normal vision. The range of normal is difficult to define in children before school age because it varies much depending on the test used, the tester, and the test situation. Deviations from normal can be measured more reliably when the optotype acuity test can be used starting at age 13 to 14 months (at the earliest in well-functioning toddlers) and much later in many visually impaired children with other handicaps. As long as visual acuity can only be measured as grating acuity and it is below six cycles per degree, it often is impossible to guess what kind of visual image the infant or child is using as a source of information. Improvement of visual acuity occurs in most visually impaired children with stable conditions.

If an infant has *central scotoma,* which is common in children with many retinal disorders, optic atrophy, or periventricular leukomalacia (PVL), fixation becomes *extrafoveal fixation,* that is, the infant seems to look past the adult when looking at an adult person's face. This often causes a negative response in adults who need repeated confirmation that the infant is looking at them and is interested in interaction. Adult caretakers are taught to observe nonvisual cues of responses so that they begin to understand the infant and are able to react positively toward the infant. When supported by early intervention services, the adults begin to understand that the problem in interaction is *their* problem caused by cultural expectations, not a dysfunction of the infant. The infant is using the best vision available for interaction.

Planning of eye movements, i.e., the visual map of the environment, may be of good quality, but execution of eye and hand movements may be slow, and grasping may take a long time. When still of school age, these children have to use early reflexes to bring their head and eyes in the direction of the visual target or their eyes will catch a target by chance. The motor response of the arm may be so slow that the child's head and eyes have passed the target several seconds before the hand is approaching the target. If the delays are not understood, therapists and teachers do not facilitate the child's movements properly. Because many of these children do not talk but are assisted to respond by pointing at letters, sentences, or pictures, it is essential that communication be recorded on video and carefully analyzed by the pediatric low-vision team.

Refraction of small prematurely born infants and of infants and children with cloudy media often is difficult at best, if not impossible. Refractive errors of infants can be roughly assessed by using strong corrective lenses and observing the effect on the infant's behaviors. At the beginning of school age, many well-functioning children with low vision can be tested using subjective test situations. If refractive error is not corrected, all functional test results and observations may be wrong.

Changes in refraction may be toward emmetropia as in normal infants, may not occur at all, or may occur only in one eye. The last condition may lead to anisometropia and a risk of anisometropic amblyopia.

Refraction and how it has been corrected are important pieces of information to be reported to therapists and teachers. Causes of undercorrection or overcorrection and the distances where the image is thought to be clearest should be carefully explained.

Aphakia affects the visual development of many infants who have required lensectomy to repair retinal detachments. Because binocularity seldom is possible with unilateral aphakia, correction with two pairs of spectacles over the basic correction with contact lenses may be used to teach the child to use both eyes, thus avoiding amblyopia. In one pair, the right eye is corrected for near; in the other pair, the left eye is corrected for near. If the infant or child explores objects at 10 to 12 cm, the near add is 10 diopters, *not* 3 diopters. The "distance" correction is fitted to fill the needs of the infant, i.e., first an add of 2 to 2.50 diopters, at a later age less, and in school-aged children, a correction for seeing the blackboard, which often is a distance of 2 m or less. Before that, details at far distances are observed using telescopes or in the classroom with the video camera of the closed-circuit television. Many pediatric ophthalmologists who do not take care of visually impaired infants and children have criticized this practice of correcting distance vision for viewing closer than infinity. They insist that distance correction should be the full correction of cycloplegic refraction in every case. Fitting glasses is a task different from measuring refraction: glasses are fitted for use at the distance where the most important information to the child is located. In severe low vision, details at distance are not seen with distance correction but require magnification. Full distance correction blurs details at intermediate distances if the child cannot accommodate. Before school age, children cannot tell what the most comfortable correction is, so we must use our knowledge of physiologic optics and fit the glasses for distances that are important to the child's function.

Children's teachers and therapists should learn the most common clues of improper refractive correction. Presently it is possible to notice a school child lifting the reading part of the bifocal lens in front of the eye and moving it a bit away from the eye to look at the blackboard, which means undercorrection by several diopters. On the other hand, teachers and therapists need to be informed that highly myopic children use their eyes as magnifiers when they look at near distances without their glasses. Use of a +5 diopter lens as a field lens by aphakic children with moderate low vision also can be taught.

Communication and interaction are the most important vision-related functions. Visual function at low contrast levels is crucial in communication. Our expressions are low-contrast visual information in motion. We can assess low-contrast vision with the Hiding Heidi test (GoodLite) by measuring the distance and contrast at which the infant responds to the picture of the Heidi face. If the infant responds with a smile, we know that the child not only has seen the picture but has perceived the expression at low contrast and responded to it with a normal social smile. This sequence of brain functions tells us that the infant has had good enough vision for early communication and has developed normal emotional responses to friendly smiling faces.

If an infant only responds to high-contrast Heidi pictures at close distances, the adult caregivers need to accentuate their faces to be visible to the infant. This often requires thorough explanation of visual functions and use of demonstration glasses by the caretakers to clarify that the infant can see visual communication only when the caretakers use strong makeup and are close to the child.

Spatial awareness and eye–hand coordination (coordination of vision and motor functioning) require rich experiences of small spaces that the infant or child can explore with all senses and measure with his or her own body. Normally sighted infants receive this information when crawling around their home and exploring objects and spaces of varying sizes: so big that the child can snuggly get in them or so small that only his or her hand or a finger is small enough to explore.

Visually impaired infants who have motor problems, hearing impairment, and developmental delays benefit from "little rooms" that are especially made for them so that they can easily reach the walls of the box. For children who have useful vision, the little room needs to have accentuated visual structure. That is made possible by cutting narrow slits close to the upper edge of a regular brown box. The slit gives a visual boundary to the space. The walls of the box are decorated with visuotactile elements to entice the infant or child to explore (Fig. 33-3). Objects hanging from a thick elastic band above the infant help the development of object permanence and exploration with both hands and mouth.

Infants and children who have poor function of their hands and arms need to get help so they can bring objects into their mouth. We have all learned to see by grasping objects and by exploring them with our hands and mouth. Without that experience, visual information remains distant and abstract. Confirmation through tactile, haptic, and kinesthetic information of the concrete form and its surface qualities is lacking. There are numerous children with severe tetraplegic conditions who have never explored anything

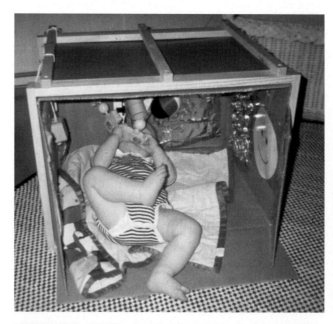

FIGURE 33-3. A little room that is made to fit the size of the child, i.e., his range of reaching, is an inexpensive and effective multisensory playing area. The infant can measure it with his own body, touch, see, smell, and listen. The toys hanging from a thick rubber band do not disappear and help to develop the concept of object permanence.

with their mouth before they come to school. Training of visual and compensatory functions fits well in the early intervention therapies and therefore should be an integral part of motor training, especially during the first year.

Some children with motor problems also have stereoagnosia, which is loss of haptic information. This makes the use of hands ineffective and is an important additional problem that needs to be considered in training and special education. Because hands function as the "other eyes" in the life of visually impaired children, stereoagnosia should be assessed at the time of diagnosis of vision impairment, and supportive training should always be a part of the early therapies and of school.

Body awareness and the possibility of seeing one's own body parts facilitate both development of perception of space and development of motor functions. Physiotherapy should be instituted in the early intervention activities of all visually impaired infants, except in the rare case when motor development reaches normal milestones without special therapy. Physiotherapy of visually impaired infants is a special area of neurodevelopmental therapies (NDT). If a local therapist does not have that training, a therapist with NDT training should function as an itinerary teacher until the local therapist has learned the special needs of the infant.

Everybody around the infant can support the development of the infant by learning the special features of early care of visually impaired children. This is described nicely by Patricia Sonksen and Blanche Stiff (6) in their book, *Tell Me What My Friends Can See.* The pictures in this book are a good guide for parents and therapists of young infants, and this approach should be introduced into the routines at the hospitals.

Motor development of visually impaired infants and children is at risk because poor vision does not give the drive to move and grasp as normal vision does. Movements are planned in visual space, auditory or kinesthetic space, or a space that combines all three sources of information. By structuring the play and therapy areas so that the infant or child can grasp objects visually and then get close enough to grasp them with his or her hands, we lay good foundation for movement in space.

Inactivity is often a typical feature in the behavior of a visually impaired baby and child. In a normal infant, visual information stimulates brain functions. When eyes are opened, visual information flows into the ascending reticular formation, which in turn activates the brain cortex and causes arousal. The child wakes up. If an infant is unaware of the visual world around him or her, this unawareness affects the infant's wakefulness and motor functions. Often an infant is thought to be sleepy because he or she does not open the eyes. The correct interpretation may be that opening the eyes does not change the image enough to be stimulating. Some infants move very little, and the usual reflexive movements are sparse. If an operation results in clearer vision, it should be used effectively in physiotherapy to teach body awareness and motor functions as long as the infant has vision.

Motor development and vision are closely related. When a normally sighted infant sees his or her hand and brings it into the mouth, the early asymmetrical tonic neck reflex is counteracted. If a visually impaired infant does not see his or her hands, there is no incentive to explore them with the mouth and the early reflex pattern may remain. Therefore, playing with the infants' hands, guiding them to meet in the midline, and bringing them into the mouth are important moments in play therapy.

Some newborn infants keep their head turned on the shoulder until they become aware of vision and aware of their hands. Sometimes this is misdiagnosed as torticollis. It disappears sooner if the physiotherapist uses high-contrast objects or a light box to get the gaze moving to the midline of the body and repeatedly brings the hands to the midline. In the assessment of motor development, we need help from the child's own therapist and an experienced therapist who has observed the variation of motor development in visually impaired children.

Orientation in space is an important area of special education from birth to adult. Details of spatial landmarks may appear blurred, and some may not be seen at all. Training of orientation can be started early by structuring children's playmats so that there are strong enough visuotactile details to be perceived using an impaired system. The visual and tactile components are designed so that they coincide. This makes it easier for the child to integrate information from the two modalities that help each other rather than competing for representation in the cortical functions (7).

A visually impaired child must see details at long distances when orienting in an unknown place. Telescopes are a solution, but teaching their use often is difficult even if the child has good motor functions. Looking through a telescope is difficult, so we fix the telescope first on a stand at a window and place a bird feeder outside so that there is something interesting to see through the telescope. It is very difficult to motivate the child to explore the environment with a telescope. Without having seen something, it is difficult to understand what one sees through the telescope. By getting close to an interesting landmark and studying it in detail, then getting farther away and looking at it with a video camera while zooming in and out, the child will get an idea of how he or she can check landmarks and other interesting details in the environment using the telescope.

Orientation in space may be disturbed because of loss of depth perception and/or loss of spatial awareness caused by specific cortical lesions. In some cases, symptoms may be observed as soon as the infant starts to move or when a child moves in unknown surroundings. Therapists should be aware of this group of difficulties and train compensating strategies early on.

Incidental learning is an important area of learning in childhood. Children learn to understand and perform many functions by copying activities that they see during the day. Normally sighted children keenly observe relationships between visual and auditory information, and they learn to recognize places where they are brought and relationships and moods of family members and other important persons. Therefore, we should assess how much vision there is for incidental learning. A child's own therapist(s) and early intervention specialist can make relevant observations at home and in therapy situations: how far does the child recognize objects and persons, and how interested is the child in observing what happens around him or her? Often it takes time to learn what plays the most important role: the quality of visual information, the quality of visual memory, or the child's capability to direct attention.

Language development is related to what the child can perceive visually. If the infant is not supported to explore objects and surroundings tactfully and through auditory information, many concepts remain rather empty of real content. On the other hand, a visually impaired child who has received explanations on what was going on around him or her may learn to use language as an effective compensatory function.

Infants and children who have auditory impairment or who have impaired higher auditory functions such that they hear but cannot decode the sounds to form words need to have sign language early on as their avenue of communication. This seems to be poorly understood in many countries and leads to frustration in children who do not have means to express themselves through speech and who do not have visual or tactile sign language. It should be kept in mind that there are children who have specific loss of motion perception although vision otherwise may be close to normal. In such a case, visual sign language and lip reading are not perceived and need to be replaced with tactile signs.

When a visually impaired child cannot speak, objects, pictures, and other visual materials are used in communication, often before anybody has been able to measure visual acuity, contrast sensitivity, perception of pictures, or picture comprehension. The low-vision team should keep an eye on the methods used in communication and evaluate vision required for each technique.

Picture perception can develop later than in normally sighted children, even if there is no specific cortical lesion. When objects and pictures are seen as blurred, it is difficult to develop the concept of pictures representing objects. Drawing around objects is an effective way of helping the child to understand pictures.

Diurnal rhythm of many visually impaired infants is irregular and therefore causes constant strain to the parents who are deprived of rest. Often an infant or older child needs to be taken to the hospital for a "sleep training course" so that the rest of the family gets a break and can rest while the visually impaired child is getting accustomed to a regular rhythm of activities during the day and inactivity during the night. Melatonin has been used with good results in some, but not all, cases.

Infantile spasms and epilepsy are common problems of visually impaired children with brain damage. Their presence affects the assessment situations so often that ophthalmologists should always receive a thorough explanation from the child's pediatric neurologist on the nature of the disorder and on medications. Medications cause drowsiness and effectively decrease the time when the infant can explore and learn, thus causing delays in all areas of development. Because abnormal brain activity is so common, it is important that everyone in the early intervention team be trained to observe signs of seizures, changes in oculomotor activity, unusual repetitive motor activity, or shorter or longer absence, which should not be taken as a sign of losing interest if the child loses consciousness.

"Blindisms" (stereotypic behaviors) have decreased among visually impaired infants but are still a problem among infants and children with retinopathy of prematurity and Leber congenital amaurosis. Visually impaired infants with other conditions also may start pressing on their eyes, which may develop into eye poking. The causes are not obvious, but self-stimulation seems to be more frequent when the infant is not occupied by play or interaction. Eye poking causes pressure atrophy of fat tissue in the orbit and of the bony rim of the orbit. Often the skin around the eye becomes darker.

A deep-set eye is a cosmetic problem that may disturb the child later in life. It also is possible that eye poking leads to detachment of the retina. Because a child usually does not tell anybody about changes in vision, retinal detachment usually is noticed so late that surgical results are poor. One symptom of which we should be aware is hitting of the forehead: if an infant or child hits his or her forehead and then quiets as if watching something in front of him or her, the interesting phenomenon to watch might be lights, flashes, or shadows produced by movement of the detaching retina.

Rocking of the head or body, jumping, and waving hands are other stereotypic behaviors that may develop in otherwise well-functioning infants. Because they are later problematic in social situations, it is wise to help the child back toward normal motor development. Increased activity of hands, exploration of the environment, and changing the stereotypic movements to normal play activity as soon as they start usually diminish them. Eye poking may disappear if glasses with side shields are used, but they must be introduced immediately when eye pressing starts, otherwise the little fingers find their way around the edge of the glasses.

The first signs usually are not noticed by the parents. Therefore, people involved with the care of visually impaired infants need to be active in observing each infant and helping the parents to prevent development of mannerisms.

Depression is common among disabled children. Nearly every child with chronic illness or impairment goes through a more or less clearly expressed depression around the age of

9 years (8). This happens when the children become aware that parents and medical experts are unable to make them like their peers and that they have to include their impairment and disability as a special feature in their self-image. Because the depressive period is so common, it should be remembered during the vision assessment and it should be known at the school. Information about the impairment should be given with an accepting tone, stressing the fact that the child is healthy with a functional problem. The school and the low-vision services should work together to help the child through this difficult time.

Integration of visual, tactile, kinesthetic, and auditory information occurs in normally developing infants and children without any special training. During early development, there is constant competition among different modalities of use of the cortical structures. If one of the senses has weak representation because of poor quality of information, it may not get its usual role in the higher integrated functions.

Infants born prematurely, especially very small premature infants, may have severe problems in learning to integrate information from the impaired visual system with information from the hypersensitive tactile and auditory systems and poorly functioning motor functions. More than 70% of visually impaired infants and children treated in the retinal services have at least one other impairment or chronic disorder that affects the use of vision and learning through vision. Many infants have more than four severely disabling functions. Training of visual functions and use of vision to support development of other functions become complicated when several therapies need to be combined. Therapists are in need of continuous support from the ophthalmologist. The child's pediatrician or pediatric neurologist works in puzzling situations caused by unusual responses of the infant and the many restrictions in activities that the therapists would like to use in training of the infant or child.

Compensatory Modalities

Hearing, touch, kinesthetic, and haptic information combined with movements are the source of information that cannot be received via vision. If the hands are normal, their sensitivity can be trained to explore forms and surface qualities and to combine that information with visual information. This requires structured play situations and use of educational toys. In the early intervention plan, hands should be mentioned as a specific area of teaching and training.

Hearing is the most important compensatory sense in communication. Therefore, it is important to follow its development as closely as vision development. It should be known that the responses of severely visually impaired infants differ from responses of sighted infants: a severely visually impaired infant does not turn the eyes toward the sound source but quiets to learn more about the new sound.

A combination of visual and auditory information needs to be trained in a visually impaired infant more so than in a normally sighted one. All infants throw toys and listen to the echoes to build their auditory space within their well-functioning visual space during the last months of the first year. When the visual space is limited, training of the auditory space is more difficult and more important as a compensatory function, so visually impaired infants should have numerous play situations where they can experiment with different sounds. Such a simple thing as a grandfather's clock with its low tick-tock is an excellent auditory lighthouse that helps the infant and child to localize the direction in which he or she is moving.

EARLY INTERVENTION

Early intervention in vision care includes all of the special features of care and the special education that an infant or a child needs because of a vision disorder. Most visual impairments of children are caused by disorders that affect vision before, at, or soon after birth. Therefore, early intervention often is believed to mean intervention during the first year. However, visual impairment may start affecting a child's life later so that the child may have had normal or nearly normal vision during the first year or years. Thus, early intervention may be needed at any age; its content depends on the age of the child and the type and severity of the disorder.

Early Intervention in Infancy

Early intervention in infancy varies in its content, depending on the cause of impairment and the general health of the infant. An early intervention team needs to be ready to support an infant and his or her family when the child has an uncomplicated retinal disorder. It also is important in the brain-damaged infant after a nonaccidental injury. Ideally, in each case the support matches the needs of the family. In reality, supporting services may be late to start and are rather limited in many cases. Even in the best surgical services, the quality of early intervention does not always match the quality of surgery.

Functional assessment of vision and the general health of the infant are the starting points in the planning of early intervention. Functional assessment of vision is based on the findings during clinical examination and enlarges to cover many neuropsychological test situations that need to be modified for pediatric evaluation. The most important findings of the clinical examination to be reported to the low-vision team are as follows:

- Structure of the eye and the optic nerve
- Structure of the visual pathways when investigated with echography, computed tomography, or magnetic resonance imaging
- Refractive error of both eyes and whether correction is equal to the measured refraction or there is undercorrection or overcorrection

- Whether the infant uses eyes binocularly or alternatingly, or uses only one eye
- Oculomotor functions, alignment, or nonalignment of the eyes, and type of fixation
- Visual anticipation
- All values measured during the clinical examination, including grating and optotype acuity, contrast sensitivity, size of the visual field, and electrophysiologic findings

Assessment of an infant's functioning in general and evaluation of functional vision for early intervention should be a calm, encouraging, yet realistic and positive experience for the parents. It is unfortunate that the clinical examination of young infants is often performed by residents who have little or no experience with infant development and limited experience in examination techniques. Their evaluation of the situation is usually less optimistic that what is later found by the early intervention team. Because untrained residents are not allowed to operate, we should use experienced physicians for the assessment of the infant's/child's functioning. Intervention would then be based on a thorough, experienced examination, and the physician would be more likely to have an understanding of parents situation and cultural background.

Support and assessment by the early intervention team often starts after some delay. Although early intervention should be a part of clinical care, in many hospitals the child and family are referred to the early intervention services outside the hospital. Parents may not have the strength to contact the early intervention services for several weeks, sometimes months, at a difficult time in the care of their child.

Ideally, early intervention should be an integral part of the diagnostic examinations and therapies, and supporting functions should be started as soon as there is a suspicion of visual impairment, not first when a "confirmed diagnosis" is available, which may take years. In pediatric orthopedics, supportive training precedes an operation and starts only a few hours after the child has been operated on. This approach would be a good model in ophthalmology.

Because counseling and training the parents take time, these processes should be started without delay, even if the infant is in such poor condition that very little training of vision and other functions of the infant is possible.

Infants who have disorders that, according to the textbooks, lead to death before the age of 2 to 3 years should not be denied early intervention. Many of these infants survive beyond the range reported for their conditions and therefore need all supportive measures available in the local services.

Vision has an important organizing role in early communication and learning. It gives an effective overview of many situations. An infant can use visual information by repeatedly looking at objects, persons, and the environment. Objects can be visually explored from different angles and the environment observed thousands of times during each day. In contrast, auditory information is heard once and disappears: its relation to the sound source is detected through vi-

sion or sometimes from vibration of the surface of the source. Visual information is constantly combined with information from other modalities, and its use requires development of numerous brain functions that need to be determined as a part of a thorough assessment of all visually impaired infants.

When a child is learning about the environment using compensatory techniques, it takes much more time than visual exploration. For example, a child may stand on door steps for several minutes, moving the door back and forth and listening to the weak sounds that he or she can hear. Or a child may explore an interesting object tactfully using hands, lips, and tongue to learn about the small differences in the surface qualities. Autistic children have similar behaviors as visually impaired children; thus, visually impaired children often are diagnosed as having "autistic features" even though they are skillfully using techniques that compensate for loss of visual information.

When we observe and assess an infant's visual development, we need to assess both peripheral and central visual function. The peripheral pathways develop rapidly during the first year, and although there is variation in the speed of myelination of the pathways and in the development of individual visual functions, this variation is known. Use of vision requires development of attention, which may vary and often is a greater problem than the basic visual functions in children with brain damage.

In the following text, contents of intervention are discussed at different ages of infants and children. At each age, the functions mentioned earlier and the special problem areas of each infant and child will be covered. To avoid repetition, the most common and important problems are discussed at each age level.

0–3 Months

Severe vision impairment affects brain development. Visual functions are not normally represented in cortical functions, whereas tactile and auditory functions dominate. Therefore, training of vision should be started as soon as there is a suspicion of low vision. Training will not have been harmful if it is shown later that visual development is normal. The delay in development may have been temporary and training may have helped the infant to get on the normal path of visual development.

Vision training has a special connotation is the United States because of the practices of some behavioral optometrists. Therefore, in this text, I will use "training of visual functions" instead of "vision training." In Europe, it is a proper term for training an infant or child to best use his or her impaired vision and to develop compensatory strategies in tasks that cannot be performed like a sighted child.

Training of visual functions has two different stages:

1. If an infant does not respond at all to visual stimuli or responds only very weakly, the infant is made aware of visual information by using high-contrast objects and optimal lu-

minance levels and, if nothing else works, flickering high-contrast visuotactile pictures. This is the stage of passive stimulation. To be effective, the information must be in the form of patterns, not diffuse light of different colors.

2. After short passive stimulation, *active stimulation* is used in the same session. If the child does not yet grasp anything, the little hand or foot is guided to touch and then hold an interesting object, moving it slowly in front of the eyes. Combination of visual information with motor activity is the cornerstone of development of vision for moving and spatial concepts.

Eye movements, saccades, and pursuit movements are difficult to learn if there is nothing to look at. Objects with good contrast need to be close enough and at the optimal luminance level to facilitate visual search and fixation. Sometimes it is helpful to dim the lights in the room and shine a focal light on the toy within reach of the infant. Simple things such as a balloon also work well in early stimulation. If a balloon is tied to the hand or foot of the infant, it moves when the hand or foot moves. Thus, the infant experiences the sequence "I did something and something happened, I did the same thing and again it resulted in the same thing happening." Such an experience is an effective learning situation.

If no responses to visual stimulation can be elicited during the first few therapy sessions, it should be stressed during the discussion with the parents that development of vision may be delayed and may start when visual pathways are stimulated. If an infant is called blind, parents have no motivation to continue play situations that stimulate vision.

Interaction and communication are the most important functional areas to assess and support. Infants who have loss of central vision due to retinal scars (e.g., toxoplasmosis) or damage to the visual pathways must use the part of the visual field next to the edge of the central scotoma and will seem to look past the person upon whom they fix. Therefore, they do not have "normal eye contact." In the beginning, the area of retina used for fixation, the preferred retinal locus, varies, but soon the infant may start using a certain area or several different areas of the retina in different visual tasks.

We experience eye contact with an infant to be positive and important. Therefore, loss of normal eye contact can be emotionally difficult for the parents and other persons taking care of the infant. Abnormal eye contact needs to be discussed with parents and caretakers and early interaction supported by visual communication close to the infant, and by nonvisual communication.

Infants who are in incubators or in intensive care units during the perioperative period should be held on the lap soon after surgery and as often as possible. The infants often are so sleepy that their visual activation is not feasible. When they start to awake, simple pictures can be placed in the incubator or crib. When strong visual stimuli are introduced, infants need to be carefully monitored for increase in heart rate or breathing to ensure that the infant is not overstimu-

lated. Inhibitory mechanisms are not well developed in young infants, so signs of too strong stimulation need to be watched. Simple geometric forms with good contrast interest young infants. If the pictures are made of plastic they are easy to wipe clean. Tiny infants do not touch these; thus, they remain in good condition for years in intensive care units.

Infants with poor vision may not look around and may not lift their heads. Delay in head lift delays development of motor functions of the arms and shoulders, and the infant often dislikes to be on his or her stomach. Therefore, training of head lift is a special activity in physiotherapy for these young infants.

In play situations, the infant's hands are brought to the midline. This helps many infants to bring the eyes to the midline and to look at the person in front of them. During clinical examinations and therapies, parents have an opportunity to see how close playthings should be presented to their child. The responses to visual stimulation may be weak; thus, parents may need the support of video recordings showing how the infant clearly enjoys interaction.

When an infant is able, saccade testing of grating acuity with LEA Gratings or Teller acuity cards and contrast sensitivity with the Hiding Heidi test should be performed. The low-contrast Heidi pictures demonstrate to the parents and the caretakers the contrast levels to which the infant responds and at which distances. Observation of the test situation usually motivates everyone to communicate closely enough and to increase contrast on their faces with makeup (also men can use brown contour pen).

Poor eye contact usually is the most disturbing experience for parents. They may not be able to specify what it is that makes them feel that the infant is not interested in them. Therefore, the role of eye contact in early interaction needs to be explained repeatedly. The parents should be helped to notice their negative feelings and sadness when the infant does not respond like a sighted infant and to observe and correctly interpret the responses of a severely visually impaired infant who uses auditory information more than a sighted infant.

If interaction with an infant is difficult, it is avoided. The infant then spends more time in the crib than a sighted infant would, although he or she may need to spend *more* time with parents than a sighted baby does. Often a person who stimulates the infant, i.e., a therapist or early intervention specialist, should show the parents how to communicate and play with the infant. If acceptance of the infant's situation is delayed, it affects the general development of the infant and the well-being of the parents, sometimes leading to depression in both the infant and a parent, usually the mother.

Parents have such a central role in the development of an infant that they should get more attention, proper guidance, and support during the important formative years and especially during the first months of shock, worries, and disappointment. Parents of healthy infants can become frustrated with seemingly minor practical problems. When an infant requires repeated hospital care and complicated care at home, such as tube feeding or care of contact lenses, and does not reward the parents with normal interaction, parents will require support and practical help. This need does not decrease as the child matures but rather continues until the parents have learned to know their child and have become special therapists and special educators of their own child. In some cases this never happens. In such a case, the infant/child needs continuous, frequent support by a person who understands the effects of visual and other impairments on interaction and development.

Early intervention also considers the other members of the family and all other persons who take care of the infant. Involvement of siblings, grandparents, and neighbors in the activation and support of the family is important from the start and throughout childhood because several new crises will be met as the child grows. These should be noticed and addressed during later assessments.

4–6 Months

A normally sighted infant becomes visually aware of his or her hands at the age of 3 months and spends hours admiring his or her fingers at different distances, training stereo vision, accommodation, convergence, and concepts of egocentric space. When an infant is visually impaired, details of the hands may not be sufficiently visible to interest the infant and thus an important play situation does not spontaneously occur. The small fingernails can be accentuated with bright nail polish and hands made more clearly visible with striped half-mittens (fisherman's mittens that do not cover fingers). Children also can watch their hands against the illumination of a light box.

Seeing the hands, bringing them into the mouth, and tasting them is an important multimodal learning experience that during the first year gives most accurate information about structures and surface qualities (5). Mouthing remains an effective way to explore at school age. It is not a sign of autism. Severely visually impaired adult people also use their tongue to feel details that cannot be felt well enough with the fingertips.

A severely visually impaired infant needs guidance in learning to reach out and explore. Although it is a typical function in the next period of 6 to 9 months, its foundation is laid during this period of 3 to 6 months. Patricia Sonksen and Blanche Stiff's book, *Show Me What My Friends Can See*, contains nice examples of how to guide hands and arms to reach out. As long as the hands and arms move aimlessly at the shoulders, they should be guided often to touch each other in the midline. Bringing hands to midline, thus creating a concept of midline, is an important step in motor development. In some children, bringing hands to midline helps them to bring their gaze to midline.

At this age, functional assessment should include assessment of vision for communication and awareness of one's own body and the immediate surrounding space.

At the age of 3 months, eyes of normally developing children usually are working together, although strabismus still occurs, especially when infants are tired. Visually impaired children may develop binocularity, but it is rare. In many cases, one of the eyes sees better than the other, thus, functional amblyopia may develop in the more poorly sighted eye.

Therapy situations should be used for diagnostic observations and assessment of amblyopia training. Oculomotor functions, tracking, and saccades are trained as a part of therapies by using high-contrast toys to attract the infant's attention. Sometimes toys that the infant moves by himself or herself elicit better tracking movements than toys shown to the infant.

In parent–infant interaction, *visual sharing* starts normally at this age. The infant sees something interesting, looks at it, looks at the parent, and then looks at the interesting object. The parent responds to the cue, looks at the object, tells the child what the object is, and may ask whether the infant might like to play with it. Sharing also may start from the adult looking at something. The infant notices it and looks at the same object, which then is described to the infant when the adult person notices the child's interest. Sharing interest is an important part of interaction; thus, we need to observe whether it is possible to the visually impaired infant. This kind of incidental learning and communication is not available to most visually impaired infants. Their world is smaller than that of their peers, and they cannot see objects or facial expressions well enough *to initiate visual sharing*. It can be trained by showing objects that the infant knows and by telling the infant: "I have a soft brush. Would you like to have it for a while?" Or, "Are you looking at your mug, would you like to drink?" Infants start to understand this kind of questions quite early, not word by word but the intention to share a common interest and learn to initiate interaction by looking at objects.

Refractive errors in healthy children progress toward emmetropia. Among visually impaired children, this development is rare; thus, large refractive errors typical to the early part of the first year may remain. If accommodation does not develop, an infant's vision for communication is disturbed. Thus, accommodation needs to be measured at least every other month during the first year as part of the assessment of functional vision until it appears. When insufficient accommodation is diagnosed, a "reading add" of +2.0 to +10 is prescribed for near-vision tasks. These near corrections need to be used during all tests at near, including grating acuity and Hiding Heidi tests.

Visual information stimulates infants to reach for, and move toward, interesting objects. If an infant's visual sphere is limited, motor development is slow, but it can be kept within normal milestones with physiotherapy and occupational therapy, preferably given by a therapist with training in neurodevelopmental therapy (NDT).

Orientation in space requires stronger contrasts if a child's vision is impaired. The usual pastel colors are not good in the crib or as the colors of the play mat and toys. If the mother or someone else has time to sew a play mat with high-contrast visuotactile details, it becomes a useful plaything for developing orientation in space. "Strong contrast" does *not* mean black and white stripes. Good contrast can be created by choosing light and dark shades of any color that parents like. Another play situation that activates the infant to explore space is the *resonance board* with clear visuotactile markings on it. Often the resonance board is the first gift the father can make for the infant, and it may strengthen the bond between them.

7–12 Months

In a normally sighted infant, visual and motor activities increase by the beginning of the second half of the first year. The infant's eyes "are everywhere," as are the hands that have a nearly compulsive desire to grasp everything within reach. The infant notices tiny crumbs on the floor and starts to develop a pincer grasp to pick them. This activity can be used to measure detection acuity at home during therapy or play. When the infant sits on the floor, a few small sweets are placed behind his or her back. When the infant is turned on his or her stomach and placed so that the sweets are close to the eyes, the infant usually stops moving for a moment, looks at the sweets, supports himself or herself on one arm and hand and reaches with the other hand toward the sweets to pick them up.

A severely visually impaired infant may not yet be able to support himself or herself on one arm. Also, visually impaired children with motor problems need a modification of the test situation. Infants who can sit in a high chair can be tested by placing sweets on a table. If the infant does not yet sit but can stand supported, the sweets can be placed on the tray of the supporting stand. Placing the sweets is done either before the infant is brought to the place or as a game. Have a few sweets in both hands, tell the child that something will appear on the table or tray while moving both hands above the table. Now and then drop a sweet from your hand without stopping the movement. When you have dropped a few sweets, the infant may spontaneously pick them up. If not, search together with the infant for what might be on the table.

If the small sweets cannot be noticed, try larger sweets and cereals. Notice that contrast between the color of the sweets and the surface of the table is an important factor. It is better to use dark small objects on a light-colored surface than vice versa. Small white objects on a dark surface may give a falsely optimistic sense of visual acuity. If the child has uncorrected refractive error or cannot accommodate, the blurred image of a small white object may be quite a large blurred ring and thus much more easily noticeable than the object is when it is seen clearly.

Vision can be assessed using detection tests: grating acuity tests as discussed earlier and now the Cardiff test. Contrast sensitivity is assessed with the Hiding Heidi test and visual field using confrontation. If visual field defects such as hemianopsia are noticed, training of the poorer functioning side is started immediately by making the infant aware of objects on that side and by moving interesting things from the better functioning side to the poorer functioning side. In some cases, the measured difference in the use of field halves is not due to visual field loss but rather to loss of attention. With training, the difference may disappear or at least decrease in a few months.

Development of spatial concepts uses a combination of visual information and the size and reach of the child. Use of a "little room" is particularly important at this age.

Visual impairment makes some motor skills difficult to learn; therefore, training of basic motor skills, saving responses (or catching one's balance), and overall balance should continue as a part of physiotherapy to support later specific mobility training for safe movement when the child starts to walk. Our balance usually is dependent on the function of the inner ear, information from the peripheral visual field, and proprioceptive information from the lower extremities and trunk. An infant who is learning to sit unsupported does not yet get much information from proprioception, and if peripheral visual field does not function well, balance depends on the function of the inner ear. In such a situation, saving responses require a lot of training.

Moving is often a frustrating effort at the age of 7 to 8 months if the arms and legs are not yet strong enough to support the weight of the body. Training in water, baby swimming, or playing in the bathtub develops motor functions, also oculomotor functions.

Toward the end of the first year, problems in cognitive vision start to become noticeable. If an infant does not recognize family members by their faces but does recognize them by their voices, the infant may have a specific loss of the cell groups responsible for face recognition. Some infants have no recognition of facial expressions and therefore cannot understand the emotional content of visual communication. These two deficits in cognitive visual functions are the socially most important ones and therefore should be assessed during therapies and discussed during each ophthalmologic examination.

Of the more than 30 different higher visual activities that could be damaged, the common ones are capability to track a moving object, to perceive motion, or to see an object that does not move, or different problems with parietal visual functions, eye–hand coordination, orientation in egocentric space, and eye movements. A clumsy infant should always be carefully assessed as early as possible.

Training of cognitive vision tests can be a part of early intervention therapies so that test situations are familiar and thus possible earlier than without training. During training, it becomes obvious which tasks are more difficult than usual at a similar age, and these functions can be specifically trained. Training of cognitive functions usually needs to continue until school age or even later. The earlier it is included in the therapies, the better are the possibilities that training will benefit the development of brain functions. For example, training of perception of orientation of lines includes training of hand movements, first moving the fingers along visuotactile lines and then along visual lines, and rotations of wrists that often are poorly developed in visually impaired children because of lack of use.

Picture perception is an especially difficult area for many visually impaired children at this age. Drawing with high-contrast ink and filter pens should be a part of daily play situations. The pictures can be of common objects to clarify the relationship between objects and pictures, but they also can be pictures from fairy tales to develop imagination. Infants can perceive and understand a picture much better when they have seen it appear on paper and have the different details described by an adult.

Early Intervention for Toddlers and Preschoolers

Vision plays a central role in the communication of a toddler. If we bring together five to six toddlers for the first time, it takes them less than half an hour to decide who is the boss, who is the last, and what the ranking order is between these two. There has been no discussion because there is no speech yet, but body language and expressions make the status of each child clear. When a visually impaired toddler is brought to a day care center, limitations in visual communication must be described to the personnel, e.g., poor contrast sensitivity and visual acuity, loss of central visual field, or cognitive problems in recognition of facial features and/or expressions. A teacher's aide with good communication skills should function as the interpreter, structuring the play situation of the visually impaired child and explaining to the other children when the visually impaired child does not respond typically. Personnel in day care centers are given information about problems that noise causes when the auditory channel is the dominant distance sense: that the child may need special lighting, that limited vision of the child is to be kept in mind when pictures and objects are presented to a group of children, and that the families of the other children need to be given information about vision impairment.

The clearer the description of vision for communication, the easier it is to integrate a toddler into a group of toddlers. Because there still are day care centers that refuse to adapt their programs to meet the needs of children with impairments, the attitudes of the personnel should be investigated

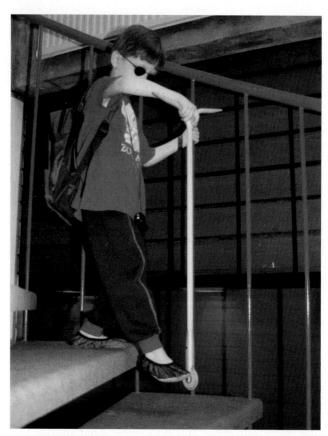

FIGURE 33-4. When a visually impaired child has learned to walk, training becomes even more intensive. Specialized training includes moving up and down stairs, in a forest, on rocks and soft sand, and with or without a cane.

in detail. Otherwise, a visually impaired toddler may be experienced as a child with "autistic behaviors" or intellectual disabilities when his or her responses differ from those of his or her sighted peers.

Many visually impaired children have some problems in learning to walk. When they learn to walk, their therapies should not be discontinued simply because they have reached a milestone in motor functions appropriate to the age. It should be stressed to the pediatric rehabilitation team that, at this age, a visually impaired child needs *more* training in mobility than ever before. Well-planned pediatric orientation and mobility training are key to integration into local school and society. If no instructor is available locally, a child's therapist should have good support by an itinerary instructor so that the child is taught proper strategies in orientation and moving (Fig. 33-4).

Children Who Become Visually Impaired at Preschool Age

A small number of children who see normally or near normally during the first year of life become visually impaired later on. Some of them also become severely, multiply handicapped before school age. Encephalitis, tumors, and accidents may cause dramatic losses of vision. Rheumatoid arthritis may cause few or no symptoms in joints before severe symptom-free uveitis has resulted in cataracts in both eyes. Numerous rare syndromes affect vision and other functions of the child. The severity of vision loss varies; therefore, both treatments and early intervention are highly individual.

Children who become severely disabled require special attention because their integration into day care, kindergarten, and other preschool functions may become a problem. Teachers and therapists might experience the care of these children as too difficult and the risks of errors too high. Therefore, the functional assessment of these children is very important. The assessment of these children resembles the assessment of infants because their caretakers, therapists, and special teachers are key persons in the evaluation of visual functions and general development. The low-vision team members can help by providing the basic clinical information and making sure that the anatomy of the eyes and visual pathways is well recorded and described to the people involved with the care of the child. They can demonstrate the test situations and training of visual functions that seem feasible in the beginning and modify them later to fit the changes in visual functions.

If a multisensory room is used, it should be assessed in terms of visual sphere of the child, contrasts, and luminance level. Many multisensory rooms that are pleasant to the personnel may be designed such that almost no visual information makes sense and gives structure to a severely visually impaired child. The size of the visual and cognitive sphere of these children needs to be explained because people do not understand their limitations if a child has normal-looking eyes and seems to look around.

Many multidisabled children are awake and aware for long periods of time. Although they may sleep a major part of the day, instructional and entertaining materials should be developed for each child that would allow further observations on what the child may see and remember.

School Age

School age brings a major change in the life of a visually impaired child and his or her family. Most children go to school in a regular local school integrated into the mainstream education programs. Ideally, each visually impaired child has an individual educational plan (IEP) that covers all the needs of special learning techniques and plans as to who is going to teach them. The number of children who do not have this ideal school situation is larger than we like to believe. This is caused by criteria for services that restrict children without very severe visual impairment. Many communities include only children with visual acuity less than 20/60 or 20/200 and/or visual field loss so that the remaining field does not extend to further than 20 or 10 degrees from the fixation point.

Ophthalmologists can support the education of visually impaired children by writing clear reports stating that a child with better than 20/63 or 20/200 visual acuity may be visually impaired because of loss of other equally important visual functions. When the child's needs are well described, it usually is possible to arrange special education to meet the needs. Children at the schools for physically handicapped and in the schools for the deaf should have thorough assessments, not only visual acuity screening. Likewise, all children with intellectual disabilities need to be assessed at the ages when normally functioning children have vision screening.

During the short visits of the family of the visually impaired child, the doctor gets too little information about the large number of special arrangements and concerns that the visual impairment of the child causes (Fig. 33-5).

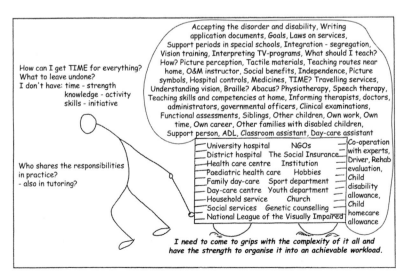

FIGURE 33-5. The numerous duties, connections to different administrative offices, and organizations that the parents of visually impaired children must address are depicted in this drawing by a mother of two well-functioning children with achromatopsia. If a child has several impairments, the number of connections to offices and people nearly doubles. The original drawing with the Finnish texts was drawn by the mother for the journal of the parent association. (Modified from the Web page *www.lea-test.fi*, with permission from Leena Herranen.)

The parents must tolerate repeated contacts with a great number of strangers, some of whom become well known later on during the school years. If the family or some of the contact persons move, the whole history of the child must be retold and explained to new persons. Decisions on visual devices often are made late, so there is insufficient time to train in their use before school starts. Services must often be negotiated several times. The parents themselves must learn a lot about early intervention and special education to be able to ask for the services to which the child is entitled. The process can be frustrating to parents. There are days when a parent may ask whether they exist to serve the rehabilitation offices or vice versa.

In the teenage years, there often are problems related to the well-being of the siblings, who may find themselves receiving less attention in the family than the impaired child. Their situation should be considered in the rehabilitation plans that are a part of the individual educational plans.

VISUALLY IMPAIRED CHILDREN WITH MULTIPLE IMPAIRMENTS

Visually impaired children who have other impairments and disabilities make up more than half of all children with vision impairment (1). The largest groups among visually impaired, multiply disabled children are those with:

- intellectual impairment,
- hearing problems, and/or
- motor impairment

Among those infants who survive, a great number of children have more than two impairments and a few have more than four. This chapter on children with multiple impairments is within the chapter of rehabilitation, although specific test situations are discussed in other areas of the text.

Because the possible combinations of the different impairments and malformations are numerous, only the common types are covered in this chapter. The following problem areas are common in all countries:

- Visually impaired children with delays in cognitive development; trisomy 21 is the most common cause
- Dual sensory impairment in otherwise healthy children, such as Usher syndrome
- Vision impairment in hearing impaired, multiply impaired children, such as those with rubella or other syndromes
- Vision impairment in children with motor problems unrelated to the cause of the vision impairment and no brain damage
- Vision impairment caused by brain damage that also causes motor impairment

Multiply impaired infants and children are remarkably alike in all countries. In some developing countries, severely, multiply impaired infants do not survive; therefore, the as-

sessment and teaching of severely, multiply impaired children is not as great a problem as it is in the industrialized countries. However, children with Usher syndrome, children with cerebral palsy and other motor problems, and visually impaired children with intellectual disabilities are found in all countries.

Management of early intervention of multiply impaired children requires cooperation among several intervention programs, clinics, hospitals, and a large number of specialists in different fields. Quite often it is necessary to carry out the evaluation together with the representatives of several teams, e.g., the vision team, representatives for the school for the deaf or for children with motor problems, the resource center for the visually impaired, the local peripatetic teacher, and a representative for the organization paying for the devices and services. This is always a challenging task. Involvement with so many people in the care of their child often is felt to be an additional impairment by the parents. If several people give advice on the same problems, it is unavoidable that misunderstandings occur.

Planning of early intervention and later planning of different services require a transdisciplinary approach in the assessment of vision and other functions. A transdisciplinary working model means that the different specialists not only work together but they train together so that the usual assessment situations can be addressed by several specialists. These children often require a long time to become accustomed to function in a new environment, so clinical measurements may give poor results. It is better to arrange test situations in places where the child is accustomed and feels safe and relaxed. The child's communication may require special devices and techniques, so direct communication with the child may not be possible. Tests used in the assessment must be trained for at school and at the day care center for extended periods before the tests can be properly used. There is such a great variation in the visual functions of these children that the functions must be assessed several times before the range of variation has been observed.

Infants and Children with Intellectual Disabilities

Trisomy 21 (Down syndrome) is the most common cause of intellectual disability associated with anterior visual pathway disorders in children. If the developmental delay is mild to moderate, it does not affect the assessment and early intervention in any notable way. The techniques are chosen to suit the communication and cognitive abilities of the child, i.e., tests are those used for younger children.

Quite often, training for the test situations is needed in the day care center or classroom for weeks or even months before formal testing is possible. Training for testing becomes an integral part of early intervention. Often we start with such simple exercises as moving a finger along a straight line. Because the concepts of "similar" and "different" are taught comparing colors and forms as a component of standard teaching programs, it is easy to include the colors and forms used in vision testing in classroom teaching. Measurement of visual field is based on observations in play situations, and confrontation fields can be performed as a game.

In each group of children with different developmental delays, specific features should be assessed and then trained or compensated. For example, many children with trisomy 21 have strabismus, which should be treated early, and they may have poor accommodation and need "reading glasses" at the age of 4 months.

When an infant has severe brain damage and is unresponsive to visual stimulation during clinical examination, strong visuotactile stimuli can be used to elicit responses in therapies and play situations. Because there is a danger of overstimulation, the child's condition must be carefully observed. Measurements of heart rate, breathing rate, motor activity, and sweating are useful in the observation of these children who are the most difficult to assess. Often we have to record breathing and pulse for long periods to find a change that coincides with auditory, tactile, or visual information or a change in the child's physical position. This does not always prove that there is a causal relationship between the change and the subjective perception of sensory information. The effect may be at a lower level in the brain. Recording of pulse is the easiest way to observe the child's status when strong sensory stimuli are used. Because the inhibitory mechanisms may not be effective, a strong stimulus may cause an abnormally strong arousal in the brain when the stimulus is suddenly transferred through the damaged pathways. Stimuli such as the Disco Heidi or loud music with beating rhythm should be used only while carefully observing the child's behaviors.

Children with Dual Sensory Loss

Dual sensory loss has become the name for impairment of both vision and hearing. Often it is limited to children with Usher syndrome and children with coloboma and microphthalmia of different etiologies. However, the group is much larger. Children born as small premature infants and children who have lost hearing in one ear because of infection, accident, or an inherited disorder can have dual sensory loss that affects their orientation in space. They cannot use auditory orientation to compensate for losses in visual orientation in space. This difficulty with visual orientation in space can occur with monoaural or single-sided hearing loss. The use of a bone-anchored hearing device implanted in the temporal bone on the side of the impaired ear may slightly improve sound localization capabilities in some situations but does not give the person good enough auditory orientation to compensate for the vision loss.

Children with Retinitis Pigmentosa

Usher syndrome is known in all parts of the world. It is common in Nordic countries, so there has been interest in

developing services for deaf-blind people at all ages. Definition of deaf-blindness has been discussed for more than 30 years, but there still is no consensus. In our practical work, we have used common sense and consider all functions of all visually impaired children with hearing loss. In hearing impaired children and teen-aged youngsters, vision needs to be assessed regularly and the progressive nature of retinal degenerations understood in the special education of deaf children. Deaf children need to develop their communication skills so that they will be able to function if they lose their vision in their forties or fifties. Their written language skills need to be so good that they can read Braille as the mode of communication when visual sign language is lost. Tactile sign language is too slow and there are too few people who master it.

A cochlear implant improves the auditory functions in Usher type I patients, but they still have dual sensory impairment.

The visual problems of hearing impaired children are the same as those of hearing children, but communication during testing is a special feature in assessing deaf children. Deaf children are amazing in their ability to understand poor sign language. They seem to find it amusing that a "grownup" doctor cannot express him/herself any better. Therefore, it is possible to have direct communication with a deaf child even with rudimentary capabilities in sign language. However, a person with good communication in sign language needs to be available, either an interpreter accustomed to ophthalmologic examinations or a teacher with similar good communication capability (if an interpreter is not available), to ensure that information is correctly understood by both parties.

Retinitis pigmentosa may be the only retinal disorder in both normally hearing and hearing impaired children. However, it is possible to have both retinitis pigmentosa and another retinal disorder. A child may have lost hearing and have retinopathy due to maternal rubella. Rubella retinopathy is a stable condition. However, if the child also has inherited retinitis pigmentosa, the development of visual field defects and night blindness may occur at an earlier age than usual. Thus, retinitis pigmentosa and sensory hearing loss occurring in a child may represent Usher syndrome or may be two separate conditions. Hearing impairment also can be caused by an infection or trauma. The appearance (phenotype) may be the same in all of these cases, but they have differences in terms of prognosis and genetic counseling. In a sporadic case of dual sensory impairment in a 10-year-old child with asymmetrical loss of visual field, the likely cause is recessive retinitis pigmentosa combined with an unrelated disorder or disease causing hearing loss and possibly some damage to the retina. In Usher syndrome the changes usually are symmetrical.

In hearing impaired children, retinitis pigmentosa should always be remembered when the diagnosis of severe hearing loss is made during the first year of life. It also should be kept in mind in an older child with a less severe hearing loss. Retinitis pigmentosa and related retinal disorders start to affect retinal functions during the first year of life, but functional changes usually are not detected before age 18 months. However, in families with an older child diagnosed with retinal degeneration, the parents may notice a decrease in the speed of dark adaptation during the first year of life.

Vision for communication of hearing impaired children needs to be assessed early, because visual communication is so important in the life of deaf infants and young children. Hiding Heidi low-contrast pictures can be used to measure the distances at which the infant responds to facial features at different contrast levels. In some countries, deaf children use either sign language or lip reading supported by finger spelling, or they use both techniques. There are still many places where deaf children are not allowed to use sign language and parents are not taught to sign, so little infants have to try to understand lip reading without hearing the words.

Communicative information is visual information in motion; therefore, it would be important to measure motion perception but presently there are only experimental tests. Retinitis pigmentosa may affect motion discrimination quite early, but rarely before school age. How much motion perception can change without affecting lip reading or finger spelling is not known. If a youngster complains that seeing finger spelling has become more difficult, changes in motion perception should be kept in mind and signing modified for optimal clarity. On the other hand, motion perception seems to be present in ring scotomas that do not respond to the brightest Goldmann stimuli.

Visual communication usually is undisturbed in most children with retinitis pigmentosa through primary or grade school. Problems occur in high school, college, or in young adulthood. Many people with Usher syndrome have a useful person-to-person communication field until their forties and sometimes to retirement age. Group communication may be disturbed already in the teenager with an advancing ring scotoma.

Contact with other children having similar or more severe problems helps the child to get a realistic picture of his or her situation and often gives the parents much needed emotional support. These contacts can be accomplished at weekend gatherings and during holiday camps. Young, well-adapted adults with Usher syndrome are important role models for children. Children with Usher syndrome and their classmates usually appreciate their visits to schools.

Everyone related to the care or teaching of children with vision impairment should be able to recognize certain typical behaviors caused by visual field changes or loss of dark adaptation. For example:

- If a child who previously has run up and down the stairs starts to look at his or her feet when going downstairs, sensitivity of the lower part of the visual field may have decreased and should be reassessed.

- If a child misunderstands spoken information in twilight or does not pay attention to signing in twilight, visual adaptation to low luminance levels may have become delayed or decreased. The child also may have started to avoid playing outside in the evening, which should not be interpreted as avoiding group activities.

- If a teenager walks backward when someone starts to sign to him or her, the likely explanation is a limited visual field rather than emotional problems.

When adaptation to lower luminance levels slows in a teenager, retinal changes also may cause photophobia. Photophobic children may need to avoid going outside on sunny days because it may take too long before they start seeing again in the classroom. At some schools, all children stay inside during the whole morning and during the afternoon, with a longer break for their lunch. Corridors should have sufficient illumination, and a child may need to have a torch or flashlight available when he or she is sent to get something from a poorly lit place. Both teachers and classmates should learn to live with the child with a limited visual field, clumsiness, and slow visual adaptation.

Rehabilitation often focuses only on the child. Yet people around the child also are in need of education and may require help to deal with their emotions and to make sensible decisions.

Hearing impaired children with retinitis pigmentosa have much in common with normally hearing children with diffuse retinal degenerations. Deaf children with retinitis pigmentosa are members of their deaf community, however. So we should learn about deaf culture in order to understand their communication and ways of thinking. Like any language, sign language opens a door to a different culture and teaches us an effective, logical way to express thoughts. Studies of sign language can be recommended to all teachers, therapists, and doctors as part of their training in communication.

When discussing the child's activities, we should remember the great variation in the progression of the visual loss in retinitis pigmentosa (see Chapter 10). There are people with retinitis pigmentosa who can play badminton in their thirties and other persons in the same family who have small tubular fields by age 20. Careful assessment of functional vision is essential if we want to give the child, the family, and the school correct information for planning the individual educational plan and the future.

The size of the visual field can be assessed starting in early infancy using Sheridan balls, but this test does not reveal changes related to retinitis pigmentosa. The early changes are in the "midperiphery" of the visual field. Small patches of diminished function are difficult to measure before the age of 4.5 to 5 years. If a child is given the opportunity to watch Goldmann perimetry of an older child, it is easier to teach him or her to keep looking at the fixation target straight ahead and to respond to peripheral stimuli.

Goldmann perimetry depicts the development of visual field changes fairly well. First there is a decrease in the size of the isopters I/4 and III/4, and there are small patches of decreased sensitivity. Later there is further loss of function in the midperiphery of the visual field, and the ring scotoma develops and becomes "absolute." An "absolute" scotoma is absolute only in Goldmann perimetry at low luminance levels. In daylight, there can be quite good function in the area of the ring scotoma. Loss of sensitivity in the midperiphery may cause problems in perception of motion, so ball games may become difficult in some but not all children with retinitis pigmentosa. In Finland, one of the best young goalkeepers in ice hockey has a good-sized ring scotoma in the lower visual field as measured with Goldmann perimetry, with only slightly decreased flicker sensitivity in the area of the scotoma. A relative ring scotoma may become absolute at low luminance levels, i.e., the visual field may shrink suddenly when the child enters a dark place.

When the ring scotoma becomes larger with time, there is only a "tubular" visual field in the middle and a small peripheral crescent of visual field remaining when measured with Goldmann perimetry. In actuality, the tubular field is not like a tube as often erroneously described but a cone that allows larger areas to be seen at longer distances. In daylight it can be several degrees larger than at the 10 cd/m^2 (candelas/meter^2) luminance in Goldmann perimetry.

Goldmann perimetry requires good cooperation of a hearing adult patient. It is a very demanding task to measure the visual fields of a 5- or 6-year-old deaf child. The instrument is first introduced on both sides, so the child can look through the peephole and see the eye of a parent. The child also can see how the tester moves the light. The parents can be tested briefly to demonstrate difficulties in responding correctly. After that, they appreciate the performance of their child much more and understand the test results better.

The interpreter for a deaf child in this test situation must be a person with experience in visual field testing and communication with young deaf children in general. If an interpreter is not available, sometimes the child's own teacher is the interpreter. In this case, it often is necessary to briefly measure the visual field of the teacher as an introduction, otherwise interpretation may not be exact. Parents should not function as interpreters during such a difficult test.

No visual communication is possible after the deaf child puts his or her chin on the headrest. Therefore, I usually tell the child that I will tap him or her on the knee in case fixation is not on the fixation target. This helps the child to hold fixation stable. The first examination is more like a training session than a test. During the second measurement, at least one visual field is measured reliably and during the third examination the other. There is a tendency for the largest isopters to move slightly outward between the ages of 5 and 9 years, after which they may remain stable for some years. This "improvement" does not mean real enlargement of the visual field but is a sign of improved cooperation.

The time available for Goldmann perimetry is limited. As soon as the child becomes bored, the thresholds start to vary. Therefore, it is wise to limit the test to the isopters IV/4 and I/4. If the distance between these two isopters is larger than normal, there is loss of function in the midperipheral field.

Presently, we do not use standardized techniques for measurement of the scotopic visual field except at a few university clinics, even though Goldmann perimeters have the ability to measure at lower luminance levels. If the child seems to have problems following instructions in dim light, confrontation fields can and should be measured at low mesopic luminance levels.

In assessment of visual fields and all other visual functions in children with rod-cone degenerations, we should consider the amount of light to which the child was exposed before the measurement. If the child comes for the examination on a sunny day, visual acuity and contrast sensitivity may be worse than on a cloudy day, and the difference may be even more marked in the visual fields.

Demonstration of ring scotoma by a youngster makes it easier to understand recordings of Goldmann visual fields. When the child shows where he sees his finger movements, e.g., they are visible at the level just in front of his ears, look different in the midperiphery, and are again better seen in the center of the visual field, we remember the structure of his visual field much better than we can remember laboratory results. It is advisable to ask each child to describe the visual fields as observation of finger movements at several different luminance levels to learn about the effect of changes in illumination. All clinical visual field tests, except finger perimetry, are performed at low luminance levels that overestimate visual field losses in most diffuse retinal degenerations.

The concept of communication field should be taught to deaf children in the early teenage years. Each deaf youngster should be able to tell the interpreter the distance at which the interpreter needs to stand and which size of signing field is comfortable at that distance. If adult persons, teachers, therapists, and parents remember to ask the child where they should stand when signing, the child becomes accustomed to expect proper signing during interpreting.

Children with Colobomas

Typical features of these children are microphthalmia, colobomas of the retina, iris, and/or the optic nerve, cataracts of different kinds, corneal cloudiness, and deviations in the structure of the entire anterior chamber of the eye. In order to understand these numerous deviations from normal development, parents and caretakers usually appreciate a short summary of the development of the eye.

Because malformations are an important cause of vision impairment, it is good to have a three-dimensional model of the eye and a description of the structural changes with a draft drawing depicting them. A drawing often makes it possible to understand the effect of the structural changes on the function of the eye. Equally important is to know if there is hypoplasia of the optic nerve.

Large refractive errors and the need for glasses are common in the group of children with colobomas. Microphthalmic children also may have high refractive errors.

Prematurely born children with colobomas may have retinopathy of prematurity and changes in the visual pathways due to periventricular leukomalacia. Because the motor pathways are located close to the ventricles, these children may have obvious motor problems, or their motor defects may be so mild that they remain undiagnosed until the assessment of the visual pathways leads to a more careful neurologic examination and minor disturbances in the motor functions are detected. For the planning of sports and other physical activities, it is good to learn about even minor motor problems.

Auditory impairment and disability and communication problems vary as much as vision impairment and disability vary. It is essential to become familiar with the child's communication techniques and level when planning the assessment of visual functioning. In the beginning of the assessment, the possibility of loss of the upper visual field in children with colobomas is investigated. Therefore, measurement of the extent of the visual field is one of the first tests. If the child is binocular and the field defects are not symmetrical, the functional visual field may be normal. The next test is to determine the sphere for visual communication by using the Hiding Heidi test. By testing first at the usual communication distance, it is possible to quickly measure the contrast at which the child can perceive the Heidi face at different contrast levels.

In visual communication with hearing impaired children with colobomas that cause visual field defects, the same rules apply as in communication with deaf children with retinitis pigmentosa, except that signs that appear high up in the visual field may need to be avoided or the child is guided by the signer's gaze to look up before the gesture is made. It also is important to use sign language at the level of the child's face.

Measurement of visual acuity, reading acuity, contrast sensitivity, and color vision for planning of the rehabilitation usually are easy once the communication is fluent. Problems of visual adaptation are rare but worth observation at both high and low luminance levels. If the colobomatous area is large, the white scleral surface may reflect light within the eye, and the child may use sunglasses. Measurement of the visual field is done with perimetry, campimetry, or a confrontation technique, depending on the communication level of the child. If the child has poor contrast sensitivity, facial expressions may appear so blurred that the structure and content of facial expressions are not well known by the child. The Heidi Expressions Game can be used to make the child aware of the structure

of different expressions. The use of the Heidi Expressions Cards can be combined with tactile exploring of facial expressions and drawing of the different expressions. When the expressions are learned at high contrast, then the low-contrast cards can be used to train the child to watch for low-contrast information. Magnifying mirrors are good tools for studying expressions.

If the child uses a hearing aid, we need to learn how well the child can handle it or whether it is turned off most of the time. During communication with a hearing impaired child, we must remember to pay attention to the microphone, the rhythm and speed of our speech, and the vocabulary at the same time as we take care of the quality of the visual information. Experimentation with one's voice and facial expressions is a part of visual assessment of these children. Difficulties in listening to voices vary, therefore pronunciation always means a lot, similarly the visibility of the lip movements. In the communication with these children there is no place for a hanging moustache or dazzling trinkets. The brown contrast pen to accentuate lips can be used by male doctors, teachers, and therapists to facilitate lip reading. If the child's limited visual sphere is demonstrated to the therapists and teachers by showing how far they can go until the child loses visual information conveyed by facial expressions, they will be motivated to get close enough and to use makeup or a contrast pen in order to give the child an opportunity to see their expressions.

The needs of children with dual sensory impairment are so individual that group communication often is time consuming and complicated. A child with dual sensory disability in a regular school class is a challenge. In all teaching, it is important to obtain feedback on what the children have heard and seen during the lessons and to carefully ascertain the content of information that the children have received. When both distance senses are impaired, the child may miss a key word and then misunderstand a sizable part of a lesson.

The many other disorders of these children should be taken into account during therapy and teaching. For example, the child may have problems in swallowing, gut function, and the heart. With so many deviations from the norm, it is important to find the strengths of the child to help him or her in developing a positive self-image.

Because of their multiple problems, children may make numerous visits to different clinics during preschool and school age. A child's teacher can be very helpful to the family if he or she insists that the child needs to participate in the educational activities as much as possible and, therefore, the visits at the different clinics need to be combined into as few visits as possible. This decreases the stress to the child and the parents who otherwise may spend long hours waiting for the examinations. Schools should send with the child their reports to the hospitals on observations and measurements of functional vision. When the child comes to the eye clinic, information about the use of vision at school and during hobbies and about worries and problems can be very helpful and makes the doctors think more about the function of the child than simply the disease of the right or the left eye.

Children with Motor Problems

Special problems of the child with difficulty moving are related to the increased need for the child to plan the routes for longer distances than a normally moving child with visual impairment needs to master. Wheelchair users especially need instructions in the use of telescopes and recognition of landmarks for their mobility. The use of telescopes may be problematic if the hands do not function normally. In this case, a small telescope fitted on the distance glasses may be a good solution.

Another problem that often must be solved is modification of a keyboard so that the child can see the keys without difficulty. Keys are easier to locate if the keyboard is divided into three or four areas with different background colors of the keys. Then the child does not need to see the letters and numbers clearly when he or she knows that a certain letter is the left, the middle, or the right one within a certain color area.

Ergonomic evaluation should cover the needs related to visual and motor impairment.

CEREBRAL VISUAL IMPAIRMENT (CVI)

Cerebral visual impairment has so many different combinations of the possible losses of individual cortical and subcortical functions that an overall description of early intervention and planning of special education is not possible. The low-vision team and the child's neurologist assess all functions and decide how each of them may be possible to train and which compensatory functions will be important to develop. After a child's anterior visual impairment has been assessed, cortical functions are evaluated by determining whether the child displays (i) increased crowding, (ii) contrast sensitivity problems, (iii) color vision defects, (iv) photophobia, (v) visual field loss, (vi) motion perception changes, (vii) oculomotor problems, (viii) deviation from normal in perception of length and orientation of lines, (ix) difficulties in recognition of facial features, (x) difficulties in recognition of facial expressions, (xi) problems in perception of depth, (xii) problems in form perception, (xiii) problems in perception of surface qualities, (xiv) problems in picture perception and comprehension/understanding, (xv) difficulties in composing a whole picture of its parts, (xvi) problems in spatial awareness and orientation in space, (xvii) problems in eye–hand coordination (vision–hand coordination), and (xviii) simultan agnosia.

The effect of posture on the use of vision is assessed in all children with motor problems. For the planning of early in-

tervention and special education, it is not sufficient to tell that a child has "cerebral visual impairment" or "cortical visual impairment" but to carefully describe which cortical and subcortical functions are affected and to what degree.

In planning training and special education, neuropsychological testing is important in each case of CVI, although the functions also are observed and described during therapies, at school, and at home. A vision teacher can help by writing a résumé of the student's visual functions to help the neuropsychologist in the choice of tests and in the evaluation of test results.

In the care of children with CVI, it is essential to accept that we cannot see the world from the same perspective as the child does. Therefore, it is wise to ask the child's opinion on every aspect of schooling, devices, and therapies. Children are honest and very good observers. However, they are loyal and seldom criticize any of the adults around them even if there was good reason to do so.

The number of children with CVI is increasing in all western countries because the small premature infants and the older children with brain trauma or infections survive. Therefore, it is important that ophthalmologists, pediatricians, therapists, and teachers be aware of the need to observe the behaviors of children and that every visual cognitive function may be lost without changes in other visual functions. Whenever the profile of visual functions is uneven, all cognitive visual functions should be thoroughly investigated so that correct information is given to schools and therapists. A child may need special education as a blind student in only one limited area such as geometry, where orientation of lines cannot be visually perceived. Children who simultaneously use techniques of sighted and techniques of blind are difficult to understand, so the reports should describe each child's functions in detail. Solutions that work for one child should be made known to therapists and teachers. For example, if a child does not recognize faces, he or she can be taught to nicely say to a person whom he or she does not recognize: "My name is . . ., what is your name?" A child with poor spatial orientation may benefit from video recordings of the routes to be learned outside the time spent during training sessions. If the child has difficulties in remembering the landmarks of a route, it may help to write a song of the landmarks with a well-known melody. We need to use common sense and our basic knowledge on the functions of the brain in training children with CVI and other forms of vision loss.

One's ability to reach for the unconventional and to "think out of the box" is the only limiting factor in finding solutions in everyday tasks and activities of visually impaired children.

REFERENCES

1. Rosenberg T, Flage T, Hansen E, et al. Incidence of registered visual impairment in the Nordic child population. *Br J Ophthalmol* 1996;80:49–53.

2. Stern GK, Hyvärinen L. Addressing pediatric issues. In: Fletcher D, ed. *Low vision rehabilitation, caring for the whole person.* Hong Kong: American Academy of Ophthalmology 1999:107–120.

3. *Management of low vision in children. Report of a WHO Consultation, Bangkok, July 23–24, 1992.* WHO PBL 93.27.

4. *International classification of functioning, disabilities and health.* Geneva: World Health Organization, 2002.

5. Hyvärinen L. Assessment of visually impaired infants. In: Colenbrander A, Fletcher DC, eds. *Low vision and vision rehabilitation. Ophthalmol Clin North Am* 1994;219–226.

6. Sonksen PM, Stiff B. *Show me what my friends can see. A developmental guide for parents of babies with severely impaired sight and their professional advisors.* London: Institute of Child Health, 1991.

7. Hyvärinen J, Hyvärinen L. Blindness and modification of association cortex by early binocular deprivation in monkeys. *Child Care Health Dev* 1979;5:385–387.

8. Lagerheim, B. "Why me?"—a depressive crisis at the age of nine in handicapped children. In: Gyllensvärd Å, Laurén K, eds. *Psychosomatic diseases in childhood.* Stockholm: Sven Jerring Foundation, 1983.

SUGGESTED READINGS

1. Adelson E, Fraiberg S. Gross motor development in infants blind from birth. *Child Development* 1974;45:114–126.

2. Aitken S, Bower TG. Developmental aspects of sensory substitution. *Int J Neurosci* 1983;19:13–19.

3. Andersen ES, Dunlea A, Kekelis LS. Blind children's language: resolving some differences. *J Child Lang* 1984;11:645–664.

4. Ashmead DH, Hill EW, Talor CR. Obstacle perception by congenitally blind children. *Percept Psychophys* 1989;46:425–433.

5. Baird SM, Mayfield P, Baker P. Mothers' interpretations of the behavior of their infants with visual and other impairments during interactions. *J Vis Impair Blind* 1997;91:467–483.

6. Barraga NC, Collins ME. Development of efficiency in visual functioning: rationale for a comprehensive program. *J Vis Impair Blind* 1979;73:121–126.

7. Chapman EK, Tobin NJ, Tooze FHG, et al. *"Look and think". A handbook for teachers. The Schools Council Visual Perception Training Project of Blind and Partially Sighted 5–11 Years Old.* London: University of Birmingham Schools Council Publications, 1979.

8. Fielder AR, Best AB, Bax MCO. *The management of visual impairment in childhood.* Mac Keith Press, 1993.

9. Hill EW, Dodson-Burk B, Smith BA. Orientation and mobility for infants who are visually impaired. *Re:View* 1989;21:47–60.

10. Hof-van-Duin J, Heersema DJ, Groenendaal F, et al. Visual field and grating acuity development in low-risk preterm infants during the first 2,5 years after term. *Behav Brain Res* 1992;49:115–122.

11. McConachie HR, Moore V. Early expressive language of severely visually impaired children. *Dev Med Child Neurol* 1994;36:230–240.

12. Porro GL. *Vision and visual behaviour in responsive and unresponsive neurologically impaired children.* Utrecht: Brouwer Uithof, 1998.

APPENDIX A

LOCALIZED AND IDENTIFIED GENES ASSOCIATED WITH RETINAL DISORDERS AS CATEGORIZED TO INHERITANCE PATTERN

BRONYA J.B. KEATS
DEBORAH COSTAKOS
J. BRONWYN BATEMAN

Genes that are associated with retinal disorders are categorized according to inheritance pattern in Tables A-1, A-2, and A-3. Table A-4 lists disorders in which nonretinal ocular anomalies are found. Cross-referencing to chapters is given where applicable.

Retinal disorders that are tabulated in chapters are not duplicated here. They are retinitis pigmentosa (Tables 7-1, 10-1), cone rod dystrophies (Table 7-3), congenital stationary night blindness and achromatopsia (Table 7-4), Usher syndrome(Table 11-2), albinism (Table 6-1), lysosomal storage disorders (Tables 6-2, 6-3, Appendix A, Table A-4, mitochondrial disorders (Chapter 9), peroxisomal biogenesis disorders (Chapter 9), retinoblastoma (Chapter 14), and phakomatoses (Chapter 15, Appendix A, Table A-4).

TABLE A-1. AUTOSOMAL DOMINANT

Disease	Location	Gene	Protein
Alagille syndrome	20p12	JAG1	Ligand for Notch1
Best disease (juvenile-onset vitelliform macular dystrophy) (Chapter 7)	11q13	VMD2	Bestrophin
Cerebral cavernous malformation	7q21–q22	CCM1	Novel
Doyne honeycomb retinal dystrophy	2p16	EFEMP1	EGF-containing fibulin-like extracellular matrix protein-1
Familial adenomatous polyposis (congenital hypertrophy of RPE)	5q21–q22	APC	Novel
Familial exudative vitreoretinopathy 1 (Chapter 28)	11q14–q21	FZD4	Frizzled 4
Familial exudative vitreoretinopathy 3 (Chapter 28)	11p13–p12	EVR3	Novel
Fundus Albipunctatus	6p21.1-cen	RDS	Peripherin
Fundus Dystrophy (Sorsby macular degeneration)	22q12.1–q13.2	TIMP3	Tissue inhibitor of Metalloproteinase-3
Marfan syndrome (Chapter 24)	15q21.1	FBN1	Fibrillin-1
Neurofibromatosis 1 (Chapter 15)	17q11.2	NF1	Neurofibromin
Neurofibromatosis 2 (Chapter 15)	22q12.2	NF2	Merlin (tumor suppressor)
Ocular coloboma	7q36	SHH	Sonic hedgehog transcriptional regulator
	11p13	PAX6	
Open angle glaucoma	1q24.3–q25.2	MYOC	Trabecular meshwork-induced glucocorticoid response protein
Papillorenal syndrome (Chapter 1)	10q24.3-q25.1	PAX2	Transcriptional regulator
Patterned dystrophy of the RPE	6p21.1-cen	RDS	Peripherin
Pseudoxanthoma elasticum (PXE)	16p13.1	ABCC6	ATP-binding cassette (ABC), subfamily C, member 6
Spinocerebellar ataxia 7	3p21.1-p12	SCA7	Ataxin-7
Spondyloepiphyseal Dysplasia congenita	12q13.11–q13.2	COL2A1	Type II collagen, α1 chain
Stargardt-like macular dystrophy	6q14	ELOVL4	Novel

(continues)

TABLE A-1. *(continued)*

Disease	Location	Gene	Protein
Stickler syndrome (Chapters 1, 24)			
Type 1	12q13.11–q13.2	*COL2A1*	Type II collagen, α1 chain
Type 2	1p21	*COL11A1*	Type XI collagen, α1 chain
Tuberous sclerosis (Chapter 15)	9q34	*TSC1*	Hamartin
	16p13.3	*TSC2*	Tuberin
von Hippel-Lindau syndrome (Chapter 15)	3p25	*VHL*	Novel (tumor suppressor)

ATP, adenosine triphosphate; EGF, epidermal growth factor, RPE, retinal pigment epithelium.

TABLE A-2. AUTOSOMAL RECESSIVE

Disease	Location	Gene	Protein
Abetalipoproteinemia (Chapter 10)	4q22–q24	*MTP*	Microsomal triglyceride transfer protein
Alstrom syndrome	2p13	*ALMS1*	Novel
Bardet Biedl (Chapter 10)	11q13	*BBS1*	Novel
	16q21	*BBS2*	Novel
	15q22.3–q23	*BBS4*	Novel
	20p12	*BBS6 (MKKS)*	Chaperonin family
	4q27	*BBS7*	Novel
	14q32.1	*BBS8*	Tetratricopeptide repeat protein
Bothnia dystrophy (Chapter 7)	15q26	*RLBP1*	Retinaldehyde-binding protein-1
Cohen syndrome	8q22–q23	*COH1*	Novel
Congenital disorder of glycosylation type Ia (CDG Ia)	16p13.3–p13.2	*PMM2*	Phosphomannomutase-2
Enhanced S-cone (Goldmann-Favre) syndrome (Chapter 7)	15q23	*NR2E3*	Retinal nuclear receptor
Fundus albipunctatus	12q13–q14	*RDH5*	11-*cis* retinol dehydrogenase
HARP syndrome	20p13–p12.3	*PANK2*	Pantothenate kinase-2
Hyperoxaluria type 1 (Chapter 9)	2q36–q37	*AGXT*	Alanine: glyoxylate aminotransferase
Knobloch syndrome (Chapter 1)	21q22.3	*COL18A1*	Type XVIII collagen, α1 chain
Leber congenital amaurosis (Chapters 7 and 13)	1q31–q32.1	*CRB1*	Novel
	1p31	*RPE65*	RPE-specific 65-kDa protein
	6p21.3	*TULP1*	Tubby-like
	17p13.1	*GUCY2D*	Photoreceptor guanylate cyclase
	19q13.3	*CRX*	Photoreceptor-specific homeobox
	17p13.1	*AIPL1*	Arylhydrocarbon receptor interacting protein-like 1
	14q11	*RPGRIP1*	Novel
Neuronal ceroid lipofuscinosis (Batten) (Chapter 10)			
Infantile	1p32	*CLN1*	Palmitoyl-protein thioesterase
Late infantile	11p15.5	*CLN2*	Lysosomal peptidase
Juvenile	16p12.1	*CLN3*	Novel
Variant late infantile	13q21.1–q32	*CLN5*	Novel
Variant late infantile	15q21–q23	*CNL6*	Novel
Newfoundland rod-cone dystrophy (Chapter 7)	15q26	*RLBP1*	Retinaldehyde-binding protein-1
Oguchi (Chapter 7)	2q37.1	*SAG*	Arrestin
	13q34	*RHOK*	Rhodopsin kinase
Pseudoxanthoma elasticum (PXE)	16p13.1	*ABCC6*	ATP-binding cassette (ABC), subfamily C, member 6
Refsum disease (Chapter 9)	10pter–p11.2	*PAHX*	Phytanoyl-CoA hydroxylase
	6q22–q24	*PEX7*	PTS2 receptor
Senior-Loken syndrome	2q13	*NPHP1*	Novel
	3q22	*NPHP3*	Novel
	1p36	*NPHP4*	Novel
Stargardt disease/fundus flavimaculatus (Chapter 8)	1p21-p13	*ABCA4*	ATP-binding cassette (ABC) transporter
Walker-Warburg syndrome	9q34.1	*POMT1*	O-mannosyltransferase

RPE, retinal pigment epithelium.

TABLE A-3. X-LINKED

Disease	Location	Gene	Protein
Adrenoleukodystrophy (Chapter 9)	Xq28	*ABCD1*	ATPase-binding cassette protein
Alport syndrome	Xq22.3	*COL4A5*	Type 4 Collagen, α5 chain
Choroideremia (Chapter 7)	Xq21.2	*CHM*	Rab escort protein (REP-1)
Coats disease (Chapter 29)	Xp11.4	*NDP*	Norrin
Familial exudative vitreoretinopathy 2 (Chapter 28)	Xp11.4	*NDP*	Norrin
Incontinentia pigmenti	Xq28	*NEMO*	I-kappa-B kinase component
Menkes	Xq12-q13	*ATP7A*	Copper transporting ATPase
Norrie disease	Xp11.4	*NDP*	norrin
Retinoschisis (congenital) (Chapter 25)	Xp22.2-p22.1	*RS1*	retinoschisin

TABLE A-4. OCULAR FINDINGS IN MULTISYSTEM DISORDERS

Disease	Cornea	Lens	Retina	Optic Nerve	Inheritance	Gene	Protein	Location
Sphingolipid storage								
Niemann-Pick A	+	+	CRS	+	AR	*SMPD1, NPD*	Sphingomyelin phosphodiesterase-1	11p15.4-p15.1
Fabry	+	+	V	−	XR	*GLA*	Galactosidase	Xq22
GM$_1$-I gangliosidosis	+	−	CRS	−	AR	*GLB1*	Beta galactosidase	3p21.33
Tay-Sachs (GM$_2$-I)	−	−	CRS	+	AR	*HEXA*	Hexosaminidase A	15q23–q24
Sandhoff (GM$_2$-II)	−	−	CRS	+	AR	*HEXB*	Hexosaminidase B	5q13
Krabbe	−	−	−	+	AR	*GALC*	Galactosyl-ceraminidase	14q31
Metachromatic leukodystrophy	−	−	−	+	AR	*ARSA*	Arylsulfatase A	22q13.31-qter
Multiple sulfatase deficiency	−	−	D, CRS	+	AR	*SUMF*	Sulfatase modifying factor	3p26
Oligosaccharide storage								
Sialidosis (Mucolipidosis I)	+	+	V	−	AR	*NEUI, NEU, SIAL1*	Neuroaminidase, sialidase	6p21.3
Mannosidase A	+	+	−	−	AR	*MANBA*	Mannosidase beta A	4q22–q25
Mannosidase b	+	+	−	−	AR	*MAN2B1*	Mannosidase B	19cen–q12
Mucopolysaccharide storage ridoses								
Hurler (I-H)	+	−	D	+	AR	*IDA, IDUA*	Iduronidase-alpha	4p16.3
Scheie (I-S)	+	−	D	+	AR	*IDA, IDUA*	Iduronidase-alpha	4p16.3
Hunter (II)	−(?)	−	D	+	XR	*IDS*	Iduronidase 2-sulfatase	Xq28
Sanfilippo (III)	−	−	D	+	AR	*NAGLU*	N-acetylglu-cosaminidase	17q21
Morquio A (IV)	+	−	−	+	AR	*GLNS, MPS4A*	Galactosamine (N-acetyl)-6-sulfate sulfatase	16q24.3
Maroteaux–Lamy (VI)	+	−	−	+	AR	*ARSB*	Arylsulfatase B	5q11–q13
Wolman	−	−	+	+	AR	*LAL*	Lysosomal acid lipase	10q24–q25

(continues)

TABLE A-4 *(Continued)*

Disease	Cornea	Lens	Retina	Optic Nerve	Inheritance	Gene	Protein	Location
Amino Acid Metabolism								
Cystinosis	+	−	D	−	AR	CTNS	Cystinosin	17p13
Homocystinuria	−	+	−	−	AR	CBS	Cystathionine beta synthase	21q22.3
Gyrate atrophy	−	−	D	+	XR	OAT	Ornithine aminotransferase deficiency	10q26
Tyrosinemia	+	−	−	−	AR	FAH	Fumarylacetoacetase	15q23–q25
Hyperlysinemia	−	+	−	−	AR	AASS	Alpha-aminoadipic semialdehyde synthase	7q31.3
Methylmalonic aciduria	+	−	−	−	AR	MCM	Methylmalonyl-CoA mutase	6p21
Carbohydrate Metabolism								
Galactosemia I	−	+	−	−	AR	GALT	Galactose-1-phosphate uridyl transferase deficiency	9p13
Galactosemia II	−	+	−	−	AR	GALK1	Galactokinase	17q24
Metal Metabolism								
Wilson disease	+	+	−	−	AR	AT7B	ATPase	13q14.3–q21.1
Central Nervous System								
Optic atrophy with deafness-dystonia syndrome	−	−	−	+	XR	TIMM8A	Inner mitochondrial membrane translocase 8 homolog A	Xq22
Phakomatoses								
Neurofibromatosis	−	+	+	+	AD	NF1	Neurofibromin	17q11.2
von Hippel-Lindau	−	−	V	+	AD	VHL	von Hippel Lindau	3p25
Other								
Wolfram syndrome	−	−	−	+	AR	WFS1	wolframin	4p16.1

Source: www.sph.uth.tmc.edu/Retnet/disease.htm and www.ncbi.nlm.nih.gov/omim/)
CRS, 'cherry-red' spot; V, vascular abnormality; D, retinal degeneration; AR, autosomal recessive; XR, X-linked recessive; AD, autosomal dominant.

APPENDIX B

HEMORRHAGES

MICHAEL T. TRESE
ANTONIO CAPONE, JR.
MARY ELIZABETH HARTNETT

Hemorrhages within the posterior segment of the eye can involve the vitreous, subhyaloid space, inner retina, subretinal space, and choroid. Unlike the case in adults, the determination in children is not always easy or as helpful. History and specific patterns of hemorrhage become essential in determining the diagnosis. Long-standing hemorrhage can become khaki-colored as hemoglobin is lost.

The following are examples of conditions with various hemorrhages in infants and children. The reader is referred to specific chapters for greater detail.

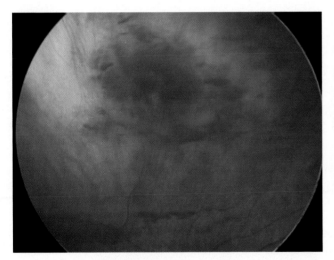
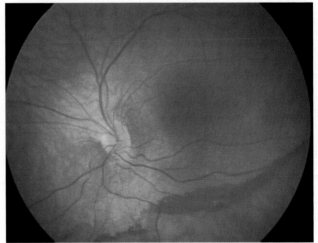

FIGURE B-1. A: Preretinal hemorrhage in a 2-year-old boy with congenital retinoschisis. **B:** Same eye as shown in **A.** Hemorrhage has tracked through an inner retinal break. The intraschisis blood indicates the posterior extend of the schisis cavity (see also Chapter 25).

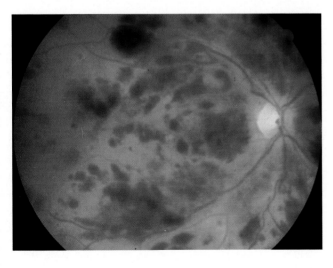

FIGURE B-2. Leukemic retinopathy with numerous blot hemorrhages in a child with thrombocytopenia.

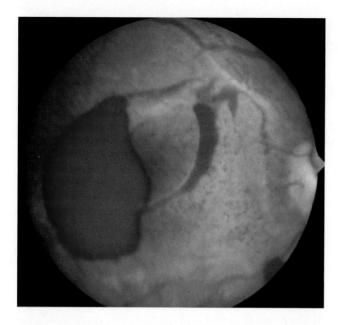

FIGURE B-3. Nonamblyogenic sublaminar hemorrhage due to nonaccidental trauma (shaken baby syndrome) in a 3-month-old infant (see also Chapter 32).

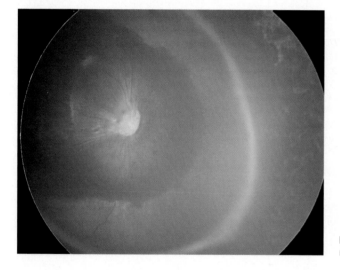

FIGURE B-4. Subretinal blood in a stage 4 retinopathy of prematurity–related retinal detachment (see also Chapter 27).

APPENDIX C

MACULAR ABNORMALITIES

MICHAEL T. TRESE
ANTONIO CAPONE, JR.
MARY ELIZABETH HARTNETT

Macular disease in children can be difficult to discern at a glance. In early disease, a reduced foveal reflex may be all that is noted. It is helpful to look at the periphery to determine if, for example, cystoid foveal change is associated with peripheral retinoschisis (suggesting congenital retinoschisis) or if exudates are associated with telangiectasia in the far periphery (suggesting Coats' disease).

The following are examples of conditions affecting the macula in infants and children. The chapters in which information regarding the disease can be found follow in parentheses.

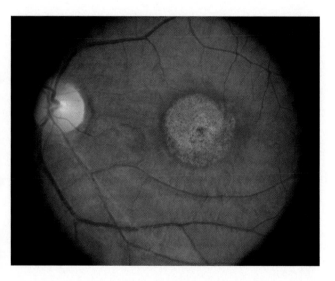

FIGURE C-1. Cone-rod dystrophy from a member of a family with autosomal dominant inheritance pattern (see also Chapter 7).

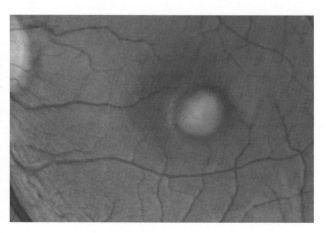

FIGURE C-2. Best disease. The left macula of a 19-year-old man with Best disease. Note the vitelliform lesion in the macula. The other eye demonstrates a smaller vitelliform lesion than the left eye. Visual acuity is 20/30 OD and 20/40 OS (see also Chapter 7).

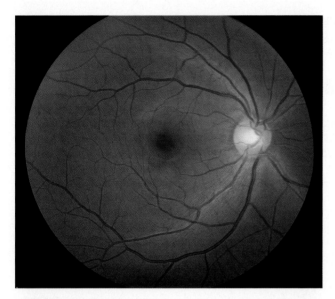

FIGURE C-3. Solar retinopathy with characteristic small round foveolar reddish-brown lesion. Right macula of young man who gazed at the sun when he was under the influence of cocaine. Color image appears to be a macular hole, but optical coherence tomography showed good foveal contour with greater reflectance in the fovea at the level of the retinal pigment epithelium. (Color images performed by Kelly Shields, B.S., C.R.A.)

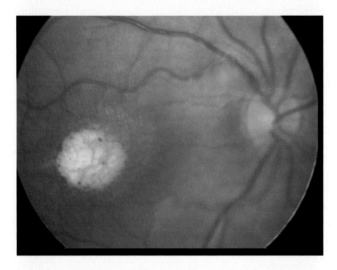

FIGURE C-4. Punched-out lesion showing chorioretinal atrophy in congenital toxoplasmosis (see also Chapter 16).

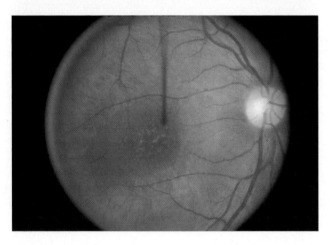

FIGURE C-5. Macular cysts in a child with congenital retinoschisis (see also Chapter 25).

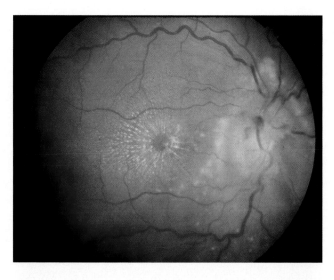

FIGURE C-6. Leber neuroretinitis with disc edema and macular star (see also Chapter 16).

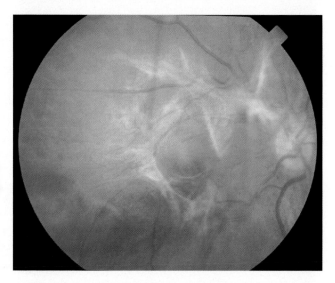

FIGURE C-7. Combined hamartoma of the vitreous, retina, and retinal pigment epithelium.

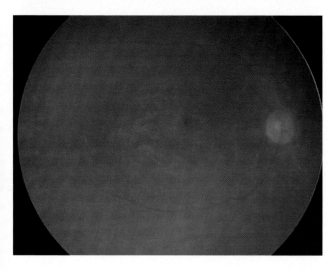

FIGURE C-8. Neuronal ceroid lipofuscinosis in a 3-year-old boy with poor motor and speech development and a recent history of seizures. Note disc pallor and retinal arterial attenuation. Periphery is remarkable for subtle diffuse pigmentary attenuation (see also Chapter 10).

APPENDIX D

PIGMENTARY ABNORMALITIES

MICHAEL T. TRESE
ANTONIO CAPONE, JR.
MARY ELIZABETH HARTNETT

The following are examples of abnormalities of pigmentation in infants and children. The reader is referred to specific chapters for greater detail.

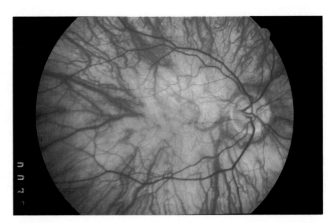

FIGURE D-1. Albinotic fundus in an African-American adolescent (see also Chapter 6).

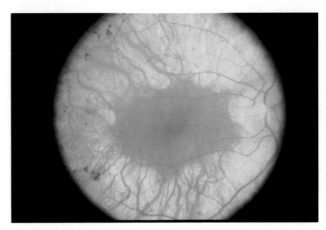

FIGURE D-3. Choroideremia. Note sparing of the macula (see also Chapter 7).

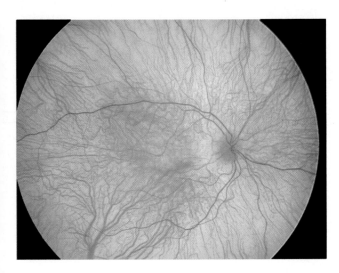

FIGURE D-2. Albinotic fundus in a Caucasian infant (see also Chapter 6).

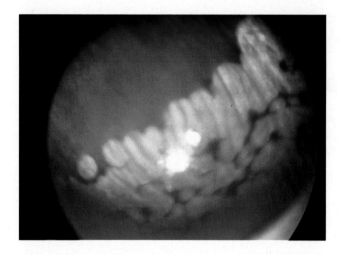

FIGURE D-4. Peripheral lacunar retinal pigment epithelium defect in gyrate atrophy (see also Chapter 6).

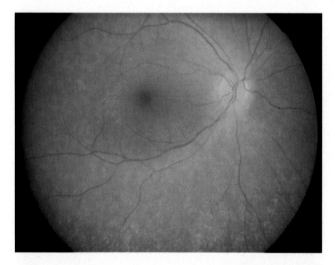

FIGURE D-5. Retinitis pigmentosa in a young adult. Note narrowed arterioles and pigmentary changes beyond arcades (see also Chapter 7 and 10).

APPENDIX E

POSTERIOR SEGMENT MASSES

MICHAEL T. TRESE
ANTONIO CAPONE, JR.
MARY ELIZABETH HARTNETT

The following are examples of posterior segment masses. The reader is referred to specific chapters for greater detail.

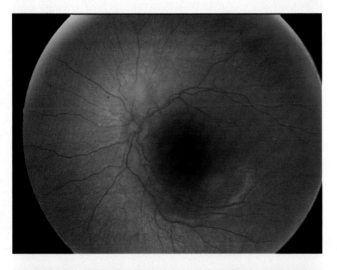

FIGURE E-1. Two retinal astrocytic hamartomas in a child with tuberous sclerosis (see also Chapter 15).

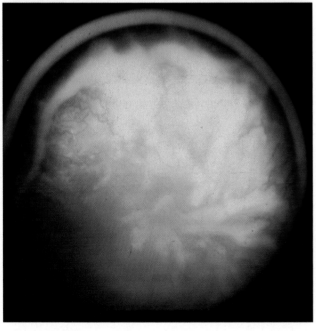

FIGURE E-2. Familial exudative vitreoretinopathy with extensive subretinal lipid (see also Chapter 28).

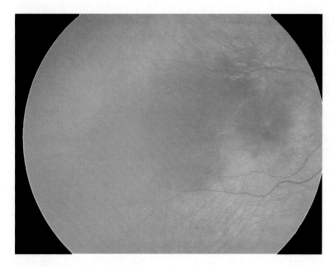

FIGURE E-3. Large flat posterior pole nevus.

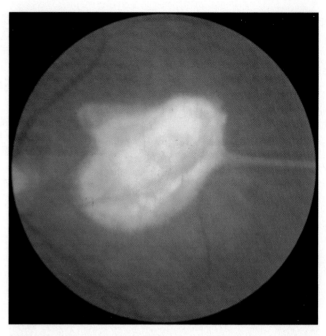

FIGURE E-4. Submacular toxocara canis granuloma (see also Chapter 16).

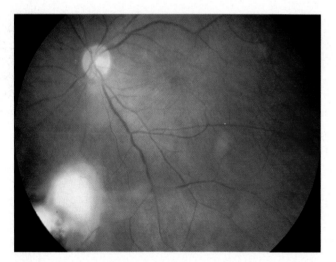

FIGURE E-5. Retinochoroiditis from toxoplasmosis (see also Chapter 16).

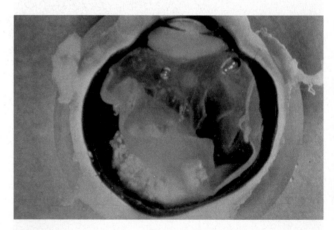

FIGURE E-6. Pathology showing retinoblastoma (see also Chapter 14).

APPENDIX F

FUNDUS FLECKS AND WHITE SPOT SYNDROMES

MICHAEL T. TRESE
ANTONIO CAPONE, JR.
MARY ELIZABETH HARTNETT

The following are examples of flecks or multiple white spots. The reader is referred to specific chapters for greater detail.

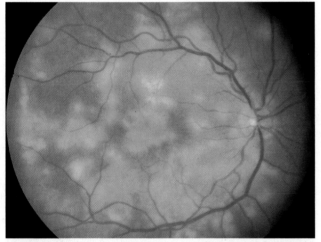

FIGURE F-1. Acute posterior multifocal placoid pigment epitheliopathy (AMPPE) in a 17-year-old boy with antecedent viral upper respiratory infection.

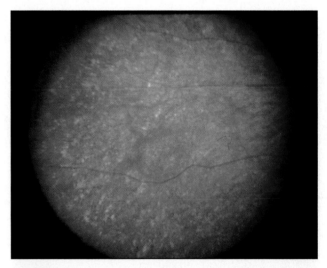

FIGURE F-2. Retinitis punctata albescens (see also Chapter 7).

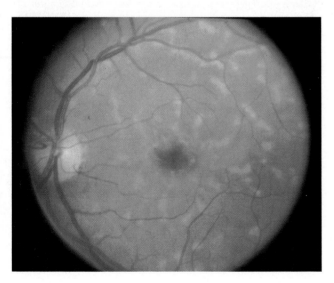

FIGURE F-3. Pisciform flecks in Stargardt flavimaculatus (see also Chapter 8).

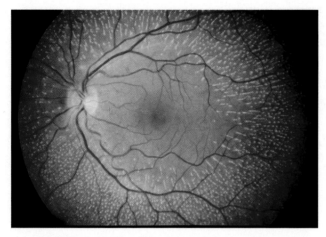

FIGURE F-4. Fundus albipunctatus (see also Chapter 7).

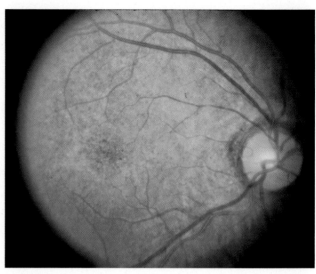

FIGURE F-5. Congenital rubella retinopathy (see also Chapters 16 and 18).

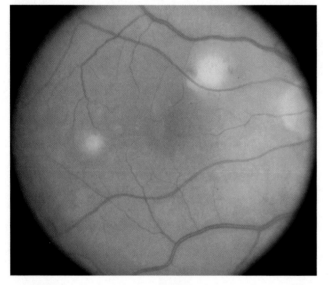

FIGURE F-6. Candida chorioretinitis (see also Chapter 16).

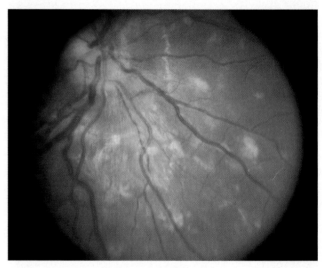

FIGURE F-7. Example of sarcoid choroiditis (see also Chapter 17).

APPENDIX G

ABNORMAL VASCULAR PATTERNS

MICHAEL T. TRESE
ANTONIO CAPONE, JR.
MARY ELIZABETH HARTNETT

The following are examples of abnormalities in vascular patterns. The reader is referred to specific chapters for greater detail.

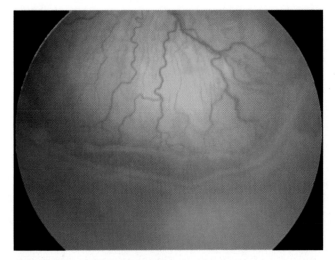

FIGURE G-1. Double demarcation line in retinopathy of prematurity (see also Chapters 26 and 27).

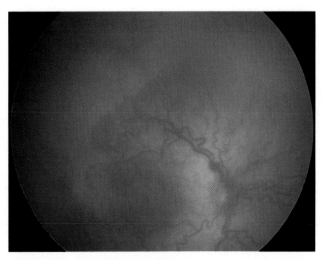

FIGURE G-2. Flat velvety stage 3 retinopathy of prematurity in zone 1 (see also Chapters 26 and 27).

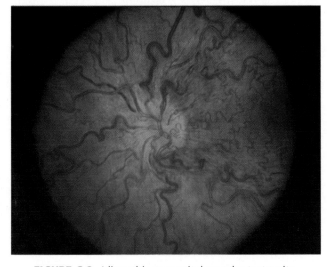

FIGURE G-3. Idiopathic congenital vascular tortuosity.

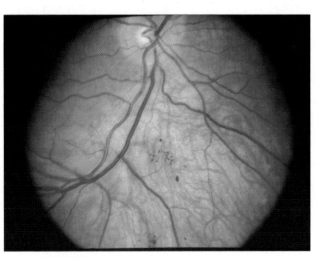

FIGURE G-4. Retinal cavernous hemangioma.

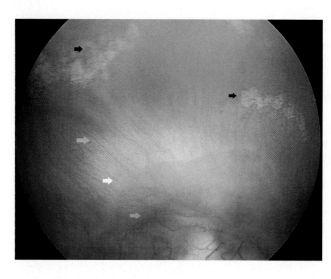

FIGURE G-5. Stage 3 zone 1 retinopathy of prematurity following incomplete laser. Wide-angle fundus image demonstrating the anterior edge of flat stage 3 retinopathy of prematurity *(white arrow)*, bordered posteriorly by evolving shunt vessels *(green arrow)*. Prominent choroidal vessels are visible through pale premature retinal pigment epithelium *(blue arrow)*. Anterior placement of laser scars results in broad "skip area" of untreated avascular retina extending back to shunt vessels *(black arrows)* (see also Chapters 26 and 27).

Incontinentia pigmenti is reported to occur in 1 in 40,000 persons worldwide. It is X linked and autosomal dominant. It usually occurs in females and is lethal in males (see Appendix A). There can be variable expressivity of defects involving several systems: skin, eye, teeth, and central nervous system. Four stages that affect the skin of the torso at different ages of the patient are described. When cutaneous findings are noted, a funduscopic examination should be performed to detect possible peripheral retinal nonperfusion and intravitreous neovascularization. Prompt laser treatment of the nonperfused retina, similar to that performed for severe retinopathy of prematurity (see Chapter 22), can prevent retinal detachment and reduce blindness (Table G-1).

TABLE G-1. FINDINGS IN INCONTINENTIA PIGMENTI TYPE 2 (BLOCH-SULZBERGER SYNDROME)

System	Reported Incidence	Defects
Cutaneous	Up to 100%; carriers may only have hypopigmented lesions (stage 4); nail dysplasia reported in 40%–60%; thin sparse hair, alopecia, wooly nevus	Stage 1: Vesicular stage beginning at birth and sometimes recurring in childhood with fever Stage 2: Verrucous stage with papules and plaques occurring between 2 and 8 weeks of age Stage 3: Hyperpigmentation occurring between 12 and 40 weeks of age Stage 4: Hypopigmentation from infancy through adulthood
Ocular	33%	Retinal hypopigmentation, peripheral nonperfusion with intravitreous neovascularization (both considered nearly pathognomonic), retinal detachment, microphthalmia, leukocoria, cataracts, and strabismus
Dental	65%–90%	Delayed eruption of teeth, abnormally shaped or sized teeth and/or jaw
Central nervous system	10%–40%	Mental retardation, seizures, strokes, microcephaly
Structural	14%, usually associated with severe neurologic disorders	Asymmetry, scoliosis, spina bifida

From Chang C. Incontinentia pigmenti. In eMedicine.com [online] 2002. Cited March 16, 2004. Available from: *http://www.emedicine.com/neuro/topic169.htm*

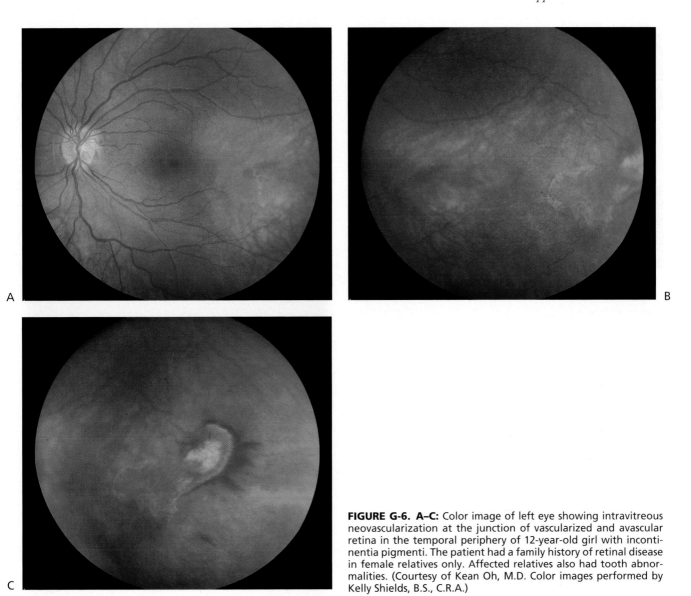

A

B

C

FIGURE G-6. A–C: Color image of left eye showing intravitreous neovascularization at the junction of vascularized and avascular retina in the temporal periphery of 12-year-old girl with incontinentia pigmenti. The patient had a family history of retinal disease in female relatives only. Affected relatives also had tooth abnormalities. (Courtesy of Kean Oh, M.D. Color images performed by Kelly Shields, B.S., C.R.A.)

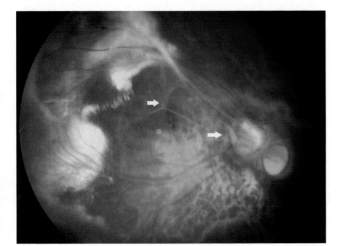

FIGURE G-7. Subretinal lipid accumulation and transvitreous traction evidenced by transvitreous strands *(left arrow)* and traction on epipapillary ring of condensed vitreous *(right arrow)* in the left eye of a 13-year-old adolescent with familial exudative vitreoretinopathy (see also Chapter 28).

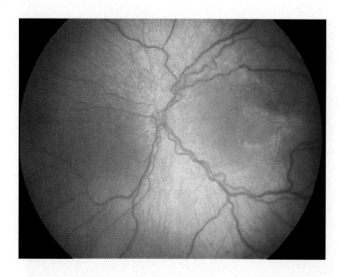

FIGURE G-8. Temporal Plus disease and nasal pre-Plus disease in an infant with retinopathy of prematurity (see also Chapters 26 and 27).

APPENDIX H

RETINAL DETACHMENT AND RETINOSCHISIS

MICHAEL T. TRESE
ANTONIO CAPONE, JR.
MARY ELIZABETH HARTNETT

The following are examples of retinal detachment and retinoschisis. The reader is referred to specific chapters for greater detail. Wide-angle images are taken with the Retcam wide-angle, contact fundus camera (for greater details on imaging, see Chapter 5).

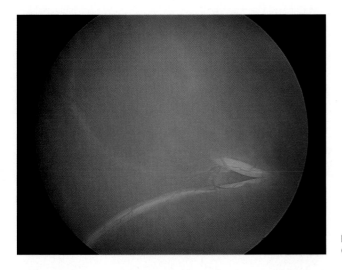

FIGURE H-1. Exudative retinal detachment in Coats disease (see also Chapter 29).

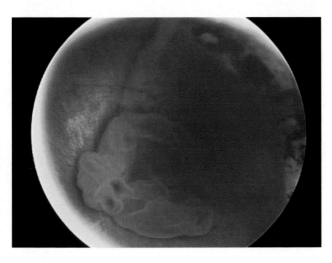

FIGURE H-2. A 360-degree giant retinal tear (see also Chapter 24).

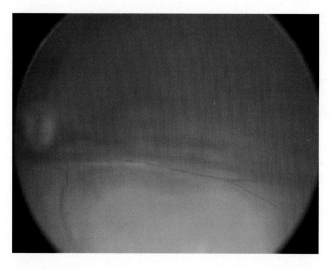

FIGURE H-3. Inferior bullous congenital retinoschisis in a 2-year-old boy (see also Chapter 25).

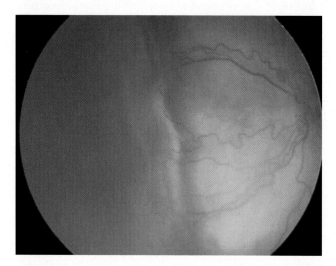

FIGURE H-4. Stage 4A exudative retinopathy of prematurity-related retinal detachment with extensive Plus disease (see also Chapters 26 and 27).

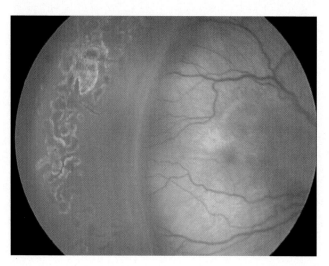

FIGURE H-5. Stage 4A retinopathy of prematurity developed posterior to a laser skip-area. The retina posterior to the ridge is shallowly detached, even though the macula appears attached clinically in this image.

OPTIC NERVE ABNORMALITIES

MICHAEL T. TRESE
ANTONIO CAPONE, JR.
MARY ELIZABETH HARTNETT

The following are examples of optic nerve conditions or abnormalities. The reader is referred to specific chapters for greater detail.

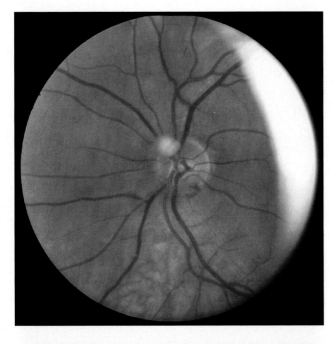

FIGURE I-1. Bergmeister papilla (see also Chapter 1).

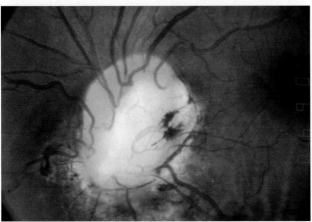

FIGURE I-2. Coloboma of the optic nerve (see also Chapter 1).

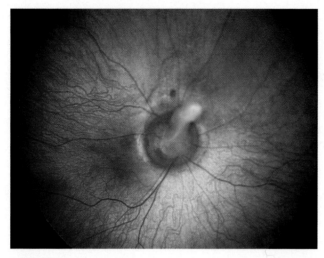

FIGURE I-3. Morning glory disc with central fibrotic stalk (see also Chapter 1).

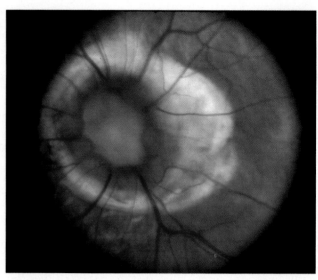

FIGURE I-4. Morning glory disc without a central fibrotic stalk (see also Chapter 1).

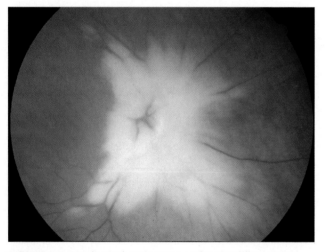

FIGURE I-5. Myelinated optic nerve and peripapillary retina.

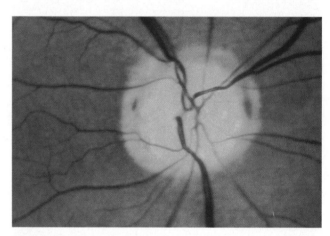

FIGURE I-6. Optic nerve head drusen.

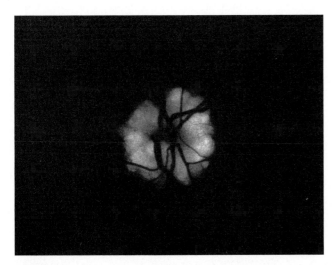

FIGURE I-7. Optic nerve head drusen autofluorescence.

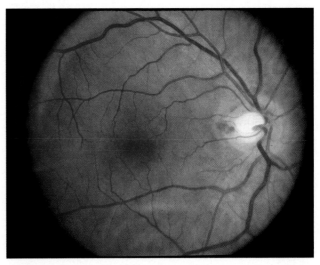

FIGURE I-8. Optic nerve head hemangioma.

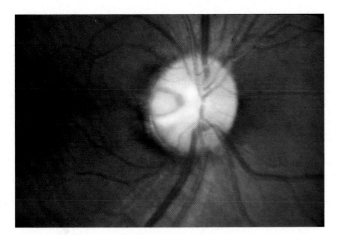

FIGURE I-9. Optic pit (see also Chapter 1).

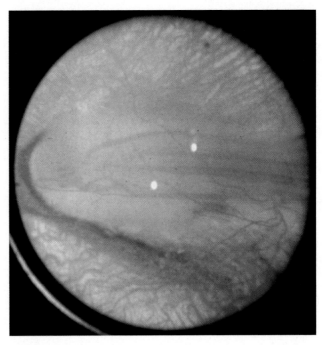

FIGURE I-10. Dragged disc and subretinal pigment in retinopathy of prematurity (see also Chapters 26 and 27).

INDEX